Clinical Neurology

Clinical Neurology

BERNARD J. ALPERS, M.D., Sc. D. (MED.)

Professor of Neurology, Jefferson Medical College, Philadelphia;
Neurologist to the Jefferson, Pennsylvania,
and Wills Hospitals, Philadelphia

244 Illustrations

FOURTH EDITION

F. A. DAVIS COMPANY... *PUBLISHERS*

PHILADELPHIA

1958

PRINTED IN THE UNITED STATES OF AMERICA

To

L. S. A.

Preface to Fourth Edition

Since the last edition of this text, neurology has seen expansion in the fields of epilepsy, vascular diseases, encephalitis, neuritis and infantile palsies, to mention only a few of the conditions which have occupied investigators. Hardly a field of clinical neurology has failed to feel the effects of vigorous investigation. In this new edition an effort has been made to bring all the material up to date and to embody in the text all new diagnostic and therapeutic information. The discussion of many sections has been revised and new material has been added as indicated by research and experience.

As in the first and subsequent editions the objective of this book is to provide a text that will give the student, internist, and general practitioner a background for recognition of neurological disorders as well as understanding of unusual manifestations of a neurological basis occurring in the course of almost any illness.

My thanks are due to many friends who have offered helpful criticisms, and especially to members of my staff for their generous help.

Bernard J. Alpers

Preface to First Edition

The primary purpose of this book has been to present the subject of neurology in such a manner as to make it intelligible to medical students and general practitioners. To do this, one of two courses was open: either to describe syndromes in the most general of terms, or to give a concise or detailed account of all the neurological conditions to be encountered in practice. I have chosen the latter method, and have tried to make the description of disease as inclusive as possible. It may be that in doing so, too much space has been given to relatively uncommon conditions, but an attempt has been made to avoid this as much as possible. The effort has also been made to indicate how the diagnosis of a condition is constructed and tables of differential diagnosis have been added in the hope that they may help in orientation.

The writing of a book, no matter how modest, must inevitably involve many collaborators. In this respect, the present publication has been no exception. The author is indebted in many ways to his secretary, Mrs. Esther I. Kahn, who has been of inestimable help in collecting material and in managing details. To Miss Mary E. Smyth, who typed the manuscript and prepared the index, I am sincerely grateful for painstaking and careful work. Finally, all the members of my staff have helped in many ways, particularly Dr. Francis M. Forster, who read the proof and offered many valuable suggestions.

BERNARD J. ALPERS

CONTENTS

Contents

Contents

Clinical Neurology

1

Examination of the
Nervous System

I. INTRODUCTION

An adequate examination of the nervous system is essential to even an elementary understanding of its diseases, yet it is precisely this feature which is almost universally neglected among practitioners of medicine. A tap of the patellar tendons with a stethoscope in order to elicit the patellar reflexes, a flash of light in the eyes for pupillary reactions, and a neurological examination is completed for the average practitioner or student. The neurological examination of a patient is a long and complex matter, and it is usually taught in this fashion. Hence it has come to be regarded by most physicians as hopelessly beyond their reach, or if within it, as too complex and mysterious to be attempted except by the initiated. This shrinking from an adequate neurological examination results often in lack of recognition of neurological syndromes; sometimes to the detriment of the patient. It is of the highest importance, therefore, to indicate to those who are not neurologists, how to examine the nervous system, and how to utilize the data so collected. For this reason this chapter will be devoted to a description of a full examination of the nervous system, followed by an account of an adequate examination for the student and the general practicing physician.

An examination of the nervous system requires systematic investigation of the cranial nerves, motor system, cerebellar system, reflex system, and sensory system. For special purposes investigations may be made of the endocrine and vegetative systems.

II. THE HISTORY

No examination can be complete without a history and no history can be too complete. The diagnosis of any medical disease involves the careful collection and sifting of evidence, in which the taking of a history is the first logical step.

The recording of a history may follow two general lines: the patient may recite without guidance or help from the physician his entire story, or he may be guided in his presentation of evidence by leading questions from the examining physician. A good history combines the two approaches.

It is good policy to let the patient recite his own story and to follow this by pointed inquiries concerning pertinent points and information which have been omitted. Any medical history is always better the greater the experience of the physician, a point which is particularly true of neurological diseases. The greater the orientation in things neurological, the more pertinent and thorough will be the history. Despite this, much can be overcome by aggressive curiosity and by the guiding principles that no patient must be taken at this proffered value in the recital of his story and no symptom must be left unanalyzed.

All patients approach the physician with some degree of fear; hence their offer of evidence as given in the history will vary with their own personality makeup. Some will make light of symptoms and offer little information; others will make too much of symptoms and offer too much confusing evidence; others will attempt to define their symptoms in diagnostic terms and by interpretations of their own; the rare patient will present his evidence logically and carefully. Because of the patient's anxiety concerning his illness his ability to recite his symptoms logically will be impaired. In this he will need the guidance of the physician.

The Family History: This is usually of little significance in nervous diseases except in those cases in which there is a definite familial disease as for example in Friedreich's ataxia, some forms of myopathy, hereditary paraplegia, amaurotic family idiocy, and other disorders. The family history is important in congenital neurosyphilis. It is also important in idiopathic epilepsy.

The Developmental History: This becomes important in all cases of diseases of the nervous system occurring in infancy and childhood. The health of the mother during pregnancy may give substantial clues as to the cause of the condition in question. Infections of various sorts may be transmitted across the placental membrane, while poor health in the mother may result in prematurity or inferior development of the infant. The health of the mother is of great importance during pregnancy and great care is required to determine whether there has been evidence of avitaminosis, infection (rubella), or bleeding. Persistent vomiting, fear, hypertension, and bleeding should all be inquired about specifically.

Particular attention should be directed toward ascertaining whether the child was premature or born at term. If premature the exact details as to prematurity are essential. The duration and nature of the delivery should be investigated. Prolonged or precipitate delivery, natural, or forceps birth are all important. The type of anesthesia and its duration should be investigated, especially in the case of barbiturates. The weight of the infant at birth and the condition on delivery are important, particular inquiry being made concerning cyanosis, convulsions, and apnea. If initiation of breathing was difficult it is essential to know the duration of the period of apnea and whether incubation or the use of the respirator was necessary. It is important to know also whether the infant was breast or bottle fed and whether sucking either the breast or nipple was difficult or impossible. The rapidity of gain of weight, a tendency not to gain, or to vomit should be looked into. Further developmental details concern the appearance of dentition; the age of development of sitting, standing, creeping, and holding up the head; the appearance of talking; the development of toilet habits; the development of skilled acts; and in older children the school record and the occurrence of childhood diseases.

The inquiry into the development of the infant or child can be as detailed as one wishes to make it, but a bird's-eye sketch will suffice in most cases. No study of the development of the child is complete without inquiry into personality structure. For this it becomes necessary to examine carefully the home environments with particular reference to the parents. Inquiry should be made as to whether the child was planned for and what the parents' preparation for childbirth was; whether there are other children in the family; what the personality of the father and mother is, what their reactions are to the child, whether over-protective or otherwise, what the infant's routine is, and other pertinent features of personality development in order to obtain a sketch of this aspect of the problem.

III. ETIOLOGY AND SYMPTOMATOLOGY

The Onset of the Disease: This is a point of great importance, since an analysis of the method of development of the illness gives important information concerning its nature. An abrupt or apoplectic onset of symptoms is found in cerebral hemorrhage and embolism, in some forms of brain tumor, in meningitis, particularly in the fulminating form of meningococcus meningitis, in head injury, and in infections such as encephalitis, to choose random examples. The mere reporting of such an onset, however, is not sufficient. It is important to know, for the purposes of differential diagnosis, whether the onset was with fever, pain, injury, convulsions, or loss of consciousness. The acute development of paralysis of the legs with pain is something quite different from that without pain; in the former instance the orientation is toward neuritis, in the latter toward poliomyelitis.

The occurrence of headache with fever suggests meningitis, systemic disease, or meningoencephalitis; without fever the orientation is totally different and suggests aneurysm, tumor, subarachnoid hemorrhage, etc. By a careful analysis of such details it may be possible to obtain clues to diagnosis. It may even become apparent on careful questioning that while the onset of the immediate symptoms was abrupt, evidences of abnormality may have been present for a greater or lesser time before the acute onset. This is apparent in the history of high blood pressure and of transient attacks of vertigo or headache preceding the apoplectic onset of cerebral hemorrhage; or in the history of disregarded headaches preceding the acute onset of brain tumor; or in cases of spinal cord tumor with sudden development of paraplegia, and with a history of trunk or leg pains in the past, obtained only by specific inquiry.

In other instances the onset of the illness may be slow and the development gradual. In such cases it is important to determine whether the development has been steadily progressive or whether it has been broken by periods of complete or incomplete remission of symptoms. Slow onset or development of a disease may take place over a period of months or years and its beginnings may be so indefinite as to be lost in the past. Slight memory disturbances, increased irritability, mild personality deviations, all these may be so slight at first as to be disregarded; their true nature being apparent only when the disease has become well advanced. It is essential therefore that they be recognized early, a capacity which is possible only for a practiced eye and ear.

Progression of a Disease: The determination of progression of a slowly developing disease is also essential, since progression implies continued activity regardless of the cause of the disorder. It is important to know whether progression has been maintained over a long period of time to the present, or whether there have been letups in the progression, with leveling off of symptoms for varying periods of time only to be followed by more progression, or whether there have been remissions for longer or shorter periods. It is equally important, moreover, to determine whether the progression of symptoms has been rapid or slow.

In senile dementia the symptoms as a rule develop gradually and progress without letup. The same holds true for cerebral arteriosclerosis, general paresis, and cases of brain tumor. Paralysis agitans, on the other hand, develops slowly and progresses gradually with periods of leveling off so that there are usually more or less lengthy periods before new symptoms develop. Inflammatory disorders such as some forms of encephalitis may develop and unfold over a short period, becoming static or fixed in their manifestations. Rapid progression of symptoms is found in malignant forms of brain tumor, in amyotrophic lateral sclerosis, in some forms of general paresis, and in encephalitis, to choose random examples.

The development of a disease with remissions is of the greatest importance in proper orientation toward the correct diagnosis. It is important to determine whether remissions of symptoms have been complete or incomplete and if complete, the duration of the complete remission. The outstanding example of development with remission or improvement of symptoms is multiple sclerosis, but remissions occur in other diseases as well. They develop in general paresis, in myasthenia gravis, in some cases of brain tumor, and rarely in spinal cord tumor.

Having determined the method of onset of the illness it is then possible to proceed to an analysis of the main complaints. In this approach it is essential to be on guard against taking the patient's word for any symptom. Careful analysis of the various symptoms of which he complains will help greatly in establishing a diagnosis. Thus patients frequently complain of numbness of a limb or limbs when they mean weakness; or they often complain of dizziness but do not mean vertigo in the true sense of the word.

Pain: The complaint of *pain* must be analyzed carefully. Any complaint of pain in any part of the body should be analyzed along the following lines: (1) The exact location of the pain; whether it is distributed along a peripheral nerve or spinal root distribution, or along neither, as in central pains due to lesions of the thalamus or spinothalamic tract; (2) the duration of pain; whether it is constant or intermittent; (3) the nature of the pain with particular reference to its intensity It is often difficult for patients

to describe this feature of the pain but a little patience will elicit helpful information. It is helpful to know whether the pain is *deep* or *superficial, lancinating* and *radiating* from one part to another, or whether it appears all at once in all parts of a limb. (4) The factors which relieve the pain; whether it is relieved by drugs and if so, in what dosage; or whether it is relieved by heat, posture, climate, etc. (5) The factors which aggravate the pain, whether movement, posture, climate, etc.

Headache: Similarly, a history of *headache* must be analyzed carefully with particular reference to (1) its location. It is essential to know whether a headache is generalized or whether it is chiefly frontal, occipital, or felt only on one side of the head. (2) Its nature; whether it is deep or superficial, severe or mild, constant or intermittent, periodic or irregular in appearance. (3) Its incidence. (4) The factors which relieve it. (5) The factors which aggravate it (*v.* Headache, Chap. 4).

Convulsions: The problem of *convulsions* also requires careful analysis. In this connection it is important to determine (1) the nature of the convulsion, with particular reference to auras, whether it is generalized or focal, whether it is associated with tonic or clonic movements, or with sensory disturbances of any sort. This information is obtainable only from relatives or friends of the patient since the latter is usually unaware of the nature of grand mal attacks unless he has been informed of them. Petit mal or minor attacks, uncinate fits, motor or sensory jacksonian fits, psychomotor attacks, can usually be described by the patient himself. (2) The association of loss or impairment of consciousness. This is an extremely important factor and one on which depends important decisions relative to diagnosis. It must always be inquired about specifically. If there is doubt as to whether it is present during a convulsion, the presence of a fall during the attack, or of tongue biting, or incontinence will help greatly in reaching a decision. (3) The occurrence of the attacks; whether they occur chiefly during the day or night, or both, whether they occur in relation to meals or with hunger, fatigue, or excitement, or whether they develop chiefly around the time of the menses. In this connection it is important to inquire into the spacing of the attacks and their frequency. (4) The onset of the attacks; it is essential to know whether the attacks have been present from birth, or whether they developed during infancy, puberty, or adult life. Inquiry should be made into the development in relation to head injury, infantile encephalitis, meningitis, syphilis, hypertension, etc. (5) The reaction of the attacks to medication. Most persons with convulsions have had some medication before seeing the physician and a knowledge of the nature of the drugs used and their effects is important.

Vertigo: Another symptom requiring careful analysis is vertigo (v. Vertigo). Most patients, even those of good intelligence, do not mean vertigo when they complain of dizziness. It is necessary therefore to determine whether true subjective or objective vertigo is present, whether there is a sensation of rotation of the patient or of objects in the environment, whether there are lurching, nausea, or vomiting, or whether by dizziness the patient means only a sense of faintness or giddiness, or some nondescript sensation which he finds difficulty in elucidating. Careful analysis of the complaint of dizziness will be repaid by a clearer conception of the disease in question.

Numbness: Another complaint requiring some analysis is *numbness*, which many patients use synonymously with weakness. It is therefore necessary to require the patient to define carefully what is meant by numbness; in most cases it

will be clear that weakness of a limb or part of a limb is meant. It is of the utmost importance to determine whether the numbness has developed all at once in the affected part, whether it has progressed from one part of the limb to another, or whether there has been a march of the sensation, as in sensory jacksonian seizures.

Vision: *Blurred vision* covers a variety of meanings and must be looked into carefully. It may mean actually what it is supposed to mean; it may be used to refer to double vision which the patient will not indicate unless it is inquired after specifically; it may refer to indistinct vision because of a scotoma in the visual field; or it may be used to indicate the sensation of blurring associated with a hemianopic field defect. All these can be determined by proper questioning. Diplopia especially must be analyzed carefully so that it becomes certain whether true double vision is present. Inquiry must be made therefore in order to determine the position of the objects in relation to one another, the position of the false image, and whether the diplopia is present with monocular vision as is the case in hysterical subjects.

These are but samples of the method of inquiry into specific symptoms of presentation in neurological disorders. They serve to emphasize the essential fact that no patient must be taken at his face value in the recording of his complaints. All symptoms must be analyzed carefully and *in extenso* in order to reach an accurate diagnosis.

When the history of the present illness has been completed, details of the occupational, educational, marital, and past medical histories must be covered in order to determine whether these offer factors of any importance in the illness. Not only must physical factors such as exposure to lead, arsenic, carbon disulfide, cold, and other hazards be investigated, but it is important as well to determine whether in white-collar occupations the work is interesting and congenial, whether the patient works under tension and pressure, and whether his work history indicates good adjustment on this score. The per-

tients some degree of anxiety which is responsible for the development of reactions which may often obscure the symtoms of the structural illness. These may in some instances become so pronounced as to dominate the picture. It is impor-

Table 1—Personality Study
(After Strecker and Appel)

Health	Energy	Feelings	Social Attitudes	Family Relationships			Type
Good	Much	Tense	Outgoing	Affectionate			Athletic
Delicate	Little	Calm	Friendly	Demonstrative			Intellectual
Size	Fatigue	Excitable	Withdrawing	Characteristic			Social
Inferiority	Quick	Nervous	Reserved				Artistic
How stand:	Slow	Temper	Sensitive				Mechanical
Sickness		Exaggerations	Self-conscious				
Pain		Even	Easily hurt		F	M	Interests
Alcohol		Moody	Suspicious				
		Cheerful	Communicative	Looks like			Diversions:
		Worry	Decisive	Temperament			Amusements
		Pessimistic	Indecisive	like			Hobbies
		Irritable	Doubts	Understood			
		Angry	Determined	best by			Work:
		Fears	Wilful	Gets on			Attitude toward
		Serious	Obstinate	best with			
		Jovial	Stubborn	Closer to			Goals or Ambitions:
			Orderly				Ideals, Religion
			Neat				Who admire, envy
			Controlled	Disciplined by:			change with
			Controlling	Frequency			
			Dominating	Severe			Assets
			Executive	Average			
			Gets own way	Family constellation			Liabilities
			Yielding	Relation with siblings			
			Flexible	Dependent			Difficulties (strains,
			Adaptable	Independent			sadness) in life:
			Contrary	Antagonistic			How met
			Disciplinary	Jealous			
			Dogmatic				
			Cold—stern				

tinent factors in the past history will depend on the nature of the illnesses from which the patient has suffered so that no specific points can be indicated.

IV. PERSONALITY

No history of the patient's illness can be regarded as complete without at least brief inquiry into his personality structure. Illness invariably evokes in all pa-

tant to know therefore the manner of person who has developed the illness being probed. For this purpose a brief personality survey must be made.

An investigation of the family background with especial reference to physical environment, the patient's place in the family, the personality of father, mother, and other members of the family, and the patient's relationship to them can be covered briefly but adequately. The educational history and the patient's adjustment to school should be touched on, as well as the occupational history and an account of various positions and of adjustment to work. An account of the marital history and of the adjustment of the patient to his wife and children will give valuable information and can, of course, become extremely detailed if the history warrants it. Finally, a brief personality sketch of the patient should be recorded, special effort being made to determine his main types of reaction. For this purpose the chart on preceding page is very useful since it covers the main points in a personality study and permits a rapid survey of the patient's reactions.

Having determined the main features of the history, the patient is then ready for examination.

V. INTELLECT AND SKILLED ACTS

Since one's first contact with the patient is through the account of his illness, the physician is offered at the outset an opportunity to study various features of importance in the examination. The *facial expression* may be noted and impressions gained as to facial mobility, anxiety, as to whether the patient has a blank or rigid facies. The general *intellectual level* of the patient may be roughly estimated by his vocabulary, the manner of presentation of the material having to do with his illness, by his occupation, and activities. This can be tested further by directing questions at him concerning general knowledge and culture.

Memory can be tested by the manner in which the patient recalls the details of his life, as well as by history obtained from relatives or fellow workers. It can be determined further by asking the patient to repeat a number of digits both forward and backward and by recounting a simple story, asking the patient to re-

peat as many of its details as he can recall. Simple arithmetical problems should be given in order to see how they are handled. Orientation for time and place may be tested in those cases where it is indicated by inquiring as to where the patient is and asking him to identify faces, time, etc. The *speech* can be examined during the course of the history taking and it can be readily determined whether dysarthria or aphasia is present (*v.* Chapter 2). In proper cases test phrases may be given. The *mood* and general reaction of the patient to his illness can be determined by observation during the routine examination so that anxiety, depression, excitement, suspiciousness, etc., may be readily determined.

VI. THE CRANIAL NERVES

Olfactory: The olfactory nerve does not as a rule require investigation for routine purposes. It is examined by closing one nostril and asking the patient to smell coffee or lemon extract with the other. Tobacco, peppermint, asafetida, vinegar, or other aromatic substances may be used.

Optic: This is tested by a direct examination of the optic nerve and by investigation of visual acuity and the visual fields. The *optic nerve* is examined by means of an ophthalmoscope. Every physician should learn its use, since information can be obtained from the fundus oculi which is of great value in internal diseases. A description of the normal fundus can be found in any standard text of ophthalmology. The *visual fields* for accurate study must be examined by means of a perimeter. Gross visual field defects may be detected, however, by means of the confrontation test. This is performed by having the patient face the examiner at a distance of two or three feet, asking the patient to cover one eye with his hand, and to fix his gaze on the examiner's nose. The examiner's finger is then brought in

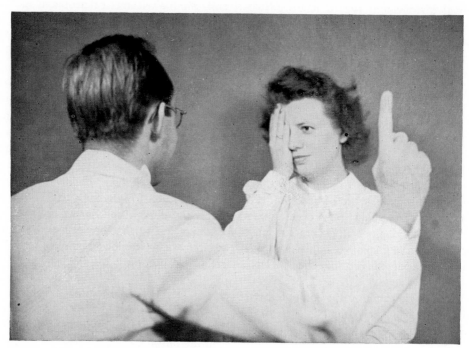

Fig. 1—*Confrontation method* of determining the visual fields.

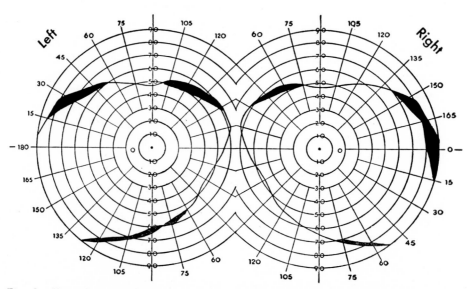

Fig. 2—*Normal visual fields* showing the characteristic flattening above and on the nasal sides.

along the main axes of the visual field; nasal, temporal, superior, and inferior, the patient calling out as soon as the examiner's finger is seen. A corsage pin with hemianopic field defects may be disclosed. Scotomas may be detected also by this method; the patient's position in relation to the examiner remains as de-

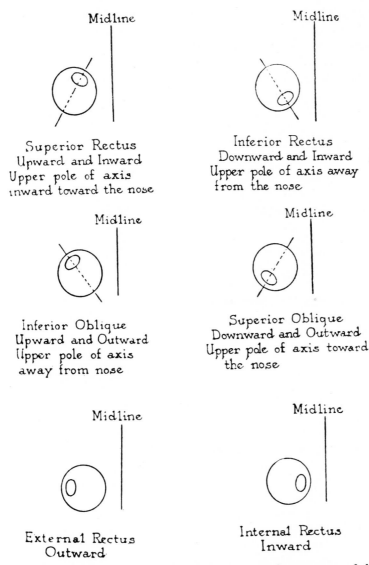

Superior Rectus
Upward and Inward
Upper pole of axis
inward toward the nose

Inferior Rectus
Downward and Inward
Upper pole of axis away
from the nose

Inferior Oblique
Upward and Outward
Upper pole of axis
away from nose

Superior Oblique
Downward and Outward
Upper pole of axis toward
the nose

External Rectus
Outward

Internal Rectus
Inward

Fig. 3—*Normal ocular movements*, **illustrating the principal movements of the various ocular muscles.** *(Riley, Arch. Ophth. 4:640, 1930.)*

a white head may be used for more accurate determinations. The fields may be mapped out by means of a flashlight, in some instances with visual loss. By means of the confrontation test gross scribed, the patient being asked as the finger approaches to indicate where vision is lost in the visual field. *Visual acuity* is tested by means of the standardized charts for testing vision.

Ocular Nerves: All the ocular nerves are examined together.

1. *Pupillary Reflex:* This is tested preferably in the darkness, or shade, by flashing a light in the pupil and examining the size, regularity, shape, and reaction of the pupil. Normally the pupils are equal in size, regular in outline, and react promptly to direct light flashed into the eye. Under normal circumstances the pu-

one eye and observing movement in all axes. Limitation of movement is looked for. Convergence is tested by asking the patient to look at the finger at a distance and on close examination. As the finger approaches the patient's nose from a distance the eyes normally are seen to converge inward and to maintain this converged position.

Trigeminal: The *motor* portion of the

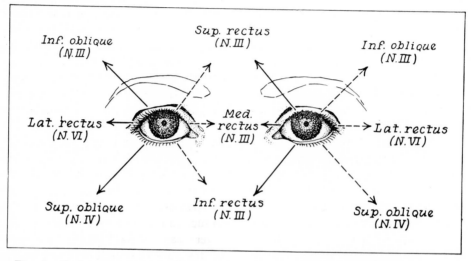

Fig. 4—*Ocular movements* indicating the movements of the various ocular muscles.
(Modified, *Spurling. Charles C Thomas, Springfield, Ill.)*

pil reacts quickly to light, the contraction being maintained for a very brief time and then relaxing as the sphincter of the iris fatigues with continued application of the light. A routine examination should include also a study of the *consensual reaction.* Under normal circumstances flashing a light in one pupil results in a prompt contraction of the opposite pupil as well. This is known as the consensual reaction. The *accommodation* reflex may be tested by watching the size of the pupil as it accommodates to near and far vision.

2. *Ocular Movements:* Conjugate movements are tested by asking the patient to look to either side as far as he can or to follow the finger to either side as well as up and down. Individual eye muscle movements are tested by covering

nerve is tested by asking the patient to clench his teeth, the examiner feeling the masseters and temporals in order to determine force of contraction and the muscle bulk. The pterygoids may be tested by having the patient press laterally with the jaw against the examiner's finger, the mouth being partially open. Deviation of the jaw due to masseter paralysis, or weakness, is tested by asking the patient to open the mouth, weakness being manifested by deviation of the jaw to the weak side. The *sensory portion* of the nerve is tested by taking the corneal reflex with a hair stimulator. The corneal reflex is extremely important under some circumstances, but as ordinarily taken in routine fashion it has little value since in most instances it is taken not by stimulation of the cornea but of the sclera. It must be taken in such a fashion as to be invisible to the patient since the latter will naturally blink on seeing an object approach the eye. For this purpose a fine hair mounted on an applicator can be curved in such a way as to stimulate the cornea directly without being seen by the patient. The response consists of a rapid and forceful contraction of the eyelid similar to that experienced when a foreign body enters the eye. When no response is obtained there is no contraction of the eyelid; this should always be checked by asking the patient whether the stimulus was felt. Facial sensation is examined by testing the skin of the face for touch, pain, and temperature sensations. The mucous membranes of the nose and mouth, and the anterior portion of the tongue, may also be tested.

Facial: This nerve is examined by asking the patient to wrinkle the forehead, to frown (frontalis muscle), to close the eyelids tightly, or to wink (orbicularis palpebrae muscle), to open the mouth, retract the mouth, blow out the cheeks and pucker the lips, screw up the nose, whistle, etc. (muscles of facial expression). By these various simple maneuvers the several muscles innervated by the facial nerve are tested and weakness or paralysis of the facial muscles is easily detected. In addition to innervating the muscles of the face the facial nerve supplies taste innervation to the anterior two-thirds of the tongue. This need not be tested routinely but in cases of peripheral facial paralysis it becomes necessary to determine whether the taste fibers are involved. This is tested by having the patient protrude the tongue and by rubbing into the tongue sugar, salt, and quinine at different times. The patient is asked to detect the materials used without pulling the tongue back into the mouth, an easy performance for the normal subject.

Auditory: Examination of the auditory nerve is carried out by testing the cochlear and the vestibular portions of the nerve.

1. *Cochlear:* This portion is concerned with hearing, which may be tested by observing the patient's ability to hear the spoken voice or a whisper. It may also be tested by simple tuning fork procedures, using a C 256 or a higher pitched turning fork. This is set in vibration, placed on the mastoid process, and the patient asked to let the examiner know when the vibration has ceased. At this point it is placed next to the ear and the patient asked whether the tuning fork is still heard. Under normal circumstances air conduction (AC) is greater than bone conduction (BC) and the fork will be heard after it is no longer heard on the bone. Measurement may be made of the times over which the tuning fork is heard over the bone as compared with air, but for routine purposes this is not necessary. In conduction deafness, bone conduction is longer than air conduction. Lateralization tests are also used. A tuning fork is placed on the forehead, and one ear completely occluded by the examiner's finger, the patient being asked to tell on which side the vibration is heard loudest. Normally it is always heard best on the occluded side. In conduction deafness the tuning fork is referred to the diseased ear, while in nerve deafness it is not heard on the affected side even with occlusion.

For more precise examination of audition, the *audiometer* is used. By means of this special instrument the degree of hearing loss and the amplitudes in which it is affected may be accurately measured.

2. *Vestibular:* This portion of the nerve is tested by means of pass pointing tests. The patient is asked to raise his arm and to bring the index finger down on the examiner's finger with the patient's arm outstretched. This is done first with the eyes open and closed. It is also car-

ried out in the horizontal plane. Normally the patient's finger touches the examiner's without difficulty, with eyes open and closed. In vestibular disease the finger pass points to one side or the other consistently. The function of the vestibular portion of the auditory nerve is often investigated by means of the *Bárány tests,* which consist of stimulation of the semicircular canals and recording of the responses obtained. The test is carried out by the injection of cold water (18° to 20° C.) slowly into the external auditory canal with the patient sitting upright, the injected water being caught in a kidney basin under the ear.

After the injection of 100 cc. of water, observations are made concerning the following features: (1) nystagmus, (2) pass pointing, (3) the occurrence of vertigo, nausea, or vomiting. With the patient in the upright position the vertical canals are stimulated. The responses of the horizontal canals are tested by bending the head forward, observations being made on the factors mentioned. After irrigation of the ears normal responses of a definite sort are observed. Thus after irrigation of the right ear there are noted (1) vertigo within two minutes after irrigation is begun; (2) lateral and rotary nystagmus to the left; (3) pass pointing to the right; (4) nausea and sometimes vomiting; (5) increase of the nystagmus to the right side with the head flexed, and (6) intensification of the vertigo, nystagmus, and pass pointing on return of the head to the upright position. After irrigation of the left ear the subjective reactions such as nausea, vertigo, and vomiting remain the same but the nystagmus is to the right and the past pointing chiefly to the left.

Under some circumstances no responses are obtained from the semicircular canals of one ear as in cerebellopontine angle tumor. In other cases the responses may be perverted, nystagmus occurring to the wrong side. In posterior fossa tumors the subjective responses such as nausea, vertigo, and vomiting are completely absent or decreased. In tumors above the tentorium they are often greatly exaggerated.

The vestibular portion of the auditory nerve is examined also by looking for *nystagmus.* This consists of a to-and-fro movement of the eyeballs usually in the horizontal plane but sometimes in the vertical plane. It is examined by asking the patient to look to one side, the eyeballs moving to the extreme positions. True nystagmus is characterized by a sustained movement consisting of two components, a fast jerk to the side of the deviation and a slow jerk back to the midline. At times a rotary element is seen, the eyeballs moving in a rotary fashion, especially in disease of the peripheral vestibular apparatus. At times vertical nystagmus is elicited on looking upward and sometimes on downward gaze. It consists of a straight up-and-down movement of the eyeballs in a vertical plane.

Glossopharyngeal: This nerve is tested routinely with the vagus nerve. Its chief function is sensory, supplying the pharynx and posterior third of the tongue with taste fibers. Its only motor function has to do with movement of the pharynx by means of the stylopharyngeus muscle whose rôle in this function is so minor that it can hardly be tested.

Vagus: The vagus nerve has many functions. It is the chief motor nerve of the pharynx and larynx. It is tested routinely by observing pharyngeal movements. This is best done by asking the patient to phonate by saying "ah." Under normal circumstances the soft palate and uvula will be pulled up in the midline. In case of weakness of one side, the palate will be pulled up on phonation to the healthy side while the diseased side droops; in cases of bilateral paralysis there will be no palatal movement. The pharyngeal reflex may be tested by touching the back of the pharynx with a throat stick, with ensuing contraction of the palatal muscles under normal conditions.

The larynx may be tested by studying the timbre of the voice, the vocal musculature being supplied through the vagus by the recurrent laryngeal nerve. In case of hoarseness or aphonia, direct mirror laryngoscopy is advisable.

The vegetative functions of the vagus nerve such as pulse, respiration, etc., may also be tested.

Spinal Accessory: This nerve innervates the sternomastoid and trapezius muscles. It is tested by asking the patient to shrug his shoulders against resistance and by turning the head against resistance.

Hypoglossal: This is the motor nerve of the tongue. It is tested by asking the patient to protrude the tongue. Under normal circumstances the tongue is protruded in the midline. In paralysis of the tongue, there is deviation to the paralyzed side. Power of the tongue may be tested by asking the patient to press the tongue against each cheek, the force of the protrusion being tested by the finger of the examiner pressing against the tongue.

For ordinary routine purposes examination of the pupillary reflexes, ocular movements, facial innervation, pharynx and tongue movements are most important, and are sufficient for most examinations in a busy general practice.

VII. MOTOR SYSTEM

Examination of the motor system has as its object (1) the determination of muscle power; (2) the study of muscle bulk; (3) the determination of muscle tone.

For the determination of weakness or strength of the muscles a few simple maneuvers are sufficient; if more complex studies are necessary they may be carried out on the muscles indicated. Thus, routine examination of the muscles of the shoulder and pelvic girdles is not necessary, but in cases of shoulder pain or weakness, or of leg pain, or weakness, careful examination of these muscles is essential.

Hands and Arms: The *hand grips* are tested by asking the patient to squeeze the examiner's fingers, it being first determined whether the patient is right- or left-handed. The power of the hand grips is determined by the force required to withdraw the fingers from the clenched fist; or the patient may be asked to fix the tightly clenched fist at the wrist, the examiner attempting to loosen the fixed wrist. Power in the *arms* is tested by asking the patient to flex and extend the forearm against resistance. When there is a history of neck, shoulder, or arm pain, examination of the shoulder girdle muscles is essential.

Legs and Feet: The legs are similarly tested by asking the patient to flex and extend them against resistance. Dorsiflexion of the feet is tested by asking the patient to push the partially flexed foot against the examiner's hand, and plantar flexion by pushing down against the examiner's hand, or dorsi- and plantar flexion of the feet may be tested by asking the patient to walk on the heels and toes.

Movements of the shoulder and pelvic girdles need not be tested routinely.

While the musculature is being examined for evidence of weakness, search should also be made for change in *muscle tone,* such as flaccidity, spasticity, or rigidity. If a change of muscle tone is found, it should be determined whether this is focal or general.

Search should also be made for *muscle atrophy*, and, if found, its distribution should be determined. *Muscular fasciculations* should always be sought for whether or not atrophy is present.

Involuntary movements such as chorea, athetosis, tics, or hemiballism should be looked for.

To one who is well versed in the routine examination of the nervous system all this and more can be performed in examination of the motor system very quickly and accurately. For ordinary routine purposes in which the neurological examination is part of a general physical survey of the patient, examination of the motor system may be confined to studying the power of the arms and legs, the other factors mentioned being reserved for cases with definite findings (*v.* Chapter 2).*

VIII. CEREBELLAR SYSTEM

Routinely, some survey should be made of the cerebellar system, the function of which is to perform smooth coördinated movements. For this purpose tests are devised to determine the cerebellar functioning of the limbs and trunk.

1. Arms

Finger-Nose Test: The patient is asked to place the index finger of each hand on the nose. This is normally performed smoothly and easily. This test may be varied by asking the patient several times quickly to touch the nose in rapid succession.

Finger-Finger Test: The patient is asked to place the index finger of his hand on the examiner's index finger. This may be repeated several times in rapid succession.

Pronation-Supination Test: With the arms extended in front of him the patient is asked to pronate and supinate rapidly, using the elbows as a fulcrum. Under normal circumstances the movements are

*See pp. 23-28 for Table of Muscle Innervation.

of equal amplitude, smooth and even, and there is no tendency on the part of the arms to drift outward or inward during the movement. The beat and rhythm are well maintained.

Patting Test: The patient is requested to pat rapidly with each hand the examiner's hand or his own leg. Under normal conditions this is performed smoothly with even amplitude and a smooth rhythm. In cerebellar disease there is irregularity of amplitude and rhythm.

2. Legs

Heel-Knee Test: With the patient in the supine position the heel of one foot is placed on the opposite knee. This is done smoothly, without tremor and with accuracy.

Heel-Toe Test: The patient is asked to walk heel to toe along a straight line. This can be done normally without faltering or loss of balance.

3. Trunk

Gait: Testing the gait constitutes a good method of determining trunk coordination. In order to do this the patient should be given plenty of room and asked to walk briskly with the eyes open and closed, and to turn quickly.

He may be asked also to walk around a chair, to sit and rise quickly from a chair.

The patient may be asked also to arise from a reclining posture without a pillow and with the legs widely separated.

The *station* is also tested routinely, the patient being asked to stand with the feet close together, first with the eyes open, then with the eyes closed.

For ordinary purposes the finger-nose, heel-toe, gait and station, and pronation-supination tests will suffice to determine cerebellar function.

IX. REFLEX SYSTEM

1. Pupillary Reflex: This has already been described under the cranial nerve section.

2. Corneal Reflex: This may be tested by means of a curved hair attached to a stick, enabling the examiner to touch the cornea without the stimulating hair being seen. The result is a quick wink reflex.

3. Biceps Reflex: This is examined by placing the elbow of the arm to be examined in the hand of the examiner, the examiner's thumb being placed over the biceps tendon and struck briskly with a

tended, the triceps tendon being tapped by the reflex hammer, an extension movement of the arm resulting. In the supine position the arm is drawn across the chest, the forearm slightly flexed and the triceps tendon tapped just above the olecranon.

6. Patellar Reflex: This is taken by tapping the patellar tendon with the leg partly extended. If it is taken with the patient in bed, placing a rolled pillow

Table 2—Important Deep Tendon Reflexes

	Elicited by	Response	Segmental Level
JAW	Tapping mandible in half open position	Closure of jaw	Pons
SCAPULO-HUMERAL	Tapping vertebral border of scapula	Contraction of teres minor infraspinatus, etc.	C5 and C6
TRICEPS	Tapping triceps tendon	Extension at elbow	C7 to D1
BICEPS	Tapping biceps tendon	Flexion at elbow	C5 and C6
RADIAL	Tapping styloid process of radius	Contraction of supinator longus	C5 and C6
KNEE	Tapping patellar tendon	Extension at knee	L3 and L4
ANKLE	Tapping tendo Achilles	Extension at ankle	S1 and S2

reflex hammer. The result is a flexion of the arm.

4. Brachioradial Reflex: This is elicited by tapping the lower third of the radius with the forearm midway between pronation and supination. The result is flexion of the forearm on the arm, and usually also flexion of the fingers and hand. This is one of the most important reflexes of the arm but it is often neglected. With a lesion in the fifth cervical segment tapping of the radius causes only flexion of the hand and fingers but not of the forearm (inversion of the radial reflex). A similar response may be elicited in normal persons and has been found also in myopathies.

5. Triceps Reflex: This is taken by holding the arm of the patient supported under the elbow with the arm partly ex-

under the knees facilitates taking the reflex.

7. Achilles Reflex: This may be taken with the patient lying on his face, the knee flexed, the foot held slightly dorsiflexed by the examiner's hand, and the Achilles tendon struck in order to produce plantar flexion. This is the ideal method of eliciting this reflex. It may be taken also by asking the patient to kneel on a chair with a soft pad while the Achilles tendon is struck. It may be taken also with the patient on his back, and the legs flexed and everted, the Achilles tendon being struck while the foot is held dorsiflexed.

8. Plantar Reflex: For routine purposes the sole of the foot is stimulated by a blunt object carried along its outer and inner sides. The normal response is flexion of the toes.

9. Abdominal Reflexes: These are taken by running an object such as the blunt end of an orange stick, a pin, match, key, brush, or the finger nail, along the upper and lower abdominal quadrants on either side. A normal response consists of movement of the abdominal musculature and a pull of the umbilicus toward the stimulated side. Medium tension of the abdominal musculature is most favorable for the response.

10. Cremasteric Reflex: This is examined by stimulating the inner side of the thigh by means of an orange stick, the response being retraction of the testicle on the stimulated side.

For routine purposes examination of the biceps, patellar, Achilles, plantar and abdominal reflexes is sufficient.

11. Additional Reflexes: The *orbicularis oculi reflex* is elicited as follows: The skin at the outer corner of the eye is held between the thumb and index finger, pulling it back slightly, and the thumb is tapped lightly with a reflex hammer. There follows a reflex contraction of the orbicularis oculi muscle. Diminution of the reflex is found in facial palsies of peripheral origin. It is preserved in central facial palsies. The response obtained is a deep muscle reflex. The *jaw reflex* is elicited by tapping the mandible with the jaw half opened, the lower jaw moving briskly upward. It has slight clinical significance, but it may be increased on bilateral supranuclear cerebral lesions. The *scapulohumeral reflex* is elicited by tapping the vertebral border of the scapula with resulting contraction of muscles of the shoulder girdle and arm. Many muscles are brought into play, especially the deltoid, pectoralis major, infraspinatus and teres minor. Adduction of the arm occurs. Unilateral absence of the reflex is found in lesions of the fifth cervical segment. The *adductor reflex of the thigh* is obtained by placing the finger on the medial condyle of the femur with the leg slightly abducted. When the finger is tapped adduction of the leg follows. The *bi-*

Table 3—Important Superficial Reflexes

	Elicited by	*Response*	*Segmental Level*
CORNEAL	Touching cornea with hair	Contraction of orbicularis oculi	
PHARYNGEAL	Touching posterior wall of pharynx	Contraction of pharynx	
PALATAL	Touching soft palate	Elevation of palate	
SCAPULAR	Stroking skin between scapulae	Contraction of scapular muscles	C5 to D1
EPIGASTRIC	Stroking downward from nipples	Dimpling of epigastrium ipsilaterally	D7 to D9
ABDOMINAL	Stroking beneath costal margins and above inguinal ligament	Contraction of abdominal muscles in quadrant stimulated	D10 to D12
CREMASTERIC	Stroking medial surface of upper thigh	Ipsilateral elevation of testicle	L1 and L2
GLUTEAL	Stroking skin of buttock	Contraction of glutei	L4 and L5
BULBO-CAVERNOSIS	Pinching dorsum of glans	Contraction of bulbous urethra	S3 and S4
SUPERFICIAL ANAL	Pricking perineum	Contraction of rectal sphincters	S5 and coccygeal

ceps femoris reflex is best elicited with the patient lying on the side opposite the one being examined, the leg being bent at the hip and knee. The finger is placed on the hamstring tendon and is tapped with a reflex hammer. Contraction of the muscle results. The *pharyngeal reflex* is elicited by touching the posterior wall of the pharynx, contraction of the pharynx resulting. The *scapular* reflex, elicited by stroking the skin between the scapulae, results in contraction of the scapular muscles. The *gluteal reflex* results in contraction of the glutei on stroking the skin of the buttock.

X. SENSORY SYSTEM

A complete sensory examination includes the investigation of touch, pain, heat, cold, position, and vibration senses. Of these, pain, position, and vibration senses suffice for a routine examination. The others may be investigated whenever indicated. For an accurate sensory examination the patient should be examined in a quiet room where he is not distracted by extraneous stimuli and preferably when he is fresh and not fatigued. The examination should not be too lengthy, since fatigue sets in rapidly and the replies become increasingly inaccurate under such circumstances. In routine examinations sensation is usually tested at the end of the examination. If sensory changes are found the examination should be repeated alone.

Examination of sensation consists of two portions: (1) *Qualitative*, to determine what elements of sensation are affected, (2) *quantitative*, to determine the degree of involvement of sensation when it is impaired, and (3) *regional*, to map out the areas of sensory impairment or loss. In the normal subject only the qualitative aspects of sensation are studied, it being determined that sensation is well appreciated over the body surface and is equally felt over both sides of the body, limbs, and face. In cases of sensory impairment, whether sensation is lost or decreased, it becomes necessary to investigate the degree of sensory loss and the distribution of this loss. Complete sensory loss is spoken of as *anesthesia* (touch), *analgesia* (pain), etc.; partial sensory loss is referred to as *hypalgesia*, etc. In some instances sensation is more keenly felt than normal; this is referred to as *hyperesthesia, hyperalgesia,* etc. It is extremely important in every case of sensory loss to determine the exact distribution of the loss in order to determine whether the loss corresponds with peripheral nerve or with root distribution; whether it is a complete sensory level as seen in transverse spinal cord lesions, or a hemianesthesia, or a dissociated sensory syndrome (*v.* Chapter 3).

Touch: This sense is tested by means of a cotton wisp on an applicator, or by a camel's-hair brush, or even by the examiner's finger, which is brought gingerly and lightly down on the skin.

Pain: It is tested by a pin with which the patient is pricked over various parts of the skin's surface. The qualitative aspect is examined by determining whether the patient appreciates correctly the pin prick over various parts of the body, the patient being asked to determine whether he can feel the pin point or the head of the pin over various parts of the body.

Heat and Cold: They are tested by means of test tubes containing hot water and cracked ice. These are extremes of temperature which suffice for routine neurological examination. The patient with the eyes closed is asked to identify hot and cold over various parts of the body.

Vibration Sense: This is examined by means of a C 128 tuning fork applied over the elbow, wrist, ankle, and shin. The tuning fork is set in active vibration and the patient, with the eyes closed, is asked to identify the sensation. He is also asked to determine when the vibration ceases, the examiner interrupting the vibration as he desires. In doubtful instances a rough quantitive test may be made, the patient being asked to determine how long he feels the vibration over the back of the hand or tibia. Rough clinical tests on a C 128 tuning fork indicate that vibration is felt over the back of the hand for an average of fifteen to twenty seconds, and over the tibia for seven to ten seconds in young subjects. In patients over fifty vibration sense is often lost in the legs.

Position Sense: It is examined by grasping the sides of the thumb or great toe and gently moving it, the patient being asked to determine whether the digit is pointed up or down.

Special sensory examinations consist of the determination of *two-point discrimination,* which is examined by means of a calibrated compass. The patient is asked to indicate whether he feels one or two compass points over various parts of the body. The test is important in diseases of the sensory cortex and in peripheral nerve disease but it is difficult to interpret because it is not well standardized. *Spot localization* is tested with the patient's eyes closed, by touching a spot on the skin, the patient being asked to indicate the spot touched by placing his finger on it.

Graphesthesia consists of the ability to recognize numbers or letters traced on the skin with a blunt object. The patient is asked to identify the number or letter so drawn.

Differences in texture and weight may be tested by asking the patient to identify various textures of cloth and to determine the difference in the weight of standardized blocks.

Stereognosis is tested by asking the patient, with the eyes closed, to identify the size and shape of an object placed in the hand. This ability is lost in some cases.

XI. SPECIAL EXAMINATIONS

Since special examinations of various sorts are often required in a study of the nervous system, some consideration of the technics employed in their use seems to be indicated.

Lumbar Puncture: Examination of the spinal fluid is often necessary and is obtained with the patient lying on the side. The proper position of the patient is absolutely essential for a good lumbar puncture and constitutes the most important part of the procedure. The patient is placed on a hard surface such as a stretcher or is brought out to the edge of the bed. The knees should be drawn up on the abdomen and clasped firmly by the hands. The shoulder on which the patient lies should be drawn under and the subject should lie squarely on the bed. The head and body should be acutely flexed.

The back is prepared with iodine and then cleaned off with seventy per cent alcohol from the level of the anterior superior spine to the uppermost lumbar vertebra. Sterile towels should be placed under the back and over the buttocks, or a surgical drape may be used.

The puncture should be performed under sterile precautions, with careful preparation of the hands and with sterile rubber gloves. The lumbar puncture needle should be sharp and should be as small as consistently possible with good pressure readings. The tap is best made between the fourth and fifth or third and fourth lumbar vertebrae, the latter being preferred because of frequent anomalies involving the former.

Procaine is injected into the skin as a local anesthetic. The lumbar puncture needle may be inserted in the midline or about 1 cm. to one side of the midline and is directed slightly upward. Entrance into the subarachnoid space is felt as a "give" before the needle as it penetrates the dura, the subarachnoid membrane lying immediately below it. If the puncture has been performed without trauma, a clear fluid is obtained on withdrawal of the stylet.

The manometer for measuring pressure of the spinal fluid should be attached at this point without loss of any of the spinal fluid. A water manometer is by far preferable, but a mercury manometer may be used if no water manometer is available. The level of the fluid column should be measured after it has come to rest. If the patient is tense this may require four or five minutes, or longer; if he is relaxed an accurate pressure reading may be taken within this time.

In cases of suspected block of the spinal subarachnoid space a Queckenstedt test may be performed. It should never be performed in cerebral cases, especially if a brain tumor is suspected. The test is performed with the aid of an assistant, who makes pressure for ten seconds on one jugular vein, then the other, and then on both jugulars simultaneously. The rise of pressure at the end of ten seconds is recorded, the pressure released and the level of pressure recorded at the end of ten seconds after release of the pressure. In normal cases with no block of the subarachnoid space a rapid and high rise of the spinal fluid follows bilateral jugular compression (to 400 or 500 mm. of water) provided the lumen of the needle is well in the subarachnoid space. Fall of the fluid to its original level takes place in ten to fifteen seconds after release of the pressure.

The test is completed by asking the patient to strain and then to cough when a similar rise in pressure occurs. The elevation of pressure on compression of the jugular veins is due to increase in intracranial pressure by blockage of venous escape from the skull; if a block is present in the subarachnoid space no rise occurs or only an imperfect rise. Coughing and straining, however, will still cause a rise in pressure despite a block because of elevation of the spinal pressure from increased abdominal pressure and blockage of escape of blood from the spinal veins (v. Spinal Cord Tumor).

After the hydrodynamics are completed the manometer is detached and enough fluid removed for routine examination which should consist of cell count, globulin, Wassermann reaction, colloidal gold reaction, total protein estimation, and sugar reduction. Special studies, such as culture of the spinal fluid, chloride estimation, and smear, should be made as indicated. The level of the spinal fluid pressure is taken routinely after the fluid is withdrawn.

The puncture wound is covered with a sterile dressing and the patient instructed to lie flat, but not necessarily on his back, for twenty-four hours in order to avoid a lumbar puncture headache. The diet after puncture needs no restrictions. The patient may be allowed to get up twenty-four hours after lumbar puncture.

Cistern Puncture: This is necessary under some circumstances. The hair should be shaved to the level of the occipital protuberances. The patient is placed on his side, with the head sharply flexed, the chin on the chest and the head absolutely straight. Rotation of the neck of any degree must be avoided. The back of the neck is prepared with iodine and alcohol and the patient's head and shoulders draped with sterile towels. The cistern puncture is then performed under strict aseptic precautions. A lumbar puncture needle is used.

The spine of the second cervical vertebra is identified and the thumb of the left hand held firmly down on this spine. The needle is then directed along the knuckle of the flexed left thumb, the point coming directly in the center of the depression above the second cervical spine. The needle is then directed in the midline slightly upward along a line transecting the external auditory meatus and the bridge of the nose. After two or three resistances are penetrated a sudden "give" is felt, indicating entrance of the needle into the cisterna magna. This is reached in thin-necked persons at a depth of about 4 cm., and in thick-necked persons at about 5 cm. If blood is encountered the needle should be withdrawn and no further attempts made. If the neck has been in good position, and the needle held strictly in the midline in the direction indicated, the cistern will be reached without difficulty.

Encephalogram: This is necessary for many reasons and is carried out as follows: The meal preceding the test is withheld. Sedation, usually a barbiturate, is given $2\frac{1}{2}$, $1\frac{1}{2}$ and $\frac{1}{2}$ hours before the procedure is carried out. Dilaudid or morphine may be given if the patient is inadequately controlled by barbiturates. With the patient under the influence of sedation, the procedure is carried out in the roentgenographic department with the patient sitting up and straddling a chair, the arms and chin resting on a pillow thrown over the back of the chair. Lumbar puncture is carried out in the usual fashion and 15 cc. of spinal fluid is allowed to run into a graduated beaker. Ten cc. of air is then drawn through sterile gauze into a sterile syringe and injected into the subarachnoid space. Ten cc. of fluid is again allowed to flow out and is replaced by an equal quantity of air. The procedure is continued until 100 cc. of air has been injected. For children and infants less air is injected. If there is any question as to the adequacy of injection the needle is left *in situ* and a spot film of the skull taken in order to determine whether the ventricles are well visualized or not.

Temperature, pulse, respiration, and blood pressure readings are taken before fluid is withdrawn, and the last three recorded every five or ten minutes thereafter. If an appreciable fall is noted, caffeine sodium benzoate is given subcutaneously ($3\frac{1}{4}$ gr.) and repeated if necessary. Epinephrine may be given if signs of collapse develop. After the necessary films are taken the patient is returned to bed on a stretcher and placed in the Trendelenberg position for twenty-four hours. Carbon dioxide and oxygen are given immediately on return to bed by mask inhalation.

Myelogram: Pantopaque is injected into the spine for the purpose of creating a contrast medium against which one may visualize defects in the spinal canal. It may be injected by the lumbar or cistern routes. *Lumbar* injection is carried out with the patient on a fluoroscopic table in the roentgenographic room. Lumbar puncture is carried out in the usual fashion and 10 cc. of spinal fluid is collected. Pantopaque which has been previously warmed by immersion of the ampoule in warm water is now removed from its warm bath and the contents (10 cc.) poured into the barrel of a syringe which is attached to the lumbar puncture needle. The Pantopaque is injected slowly until 5 to 10 cc. is injected. The column of iodized oil is then studied under the fluoroscope on a tilt table and spot films taken. For *cisternal* injection a routine cistern puncture is carried out and Pantopaque injected as by the lumbar route.

For lumbar lesions, such as spinal cord tumor or herniated disc, lumbar myelography by the lumbar route is sufficient. For cervical and thoracic lesions, cisternal myelography is more accurate.

Table 4—Muscle Innervation

(After Raezer)

ORDER OF ARRANGEMENT: *Muscle action; muscles with spinal cord segments* (C—cervical, T—thoracic, L—lumbar, S—sacral) ; *cord of plexus—peripheral nerve.* Asterisks (*) indicate the muscles chiefly responsible for the movement in question.

UPPER EXTREMITY—BRACHIAL PLEXUS—C5 to T1

1. FLEXORS AND LATERAL ROTATORS OF HEAD:
   * *a   Sternocleidomastoid m.—medulla and C2, C3, C4—Cranial Nerve XI
   * b. Posterior neck m.—C2, C3, C4 and nerves
     * i   Longus capitis
     * ii Rectus capitis anterior
     * iii Longus colli

2 EXTENSORS OF HEAD:
   * a. Trapezius m.—medulla and C2, C3, C4—Cranial Nerve XI
   * b. Posterior neck m.—C2, C3, C4 and nerves
     * *i   Longissimus capitis
     * ii Semispinalis capitis

3. ELEVATORS OF SHOULDERS: Test: Shrugging of shoulders
   * *a. Trapezius m.—same as 2a
   * b. Elevators of scapula—C3, C4, C5—dorsal scapular n.
     * i   Levator scapulae
     * ii Rhomboidei

4. RETRACTORS OF SHOULDERS:
   * *a. Trapezius m.—same as 2a
   * b. Rhomboidei—same as 3b

5. LATERAL ABDUCTORS OF ARM: *Above 90° angle* (also fix scapula below 90°)
   * a. Trapezius m.—same as 2a
   * b. Anterior serratus m.—C5, C6, C7—long thoracic n.

6. FORWARD THRUSTING OF ARM: Test: Patient extends arms forward placing the palms against a wall and pushes body toward the wall keeping the arms extended. Examiner observes scapula for "winging" (separation of scapula from back) with the inferior angle of the scapula pulled up and in
   * a. Anterior serratus m.—same as 5b

7. ADDUCTORS OF HUMERUS:
   * *a. Latissimus dorsi m.—C6, C7, C8—posterior cord of brachial plexus—thoracodorsal n.
   * *b. Pectoralis major m.—C5 to T1—lateral and medial cords—anterior thoracic n.
   * c. Teres major m.—C5, C6—posterior cord—subscapularis n.
   * d. Teres minor m.—C5, C6—posterior cord—axillary n.
   * e. Coracobrachialis m.—C5, C6—musculocutaneous n.

8. FLEXORS OF HUMERUS: Test: Arm at side pushing forward against resistance—"punching" action
   * *a. Pectoralis major and minor m.—same as 7b
   * b. Deltoid m.—C5, C6—axillary n.
   * c. Subscapularis m.—C5, C6—posterior cord—subscapularis n.
   * d. Coracobrachialis m.—same as 7e

9. EXTENSORS OR RETRACTORS OF ARM: Test: Arm and elbow at side pushing back against resistance—"swimming" action
   * *a. Latissimus dorsi m.—same as 7a

10. ABDUCTORS OF ARM: Test: Arm laterally abducted *up to 90° angle*
    * a. Initiator of abduction—C5, C6—suprascapular n.
      * i   Supraspinatus m.
    * *b. Deltoid m.—same as 8b

TABLE 4—*Continued*

11. MUSCLES OF RESPIRATION:
    a. Normal respiration:
       i Diaphragm—C3, C4, C5—phrenic n.
       ii Intercostals ⎫
       iii Subcostals   ⎬T1 to T12—intercostal n.
       iv Levator costorum ⎭
       v Scaleni—C4, C5—cervical nerves
    b. Accessory muscles of respiration:
       i Sternocleidomastoid M.—same as 1a
       ii Trapezius m.—same as 2a
       iii Anterior serratus m.—same as 5b
       iv Latissimus dorsi m. (coughing)—same as 7a
       v Pectoralis major and minor—same as 7b
       vi Rhomboidei m.—same as 3b
       vii Supraspinatus m.—same as 10a

12. MEDIAL OR INWARD ROTATORS OF ARM: Test: Arm extended at side and rotated inward against resistance:
    a. Pectoralis major m.—same as 7b
    b. Latissimus dorsi m.—same as 7a
    c. Teres major m.—same as 7c
    d. Subscapularis m.—same as 8c
    e. Deltoid m.—same as 8b

13. LATERAL OR OUTWARD ROTATORS OF ARM: Test: Arm held at side and laterally rotated against resistance:
    a. Teres minor m.—same as 7d
    b. Infraspinatus m.—same as 10a
    c. Deltoid m.—same as 8b

14. FLEXORS OF FOREARM (elbow):
    a. Chief flexors: C5, C6—lateral cord—musculocutaneous n.
       *i Biceps brachii
       ii Brachialis
       iii Coracobrachialis
    b. Accessory flexors:
       i Brachioradialis—C5, C6—posterior cord—radial n.
       ii Pronator teres—C6—median n.
       iii Palmaris longus—C6—median n.

15. EXTENSORS OF FOREARM (elbow):
    a. Triceps brachii m.—C6, C7, C8—posterior cord—radial n
    b. Anconeus—same as triceps

16. PRONATORS OF FOREARM (rotation of forearm inward):
    a. Pronator teres—C6—median n.
    b. Pronator quadratus—C7, C8—median m.
    c. Flexor carpi radialis—same as pronator teres

17. SUPINATORS OF FOREARM (rotation of forearm outward)
    a. Supinator m.: C5, C6—posterior cord—radial n
      (arm extended)
    b. Biceps brachii: Same as 4a
      (arm flexed)

18. FLEXORS OF WRIST:
    a. Main flexors: C6—median n.
       i Flexor carpi radialis
       ii Palmaris longus
       iii Flexor digitorum sublimis
    b. Accessory flexion:
       i Flexor carpi ulnaris—C8, T1—ulnar n.
       ii Flexor digitorum profundus—C6, T1—median and ulnar nerves

TABLE 4—*Continued*

19. EXTENSORS OF WRIST: All innervated by C6, C7, C8—radial n.
    a. Extensor carpi radialis longus ⎫
    b. Extensor carpi radialis brevis ⎬ extend wrist
    c. Extensor digitorum communis extends all phalanges of fingers
    d. Extensor digiti quinti proprius—extends phalanges of little finger
    e. Extensor carpi ulnaris—extends ulnar side of wrist
    f. Extensor pollicis brevis—extends proximal phalanx of thumb
    g. Extensor pollicis longus—extends distal phalanx of thumb
    h. Extensor indicis proprius—extensor of index finger
20. ADDUCTORS OF WRIST: Movement of wrist toward the ulna bone
    a. Flexnor carpi ulnaris—same as 18b
    b. Extensor carpi ulnaris—same as 19e
21. ABDUCTORS OF WRIST:
    a. *Flexor carpi radialis:* Same as 18a
    b. *Extensors which abduct:* Same as 19
        i Extensor carpi radialis longus and brevis
        ii Extensor pollicis longus and brevis
    c. *Abductor pollicis longus* (abductor of base of thumb):
        C6, C7, C8—radial n.

HAND

I   MOVEMENTS OF THUMB:
    1. *Abduction of thumb:*
        a. Abductor pollicis brevis (abducts first metacarpal)—C6, C7—median n.
        b. Abductor pollicis longus—C6, C7, C8—radial n.
    2. *Extensors of thumb:* C6, C7, C8—radial n.
        a. Extensor pollicis longus and brevis
    3. *Adductor of thumb:* (pure adduction of thumb when thumb is on a plane with the hand)
        a. Adductor pollicis—C8, T1—ulnar n.
    4. *Flexor of Thumb:* C6, C7—median n.
        a. Proximal phalanx—flexor pollicis brevis
        b. Terminal phalanx—flexor pollicis longus
    5. *Opposition of thumb to fingers:* C6, C7—median n
        a. Opponens pollicis—assisted by
            i Flexor pollicis brevis—4a
            ii Adductor pollicis—3
II MOVEMENTS OF SMALL FINGER: C8, T1—ulnar n.
    1. *Abductor of little finger:*
        a. Abductor digiti quinti
    2. *Flexor of little finger:*
        a. Flexor digiti quinti
    3. *Opposition of little finger to thumb:*
        a. Opponens digiti quinti
    N.B. All 3 of the above muscles act only on the metacarpophalangeal joint
III. MOVEMENTS OF FINGERS:
    1. *Flexor of metacarpal:* Phalangeal joints—C6—median n
        a. Flexor digitorum sublimis
    2. *Flexor of distal interphalangeal joints:* C7 to T1—median and ulnar n.
        a. Flexor digitorum profundus
    3. *Extensor of all joints of 4 fingers:* C6, C7, C8—radial n.
        a. Extensor digitorum profundus
        b. Extensor digiti quinti proprius
        c. Extensor indicis proprius
    4 *Accessory extensors of interphalangeal joints and flexors of metacarpophalangeal joints*
        a. lateral 2 lubricales—C7 to T1—median n.
        b. Medial 2 lumbricales—C8, T1—ulnar n.
        c. Interossei m.—C, T1—ulnar n.

TABLE 4—*Continued*

5. *Ab*ductors (spreading) and *ad*ductors (approximating) of fingers—C8, T1—ulnar n
   a. Interossei m.
      i   4 volar interossei *ad*duct
      ii 4 dorsal interossei *ab*duct
6. *Thenar eminence of hand:* Muscles at base of thumb—C6, C7, C8, T1
7. *Hypothenar eminence of hand:* Muscles at base of little finger—C8, T1

SUMMARY OF MUSCLE INNERVATION
UPPER EXTREMITY

1. All movements of head and neck are initiated through the medulla and C2, C3, and C4—cranial nerve XI and respective cervical nerves.

2. Shrugging and retraction of shoulders mediated through the medulla and C2, C3, C4, and C5—cranial nerve XI and respective cervical nerves.

3. Paralysis of deltoid alone with normal flexion of wrist and metacarpophalangeal joints localizes the lesion to the fifth (5) cervical cord segment.

4. Abduction and lateral rotation of arm; flexion of the elbow and supination of the forearm are all carried out through the fifth (5) and sixth (6) cervical cord segments *only.*

5. Flexion of metacarpophalangeal joints of the 4 fingers is mediated by only the sixth (6) cervical cord segment.

6. Retraction of arm (swimming action) is initiated through C6, C7, and C8—thoracodorsal nerve.

7. Retraction of the arm, extension of the elbow, wrist and all the fingers, abduction of the wrist and thumb and pronation of the forearm are all mediated through the sixth (6), seventh (7) and eighth (8) cervical cord segments.

8. Flexion of the terminal phalanges of all *5* fingers is initiated through the seventh (7), eighth (8) cervical, and first (1) thoracic cord segments.

9. The muscles of the hypothenar eminence of the hand and interossei are innervatedl by C8 and T1 only through the ulnar nerve.

10. Adduction, flexion and medial rotation of humerus initiated through C5 to T1 and al portions of the brachial plexus.

The ten summary movements noted above will be seen to follow a natural progression of movement. This will be made more clear if one performs these movements for himself in the order in which they are written. Furthermore this will aid greatly in fixing the above pattern and make memorization less arduous.

It should be noted that No. 10 is a set of movements that include the whole brachial plexus and hence are always involved to a greater or lesser extent with any lesion of the brachial plexus, or cord segments from C5 to T1.

LOWER EXTREMITY
LUMBROSACRAL PLEXUS—L1 TO S2

1. FLEXORS OF HIP JOINT: L2, L3 and L4
   *a. Iliopsoas m.—L2, L3 and L4—ant. rami of L2, L3 and L4 and femoral n.
   b. Rectus femoris ⎫
   c. Pectineus m.   ⎬ L2, L3 and L4—femoral n.
   d. Sartorius m.   ⎭
   e. *Ad*ductor longus and brevis ⎫
   f. *Ab*ductor magnus   ⎬ L3 and L4—obturator n.
   g. Obturator externus   ⎭
2. ADDUCTORS OF THIGH: L2, L3 and L4
   a. Adductor magnus   ⎫
      i Adductor longus ⎪
      ii Adductor brevis ⎬ L2, L3 and L4—obturator n.
   b. Gracilis   ⎪
   c. Obturator externus ⎭
   d. Sartorius m. ⎫ L2, L3—femoral n.
   e. Pectineus m. ⎭

TABLE 4—*Continued*

3. EXTENSION OF KNEE: L3, L4 (±L5, S1)
     *a. Quadriceps femoris—L3, L4
     b. Tensor fascia lata—L4 (L5 and S1)—superior gluteal n.

4. ABDUCTORS OF FEMUR: L4, L5, S1 (S2)
     a. Gluteus medius ⎫
     b. Gluteus minimus ⎬ L4, L5, S1—superior gluteal n.
     c. Tensor fascia lata ⎭
     d. Superior and inferior gemelli m. ⎫
     e. Obturator internus m. ⎬ S1, S2—anterior rami n
     f. Pyriformis m. ⎭

5. EXTENSORS OF HIP:
     a. Gluteus maximus—L5, S1, S2—inferior gluteal n.
     b. Biceps femoris m. ⎫
     c. Semitendinosus m. ⎬ L5, S1, S2—sciatic n.
     d. Semimembranosus m. ⎭

6. LATERAL ROTATORS OF THIGH: L2 to S2
     a. Sartorius—same as 2d
     b. Adductor magnus, longus and brevis—same as 2a
     c. Obturator externus—same as 2c
     d. Gluteus maximus—same as 5a
     e. Biceps femoris (when knee is flexed)—same as 5b
     f. Inferior gemellus m.—same as 4d
     g. Pyriformis m.—same as 4f
     h. Obturator internus m.—same as 4e
     i. Superior gemellus m.—same as 4d

7. MEDIAL ROTATORS OF FEMUR: L4, L5, S1
     a. Tensor fascia lata—same as 3b
     b. Gluteus medius and minimus—same as 4a and 4b
     c. Adductor magnus m.—same as 2a

8. FLEXORS OF KNEE: L2 to S2
     a. Sartorius—same as 2d
     b. Gracilis—same as 2b
     c. Biceps femoris—same as 5b
     d. Semitendinosus ⎫
     e. Semimembranosus ⎬ same as 5c and 5d
     f. Gastrocnemius—S1, S2—tibial n.

9. DORSI-FLEXORS OF ANKLE (foot): L4, L5, S1—deep peroneal n
     a. Tibialis anticus m.
     b. Extensor digitorum longus m.
     c. Peroneus tertius
     d. Extensor hallucis longus

10. EXTENSORS OF TOES: L4, L5 and S1—deep peroneal n.
     a. Extensor digitorum longus and brevis
     b. Extensor hallucis longus

11. PLANTAR FLEXORS OF FOOT: L4, L5, S1, S2
     a. Peroneus longus and brevis—L4, L5, S1—superficial peroneal n
     b. Gastrocnemius m.—S1, S2—tibial n.
     c. Soleus
     d. Flexor digitorum longus ⎫
     e. Flexor hallucis longus ⎬ L5, S1, S2—tibial n.
     f. Tibialis posticus

TABLE 4—*Continued*

12. INVERSION OF FOOT: L4, L5, S1
    a. Tibialis anticus—L4, L5, S1—deep peroneal n.
    b. Tibialis posticus—L5, S1—tibial n.

13. EVERSION OF FOOT: L4, L5, S1
    a. Peroneus tertius—L4, L5, S1—*deep* peroneal n.
    b. Peroneus longus and brevis—L4, L5, S1—*superficial* peroneal n.

14. MEDIAL ROTATORS OF FOOT (with knee flexed and foot flat on floor): L4 to S2
    a. Semitendinosus } same as 5c and 5d
    b. Semimembranosus }
    c. Sartorius m. } same as 2b and 2d
    d. Gracilis m.   }
    e Popliteus m.—L4, L5, S1—tibial n.

15. LATERAL ROTATOR OF FOOT WITH KNEE FLEXED:
    a. Bicep femoris m.—L5, S1, S2—sciaticus n.

16. PLANTAR FLEXORS OF TOES: L4 to S2
    a. Flexor digitorum longus   }
    b. Lumbricales (same action as in hand) } L5 to S2—tibial n.
    c. Flexor hallucis longus   }
    d. *Ab*ductor hallucis longus }
    e. Flexor digitorum brevis   } L4, L5, S1—medial plantar n. (branch of tibial)
    f. Flexor hallucis brevis   }
    g. Flexor digiti quinti brevis } S1, S2—lateral plantar n.—branch of tibial n.
    h. Interossei   }
    i. Quadratus plantus m.

17. EXTERNAL ANAL SPHINCTER: S3, S4—pudendal n.

SUMMARY OF MUSCLE INNERVATION
LOWER EXTREMITY

1 Flexion of hip, sitting up and adduction of femur mediated by L2, L3, and L4.

2. Extension of knee mediated by L3 and L4 (exception—tensor fascia lata—L4 to S1).

3. Therefore—dissociation in strength between flexion of the hip and adduction of the thigh on the one hand and extension of the knee on the other—points to an exquisite lesion of L2 or L4 (sartorius muscle will be weak if such is the case).

4. Abduction and medial rotation of femur, dorsiflexion of foot, extension of toes, inversion and eversion of foot are all innervated by L4, L5 and S1.

5. If patient can adduct (L2, L3 and L4) the femur, and has poor abduction of the femur—a lesion of L5 and S1 is indicated.

6. Poor abduction of femur associated with normal strength in the gastrocnemius, soleus and muscles of lateral half of foot isolates the lesion to L5.

7. Atrophy of muscles on the lateral half of the sole of the foot with some atrophy and weakness of the calf muscles (gastrocnemius and soleus muscle) and good flexion of *all* the toes—the lesion may be postulated to involve S1 and S2 with sparing of L5.

8. Ability to walk on heels reflects integrity of L4, L5 and S1.

9. Ability to walk on toes reflects integrity of L5, S1 and S2.

10. Injury to common peroneal nerve (especially over head of fibula) results in loss of dorsiflexion and loss of ability to evert the foot—foot is inverted with plantar flexion.

11. Injury to the deep peroneal nerve produces weakness or paralysis of dorsiflexion of foot with ability to evert the foot intact.

12. Injury to superficial peroneal nerve leaves dorsiflexion of foot intact and produces weakness or paralysis of eversion of the foot.

Generally: The anterior thigh muscles represent the upper lumbar cord segments and nerves; anterolateral aspect of the lower leg, the lower lumbar cord segments; the posterior thigh and leg, the lower lumbar and upper sacral cord segments; and the sole, the upper sacral cord segments. The external anal sphincter tone is supplied by the third and fourth sacral cord segments.

2

Interpretation of Neurological Symptoms and Signs

An exhaustive survey of the meaning of neurological symptoms and signs would lead too far afield, yet some consideration of this aspect of the neurological examination is essential for the reason that the attainment of a logical diagnosis begins with a recognition of abnormal signs, followed by their proper analysis and their grouping into a proper diagnosis. The chief abnormal findings which may be encountered therefore in a neurological examination merit some description.

I. CRANIAL NERVES

Olfactory: *Anosmia,* or complete loss of smell, is found most commonly as a result of local disease. It occurs with meningiomas involving the olfactory groove; with trauma affecting the ethmoid plate, and is associated with laceration of the base of the frontal lobe. It is frequently overlooked by the patient, who may be totally unaware of a complete loss of smell. *Hyposmia,* or decrease of smell, is associated with the same causes as loss of smell but is of little clinical importance since the finding is so common in normal subjects due to nasal obstruction, previous catarrh, etc. Repugnant smells are found as a part of uncinate fits in epilepsy and indicate a lesion involving the uncus in the temporal lobe. They are often associated with repugnant tastes and smacking movements of the lips.

Optic: Disease of the optic nerve is characterized by (1) disturbance or loss of visual acuity, (2) visual field defects, (3) changes in the fundus oculi involving the nerve and retina. The optic nerve may be the seat of primary or secondary optic atrophy, the former resulting from direct injury (inflammation, compression, etc.) of the nerve between the retina and optic chiasm, and the latter from previous infiltration of the nerve which has been replaced by organization of tissue.

Disease of the optic nerve usually is characterized by a partial or complete loss of vision. A history of involvement of the optic nerve is characterized by an account of visual loss. This is usually slowly progressive in the case of tumors which compress the optic nerves, or in such conditions as multiple sclerosis and syphilis. In other instances, as in encephalomyelitis, acute multiple sclerosis, and retrobulbar neuritis, the visual loss is acute.

Primary Optic Atrophy: This results from many causes, most of which are of primary concern to the ophthalmologist and require no mention here. The important neurological conditions associated with primary optic atrophy are: (1) *Tumors* such as pituitary tumor, tumors lying above the sella turcica (suprasellar), sphenoid ridge tumors, olfactory groove meningiomas, aneurysms; (2) *inflammations,* including central nervous system syphilis (tabes dorsalis, general paresis), encephalitis, encephalomyelitis, and some forms of neuritis; (3) *degenerative conditions* such as multiple sclerosis, Friedreich's ataxia, Marie's cerebellar ataxia; (4) *intoxications* due to arsenic (tryparsamide), lead, nicotine, quinine; (5) *miscellaneous conditions* such as exsanguination, trauma, aneurysm, etc.

ma continues and exudates may develop as the process becomes older.

The choked disc eventually becomes organized and replaced by connective tissue, the edema receding and the nerve head becoming visible as the organization proceeds. Eventually secondary optic atrophy develops, the nerve head appear-

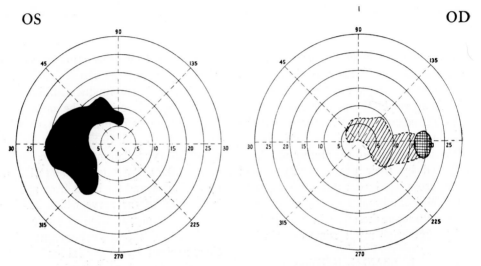

OS   OD

Fig. 5—*Absolute paracentral scotoma* in left eye and *relative central-paracentral scotoma* in right eye in a patient with multiple sclerosis.

Secondary Optic Atrophy: It develops in optic nerves which have been previously inflamed or edematous, in which organization has occurred. It may follow optic neuritis, retrobulbar neuritis, choked disc, and vascular obstructions.

Choked Disc or Papilledema: This is an important condition affecting the optic nerves and is considered in the chapter on Neuritis. It is characterized by swelling and edema of the optic nerve head associated with dilatation of the veins. The nerve head is elevated above the level of the retina, the edges of the nerve are at first obscured and then completely obliterated, and the nerve head eventually becomes completely obliterated. The surrounding retina shows no changes at first but later hemorrhages appear as the ede-

ing grayish or grayish white, and the edges indistinct in outline. The elevation of the nerve head in choked disc is measured by first focusing the ophthalmoscope clearly on the retina at some distance from the disc elevation and then focusing the ophthalmoscope on the edematous nerve head to the point of greatest clarity. The difference between the original and the last reading represents the elevation of the choked disc which is measured in diopters of swelling (1D, 2D, etc.). About 3D of swelling is equivalent to 1 mm. of elevation of the nerve head.

Choked disc is caused by tumor of the brain in the vast majority of instances, but it may be caused by other conditions such as subdural hematoma and brain abscess, and rarely by tuberculous meningitis, multiple sclerosis, and encephalitis.

Visual Field Defects: These are found in almost all optic nerve afflictions. When the optic nerve is involved anywhere from the retina to the optic chiasm, the visual defect is usually a *scotoma*, which may be central or paracentral or both, the size depending on the degree of nerve damage. Sector defects may be seen, or even unilateral defects obliterating an upper or lower field. In disorders involving the optic chiasm, tract, or radiation the defect is a *hemianopsia*. These may be congruous or incongruous. In an incongruous field defect one field is affected more than the other. In a congruous defect they are equally affected (*v*. Neuritis).

Hemianopsias may be (1) bitemporal, or (2) homonymous. *Bitemporal hemianopsia* is characterized by a loss of both temporal fields of vision and is due to compression or disease of the optic chiasm, particularly those fibers within it which are derived from the nasal sides of

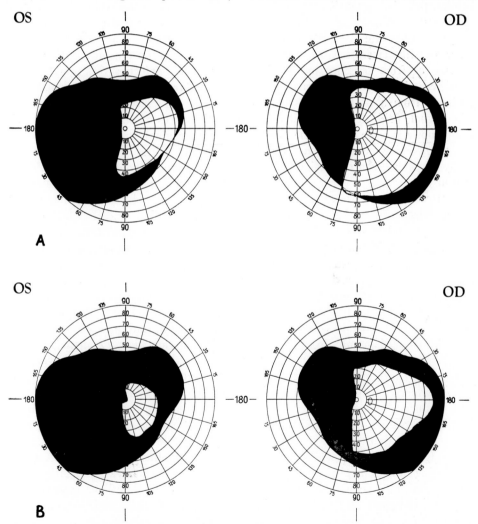

Fig. 6—A, *Congruous left homonymous hemianopsia. B, Incongruous left homonymous hemianopsia.*

the retinae. The presence of bitemporal hemianopsia indicates a lesion in or above the sella turcica. In the majority of instances this lesion is a primary pituitary tumor growing within the sella turcica, expanding upwards to compress the optic chiasm. In other instances the condition is due to lesions lying above the sella turcica and compressing the optic chiasm (meningioma, adenoma, hypophyseal stalk tumor, aneurysm, arachnoiditis). Lesions at the side of the sella turcica (parasellar) may cause bitemporal hemianopsia by extension medially to compress the chiasm. Bitemporal hemianopsia may in rare instances result from trauma with laceration of the optic chiasm, or from pressure by a dilated third ventricle due to internal hydrocephalus from a posterior fossa tumor. The visual field defect in bitemporal hemianopsia is often through the fixation point, involving central vision, but in many instances central vision may be spared.

HOMONYMOUS HEMIANOPSIA: This is characterized by loss of the temporal field of one eye and of the nasal field of the other. It is considered in detail in Chapter 3. Briefly, it may involve the entire homonymous half fields, or less commonly it may produce a quadrantic defect (quadrantanopsia). The field defect may spare or involve central vision. Homonymous hemianopsia results from disease of the optic tract or radiation from the optic chiasm to its termination in the occipital lobe. Tumors, aneurysms, and injuries may produce a homonymous hemianopsia in the optic tract between chiasm and the primary visual centers in the midbrain, Rarely, such defects occur from infiltrating tumors involving the primary centers (external geniculate bodies).

In the temporal and occipital lobes, homonymous hemianopsia may result from a variety of conditions: encapsu-lated tumor, glioma, abscess, softening, hemorrhage, multiple sclerosis, encephalitis, etc. Distinction between a hemianopsia caused by a temporal or occipital lobe lesion is not possible. The hemianopic cut is likely to be more clean cut and to involve central vision in temporal lobe lesions because the fibers of the optic radiation are more closely packed in the temporal lobe and spread out more widely in the occipital lobes. This distinction is not definite, however, since a lesion of sufficient size is capable of interrupting all the visual fibers in the occipital lobe. In the last analysis, it is not possible to distinguish between a temporal and occipital lobe process purely on the basis of the visual field defects.

Ocular: Diseases of the ocular nerves produce (1) changes in the pupils, (2) disturbances of ocular movements (ophthalmoplegias).

Abnormalities of the *pupils* are found in diseases involving the oculomotor nerve. The *normal pupil* is round, centrally placed, regular in outline, equal in size to its fellow, and responds promptly to light, accommodation and consensual reactions. *Unequal, irregular pupils* reacting slowly to light are found in syphilis of the nervous system, chronic alcoholism, encephalitis, and not infrequently in cerebral arteriosclerosis. A pupil may be said to be slow and sluggish in its reaction when it contracts slowly or imperfectly to direct light, or when after contraction it relaxes almost immediately. The arc of contraction is smaller in sluggishly reacting pupils. *Argyll Robertson pupils* are found in tabes dorsalis particularly, and less frequently in general paresis and other forms of neurosyphilis. They are almost always indicative of neurosyphilis, but they have been described also in encephalitis, multiple sclerosis, infiltrating tumors of the midbrain, and chronic alcoholism. Isolated loss of the light reflex (not typical Argyll Robertson pupils) has been described in diabetes mellitus, trauma of the eyeball and orbit, and syringomyelia. Argyll Robertson pupils are characterized by the following features: They are contracted and small in typical cases, but they may be dilated. They are irregular in outline, often unequal, and they fail to react to light or consensual reactions. In typical instances they respond to accommodation, but the reaction may be so slight that it is difficult to see. In other instances the pupils fail to react to accommodation. They respond poorly to painful stimuli and they dilate but slightly with mydriatics. Unilateral Argyll Robertson pupils are sometimes found in neurosyphilis. The pathogenesis of the Argyll Robertson pupil has been explained on the following bases: (1) It is due to interruption of the afferent limb of the reflex arc in the posterior commissure (Merritt and Moore); (2) it is due to a lesion at the synapses between the cells of the sphincter of the iris and the reflex collaterals surrounding these cells (Spiegel). *Unilateral dilated pupil* failing to react to light (Hutchinson's pupil) is found at times in subdural hematoma and extradural hemorrhage, but is neither a constant nor an invaluable sign. It may develop also as a result of irritation of the cervical sympathetic pathway from its peripheral course in the neck to its central portion.

Horner's syndrome is the result of paralysis of the cervical sympathetic trunk and is characterized by contraction of the pupil, partial ptosis of the eyelid, enophthalmos and inconstantly, a loss of sweating over the affected side of the face. It may be due to (1) lesions affecting the cervical sympathetic trunk in the neck; gunshot or stab wounds, disease of the cervical glands, tumors,

aneurysms, etc.; (2) spinal cord (segments C-8 to T-1) or spinal root (C-8 to T-1) lesions such as extramedullary tumors, trauma, pachymeningitis and other extramedullary processes, intramedullary lesions such as syringomyelia, intramedullary tumors, hematomyelia, syphilitic meningomyelitis; (3) brain stem lesions such as syringomyelia and infiltrating tumors.

Paradoxical pupil is a dilation of the pupil on stimulation by light and is found at times in tabes dorsalis. The *tonic pupil* of Adie's syndrome is usually found in women, is often unilateral (80%), is usually larger than its fellow, is sometimes bilateral, responds poorly to light but relaxes in the dark, after which it can be made to respond to light, and to react normally to mydriatics. It may be associated with loss of the Achilles and/or patellar reflexes. The most important feature of the myotonic pupil is its behavior on convergence. "If the patient fixes a near object and continues to gaze at it intently, the pupil, sometimes after a delay of several seconds, contracts slowly and with increasing slowness through a range, often greatly in excess of the normal; contraction down to pinhead size is not uncommon; the larger abnormal pupil then becomes smaller than its fellow" (Adie). It has been found that the abnormal pupil manifests marked constriction after instillation of 2.5 per cent *methacholine,* while the normal pupil fails to react.

Disturbance of movement of the eyeballs is found regularly in disease involving the ocular nerves. These are spoken of as ophthalmoplegias and are discussed in diseases of the cranial nerves (*v.* Neuritis).

Trigeminal: The trigeminal nerve is composed of both motor and sensory portions; hence motor and sensory manifestations may be found alone or in combination. *Motor* weakness can be elicited by palpation of the masseters and temporals when atrophy of the affected masseter and temporal can be detected. Weakness can also be elicited by having the patient bite on a tongue depressor, which can be pulled away easily from the affected side and not at all from the normal side. Deviation of the jaw can be noted also if the masseters and pterygoids are weak on one side, the deviation being toward the paralyzed side Because of the deflection of the jaw the tongue appears to be deviated as well, but this is not the case, since a line drawn through the incisors will be found to cut through the tip of the tongue.

Motor weakness involving the masseter, temporal, and pterygoids which are supplied by the trigeminal nerve, may be the result of a peripheral lesion such as trauma, skull fracture, or tumor. It may also result from a tumor of the cerebellopontine angle which compresses the trigeminal nerve at its exit from the pons, from an infiltrating tumor of the pons, or from encephalitic or other processes involving the motor nucleus of the trigeminal nerve in the pons.

The Sensory Division of the Trigeminal Nerve: This supplies the face and head to the vertex, the cornea, and the mucous membranes of the nose, mouth, hard and soft palate, and tongue to the midline. Complete interruption of sensory function is rare, but it may develop with tumors of the gasserian ganglion, or with inflammatory disease of this ganglion. In such instances it is associated with pain in the face along the branches of the trigeminal nerve. Incomplete sensory syndromes involving the face are found in infiltrating tumors of the pons, or in connection with other conditions which affect the sensory trigeminal nucleus, such as multiple sclerosis and encephalitis. A special type of sensory involvement of the face is seen in lesions affecting the descending root of the trigeminal nerve,

as in occlusion of the posterior inferior cerebellar artery. In such conditions the sensory loss is in a so-called onion peel arrangement and does not conform to the anatomical outlines of the trigeminal nerve. Sensory loss of the individual branches of the trigeminal nerve occurs under many circumstances: herpes zoster, injury, disease of the gasserian ganglion.

One of the early manifestations of sensory loss of the trigeminal nerve is loss of the *corneal reflex.* This may be the only manifestation of involvement of the sensory branch. It occurs early in many cases of cerebellopontine angle tumor. It is found in hemiplegia, in thalamic syndromes, in infiltrating tumor of the pons, encephalitis, multiple sclerosis, tumor of the gasserian ganglion, herpes zoster ophthalmicus, after section of the trigeminal nerve for trigeminal neuralgia, and in any disorder affecting the gasserian ganglion, the sensory nucleus of the trigeminal nerve in the pons, or in local conditions of the eye.

Facial: Involvement of the facial nerve occurs frequently in disease of the nerv-

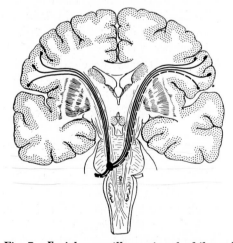

Fig. 7—*Facial nerve* illustrating the bilateral innervation of the upper portion of the facial nerve (solid lines) and the unilateral innervation of the lower portion (broken lines), thus accounting for central facial weakness.

ous system. Careful distinction must be made between central and peripheral nerve involvement.

A *central* facial weakness is characterized by weakness of movement of the lower portion of the face on the side opposite the lesion. It is due to the fact that the upper portions of the face receive innervation from both motor areas, while the lower portion is innervated only from one side of the brain: the opposite motor cortex. It is recognized by a slight drooping of the corner of the mouth on the affected side, with accompanying drooping of the upper lip, a slight smoothness of the nasolabial fold, weakness in retraction of the corner of the mouth on the affected side, and a flattening of the angle of the mouth on opening it. When the sign is well pronounced it is easy to detect, but slight differences require careful scrutiny and are sometimes difficult to recognize. In the usual case of central facial weakness the forehead can be wrinkled normally and closure of the eyelid is normal. In acute cases of facial weakness, as in acute hemiplegias, a slight weakness in

wrinkling the forehead and in closing the eye is at times seen. In such instances the weakness in the lower portion of the face is always more pronounced, while that of the upper portions tends to disappear within a few days as a rule. While voluntary facial expression is weak in central palsies, *emotional expression* remains intact or may even be exaggerated. In lesions of the thalamus, however, emotional expression may be lost, while voluntary movements are intact. This dissociation of voluntary and emotional expression is important in differentiating a deep-seated from a cortical lesion.

Central Facial Weakness: This may result from lesions involving the motor innervation to the face anywhere between the face area in the opposite motor cortex and the nucleus of the facial nerve in the pons, involving the corticobulbar pathway which contains the fibers of all the motor cranial nerves between motor cortex and their nuclei in the brain stem. Thus a central facial weakness may result from a lesion in the face area of the opposite motor cortex, resulting

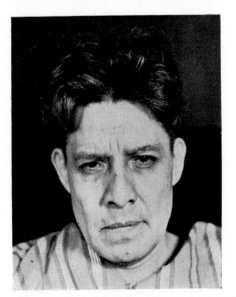 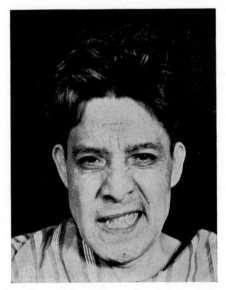

Fig. 8—*Central facial weakness* showing the drooping of the right corner of the mouth with the face in repose and the weakness of retraction of the mouth on voluntary effort.

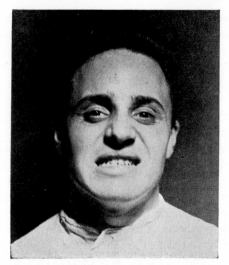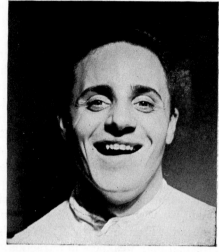

Fig. 9—*Central facial weakness* showing good retraction of the corners of the mouth on voluntary movement but with definite weakness of the left corner of the mouth on laughing.

from a variety of lesions: tumor, encephalitis, multiple sclerosis, vascular lesions, etc. It may be involved alone or in conjunction with weakness of the hand, arm, or other parts of the body. Central facial weakness existing alone, or with other focal weakness (faciobrachial monoplegia, etc.), is usually the result of a focal lesion of the opposite motor cortex, but may represent the residual of an old hemiplegia. In the majority of instances central facial weakness is associated with a hemiplegia, and is due to simultaneous interruption of corticospinal and corticobulbar pathways.

Peripheral Facial Paralysis: This differs from central facial weakness in the involvement of all portions of the facial musculature. It results from a lesion of the facial nerve anywhere along its peripheral course from the facial nucleus in the pons to its distribution in the face (*v.* Neuritis). The lesion producing the paralysis is ipsilateral to the paralysis. All portions of the face on the affected side are paralyzed. Wrinkling of the forehead, closure of the eyelid, movements of the muscles of fa-

cial expression are impossible; taste is at times lost on the anterior two-thirds of the tongue on the affected side; tenderness of the nerve trunks of the face may be present, and reaction of degeneration may be elicited if regeneration fails to ensue. While a complete discussion of peripheral facial paralysis follows, brief mention may be made here of its general implications. It may result from involvement of the facial nucleus in the pons as in poliomyelitis, encephalitis, or infiltrating tumors of the pons. It may be involved as a result of disease of the nerve within the skull, as in cerebellopontine angle tumors, meningitis (syphilitic, tuberculous), or subarachnoid hemorrhage; or, it may ensue from disease of the facial nerve at any point after its emergence from the skull as the result of neuritis, fracture of the skull, tumors of the neck, herpes zoster, etc. The features of the disease of the nerve at its various points of involvement are considered later. Facial nerve paralysis resulting from involvement of the facial nucleus is characterized by signs of anterior horn cell involvement — atrophy of the muscle, fasciculations, paralysis, etc. (*v.* Chapter 3). Involvement of the nerve trunk is featured by the usual signs of neuritis involving a motor nerve (*v.* Chapter 3).

Acoustic: The acoustic nerve is composed of cochlear and vestibular divisions, the former having to do with hearing, the latter with equilibrium. Disease of the *cochlea* is characterized by nerve deafness, the main features of which are loss or impairment of hearing, loss of air con-

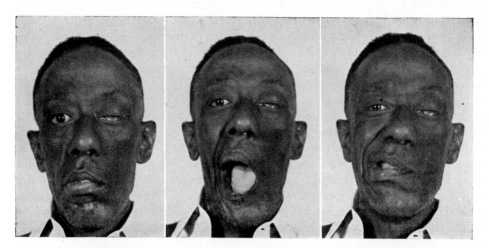

Fig. 10—*Peripheral facial paralysis* showing the involvement of all facial muscles of the left side, with inability to wrinkle the forehead and to close the eyelid and paralysis of the muscles of facial expression.

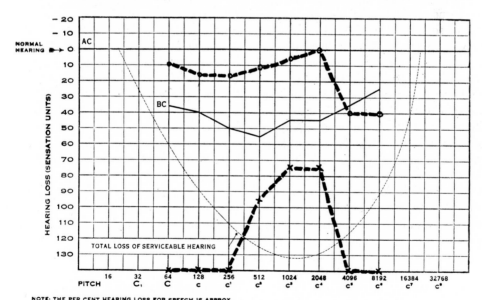

Fig. 11—*Audiometer chart.* There is a characteristic nerve deafness involving the left ear as revealed by the loss of hearing of the higher frequencies.

duction, and failure to lateralize sound to the affected ear. Usually there is an associated history of tinnitus, but this is sometimes lacking. Tinnitus may be present for some time before deafness ensues. Nerve deafness is practically always the result of disease of the peripheral portion of the auditory nerve. Theoretically, it is possible as a result of central lesions involving the auditory pathways in the brain stem and the termination of the cochlear fibers in the temporal lobe. Actually this occurs extremely rarely due to the fact that the auditory pathways are both crossed and uncrossed and a very extensive lesion is required in order to cause loss of hearing. Loss of hearing may be tested much more accurately by the audiometer than by tuning-fork tests. By this means notes of standard pitch and varying intensities are sent through the ear. Nerve deafness is indicated by a loss of hearing in the higher frequencies.

Special forms of hearing disturbance are found in Meniere's disease. Distortion of sound in the affected ear is common. Diplacusis is sometimes present, and the recruitment phenomenon is characteristic (*v*. Meniere's Disease).

The *vestibular* portion of the auditory nerve is frequently affected in diseases of the nervous system. Its outstanding feature is vertigo, a subjective sensation requiring careful analysis (*v*. Vertigo). Loss of hearing in neurological disorders is found in Meniere's disease, cerebellopontine angle tumors, cranial trauma, otosclerosis, syphilitic meningitis, and tabes dorsalis, to choose random examples.

Nystagmus: This is found in disease of the vestibular portion of the auditory nerve, as well as in other conditions. A consideration of its features is desirable at this point.

DEFINITION : Nystagmus is an involuntary oscillation of the eyeball. It is usually bilateral, the two eyes moving synchronously, but unilateral nystagmus may occur.

Nystagmus may be *rhythmical* or *pendular*. In rhythmical nystagmus, there are alternate slow and quick ocular movements, the rapid movement being in the direction of gaze, followed by a slower return movement. In pendular nystagmus, there are more or less regular to-and-fro movements of equal range and velocity.

Nystagmus may be horizontal, vertical, oblique, rotatory, or mixed in form, and may be directed to the right, left, upward, or downward. It may be slow, medium, fast, and may vary from 10 to 1000 oscillations per minute. It may be transient or sustained. Nystagmus may be congenital or acquired, spontaneous or induced, and may be present at rest, on fixation, or on deviation of the eyeballs.

The fast component in rhythmical nystagmus is of cerebral origin. It is said to disappear with anesthesia and to return with the return of consciousness. The precise portion of the cerebrum which regulates the quick component in nystagmus is not definitely known. It is said to be in the occipital lobe, with communication to the second frontal convolution (Fox and McIntyre). On the other hand, "It has been shown that the only part of the central nervous system essential for the production of the slow and quick phases of nystagmus is that portion situated between the oculomotor nuclei above and the vestibular nuclei below" (de Jong). The slow component in nystagmus is compensatory and is of peripheral or vestibular origin. Its purpose is to preserve the image on the retina.

CLASSIFICATION : Many classifications of nystagmus have been offered. The usual grouping is into ocular, vestibular, and central types. The following grouping, based on the studies of de Jong, covers the problem well:

1. *Induced nystagmus.*

    (*a*) *Optokinetic nystagmus* (optic, optomotor nystagmus): This form of nystagmus is elicited when a drum with vertical stripes is rotated rapidly before the eyes, or where a person in a rapidly moving vehicle directs his eyes on fixed objects (railway or elevator nystagmus). The nystagmus is fine, rapid, and rhythmical, and is horizontal. Optokinetic nystagmus is a physiological response, and its absence is significant. It has been found absent in lesions of the opposite temporal and parietal lobes between the visual cortex and the second frontal convolution. It has been found absent in cases of homonymous hemianopsia especially when objects are moving from the blind to the normal field.

    (*b*) *Labyrinthine nystagmus:* This follows stimulation of the semicircular canals. The nystagmus is the result of movement of the endolymph with resulting stimulation of the vestibular nerves. Labyrinthine nystagmus is characterized by a quick and slow component and must be regarded as a reflex response to movements of the head or body, or to stimulation of the labyrinth. It may be horizontal or rotary, or both. Labyrinthine nystagmus can be produced by rotation in a Bárány chair, by thermal or caloric stimulation, by douching the external auditory canals, by galvanic stimulation, and by compression.

    (*c*) *Reflex acoustic nystagmus:* This form of nystagmus results from loud auditory stimuli.

    (*d*) *Reflex sensory nystagmus:* This form of rhythmical nystagmus follows stimulation of the skin, in the neighborhood of the ear, on pressure on the tragus.

    (*e*) *Chemical, or toxic, nystagmus* follows the use of drugs.

2. *Pathological nystagmus.*

    (*a*) *Optic origin.*

        (1) *"Ocular" nystagmus:* This is pendular, oscillating, and coarse and slow. The movements are usually horizontal, occasionally vertical, and rarely rotary. This form of nystagmus is seen in subjects with deficient vision since birth, in those whose vision has failed before fixation is learned, in subjects whose fixation is defective, in the colorblind, and in persons with an increased sensitivity to light. It is seen in congenital cataract, ophthalmia neonatorum, interstitial keratitis, congenital corneal leukoma, chorioretinitis, high-grade myopia, and albinism. The nystagmus results from an effort to attain fixation despite defective vision.

        (2) *Occupational nystagmus:* This is oscillating or pendular, fine, rapid, often vertical, and increased on upward gaze. Fixation is defective. It is seen in miners and in others who work in poor light, such as compositors, draftsmen, jewelers, train dispatchers, crane workers, and painters. "It most often develops after long exposure to poor illumination, especially after working in a stooped attitude with the eyes deviated upward, and it is probably the result of insufficiency of binocular fusion" (de Jong).

        (3) *Spasmus nutans.*

    (*b*) *Neuromuscular origin:* Unsustained nystagmoid jerks are seen in a large number of normal persons on extreme deviation of the eyes. This is referred to as "end-position nystagmus" and has no clinical significance. Exaggerations of this type of nystagmus are seen in the following:

        (1) *Paretic nystagmus,* which develops on attempts to use a paretic ocular muscle.

        (2) *Fatigue nystagmus,* which follows excessive use or increased fatigability of certain ocular muscles.

        (3) *Nystagmus of eccentric fixation:* This occurs on deviation of the eyes beyond the limits of the binocular field. It is jerky and occurs in 50 to 60 per cent of normals.

(4) *Latent nystagmus:* This occurs on covering one eye in subjects with poor visual acuity or without binocular vision especially patients with amblyopia resulting from strabismus. It occurs in the covered eye and is in the direction of the open eye.

(c) *Labyrinthine nystagmus:* This may result from disease of the labyrinth or of the vestibular nerve.

(d) *Central nystagmus:* This develops from lesions in the brain stem or the posterior longitudinal bundle. It varies in type, degree, rate, and direction, but it is always rhythmical. Vertical nystagmus is said to be pathognomonic of a brain-stem lesion, but it has been shown to be due to labyrinthine disease as well. Central nystagmus may result from many diseases, too numerous to be listed here.

(e) *Miscellaneous types.*

(1) *Toxic nystagmus:* This results from the use of barbiturates, acetanilid, disphenylhydantoin, lead, nicotine, chloroform, quinine, and alcohol.

(2) *Congenital nystagmus:* This dates from birth and must be differentiated from ocular nystagmus, which does not develop until fixation is attempted.

(3) *Nystagmus with cervical cord disease:* Nystagmus occurs at times with diseases of the cervical portion of the spinal cord, usually above C4.

(4) *Voluntary nystagmus:* This is oscillating, unilateral or bilateral, rapid, and usually horizontal. The movements are increased by fixation, convergence, or increasing the width of the palpebral fissure.

Glossopharyngeal: The glossopharyngeal nerve is rarely diseased alone, but when present is characterized by loss of taste over the posterior third of the tongue, and over the palate and pharynx. This has been observed in syphilitic meningitis and in infiltrating tumors of the brain stem. Pain in the throat is found in glossopharyngeal neuralgia, a rare disease characterized by severe paroxysms of pain initiated by swallowing (*v.* Neuritis).

Vagus: The vagus nerve, associated as it is with many vital activities, may theoretically show numerous disturbances of function. From a practical viewpoint, disturbances of swallowing and phonation are the most important features of vagus dysfunction. Bradycardia may be found in increased pressure but is not constant. *Aphonia* or *hoarseness* may result from involvement of the nucleus ambiguus portion of the vagus innervation in the medulla, from involvement of the vagus nerve in the posterior fossa, or from recurrent laryngeal paralysis. It is found in syringobulbia, infiltrating tumors of the brain stem, occlusion of the posterior inferior cerebellar artery, multiple sclerosis, encephalitis, poliomyelitis, amyotrophic lateral sclerosis, and other conditions. It is associated with abductor paralysis of the vocal cord. *Swallowing* weakness or paralysis occurs under a variety of circumstances. It may be found in hemiplegia, due to involvement of the corticobulbar pathway, and is associated in these circumstances with paralysis or weakness of the soft palate. Swallowing in such conditions is never lost, but only impaired. It may result also from involvement of the muscles of deglutition from a lesion of the nucleus ambiguus in the medulla, from causes similar to those mentioned in disease of the glossopharyngeal nerve. In such instances the palate moves poorly and there is loss of power of the middle and inferior constrictors of the pharynx, with regurgitation of food through the nose due to inability to close the pharynx on swallowing. In some instances of difficulty in swallowing the palate is capable of moving well while the inferior pharyngeal constrictors fail to

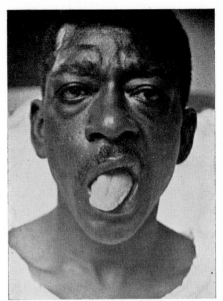

Fig. 12—*Lingual paralysis* showing the deviation of the tongue to the right side in a case of right hemiplegia.

function. Loss of function of the latter is seen in weakness or loss of movement of the Adam's apple in attempted swallowing.

Involvement of the vagus nerve at the various levels of its course is discussed later (*v.* Neuritis).

Spinal Accessory: This nerve is not often diseased, but when it is there results disturbance of function of the sternomastoid and trapezius muscles (*v.* Neuritis).

Hypoglossal: The hypoglossal nerve, like the facial nerve, may show evidence of central or peripheral involvement. *Central* weakness of the hypoglossal nerve is characterized by a deviation of the tongue to the affected side, the tongue being pushed over by the action of the healthy muscles of the opposite side. Such disturbances are seen in involvement of the tongue fibers anywhere from their origin in the opposite motor cortex to its nucleus in the medulla. It is often found in conjunction with hemiplegia.

whatever may be its origin. Rarely it is seen as a single symptom of focal motor cortex disease. It is unassociated with atrophy or muscle fasciculations.

Peripheral weakness is characterized by atrophy of the tongue associated with muscle fasciculations. In early cases the atrophy can be detected as an indentation or scalloping along the edges of the tongue, associated with fine fasciculations. As the process becomes more advanced, atrophy of the muscle of the tongue becomes more apparent, the tongue shrinking perceptibly on the affected side. With the tongue in the floor of the mouth, a curvature can be seen toward the healthy side; muscle fasciculations are active when the process is well developed. Weakness of the tongue can be demonstrated by pressing the tip of the tongue against the cheek. In severe cases the tongue cannot be protruded. The process develops, as a rule, as a result of disease of the nucleus of the hypoglossal nerve in the medulla, as for example in amyotrophic lateral sclerosis, progressive bulbar paralysis, and syringobulbia.

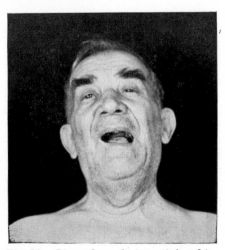

Fig. 13—*Lingual paralysis,* peripheral in origin, as indicated by the inability to protrude the tongue. Atrophy is visible, indicated by the corrugation and indentation of the tongue.

II. INTELLECTUAL FUNCTIONS AND SKILLED ACTS

No examination of the nervous system is complete without a survey of the intellectual functions and skilled acts, and since the examination begins with history taking, an analysis of these functions can be made at the very outset.

problems, often changes in personality and mood changes. This type of reaction is seen in a number of conditions and is indicative chiefly of involvement of the frontal lobes. It is found in cerebral arteriosclerosis, senile dementia, brain tumor, in some forms of encephalitis, and indeed in any condition which causes dif-

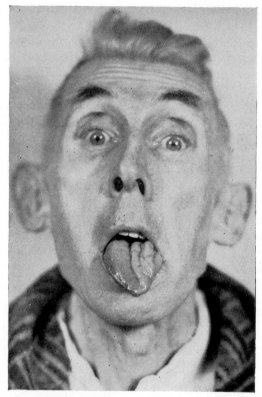

Fig. 14—*Hemiatrophy of the tongue* in a patient with amyotrophic lateral sclerosis.

The responses of the patient must be analyzed carefully. Slow, hesitant replies are of great significance, provided it can be determined that they are not normal for the individual in question. The *organic mental reaction* appears in a number of syndromes and is characterized by loss or impairment of memory especially for recent events, difficulty in concentration, impairment of ability to comprehend abstract concepts and to synthesize ideas, difficulty with simple arithmetical

fuse or extensive destruction of the cerebral cortex.

Most of the information referable to the organic type of mental reaction is often obtained from the family or relatives, but much information concerning it can be gleaned from observation of the patient himself. The reactions are annoyingly slow and deliberate and the patient tantalizingly retarded.

Memory loss can be tested by a few simple tests such as the ability to repeat five or more figures forward and backward, the repetition of a simple story such as the cowboy story in the Binet-Simon test, and the ability to recall essential facts in the life of the patient and the history of his illness. Simple arithmetical problems are impossible and errors in calculation may be elicited by the serial seven test which consists merely of asking the patient to subtract seven from one hundred and from the result until nothing is left.

Personality changes are found often in organic brain disease affecting particularly the frontal lobes. They are not in themselves indicative of frontal lobe disease, but they occur with disorders of these areas frequently. The fundamental feature of the reaction is a change in the normal mode of reaction of the affected person. Mistakes in judgment, loss of the niceties of social behavior, coarse behavior, sexual excesses and indiscretions, and many other nonspecific forms of reaction are encountered. The type of reaction varies widely for each patient, but the important fact is, that, as compared with the premorbid personality, there is a change in the reactions of the patient.

Emotional disturbances of various sorts may be found in organic brain disease: Emotional lability, depression, excitements, apathy, and confusional reactions. They have no localizing significance.

Among the skilled acts which may be disturbed is *speech*. This may be manifested by aphasia or loss of speech, or dysarthria, which refers merely to disturbance in enunciation. *Aphasia* (*v.* Chapter 3) may be detected readily by an inability on the part of the patient to find words, a difficulty of which he is usually aware. Severe loss of words is readily recognized, but an occasional deficit may be missed. There may also be a lack of understanding of words or an inability to read.

Dysarthrias may be manifested by a mere slurring of speech, a difficulty in clear enunciation of words, noted in cases of multiple sclerosis. In early stages of the disturbance the deficit may not be apparent to the patient and too much weight must not be given to denial of the speech disorder by the patient or his family. Slurred speech is also evident in general paresis and may be elicited by means of test phrases such as "Massachusetts artillery, particular statistics, truly rural, Irish constabulary, round the rugged rock the ragged rascal ran, etc."

Special types of dysarthria are seen in cases of bulbar or pseudobular paralysis, the speech having a nasal quality due to failure of contraction of the pharyngeal and lingual muscles during speech. Severe dysarthrias are found in cerebellar disease of various types; here the speech becomes almost unintelligible because of the dyssynergia of the muscles concerned with speech. Severe dysarthrias are noted in progressive lenticular degeneration, Huntington's chorea, cerebral diplegia, congenital double athetosis, and other conditions.

III. MOTOR SYSTEM

The method of routine examination of the motor system has been indicated in Chapter 1. Examination of the muscles for abnormalities is concerned with a search for disturbance of muscle bulk, muscle power, muscle tone, and involuntary movements.

1. Changes of *muscle bulk* may manifest themselves either as atrophy or hypertrophy. Atrophy of muscles is almost always the result of disease of the peripheral pathways, either of anterior horn cells or peripheral nerve; it may result from cerebral involvement. When due to peripheral disease its distribution is segmental in the case of anterior horn cell disease or along the distribution of pe-

ripheral nerves in case of involvement of these structures. When it is of cerebral origin it is as a rule associated with old hemiplegias and is said also to occur with parietal lobe disease. It has, therefore, in central disorders a hemiplegic distribution. It is best seen in such circumstances in infantile hemiplegias, the muscles and bones of the affected side being smaller than those of the normal side. Involvement of the muscles of only the hand or arm may be found in central cortical disease. The precise location of the cortical lesion associated with muscle atrophy is still unsettled. The motor cortex is involved in most cases, but implication of the postcentral gyrus has been demonstrated in others. The reason for the atrophy in instances of this kind is unknown, but the presence of atrophy suggests a trophic function of the cortical areas concerned. That associated with infantile hemiplegia is largely due to lack of use.

In instances of muscle atrophy careful search must always be made to determine the exact distribution of the atrophy; whether it is segmental or generalized. It is important to determine, for example, whether it is confined to the small muscles of the hand or hands, to the shoulder girdle or thigh, or whether it is diffuse. Muscle fasciculations or fibrillations should always be searched for carefully. Electrical studies in order to determine whether reaction of degeneration is present are not always necessary but are desirable in order to determine the degree of involvement of the peripheral innervation of the muscle in anterior horn cell or peripheral nerve disease.

Muscle fasciculations or *fibrillations* are indicative of anterior horn cell disease but they are seen at times in peripheral nerve disease under special conditions. In such instances there is associated disease of the anterior roots and anterior

horn cells. This occurs in special types of neuritis as in acute infectious polyneuritis, at times in diabetic neuritis when the entire reflex arc is affected, in porphyrinuric neuritis, etc. They are seen also inconstantly in neurotic subjects, in fatigue, and on exposure to cold. They are seen so predominantly in anterior horn cell disease that for all practical purposes they may be said to be indicative of this disease, occurring in poliomyelitis, progressive spinal muscular atrophy, amyotrophic lateral sclerosis, syringomyelia, infiltrating spinal cord tumor, etc. They are seen as irregular fine or coarse twitchings of parts of muscles, appearing irregularly and unassociated with movement of the affected muscle at the joint. They are associated with atrophy of the muscles due to interruption of muscle innervation, but they are not always seen in atrophied muscle due to anterior horn cell disease because there may be no muscle present to fibrillate. Fasciculations may be seen early in anterior horn cell disease with little or no atrophy. They are often inconstant, and can be seen in muscles at one time and not at another. At times they are abundant; again they require careful search. They may be brought out on mechanical stimulation of a muscle by tapping, or by placing the muscle on stretch. Their mode of origin is not known. They are not consistently obliterated by nerve block and by spinal anesthesia and appear to be completely obliterated by curare, by section of the nerve (Forster and Alpers), and by injection of local anesthetic directly into the muscle. They are increased by acetylcholine and neostigmine. A metabolic factor may be present in muscle fasciculations, since it has been found that thyroidectomy tends to delay, and feeding with dessicated thyroid to decrease, the time before onset of fibrillations in rabbits. Not all atrophy is associated with muscle fasciculations. The atrophy due to primary muscle disease, as in the myopathies, the atrophy of peripheral nerve disease or injury, and that of cortical involvement, is not associated with fasciculations. Hence their demonstration is indicative of anterior horn cell disease. The cause of atrophy of denervated muscles due to anterior horn cell disease is not clear, but two theories prevail: (1) That it is the result of overactivity due to the muscle fasciculations: (2) that it is the result of disuse.

Muscle fasciculations are sometimes seen in *neurotic subjects* with great tension and anxiety. They may be diffuse or focal and may even involve the face and tongue. They are indistinguishable from fasciculations associated with an-

terior horn cell disease, but they are never found with atrophy or reflex changes. They are not indicative of disease of the anterior horn cells. They may persist for some time and disappear, only to recur at varying intervals. Sometimes they are associated with painful muscle cramps.

Muscle fasciculations must not be confused with *myoclonus,* which is a muscle twitch or contraction of the muscle capable of producing movement of the affected muscle. It is a rapid, coarse muscle jerk which may be isolated or multiple, involving a large part of the muscle belly.

Muscle atrophy is found not alone in anterior horn cell disease. It is found also in peripheral neuritis of various kinds, the degree and distribution of the atrophy depending on the degree of injury of the

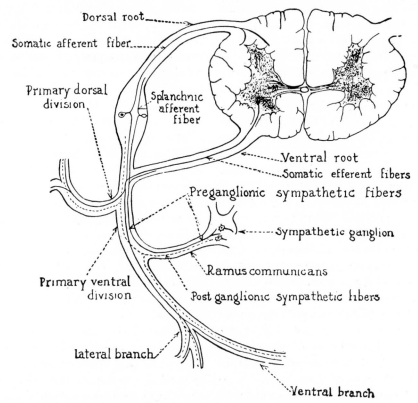

Fig. 15—*Reflex arc,* showing the relative relationships of posterior and anterior roots and the fibers of the sympathetic nervous system. (*Stookey: Nelson Loose Leaf Surgery, Vol. 2.*)

nerve trunks. In neuritis it is associated with tenderness of the muscles and nerve trunks, loss of reflexes, and often with sensory disturbances.

Atrophy is found also in peripheral nerve injuries and in arthritis. In the latter instance it is seen in the muscles surrounding the joints involved. It is found also in muscles which have not been used for some time (atrophy of disuse), as, for example, in muscles which have been in a plaster cast or in hemiplegic limbs deprived of movement. In chimpanzees marked atrophy of the hemiplegic muscles follows after ablation of Area 4 (Fulton), and affects particularly the distal muscles. It does not occur after ablation of other areas including the postcentral convolution.

Muscle atrophy is found in myopathies, in which case it may be diffuse or focal (scapulohumeral, etc.). In such instances it is unassociated with fasciculations or with reaction of degeneration.

Muscle *hypertrophy* is found in some forms of myopathy, as in pseudohypertrophic muscular dystrophy and in true hypertrophy. In cases of the former condition it is usually associated with atrophy of other muscles. The hypertrophied muscles have a hard, firm, rubbery consistency, and despite their appearance are usually weak. Mild degrees of muscle hypertrophy are found also in overuse of a limb in case of lack of use of the opposite limb. True muscle hypertrophy is found in association with some forms of congenital disease of the nervous system, in congenital hemihypertrophy involving one-half of the body, in hemihypertrophy involving half of the face, and in the generalized hypertrophy of the muscles found in the infant Hercules form of muscular dystrophy.

2. Changes of *muscle tone* must be searched for in any routine examination of the muscle system. There may be in-creased muscle tone (spasticity or rigidity), or decrease or loss of muscle tone (hypotonia), or flaccidity. Interruptions of the corticospinal pathway result in *spasticity,* a condition characterized by an increase in the muscle tone, associated with increase of reflexes, and with pathological reflexes such as the Babinski sign (*v.* Chapter 3, Upper Motor Neuron).

There is much doubt as to whether the spasticity of pyramidal lesions is the result of pure corticospinal interruptions or whether it is due to extrapyramidal mechanisms. Interruptions of the extrapyramidal system result in a state of increased tone referred to as *rigidity.* Spastic muscles on passive movement are associated with an increase of resistance to movement followed by a sudden or gradual release of resistance (clasp-knife reaction); rigid muscles on the other hand reveal a plastic reaction, with an even steady resistance to passive movement similar to that of bending a lead pipe; hence the term "lead pipe rigidity" given to this form of increased tonus (*v.* Chapter 3, Extrapyramidal System).

The presence of spasticity gives no clue as to localization of the lesion producing it. It is indicative only of a lesion causing interruption of the corticospinal pathway anywhere along its course. Thus, spasticity may result from interruption of this pathway in the cerebral hemisphere, in the internal capsule, in the brain stem, or spinal cord. Generally speaking the farther the lesion from the cortex the more probable is the occurrence of spasticity.

Interruption of the corticospinal pathway is by no means invariably associated with spasticity. In some instances, decreased muscle tone or flaccidity follows, but the mechanism of its production in the human has not yet been demonstrated. The flaccidity associated with cortico-

spinal disease resulting in a flaccid hemiplegia may last a few days to a few weeks,
or may persist throughout the course of
the hemiplegia. In monkeys and chimpanzees flaccid hemiplegia is produced by
ablation of Area 4 of the motor area, while
spasticity follows ablation of both the
motor and premotor areas (Areas 4
and 6).

Flaccidity is also produced in cats by
section of the pyramid in the medulla.

Evidence has accumulated to indicate
that in the human, too, flaccidity results
from ablation of the motor cortex and
that the spasticity and increased reflexes
found in corticospinal disease are the result of extrapyramidal rather than pyramidal or corticospinal mechanisms,
these extrapyramidal mechanisms acting
apparently unopposedly against the destroyed corticospinal tract. As yet, however, the parallelism between motor

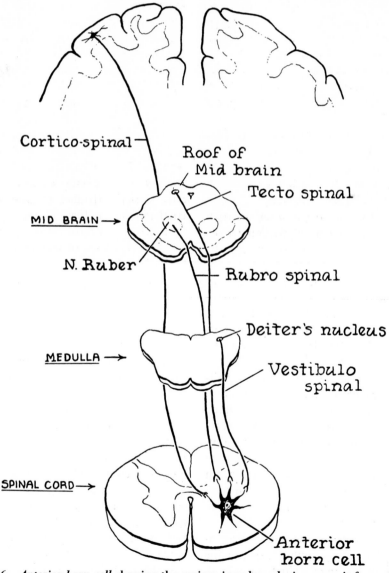

Fig. 16—*Anterior horn cell* showing the various impulses playing upon it from above.

cortical ablations in chimpanzees and lesions of the corticospinal pathway in man are imperfect. There is no doubt, however, that flaccid paralysis from a corticospinal lesion in man may occur in capsular lesions.

Hypotonia or *flaccidity* is characteristic of peripheral involvement and is invariably associated with disease of the an-

Posterior column disease, particularly tabes dorsalis, is associated with hypotonia of the muscles and hyperextensibility of the joints, but it is probable that in tabes, at any rate, the hypotonia is due to the associated disease of the posterior roots. Experimental injury of the posterior columns in monkeys results in some degree of hypotonia.

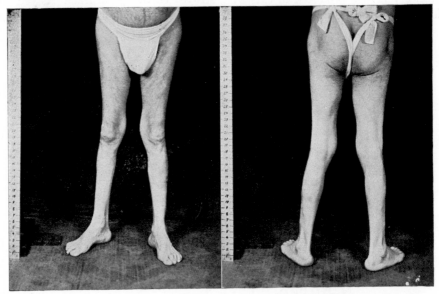

Fig. 17—*Anterior horn cell atrophy* involving the thigh and leg muscles, due to poliomyelitis. Note the pes cavus from involvement of the intrinsic foot muscles.

terior horn cells and peripheral nerves. The muscles are toneless, loose, their normal rounded contour is replaced by a flattened appearance, and the affected limbs are hyperextended at the joints and flail-like in their looseness. Disease of the posterior roots (radiculitis) is associated with hypotonia. Section of these roots results in flaccidity of the muscles denervated and the hypertonicity of decerebrate rigidity can be abolished by posterior root section. Hypotonia is found also in cerebellar lesions, where it is more likely to be associated with acute injuries, or disease of the cerebellum than with chronic conditions. It is less commonly seen in the human than in the experimental animal.

3. Changes of *muscle power* are invariably associated with disease either of the upper or lower motor neuron, or of the muscles. The degree of weakness depends on the degree of injury of the anterior horn cells, peripheral nerves, motor pathways, muscles, or other motor units anywhere in the neuraxis. The weakness may be partial, in which case it is referred to as *paresis,* or it may be complete when it is of course designated as *paralysis.* The weakness of anterior horn cell disease is segmental in character and associated with flaccidity, atrophy, fasciculations, and loss of reflexes; that of peripheral nerve disease follows the distribution of the affected nerve or nerves, is often as-

sociated with pain and sensory disturbances, and is accompanied by loss of reflexes; that of upper motor neuron disease is hemiplegic in character, involving face, arm, and leg as a rule, and is associated with spasticity, overactive reflexes, pathological reflexes, and is without sensory changes (*v.* Chapter 3). Apparent weakness is found in disease of the extrapy-

result also from interference with nervous impulses at the myoneural junction, as in myasthenia gravis and botulism. In some disorders, such as family periodic paralysis, a generalized but transient paralysis of the muscles develops as the result of mechanisms as yet unknown. Similarly, generalized attacks of muscular weakness, induced by emotional excitement of

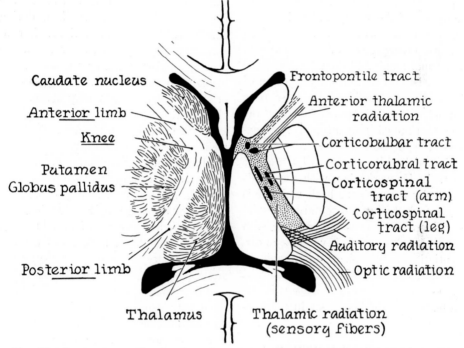

Fig. 18—*Internal capsule* showing the relative position of the corticospinal and corticobulbar tracts as well as the three divisions of the internal capsule and the optic and auditory radiations.

ramidal system; however, it is the result not of true weakness, but of slowness in initiating movement.

Not all weakness is associated with denervation of the muscles, either from peripheral or central disease of the nervous system. Primary disease of the muscles (myopathies) is invariably associated with weakness either local or generalized, and may be partial or complete. The weakness of primary muscle disease is fully as great as in disease of the nervous system. Marked weakness may

any sort, and resulting in complete transitory collapse, are found in the cataplectic attacks of narcolepsy. Here, too, the mechanism of their production is unknown.

Loss of movement is by no means indicative of paralysis, a simple fact which is sometimes overlooked. Loss or decrease of movement is seen characteristically in paralysis agitans, unassociated with paralysis or motor weakness of any degree. This is first seen in early cases in a loss of the normal arm swing and later in loss of almost all voluntary movement. Loss of movement may result from contractures or from fixation of joints by trophic or other processes. It may be associated also with catatonia and with hysteria, the latter without organic changes of any sort.

Accessory or *associated* or *synkinetic* movements are seen under some circumstances, especially in disease of the corticospinal system. Flexion movements of the fingers of the paralyzed hand may be observed in cases of hemiplegia when a patient squeezes the examiner's hand with the normal hand, and dorsiflexion of the paralyzed foot often occurs on flexion of the paretic leg. Dorsiflexion of the paretic foot in hemiplegia is seen on flexion of the knee (Strümpell phenomenon); pronation of the paretic forearm is found on extension of both arms upward (pronator sign). In Hoover's sign, with the hands held under the patient's heels while he is on his back, lifting the sound leg results in an increased downward pressure with the paralyzed leg. This is valuable in differentiating a hemiplegia of organic or structural origin from one of hysterical origin since the downward pressure of the paralyzed leg will be absent in the hysterical patient.

IV. INVOLUNTARY MOVEMENTS

Involuntary muscular movements occur in a variety of forms and under many circumstances. They consist of the following forms: Tremor, chorea, athetosis, tics, spasms, muscle fasciculations, myokymia, and myoclonus. The problem of muscle fasciculations has already been described in connection with the finding of muscle atrophy. Many of the involuntary movements listed are discussed subsequently (*v.* Diseases of Extrapyramidal System).

1. **Tremor:** This occurs under many circumstances. It may be defined as an involuntary, purposeless movement af-fecting the limbs most frequently, at times the head and neck, and rarely the trunk. For its physiological features refer to the chapter on Extrapyramidal Diseases.

Fine rapid tremors of the extended fingers are found in general paresis and are associated as a rule, but not always, with tremors of the tongue, eyelids, and lips. Fine tremors of the extended fingers are found also in hyperthyroidism, during emotional excitement, in fatigue, after injections of epinephrine, after the ingestion of amphetamine, or ephedrine, and in many neurotic states. Coarse tremors of the fingers are commonly observed in chronic alcoholism, reaching their severest degree in delirium tremens, where the tremors are violent and involve not only the limbs but the face and trunk as well.

Excessive use of tobacco results at times in finger tremors. A coarse type of tremor of the hands and fingers is found also in rare instances as a familial tremor, occurring chiefly in males, and making its appearance often early in life during adolescence. Senility is associated with a coarse tremor of the fingers and often of the head, resulting either in a nodding tremor of the head (affirmative type), or a rotary tremor (negative type). Senile tremors assume many forms. They may be present on rest or movement or both. Similar tremors are seen in cerebral arteriosclerosis. Excessive use of coffee and tea, mercury, manganese and lead poisoning, bromidism, barbiturate poisoning, cocainism, and morphinism are associated with tremors. Tremor is seen also in weakened limbs.

Disease of the cerebellum or its pathways results in tremor referred to as intentional tremor, which is characterized by appearance of the tremor on voluntary movement and its increase on continued motion in approaching a goal. Tremors of this type are seen in cerebellar disease such as tumor or softenings. They are particularly pronounced in disease of the superior cerebellar peduncles as seen in thrombosis of the superior cerebellar artery, or in interruptions of the cerebellar pathways and red nucleus in mesencephalic lesions as in Benedikt's syndrome (*v.* Vascular Diseases). Multiple sclerosis is often associated with an intentional type of tremor.

Extrapyramidal diseases of many sorts are usually, but not always, associated with tremor. The tremor of paralysis agitans involves the limbs, outstandingly, especially the fingers and hands, but it may also affect the head and lips. It is fine or coarse, usually of the pill-rolling type, and may be static or present when the limb is at rest, intentional, or evoked on movement, or both. Progressive lenticular degeneration (Wilson's disease) is also associated with tremor simulating closely that of paralysis agitans. A peculiar coarse tremor of the arms and hands, seen on abduction of the arms, characterized by a wing-flapping movement, is seen in this disease.

2. Choreiform Movements: These occur in Sydenham's chorea, Huntington's chorea, symptomatic chorea from various causes, senile chorea, and a variety of other conditions. They are characterized by abrupt, involuntary movements. For their general physiological characteristics refer to the chapter on Extrapyramidal Diseases.

3. Athetosis: This is characterized by the presence of slow, snakelike movements in contrast to the abrupt movements of chorea. It occurs under many circumstances. Symptomatic athetosis is found in cerebral arteriosclerosis, syphilis of the nervous system, encephalitis, and degenerative diseases of various kinds, the lesion responsible for the movement being in the basal ganglia. Athetosis is seen also in cerebral diplegia, infantile

hemiplegias, and in double athetosis, the last named being associated with the condition known as status marmoratus. Pseudoathetosis, characterized by athetoticlike movements, is seen in tabes dorsalis, subacute combined degeneration, and peripheral neuritis.

4. Myoclonic Movements: These are clonic, rapid contractions of the muscles of the extremities and trunk resulting, as a rule, in no movements of the affected limbs. They occur in generalized or focal varieties and are found in encephalitis, cerebral vascular disease, and in special forms of myoclonia such as paramyoclonus multiplex and myoclonus epilepsy (*v.* Extrapyramidal Diseases). A rare form of myoclonus affects the diaphragm in postencephalitic states.

5. Spasms: Spasms of various kinds are seen in nervous disorders. Habit spasms of many sorts are common, involving face, limbs, or trunk. Spasmodic torticollis is a variety of spasm involving the neck muscles, resulting in movement of the head. Hemispasm of the face, associated with organic lesions of the facial nerve, or occurring as a habit spasm, is sometimes seen. Blepharospasms are found following encephalitis and consist of spasmodic contractions of the eyelids. Spasms of the tongue and spasms of swallowing are seen at times, the former in states of emotional instability, or in conjunction with reflex irritation from throat, teeth, or mouth infections, and the latter in neuroses. A special form of spasm is seen in the head-nodding of spasmus nutans seen in rachitic children.

6. Convulsions: These occur under many circumstances. They vary greatly both as to variety and cause and are discussed in detail later (*v.* Epilepsies).

V. DISTURBANCES OF STATION

Standing is a postural reflex which is dependent on reflexes mediated through the medulla oblongata and influenced to a marked degree by tonic neck and labyrinthine reflexes. Hence, interference with any of the mechanisms responsible for the maintenance of local, segmental, or general static postural reflexes will cause interference with the act of normal standing.

Disturbances of *station* are characterized by an inability to maintain normal equilibrium in standing, either with the eyes open or closed. The majority of such disturbances are due to interference with the mechanisms chiefly responsible for the maintenance of station; namely, the posterior column system, the cerebellum and its pathways, and the vestibular system. In other instances station may be greatly impaired because of weakness or deformities of a leg, primary myopathies, and nerve injuries.

The station difficulties found in disease of the *posterior columns* (tabes, syringomyelia, subacute combined degeneration, Friedreich's ataxia, etc.) are dependent on loss or impairment of deep sensation; particularly of muscle, tendon, and joint sensations, manifested by a loss of position sense in the joints. The fundamental difficulty lies in a loss of proprioceptive impulses from the joints, tendons, and muscles. In disturbances of posterior column function, *Romberg's sign* is positive and is characterized in classical instances by an increased inability to stand steadily with the feet together, the difficulty being increased with the eyes closed. Often the patient with posterior column disease is unable to stand with eyes both open or closed, the disability being increased on closing the eyes. A Romberg sign may be regarded as positive only if there is actual loss of balance during the maneuver, with a shift in the position of the feet in order to maintain equilibrium. Swaying of the trunk without loss of equi-

librium cannot be regarded as a positive Romberg sign. Various degrees of loss are encountered; in mild cases a mere shifting of balance is seen; in severe cases a complete collapse and fall. Not all posterior column disease is associated with a positive Romberg sign; mild degrees of posterior column impairment with little disturbance of position sense are often found without Romberg's sign or without station disturbances.

Though there may be no interference with station in the Romberg position in early or mild cases, definite difficulties in maintaining balance may be brought out by asking the patient to maintain his balance on one leg with the eyes open or closed. This is well done by normal subjects but difficult or impossible for the patient with even slight disease of the posterior columns.

Disturbances of station are found also in diseases of the cerebellum or its pathways. In those cases of cerebellar disease associated with truncal incoördination there is inability to stand with the feet close together either with the eyes open or closed. Indeed, such station becomes impossible in advanced cases even with the legs widely separated. No such disturbance of station occurs in cerebellar disease without truncal involvement. The disability in cerebellar disease, unlike that of posterior column disease, is not affected by closing the eyes and is not dependent on loss of deep sensation.

Difficulties in standing are encountered in cases of weak or paralyzed limbs due, of course, to inability to support the weight on the weakened limb. Deformities of the lower extremities due to joint disease (arthritis, Charcot joint) interfere with proper station. Weakness due to myopathies may render erect posture impossible, or may cause difficulty in maintaining the erect position due to weakness of the trunk muscles.

Interference with standing is found in disease of the labyrinths, the vestibular pathways, or any disorders which cause vertigo, and results in such instances from interference with spatial orientation and the false sense of motion associated with the sensation of vertigo. Patients with dizziness are unable to stand even with the legs widely separated and they cannot walk a straight course.

VI. DISTURBANCES OF GAIT

Impairment or loss of the normal act of walking is encountered in a wide variety of conditions in neurological disease. The act of normal locomotion is influenced by a number of bodily mechanisms. It is the result of integration of many types of reflexes. It is dependent on simple reflex mechanisms at the spinal cord level, on righting reflexes in order to maintain the proper position of head, limbs, and trunk against gravity, on postural or standing reflexes to hold the body erect by increasing and maintaining extensor tone in the necessary extensor muscles, and on neck and labyrinthine reflexes for the proper maintenance of muscle tone, and for proper spatial orientation. Under these circumstances, walking may be abnormal as the result of disintegration of spinal cord reflex mechanisms, brain stem disorders, vestibular and cerebellar disturbances, proprioceptive mechanisms involving the posterior columns, and cortical disintegration.

In the analysis of gait disorders, great importance is placed on the occurrence of vertigo. A history of difficulty in walking during dizziness is to be expected, and is the direct result of the sense of false motion associated with the dizziness. On the other hand, gait disturbances without dizziness indicate difficulties referable to other parts of the proprioceptive system—the cerebellar or posterior column systems. In any history of disturbance of gait it is therefore important to be certain whether the unsteadiness in walking is associated with dizziness or is independent of it.

Steppage Gait: Walking is abnormal in diseases involving the peripheral pathways from the anterior horn cells to the motor peripheral nerve pathways. A common variety is seen in the *steppage gait* associated with foot drop and due either to a lesion of the external popliteal nerve or to its innervation from spinal cord segments L-5 to S-1. The leg is flaccid and the gait characterized by foot drop, a high elevation of the thigh and leg in order to clear the dropped foot from the ground. The condition is sometimes bilateral, due to diseases involving the cauda equina, or in bilateral involvement of the spinal cord segments as in poliomyelitis, or in cases of peroneal muscular atrophy, progressive muscular dystrophy, peripheral neuritis, or spinal cord tumor. Unilateral foot drop is seen in sciatic neuritis or in secondary sciatica (*v.* Neuritis).

A special form of gait due to peripheral mechanisms is that seen in cases of sciatica. In such instances, the knee and hip are flexed on the painful side, the pelvis drops toward the painful side, and the gait is carried out with short steps, and with the limb flexed as described in order to avoid stretching the sciatic nerve.

A peculiar gait, also of peripheral origin and due to pain, is that seen in cases of peripheral neuritis (alcohol, arsenic, beriberi), in causalgias due to nerve injuries, or in vasomotor disorders (erythromelalgia), associated with painful hyperesthesias of the soles of the feet. In such cases weight bearing is painful; hence the gait is with short steps, with an effort to avoid weight bearing on the feet, giving the gait a limping, halting character, with the feet rotated in such a position as to avoid walking on the painful portions, or to utilize the less painful parts of the skin surface.

Waddling Gait: It is seen in cases of muscular dystrophy and is characterized by a wide base, lordosis, and a peculiar waddle with lateral movement of the pelvis due to weakness of the gluteal muscles.

Hypotonic Gait: This, with hyperextension of the knees and loose, flail-like joints, is seen in tabes dorsalis and in the myopathies.

In addition to the gait disturbances which develop from interference with peripheral mechanism are those which follow disease of the posterior column system. Outstanding among these is the gait of tabes dorsalis which is broad based in order to shift the center of gravity, with the legs lifted high in walking, slapped down firmly on the ground in order to elicit what proprioceptive reflexes may be present, and with the eyes carefully watching the feet in walking. The ataxia is greatly increased in the dark and with the eyes closed. Similar types of gait are found in any disease of the posterior columns.

Cerebellar Gait: This is characterized by an inability of truncal, pelvic, and limb muscles to move in unison. In consequence the patient with cerebellar disease walks with a widened base, with the pelvis held stiffly and somewhat tilted anteriorly, the trunk and limbs moving seemingly independent of the pelvis. The result is a disorganized gait, with marked ataxia, with legs thrust forward from the hip in mechanical fashion without direction or coördination, with lurching and staggering. So incoördinate is the performance that patients with cerebellar disease are often accused of intoxication because of the incoördinate performance.

Patients with this sort of gait have, as a rule, destructive lesions of the vermis. Frequently in cases with cerebellar gait the head is held stiffly and anteriorly flexed, particularly in midline cerebellar tumors and in those which obstruct the fourth ventricle. A staggering and reeling gait is encountered also during acute vestibular disease, as in labyrinthitis, or in interruption of the vestibular pathways in the brain stem.

The Corticospinal System: Disease of the corticospinal system is associated with special gait disorders. Chief among these is the *hemiplegic gait*, with arm spastic and flexed and leg spastic, extended, circumducted, and scraping along the ground, particularly the forward portion of the foot. The pattern is so characteristic that it can hardly be mistaken for anything else. It may occur in any of the diseases responsible for the production of hemiplegia (*v.* Vascular Diseases). Bilateral disease of the corticospinal pathways results in a *spastic gait*, characterized by a shuffling type of gait in which the legs are stiff, extended and scraping over the surface without being lifted from the ground. In some types of spastic gait the legs, spastic while attempting to walk, are quite limber on recumbency. In cerebral diplegia the severe spasticity of the legs results often in a *scissors gait*, in which the legs in walking cross over in front of one another as each is put forward, resulting in a scissorslike action, due to the marked spasticity and the pronounced adductor hypertonicity. The gait in such cases is chiefly on the balls of the feet, with the feet in extension.

Basal Ganglia: Gait disorders are seen in basal ganglia disorders, especially in *paralysis agitans*. In early cases there is seen only a loss of automatic swinging of one of the arms while walking, with some flexion of the affected limb. In advanced cases the head and body are flexed, the arms and legs are flexed and rigid and the gait slow and shuffling. Initiation of the act of walking is slow, so that there may be a long latency between arising from a chair and the beginning of the walking act. Often the gait is propulsive, the patient shooting forward without control, walking with increasing rapidity as he continues in his gait. At times retropulsive gaits are seen. In *dystonia musculorum deformans* the gait is characterized by severe contortions, giving a ludicrous, bizarre appearance to the act.

Hysterical Gaits: These are not easily described but are characterized chiefly by their bizarre character. Any sort of bizarre performance may be encountered in hysteria. Astasia abasia, or a complete inability to stand or walk, is seen in hysteria.

Short-stepped, shuffling sorts of gaits *(Marche a petit pas)* are seen in senile cases and in cerebral arteriosclerosis.

VII. DISTURBANCES OF COÖRDINATION

The smooth coördination of muscular movement is impaired or lost under many different circumstances in diseases of the nervous system. Since normal coördination depends upon the proper functioning of agonists and antagonists it follows that any disorder which interferes with this function will cause incoördination. *Weakness* of a muscle or limb will result in loss of coördination of movement due to the muscular imbalance created by the weakness. A paretic arm finds difficulty in performing smoothly the finger-nose test or in rapidly pronating and supinating the arm. A special form of incoördination is seen in the impairment of the finer movements of the thumb and fingers, particularly the index finger, in cases of disease of the corticospinal pathways. Fine movements, such as buttoning clothes and picking up small objects, are lost.

Table 5—Differentiation of Cerebellar and Posterior Column Incoördination

	Cerebellar	*Posterior Column*
SENSORY DISTURB-ANCES	Absent	Always present. Loss or impairment of position and vibration senses
VISION	Symptoms not increased by shutting out vision	Symptoms increased by obliteration of vision
DYSMETRIA	Reaches goal with tremor, or overshoots and finally settles on it	Overshoots goal and fails to find it with eyes closed
TREMOR	On voluntary movement	Incoördination tremor
GAIT	Wide-based, pelvis fixed, trunk and limbs moving asynchronously	Wide-based, steppage with eyes watching feet and ground
STATION	Romberg's sign not present, but unsteadiness in standing with eyes open and closed	Romberg's sign present

Incoördination is found strikingly in *posterior column* ataxia due to interruption of the posterior columns, or its brain stem prolongation, the mesial fillet. It is dependent on loss of proprioceptive impulses from muscles, tendons, and joints, is accompanied by loss of position and/or vibration senses, and is increased on closing the eyes. The ataxia of posterior column disease is characterized by dysmetria and coarse tremor. It is seen especially strikingly in the characteristic gait. Movements are characterized by an inability to measure distance properly; hence there is often an overshooting of the goal. Tremor accompanies the movement (*v.* Chapter 3). It is found in any form of posterior column disease.

A special form of incoördination known as *asynergia,* or *dyssynergia* is found in cerebellar disease and is not dependent on disturbance of sensation. It is characterized by dysmetria, inability to perform movements smoothly (pronation-supination movements of the arms, rapid patting with the hands), by disturbances of gait, etc. (*v.* Chapter 3). Cerebellar dyssynergia may be pronounced and may involve all the limbs, it may be slight and be elicited in a single limb, or it may affect severely the trunk and limbs, or the trunk alone. Slight degrees of dyssynergia are seen in the pronation-supination test in the performance of which the patient is clumsy, the arm swinging out more than normally, the patient overpronating or supinating, losing the beat of the rhythmic movement of the test. In severe cases no rhythmic movement is possible. The cerebellar gait, which is but an expression of the dyssynergia of the trunk muscles, has been described. It is essential to recognize the fact that dyssynergia, which is the expression of cerebellar disease, may be found involving only the limbs, only a single limb, the limbs of one side only, or the trunk alone, or in conjunction with involvement of the limbs.

Disease of the *labyrinths,* the vestibular nerve, and the vestibular pathways in the brain stem is associated with incoordination characterized by dysmetria, past pointing, nystagmus, and vertigo. Efforts to reach an object or goal as in the finger-nose test result in overshooting the mark and in passing beyond it. In such cases vertigo is always present.

Table 6—Pathologic Reflexes of Lower Extremity

Reflex	Stimulus	Response
BABINSKI	Stroking outer edge of sole of foot	1. Extension of great toe 2. Flexion of small toes 3. Spreading of small toes 4. Flexion of leg
CHADDOCK	Stroking lateral aspect of dorsum of foot and external malleolus	Extension of great toe
OPPENHEIM	Firm downward stroking of medial aspect of tibia	Extension of great toe
ROSSOLIMO	Tapping balls of toes	Plantar flexion of toes
MENDEL-BECHTEREW	Tapping dorsum of foot on outer surface	Plantar flexion of toes

VIII. REFLEX DISTURBANCES

The common reflexes which should be examined routinely in a nervous system examination have been referred to in Chapter 1.

Loss of Tendon Reflexes: This occurs most frequently in cases of interruption of the reflex arc whether it be in anterior horns, anterior roots, peripheral nerve, or posterior roots. The features which distinguish interruption of the reflex arc at its various levels are described in Chapter 3. Loss of reflexes may occur also in the myopathies, usually in advanced stages of the disease associated with muscle atrophy. In advanced stages of myasthenia gravis no reflexes can be elicited. The reflexes are lost temporarily during the periods of paralysis of family periodic paralysis. They are lost also in Friedreich's ataxia, and in instances of spinal shock in which there has been an acute transection of the cord, or in an acute compression with resulting flaccid paralysis and loss of reflexes. The stage of spinal shock may persist for two weeks to two or three months and be replaced by spasticity and overactive reflexes, or it may persist indefinitely. The tendon reflexes disappear also in many toxic infectious conditions such as pneumonia, meningitis, typhoid fever, etc., in which there is profound systemic prostration. Increased intracranial pressure of a high degree, especially in posterior fossa tumors, is found to be associated with loss of the tendon reflexes. Rarely, in normal subjects no patellar reflexes may be elicited or there may be loss of all tendon reflexes.

Increase or Exaggeration of Tendon Reflexes: These occur in the vast majority of instances as a result of disease of the corticospinal pathways. In such instances, as in hemiplegias or paraplegias, a slight tap on the tendon causes a marked response. Overactive reflexes are sometimes but not consistently found in extrapyramidal disease such as paralysis agitans. The exaggerated reflexes of corticospinal disease are associated with abnormal reflexes such as the Babinski sign. Increase of reflexes is seen often in neurotic subjects, but it is not accompanied by abnormal responses. A false exaggeration of reflexes is seen in instances of atrophy and weakness of a muscle so that the muscle which normally acts in opposition responds unopposedly when the reflex is taken. Thus in atrophy of the triceps muscle, tapping the biceps tendon often results in exaggeration of the biceps reflex due to lack of restraint from the braking action of the triceps; the same holds true

in weakness and atrophy of the hamstrings, so that tapping of the patellar tendon causes a false increase of the patellar reflex.

Babinski sign: Associated with increased reflexes are various types of abnormal reflex, seen in disease of the corticospinal system. Chief among these reflexes is the *Babinski toe sign,* consisting of extension of the great toe, and spreading and flexion of the small toes on stroking the outer edge of the sole of the foot. This sign is pathognomonic of corticospinal disease. It is never present in normal subjects except in infants during the first six months of life. While a Babinski sign always indicates disease of the corticospinal pathway, it does not follow that it is always present with interruption of this pathway. It is not unusual to find disturbance of the corticospinal pathway without a Babinski sign but with all other evidences of involvement of this system present. In some cases, as in subacute combined degeneration, the Babinski sign may be the only evidence of corticospinal disease save for exaggerated reflexes; or it may be the only residual of previous more extensive disease of this system. Care must be taken to avoid interpretation of a voluntary extensor toe response as a Babinski sign. The toe extension in corticospinal disease is slow and usually disappears soon after the stimulus is removed; that of a voluntary response is faster and associated with rapid withdrawal of the leg. Transient Babinski signs may be found following a focal or generalized convulsion, in coma, and in uremic states.

None of the other signs which have been described in corticospinal tract disease appears with the same constancy as the Babinski sign.

Oppenheim's Sign: Extension of the great toe on firm downward stroking

Table 7—Pathological Hand Reflexes Resulting from Lesions of the Pyramidal Tract

Name	Stimulus	Response
PALM-CHIN REFLEX (*Marinesco-Radovici*)	Stimulation of hypothenar region (ulnar, median)	Contraction of muscles of chin and elevation of corner of mouth
THUMB-ADDUCTOR REFLEX ("*Babinski of the hand*") MARIE-FOIX	Superficial stroking of hypothenar region (ulnar)	Adduction and flexion of thumb; sometimes flexion of adjacent digits and extension of little finger
EXTENSION-ADDUCTION REFLEX (*Dagnini*)	Percussion of dorsum of hand (radial)	Slight adduction and extension of wrist
"MENDEL-BECHTEREW OF THE HAND"	Percussion of dorsal aspect of carpus and metacarpus (radial)	Flexion of fingers
"ROSSOLIMO OF THE HAND"	Percussion of palmar aspect of metacarpophalangeal joint	Flexion of fingers
HOFFMAN'S SIGN	Snapping nail of middle finger (median)	Flexion of thumb and fingers
TRÖMNER'S SIGN	Tapping palmar surface of tip of middle or index finger	Flexion of fingers and thumb
GORDON'S SIGN	Compression of region of pisiform bone (ulnar)	Extension of flexed fingers
CHADDOCK'S SIGN	Pressure on tendon of palmaris longus muscle	Flexion of wrist; extension of fingers

Synkinesis of Upper Extremity in Cases of Pyramidal Lesions

Name	Stimulus	Response
WARTENBERG'S SIGN	Active flexion of fingers about a stick	Flexion and opposition of thumb
SIGN OF KLIPPEL AND WEIL	Passive extension of fingers (when there is some contracture in flexion)	Flexion and opposition of thumb
SOUQUES' SIGN OF INTEROSSEOUS MUSCLES	Active elevation of extended arm	Extension and adduction of fingers
STRÜMPELL'S SIGN	Active flexion of elbow	Pronation and flexion of hand
BRACHIOBRACHIAL SYNKINESIS	Extension of flexed elbow of normal side by examiner, against patient's resistance	Flexion of elbow on paralyzed side
STERLING'S SIGN	Active adduction of shoulder on normal side against resistance by examiner	Adduction of shoulder on paretic side

along the medial side of the tibia is indicative of corticospinal disease but is not constant; indeed, it is infrequently encountered. When found without a Babinski sign it has the same significance as the latter.

Chaddock's Sign: The same is true of Chaddock's sign, which consists of extension of the great toe on stroking the dorsum of the foot on its outer edge.

Gordon's Sign: Extension of the toe on firm compression of the calf; it appears in corticospinal disease.

Rossolimo Sign: It consists of plantar flexion of the toes on tapping the balls of the toes. This sign is regarded as indicative of pyramidal tract disease, but it is often absent in disease of this system, it has been described in normal subjects, and it is an unreliable indicator of pyramidal disease when found alone without a Babinski sign or evidence of weakness. It appears relatively late after pyramidal tract disease, developing about six weeks after involvement of this system, becoming more pronounced with time and as muscle tone increases. It is found in children from two to three months to two to three years of age. A similar flexion of the toes is seen in Mendel-Bechterew's sign, elicited by tapping the dorsum of the foot on its outer surface over the cuboid bone. It is much less common than the Rossolimo sign and it is doubtful whether it can be regarded definitely as a sign of pyramidal disease.

In the upper extremity the *Hoffman sign* is said to be indicative of corticospinal disease. It is elicited by lightly flicking the terminal phalanx of the middle finger, or by snapping the nail of the middle finger, the resulting response being a flexion and adduction movement of the thumb and flexion of the fingers. The sign is of doubtful value since it is often present in tense normal subjects and is frequently absent in the presence of well-pronounced disease of the corticospinal system. The Hoffman sign must be regarded as an exaggerated form of the finger flexor reflex, indicative of a state of increased muscle tone. This may in many instances be due to a pyramidal lesion, but it is often functional and it is not infrequently lacking in the presence of pyramidal tract disease. It is an index of increased muscle tone rather than of corticospinal disease as such. It is definitely not pathognomonic of pyramidal tract disease, as is so often assumed. Other abnormal hand reflexes are listed in Table 7.

Trömner Reflex: This is a modification of the finger flexor reflex and is elicited as follows: The patient keeps his fingers flexed while the examiner taps with his middle finger the palmar surface of the tip of the middle or index finger of the patient. A positive response is indicated by flexion of all the fingers including the thumb. The sign was regarded erroneously as indicative of corticospinal disease. It is not indicative of this, but rather of increased muscle tone of the fingers.

Hoffmann Reflex: This too is a finger reflex. It is elicited as follows: The examiner holds the middle finger of the patient between his own second and third fingers, and nips the nail of the patient's finger with a flick of the thumb. The reflex is positive when flexion of the thumb and fingers follows.

Finger-Thumb Reflex (Mayer): This reflex consists of opposition and adduction of the thumb combined with flexion at the metacarpophalangeal joint on firm passive flexion of the third to the fifth finger at the proximal joints. The reflex is positive in normal persons and absent in patients with corticospinal lesions. When lost on one side it constitutes an important sign of a pyramidal tract lesion.

Reflexes of Defense (Reflex of Spinal Automatism): After transection of the spinal cord, there develops first a state known as spinal shock, during which all reflex activity below the level of the lesion is lost. As recovery ensues, reflex activity returns and is seen first in a return of the flexion reflexes of the toes and feet, followed in the course of time by flexion of the entire lower extremity. One form of this flexion reflex has been described as the reflex of defense.

These are seen in transecting lesions of the spinal cord. They are in effect flexion reflexes. They are elicited by stimulating the skin of the trunk of limbs below the level of the lesion by pinching, pin prick, scratching, application of cold, stroking the sole of the foot, or by the use of any noxious stimulus. The result is a massive reflex movement of flexion of the thighs and legs with dorsiflexion of the foot and toes. The movement is sometimes mistaken by the patient for a voluntary movement and as an indication of improvement.

Defense reflexes are seen most commonly in instances of complete interruption of the spinal cord by transection due to injury, compression, vascular disease. etc. They appear, however, without complete interruption, in the presence only of bilateral pyramidal tract disease, as in spastic paraplegias. A type of defense reflex is seen in cases of spastic paraplegia in extension, in the course of which there may spontaneously develop flexion of the legs with subsequent return to extension. The Babinski sign may be regarded as a fraction of a flexion reflex. In spastic paraplegia, stimulation of one leg will often result in flexion of this leg with crossed extension of the opposite limb. This is known as *Phillipson's reflex*. In spinal man, that is, in a subject in which the spinal cord has been transected from some cause, there ensues on scratching or stimulating any part of the legs a *"mass reflex"* characterized by flexor spasm of the ventral abdominal wall and lower extremities, evacuation of the bladder, and sweating from an area of skin varying with the level of the lesion. This is due to diffuse spread of sensory impulses throughout the spinal cord instead of being restricted to well-defined channels.

Postural Reflexes: These appear under certain conditions in man but are of greater physiological than clinical significance. Tonic neck and labyrinthine reflexes are extremely important in the maintenance of posture. In decerebrated animals destruction of the labyrinths permits a study of the tonic *neck reflexes*, whereby it is possible to demonstrate that rotation of the head causes an increase in extensor tonus of the limb toward which the jaw points ("jaw limb") and relaxation of the limb toward which the vertex is rotated ("skull limb"). Furthermore, flexion of the head toward one shoulder causes extension of the "jaw limbs" and relaxation of the "skull limbs"; extension of the head causes extension of the forelimbs and flexion of the hind limbs; and flexion of the head causes flexion of the forelimbs and extension of the hind limbs. Counterparts of these reflexes are seen in some conditions in the human, particularly in newborn infants in whom the pyramidal tracts are not yet developed, in some cases of cerebral diplegia, in longstanding hemiplegias, in tuberculous meningitis, and in cases of decerebrate rigidity in man. Tonic neck reflexes are found in infants until the twelfth week of life. In children of over five to six months of age with fixed or progressive lesions of the nervous system, the presence of tonic neck reflexes has been found to be of serious prognostic import, indicating a seriously inadequate nervous system. A special neck reflex occurring in infants has been described by Landau. If an infant during the second year is supported under the chest by one hand, the neck extends, the back arches, and the extremities extend. If the head is passively flexed in such a case the extension of trunk and limb vanishes and the baby folds up like a jackknife. Another special reflex is the *Moro reflex*, in which all four extremities are thrown into sudden rigid extension if the supporting surface on which the infant lies is suddenly jarred or shaken. It is present in infants for about the first three months of life.

Tonic *labyrinthine reflexes* are studied in decerebrate animals after section of the cervical roots, thus eliminating the neck reflexes. Under such conditions it can be demonstrated that marked changes occur in posture and muscle tonus with the variation of the body in space, maximal extension occurring in the supine position with the snout about 45 degrees above the horizontal plane and minimal extension with the snout 45 degrees below the horizontal. The reflexes are dependent upon intact labyrinths, taking their origin in the otoliths, and disappear completely after bilateral labyrinthectomy. These reflexes are undoubtedly of importance in the human but have been investigated in few clinical conditions and are therefore as yet of little significance in clinical diagnosis. The same may be said of the *righting reflexes*, which are the mechanisms whereby the animal attempts to bring body and head into normal position by means of labyrinthine, neck, optical, body-to-head, and body-to-body reflexes.

Of greater clinical significance is the *grasp reflex* which is found in paretic limbs. It is characterized by an inability to relax the muscles after a voluntary grasping of an object. The reflex is not found in cases of complete paralysis. Two components of the reflex have been estab-lished: (1) Volitional grasping movements in response to objects seen or contacts felt in the palm of the hand, and (2) reflex tonic grasping in response to stretching the flexor muscles of the fingers (Walshe and Hunt).

The stimulus required for the reflex appears to be stretch of the flexor muscles of the fingers since there is no difficulty in opening the clenched fist when it is empty. Similarly the patient with forced grasping is able to open the fingers of the clenched hand even when it contains an object which is not being pulled away and therefore no stretch is being exerted on the flexors of the fingers. The grasp reflex is unaffected by loss of sensation of the skin of the hand and by visual stimuli since it is found with undiminished intensity after local anesthesia of the hand and after blindfolding. It is present without hypertonicity of the muscles. It is regarded by most observers as a purely reflex phenomenon but some believe a volitional element is present. It varies with the position of the body in space in monkeys and is therefore part of the righting reflex mechanism. It is also in monkeys influenced to some extent by neck and labyrinthine reflexes. In chimpanzees it is present transiently in unilateral ablation of Area 6 (premotor) and of Areas 4 and 6 (motor and premotor); it is permanently present in bilateral ablation of Areas 4 and 6.

The grasp reflex and forced grasping have been found in humans in cases of lesions of the opposite frontal lobe. It has been found in association with tumors of the opposite premotor cortex (Area 6 of Brodmann) and when present in a human subject must be regarded as indicative of a frontal lobe lesion. It is a normal phenomenon in infants.

The *superficial reflexes* are disturbed in many conditions. The *abdominal reflexes* are lost in hemiplegia on the side of the weakness. They are lost bilaterally in multiple sclerosis and not infrequently disappear early in the disease. They may be lost also in transverse lesions of the spinal cord, the lower abdominals being lost in lesions of the lowermost thoracic segments (T-11 to T-12) and the upper abdominals in segments slightly higher (T-8 to T-10). The *corneal reflex,* when lost, is a sign of great significance. It may be absent as the result of local disease of the cornea. It is always absent or decreased in cases of fresh hemiplegia and it is absent in lesions which involve the sensory trigeminal nucleus in the pons from whatever cause (multiple sclerosis, encephalitis, tumor of the pons), in lesions of the trigeminal root or ganglion. It is often lost early in cerebellopontine angle tumors.

Additional Reflexes: The *orbicularis oculi reflex* is elicited as follows: The skin at the outer corner of the eye is held between the thumb and index finger, pulling it back slightly, and the thumb is tapped lightly with a reflex hammer. There follows a reflex contraction of the orbicularis oculi muscle. Diminution of the reflex is found in facial palsies of peripheral origin. It is preserved in central facial palsies. The response obtained is a deep muscle reflex. The *jaw reflex* is elicited by tapping the mandible with the jaw half opened, the lower jaw moving briskly upward. It has slight clinical significance, but it may be increased on bilateral supranuclear cerebral lesions. The *scapulohumeral reflex* is elicited by tapping the vertebral border of the scapula with resulting contraction of muscles of the shoulder girdle and arm. Many muscles are brought into play, especially the deltoid, pectoralis major, infraspinatus and teres minor. Adduction of the arm occurs. Unilateral absence of the reflex is found in lesions of the fifth cervical

segment. The *adductor reflex of the thigh* is obtained by placing the finger on the medial condyle of the femur with the leg slightly abducted. When the finger is tapped adduction of the leg follows. The *biceps femoris reflex* is best elicited with the patient lying on the side opposite the one being examined, the leg being bent at the hip and knee. The finger is placed on the hamstring tendon and is tapped with a reflex hammer. Contraction of the muscle results. The *pharyngeal reflex* is elicited by touching the posterior wall of the pharynx, contraction of the pharynx resulting. The *scapular reflex,* elicited by stroking the skin between the scapulae, results in contraction of the scapular muscles. The *gluteal reflex* results in contraction of the glutei on stroking the skin of the buttock.

IX. SENSATION

The methods of performing a sensory examination have been described (Chapter 1) and the various types of abnormal sensory patterns are indicated (Chapter 3) at peripheral, radicular, spinal cord, brain stem, thalamic, and cortical levels.

X. ELECTRICAL REACTIONS

The neurological examination makes use in many instances of the electrical response of muscles. This is not a routine feature of any examination, but it is one which becomes important under special circumstances and its uses and interpretations are therefore important to know. Its chief value lies in the examination of muscles and motor nerves in order to determine whether normal reactions are elicited after anterior horn cell disease, peripheral nerve disease, or disease of the muscles.

Normally, muscles react to faradic stimulation through stimulation of the motor nerve at its "motor point." The result on stimulation of this point is a maximal contraction of the muscle. Galvanism causes contraction of a muscle at the moment of closure and opening of the current as well as during its flow if the current is strong enough, in contrast to the case in stimulation of a motor nerve fiber which responds during opening and closing of the current but not during its flow. Thus, even after degeneration of a nerve, galvanism can still elicit response in the muscle directly. Advantage is taken of these reactions in the human. Normally, a healthy muscle when stimulated by a galvanic current contracts on closure of the current and again on opening it, remaining relaxed during the period of flow of current. The contraction thus elicited is greater with the negative pole (cathode) than with the positive pole (anode); hence the normal formula reads CCC (cathode closing contraction) > ACC (anode closing contraction). If the current is made strong enough contractions are obtained on opening currents.

Abnormal electrical reactions are found in many diseased states. Most important is the *reaction of degeneration* (RD). This is indicative of interruption of the nerve supply to a muscle and occurs as a result of a lesion anywhere along the efferent reflex pathway. It is found, therefore, in loss of innervation to the muscle from anterior horn cell disease (poliomyelitis, amyotrophic lateral sclerosis, progressive spinal muscular atrophy, syringomyelia, etc.), or from disease of the peripheral motor nerve (neuritis, nerve injury, etc.).

Complete Reaction of Degeneration: This is characterized by (1) loss of faradic and galvanic irritability of the nerve; (2) loss of faradic irritability of muscle; (3) persistence of galvanic irritability of muscle; (4) qualitative changes in contraction so that ACC = CCC or ACC > CCC and COC =

AOC; (5) a slow, long-drawn contraction of the muscle on stimulation. The chronaxia of such muscles is delayed greatly. A reaction of degeneration develops as a result of degeneration of the nerve supply to a muscle and is therefore of serious significance. It remains permanent unless the nerve supply is replaced by regeneration or suture. A reaction of degeneration does not indicate necessarily inability of the muscle to recover its function. It indicates complete degeneration of the nerve supply and in this sense is of very serious prognostic significance. Most cases with reaction of degeneration fail to show recovery but it does not follow that this is invariably the case. A reaction of this type associated with anterior horn cell disease indicates no recovery, since there is no possibility of regeneration of the anterior horn cells and therefore the nerve supply to the muscle is lost. The condition is different in disease or injury of a peripheral nerve, whether it be cranial limb or trunk, since peripheral nerves possess the power of regeneration. A reaction of degeneration in such a case, though indicating complete interruption of nerve supply, is still compatible with recovery provided regeneration of the nerve takes place. Recovery in such instances is likely to be slow and incomplete, and in many instances fails to develop, but it is still theoretically and practically possible.

Partial Reactions of Degeneration: These occur under many circumstances and are characterized by (1) a sluggish contraction to galvanism, ACC being greater than CCC, (2) a diminished reaction to faradism. Reactions of this nature indicate partial interference with the nerve supply to a muscle.

Hyperexcitable electrical reactions are found in tetany, both for faradic and galvanic stimulation. Quantitative decrease

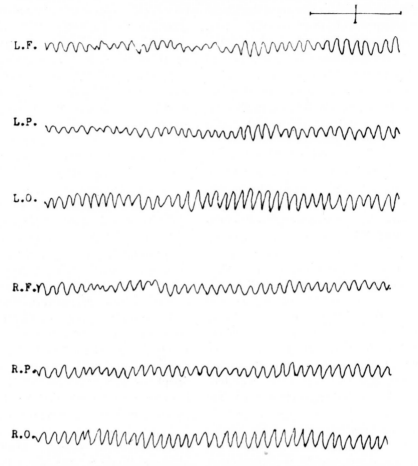

Fig. 19—*Electroencephalogram*, showing normal 8-10/sec. rhythm in frontal, parietal and occipital areas of the cortex.

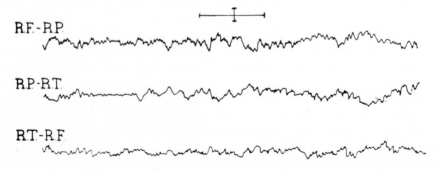

Fig. 20—*Electroencephalogram*. The record shows out of phase activity between the tracings right frontal to right parietal (R.F.-R.P.) and right parietal to right temporal (R.P.-R.T.) indicating a lesion beneath the right parietal electrode. At operation an astrocytoma was found in this location.

of excitability both for galvanism and faradism is found in the myopathies A special form of electrical reaction is seen in myasthenia gravis and is known as the myasthenic reaction. It is characterized by diminution and eventual loss of the muscle on repeated faradic stimulation, only to have the excitability reappear on rest. This is characteristic of the fatigue reaction in myasthenia gravis. In advanced stages of the disease the muscles react only feebly for a short time or they may not react at all. A myotonic reaction is seen in myotonia dystrophica and is characterized by persistence of the muscle contraction long after faradic stimulation has ceased.

Electroencephalography: Electroencephalography, a term coined by Berger, consists of the amplification, recording, and analysis of the electrical potentials of the brain. This is dependent upon the fact that functioning cells undergo electrical, thermal, mechanical, and chemical changes. In the nervous system, the electrical changes predominate. The electrical activity, as recorded from the scalp, is not that of the individual neurons but represents rather a synthesis of the activity of many neurons. For this reason, cutaneous sensory stimulation does not alter the scalp record, nor does the induction of motor activity change the record as noted by scalp electrodes. The basic resting rhythm is altered by opening the eyes and alteration in attention.

The electroencephalogram (EEG) must be used in conjunction with the clinical history and examination, as well as with all available evidence for its proper interpretation. There are few instances in which it has absolute value and diagnosis of cerebral disease by means of the EEG alone should be avoided. The EEG is a laboratory test, and should be used like all other such tests. Even in epilepsy where it has perhaps its greatest

value, it is not absolute in its significance. Negative EEG records occur in patients with all types of seizures. Hence the EEG cannot replace a careful and complete clinical study.

Essentially the *technic* consists of the application of suitable electrodes to the scalp, with amplification and recording of the obtained potentials. Since the electrodes obtain alternating potentials, they need not be nonpolarizing. The electrodes in common usage are solder or metal discs applied to the scalp with collodion or similar paste material. Needle electrodes are not in general usage. During the course of neurosurgical procedures, direct contact through silver or silver chloride electrodes may be utilized to obtain cortical potentials.

Since the average voltage of the cortical potentials is about thirty millionths of a volt, amplification is necessary for clinical readings. The most satisfactory method of amplification at the present time is the use of vacuum tube amplifiers.

Electroencephalographic records are obtained over relatively long periods of time, thus demanding a constant, yet inexpensive, method of recording. This purpose is answered by electromagnetic ink writers, which faithfully reproduce waves between frequency ranges of one in three seconds to fifty a second.

While there is considerable variation from clinic to clinic in the application of electrodes, in general eight grounded electrodes suffice in the study of patients suspected of epilepsy. These are usually placed one each over the frontal, parietal, occipital, and temporal lobes of each side, and anterior temporal areas and ears. For localization purposes, a greater number of electrodes is employed.

Tracings may be obtained by reading from scalp electrode to ear electrode, and from scalp electrode to scalp electrode. The scalp-to-ear records were formerly considered monopolar tracings, the ear being considered electrically silent. However, the ear electrodes pick up much temporal lobe activity, and therefore such records are not monopolar. All tracings should include scalp-to-scalp tracings and scalp-to-ear tracings.

Electroencephalographic studies are carried out in quiet rooms, which have been adequately shielded against electrical

ied, and it has been found that at birth frequencies of one to three per second predominate. With increasing age, the trend is toward faster frequencies, so that by fourteen years adult type records are obtained with some childhood features persisting. The frontal and parietal regions are not uncommonly the last to assume adult type records; in normal persons this occurs no later than at nineteen years.

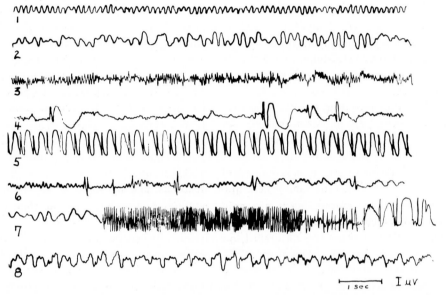

Fig. 21—Normal and abnormal cerebral rhythms. 1. Normal alpha rhythm. 2. Slow irregular waves. 3. Fast waves or discharges. 4. Spike and wave, petit mal variant. 5. Spike and wave, petit mal discharge. 6. Spike discharges. 7. Grand mal discharge. 8. Psychomotor discharge at 4—6/sec. (List, Carl *et al.*: Radiology 45:1 [July] 1945.)

artefacts. The patients must be comfortable, quiet, and relaxed, with eyes closed, but not asleep except for specific purposes as noted below.

The most characteristic feature of *normal* adult *records* taken under testing conditions is the eight-per-second to twelve-per-second rhythm. This is usually seen best in occipital tracings and least in the frontal records. In the sensory motor regions, a frequency in the neighborhood of twenty-five per second may be detected.

The effect of age upon the electroencephalograph has been extensively stud-

The electroencephalographic pattern is considered characteristic for each subject. There are, however, wide variations in individual patterns. Normal records have been divided into four groups, dependent upon the degree of alpha (ten-per-second) activity. One commonly encountered type of normal record is of low voltage with fast frequencies in all leads.

When, during recording, the subject opens his eyes, a prompt flattening of cortical activity ensues. The same effect is produced by mental attention, such as that produced by the computation of a difficult problem. In the early stages of sleep—drifting—a flattening of the ten-per-second activity occurs. As sleep deepens, fourteen-per-second to sixteen-per-second spindle waves appear, followed by high voltage, slow waves with frequencies ranging from one half to three per second.

Electroencephalography has been especially helpful to the clinician under two conditions: (1) In the diagnosis of epilepsy and the differential diagnosis of the type of convulsive disorder, and (2) in the localization of lesions of the cerebrum.

During epileptic seizures, certain electroencephalographic patterns are encountered. Thus the grand mal seizure is characterized by fast, high voltage spikes, In petit mal attacks, three-per-second rounded waves followed by fast spikes are most frequently seen; and in psychomotor seizures, square-topped, four-per-second to six-per-second waves are usual. During interseizure records in epileptic patients, isolated spikes of the grand mal type may be encountered, or the spikes may occur in short groups without clinical evidence of a seizure, which is evidence of a larval grand mal attack. Likewise, short bursts of the alternating wave and spike, or spikes in the temporal lobe may be encountered. The wave and spike may be produced by hyperventilation in patients with petit mal epilepsy. In addition to the determination of the presence of an abnormal electroencephalographic pattern, the electronencephalogram contributes to the localization of the seizure. Seizures may be found to have their inception in one area of the cortex and to spread from this region. If this area is constant in the same person, a focus of discharge may be said to be present.

In recent years, various methods of inducing electroencephalographic abnormalities have been described. These are usually referred to as "activation technics." Hyperventilation has long been recognized as an activation technic for producing petit mal seizures and discharges. Gibbs has advocated recording during sleep as being advantageous in bringing out abnormal discharges in all types of epilepsy, most particularly in psychic seizures. By this technic, he has demonstrated a temporal lobe focus for psychomotor seizures in some patients. The intravenous injection of Metrazol has been found efficacious by Walker, Jasper, and others in indicating foci of epileptogenic activity. Photic stimulation is used for similar purposes.

Gross lesions of the cerebrum, when they lie within the range of electrodes, may be localized by means of electroencephalography. For this purpose, unipolar and bipolar recordings are used. Gross lesions, such as hemorrhages and tumors, produce slow, one-half-per-second to three-per-second waves, or high voltage may produce slower than normal waves in relation to the electrode over the lesion. When recordings are made in series, these waves appear out of phase.

The EEG is of great help in the diagnosis of brain tumor. As would be expected, the best results in localization are obtained when the tumor lies close to the surface. Various investigators have obtained accurate localization under these conditions in as high as 90 per cent of cases. Deep-seated cerebral lesions are less frequently localized as are parasagittal lesions. The role of electroencephalography in localization of infratentorial lesions is still debatable, but the best evidence to date indicates that little may be expected of this technic when the lesion is in the posterior fossa.

The EEG may be helpful in head injuries (v. Cranial Trauma).

While earlier studies and correlations between the electroencephalographic pattern and the personality of the subject were for the most part fruitless, the application of the Fourier analyzer and the study of the large groups of persons in different social strata by Gibbs and his collaborators suggest that such correlations exist but are, for the most part, applicable only to groups and not to individual records.

The results of study of the so-called "functional psychoses" — manic-depressive, schizophrenia, and involutional melancholia—are inconclusive. Thus, while there are more frequent abnormalities in the total group, it is impossible to diagnose the presence of a psychosis, much less its type, by the record of an individual patient.

Abnormalities of the electroencephalogram are more common in psychoses associated with organic brain disease. Thus in paresis, both abnormally fast and abnormally slow frequencies are found.

Attempts to correlate the electroencephalographic patterns with the intelligence level in feebleminded subjects have not been successful. The greater incidence of abnormalities in those with very low intelligence is more likely correlated with the underlying cerebral pathology than with the intelligence level.

In the field of psychiatric disorders, the greatest service has been rendered by the electroencephalogram in the study of behavior problem children. The high frequency of abnormalities has now been well established, and in many instances the abnormalities are similar to those occurring during psychomotor seizures.

XI. CEREBROSPINAL FLUID

Since a study of the cerebrospinal fluid constitutes such an important part of the neurological examination, some knowledge of its normal and abnormal characteristics is necessary. The normal circulation of the cerebrospinal fluid may be found adequately considered in any phys-iological text, to which the reader is referred.

Cerebrospinal fluid may be obtained by one of three routes: (1) Lumbar puncture, (2) cisternal puncture, (3) ventricular puncture. The lumbar route is by far the most common and for ordinary purposes is the route of choice. Cisternal puncture is necessary in cases of unsuccessful lumbar tap, and for the introduction of foreign substances (Lipiodol) or medication. Ventricular puncture is performed as a rule for purposes of ventriculography.

Routine Examination of the Cerebrospinal Fluid: This should include a study of (1) pressure, (2) cell content, (3) sugar estimation, (4) globulin, (5) total protein, (6) Wassermann reaction, (7) colloidal gold reaction. The normal *pressure* range in a water manometer is 100 to 200 mm. Pressures of over 200 mm. are definitely elevated; those of 190 to 200 mm. are borderline. The *cell* content of the spinal fluid varies normally from one to six lymphocytes; six to ten cells are borderline; a cell content of ten cells or more is definitely abnormal. The spinal fluid normally has a *protein* content of 25 to 45 mg. *Globulin* is present in slight amounts. The *sugar* content varies from 50 to 80 mg. The *Wassermann reaction* is negative in normal cases. In some instances the spinal fluid is examined for *chlorides*, which range normally from 725 to 750 mg. The *colloidal gold* test is valuable in some disorders but need not be done routinely. It reads normally as follows: 0000000000 (0^{10}).

Smear and Culture of the Spinal Fluid: These are indicated in instances of nervous system infection. Bacteria may be demonstrated by smear in many infections of the meninges (Pneumococcus, Streptococcus, Meningococcus, Staphylococcus, etc.), but failure to demonstrate them does not indicate their absence. They are often difficult to demonstrate. The tubercle bacillus is noteworthy in this respect. Both smear and culture of the spinal fluid must be made in cases of meningeal infection in order to identify the invading organism. This must be done before sulfonamide and antibiotic therapy is begun. Sterile spinal fluids in cases of meningitis are found often and in brain abscess, and in sympathetic meningitis, and syphilis. Smears and cultures will reveal no changes in meningeal exudates due to virus meningoencephalitis or encephalitis, since viruses require living tissues for their culture. Parasites, yeasts, and fungi may be found on smear in rare cases.

Abnormalities: Abnormalities of the spinal fluid are found under many circumstances, so that a search for such variations constitutes one of the most important features of the routine examination of the nervous system in cases in which spinal fluid studies are indicated.

1. Pressure: Disturbances of cerebrospinal fluid pressure are found in many conditions. *Increased pressure* is found in (1) brain tumor, but it is not an invariable accompaniment of tumor. Many tumors are associated with a normal cerebrospinal fluid pressure (*v.* Brain Tumors). It is practically always elevated in posterior fossa tumors, especially those involving the cerebellum; and in most instances of tumor involving the cerebral hemispheres. It is usually normal in tumors in or near the pituitary region. (2) In conditions simulating brain tumor such as subdural hematoma, brain abscess, and brain cysts. (3) Brain edema resulting from acute infections (meningitis, encephalitis), head injury, cerebral hemorrhage, or thrombosis, subarachnoid hemorrhage, alcoholism, uremia, and a large number of other conditions. (4) Interference with cerebrospinal fluid circulation, as in internal hydrocephalus from

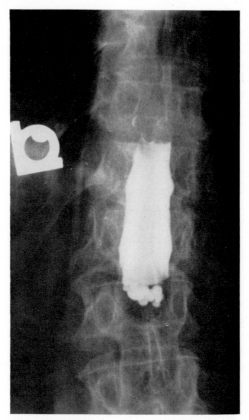

Fig. 22 — *Pantopaque myelogram* revealing **complete block due to extramedullary meningioma.**

various causes (*v.* Hydrocephalus). It is essential to recognize the fact that substantial increase of cerebrospinal fluid pressure may develop in conditions associated with brain swelling and edema and that such increases may develop in the course of many diseases.

Decreased pressures below 100 mm.: These are found in states of dehydration or in instances in which the spinal fluid column has been shortened as a result of block along the subarachnoid space in cases of spinal cord tumor, or other conditions which may produce such block. It must be recognized also that the spinal fluid pressure may be low merely due to the fact that the spinal puncture needle is not in free communication with the subarachnoid space owing to partial obstruction by arachnoid membrane, or other tissues during the course of lumbar puncture. *Obstruction* of *normal hydrodynamics* of the cerebrospinal fluid is seen in instances of blockage of the subarachnoid space due to spinal cord tumor, pachymeningitis, arachnoiditis, dislocation of a vertebra, spinal cord abscess, or any other condition which blocks the subarachnoid space, interfering thus with the free circulation of fluid. Normally, with a manometer attached to a needle in the lumbar subarachnoid space, pressure on the jugular veins causes a rapid rise and fall in the fluid in the manometer; straining causes a similar rise. This is known as the Queckenstedt test. In conditions of complete block of the subarachnoid space no rise in pressure results on compression of the jugular veins, while straining causes an increase (positive Queckenstedt). Partial blocks result in an inadequate rise and slow fall after jugular compression (*v.* Spinal Cord Tumors).

2. *Appearance:* The cerebrospinal fluid is normally colorless. It is at times turbid due to accumulations of cells, either red or white cells. In cases of subarachnoid, cerebral, or ventricular hemorrhage, it is bloody, the supernatant fluid in such cases being yellow. Under other circumstances it is xanthochromic or yellow in color. This is most frequently the result of blockage of the spinal fluid in the subarachnoid space of the spinal canal. In such instances it is associated with an increase of protein. In rare instances one sees the Froin syndrome consisting of xanthochromic fluid with high protein content and coagulation of the fluid in standing. Xanthochromia may be found also in association with brain tumor, brain abscess, subdural hematoma, tuberculous meningitis, old meningeal or cerebral hemorrhage, and other conditions.

3. *Cells:* The cell content of the cerebrospinal fluid is increased in so many conditions that it is impossible and pointless to enumerate them. A white cell content of over six cells is abnormal, while red cells in any amount are of pathological significance, if they are not the result of a traumatic puncture.

Acute meningeal infections are invariably associated with cell increase (*v.* Meningitis), the type and number of cells depending on the cause of the meningitis. Acute encephalitis in many forms is found to be associated in its early stages with a cell increase which usually disappears within short order. This is the case with encephalitis lethargica, St. Louis and Japanese encephalitis, equine encephalomyelitis, and poliomyelitis. Chronic infections of the nervous system are often associated with cellular increases in the spinal fluid as in general paresis, tabes dorsalis, meningovascular syphilis, and brain abscess. Red cells are found in the spinal fluid under many circumstances (*v.* Subarachnoid Hemorrhage). For the spinal fluid changes in the different neurological conditions the student is referred to the specific disease in question.

4. *Protein:* An increase of protein is found under many circumstances. It occurs in acute meningitis of all forms. It is found also in the chronic meningitis of syphilis, in meningeal hemorrhage, in some tumors of the brain, in acute inflammations of the brain, in degenerative diseases of various sorts, and in blockage of the spinal subarachnoid space due to spinal cord tumor, or to other causes of obstruction. It is increased also in encephalitis, poliomyelitis, multiple sclerosis, cerebral arteriosclerosis, and degenerative diseases of the spinal cord. It may be decreased in instances in which there is an excessive formation of fluid. An increase of cerebrospinal fluid protein is there-

fore found in many neurological conditions, but it is of diagnostic significance in relatively few. Thus in many diseases it is an expected and accessory finding which helps little if at all in diagnosis. This is true of meningitis, encephalitis, meningeal hemorrhage, and a number of other diseases in which the diagnosis is not dependent upon the protein increase of the spinal fluid.

While a protein increase is not always important, it is nevertheless always ab-

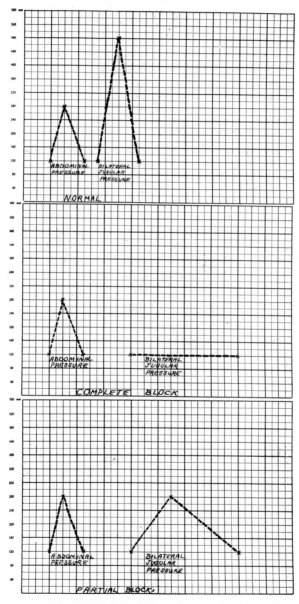

Fig. 23—*Subarachnoid block* shown in diagrammatic form. In top panel is shown the rapid rise and fall of spinal fluid pressure on abdominal straining and bilateral jugular compression. In the middle panel is shown a failure of increase of spinal fluid pressure with complete block. In the lower panel is shown the delayed rise and fall of spinal fluid pressure on jugular compression in partial subarachnoid block.

normal. Under some circumstances it is of diagnostic importance. This is true in cases of suspected spinal cord tumor in which it is increased and usually associated with subarachnoid block. It is also of diagnostic importance in cases of acute infectious polyneuritis (*v.* Neuritis) in which it is increased without an associated increase of cells. In suspected brain tumor an increase of protein may help in pursuing the diagnosis in cases with few helpful signs. It is increased especially in cases of brain tumor which lie close to the surface, abutting onto the ventricular surface, or found in the cerebellopontine angle.

5. Sugar: The sugar content of the cerebrospinal fluid may be increased or decreased. Increases of sugar are of relatively little diagnostic value. They occur in lethargic encephalitis but the diagnosis can hardly be said to depend on the finding and in the last analysis it is of little value in arriving at a diagnosis of the condition. Increases in sugar have been found in general paresis, and among normal subjects. Decreased sugar contents are found in some forms of acute meningitis and may be totally absent in meningococcus meningitis. A decreased sugar content of the cerebrospinal fluid is in itself of little diagnostic significance unless accompanied by other abnormalities such as increase of cells.

6. Chlorides: The chloride content of the cerebrospinal fluid is decreased in many acute infections. In few of them, however, does it reach the low level attained in tuberculous meningitis (650 mg. or lower). A chloride content of 650 mg. or less must always be regarded first as possible tuberculous meningitis in a case with lymphocytic increase in the spinal fluid. Levels as low as this, however, may be found in other forms of meningitis, but never as consistently as in the tuberculous type. They are found in enceph-

alomyelitis, lymphocytic choriomeningitis, brain tumor, cerebral hemorrhage, general paresis, and uremia.

7. Colloidal Gold: The colloidal gold curve of Lange has little diagnostic significance in most nervous diseases. It is abnormal in many, but of significance in few. The orthodox reading of the colloidal gold curve is as follows: (1) First zone or paretic curve 5555543210; (2) second zone or tabetic curve 1233321000; (3) third zone or meningitic curve 0000012310. Since any of these curves may occur in a number of conditions they fail to have specific importance. The greatest value of the colloidal gold curve is in neurosyphilis, particularly in general paresis, in which the paretic or first zone curve (5555543210) is found in ninety per cent of untreated cases. Such a curve, however, is found also in other forms of neurosyphilis, at times in brain tumors, tuberculous meningitis, and multiple sclerosis. It is, therefore, not pathognomonic of paresis. The colloidal gold curve is also abnormal in many cases of multiple sclerosis in which it has diagnostic value. Apart from neurosyphilis and multiple sclerosis the test must be regarded as an adjunct to other spinal fluid tests, having little or no specific diagnostic significance in those conditions in which it is found to be abnormal. Thus it is abnormal in some cases of meningitis but it cannot be regarded as of significance in such instances, for the diagnosis of meningitis could never be made on the basis of an abnormal colloidal gold curve. The same holds true of the many other neurological conditions in which it is found to be abnormal. A negative colloidal gold curve (0^{10}) by no means excludes organic disease of the nervous system; a positive curve on the other hand signifies structural disease but it gives no information in the great majority of cases as to the nature of the offending disease.

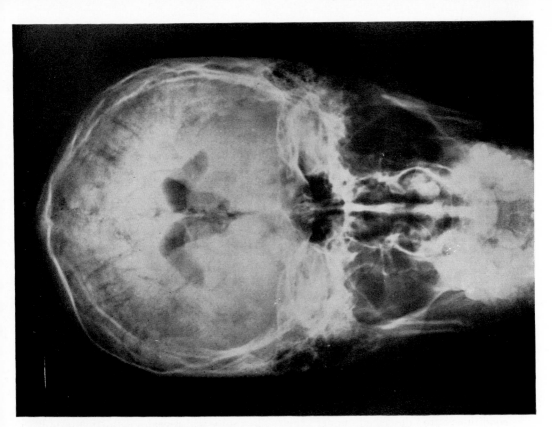

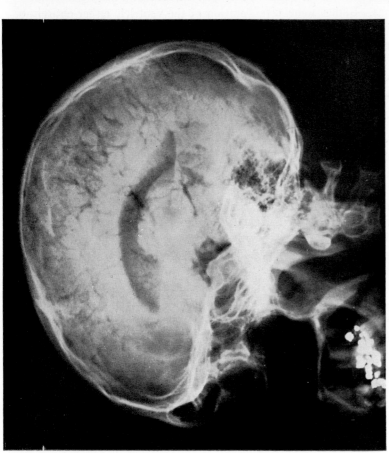

Fig. 24—*Normal encephalograms, showing the typical butterfly appearance of the anterior horns, the third ventricle in the midline and the lateral ventricle in the lateral view. The fourth ventricle is not clearly shown. There is no displacement on distortion of the ventricular structures.*

XII. ACCESSORY EXAMINATIONS

After a thorough and complete clinical examination of the nervous system it may still be impossible to arrive at a diagnosis. For this reason many accessory procedures are available. *Spinal fluid* study has already been referred to. *Roentgenologic study of the skull* is an important part of most neurological examinations and for this reason is carried out frequently. It is not a routine procedure in every case, but should be carried out in cerebral cases wherever indicated. The abnormalities to be found in roentgenograms of the skull are too numerous to be mentioned in a brief survey. The pertinent findings will be considered under their respective diseases. *Roentgenologic studies of the spine* are important under many conditions as well. Here, too, the findings in pertinent conditions are described under their appropriate headings. Under some circumstances air is injected into the nervous system. This procedure is known as *pneumography*. It is of two main types: (1) Encephalography or (2) ventriculography, to outline the cerebral ventricles and subarachnoid spaces; myelography is used to outline the spinal subarachnoid space.

Encephalography is carried out by the removal of cerebrospinal fluid and the injection of an equivalent amount of air through a lumbar puncture needle. The procedure is extremely painful and often disables patients for several days due to severe headache. By the introduction of air the cerebral ventricles, subarachnoid spaces, and basilar cisterns are clearly outlined. Abnormal variations in the appearance of the ventricles or subarachnoid channels are readily detected.

Encephalography is performed in a number of conditions. Its main general indications are (1) to determine in doubtful cases whether a brain tumor is present and if so where it is located. In cases of this type it must never be performed in the presence of choked discs, or in the presence of increased intracranial pressure without choked discs. It should be avoided under all circumstances in a suspected case of posterior fossa tumor. If a brain tumor is present it will be detected by encephalography provided it is located in the cerebral hemispheres or in the cerebellum or ventricular system. Tumors lying within the sella turcica or suprasellar or parasellar tumors may be poorly shown or not visualized at all. In suprasellar tumors, encephalography may help in diagnosis by the demonstration of incomplete filling of the prechiasmal or chiasmal cisterns. In tumors involving the cerebral hemispheres encephalography will reveal a distortion or obliteration of the ventricle either entirely or in part on the side of the tumor, with a pushing over of the ventricle to the opposite side and hence a shift of the midline structures. These are the main features of the deformities; the specific areas of deformation will depend on the location of the tumor. In frontal lobe tumor the anterior horn of the lateral ventricle will be obliterated or encroached upon: in temporal lobe tumors the inferior horn; in parietal lobe tumors the body and posterior horn, etc. Tumors of the vermis of the cerebellum occlude the fourth ventricle; hence encephalography will reveal internal hydrocephalus involving the lateral ventricles and the third ventricle, with failure of visualization of the fourth ventricle. In third ventricle tumors the lateral ventricles alone are dilated or there may be dilatation of the lateral ventricles and a portion only of the third ventricle. Cerebellopontine angle tumors show only in-

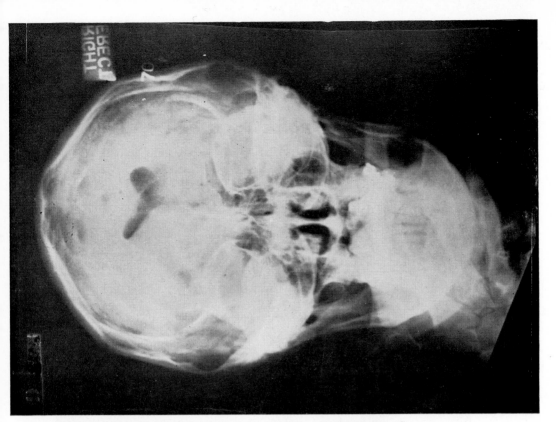

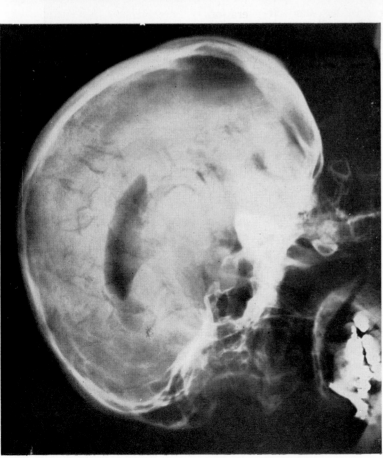

Fig. 25—*Encephalogram of a left frontal lobe tumor*, showing encroachment on the anterior horn of the left lateral ventricle in both A P and lateral views and the shift of the midline structures to the right side.

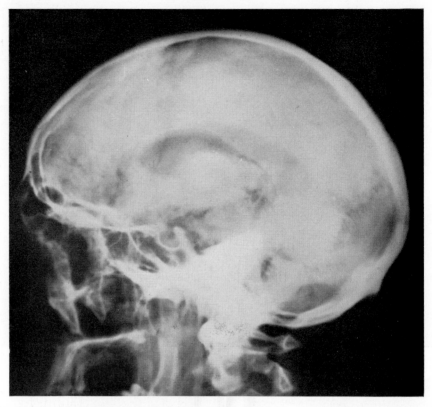

Fig. 26—*Ventriculogram* revealing the cutting off of the posterior horn and part of the body of one lateral ventricle in a parietal lobe tumor.

ternal hydrocephalus. Brain stem tumors show no deformities of any significance. (2) In cases of old head injury in which the problem of persistent cerebral symptoms leads to the investigation of the brain in order to determine whether permanent damage, either local or general, has followed the head injury. Encephalography in such cases may reveal a cerebral cicatrix, subdural hematoma, cortical atrophy, arachnoiditis, or it may disclose nothing at all. Cerebral cicatrix will be indicated by a dilated ventricle on the side of the scar, with a pulling over of the ventricle due to the traction exerted by the scar. Subdural hematoma is revealed by encroachment on the ventricle, displacement of the midline structures, and

at times by the presence of subdural air. Cortical atrophy is often diagnosed, frequently when it is not present. It is easy to be deceived by the appearance of the cortical gyri in an encephalogram; mere widening of the gyri as seen by accumulation of air in the gyri is not enough to make a diagnosis of cortical atrophy. If dilatation of the ventricles is present at the same time, cortical atrophy can be diagnosed safely. Focal atrophy involving one or only a few gyri may be present without dilatation of the ventricle. It is difficult to diagnose this by encephalogram. The clinical findings and EEG will help in such instances. Arachnoiditis is often diagnosed by encephalogram due to failure of air to enter the cortical subarachnoid spaces. This, too, must be interpreted with great caution; failure of air to fill the subarachnoid channels may often be due to technical faults. (3) In cases of symptomatic epilepsy occurring in adults or children, encephalography is used widely, but has been rendered unnecessary in many instances since the advent of the electroencephalogram. Encephalogram, however, should be used in all cases of symptomatic epilepsy if there seems to be a possibility of establishing a cause for the convulsions in central nervous system disease. (4) In a variety of other conditions: birth injury, porencephaly, degenerative diseases of the brain which simulate brain tumor, etc.

Ventriculography: This is carried out by the injection of air directly into the

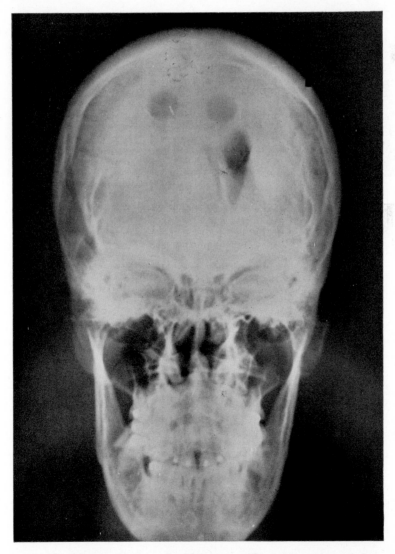

Fig. 27—*Ventriculogram* showing the almost complete obliteration of the anterior horn of one side with a deviation of the midline structures. Diagnosis: Right frontal lobe tumor.

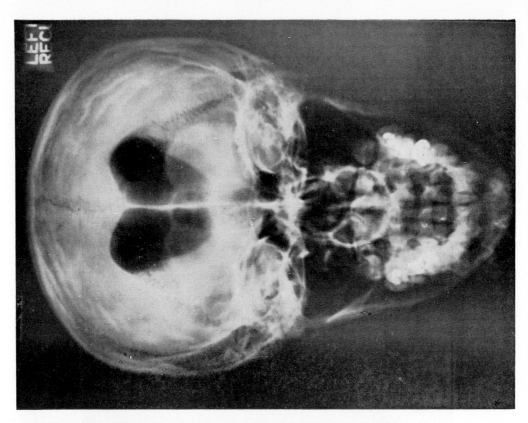

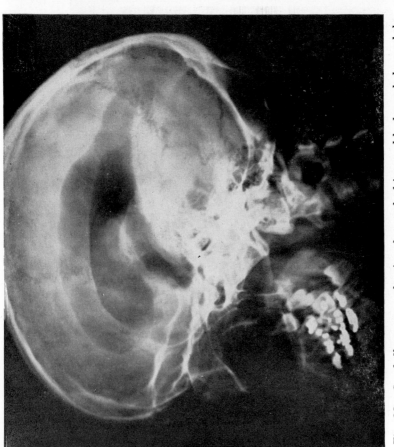

Fig. 28—*Cerebellar tumor, showing the marked internal hydrocephalus and the failure of filling of the fourth ventricle.*

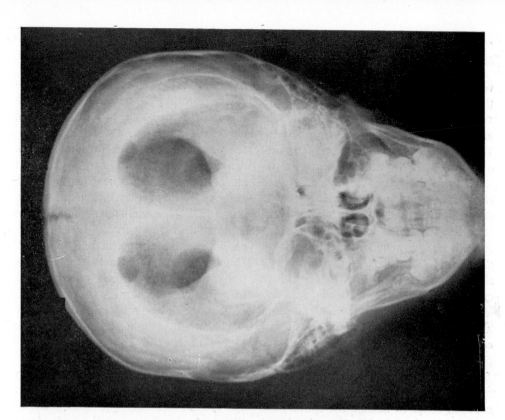

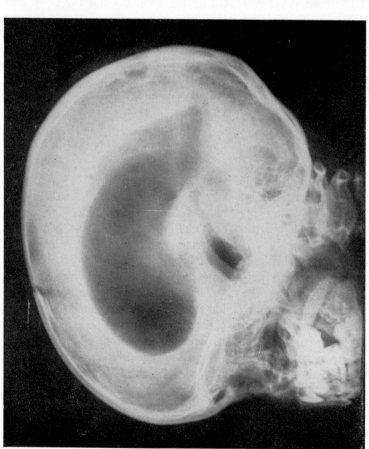

Fig. 29—*Ventriculograms in a case of tumor of the vermis of the cerebellum in a child, showing the internal hydrocephalus and the obliteration of the fourth ventricle.*

ventricles through trephine openings in the skull. By means of this method the ventricles are clearly outlined but the subarachnoid pathways are not visualized. The method is used outstandingly in cases of brain tumor in which localization of the tumor is impossible by the usual clinical means. Like encephalography it depends upon deformities of the ventricular system for its efficacy, the deformities so produced being the same as in encephalography. Ventriculography should always be used in preference to encephalography in cases of increased intracranial pressure. It may be used also in those instances in which encephalography seems undesirable for other reasons.

Myelography: *Air myelography* is a method of air injection into the spinal canal in order to outline the spinal subarachnoid space. It has been developed in order to avoid the use of irritating contrast media such as iodized oil, its greatest field of usefulness being as an aid in the diagnosis of spinal-cord tumors or of other obstructions of the spinal subarachnoid space. The method requires great technical skill in the interpretation of the results, but in experienced hands it seems to be extremely useful. Tumors, herniated nucleus pulposus, and other deformities can be outlined by the column of air in the spinal canal. The method has the advantage of being followed by the complete absorption of the air in the spinal canal.

In many instances of suspected spinal-cord tumor and herniated nucleus pulposus, it is desirable to examine the subarachnoid space of the spinal canal by a contrast medium because routine examination, spinal fluid studies, and Queckenstedt tests fail to reveal evidence of the suspected lesion. This is a more practical and widely used method than air myelography. For this reason *Pan-*

topaque has been developed. This substance is of high specific gravity, with the unfortunate sequel of root irritations, meningeal irritation, and back pain following its use sometimes for long periods. A sterile meningitis follows its use, with an increase of cells in the spinal fluid. Its effects may be very irritating. It is introduced into the spinal subarachnoid space in amounts varying from 5 to 10 cc., depending upon the circumstances of its use. In cases of suspected herniated nucleus pulposus 5 cc. or more is usually used; in spinal-cord tumor less may be used. It may be introduced into the lumbar region or by the cisternal route, the course of the oil being followed carefully by the fluoroscope after its introduction, by tilting the head down on a tilt table if the oil is introduced into the lumbar subarachnoid space and by tilting the head up and the body down if injected into the cistern. In cases of complete blockage of the subarachnoid pathways a complete arrest of the oil can be seen by fluoroscope and by roentgenograms. In incomplete block some of the oil escapes around the block. Herniated nucleus pulposus can be detected by this means as an irregular knoblike projection. Errors in interpretation of apparent blockage of the oil are common, so that care must be exercised in accepting the results. False blocks are not uncommon, tumors blocking the subarachnoid space may not be seen in some instances, and incomplete blocks are sometimes seen but cannot be confirmed on exploration.

The use of Pantopaque is not without hazards. Its introduction into the spinal canal is associated with a meningeal reaction, causing increase of cells in the spinal fluid and fibrosis of the overlying meninges (Tarlov). A chronic arachnoiditis may develop following its use. Neurological symptoms, such as pains, bladder retention, and even weakness of muscles, may develop following its introduction into the spinal canal, either immediately or after several weeks.

Arteriography: This is sometimes used in the diagnosis of brain tumor and aneurysms. It is carried out by the injection of 10 cc. of Thorotrast or other similar material into the carotid or vertebral arteries, followed immediately by roentgenograms and again two seconds later. The first films outline the arterial trunks (arteriogram), the second the veins (phlebogram). The method reveals the presence of tumor, aneurysm, or vascular anomalies by the distortion of the normal vascular outline.

The contrast material (Diodrast or Thorotrast) is introduced by percutaneous puncture of the internal carotid artery or by exposure of the artery. By this means the anterior and middle cerebral circulation is visualized. Injection of the vertebral artery may be carried out for visualization of the posterior cerebral and brainstem circulation.

Arteriography is being used with increasing frequency and is now practiced often in preference to air injection. It is particularly useful in the demonstration of cerebral aneurysm, vascular anomalies of various types, thrombosis of the internal carotid artery and other vascular conditions. It is also valuable in the diagnosis of brain tumor involving the cerebral hemispheres, by the displacement of arteries or the demonstration of abnormal arterial patterns.

A morbidity of 4.6 per cent and a mortality of 0.8 per cent has been recorded in 500 consecutive arteriograms (Kaplan and Walker).

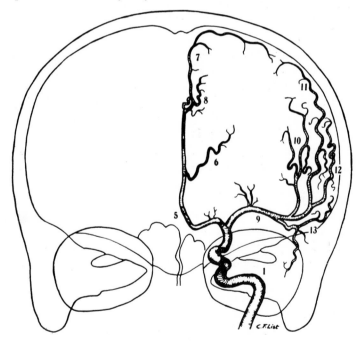

Fig. 30—Schematic drawings of normal arteriograms of the internal carotid artery: Anteroposterior posterior projection. 1. Internal carotid artery. 2. Ophthalmic artery. 3. Posterior communicating artery. 4. Anterior choroidal artery. 5. Anterior cerebral artery. 6. Frontopolar artery. 7. Callosomarginal artery. 8. Pericallosal artery. 9. Middle cerebral artery. 10. Ascending frontoparietal artery. 11. Posterior parietal artery. 12. Angular artery. 13. Posterior temporal artery. (List, Carl, et al.: Radiology 45:1 [July] 1945.)

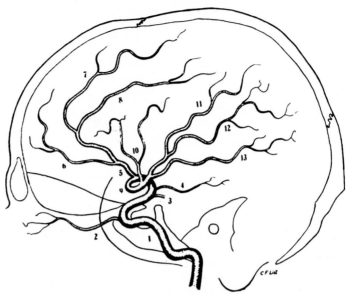

Fig. 31—Schematic drawings of normal arteriograms of the internal carotid artery: Lateral projection. 1. Internal carotid artery. 2. Ophthalmic artery. 3. Posterior communicating artery. 4. Anterior choroidal artery. 5. Anterior cerebral artery. 6. Frontopolar artery. 7. Callosomarginal artery. 8. Pericallosal artery. 9. Middle cerebral artery. 10. Ascending frontoparietal artery. 11. Posterior parietal artery. 12. Angular artery. 13. Posterior temporal artery. (List, Carl, *et al.*: Radiology 45:1 [July] 1945.)

Hemiplegia with or without aphasia and sensory changes has been reported in 2 to 10 per cent of cases. Convulsions may develop but are rare.

Injection of the superior sagittal sinus (sinogram) by a trephine opening is used to demonstrate blockage of this or other sinuses by tumor or thrombosis.

Electromyography: Records of the activity of muscles is obtained from the electromyogram which is recorded directly from muscles by means of a needle electrode, the electrical potentials being amplified and recorded on a cathode-ray oscillograph. Electromyography has been used in clinical disorders involving the muscles and in various diseases associated with denervation, such as amyotrophic lateral sclerosis. It is of relatively little help in its present state of development in the establishment of a diagnosis. The diagnosis of amyotrophic lateral sclerosis, for example, cannot be made on the electromyogram alone, though it may give information regarding the degree of denervation in the muscle.

3

The Topical Diagnosis
of Nervous Disease

Neurological diseases become intelligible only if some general idea of the symptoms arising from the areas diseased is possible. The mere thought of localization in the nervous system is enough to send the average physician into a frenzy. Actually, the step is the next logical procedure after examination, and the practitioner of medicine should be capable at least of determining the larger categories of neurological localization.

I. SYMPTOMS OF DEFICIT

Those symptoms which arise from disease of any part of the central nervous system are the expression, not of the diseased or degenerated areas, but of other portions of the brain or spinal cord, the action of which becomes unopposed after the involved areas are thrown out of action. In other words, disease of any portion of the nervous system resulting in loss of cells, axis-cylinder destruction, or destructive processes of any sort, cannot produce positive symptoms. This was pointed out clearly by Hughlings Jackson, to whom belongs the credit for crystallizing this seemingly obvious principle. The spasticity, paralysis, and reflex changes which are found in a hemiplegia cannot be the expression of an area of destruction of the internal capsule or of any portion of the corticospinal system, since it is obvious that *a destroyed area cannot give rise to impulses.* In a hemiplegia, the impulses conveyed through the corticospinal system are completely interrupted. It follows, therefore, that the signs and symptoms of a hemiplegia must be the expression of other portions of the brain or brain stem which act unopposed after the destroyed area has been shunted out of action, or it follows as the result of liberation of the diseased area from the control of higher centers. The same holds true for extrapyramidal symptoms associated with paralysis agitans. The diseased basal ganglion cells cannot give rise to the positive manifestations of the disease, such as rigidity, tremor, postural changes, etc. These must result from the action of other parts of the nervous system which probably normally act in unison with the diseased areas. Other examples could be multiplied indefinitely.

The symptoms of chorea or athetosis and those of disease of any part of the nervous system must be regarded in the same light. The symptoms resulting from disease of the cerebellum, for example, result probably from unopposed action of the cerebral cortex. Positive symptoms cannot be produced therefore by negative lesions. In one sense the principle appears not to hold and that is in the case of sensory disturbances. The loss of pain sensation and of other sensory disturbances cannot be regarded as resulting from unopposed action of other areas but must be looked upon as the result of interruption of conduction of fibers with specific functions.

One can do no better than to state

the principle involved in the words of Hughlings Jackson. To take hemiplegia as an example, the spasticity in hemiplegia is not the result of the lesion. "There is evidently a duplex symptomatic condition, negative and positive, with loss of power over the muscles, there is tonic action of them. Whilst the primary cerebral lesion can account for the paralytic element—the negative condition—it cannot (nor can the sclerosis in the lateral column) account for the tonic condition of the muscles, the positive element. Negative states of the nervous centers cannot cause positive

side of the reflex arc results in common symptoms of deficit whether the interruption be at the anterior horn cell, anterior root, or motor peripheral nerve. Means of differentiation at the various levels of involvement are available, but the fact remains that lesions of the anterior horn cell and the motor system "downstream" from it have many patterns in common. All lesions on the motor side of the reflex arc produce paralysis, atrophy of the muscle or muscles affected in varying degree, loss or decrease of reflexes, and quantitative changes in the electrical reactions. The

Table 8—Differential Characteristics of Interruptions at Various Levels of Motor Reflex Arc

	Paralysis	Atrophy	Fasciculations	Reflexes	Electrical Reactions
ANTERIOR HORN CELL	Present. Segmental. Proportional to cell loss	Present. Proportional to degree of cell loss	Always present unless complete atrophy of muscle is present	Lost or decreased Never normal	Decreased or R D present
ANTERIOR ROOT	Same as anterior horn cell	Same as anterior horn cell	Same as anterior horn cell	Same as anterior horn cell	Same as anterior horn cell
MOTOR PERIPHERAL NERVE	Present. Not segmental. Proportional to disease of nerve	May or may not be present depending on various factors	Never present unless anterior horn cells are diseased by retrograde degeneration	Lost or decreased	Decreased or R D present

states of muscles, though they may permit them."

II. LESIONS OF THE LOWER MOTOR NEURON

Lesions of the lower motor neuron may involve (1) the anterior horn cells, (2) the anterior roots, (3) the peripheral nerve or, in other words, the peripheral neuron anywhere from its cell of origin (anterior horn cell) outward. They may involve also the sensory component of the reflex arc (posterior root), but this will be reserved for discussion later.

Interruption of function of the motor

specific features at various points of the motor side of the reflex arc will now be considered.

1. Anterior Horn Cell Syndrome

The features of anterior horn cell disease hold true for involvement of the anterior horn cells of the spinal cord or brain stem (motor cranial nerve nuclei), by any of the diseases which may attack them, whether it be poliomyelitis, amyotrophic lateral sclerosis, syringomyelia, progressive muscular atrophy, or other disorders. The syndrome is characterized by: (1) *Paralysis*. This is always flaccid and hypotonic, segmental in character, and either partial or complete for a particular muscle or group of muscles, depending on the number of anterior horn cells destroyed. (2) *Atrophy*. This is always present and depends in degree on the number of cells destroyed. It usually follows soon after paralysis occurs but may be delayed. (3) *Muscle fasciculations*. These occur as part of the anterior horn cell syndrome and where present lend strong support to the diagnosis of anterior horn cell disease. They are not always found, however, because of total atrophy of the muscle or obscuring by overlying fat. (4) *Loss of reflexes*. These occur as the result of interruption of the reflex arc. (5) *Reaction of degeneration*. This is merely an index of the degree of injury to the anterior horn cells. It is found also in completely interrupted peripheral nerves, whether the interruption be the result of injury or disease. (6) *Absence of sensory disturbances*. Since the anterior horn cells are purely motor in function, sensory disturbances are completely lacking.

Pathogenesis: The pathogenesis of the various features of disease of the anterior horn cells is a matter of great practical interest. The *paralysis* which invariably accompanies the disease is the direct result of loss of innervation of the muscles due to interruption of the motor fibers at their cell of origin. It is obvious that if all the cells innervating a muscle or muscles are destroyed the paralysis will be complete; if the anterior horn cell destruction is incomplete the degree of paralysis will depend on the number of cells destroyed and therefore the number of fibers interrupted. Study of the innervation ratio, that is, the proportion of nerve to muscle fibers in lower animals, indicates that in extensor longus digitorum, for example, the ratio is 1 : 165 and in soleus 1 : 120. "This means that

when one anterior horn cell to soleus is stimulated an average of 120 muscle fibers is thrown into action" (Fulton); consequently, the loss of a single anterior

Table 9—Rate of Atrophy of Skeletal Muscle
(Summary of Work Compiled from Literature)

1. DENERVATION
   (1) *Rabbits*
       Began 3-7 days.
       Established and progressed, 14-63 days. (2-9 weeks)
   (2) *Rats*
       Evident 3-10 days.
       Established and progressed, 14 days on.
   (3) *Monkeys*
       Evident 7 days.
       Established and progressed, 84 days. (12 weeks)
2. TENOTOMY
   (1) *Rabbits*
       Evident 2 weeks.
   (2) *Rats*
       Evident 7-10 days.
       Established and progressed, 17 days.
3. DISUSE
   Monkeys
       Evident 1 week.
       Established and progressed, 10 weeks.
4. ANTERIOR RAMISECTION
   Monkeys
       Evident 10 days.

horn cell by disease will result in a considerable loss of power in the affected muscle. This can be demonstrated in still another fashion. It has been demonstrated "that in the gastrocnemius a single anterior horn cell is capable, through repetitive discharge, of developing an average of 30 Gm. of tension" (Fulton); hence the loss of a single anterior horn cell will cause a respectable degree of loss of power.

Still another feature of anterior horn cell paralysis requires mention and that is its segmental character. The spinal cord is a chain of segments operating through separate reflex arcs interacting with one another. Each segment of the spinal cord is in relation to a definite sensory and motor segment of the body. From the motor side, specific muscles are innervated through specific segments of the spinal cord. Muscles may be innervated through a single cord segment, or, as is more usual, through two or three segments. Thus, through segments C5 and C6 in the cervical cord are innervated the biceps, deltoid, part of the pectoralis major, teres major and minor, serratus magnus, supraspinatus, infraspinatus, rhomboids, subscapularis, and the flexor muscles of the hand. A lesion involving these segments, therefore, will result in complete or partial paralysis of the affected muscles, or in other words, a segmental type of paralysis. The same group of muscles may be affected by simultaneous involvement of their respective peripheral nerves, but their resulting features differ from those of anterior horn cell disease. It does not follow, of course, that in disease of a specific segment or segments all the muscles innervated through these segments will be paralyzed. Some may be affected and others not. The atrophy associated with anterior horn cell disease may be so extensive and diffuse that its segmental character cannot be identified. This feature of anterior horn cell involvement therefore may be of more theoretical than practical significance.

The *atrophy* resulting from anterior horn cell disease is still unexplained in many details. It is regarded by many as resulting from constant action of the muscles associated with the fasciculations occurring in anterior horn cell disease. According to this concept therefore atrophy results from the overactivity of the muscles as a result of the constant fasciculations or fibrillations resulting from denervation. Opposed to this is the fact that (1) atrophy results from disuse in fixation of the joints, etc.; (2) in clinical cases atrophy is often advanced in instances wherein fasciculations are few. In experimental animals atrophy of skeletal muscle was found to follow lower motor neuron lesions, upper motor neuron lesions by transection of the cord, and skeletal fixation by fixing the knee and ankle joints. For at least ten days atrophy occurred from all the lesions and then tended to recover in the cord section and skeletal fixation experiments (Solandt). The findings point to the fact that disuse may be a factor in the production of atrophy. The time of development of atrophy after anterior horn cell disease has not been worked out definitely. In some instances it develops rapidly, as in poliomyelitis; in others more slowly, as in progressive muscular atrophy and amyotrophic lateral sclerosis. From a clinical standpoint it seems true that the more extensive the destruction of anterior horn cells the more rapid the atrophy.

The Problem of Fasciculations: This has already been discussed (Chapter 2), but a few more remarks seem pertinent. A compilation of the literature reveals that muscular twitchings closely resembling fibrillations may be found in cases of purulent meningitis, extramedullary tumor of the spinal cord, dementia paralytica, syringomyelia, inflammatory conditions of peripheral nerves, progressive hypertrophic polyneuritis, paralysis agitans, infectious polyneuritis, compression of peripheral nerves, and debilitating conditions such as ulcerative colitis (Swank and Putnam). Despite the fact that fasciculations have been seen in these varied conditions, it is an incontestable fact that muscle fasciculations are found in the vast majority of instances in anterior horn cell disease and only rarely in other conditions. In the many conditions in which fasciculations have been reported, anterior horn cell disease has been present in addition to the other conditions found. Their presence, therefore, must always be regarded as evidence of disease of the anterior horns until proved otherwise. While this is true from a clinical standpoint, it proves nothing from the standpoint of the mechanism of the production of fasciculations. It has been pointed out (Chapter 2) that muscle fasciculations may be present after spinal anesthesia, that they continue after peripheral nerve block (Swank and Price), and that they are obliterated by curare (Forster and Alpers) and section of the peripheral nerve (Alpers and Forster).

Whether the fasciculations are derived from the peripheral nerve or the myoneural junction is not yet known. Few observations have been made in the human on the relationship of fasciculations to atrophy but recent studies of amyotrophic lateral sclerosis indicate that muscle fasciculations appear early in the disease before weakness or atrophy is evident (Swank and Putnam). They appear also to be a rough index of the severity of the disease, for investigations show that few fasciculations indicate a slow course in amyotrophic lateral sclerosis, while many fasciculations indicate a rapid course (Swank and Putnam).

2. Anterior Root Syndrome

This is indistinguishable from that of the anterior horns.

3. Motor Peripheral Nerve Syndrome

Some peripheral nerves are exclusively or almost exclusively motor in function (radial, long thoracic nerve, etc.). Disease of such nerves may give rise to syndromes similar to those of anterior horn cell disease. The main clinical characteristics are: (1) Paralysis, which, as is the case in all peripheral nerve syndromes, is always flaccid; (2) atrophy of the muscle or muscles supplied by the affected nerve; (3) loss of reflexes; (4) reaction of degeneration provided the lesion is complete or total degeneration of

the nerve ensues; (5) absence of pain; (6) absence of sensory disturbances. They differ, however, in the following respects: (a) The atrophy is, as a rule, less extensive and severe, and develops less rapidly. In a completely interrupted nerve, however, it may be as intense as in anterior horn cell disease. (b) There are no fasciculations of the muscles. In those instances in which fasciculations are found in peripheral nerve disease, the assumption must be made that there is coexistent anterior horn cell disease. Apart from these differences the findings are similar.

4. Mixed Peripheral Nerve Syndrome

Since most nerves contain both motor and sensory fibers, the syndromes involving the peripheral nerves are of a mixed type. Not all the features of a mixed peripheral nerve syndrome are found in the same degree in all instances of involvement of the nerve. They may vary with the severity of the offending agent and the degree of damage of the nerve. The symptoms are considered in the discussion of peripheral neuritis, but may be reviewed briefly here. They consist of: (1) *Pain:* This immediately differentiates the syndrome from pure anterior horn cell involvement, since the latter is purely motor in function. The pain is felt along the distribution of the peripheral nerve affected; it is constant and usually severe, is relieved by heat, some drugs, and increased as a rule by movement. (2) *Tenderness of the nerves, muscles, and tendons:* Tenderness of the nerves is always present but it varies in degree; in some cases it is severe, in others only moderate or mild. Usually muscle tenderness is present in the region of the muscles supplied by the affected nerve, but it may be absent or very mild in degree. It must not be forgotten that while nerve and muscle tenderness is always found in nerve irritation of a mixed nerve, it is sometimes found as a result of compression of a nerve at a distance. (3) *Paralysis:* This is flaccid in nature and depends in degree on the amount of injury to the nerve. (4) *Atrophy* is not necessarily present. It depends upon several factors such as the nature of the noxious agent, the time

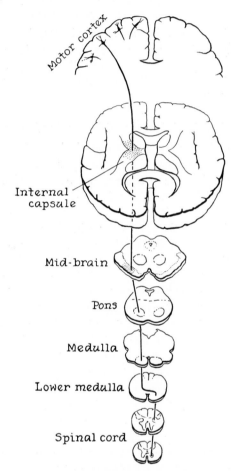

Fig. 32—*Corticospinal* tract indicating its origin and destination around the anterior horn cells.

elapsed since onset of the disturbance, and the degree of injury to the nerve. Long-standing cases will have some degree of atrophy; in others severe atrophy may develop quickly; in still others not at all. (5) *Loss or diminution of reflexes*

due to interruption of the reflex arc. (6) *No reaction of degeneration* except in complete interruption of the nerve. (7) *Sensory disturbances* in the region of the peripheral nerve distribution, involving all types of sensation (pain, touch, heat, cold, position, vibration) in complete interruption and only superficial sensation in other cases (pain, touch, heat, cold). Hyperesthesia or paresthesias may occur.

III. LESIONS OF THE UPPER MOTOR NEURON

Lesions involving the upper motor neuron may affect this neuron anywhere from the cerebral cortex to the spinal cord before its distribution to the muscles. By the upper motor neuron is meant any central neuron conveying impulses to the anterior horn cell. The most important of these is the corticospinal pathway (pyramidal tract) which takes its origin in the cells of the cortex, passes through the internal capsule, the cerebral peduncle, pons, decussates low in the medulla, and passes down the cord in the lateral columns, synapsing eventually with anterior horn cells.

Not all the fibers of the corticospinal or pyramidal tract are derived from the Betz cells of Area 4 (Fig. 33), the precentral gyrus, since it is now known that the pyramidal tract contains fibers derived from other parts of the cortex. These are known to stem from the parietal lobe in monkeys, especially from areas 3, 1, 2, 5, and 7. Other fibers arise from Area 6 of the premotor region. It is probable that the parietal lobe in the human makes important contributions to the pyramidal tract, but the precise portions making this contribution are not as definitely defined as for the monkey. "At least 50 per cent of all the fibers in the pyramids are corticospinal, originating in the precentral gyrus and the parietal lobe. This is the best known group of fibers in the pyramids. Whether the remaining 50 per cent of fibers have cortical or subcortical origin is uncertain" (Tower).

Other upper motor neuron impulses play upon the anterior horn cell. These include: (1) the rubrospinal pathway from the opposite red nucleus; (2) the tectospinal pathway from the roof of the midbrain; (3) the reticulospinal pathway from the reticular formation of the brain stem; (4) the vestibulospinal pathway from the vestibular nucleus of the same side.

Interruption of the corticospinal pathway results in paralysis of the opposite side of the body, of the face, arm, and leg. This is known as *hemiplegia*. It may result from a variety of causes which will be considered in a discussion of vascular diseases. When both corticospinal pathways are interrupted in the brain, *diplegia* results, as in the cerebral diplegia of children. If a single limb or a focal portion of the body (face) is affected, the result is a *monoplegia*. At lower levels *paraplegia* develops, involving usually the legs or the arms and legs.

Paraplegia: The term "paraplegia" is customarily used to refer to paralysis of the legs, but it could be used for paralysis of the arms as well (brachial paraplegia), or for arms and legs. It is associated as a rule with bilateral pyramidal tract involvement of the spinal cord, but it may result from focal bilateral disease of the motor cortex or even of the corticospinal pathway in the brain stem. Rare instances are recorded of paraplegias due to internal capsule involvement and to involvement of the corticospinal pathway in the pons.

Extension Paraplegia: Paraplegia in the majority of cases is an *extension paraplegia* with marked weakness of the legs, spasticity, Babinski signs, and all the other signs indicative of pyramidal tract disease. It results from gradual compression or destruction of the cord by infiltrating or destructive processes.

When it develops acutely, as in cases of spinal cord injury or in acute transection from other causes, the paraplegia is flaccid due to the syndrome of spinal shock which will be discussed later. In some instances typical spastic paraplegia is seen when the patient walks, a characteristic shuffling gait resulting due to the increased extensor tonus; on recumbency the spasticity usually persists but disappears in large part in some cases, only to be elicited again on walking.

Flexion Paraplegia: In some instances this develops, always following paraplegia in extension. In such cases the legs develop involuntary flexor spasms, elicited by touching the foot, stroking the skin, lifting the bedclothes, etc. The flexor spasms are followed by involuntary extension after a varying period of time. The result is alternating flexion and extension occurring at irregular intervals. These eventually give way to a complete flexion paraplegia. The legs are paralyzed in the final stages of the disorder; the patellar reflexes cannot as a rule be elicited because of the marked flexor rigidity which prevents extension of the leg on patellar stimulation, and the defense reflexes are greatly exaggerated in the condition. The condition is indicative of complete or near complete interruption of the spinal cord. It has been reported in spinal cord tumor, multiple sclerosis, spinal cord syphilis, and is likely to be seen in any long-standing paraplegia associated with complete or incomplete interruption of the spinal cord pathways. The flexors alone retain reflex activity in flexion paraplegia, the extensors showing little or no action. The condition is presumably the result of interruption of an extrapyramidal path in the spinal cord, or to unopposed activity of such a path, since flexion paraplegia does not result from pure pyramidal tract interruption.

If only portions of the corticospinal pathway are diseased or injured, *monoplegia* results. This is manifested by a focal loss of power in the opposite side of the body, thus resulting in facial weakness or weakness of a hand (manual monoplegia), or of an arm (brachial monoplegia), or of face, tongue, and arm (facio-lingual-brachial monoplegia). The number of possible combinations is great depending upon the area affected. Monoplegias result almost always from disease of the motor cortex, but in rare instances they may result from involvement of the corticospinal pathway in the brain stem and in rare instances even of the spinal cord. Irritative lesions of the corticospinal path produce *focal* (jacksonian) *convulsions* (*v.* Epilepsy).

Corticospinal or Pyramidal Interruption

This is characterized by the following group of symptoms:

(a) Paralysis: In a typical instance this involves the opposite face, arm, and leg. In some cases face, palate, tongue, arm, and leg may be involved. The chest and abdominal muscles of the affected side are affected and in fresh hemiplegias particularly it is possible to detect weakness of the abdominal muscles which are hypotonic and fail to contract as well as those of the healthy side The paralysis is usually spastic. This *spasticity* is in contrast to the flaccid paralysis of the lower motor neuron. It is characterized by an increase of muscle tone of a "clasp knife" variety. Thus, passive movement of a muscle results first in an increase of the muscle tone, followed, as one continues resistance, by a sudden release of the muscle resist-

Table 10—Localization of Precentral and Postcentral Gyri

Postcentral SENSORY SEQUENCE		Precentral MOTOR SEQUENCE	
Toes		Toes	
Foot		Ankle	
Leg		Knee	
Hip		Hip	
Trunk		Back	
Shoulder		Shoulder	
Arm			
Elbow		Elbow	
Forearm			
Wrist		Wrist	
Hand		Hand	
Little F.		Little F.	
Ring F.		Ring F.	
Middle F.		Middle F.	
Index F.		Index F.	
Thumb		Thumb	
Eye		Brow	Eye Movements
Nose		Eyelid	
Face		Vocalization	
Lips		Lips	
Tongue		Jaw	
Taste		Tongue	
Jaw-teeth			
Throat		Swallow	

RIGHT CENTRAL FISSURE OF ROLANDO

FISSURE OF SYLVIUS

ance. Frequently this particular reaction is not elicited, but there is felt an increased resistance of the muscle to passive movement. It is abolished through section of the posterior roots. The spasticity is selective; the muscles of the forearm, arm, and hand are flexed, the forearm is pronated and the muscles of the shoulder are adducted. The extensor muscles are more involved in the leg. The paralysis is selective in still other ways. It involves the arm and leg more than the head, neck, and trunk. In the arm, the finger and hand movements are most severely affected and the forearm, arm, and shoulder movements somewhat less. The arm is held in flexion. In the leg movements of the toes, foot and knee are most involved. The leg is held in extension. Interruption of the pyramid results in the loss of discrete control of movement (Tower).

Paralysis due to interruption of the corticospinal pathway is not always spastic, however. Under some circumstances it is completely flaccid but without atro-

phy or the other features of anterior horn cell disease. The flaccidity may be transitory, lasting from a few hours or days to weeks, or it may persist throughout the course of the paralysis. The cause of the flaccidity is not definitely known. Reference has been made (Chapter 2) to the problem of flaccidity in cortico-

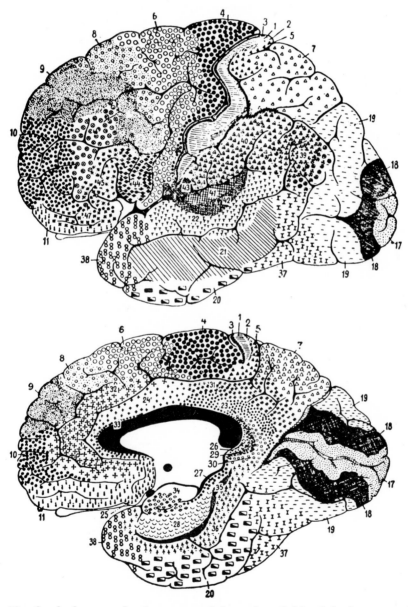

Fig. 33—*Cerebral cortex* showing a map of the various fields of the human cerebral cortex (*Brodmann.*)

spinal lesions, but a more extensive consideration of the problem seems indicated in view of its clinical importance. Most of our real knowledge concerning the problem is derived from observations on animals, and is largely the result of the work of Fulton and his associates.

The motor cortex of primates arises in the depths of the central sulcus (fissure of Rolando) and extends for a variable distance rostrally over the precentral convolution. This has been designated Area 4 in accordance with the cytoarchitectural maps of the cerebral cortex and is regarded as the motor cortex. Immediately rostral to Area 4 is Area 4s,

or the strip area of Hines, and one of the suppressor areas of Dusser de Barenne and McCulloch. Area 4s is usually situated on the more anterior portions of the precentral gyrus. Immediately rostral to Area 4s is Area 6. Physiologically, these areas differ in their responses to stimulation and in the pictures of deficit produced by ablation. Electrical stimulation of Area 4 produces simple, discrete movements of a part of the opposite half of the body. The part moved depends upon the region of Area 4 stimulated, since there is a topographical representation for the opposite side of the body, which is an inverse arrangement, so that the lower portions are

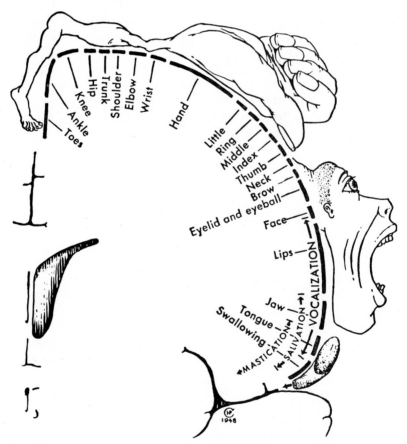

Fig. 34—*Motor homunculus*, showing the representation of the various parts of the body in the motor cortex. The face, hand, and foot areas are most widely represented. *(Penfield and Rasmussen: The Cerebral Cortex of Man. By permission of The Macmillan Co.)*

represented more superiorly on the gyrus. Thus the lower extremity is represented in man on the medial surface of the brain, while the face area is just above the Sylvian fissure. Severe electrical stimulation will produce seizures of jacksonian pattern. Electrical stimulation of Area 4s induces a prolonged, often phasic decrease in the electrical activity of the cerebral cortex and a prolonged period during which the threshold of stimulation of motor cortex is increased. There is, therefore, a suppression of cortical function resulting from the activity of suppressor cortex. Electrical stimulation of Area 6 results in simple, discrete movements of the opposite side and also postural movements. The simple, discrete movements are due to fibers from Area 6 to Area 4; and if a simple incision is made between Areas 4 and 6, the simple, discrete movements of the opposite side of the body are no longer elicitable. The postural movements are still readily elicited, however, after such a section and represent the chief function of Area 6. There is no sharp topographical distribution for parts of the opposite side; and indeed with increased electrical current, it is possible to induce bilateral postural movements.

Ablation of Area 4 alone produces in monkeys and chimpanzees a transitory, contralateral hemiplegia. This is a flaccid hemiplegia, although a short transitory period of increased muscle tone may exist. The deep reflexes are slightly increased, if at all, and in chimpanzees a positive Babinski sign is produced. The paralysis is transitory, and the permanent defect from pure Area 4 lesions is moderate and most marked in movements of the digits. Inclusion of Areas 4 and 4s in the ablation results in the addition of moderate spasticity of permanent nature to the hemiplegia and hyperactivity of the deep tendon reflexes. Ablation of Areas 4, 4s, and 6 together result in a marked contralateral hemiplegia with marked spasticity, hyperreflexia, positive Babinski sign, and a positive grasp reflex. The spasticity and grasp reflexes are dependent upon the forces of gravity. The typical posture of hemiplegia is with the arm in flexion and the leg in extension. The resistance on passive manipulation of the extremities is to extension in the arms and to flexion in the legs. This is a push against gravity as can be readily demonstrated by the observation of having a spastic hemiplegic patient assume a quadrupedal posture, the spasticity of the arm then being evident in extension and not in flexion. The grasp reflex is more readily elicited when the recumbent patient is placed on his side so that the nonparalyzed side is into the bed and the paralyzed side farthest from the earth.

It is helpful in the understanding of some of the symptoms of pyramidal tract disease to know something of the cortical projection of fibers, in addition to the corticospinal or pyramidal tract. These are in reality extrapyramidal fibers. Most of the projections arise from Areas 4, 4s, and 6. In the monkey, Areas 4s, 8, 9, 24, 2, and 19 discharge to the caudate; Areas 6 and 4 project to the putamen; and Area 6 projects to the pallidum. Areas 4, 4s, and 6 project to the substantia nigra and subthalamic region. Areas 4 and 6 are reported to project to the nucleus ruber. Area 19 discharges to the tectum. Areas 4s, 8, 24, 2, and 19 discharge to the reticular nuclei in the medulla. Other cortical extrapyramidal fibers consist of the corticopontocerebellar fibers.

Most of the understanding of these areas is based on experimental work in higher primates. There are rare cases of lesions of Area 4 alone (Neilsen and Vonderahe). There are no cases of pure Area-4s lesions in man, in fact there is only one report of the physiological demonstration of Area 4s in man (Bucy and Garol). Extensive lesions of the motor areas are not uncommon, and the human counterpart of combined ablations of Areas 4, 4s, and 6 are all too frequent.

The problem seems not to be as clean cut in the human as in the primate. The problem is difficult to control in the human. Spasticity is usual in the average hemiplegic and is associated chiefly with a lesion involving the internal cap-

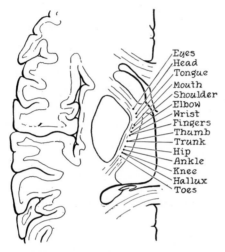

Fig. 35—*Internal capsule,* showing in diagram form the situation of the fibers to the various portions of the limbs and trunk of the opposite side of the body.

sular area. It has been observed that in cerebral lesions spasticity is marked in proportion as the lesion is situated caudally (Monakow). Instances are well known in clinical experiences, however, in which flaccid paralysis is associated with capsular lesions. Pure motor cortical lesions in the human are rare; hence, it is not possible to assert whether in the human, lesions of the motor cortex are associated with flaccidity as is the case with primates. Though the findings are not as definite in the human, the evidence appears to indicate that the spasticity resulting from lesions of the corticospinal system is the result of unopposed activity of some other portion of

the brain, an extrapyramidal portion. Hence spasticity is a manifestation of extrapyramidal rather than of pyramidal action.

"From clinical and experimental sources come several indications, as yet imperfectly understood, that a pure cortical lesion of the pyramidal system often does not produce spasticity as an accompaniment of the loss of power. They suggest the possibility that in the cerebral lesion underlying, for example, a typical spastic residual hemiplegia, analysis may ultimately reveal a second component. That is, in addition to a negative lesion of the corticospinal path, interruption of another descending path may be concerned in the production of spasticity. Such a path need not necessarily be cerebrospinal" (Walshe).

Facial Paralysis: It is present in corticospinal lesions. It involves only the lower part of the face and is shown by a slowness and weakness in retraction of the mouth, and a flattening of the normal angulation of the mouth on the affected side. Sometimes the palate is paralyzed on one side, manifested by a drooping of the affected side, with a pulling up of the palate to the healthy side on phonation. The tongue when paralyzed is pushed over to the paralyzed side on protrusion. The mechanism of production of cranial nerve palsies in hemiplegia is understandable, after a consideration of the anatomy involved in the problem. The motor nuclei of the brain stem receive innervation from the motor cortex through a special tract, the corticobulbar tract. By means of this pathway impulses are conveyed to the motor cranial nerve nuclei from above (supranuclear innervation). The tract in question forms part of the corticospinal system but is contained within it in a separate bundle. Thus, it courses through the knee of the internal capsule and is specifically located in other parts of the pyramidal tract. Fibers to the face are conveyed through this tract, the forehead and eyelids being innervated bilaterally, while the lower portion of the face receives only unilateral innervation For this reason only the lower portion of the face is paralyzed as a result of a unilateral corticospinal lesion. Other motor functions, such as phonation, chewing, etc., dependent on innervation from motor nuclei in the brain stem, receive bilateral innervation and are, therefore, not affected in corticospinal disease.

(b) Increase of Tendon Reflexes: The tendon reflexes of the paralyzed side (biceps, triceps, patellar, Achilles reflexes) are overactive in corticospinal lesions, presumably due to release of the anterior horn cells from the inhibitory effects of the corticospinal pathway. The overactive reflexes, like the spasticity, are the expression of extrapyramidal influences. Generally speaking, the tendon reflexes are increased in proportion to the spasticity of the muscles; however, muscles may be so spastic as to produce no response and the flaccidity of corticospinal disease is not infrequently associated with overactive reflexes. The reflexes may be overactive in flaccid hemiplegia due to corticospinal disease. *Clonus* of the muscles is frequently found, usually ankle clonus, but sometimes patellar, wrist, and even pectoral clonus. This consists of a repetitive movement of the muscles and is associated with increased muscle tonus. Ankle clonus is elicited by quick, vigorous dorsiflexion of the foot, with the knee held in flexion. The result in cases of corticospinal disease is a repeated clonic movement of the foot which is maintained so long as the foot is held firmly in dorsiflexion. Ordinarily, the clonus ceases when the foot is released, but in some instances it may continue

spontaneously and ceases only with vigorous plantar flexion. Spontaneous clonus at the ankle joint may develop in cases of advanced spasticity and may constitute an annoying symptom. Patellar clonus is elicited by vigorous downward movement of the patella with the leg in full extension. Wrist clonus is produced by vigorous extension of the wrist.

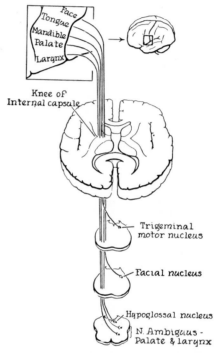

Fig. 36—*Corticospinal tract,* **showing the projection of the corticobulbar pathways on the motor nuclei of the brain stem.**

(c) Loss of Cutaneous Reflexes: An almost constant feature of corticospinal disease is the loss of the cutaneous reflexes, notably the abdominal reflexes on the side of the paralysis. They are lost bilaterally in paraplegia. In some instances of hemiplegia the abdominal reflexes are retained.

(d) Abnormal or Pathological Reflexes: The most important and the most significant of the abnormal reflex responses which follow corticospinal disease is the extensor response of Babinski (Babinski's sign). This is pathognomonic of corticospinal disease; it never occurs without it, though corticospinal disease may be found without a Babinski sign, with some or all the other features of corticospinal involvement. Both this and other pathological responses have been described (Chapter 2). Of the other abnormal toe responses—Chaddock, Oppenheim, and Gordon—the Chaddock sign may be said to have the same significance as the Babinski sign; and when found alone, it may be regarded as indicative of pyramidal tract disease. The same may be said of the Oppenheim sign, though this occurs rarely.

In many cases, all the signs listed are easily elicited. In other instances, various combinations may be encountered. Only slight weakness of one side may be present (hemiparesis). There may be only very slight weakness associated with increased reflexes with or without abnormal reflexes; or there may be a Babinski sign without other evidence of corticospinal disease; or weakness may be present with only slightly increased reflexes. These slighter and partial manifestations of corticospinal disease are even more important to recognize than the fully developed picture. It is well to bear in mind that a positive Babinski sign always means corticospinal disease, and that paralysis or weakness without increase of reflexes, abnormal reflexes, or loss of cutaneous reflexes is not structural but is probably of psychogenic origin.

IV. LESIONS OF THE EXTRAPYRAMIDAL SYSTEM

The extrapyramidal system is a part of the motor system. It is composed of the so-called "basal ganglia," and portions of the cerebral cortex which have motor functions but are not part of the pyramidal or corticospinal system. There is considerable controversy concerning what should be included in this system, but the following represent a group generally agreed upon: caudate, putamen, pallidum, corpus subthalamicum, nucleus ruber, substantia nigra. Some include the thalamus and nucleus dentatus in the cerebellum. All these nuclei are richly connected with one another (v. Extrapyramidal Diseases).

Disease of the extrapyramidal system results in disturbances of movement, as might be surmised from the motor function of the system. These are of three sorts: (1) akinetic or hypokinetic; (2) hyperkinetic; (3) mixed.

1. The Akinetic or Hypokinetic Syndrome

This is typically illustrated by the paralysis agitans group of cases. Their features will be considered in detail in a discussion of paralysis agitans. Briefly stated, they are characterized by muscular rigidity, which is different from the spasticity of corticospinal disease. The rigidity is associated with a cogwheel phenomenon which is elicited as follows: If the forearm is slowly pronated and supinated, or flexed and extended, the movement can be felt as a series of catches and releases as if the muscle were being moved over a cog; hence the term cogwheel sign. It is plastic in type, of a lead pipe variety, and uniformly resistant throughout the range of passive motion. The head and trunk are flexed, the face is fixed, movements are slow and few, accessory movements are not made, the speech is low and monotonous, and tremor is often present. The tendon reflexes are usually normal and no Babinski sign is found.

2. Choreiform Syndrome

This is seen in diseases of the extrapyramidal system in the acute chorea of Sydenham, and in the chronic progressive chorea of Huntington particularly. It is characterized by rapid, discrete, involuntary movements affecting the face and limbs, opposite muscle groups contracting simultaneously. The movements are abrupt, and completely beyond the control of the will. In some instances, they are extremely vigorous (chorea gravidarum) and in others violent and one-sided (hemiballismus). The pathological background of chorea is not definitely settled. It is presumed to be the result of disease, especially of the caudate and putamen and sometimes of the corpus subthalamicum, the choreiform movements being regarded as release phenomena in which the cerebral cortex acts unopposed by the basal ganglia. Choreiform movements have resulted from disease of many areas of the brain: cortex, thalamus, red nucleus, and striatum. No single area of the brain can be said to be diseased constantly in the choreiform syndrome, though the striatum (caudate and putamen) is most often affected. In diseases such as Huntington's chorea, it is always severely involved. Chorea may result from disease of the cortex with intact basal ganglia (Wilson), or from disease of the efferent area of the cerebellum, the dentato rubrothalamocortical pathway.

3. Athetoid Syndrome

Athetoid movements are, in contrast to chorea, slow, snaky, sinuous movements, and by blending of the involuntary movements they form a mixture of irregularly synchronous contractions of opposite muscular groups (Wilson). As is the case in chorea, opposite muscle groups contract at the same time. The site of the lesion in cases of athetosis lies in the basal ganglia, but the exact areas involved are not definitely settled. The pallidum and striatum are most frequently diseased. Of these, the pallidum is found most constantly diseased in cases

of athetosis. The symptom of athetosis must, therefore, be regarded as a release from the action of other brain areas. Separate ablation of the motor and premotor cortex results in permanent extinction of the athetosis in some cases and temporary in others.

V. DISTURBANCES OF COÖRDINATION

The problem of coördination is complex and difficult. Three systems participate in the production of smooth coördinated movement: the posterior column system, the cerebellum, and the vestibular system. All may be regarded as part of the proprioceptive system and all may be looked upon as having important functions in the maintenance of posture, the vestibular system through the labyrinthine and righting reflexes, the posterior column through the proprioceptors of muscles, tendons, and joints, and the cerebellum through its action in synergizing movements. Impulses transmitted through the posterior column system reach consciousness, while those through the cerebellar pathway do not do so directly. The former may be regarded therefore as the conscious element of the proprioceptive system and the latter as its unconscious portion. Disease of any of these systems results in disturbance of coördination.

Syndrome of the Posterior Column System: The posterior columns (gracilis and cuneatus) run the length of the spinal cord, the gracilis, or column of Goll, extending from the lowermost portions and conveying impulses from the legs and lower trunk, and the cuneatus, or columns of Burdach, extending from the midthoracic region upward and conveying impulses from the arms and upper trunk. The fibers from these columns decussate in the medulla, proceeding thence as the mesial fillet to the thalamus, whence they proceed to the cerebral cortex and particularly to the parietal lobe. They convey deep sensations from the muscles, joints, and tendons, measured clinically by position sense and vibration sense chiefly.

Lesions of the Posterior Column System: These cause *ataxia* as their outstanding symptom. This ataxia is increased by the shutting out of visual impulses. Thus, the ataxia of posterior-column disease is increased with the eyes closed, as in the Romberg test in tabes dorsalis, and in the dark, as in the gait disturbances of tabes, subacute combined degeneration, etc. The shutting out or dimming of visual impulses invariably increases the ataxia of posterior column disease. For this reason, patients with posterior column disease of whatever origin must watch their movements; their legs in walking, their arms in reaching. Because of the ataxia, the gait of posterior column disease is wide-based and unsteady (*v.* Chapter 2).

The ataxia of posterior column disease is characterized also by the fact that precision movements, such as putting the finger on the nose, or the heel on the knee or toe, produce a shooting beyond the mark accompanied by a gross irregularity of movement. This failure to reach the mark, referred to as *dysmetria,* is characteristic of posterior column ataxia. The patient so afflicted is unable to perform smooth, coördinated movement. All efforts at such movement result in ataxic performances resulting in coarse tremor and a failure to reach accurately the goal of the movement. Overshooting of the goal is therefore usual and characteristic. If the eyes are closed in finger-nose test, in a patient with posterior column atoxia, the finger will not find its goal, provided it does not touch the face. The ataxia is dependent on a sensory deficit, namely, the loss of position and muscle senses. Because

of it, there is inability to gauge the position of limbs in space.

Posterior column ataxia does not occur without sensory defects. Both position and vibration senses are usually lost in posterior column disease, but there may be loss of position sense without loss of vibration, or vibration sense may be lost without impairment of position sense. In these instances in which there is ataxia, position sense is invariably lost or impaired in the affected limbs. The severity of the ataxia is usually in direct proportion to the loss of position sense. Vibration sense may be lost in the arms or legs without ataxia, as for example in the loss of vibration sense in the legs in older subjects.

Though the symptoms resulting from deficit of proprioception are the most striking evidences of posterior column disease, other symptoms are also found associated with it, but they are not so important clinically as ataxia. They consist of astereognosis and disturbance of two-point discrimination.

Posterior column disease occurs in a wide variety of conditions, and of course has the same characteristics no matter what the condition. It is found in tabes dorsalis, subacute combined degeneration, syringomyelia, multiple sclerosis, spinal-cord tumor, and a variety of other diseases. The symptoms of posterior column disease are the same regardless of the point of interruption of the system, whether in cervical or lumbar cord, in the mesial fillet in the brain stem, or in the thalamus.

Syndrome of the Cerebellar System: The cerebellum is intimately concerned with coördination, for which purpose it has very wide connections with all parts of the body and all parts of the nervous system. It receives impulses from the trunk and limbs through the spinocerebellar pathways, and from the head and neck probably through the posterior longitudinal bundle and other paths. It is in intimate association with the vestibular system, the basal ganglia system, and it has most intimate connections with the cerebral cortex. Its precise function is a matter of controversy, though it is possible to state in general terms that it has a great deal to do with coördination.

Anatomically, the cerebellum sits

red nucleus to the anterior horn cells, fired off by impulses from the dentato-rubral pathway; and (3) a tract from the roof nuclei to the reticular formation. By means of these efferent connections the cerebellum sets off impulses in the corticospinal, rubrospinal and reticulospinal pathways, in response to impulses received in the cerebellum and transmitted through its efferent arms.

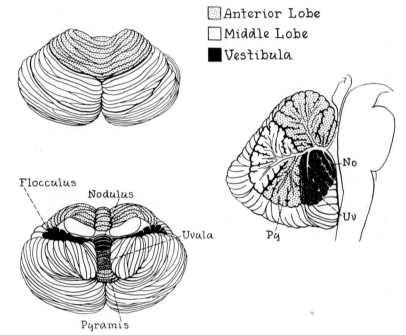

☷ Anterior Lobe
☐ Middle Lobe
■ Vestibula

Fig. 37—*Cerebellum*, showing the distribution of anterior and midde lobes and vestibular portion. (*Brown: Prec. Staff Mayo Clinic, 19:169, 1944.*)

astride the motor tracts and receives afferent impulses from all levels—from the spinocerebellar, bulbocerebellar, olivocerebellar, cortical and vestibulocerebellar connections. The information obtained by these afferent stimuli is transmitted into action by means of efferent pathways: (1) the dentato-rubrothalamocortical (superior cerebellar peduncle) pathway, the main efferent path which effects connections with the cerebral cortex and the corticospinal tract; (2) the rubrospinal tract from the

The chief symptom of deficit resulting from lesions of the cerebellum has been variously described as cerebellar ataxia, asynergia, and cerebellar atonia. Regardless of the precise primary symptom of deficit upon which all do not agree, it is nevertheless true that disease of the cerebellum results in *loss or impairment of muscle coördination* and the various symptoms which follow from cerebellar disease are the result primarily of this deficit.

The primary symptom of deficit of

cerebellar disease is *asynergy*. This consists of an inability to perform movements smoothly due to the lack of normal synergistic action between the agonists and antagonists in muscle groups. The result is a jerky, decomposed movement which is highly incoördinate. There is in cerebellar disease a true decomposition of movement. The incoördination of cerebellar disease, unlike posterior column ataxia, has no relation to vision and is the same with the eyes open or closed. *Cerebellar asynergy is not associated with sensory deficit,* and the disturbance of position and vibration senses found in posterior column ataxia is not found in cerebellar disease. In reaching for a goal, persons with cerebellar disease do so with intense incoordination, using accessory muscles of the arms or legs, describing a wide arc in their motion, but they, unlike posterior column cases, reach their goal, though they may have difficulty in holding it. Thus, in placing the finger on the nose, a person with cerebellar disease will describe a wide arc with the arm, develop coarse tremor, and with much jerking approach the nose and finally reach it, whereas a person with posterior column ataxia passes beyond it. Cerebellar dyssynergia is particularly well displayed in the cerebellar gait which is frequently described as ataxic. It is performed with a wide base, the trunk and head held stiffly, while the legs shoot out from the hips, the arms flung about without relation to movement of the legs and with considerable lurching and reeling.

Cerebellar disease is characterized also by *tremor*. This tremor is present on voluntary movement of the limb (intention tremor) and is not present with the limb at rest. It is a coarse tremor of wide amplitude and tends to increase in degree as the limb approaches the goal of its movement. It is seen best in the arm movements.

Many cases of acute cerebellar disease develop *hypotonia* of the muscles and hypermotility at the joints. This is not present in most chronic cases. Some regard the atony or hypotonia as the characteristic feature of cerebellar disease. The cerebellar *speech* is at first slow and hesitant, but later becomes completely dysarthric, due probably to an asynergia of the musculature of the pharynx and larynx. Speech disturbances appear early in cerebellar disease and are often so slight as to be missed even by intelligent patients. A slight slowness and dragging of speech characterizes the early stages of the difficulty, described often as a scanning type of speech.

Cerebellar symptoms when pronounced are easily recognized, but require experience to evaluate in minor degrees. They may be recognized by the presence of asynergia by means of tests mentioned in an earlier section, by the typical gait, and by the tremor, speech, and tonus disturbances. In pronounced cases all these features will be present. In others, only severe tremor may be found with little or no asynergia; in still others, asynergia of only a slight degree may be found in a single limb or involving only the trunk. It is essential to recognize the fact that cerebellar symptoms and signs may involve the trunk without involvement of the limbs and that the opposite condition may exist. Thus, there may be severe disturbance of gait due to cerebellar dysfunction with no evidence of limb involvement as revealed by the pronation-supination test, the patting test, or by heel-knee, heel-toe, or finger-nose performances. It is generally agreed that localization of some sort exists within the cerebellum and that disturbances of truncal coördination are associated with vermis lesions, while those of the limbs are accompanied by lesions of the cerebellar hemispheres.

Efforts to localize arm movements as distinct from those of the leg in each cerebellar hemisphere have not suc-

Generally speaking, the symptoms of cerebellar disease are the same regardless of the point of interruption of the cerebellar pathways. They are the same in disease of the spinocerebellar paths, in cerebellar involvement, and with lesions of the cerebellar peduncles.

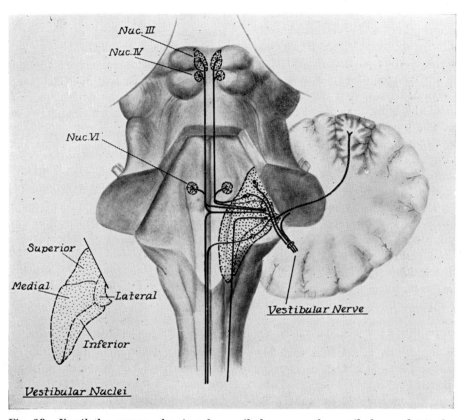

Fig. 38—*Vestibular system*, showing the vestibular nerve, the vestibular nuclei in the medulla and their connections in the brain stem.

ceeded, and some maintain that the only localization possible in the cerebellum is that of ipsilateral control of the corresponding limbs by each cerebellar hemisphere. Other evidence indicates that the lateral lobes of the cerebellum control finger and hand and to a lesser extent arm and leg motions, while the midline structures (vermis) are related to the trunk muscles.

Syndrome of the Vestibular System: Disturbances of the vestibular system may result from lesions in the labyrinths, the vestibular nerve, the vestibular pathways within the brain stem, the cerebrum, or cerebellum. The anatomy of the vestibular fibers is complex. In general, fibers pass from the labyrinth to the vestibular nerve which forms part of the auditory nerve, and are distributed to the vestibular nuclei in the medulla. From this point fibers are fed to the cerebellum, the posterior longitudinal bundle, and the spinal cord. Connections are reported also with the posterior columns and the cerebrum. Hence, the symptoms resulting from vestibular system involvement may be evoked from quite a wide area.

Interruption of the vestibular system results in the production of *vertigo,* a purely subjective sensation characterized by a disturbance of equilibrium resulting from a movement or sense of movement of the individual or his surroundings. The specific features of the types of vertigo associated with lesions in the labyrinth, brain stem, and elsewhere will be considered later (*v.* Vertigo).

Another feature of vestibular disease is *nystagmus,* which is a to-and-fro movement of the eyeballs. It may be horizontal, rotary, or vertical. True *horizontal nystagmus* is elicited by having the patient look to the right or left, the resulting movement of the eyeballs being characterized by a fast movement to the deviated side and a slow movement of the eyeballs back to the neutral position. Such nystagmus is referred to as nystagmus to the right or left, depending on whether it is elicited by deviation of the eyeballs to one side or the other. True nystagmus must be sustained and must have both a fast and slow component. Nystagmoid jerks of the eyeballs are frequently seen, consisting of a few unsustained oscillating jerks on extreme deviation of the eyes. A rotary motion is often seen in nystagmus, especially in lesions involving the labyrinth. *Vertical nystagmus* is seen at times on upward movement of the eyeballs and is a pure up-and-down movement without a rotary component. Oscillating types of nystagmus with equal components and without

fast and slow movements are found in albinos, spasmus nutans, in congenital conditions, in miners, etc.

VI. LESIONS INVOLVING SUPERFICIAL SENSATION

Deep sensation has already been dealt with. It remains to consider the disturbances of superficial sensation occurring at various levels of the nervous system. These may involve: (1) spinal roots; (2) peripheral nerve; (3) spinal cord (commissure, tract, hemisection and complete transverse syndromes); (4) brain stem; (5) thalamus, and (6) cerebral cortex.

1. Root Syndrome

The posterior roots entering the spinal cord may be involved in a variety of diseases, such as tabes dorsalis, herpes zoster, spinal cord tumor, metastatic carcinoma, pachymeningitis, tuberculosis of the spine, and a host of other conditions. The posterior root syndrome is characterized by (a) *pain.* The pain of this syndrome is referred along the specific roots shown in the chart. It is constant or intermittent and usually increased on coughing, straining, sneezing, or any mechanism which increases intraspinal pressure. The characteristics of root pain are variable and difficult to categorize. In characteristic cases the pain is intermittent, radiating along the root or roots affected. It may be a spot pain. In many cases, however, it is constant. It is always severe and variously described. The increase of the pain by any maneuver which increases intraspinal pressure (coughing, sneezing, straining, etc.) is an important feature of root pain and probably results from sudden distention with spinal fluid of the subarachnoid sheath surrounding the root, with irritation or compression of the affected root

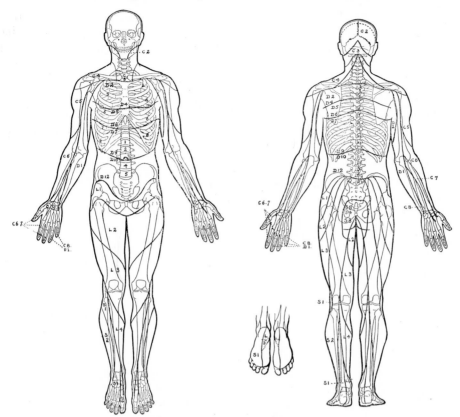

Fig. 39—*Root sensory skin innervation.* A diagrammatic view of the skin areas innervated by the posterior roots.

by the sudden wave of fluid caused by coughing or sneezing. The history of excruciating pain in root syndromes due to increasing intraspinal pressure is characteristic. In cases of acute radiculitis of inflammatory origin the pain at such times is unbearable. A similar history may be obtained in some cases of neuritis but in such instances there is not only neuritis but an associated radiculitis as well. After a diagnosis of root pain is made, careful search must follow for cause of the syndrome. (b) *Sensory disturbances* in the root distribution. These may be in the nature of hyperesthesia in irritative lesions, or there may be loss of superficial sensation (touch, pain, temperature) in the root area. Due to the fact that there is much overlapping of adjacent roots it is often difficult to map out sensory defects in root disturbances unless they are multiple.

2. Peripheral Nerve Syndrome

The full syndrome has been discussed under the section of the lower motor neuron. The sensory disturbances of the peripheral nerve are characterized by: (1) Complete loss of all forms of sensation (touch, pain, heat, cold, position, vibration) in complete interruption of the nerve; (2) partial loss of sensation in incomplete lesions. These sensory disturbances are found over the distribution of the peripheral nerve which differs from that of the roots.

3. Spinal Cord Syndrome

(a) **Commissural Syndrome:** This is the result of a lesion involving the central gray matter of the spinal cord. It is found particularly in syringomyelia, but may be found also in trauma (hematomyelia), syphilis, spinal cord tumor, and other conditions. It is characterized by a *loss of pain and temperature sen-*

sation due to the interruption of these fibers as they cross over from the spinothalamic tract. The sensory loss is bilateral, since fibers from both sides must inevitably be interrupted in such a lesion, and the deficit is segmental, involving only the fibers of the segments involved. Thus, a lesion involving the central gray matter of segments T_2 to

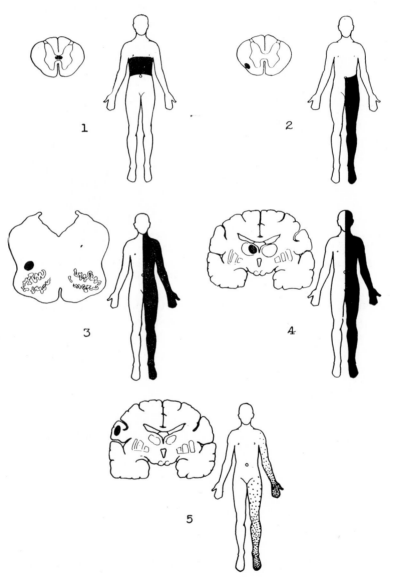

Fig. 40—*Sensory disturbance patterns.* 1. Commissural. 2. Spinothalamic tract in cord. 3. Spinothalamic tract in medulla. 4. Thalamus. 5. Sensory cortex.

T_5 will produce loss of pain and temperature sensation only in these segments. The commissural syndrome can be produced only by a lesion within the cord substance. It is anatomically impossible for an extramedullary lesion to produce the syndrome. Syringomyelia, syphilitic meningomyelitis, hematomyelia, intramedullary tumor of the spinal cord, and spinal cord concussion are all capable of producing a commissural syndrome.

the lesion. Pain and temperature sensations may not be involved with equal severity; one, usually pain, may be affected more than the other. Both intramedullary and extramedullary processes may be responsible for the condition. Intramedullary tumors, myelitis from various causes, hematomyelia, tuberculoma, and multiple sclerosis are among the intramedullary conditions which may give rise to the syndrome. The fibers

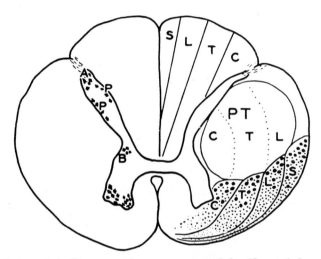

Fig. 41—*Spinal cord.* A diagrammatic arrangement of the fibers of the spinothalamic tract is clearly shown, the sacral fibers being at the outer edge. (After Walker.)

Ipsilateral impairment of pain and temperature may be found with involvement of the pain and temperature fibers in the posterior horn before they decussate in the commissure. This is usually the result of a slitlike syringomyelic cavity, and the resulting sensory disturbance may extend for a variable number of segments.

(b) Spinothalamic Tract Lesion: A lesion involving the spinothalamic tract in the anterolateral portion of the spinal cord causes a *loss of pain and temperature sensations* on the opposite side of the body, since this tract conveys only pain and temperature, and will involve all the segments below the level of

within the spinothalamic tract are arranged in laminar fashion in such a way that the sacral fibers are located at the periphery, while the fibers from higher levels are located more centrally. Hence, an intramedullary process will involve the fibers from the higher levels first and will often spare the sacral fibers. This is referred to as sacral sparing and is found with intramedullary processes. On the other hand, extramedullary processes, compressing the cord from without, results in involvement of the sacral fibers as well as those from higher levels. Extramedullary tumors are capable of producing a spinothalamic tract syndrome.

(c) Brown-Séquard Syndrome: This is seen in its purest form in a hemisection of the spinal cord. It causes:

On the Side of the Lesion: Paralysis; loss of position and vibration senses, and ataxia.

On the Side Opposite the Lesion: Loss of pain and temperature senses.

top of the level, especially in extramedullary spinal cord tumors.

(3) *Sphincter Disturbances:* There is first retention of urine in acute cases, which later develops into automatic emptying of the bladder in the course of a few days

Table 11—Causes of Root Syndrome

Infections	Compressions	Bony Deformities
Foci of infection	Extramedullary tumor	Osteoarthritis
Syphilis (*tabes, meningomyelitis*)	Intramedullary tumor (much less frequently)	Tuberculosis of spine
		Fracture of vertebrae
Pachymeningitis (*syphilitic, tuberculous*)	Metastatic carcinoma	Spondylitis ankylopoietica
	Extradural abscess	Metastatic carcinoma
	Herniated nucleus pulposus	Bone tumors
Herpes zoster		

This syndrome is not usually seen in its complete form. It is found in infiltrating tumors of the spinal cord, trauma, etc., but it may be produced also by extramedullary processes such as tumor. It is more commonly seen in incomplete or impure forms, usually as loss of pain and temperature senses on the opposite side of the body below the level of the lesion, with few evidences of ipsilateral signs.

(d) Complete Transverse Syndrome: This syndrome is of great importance and should be clearly recognized. It is found in many sorts of conditions too numerous to mention. Among them are trauma, spinal cord tumor, metastatic tumor, spinal cord syphilis, multiple sclerosis, disseminated myelitis, etc. It is characterized by:

(1) *Motor paralysis* below the level of the lesion.

(2) *Sensory paralysis* manifested as a complete loss of all forms of sensation below the level of the lesion. In some instances there is a zone of hyperesthesia at the

or weeks. Rectal incontinence is found in complete interruptions.

(4) *Trophic Disturbances:* These are manifested by trophic ulcers of the skin, trophic disturbances in the nails, etc.

The manifestations of transverse lesions of the spinal cord vary with the rapidity of development of the process. In acutely developing transverse sections as seen in spinal cord injuries, metastatic carcinoma, myelitis, etc., the manifestations are those of "spinal shock." The paralyzed muscles are toneless and flaccid, the superficial and tendon reflexes are absent, there is complete sensory loss below the level of the lesion, and retention of urine and feces. This stage may last three weeks or longer, and then pass into a second phase of reflex activity. This is manifested by a return of flexor responses characterized by flexion reflexes in response to noxious stimuli applied to the skin. A "mass reflex" is obtained often when the flexion reflexes are evoked with ease. This is characterized by flexor spasm of the legs and lower abdominal wall, evacuation of the bladder, and sweating. The tendon reflexes return during this stage. In the final stages the reflexes are again lost, the bladder and rectum empty imperfectly, bedsores develop, and death ensues. The return of bladder and rectal functions will be considered in a subsequent section.

With gradual interruption of the spinal cord, on the other hand, spinal shock is not encountered. The legs become weak and spastic, and eventually paralyzed if the process is not relieved. Flaccidity of the muscles is not found, as in the case of "spinal shock." Motor weakness usually develops before sensory paralysis in cases due to compression from without, as in extramedullary tumors, since the motor fibers appear more susceptible to injury than the sensory fibers. Gradually, however, sensory paralysis develops and with it an impairment or loss of sphincter control. The final result is a transverse syndrome

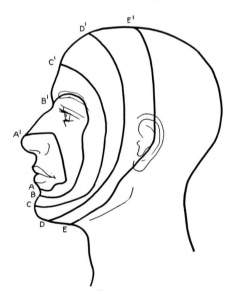

Fig. 42—*Trigeminal nerve*, showing the type of onion-peel sensory loss (pain and temperature) found in lesions within the brain stem affecting the descending root of the trigeminal nerve.

which in this instance is characterized by spastic paraplegia, sensory and sphincter loss.

Complete transverse syndromes indicate naturally a complete interruption of the motor and sensory pathways in the spinal cord. They require investigation concerning cause in every instance. The rapidity and completeness of onset give important clues concerning the etiology. In trauma the onset is immediate due to crushing of the cord. In metastatic carcinoma it is rapid and often apoplectic, usually preceded by pain. In spinal cord tumor (extramedullary) it is gradual and usually associated with root pain. In hematomyelia it is often insidious and usually painless, etc.

(e) Thalamic Syndrome: The thalamus is the end station of all forms of sensation. A complete lesion of the thalamus will cause: (1) loss of all forms of sensation involving the entire opposite side of the face, trunk, and limbs; (2) astereognosis; (3) central pains characterized by their deep, paroxysmal, excruciating nature. Partial syndromes of a hemisensory nature have been described.

(f) Cortical Syndrome: Sensory disturbances due to the involvement of the sensory parietal cortex are not as clearly defined as in lesions involving lower levels. Deep sensation (position and vibration) is more severely affected than is superficial sensation (touch, pain, temperature). They are characterized by: (1) Loss of position and vibration senses, though some deny the involvement of vibration sense. Position sense is consistently lost, while vibration sense may or may not be involved. Some investigators deny the involvement of vibration sense in lesions confined to the sensory cortex. (2) Absence of involvement of other forms of sensation, such as pain, touch, and temperature. Superficial sensation is not usually affected in lesions of the sensory cortex. Pain sensation may be decreased and is apt to be more severe in distal portions of the limbs. Touch, heat and cold are not usually affected. Pain may develop as a result of lesions of the sensory cortex and has been reported in tumors and cysts of this area. (3) Impairment of discrimination as, for example, detecting the two points of a compass, appreciating differences in texture, recognizing figures written on the skin, and appreciating differences in weight. These are the elements most severely affected in cortical lesions, for they represent a deficit of the sensory cortical function, namely, the appreciation of differences in texture, weight, and spatial differences. (4) Astereognosis, or the inability to recognize the shape or nature of objects placed in the hand, is found in lesions of the parietal lobe. The problem of astereognosis is complex, and much remains to be elucidated. Stereognosis is the ability to recognize the size, shape, weight, and other physical characteristics of objects. It is often referred to as "tactile agnosia." It is regarded by some as dependent on sensory disturbances, of which two-point discrimination appears to be the critical faculty involved (Dejerine, Campora, and Nielsen). The disturbance of deep sensation appears not to be essential, and loss of position sense is regarded as unimportant. This fails to explain adequately the cases of astereognosis in lesions of the thalamus and in the foramen-magnum tumors with disturbances of position sense. Others believe that it is not possible to speak of astereognosis unless there is intact sensation.

The precise localization of stereognostic perception is not known. "Ablation studies in trained monkeys and chimpanzees indicate that lesions of the postcentral convolutions (Areas 3, 1, 2) or the posterior parietal lobule (Areas 5 and 7) separately reduce only transiently the ability to discriminate fair differences in weight; yet total parietal lobectomy is followed, in both forms, by a permanent defect. Thus, in the monkey and chimpanzee, there is no focal representation of such functions *within* the parietal region, which is nevertheless the main area of representation of these functions. Comparable studies indicate that these functions are not focally localized in the human cortex" (Fulton).

Stereognostic perception appears, therefore, not to be focally localized in a specific portion of the parietal lobe but is dependent on the postcentral gyrus and the posterior parietal lobule.

(5) Sensory jacksonian seizures (*v.* Epilepsy).

The cortical sensory syndrome is due to a lesion of the postcentral gyrus of the side opposite to the disturbances of sensation.

VII. LESIONS OF SPHINCTERS

Loss of sphincter control occurs under many circumstances in the human, but the problem is complex and a review of the normal control of the sphincters is therefore pertinent. Disturbances of micturition are of greater practical significance than those of the bowel, and are also much more frequent.

Bladder: The bladder empties by means of a reciprocal action of its involuntary musculature, the detrusor, and the internal sphincter. These receive their innervation through the hypogastric ($T_{11, 12}$ and L_1) and sacral nerves, the former derived from the lumbar sympathetic chain, the latter from the sacral plexus by the pelvic nerves ($S_{2, 3, 4}$). The external sphincter and the voluntary muscles of the perineum are innervated by the pudendal nerves ($S_{2, 3, 4}$). The parasympathetic center for micturition in the spinal cord is in segments S_2 and S_3, the sympathetic center lying in the lumbar cord.

Stimulation of the peripheral segment of the cut pelvic nerves in animals causes powerful contraction of the detrusor muscle with relaxation of the internal sphincter. Stimulation of the hypogastric nerves for section of these nerves causes a profound depression of micturition with an atonic distended bladder. Section of the hypogastric, pelvic, and pudendal nerves is followed, after a short period of re-

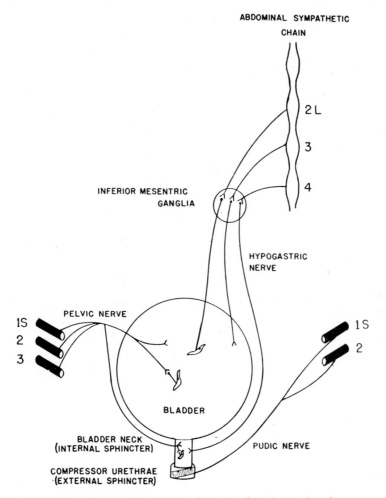

ABDOMINAL SYMPATHETIC
CHAIN

2 L

3

4

INFERIOR MESENTRIC
GANGLIA

HYPOGASTRIC
NERVE

PELVIC NERVE

1 S

2

3

1 S

2

BLADDER

BLADDER NECK
(INTERNAL SPHINCTER)

PUDIC NERVE

COMPRESSOR URETHRAE
(EXTERNAL SPHINCTER)

Fig. 43—*Innervation of bladder*, showing the central and peripheral innervations of the detrusor, and the internal and external sphincters. (*Learmonth, McLeod: Physiology in Modern Medicine*, 9th ed., p. 1128, C. V. Mosby Co., St. Louis.)

causes contraction of the internal sphincter in animals and man, accompanied by inhibition of action of the detrusor. Stimulation of the pudendal nerve causes contraction of the external sphincter. The integrity of the pelvic nerves is of paramount importance for normal micturition (Denny-Brown and Robertson), tention, by periodic discharge or "automatic micturition."

Control of the bladder musculature for the reflex act of micturition is effected by cerebral mechanisms as well as by those at the spinal cord level. Tonic control of the bladder musculature is carried out by both cerebral hemispheres, particularly by the motor cortex acting on centers in the hindbrain which in turn control the tone of the bladder (Langworthy). The cerebral control of the bladder seems to be inhibitory in function since removal of the motor cortex in animals either unilaterally or bilaterally results in overaction of the reflex of micturition. Stimulation of this area results in bladder contraction and emptying of its contents. The cortical area responsible for bladder control lies near the leg area of the motor cortex.

The normal act of micturition is dependent on a stretch reflex acting on the detrusor muscle, the normal stimulus being the stretch evoked by the volume of the contents of the bladder and by the rising intravesical pressure associated with the accumulation of urine. As a result of this stretch reflex the detrusor contracts and the sphincters relax. The internal sphincter reacts reciprocally with the detrusor and is not under separate control. The external sphincter opens later and is not under voluntary control. As a result of distention of the bladder, afferent impulses reach the spinal cord, the detrusor contracts as the result of impulses conveyed through the pelvic nerves, and reciprocal relaxation of the sphincter follows.

Types of Bladder Disturbance: Two main types are found in the human, the *atonic* and the *hypertonic* bladder. The unfortunate term "neurogenic," or cord bladder, has arisen to designate bladder disturbances of peripheral or central nervous system origin. The term is meaningless and wherever possible the precise form of bladder dysfunction should be designated. The *atonic* bladder is found particularly in lesions of the sacral segments of the spinal cord (conus medullaris) and in diseases of the cauda equina and pelvic nerves. It is characterized by an atonic bladder musculature due to loss of tone of the detrusor muscle, an in-

creased capacity of the bladder, and a loss of sensation associated with bladder distention, so that the patient is unable to tell when the bladder is full. The bladder under such circumstances may reach a very large size and may reach to the umbilicus without a sensation of distention. Destructive lesions of the sacral cord or its roots is followed, therefore, by retention of urine with distention of the bladder. This is followed by automatic emptying of the bladder which, however, never empties completely, leaving a residual of urine in the bladder. Urine in such cases is discharged in small amounts at a time but in some instances complete emptying may occur. The cystometrogram in such cases reveals an increased bladder capacity, a very slow rise in the vesical pressure during filling, and the ability to retain a large amount of fluid before sufficient stretch is produced to cause a reflex contraction of the bladder.

An atonic bladder response is found also in lesions involving the posterior roots of the spinal cord or with involvement of the posterior columns. This is seen most strikingly in tabes dorsalis, but it may develop in any condition involving the posterior roots. In this form of atonic bladder, also, the bladder capacity is greatly increased, there is no sensation of distention of the bladder, the detrusor tone is lost, and there is bladder incontinence, due to relaxation of the internal sphincter. Emptying the bladder is possible by normal volition, but the stream is feeble, residual urine is always found, and incontinence is present, due to impaired action of the detrusor. In advanced instances incontinence is severe.

The atonic bladder results essentially from interruption of the afferent and/or efferent peripheral pathways to the bladder. In contrast to it is the *hypertonic* bladder, which results from interruption of the central pathways. This may result from lesions of the spinal cord, usually transverse lesions, anywhere above the sacral segments, or from involvement of the motor cortex, or the pyramidal tract in the internal capsule, or elsewhere along its course. In lesions of the spinal cord above the sacral segments, the bladder

A similar type of bladder reaction is found in cerebral lesions or in pyramidal tract involvement in the brain or brain stem. In the completely transected spinal cord above the sacral segments there may be established an *automatic bladder*. Following the stage of paralysis and distention of the bladder there develops

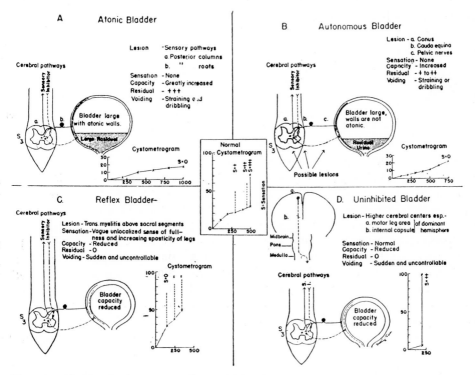

Fig. 44—*Bladder dysfunction* as illustrated by the various mechanisms which produce the several types of bladder disorder. (*White and Smithwick: Macmillan Co., N.Y., 2nd Edition.*)

capacity is reduced in contrast to the distended bladder of the atonic state. The vesical pressure rises rapidly during filling, so that relatively little urine can collect before the desire for micturition develops. Unlike the atonic bladder, sensation is not lost and bladder distention is associated with a feeling of discomfort. The bladder is emptied completely with each act of urination, and a good deal of force. The desire to micturate is uncontrollable and has to be attended to as soon as it is felt.

automatic contraction of the bladder wall with expulsion of urine but without complete emptying of the bladder. At times the automatic emptying is part of the mass reflex already described. Automatic bladder function may develop in four to five weeks after cord transection, or it may not develop at all. In many instances it fails to develop, a fact which must be given due consideration in the treatment of transverse cord lesions (*v.* Spinal Cord Injuries).

The atonic bladder may be found in

tumors of the cauda equina, or conus medullaris, in tabes dorsalis, in destructive lesions of the sacral segments of the spinal cord due to injury, multiple sclerosis, and myelitis from various causes. The hypertonic bladder is found in transverse lesions of the spinal cord, the causes of which are numerous (*v.* Transverse Syndrome), or in vascular disease of the brain, in brain tumor, and in other diseases which may affect the pyramidal tract in the brain or brain stem.

Rectum: The normal act of defecation is characterized by contraction of the rectum and reciprocal relaxation of the anal sphincter. The adequate stimulus is tension on the wall of the rectum which brings about a stretch reflex and contraction of the rectum. Active tension is more powerful than passive tension as a stimulus. The reciprocal relationship between rectum and internal sphincter is nervous in mechanism and is mediated solely through the lower sacral segments of the spinal cord ($S_{2, 3, 4}$) and its peripheral plexuses. Destruction of the sacral segments of the spinal cord or its roots results in a relaxed sphincter and continuous bowel evacuation, whereas destruction of the cord above the sacral segments causes intermittent involuntary emptying of the bowel.

VIII. LESIONS INVOLVING THE VISUAL SYSTEM

It is of great importance that lesions of the visual system be recognized for purposes of diagnosis, since many a case with visual field defects remains unrecognized for long periods of time. The pupillary and optic nerve changes will be discussed under the section on cranial nerves. Attention will be called here to disturbances in the fields of vision.

The visual fibers are distributed in orderly arrangement throughout their course. Impulses are brought to the retina from the visual field. Stimuli from the temporal field are brought to the nasal side of the retina, those from the nasal field to the temporal side. Stimuli from the upper portion of the visual field fall on the lower part of the retina, those from the lower portions on the upper part of the retina. Fibers from the temporal side of the retina (nasal field) pass through the nerve and optic chiasm uncrossed, while those from the nasal side (temporal field) cross through the chiasm. They continue to the primary optic centers, the external geniculate bodies. Thence they continue as the optic radiation, hooking around the inferior horn of the lateral ventricle as the geniculocalcarine radiation. Here the fibers are closely packed together, passing through the temporal and occipital lobes, fanning out more and more as they proceed to their final end stations in the calcarine cortex of the occipital lobe, which has an upper and lower lip. Fibers from the upper half of the retina (lower half of visual field) are distributed to the upper calcarine lip; those from the lower half of the retina (upper half of the visual field) to the lower calcarine lip.

The form of the visual fields is flattened above and restricted medially by the bony ridges of the orbit and the bridge of the nose. Hence it is not a complete circle. Its form is affected also by the width of the palpebral fissure, the size of the pupil, and the visual acuity.

The visual fields are composed of binocular and monocular portions, due to the position of the eyes in the head and the overlapping of the fields of vision. The binocular portions extend out to 60° of the visual field. In each visual field on the temporal side (60-90°) is a portion known as the temporal crescent which is concerned with monocular vision.

Experimental and clinical studies reveal the fact that the retina is projected

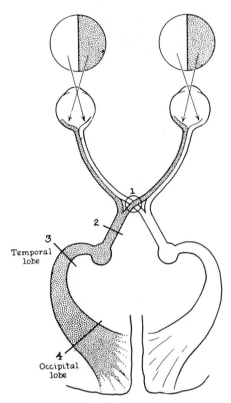

Fig. 45—*Visual fields* indicating the origin and destination of the visual pathways showing the crossed and uncrossed fibers. Lesions at 1 produce bitemporal hemianopia. Lesions at 2, 3 and 4 produce homonymous hemianopia. Lesions at 2 and 3 are more apt to produce field cuts with involvement of the fixation points.

through the tract, the primary visual centers, the radiation, and the cerebral cortex in an orderly fashion. Fibers from the upper part of the retina lie in the upper part of the optic nerve and chiasm, those from the lower retina in the lower part of the optic nerve and chiasm. The papillomacular bundle which runs from the macular region to the external geniculate body and is projected from there to the cortex lies roughly in the center of the optic nerve and chiasm and is widely distributed in the external geniculate body. In the optic chiasm the ratio of crossed to uncrossed fibers is 3:2.

The visual fibers are projected on to the striate area in the occipital lobe (Area 17, Figure 33). The macula is projected on to the tip of the occipital lobe, hence a lesion here will cause loss of central vision. Because of the frequent escape of central vision in complete hemianopsias it has been assumed that there is a bilateral representation of the macula in the striate area. Final proof for this is lacking, but the evidence supports this contention. It is believed by some that macular fibers cross in the splenium of the corpus collosum. Others assume a diffuse representation of the macula in the striate area.

Visual Field Syndromes

(a) **Altitudinal Anopsia:** This is a rare visual field defect, characterized by a loss of vision in the upper or lower halves of the visual fields. It is due to a lesion just anterior to the optic chiasm with pressure on the upper or under surfaces of the optic nerves.

(b) **Bitemporal Hemianopsia:** This common field defect results from compression or destruction of the crossed visual nerve fibers in the center of the optic chiasm coming from the nasal sides of the visual fields. It is characterized by a loss of vision in the temporal sides of the fields of vision, the loss usually extending cleanly through the fixation point, but often with sparing of central vision. Subjectively, it is noticed on the patient's part by a difficulty in seeing out of the corners of the eyes, and a tendency to bump into objects on the side. It is caused by lesions at the optic chiasm, chief among which are intrasellar tumors (pituitary adenomas). suprasellar lesions, such as meningiomas, hypophyseal stalk tumors, adenomas, arachnoiditis, aneurysm, etc. It may occasionally be caused by a tumor or aneurysm lying at the side of the sella turcica (parasellar) and compressing the optic chiasm.

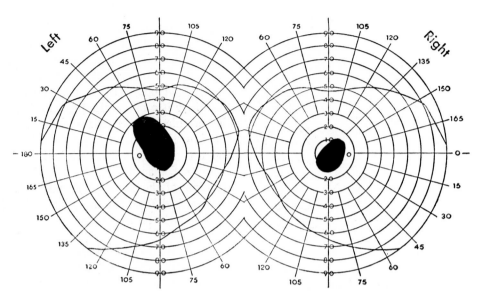

Fig. 46—*Central scotomas* in a case of multiple sclerosis, with greatly reduced
central vision.

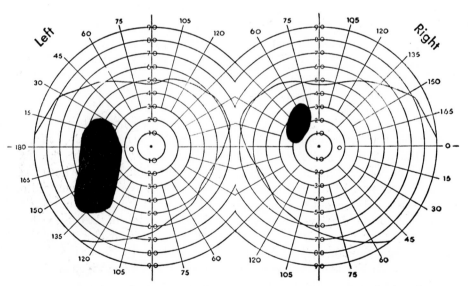

Fig. 47—*Paracentral scotomas* in both visual fields in a case of multiple sclerosis.

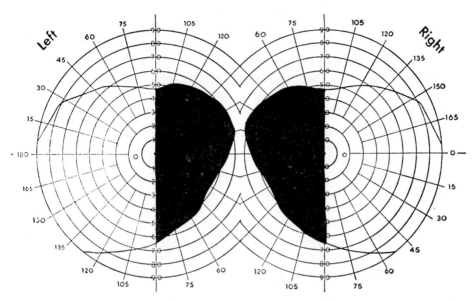

Fig. 48—*Binasal hemianopsia*, a rare form of visual field defect, in this case due to interruption of the fibers from the temporal sides of the retina by compression from sclerosed internal carotid arteries.

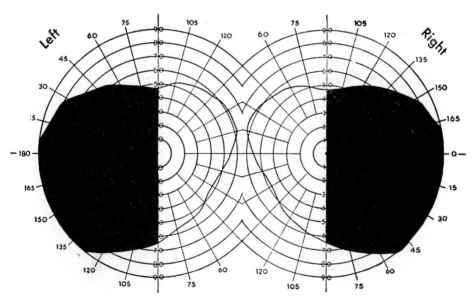

Fig. 49—*Bitemporal hemianopsia* in semidiagrammatic form, due to compression of the optic chiasm by a pituitary tumor.

(c) Homonymous Hemianopsia: This visual defect is also commonly encountered. It consists of a loss of vision in the temporal field of one eye and the nasal field of the other due to the fact that the optic tract and radiation beyond the optic chiasm contain fibers from the temporal retina (nasal field) of one eye and the nasal retina (temporal field) of the other. Homonymous hemianopsias are always referred to as left or right, and always indicate a lesion of the opposite side of the brain.

A homonymous hemianopsia occurs always in lesions of the optic tract and radiation, anywhere along the tract or radiation. Since the tract and radiation extend from the chiasm to the calcarine cortex, a homonymous hemianopsia indicates a lesion anywhere along this course which includes the tract at the base of the brain and the radiation in the temporal or occipital lobes. Chance favors the involvement of the temporal or occipital lobes, but tract involvement is not uncommon. Homonymous hemianopsia in itself has no localizing value except to

indicate involvement of the opposite tract or radiation, decision as to temporal occipital, or parasellar involvement depending upon the presence of other symptoms. Differences in the configuration of the visual fields have been used in order to indicate precise localization, but these have only very limited value. Thus homonymous field defects through the fixation point are said to indicate temporal lobe lesions since the fibers are closely packed together here, while defects with sparing of the fixation point are more likely to be due to occipital lesions. Though this is true to a limited degree it is not constant. Defects with involvement of central vision occur often in occipital lobe lesions, and sparing of central vision is not uncommon with temporal lobe lesions. It is usually asserted that a lesion of the optic tract can be differentiated from one involving the optic radiation by the following features: (1) A tract lesion tends to be incongruous, one field being affected more than the other. This is not constant, but it is true that a tract lesion is more likely if

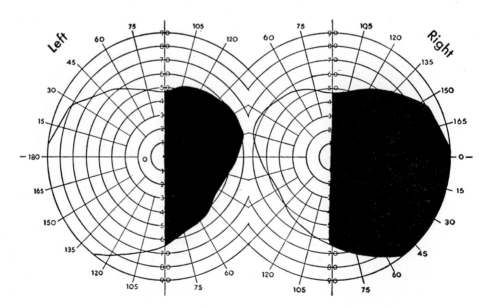

Fig. 50—*Homonymous hemianopsia* (right), due to interruption of the visual pathways in the left temporal lobe in a case of brain tumor.

OS   OD

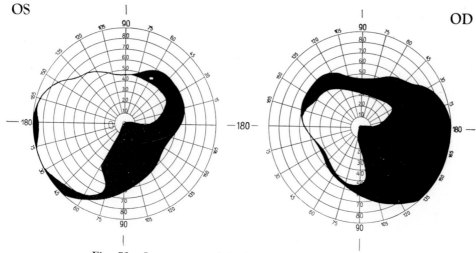

Fig. 51—*Incongruous right homonymous hemianopsia.*

the fields are incongruous. (2) The macular fibers are affected, but as has been pointed out, this may occur in lesions of the radiation if the lesion is large enough.

Under some circumstances only parts of homonymous visual fields are affected. Thus, a quadrantic field defect involving either the upper or lower homonymous quadrants sometimes is seen, and is referred to as superior or inferior quadrant anopsia. These are more likely to be found in lesions involving the temporal lobe but may occur anywhere along the tract or radiation.

Homonymous hemianopsia results from a variety of conditions such as vascular lesions, tumors, multiple sclerosis, aneurysm, etc.

IX. LESIONS OF THE CEREBRAL HEMISPHERES

Lesions within the cerebral hemispheres produce symptoms of various sorts depending upon the area affected. Some of these symptoms have already been considered (hemianopsia), and others will be discussed in subsequent sections (frontal lobe syndromes, jacksonian epilepsy). Here it remains to consider the problem of aphasia in relation to diagnosis.

1. Aphasia

Aphasia is a loss or impairment of speech due to lesions involving specific portions of the brain. It has great localization value in diagnosis, and if care is taken in examination it can be detected even by the inexperienced. The localization of the speech processes which will be mentioned shortly is structurally speaking true, but it cannot be too strictly insisted upon. Aphasia is a true speech loss and must be distinguished from a *dysarthria* which consists only of an indistinctness in enunciation of words due to interference with the peripheral speech mechanism (pharynx, larynx, etc.), as, for example, paralysis of the palate in bulbar paralysis resulting in a nasal speech due to palatal immobility, or indistinctness of speech due to weakness or paralysis of the tongue in hemiplegia, progressive muscular atrophy, amyotrophic lateral sclerosis, etc.

Normal speech depends upon various factors. It depends upon intact sensory perception (hearing and vision) and on sound vocal apparatus (muscles of pharynx, larynx, etc.). In the presence of disturbances in one or another of these spheres, speech disturbances will develop in the growing child.

(a) Tests for Aphasia: If care is taken to examine for aphasia, this type of speech defect can be picked out even by the inexperienced. The difficulty lies in the much-too-haphazard fashion in which aphasic disturbances are tested; a few objects shown to the patient hastily and a quick demand for a reply constitute the usual bedside examination of the aphasic patient. A few carefully chosen tests properly used will give a good deal of information and will not consume too much time. These are as follows:

Spontaneous Speech: If the aphasic patient can be made to speak, he will thereby produce the most valuable data of all aphasic tests. More can be learned from the spontaneous utterances than from any formal tests: Hesitancies in speech, misuse of words, substitution of words, "word hash," etc., are all apparent in the spontaneous speech. It is often difficult and even impossible to get an aphasic patient to speak spontaneously. The expressive aphasic is loathe to do so because he lacks words, while the auditory-receptive case is unable to understand one's requests. Despite this, persistence in an effort to produce spontaneous utterances by the patient will yield rich dividends and will enable the examiner to determine whether words are lost or mispronounced, whether word substitutions are made, whether consecutive ideas can be expressed, whether there is complete inability to use words, and what emotional reactions are associated with the effort to express oneself.

Auditory Receptive Tests: The understanding of the spoken word can be elicited by various simple tests. It can be done adequately in two ways: (a) By requesting the patient to follow simple commands (put out your tongue, close your eyes, etc.) and by gradually increasing the complexity of the commands until the patient is dealing with two or more

orders (close your eyes and open your mouth; or open your mouth, raise your hand and close one eye, etc.). By means of these simple tests one can learn much about the ability of the patient to understand the spoken word. (b) By lining up a number of objects which can be produced from any pocket (matches, coin, knife, key, etc.) and by specific commands determining whether the patient understands commands (show me the key, show me the coin, etc.).

Visual Receptive Tests: These can be carried out at the bedside by asking the patient to read from a paper or magazine and to interpret what has been read. It should be noted whether there is a loss of the ability to read words or whether there is only a mispronunciation of the words read. If the capacity to read is lost, it should be noted whether there is loss of recognition of letters or words, and whether the understanding of words as symbols is impaired or lost.

Writing Test: This is performed easily by asking the patient to write some spontaneous thought and also to write to dictation.

These are only a few of the available tests but they are sufficient for the bedside examination of the aphasic patient. More extensive and elaborate tests are of little clinical value but are, of course, essential for investigative purposes.

Aphasia may be grouped in the following main forms: (1) expressive (motor) aphasia; (2) receptive (sensory) aphasia; (3) expressive-receptive aphasia; (4) amnesic aphasia.

Any classification is subject to criticism partly because it is difficult to make it all inclusive and partly also because it tends to create strict categories when none such are frequently present. In this connection it is essential to recognize that the various groups listed above refer only to the predominantly affected aspect of speech. It is extremely rare to find a pure form of speech disturbance. Hence an expressive aphasia is characterized only by predominantly expressive deficits, but auditory-receptive elements are always present. The same holds true of auditory-receptive aphasia. Visual-receptive aphasia on the other hand is likely to be found in a pure or almost pure form. At times the predominance of one form of aphasic utterance overshadows only very slightly the other affected form.

(b) Expressive (Motor) Aphasia: This type of aphasia, usually referred to as motor aphasia, is characterized by a loss or impairment of power to express oneself. In a complete case total mutism develops, the patient being unable to find words of any sort, save for a very occasional single word which is usually applied in a meaningless fashion.

In less severe cases, the following features stand out:

(1) An *inability to find words* with which to express one's thoughts. This may consist of an occasional loss of a word, characterized by hesitations in speech, the exact word never being found. In such instances, the lapse may never be filled with the proper word, the patient either passing on after great effort to express himself, or bursting into tears or profanity because of his inability to express himself; or finally he may substitute another word which obviously has no connection with what he is trying to say. It is these cases which have an occasional loss of words which require recognition. In more advanced cases, words are lost in profusion, the patient being unable to find the name of familiar objects, persons, etc. As a rule, the expressive aphasic will recognize his errors and will attempt to make amends by attempting to find the correct word. In this he *fails* and as a result there is sub-

stitution of some other word. In an effort to express his thoughts the patient with expressive aphasia will attempt to form words which sound like those which he is seeking, and for this reason he will make unintelligible words, or he may substitute one letter for another in a word (hatch for catch, boat for coat, etc.). Because of the loss of words, moreover, the expressive aphasic develops at times a telegraphic style of conversation due to the dropping out of words which he cannot find. Furthermore, he uses words erroneously. Thus the language of the expressive aphasic is characterized by *frequent hesitations* in speech and *difficulty in expression*. The changes are characterized largely by breaks in the continuity of expression and of simplification of expression due to a loss of words.

(2) *A Difficulty in Writing:* Writing may be regarded as speech recorded on paper, hence the expressive aphasic will show the same disability in his writing as in his speech, the defect ranging from an occasional loss of words to a complete inability to express himself.

(3) *Retention of understanding* through hearing and vision; hence an understanding of both the spoken and written word. This is true only in a broad sense since pure forms of aphasia of any sort are rare. If examined carefully, cases of expressive aphasia will always demonstrate auditory receptive elements in their speech disturbances, characterized by difficulty in understanding what is said to them.

Expressive aphasia is the result of a lesion in the posterior part of the third frontal (F_3) convolution (Broca's area) on the left side in right-handed people, and on the right side in left-handed people. It has distinct localizing value, therefore, and its recognition is important.

(c) Receptive (Sensory) Aphasia:
In this type of aphasia, there is predominantly a disturbance or loss in the understanding of speech by ear or eye, the patient finding it difficult or impossible to understand the spoken or written word. Specifically, the outstanding features of auditory-receptive aphasia are:

Disturbances in the understanding of spoken language of a greater or lesser degree depending on the degree of destruction of the area affected. Thus, patients with auditory-receptive aphasia find it difficult or impossible to understand what is said to them. This may consist of a slight or moderate loss of understanding of words by ear, or there may be a total lack of understanding, the patient failing to respond at all to auditory stimuli. Frequently, there is some understanding of what is said, even in severe cases. Auditory-receptive aphasia occurs in the majority of instances without involvement of visual speech, but the two may exist together in varying degree. In some cases visual speech is affected almost exclusively.

In visual-receptive aphasia there is a *loss of understanding of the printed word and a failure to comprehend words as symbols.* In such instances, the capacity to identify letters is retained, but their synthesis into and meaning as words is lost. At times even individual letters fail to be recognized. In defects of a less severe degree, there may be recognition of some or most of the words in a sentence but an inability to synthesize the meaning of the sentence. Visual aphasia is practically always associated with a right homonymous hemianopsia (left homonymous hemianopsia for left-handed individuals).

Disturbances in Expression: This is characterized by the mixing of grammatical constructions, the wrong use of words, and the substitution of words and even whole phrases in a meaningless sort of

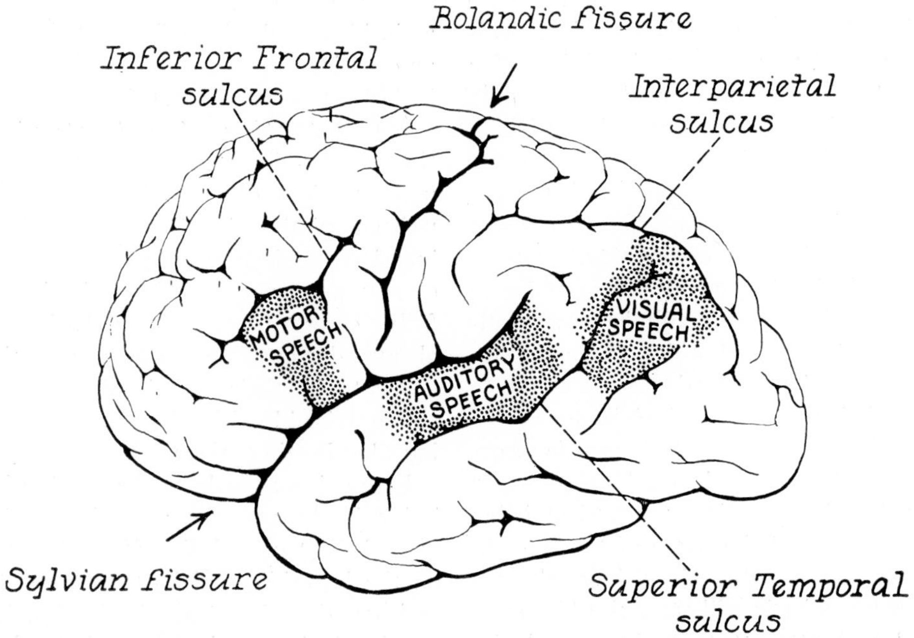

Fig. 52—*Aphasia.* A diagrammatic view of the principal speech areas in the left cerebral hemisphere of a right-handed person. Destruction of the areas indicated is associated with loss of the corresponding speech functions.

jumble. The expressive aphasic, when at a loss for a word, hesitates and fails to produce it; the auditory-receptive-aphasic person on the other hand quickly substitutes another and proceeds as if nothing were awry. Unlike the expressive-aphasic person he is unaware of his errors, largely owing to his lack of understanding of auditory impressions. Paraphrasing is common, and grammatical confusions of all sorts are characteristic. Verbal confu-' sions are common; verbal substitutions occur; whole phrases may be inserted in speech in erroneous fashion. As a result of these expressive disturbances in the auditory-receptive aphasic, speech in severe cases is likely to be more or less of a disjointed and unintelligible hash. However, it should be emphasized that there may be severe disorders of understanding with only slight disturbances in expression. The auditory-receptive-aphasic patient may hesitate for a word which he cannot find, but he quickly jumps to another or to a phrase which has no connection with the sequence of his thoughts. Difficulties in writing are as great as those of speech and are of a similar order. They may even exceed those of speaking. Writing, like speech, is profuse but confused.

Auditory-receptive aphasia results from a lesion in the posterior portion of the first temporal convolution (T_1), on the left side in right-handed persons.

(d) Expressive-Receptive Aphasia: Cases of this group are characterized by a severe loss of both expressive and receptive elements. The expressive loss is usually so great that only a few speech sounds or words remain and the capacity to make even simple sentences is lost. Complete loss of speech is not usually found, a few phrases remaining whereby the patient expresses himself, but not in a meaningful fashion. Writing is affected to the same degree as speaking in most cases but may be relatively much better preserved than motor speech. Understanding of words is greatly limited, even single words or simple phrases failing to be understood.

(e) Amnesic (Nominal) Aphasia: This type of aphasia consists essentially of a difficulty in evoking words as names for objects, conditions, or qualities. This difficulty may be so severe in some patients that speech is greatly limited. In their motor-speech performances, amnesic aphasics are slow and hesitant and in this respect resemble patients with expressive aphasia, but they show no difficulties in articulation. The amnesic-aphasic patient, unable to find the word for an object, hesitates and substitutes slang or colloquial expressions of many sorts. Outstanding in the amnesic defect is the ability of the amnesic-aphasic patient to recognize the word which he himself cannot produce, a characteristic which is not true of the expressive aphasic. Though he recognizes the correct word, and though it is repeated by himself and the examiner often, the amnesic aphasic fails to retain the correct word. The understanding of language is relatively good and reading is fair. On the receptive side, patients with amnesic aphasia are relatively much more normal than on the expressive side. Their understanding of speech and their ability to read is quite good, those defects which are present being only minor in degree.

2. Agnosia

Allied to the problem of aphasia is that of agnosia and apraxia. Agnosia implies the inability to recognize the form or nature of objects. It has been divided into many confusing categories and attempts have been made to find specific localizations for each type. It is probable that the many forms of agnosia described in the medical literature do not in themselves represent separate categories, but they are mentioned here in order to acquaint the student with the many forms described. (1) *Tactile agnosia* consists of an inability to recognize objects by touch and is referred to as astereognosis (p. 108). (2) *Auditory agnosia* refers to an inability to recognize speech sounds. A special form has been described for musical sounds and is characterized by a loss of capacity to recognize tones or melodies (music deafness, or amusia). (3) *Visual agnosia* has been divided into several categories, including an agnosia for objects, pictures, a color agnosia characterized by an inability to understand colors as qualities of objects, faulty color concept, and inability to evoke color images, none of these features being associated with color blindness or inadequate color sense; spatial agnosia featured by an inability to find one's way around familiar places though recognizing the objects in a room or house.

Other forms of agnosia are encountered. *Anosognosia* consists of ignorance of the existence of disease, and is seen usually as a lack of perception of a hemiplegia or of other paralyzed parts. There may be an imperception of the weakness with a belief by the patient that he can move the paralyzed parts, or a complete denial of the hemiplegia or paralysis. The defect is usually associated with a lesion of the opposite inferior parietal region in the vicinity of the supramarginal gyrus. *Autotopagnosia* or *somatotopagnosia* is characterized by a defect in appreciation of the body scheme. In this defect there may be loss of ability to identify the body or the relation of its various parts. There may be complete loss of identification of a part or a half of the body. In such instances the patient may feel an arm next to his body and be unaware that it is his own,

or he may be unable to identify sides of the body.

The *Gerstmann syndrome* is characterized by finger agnosia, agraphia, confusion of right and left, and acalculia. The finger agnosia is characterized by difficulty in recognizing, naming, selecting, and differentiating the fingers of either hand, the patient's own as well as those of others. The confusion of right and left is characterized by inability to recognize sides of the body, both the patient's as well as others; and the acalculia is seen in a difficulty, often profound, in performing simple arithmetical problems. It is due to a lesion involving the left angular gyrus in a right-handed person, in a region between the parietal and occipital cortex. It is caused by tumor of the brain or by a vascular lesion, and it has specific localizing value. The finger agnosia involves the three middle fingers most severely, the thumb and index less frequently and less severely, and the toes not at all. The condition occurs in a perfectly oriented subject, with no evidence of clouding of of the sensorium. Patients afflicted with the condition are usually mentally alert; they are fully oriented for time, place, and person; and there is inherent evidence of paralysis.

3. Apraxia

This form of disorder refers to an inability to perform purposeful movements or to execute the proper use of objects. Several forms are described: (1) *Limb kinetic,* characterized by absence of paralysis, slowness and awkwardness of movement, and inability to carry out a movement. (2) *Ideokinetic,* characterized by difficulty in determining what the movement shall be. (3) *Ideational,* characterized by an inability to recognize the specific movements necessary for the completion of an act. Patients so afflicted are unable altogether to strike a match and light a cigarette, or they may strike the match on the wrong side of the box, or strike with the cigarette instead of the match. (4) *Constructive,* characterized by difficulty in building with blocks, in drawing, and sometimes in writing, and by recognition on the part of the patient of his faulty constructions.

4. Clinical Significance of Aphasia, Agnosia, and Apraxia

Defects in speech of the aphasic type have an important clinical significance and indicate lesions in specific portions of the brain. Care must be taken, however, to recognize the fact that as Hughlings Jackson has said, "To locate the damage which destroys speech and to locate speech are two different things." Hence the localization of lesions causing aphasia fails to state how the speech process is elaborated. Categorically stated, *expressive aphasia* indicates a lesion in the left inferior frontal gyrus (F_3) in its posterior portion, and possibly also implicates the adjacent island of Reil. *Auditory-receptive aphasia* indicates a lesion in the left superior temporal gyrus (T_1) involving its posterior portion. *Visual-receptive aphasia* indicates a lesion in the region of the lingual gyrus. In the *expressive-receptive* group, there is involvement of frontal and temporal areas. The localization in the amnesic group is not clear.

4

Headache, Vertigo, Coma, Pain

Among the many symptoms which may develop in neurological disorders, headache is often the most baffling. If the symptom is approached logically, it may be frequently analyzed satisfactorily; hence an understanding of the natural history of headache is both useful and valuable in the analysis of this symptom.

I. HISTORY OF HEADACHE

A careful history of headache is essential for a proper understanding of the symptom. The *location* of the headache is sometimes of importance. Most headaches are generalized and are without specific significance for localization. The headache of *migraine,* however, is usually unilateral. The headache of *cerebral aneurysm* is often unilateral and often felt in the eye as well. *Pituitary tumor* headache is usually frontal or temporal in location. *Lumbar puncture* headache is occipital and appears on assumption of the erect posture. Further important details in a history of headache include a determination of *precipitating* factors in the headache. These include menstruation, fatigue, alcohol, weather changes, food, and tobacco. The *frequency* of the headache is important, as well as the *time* of occurrence, whether diurnal or nocturnal. *Associated symptoms* such as lachrymation, face pain, scotomas, stuffiness of the nose, weakness, or paresthesias are important. The *family history* as regards headache should always be investigated.

The *incidence* and *nature* of the headache may be helpful in determining its significance. A *constant* headache is quite different from *periodic* headache. The headache of brain tumor is likely to be constant, and the same is true of the headache of meningitis. On the other hand, migraine headache is periodic. Other headaches, such as those of subarachnoid hemorrhage and cerebral aneurysm, are apoplectic. *Throbbing* headaches have no specific significance. Furthermore, the actual type of headache, whether dull, sharp, etc., has no significance except that a careful description by the patient of the sensation will enable one to distinguish between headache and head pain. This distinction is essential, since it is clear that a suboccipital pain due to involvement of the occipital nerve is quite different from an occipital headache associated with a posterior fossa tumor.

Aggravation of the headache may occur with increase of intracranial pressure as in coughing, sneezing, or by compression of the jugular veins, and is found especially in brain tumors or other processes associated with increased pressure. Headache may be affected by change of posture as in lumbar puncture headache. Vascular headaches are often increased by recumbency. *Relief* of headache occurs under many conditions; hence an understanding of it in any case may yield useful information. A headache relieved by a small dose of salicylate may be regarded as mild and probably not due to increased intracranial pressure. Relief by recumbency suggests an extracranial cause. A story of relief by the ingestion of food is suggestive of hypo-glycemic headache.

A few well-placed questions, therefore, will result in information concerning headache which will be useful in diag-nosis and treatment.

II. CAUSES OF HEADACHE

The causes of headache are many. While headache may be a symptom of innumerable diseases, it may be useful to list some of the more common conditions in which the symptom is found:

1. GENERAL SYSTEM DISEASE
(a) *Acute febrile conditions:*
  Typhoid fever
  Influenza
  Grippe
  Scarlet fever
  Undulant fever
  Pneumonia
  Psittacosis
(b) *Chronic diseases:*
  Cardiorenal disease
  Hypertension
  Uremia
  Diabetes
  Gout
(c) *Toxic conditions:*
  Alcoholism
  Carbon monoxide
2. LOCAL DISEASE
(a) *Ocular:*
  Eyestrain
  Muscle imbalance
  Myopia
  Glaucoma
(b) *Aural:*
  Otitis media
  Mastoiditis
  Petrositis
(c) *Upper respiratory:*
  Sinusitis
  Tumors of sinuses
3. SKULL DISEASES
  Osteomyelitis
  Tumors of skull
4. NERVOUS SYSTEM DISORDERS
(a) *Infections:*
  Meningitis
  Meningoencephalitis:
    Syphilitic
    Tuberculous
    Virus

Meningeal abscess:
  Extradural
  Subdural
  Brain abscess
(b) *Vascular disease:*
  Meningeal hemorrhage:
    Subarachnoid
    Subdural
    Extradural
  Cerebral hemorrhage
  Cerebral thrombosis
  Cerebral embolism
  Cerebral aneurysm
  Cerebral arteriosclerosis
(c) *Brain tumors:*
(d) *Miscellaneous:*
  Allergy
  Migraine
  Posttraumatic
  Brain edema
  Hydrocephalus internus and
    externus
  Histamine
  Menopause
  Lumbar puncture headache
  Psychogenic
  Spinal anesthesia
  Cough
  Hypoglycemia

Headache occurs frequently in *infec-tions* and febrile diseases. In many of these it is so incidental as to merit little mention. In others, such as typhoid fever, influenza, and grippe, it is a prominent symptom. In psittacosis it is severe and disabling. The headache of *hypertension* is periodic and at times paroxysmal. It does not parallel the level of the blood pressure, since it may be severe with a relatively lower pressure and absent with high degrees of pressure. The headache associated with *ocular conditions* requires mention because it is often overlooked for more complex causes, and conversely, it is adhered to much too long in many cases in which the cause of the headache lies outside the eye mechanisms. It is due to refractive errors, glaucoma, infec-tions in the orbit, and paralysis of the ocular muscles. The headache of glau-coma may be quite marked and may be responsible for severe unilateral head pain. Ocular headache is usually frontal in location, is situated just above the eyeballs, is aggravated by the use of the eyes, and is associated with a drawing and tense sensation felt in the eyeballs. The headache of *meningitis* is constant and severe and is associated with evidences of meningeal irritation. *Meningoencephalitis* of syphilitic origin may be associated with very severe headache due to an accompanying acute internal hydrocephalus. The headache associated with *meningeal abscess* is usually obscured by the associated sinus disease. It is apt to be constant, severe, and may be accompanied by signs of meningeal irritation. The headache of *brain abscess* is similar to that of brain tumor. *Subarachnoid hemorrhage* is characterized by a sudden, apoplectic onset in a previously healthy young person or in a person with previous arteriosclerosis, hypertension, endocarditis, etc. It is a severe, disabling headache usually associated with prostration of varying degree. Prostrating headache often immediately precedes *cerebral hemorrhage,* but a less severe headache may precede the onset of cerebral hemorrhage for hours or days. Mild headache as a rule, but severe headache at times, may precede or usher in *cerebral thrombosis* and *cerebral embolism.*

Brain Tumor: This is as a rule severe and persistent, but headache is not an invariable symptom of tumor of the brain. It is usually deep, steady, increased by coughing and straining, and relieved at times by cold packs. It may be absent in many cases. It may appear as an early symptom—the first to usher in the disease —or it may develop late in the course of a brain tumor. Though it is rightfully regarded as one of the main features of brain tumor, it is not infrequently lacking. It is usually the first symptom in posterior fossa tumor. The headache appears to be unrelated to the level of the intra-

cranial pressure, since severe headaches may occur with normal spinal fluid pressure, while no headache may be found with high degrees of intracranial pressure. Brain tumor headache is produced by traction on intracranial, pain sensitive structures, chiefly the large arteries, veins, and venous sinuses, and certain cranial nerves (Wolff). This is of two sorts: (1) Local traction by the tumor on adjacent structures, (2) distant traction by displacement of the brain. Little can be said concerning the localizing significance of headache in brain tumor, since the headache in most cases of brain tumor is generalized. In some instances, the headache of brain tumor may be unilateral. Cerebellar tumors are usually associated with suboccipital headache and pain. Headache is almost always present with posterior fossa tumors and often lacking in supratentorial tumors. In the latter it is usually frontal and rarely in the back of the head. In the absence of papilledema the headache in two thirds of the patients immediately overlies or is near the tumor (Wolff).

Allergy: Headache may be associated at times with *allergy* and is probably the result of a local or generalized brain edema. A history of urticaria or specific allergy is usually obtainable.

Head Injury: The headaches which follow *head injury* are often disabling and baffling. They are usually generalized, often constant, and too frequently persistent. They tend to be aggravated by posture, emotional factors, and fatigue. They may and often do disappear within a short time after the injury, but some forms persist indefinitely (*v.* Trauma). They may follow injury immediately and persist; or they may disappear soon after injury and reappear weeks or months later, as in some cases of subdural hematoma. They may be associated with other symptoms such as vertigo, and they may or may not be found with signs of meningeal irritation.

The headache associated with injury of the head has been found to be associated with three mechanisms (Wolff) : (1) pain due to local tissue damage, as in those patients with tender areas in the scalp; (2) pain due to sustained neck or head muscle contraction, as in cases with a steady pressure sensation or aching pain in a circumscribed area or in a caplike distribution; and (3) pain due to dilatation of the branches of the external carotid arteries, as in those instances associated with a throbbing and aching pain occurring in attacks, usually unilateral, in the temporal and frontal regions.

The pain of subdural hematoma is due to a mechanism similar to that of brain tumor.

Menopausal Headaches: They are common but their mechanism is unknown.

Lumbar Puncture Headache: It is not common. It occurs following lumbar puncture. It may result from a loss of fluid and a settling down of the brain against the base of the skull. It develops on removal of either small or large amounts of spinal fluid and seems to bear a closer relationship to the fall in pressure associated with removal of fluid than to the amount of fluid removed. It is associated with a decrease in spinal fluid volume as evidenced by a fall in spinal fluid pressure. It is eliminated by the intrathecal injection of saline and elevation of intracranial pressure to normal (Wolff), and it is increased by bilateral jugular compression. It is caused by dilatation of and traction on pain sensitive intracranial vascular structures and it is secondary to prolonged leakage of fluid through the dural hole in the lumbar sac. It is a postural headache which appears in the erect posture, disappears in recumbency, and is unin-

fluenced by drugs. It may last a few days to a few weeks. In exceptional instances it may last three to four weeks. It is extremely disabling, is often associated with nausea and sometimes with vomiting.

Psychogenic Headache: Many headaches are *psychogenic* in origin, but before a headache is regarded as of this nature, care must be taken to exclude all physical causes and it must be clear from symptoms and motivation that a neurosis is present. Headaches of emotional origin frequently have atypical features, but this in itself should not lead to a diagnosis of headache of this nature. It may be localized in a single spot; be described as constant and intense and yet be associated with no obvious discomfort; or it may be disabling.

Tension headaches of emotional origin are frequently felt in the back of the neck and head, are often constant, and may be severe. It is usually possible to determine a relationship between the headaches and emotional conflicts or situational difficulties.

Histamine Headache: This type of headache is characterized by a unilateral headache of short duration, varying in duration from minutes to one hour or several hours. It commences and often terminates suddenly, and tends to occur at night but may occur during the daytime. The head pain characteristic of histamine cephalalgia may recur with monotonous regularity at night, week in and week out, at a definite hour. It is frequently eased on sitting up or standing, and may be aggravated by reclining. It is associated with profuse watering and congestion of the eye, stuffiness of the nostril, and often dilatation of the temporal vessels of the involved side. The pain is often described as excruciating, burning, and boring (Horton). It extends into the eye, temple, neck, and often into the face along the branches of the external carotid artery. During and after attacks, tenderness is elicited over the branches of the external and common carotid arteries. Most of the patients afflicted by histamine headache, or cephalalgia, are in the fourth and fifth decades of life. Typical attacks of headache may be induced by the injection of 0.1 to 0.2 mg. of histamine subcutaneously. There are no specific causes and no hereditary or familial characteristics.

Therapy in histaminic cephalalgia is based upon three principles: (1) determination and elimination of the sources of allergy, (2) desensitization to specific allergens, and (3) increasing tolerance to histamine (Butler and Thomas).

There is grave doubt as to whether histamine headache exists as such, or whether it is not in reality a variant of migraine. The probabilities favor the latter view because (1) the distribution and character of the pain are similar to those of migraine; (2) histamine injections may produce headache in both types; (3) both types are reduced in intensity or relieved by ergotamine tartrate or by other vasoconstrictors, such as epinephrine; and (4) both are relieved by sitting and standing positions and increased by lying down, and both are reduced in intensity by pressure on the common carotid artery (Wolff).

Spinal Anesthesia Headache: Headache not infrequently follows *spinal anesthesia* and is in many cases of this sort a true lumbar puncture headache with all the features described for headache of this nature. In other instances the headache following spinal anesthesia is not postural, as in lumbar puncture headache, but appears to bear some relationship to the spinal anesthesia itself. It may be rapidly transient or long persistent.

Sinus Disease: This is a common cause of headache, and may result from suppurative or nonsuppurative rhinitis or sinusitis. The headache of acute sinusitis results from obstruction of the nose and blockage of the openings of the nasal sinuses. The frontal sinus is most often involved, the headache in such instances being frontal, with tenderness over the sinus, with appearance of the headache on awakening and improvement after the upright posture is attained. Chronic sinus headaches may develop after acute sinusitis subsides. They are located in the frontal area with frontal sinus disease and are characterized by persistent dull headache. In ethmoid sinus disease, the headache is over the root of the nose or posteriorly over the vertex; in maxillary sinus disease, tenderness over the canine fossa is present; in sphenoid sinus disease, the headache is over the vertex or occiput. The headache of sinus disease is increased by shaking the head or by the head-down position; by straining, coughing, or a tight collar; or by anxiety, menstruation, cold air, sexual excitement, or alcohol (Wolff).

Hematogenous Headaches: These occur in hypochromic anemias, polycythemia, and leukemia.

Cough Headache: In patients with increased intracranial pressure, cough often increases the headache. In a small group of patients, headache occurs only on coughing or sneezing. The headache may be localized or generalized. Neurological examination usually reveals nothing of significance. In such patients, organic brain disease is often not found, but occasionally the symptom of cough headache may indicate the presence of a tumor.

III. MECHANISM OF HEADACHE

The investigations of Wolff and his coworkers indicate that headache may result from (1) traction on the veins that pass to the venous sinuses from the surface of the brain and displacement of the great venous sinuses; (2) traction on the middle meningeal arteries; (3) traction on the large arteries at the base of the brain and their main branches; (4) distension and dilatation of intracerebral and extracerebral arteries; (5) inflammation in or about any of the pain sensation structures of the head; (6) direct pressure by tumors on the cranial and cervical nerves containing many pain afferent fibers from the head.

Intracranial disease causes headache through one or more of these mechanisms. Traction, displacement, distention, and inflammation of cranial vascular structures are mainly responsible for headache. Processes which produce traction on the arteries or venous sinuses produce headache. Similarly, processes associated with distention and dilatation of the vessels, as in histamine headache, are also important.

IV. MIGRAINE

Migraine is a form of headache which is often unilateral, usually paroxysmal, and is associated with accompanying symptoms of a gastrointestinal, ocular, or other nature. It is estimated to occur in from 8 to 12 per cent of all patients seen in general practice (von Storch). The migraine syndrome is characterized by periodic headache, usually unilateral but commonly generalized, and associated with irritability, nausea, photophobia, vomiting, constipation, or diarrhea. It is not infrequently ushered in by scotomas, hemianopsia, and other evidences of cerebral involvement, such as aphasia, hemiparesis, and unilateral paresthesias.

Etiology: Migraine is a disease of relatively early life, is more common in women than in men, and is accompanied frequently by a history of the disease in the parents and other members of the family. The age of onset of the disease is difficult to compute but all observers agree that it appears early. In 151 of 270 cases of migraine (56%), it appeared at or before the age of sixteen years (Bassoe). It is not uncommon in children and begins in childhood more often than is recognized, at ages varying from one and one half to twelve years. Though most statistics indicate a preponderance of the disease in women, it has been claimed that this preponderance has been greatly exaggerated. Women outnumber men in seeking relief from the disease in a ratio of about three to one (von Storch), possibly because the disease is more severe in women than in men. A history of migraine in one or both parents is common, and the same is true of brothers and sisters. A similar history in the grandparents is frequently obtained. Among 270 cases, migraine was found to be present in one or both parents in 153 instances (57%), in one or more brothers and sisters in 80 cases (29%), and in one grandparent in 22 cases, or 8.1 per cent (Bassoe). Migraine heredity is found in about 65 per cent of migraine patients. "Heredity is agreed by all observers to play an important part in the production of migraine" (von Storch). There appears also to be an hereditary relationship between migraine and epilepsy. Epilepsy is found in a small percentage of cases in the forebears of migraine patients, but a history of migraine is found in a large proportion of the ancestors of epileptic patients. Of 2400 persons with epilepsy or migraine, 9.2 per cent had both, and relatives of migraine patients had epilepsy 3.6 per cent times more than a control group (Lennox).

The exact cause of migraine has not been determined but a number of factors have been indicted. Indeed, it is abundantly clear that no single process or mechanism explains all cases of migraine. It is not surprising, therefore, that a number of processes have been regarded as responsible for the condition. These include: (1) *Allergic factors:* Allergy has been implicated as a cause of migraine. The claim for this is based on (a) the occurrence of migraine in patients with hay fever and asthma, (b) the occurrence of positive skin reactions to some allergen in some patients, (c) the cure of migraine in some instances by a restricted diet, and (d) the occurrence of eosinophilia at times in migraine. (2) *Endocrine factors:* Swelling of the hypophysis, and ovarian and thyroid deficiencies have been regarded as present in many cases and beneficial results reported with estrogenic therapy, pituitary extracts, irradiation of the pituitary gland, etc. A humoral factor has been suggested in women in whom attacks frequently precede the menstrual period and cease in pregnancy. (3) *Duodenal and colonic factors* have been held responsible in some cases due to either duodenal or colonic stasis. (4) *Psychic factors* have been held responsible. These include emotional stress and anxiety, exhaustion, and other factors.

The *migraine personality* is a factor of importance in all migraine problems. It is featured essentially by the following characteristics: "childhood shyness, obedience, neatness, and reliability; also stubborn inflexibility in certain circumstances, adult perfectionism, ambitiousness, inelasticity, tension, resentment, and repetitiousness; but also efficiency, poise, and social grace" (von Storch). The result is an obsessive-compulsive type of personality structure in which two trends are noted: (a) a need for love and approval and (b) the inability to recognize and to handle properly anger in the individual himself.

No treatment of migraine is successful without a serious investigation of the personality factors involved. In essence, the migraine sufferer develops headache against a background of an obsessive-compulsive personality, with feelings of inadequacy, tendencies to perfectionism and rigidity, excessive conscientiousness, and numerous frustrations, extending far back into childhood.

Mechanism: The *mechanism* of the migraine headache has been greatly advanced by the studies of Wolff and his collaborators on the effect of ergotamine tartrate on the migraine headache. It seems clear that the headache of migraine is associated with a dilatation of arteries of the scalp, especially those of the external carotid artery, while the intracranial vessels show no change.

The preheadache phenomena of migraine, such as visual disturbances and sometimes sensory disturbances, are due to vasoconstriction, chiefly within the cranial cavity (Wolff).

The headache itself is produced primarily by distention of the cranial arteries, chiefly, but not exclusively, the branches of the external carotid (Wolff). Procedures that constrict the cranial arteries and thus reduce their amplitude of pulsation will diminish or terminate the headache. The extracranial and possibly the dural branches of the external carotid artery are the chief contributors. The face pain, which is sometimes encountered in migraine, probably results from dilatation and distention of the extracranial portion of the middle meningeal artery, the internal maxillary artery, and the trunks of the external and common carotid arteries (Wolff).

A second mechanism of pain during migraine headache involves the sustained contraction of the muscles of the head and neck.

Factors which decrease the amplitude of pulsations decrease the intensity of the headache. Ergotamine acts by a vasoconstriction of the arteries in question. Ergotamine tartrate causes an average decrease of 50 per cent in the amplitude of the temporal arteries when administered during a migraine headache and causes decrease or elimination of the headache. Histamine headache in contrast to migraine is due to a dilatation of the cerebral arteries, principally the internal carotids, vertebral and basilar arteries (Schumaker, Ray and Wolff). While the mechanism of the migraine headache is clear, the factors which cause the dilatation of the extracranial vessels are not yet known. Whether they are due to allergic, endocrine, psychic, or toxic factors remains to be determined. It is possible that no single mechanism is operative in all cases.

Symptoms: The outstanding symptom of migraine is headache; a recurrent, severe, incapacitating headache against a background of relative well-being. As a rule, the headache develops without warning, but not infrequently there may be an aura of the impending headache by various sensory phenomena, especially visual symptoms, such as flashing lights or scotomata. Fatigue, numbness, gastric pain, depression, anxiety, and even euphoria may presage the onset of an attack. For the same patient there may be a variety of auras associated with the attack of migraine.

Attacks may be precipitated by emotional disturbances, fatigue, anxiety, and other factors. The headache is usually hemicranial but it may occur in any or all parts of the head. When it is found involving one side of the head, it is apt to remain confined to the affected side, but it may affect the other side after a long period of time, or it may shift from one to the other side indiscriminately. Characteristically, the headache of migraine is confined to one side of the head, but it may on occasion be generalized. It is usually severe, but its inten-

sity may vary from time to time and be very severe on some occasions and milder on others.

The duration of the headache varies greatly; it may last for an hour or two hours, an entire day, or several days. It may be so incapacitating as to force the patient to bed, or it may be relatively mild and permit the performance of everyday duties. Not infrequently, the headache may be relatively mild and may vary in intensity from one episode to another. The frequency of the headaches varies widely. They may occur at daily, weekly, or monthly intervals, in the latter instance at the time of the menses, either before, during, or after the menstrual period. In some cases, they may recur so frequently as to seem to be constant. Associated with the headache are gastrointestinal disturbances, such as nausea or vomiting. These are not constant; nausea may be found without vomiting or both may be absent. Among 402 cases of migraine, nausea was found in 63 per cent of male patients and 70 per cent of female, and vomiting in 53 and 61 per cent, respectively (Allan).

Not as frequent as the gastrointestinal symptoms are the visual phenomena which accompany the attack. These consist of scintillating scotomata, transient hemianopsia, and fortification spectra. Visual phenomena may precede the headache and usher in the impending attack, but they usually accompany the headache. In some varieties of attack, the pain may be confined to the eye or to the vicinity of the orbit. Vertigo is not infrequently associated with attacks of headache. Tenderness of the scalp on the side of the headache is often found during an attack. Sympathetic symptoms of various types may develop. These consist of lachrymation, perspiration, pallor or flushing, tachycardia, bradycardia, urticaria, dermographia, and edema. In some instances, symptoms such as hemi-anopsia may persist for several hours after an attack.

Permanent sequelae of the migraine attack are recorded, but they are rare. Ocular and retinal hemorrhages, hemiplegia, and hemianopsia have been found to persist indefinitely after attacks of migraine (Dunning). Cerebral hemorrhage occurs at times in migraine. Occlusion of a retinal artery, either the central retinal artery or one of its peripheral branches, has been observed in the course of an attack of migraine. Occlusion of the central retinal vein has also been recorded.

Atypical Forms: Though migraine usually runs true to form and is characterized by the features outlined, it may on some occasions assume atypical forms. These include:

Ophthalmoplegic Migraine: It is characterized by the occurrence of oculomotor paralyses associated with the headache. In such instances, the headache is severe, often in the affected eye, and is accompanied by paralysis of the ocular muscles at the time of the headache or shortly thereafter. The paralysis affects usually the oculomotor nerve and is characterized by ptosis, external strabismus, and impairment of movement of the eyeball upward, downward, and inward. In other instances, external rectus paralysis develops but rarely complete external ophthalmoplegia of one side. The ocular paralyses may recover rapidly in the course of a few hours or they may persist for days or weeks, or permanently. There is considerable doubt as to whether ophthalmoplegic migraine is similar to simple migraine or whether it is the result of an associated intracranial aneurysm. The probabilities are that ophthalmoplegic migraine is due to a cerebral aneurysm, which causes the ophthalmoplegia. In support of this is the fact that instances of so-called "ophthalmoplegic migraine" have been found, after a number of years, to be associated with aneurysm, either at operation or autopsy. There still remains, however, a group of cases of ophthalmic migraine in which recurrent episodes of ocular palsy occur for years, with full recovery after each episode and with no permanent paralysis developing at any time. Arteriograms of patients with ophthalmoplegic migraine have failed to reveal an aneurysm (Alpers).

Abdominal Migraine: This is characterized by the occurrence of nausea and vomiting without headache or with relatively little headache. It occurs periodically as in the case of the headache and may persist after attacks of headache have ceased. It is not a common variety of migraine and tends to occur in children.

Menstrual migraine has attained considerable popularity, but there is considerable doubt whether any such entity occurs. In women with characteristic migraine, it was found that in only 10 per cent was there an exclusive relationship between the menstrual cycle and migraine (von Storch). There is a tendency, however, for patients with migraine to suffer onset or aggravation of their headaches before, during, or after the menstrual cycle.

Diagnosis: The diagnosis of migraine offers no difficulties in the average case, but many forms of headache which fall short of the criteria for the disease are referred to as migraine. The diagnostic characteristics of migraine in the order of their diagnostic importance are as follows (von Storch): (1) Recurrent headache, preferably, but not necessarily hemicranial in type. Recurrent paroxysmal headaches are the foundation of the disease. Constant headaches are not of a migrainous nature except under special circumstances to be considered. (2) Associated visual symptoms. (3) Gastrointestinal symptoms, usually nausea and vomiting. (4) Hereditary migraine diathesis. (5) Relief by ergotamine tartrate (found in about 85 per cent). (6) Evidence of migraine personality. Not all the criteria listed may be found in a typical case, but the presence of recurrent headache associated with one of the other features must be present before the diagnosis can be considered, and at least three features must be present for the diagnosis to be made with any degree of certainty. If adherence to these principles is maintained, relatively little difficulty will be encountered in the average case.

Considerable doubt may be cast upon a diagnosis of migraine in a patient with constant headache unless it can be shown that (a) there has been a previous history of recurrent headaches; (b) the constant headache is in reality a series of bouts of migraine headache which merge into what seems to be a constant headache; (c) there is a hereditary history of migraine. Headache may exist in migraine for several days on end, but constant headache for months on end is not usually migraine.

Ophthalmoplegic migraine offers difficulties in the diagnosis of the individual attack which simulates closely the history and findings of cerebral aneurysm. The sudden onset of headache, eye pain, diplopia, and ocular paralysis is similar in all details to that of aneurysm, but a history of a hereditary tendency, of recurrent hemicranial headaches, and of recovery from the attacks is helpful in establishing the diagnosis.

Abdominal migraine offers real difficulties in diagnosis, but a history of previous recurrent headaches and a hereditary diathesis help to establish the condition.

Many special forms of migraine have been described, but they represent no special type of the disorder. It is as fruitless to speak of facioplegic migraine as it is to refer to aphasic or hemianopic migraine. Yet facioplegic, cardiac, thoracic, and other forms have been mentioned. Precordial migraine was found to occur as a substitute for headache in 27 per cent of 880 patients with migraine (Fitz Hugh).

Treatment: No treatment of migraine is satisfactory that does not make a careful appraisal of the personality of the migraine sufferer, simultaneously with the management of the purely medical aspects of the problem. Mere manipulation of drugs is not sufficient, and the abandonment of one regimen for another must sometime come to an end. The intelligent approach to every migraine problem demands a survey of personality, social, and medical factors, with appropriate management of each.

For the migraine attack, the most efficient drug is *ergotamine tartrate* given hypodermically in doses of 0.25 to 0.50 mg. ($\frac{1}{250}$ to $\frac{1}{125}$ grain). The drug should be given as early as possible in the attack. Severe attacks may be terminated by a similar dosage of the drug given intravenously. Patients should be advised to rest one to two hours after taking the drug. The attack terminates in thirty to forty minutes after injection. Side effects of the drug, nausea and vomiting, are so distressing that many patients prefer the disease to the cure. Oral administration of the drug is not as effectual as parenteral administration, but in some cases may be very useful given in tablets of 1 mg. ($\frac{1}{60}$ grain) dissolved under the tongue several times a day (3 to 5 mg. [$\frac{1}{25}$ to $\frac{1}{12}$ grain]). Ergotamine should by preference not be given more than once in every two or three days, but it may be given daily over long periods without change in the blood pressure or without tingling, numbness, nausea, or vomiting. *Oxygen inhalation* may be used in some cases, but the results during the migrainous attack are indifferent. *Codeine* (32.4 mg. [½ grain]) may be given in repeated doses in the migraine attack. *Morphine* may be used in severe cases, but should be given sparingly and only if all other remedies fail.

Dihydroergotamine (DHE45) (1 mg. [¹⁄₆₀ grain]) is similar in its effects to ergotamine, but the relief obtained is neither as constant nor as prolonged as in the case of ergotamine tartrate. It is essentially a weak preparation of ergotamine, and its use is probably best reserved for patients who cannot tolerate ergotamine.

Intravenous *sodium nicotinate,* or *nicotinic acid,* (50 to 100 mg. [⅘ to 1⅗ grains]) is recommended for the relief of migraine in some cases, but the results are usually disappointing. The vitamin may be given daily and then maintained by oral administration (50 to 100 mg. three times daily).

Acetylsalicylic acid (0.972 Gm. [15 grains]) in repeated doses suffices to alleviate mild headaches in about one third of the cases. Acetanilid and acetophenetidin have no advantages over ordinary acetylsalicylic acid.

Potassium thiocyanate (0.194 Gm. [3 grains]) has been found to relieve the frequency and severity of migraine attacks, the best results being obtained with a cyanate blood level of 2.5 to 8.0 mg. per 100 cc. Care should be taken to watch the blood level and the reaction of the patient to the cyanate.

Neostigmine bromide has been reported to be effective in some cases of migraine (15 mg. [¼ grain] of the drug to 1 ounce of distilled water). The drug is given in doses of one drop three times daily, increasing daily until the patient takes 10 drops three times daily. This dose is maintained for one week and then reduced to a maintenance dose of 10 drops twice weekly.

A combination of *ergotamine* (1 mg. [¹⁄₆₀ grain]) and *caffeine* (100 mg. [1½ grains]) taken by mouth three to four times daily has been found to be helpful in some cases. The drug is obtainable as Cafergot. It is recommended for use at the onset of headache, the dose being one or two tablets then, followed by one or two tablets in one or two hours if necessary.

Between attacks efforts should be directed against recurrence of the headache. The *diet* should be looked into carefully and all foods eliminated to which the patient is sensitive. Unless food sensitivities are found, no dietary restrictions are necessary. On the whole, diet control is a factor of little importance in migraine. Adequate *rest* and prevention of emotional stress are important. *Vitamin therapy* has been advocated as a means of aborting and preventing the migraine attack. The vitamin regimen advocated is as follows (Palmer): Thiamine chloride, 30 to 90 mg. (½ to 1⅖ grains) intramuscularly, is given daily for a period of two weeks. After two weeks, 30 mg. is given once or twice a week for two months. "If an attack is to be terminated, 60 to 120 mg. (1 to 1⅘ grains) may be given intramuscularly or intravenously." Capsules of B complex are given during the course of the treatment, and liver is advocated intramuscularly once or twice a week. This regimen is of value only in the sense of well-being resulting from the use of the vitamin. In some cases, *histamine desensitization* is helpful. The drug is given as histamine phosphate subcutaneously in doses of 0.05 mg. twice daily for two days; then 0.066 mg. twice daily for two days, and finally 0.1 mg. daily for three or four weeks. Intravenous *histaminic acid phosphate* (2.75 mg. [¹⁄₂₅ grain] in 250 cc. of saline) daily for fifteen to thirty doses gives relief in some cases (complete relief in 40 per cent, partial in 33 per cent) (Butler and Thomas). *Endocrine* preparations should be given if there is definite evidence of endocrine dysfunction. Testosterone and diethylstilbestrol may benefit some female patients. Without such indications, endocrine medication is useless. *Surgical measures* of various types have been used in various cases. They include ligation of the middle meningeal artery, cervical sympathectomy, and section of the trigeminal nerve. Periarterial infiltration of the temporal artery and ligation of this artery are reported as affording relief in severe cases. Surgery should be used only as a desperation measure.

V. CRANIAL ARTERITIS
(Temporal Arteritis)

Definition: This is a rare condition, characterized by complaints of a systemic nature, associated with severe headaches and other cerebral symptoms.

Etiology: The disease is rare. It occurs in older subjects at an age incidence of fifty-five to eighty years, and is more common in women at a ratio of 3 to 1. The symptoms are those of a low-grade, self-limited, infectious process in an elderly person of lowered resistance (Kilbourne and Wolff). Tooth or mouth infection is not uncommon (seven out of twenty cases). The disease may be an allergic reaction. "The relatively high incidence of concomitant or preceding mouth infection plus the fact that the initial pain may occur in the teeth or jaw suggests the possibility of involvement of neighboring arteriosclerotic arteries by direct extension of local infection" (Kilbourne and Wolff).

Pathology: The vessels are tortuous, swollen, and nodular, and are associated with cellulitis of the contiguous tissues. The temporal artery is most frequently affected, but disease of the central artery of the retina, the occipital, radial, facial,

carotid, brachial, and cerebral arteries has been recorded. Microscopically, the disease is a panarteritis which cannot be distinguished from periarteritis nodosa. A typical section reveals hypertrophy of the intima, medial necrosis associated with the formation of granulomatous tissue, and the presence of foreign body giant cells, periarterial cellular infiltration, and thrombus formation. Eosinophilic invasion of the artery is rare. No cases have come to autopsy.

Symptoms: The symptoms are specific and nonspecific. Among the *nonspecific* symptoms are those of a systemic nature due to inflammation and distention of the temporal arteries. These include weight loss, anorexia, general malaise, fever, sweating, and weakness. Weight loss may be profound, and patients may show great emaciation. Sweating is constant. There is an inconstant, low-grade fever without chills in 70 per cent of the cases.

Of the specific symptoms *pain* is the most striking. It consists of a severe throbbing, steady headache associated with hyperalgesia of the scalp. Pain on mastication is present in 50 per cent of the patients and in some is an initial symptom. Facial swelling and redness of the skin overlying the temporal arteries are noted after the onset of the headache. Immediate relief may follow biopsy of the temporal artery. Prior to the onset of the headache there may be pain in the teeth, ear, jaw, zygoma, neck, and occiput. *Ocular* symptoms are common. Over a third of patients with temporal arteritis are threatened with partial or complete loss of vision. Diplopia, occlusion of the central retinal artery, and complete loss of vision have been recorded. Blindness is due to thrombosis of the central retinal artery, ischemic optic neuritis, and an indeterminate group. *Cerebral* symptoms suggesting encephalitis have been observed. Mental sluggishness, dizziness, vomiting, dysarthria, delirium, and coma have been described. Moderate *leukocytosis* (12,000-14,500) is usually present. No constant bacteriological findings are present.

The disease is self-limited, is of one to twenty months' duration, and is non-fatal. All patients show complete recovery. The condition is unaffected by treatment.

VI. VERTIGO

The problem of vertigo may be analyzed logically along the following lines: (1) Is true vertigo present? (2) What is the location of the lesion responsible for the vertigo? (3) What is the cause of the vertigo?

Vertigo may be defined as a sense of movement either of the subject or his surroundings.

Dizziness is a common complaint, but patients frequently do not mean vertigo when they complain of dizziness, giddiness, or lightheadedness. It is absolutely essential for diagnosis that a strict interpretation be placed on the term vertigo (dizziness). For true vertigo to be present there must be a sensation of turning on the part of the patient (*subjective vertigo*), or a sensation of movement of objects in the environment (*objective vertigo*). Associated with this is usually a sensation of disturbance of equilibrium with staggering and at times falling. Nausea, vomiting, tachycardia, and gastrointestinal symptoms may be present, but are not invariably found. Consciousness is not usually lost in vertigo, but there may be a fleeting sensation of confusion during an attack. In some instances of severe vertigo, as in Meniere's disease, unconsciousness may develop. Tinnitus may be present, either constant or intermittent. It occurs with peripheral and central causes, more often the former. Hearing decrease or loss is often associated with vertigo and is the result of peripheral causes involving the cochlear mechanism at its end stations or the cochlear nerve.

Mechanisms: Various mechanisms may be implicated in vertigo. These may be (1) *labyrinthine,* due to labyrinthitis; edema or hydrops of the labyrinth; or to disturbance of circulation, notably spasm or narrowing of the vestibular or internal auditory artery; (2) *peripheral nerve,* usually as the result of pressure on the auditory nerve by angle tumor, or by aneurysm, cyst, or arachnoiditis; (3) *brain stem,* resulting from the many causes which may produce vertigo from implication of the brain stem; (4) *cerebrum* or *cerebellum.*

Vertigo due to *peripheral* mechanisms is characterized by its episodic and paroxysmal nature. It appears in attacks which are featured by well-pronounced sensations of movement. Lateropulsion may be experienced, the sensation being that of forcible pushing to one or the other side. The vertigo may be subjective or objective, and is characterized further by aggravation on change of posture. Thus there is often a characteristic story of increase or appearance of the vertigo on turning to one or the other side, so that patients are as it were frozen into immobility for fear of inducing a vertiginous attack by movement of the head or body to one or the other side. Attacks of vertigo from peripheral causes may last a few to several minutes or may persist for hours, and are followed by after-effects which are extremely disturbing, particularly weakness. Unless severe, they are likely to last only a matter of minutes. Nystagmus is usually found during the attacks. It is horizontal, with a fast component toward the side of deviation of the eyes and a slow component toward the center.

There may be a rotational element in the nystagmus. Tinnitus and deafness are not always present. When present, they are rather indicative of peripheral than central disturbances. The Bárány test reveals excessively irritable responses in irritative lesions, but they may be lacking.

Vertigo resulting from the disturbance of *central* mechanisms may be distinguished as a rule from that due to peripheral causes. It is not usually episodic, is therefore more continuous, is likely to be prolonged, and is less clearly defined. It may be and often is associated with evidences of central nervous system involvement, a feature which is lacking in the peripheral cases. Thus there may be associated diplopia, ocular palsies, palatal weakness with difficulty in swallowing, hemiparesis and other indications of central nervous system disease. Nystagmus is present less frequently. It may be horizontal or vertical in type. Vertical nystagmus, when present, is characteristic of a central lesion, due usually to brain stem involvement. It may occur in peripheral lesions. Hearing is less frequently affected than in the peripheral lesions. The Bárány test is of value in central lesions only in cerebellopontine angle tumors in which the typical formula of absence of responses from the cochlea and labyrinth of the affected side and of the vertical canal of the opposite side is obtained.

The criteria for differentiation of peripheral and central vertigo are true within wide limits. Episodic attacks of vertigo, though more characteristic of peripheral lesions, are found also in central disorders. Thus, the severe episodic vertigo associated with occlusion of the posterior inferior cerebellar artery, in some posterior fossa tumors, and even rarely in cerebellopontine angle tumors.

A special form of episodic vertigo is found in the *Bruns' syndrome,* characterized by severe vertigo, headache, disturbance of vision and a feeling of blacking-out on flexion or extension of the head and associated with cysts or tumors of the fourth ventricle.

Vertigo due to central lesions is most commonly associated with disease of the brain stem, particularly the medulla, less commonly with disease of the cerebellum, and least often with involvement of the cerebral hemispheres.

Causes: They are many. An incomplete list includes the following:

Ocular:
> Muscle imbalance
> Diplopia
> Ophthalmoplegia

Aural:
> Hydrops of labyrinth (Meniere's disease)
> Obstruction of external auditory meatus
> Obstruction of eustachian tube
> Labyrinthitis and perilabyrinthitis
> Otitis media
> Mastoiditis
> Hemorrhage into labyrinth
> Embolism of labyrinth
> Cholesteatoma

Systemic:
> Cardiac disease
> Cardiorenal disease
> Arteriosclerosis
> Hypertension
> Hypotension
> Anemia
> Blood dyscrasias
> Allergy
> Nitrogen embolism (caisson disease; in airplane pilots)
> Carotid sinus syndrome
> Metabolic—gout, diabetes, hypothyroidism
> Avitaminosis
> Drugs—salicylates, nicotine, quinine, quinidine, cincophen, steptomycin, Dilantin sodium, trimethadione
> Foci of infection (teeth, tonsils, sinuses)

Neurologic:
> 1. *Vestibular nerve:*
>> Cerebellopontine angle tumor, aneurysm, arachnoiditis

2. *Brain stem:*
   (*a*) Infections:
      (1) Encephalitis
      (2) Syphilis
   (*b*) Tumors
   (*c*) Vascular:
      (1) Thrombosis of posterior infe-
         rior cerebellar artery
      (2) Thrombosis of superior cere-
         bellar artery
      (3) Hemorrhage due to trauma,
         hypertension, encephalitis,
         blood dyscrasias
   (*d*) Degenerative:
      (1) Multiple sclerosis
      (2) Syringobulbia
3. *Cerebellar:*
   (*a*) Tumor
   (*b*) Abscess
   (*c*) Vascular disease
4. *Cerebral:*
   (*a*) Tumor
   (*c*) Infections
   (*b*) Abscess
   (*d*) Vascular:
      (1) Thrombosis of cerebral vessels
      (2) Hemorrhage of cerebral ves-
         sels
      (3) Subarachnoid hemorrhage
      (4) Anoxemia
      (5) Aneurysm
   (*e*) Trauma
   (*f*) Epilepsy

Psychogenic.

The vertigo associated with *ocular* disturbances is never severe, usually fleeting, and frequently adjusted to by the
patient. That due to *aural* diseases is
almost exclusively of the peripheral type.
Vertigo is a frequent accompaniment of
hypertension and is due either to peripheral or central mechanisms in this condition. It is periodic but is not likely to be
paroxysmal unless it involves the labyrinth. *Carotid sinus* mechanisms should
never be overlooked in a search for the
cause of vertigo. *Hypotension* is fully as
important as increased blood pressure in
the production of vertigo (*v.* Postural
Hypotension). Fleeting and often ill-
defined vertiginous attacks are found in

arteriosclerosis probably due to ischemic
mechanisms involving either the central
or peripheral mechanisms, more often the
former. Vertigo in *brain tumors* is more
often associated with the posterior fossa
than with cerebral tumors. It is found
in brain stem tumors (25%) and in
cerebellopontine angle tumors. It may
be an early symptom of *multiple sclerosis,* but unless other evidences of the
disease are present, it may not be possible to establish multiple sclerosis as the
cause.

Posttraumatic vertigo is a difficult
symptom with which to cope. It is a
common sequel of head injury and may
follow concussion, contusion and laceration, subarachnoid hemorrhage, etc.
True spontaneous vertigo is uncommon.
More often the vertigo of head injury is
ill-defined, brief or prolonged, and increased with change of posture of the
head. It may last a few to several minutes, is associated with blurring of vision
and unsteadiness, and often occurs after
straining or quick change of position. It
is fleeting, however, and not of the typical labyrinthine type. Frequently, the
complaint of dizziness in posttraumatic
states is not true vertigo.

Psychogenic vertigo is usually ill-defined and is almost never true vertigo.
In some instances, however, typical episodic vertigo may be found due to psychogenic causes. Neurotics frequently
complain of dizziness, but they find difficulty in defining the symptom clearly.
As a rule, there is no true subjective or
objective vertigo, and it is one of the
distinguishing features of psychogenic
vertigo that it hardly ever conforms to
true dizziness. Psychogenic vertigo is
often described as constant.

Vascular lesions are often associated
with vertigo. In both cerebral hemorrhage and thrombosis, sudden severe vertigo may usher in the cerebral insult, or

mild vertiginous spells may precede the vascular insult for hours or days before the vascular attack. Attacks of vertigo may persist for some time after subarachnoid hemorrhage. In vascular lesions of the brain stem, sudden severe vertigo may usher in the disease. Vertigo is not a striking or characteristic feature of *encephalitis,* but if the encephalitic disease affects the proper area in the brain stem it may be prominent.

VII. MENIERE'S DISEASE

Meniere's disease is a common cause of vertigo. It is characterized clinically by vertigo, tinnitus, and progressive deafness. There is good reason to believe that the symptoms usually referred to as "Meniere's syndrome" represent a disease entity, the symptoms of which are quite characteristic. Recent evidence reveals that there is a distinct pathological background for the disorder though the conditions that may precipitate it vary. Only a few autopsy studies are available, but all indicate that Meniere's disease is due to edema or hydrops of the membranous labyrinth. Hemorrhage into the labyrinth, and toxic-infectious processes involving the labyrinth have also been suggested as causes. The syndrome occurs usually in adults and affects males slightly more than females. The *pathology* of the disease process is not understood, since the disease is not fatal and necropsy material scarce. Fourteen cases are reported in the literature, showing gross dilatation of the endolymph septum with degenerative changes in the organ of Corti. Since cause and pathology are not clear, the pathogenesis of the disorder is not specifically known. The majority of investigators believe that the symptoms are produced by disorders within the labyrinth, but some hold that the difficulty lies in the vestibular portion of the auditory nerve. The latter explains well the vertigo, but fails to provide a basis for the tinnitus and deafness. The symptoms are a combination of cochlear and vestibular involvement.

Various theories of involvement of the vestibular mechanisms have been propounded to explain the symptomatology. These assert the fact that Meniere's syndrome is the result of (1) a disturbance of water and salt metabolism resulting in the retention of water or sodium salts in the body and the production of an edema of the labyrinth (Furstenberg); dehydration and a low sodium diet are recommended on this basis; a high intake of potassium may be more important than a low intake of sodium (Talbot and Brown); during an attack there are an increase of serum potassium and a decrease of serum sodium but no increase of serum sodium; (2) a local alteration in the permeability of the capillary wall with secondary local edema involving the labyrinth and cochlea in the inner ear; histamine is recommended on this basis (Shelden and Horton); (3) a vasoconstrictor mechanism involving the labyrinth, producing a local ischemia (Atkinson); (4) a deficiency of niacin, riboflavin, and thiamine (Atkinson); (5) a physical allergy causing alteration in permeability of cell membranes and interference with water and electrolyte balance (Williams); for this, vasodilator drugs are recommended; (6) eustachian tube obstruction, with resulting secondary pressure changes in the labyrinth; and (7) bacterial toxemia. The evidence seems to be good that factors which favor a retention of fluid in the body aggravate the symptoms of the disorder, but this has not been found to be the cause by all investigators. Dehydration and a low sodium intake improve many but not all cases. The best available evidence indicates that Meniere's disease is associated with hydrops of the labyrinth.

Symptoms: They are striking and are not readily mistaken for those of other diseases. The onset is usually sudden and apoplectic but may in other instances be more gradual. A sudden attack of *vertigo* ushers in the attack, the first and subsequent attacks appearing like a bolt from the blue. Often premonitory symptoms of a vague sort characterized by a generalized uneasiness or nervousness provide warning of an impending attack and constitute a sort of aura. Hyperacusis may be present before the attack. Loudness recruitment appears to be typical of Meniere's disease (Dix and Hallpike). The dizziness develops suddenly, is associated with both subjective and objective vertigo, and frequently results in a fall and collapse. Staggering accompanies the attack, but is often not a disturbing symptom, since the vertigo is so severe that afflicted subjects lie down immediately. The vertigo may persist despite recumbency, but more often relief is obtained by lying down, the patient guarding himself against all movement, particularly of the head, in order to avoid recurrence of the attack. Rotation of the head, or the head and body, to one or both sides may precipitate severe vertigo during the height of the attack. Nausea and vomiting usually are found, the skin is cold and clammy, perspiration profuse, and the pulse rapid during the acute episode. The attack may last for several minutes or hours, or in severe cases may persist for days during which feeding is almost impossible. So severe are the attacks that sufferers with the disease live in dread lest the attacks recur. In other instances, the episodes of vertigo are not apoplectic, but are none the less disturbing.

The episodes appear at irregular intervals and are precipitated by no definite factors. Long intervals of freedom from attacks are not uncommon. Associated with the attacks of vertigo are tinnitus and deafness which are as disturbing to the patient as the vertigo but to which the patient may make an adequate adjustment. Tinnitus may precede the onset of vertigo for months or years and may involve one or both ears. It is persistent but may be inconstant, varying from time to time. Deafness is progressive and may be unilateral or bilateral. It is usually unilateral and, like tinnitus, may precede the vertigo, sometimes by years.

Auditory symptoms constitute an important feature of Meniere's disease. They develop pari passu with the vertigo as a rule, but may precede or follow it. Tinnitus is present in 90 per cent of cases. Deafness is of the perceptive type and varies with the state of the endolymphatic pressure and is always worse in the active phase. Hearing often improves between attacks of vertigo. The deafness is characterized by an excessive sensitivity to loud sounds. Diplacusis (the hearing of a single tone as if it were two tones of different pitch) is often present. Recruitment is characteristic of Meniere's disease.

Examination during an acute episode reveals horizontal or rotary nystagmus, pass-pointing, and difficulty in standing and walking. Between episodes nothing can be demonstrated on examination except the evidence of nerve deafness in one or both ears. It has been asserted that genuine Meniere's attack is invariably associated with spontaneous nystagmus. Systemic examination, as a rule, fails to reveal significant findings in sinuses, teeth, tonsils, or other possible foci of infection, or in the cardiorenal or other systems. Bárány tests are variable, and may give normal responses or may give signs of hypo- or hyper-function.

Diagnosis: This is not difficult. The history of attacks of dizziness associated with tinnitus and progressive deafness is simulated by very few diseases. The complete absence of neurological findings, except for the perceptive or nerve deafness, is important in diagnosis. The special features of the disturbances of hearing, particularly recruitment, are helpful. *Acute labyrinthitis* due to infection or toxic causes produces severe attacks of vertigo which simulate those of Meniere's syndrome, but the history of long-standing tinnitus and deafness is not obtained. Moreover, the condition is acute, tends to improve, and can usually be referred to no specific cause. In those instances in which tinnitus and hearing disturbances precede the vertigo by periods of varying duration, the diagnosis is impossible to establish until vertigo appears. *Cerebellopontine angle tumor* offers difficulties in rare instances, but usually presents no problem. Vertigo, much less apoplectic attacks of dizziness, is quite uncommon in angle tumor, but it may be found in some cases. The absence of choked disc, and of an absent corneal reflex, cerebellar signs, and of the typical Bárány findings of an angle tumor will exclude this disorder. Meniere's cases show no findings save deafness between attacks; angle tumor cases will show the signs mentioned. *Infiltrating tumors of the brain stem* may simulate Meniere's disease but are associated with numerous neurological findings indicative of their presence. *Tubal occlusion* has been regarded as a cause of vertigo similar to that of Meniere's disease, but the vertigo in such instances is usually mild and fails to resemble that of Meniere's disease. *Occlusion of the posterior inferior cerebellar artery* causes severe apoplectic vertigo and often ushers in the disease, but it is not recurrent and other evidences of the disorder are always present. *Bruns' syndrome* may resemble Meniere's disease closely. It is recurrent, is characterized by severe, incapacitating vertigo and "blackouts." It may be associated with no evidence of central nervous system involvement such as cerebellar signs or other disorders. *Multiple sclerosis* may be associated with recurrent vertigo. In a well-established case evidences of central nervous system disease are present.

Vestibular neuronitis is characterized by vertigo, usually but not always paroxysmal, and by the absence of cochlear signs and symptoms (Dix and Hallpike). It affects subjects from thirty to fifty years of age chiefly. The character of the vertigo sometimes distinguishes it from Meniere's disease, as well as the absence of cochlear symptoms. The vertigo may consist of sudden and transient seizures accompanied by sensations of blackout. Or there may be no paroxysms, but a feeling of being top heavy or off balance, especially in standing or walking. The onset is often associated with a febrile illness, or with evidence of foci of infection in the ear, nose and throat.

Treatment: The treatment of Meniere's disease is not uniform. Since concepts vary so widely concerning its nature, it follows that several forms of treatment are available. The treatment of Meniere's disease has two phases: (1) the treatment of the acute attack (2) interim treatment, directed toward prevention of further episodes.

The treatment of the *acute attack* offers serious difficulties. Once the attack is established it is difficult to control it. Vomiting is usually present and retention of medication by mouth is difficult.

If this is impossible atropine sulfate 0.4 to 0.8 mg. ($\frac{1}{150}$ to $\frac{1}{75}$ grain) by hypodermic is helpful. If medications can be retained by mouth sodium bromide 1 to 2 Gm. (15 to 30 grains) is often helpful. Ephedrine sulfate gr. $1\frac{1}{2}$ may be tried, as well as amphetamine sulfate 5 to 10 mg. Dramamine (dimenhydrinate), 50 mg. intramuscularly, is helpful. Sodium Amytal, $7\frac{1}{2}$ grains intravenously, may be of use. This may be repeated in two hours.

Of the interim treatments, that which is concerned with the limitation of fluids and of sodium intake, the Furstenberg regimen, has much to recommend it. It must be carried out carefully and painstakingly in order to be successful. The regimen as recommended by Furstenberg is as follows:

The patient takes a diet free from salt and soda. This means that no salt is used at the table or in cooking. The patient is put on a rather strict diet, as herein recommended. Ammonium chloride is given as follows: Six capsules of 0.5 Gm. each ($7\frac{1}{2}$ grains), three times a day (with each meal). This means a total of eighteen capsules, $7\frac{1}{2}$ grains each, of ammonium chloride per day. They are taken while the patient eats his food, and they must not be replaced by the chocolate-coated or the enteric-coated pills, because the latter sometimes pass through the gastrointestinal tract without being absorbed. The ammonium chloride is given in this dosage for three days and then omitted for two days. This can be carried on indefinitely without injurious effects. The patient's ingestion of fluids is not restricted, although he must not drink excessive quantities of liquid.

The diet should consist of: (1) low sodium content, *i. e.*, no salt, soda, or baking powder is to be used; (2) animal protein and cereal products unrestricted (except milk); (3) vegetables, fruits, and milk limited; (4) calories sufficient to maintain a desirable weight; (5) water unrestricted.

Another form of medical treatment, based on the vasoconstrictor concept, makes use of vasodilators. For this purpose, the following are used: nicotinic acid, 100 mg. three or more times daily; amyl or potassium nitrite, or methacholine bromide (200 mg., 2 or 5 times daily). Of these nicotinic acid by mouth is the most valuable, given in doses of 300-600 mg. daily. Its effect is produced largely by its vasodilator mechanism.

Thiamine chloride in large doses (100 mg.) is effective in some cases, especially when given in conjunction with nicotinic acid. It should be given daily, intravenously at first if the vertigo is severe, and subsequently subcutaneously or intramuscularly. It may be continued for long periods.

Histamine is recommended in some patients, especially in those with a definitely positive intradermal reaction. As a result of the histamine skin test, two groups of patients may be distinguished: histamine-positive and histamine-negative. The histamine-positive group reacts as it does because it possesses a primary vasodilator mechanism; the histamine-negative group is assumed to possess a primary vasoconstrictor mechanism (Atkinson). The former group is made worse by vasodilator drugs and the latter by vasoconstrictors. The histamine-positive group is treated by histamine desensitization, while the histamine-negative group is treated by vasodilators, such as nicotinic acid. Some believe that all the patients should receive histamine. The drug may be given intravenously in doses of 2.75 mg. of histaminic acid phosphate dissolved in 250 cc. of normal saline, given over a period of $2\frac{1}{2}$ hours at a rate of 30-40 drops per minute. Since the drug is administered slowly, there is no change in blood pressure or pulse rate. The method is particularly valuable in those patients in whom vertigo is violent and vomiting severe. One administration, however, does not prevent future attacks. The drug may be given also subcutaneously in the following fashion: 0.05 mg. twice daily for two days; 0.066 mg. for two days; 0.1 mg. daily thereafter for two to four weeks, and at less frequent intervals after this.

Magnesium sulfate intravenously in doses of 4 to 5 cc. of a 50 per cent solution is advocated by some observers, but it is not without its dangers. Its effects may be counteracted by 1 cc. of 5 per cent calcium gluconate.

Potassium salts are sometimes valuable. They may be given in convenient form as potassium nitrate (enteric coated) (7½ grains), two tablets three times daily, or as potassium chloride 6-10 Gm. daily in divided doses in aqueous solution or fruit juices.

Dramamine (50 mg.) is useful in some cases, and may be given in doses of one tablet three or four times daily.

Other suggested remedies include diethylstilbestrol, 1 mg. daily; thyroid, 15 mg. (¼ grain) three to four times daily; and Banthine, 50 mg. four times daily.

Section of the vestibular portion of the auditory nerve has been practiced in Meniere's disease. The procedure has a place in treatment of the disorder, but is rarely necessary and should be reserved for severe cases which defy treatment by other methods.

VIII. COMA

Special problems are created by patients in coma, since the situation is usually urgent and one's decision as to the cause of the coma is dependent almost entirely on the history and upon an incomplete physical survey. *Examination* of the comatose patient should include, first of all, a careful history concerning the onset of the difficulty. Unfortunately, over two-thirds of patients entering the hospital in coma come without a history, and this despite the fact that in diabetes, hyperinsulinism, poisoning, traumatic shock, exsanguination, subdural hematoma, brain tumor, meningitis, and eclampsia, coma is an emergency problem. Much can be learned concerning cause from the nature of onset. A history of trauma, alcoholism, suicidal attempt, or of status epilepticus gives valuable information concerning the cause of the coma. Much can be learned by observation of the pulse, respirations, and temperature, since stertorous breathing, bounding pulse, and temperature elevation indicate hemorrhage. The blood pressure should be taken, since hypertension may be present. Careful attention should be paid to the pupillary reactions, since pupils which fail to react to light are a bad omen in a patient in coma. Inequality of the pupils is common, but its significance is difficult to evaluate. It has no absolute value. The fundi should be examined for evidences of choked disc or neuroretinitis.

Evidences of meningeal irritation should be sought for. The breath should be smelled for evidence of diabetes, uremia, illuminating gas, or alcoholic excess. Evidences of focal brain damage, such as hemiplegia, offer valuable indications of a destructive brain lesion but give no indication as to the cause of the lesion, whether vascular, neoplastic, inflammatory, etc. The limbs of the paralyzed side drop more limply to the bed when raised and released. On forceful, painful flexion of the terminal phalanx of the finger or toe of the paralyzed side, the limb will not be withdrawn, while on the normal side forceful retraction of the limbs takes place. Examination of the urine by catheterization should be made.

Lumbar puncture is indicated if there are evidences of meningeal irritation. Blood sugar and nonprotein nitrogen estimations are important.

In summary, therefore, the examination of the comatose patient should include (1) history; (2) physical examination, with special reference to trauma, pupillary reactions, odor of the breath, neck stiffness, fractures, etc.; (3) roentgenologic studies where indicated, as in suspected extradural hemorrhage; (4) gastric lavage for all poisonings and severe alcoholics; (5) urinalysis (catheterized) and blood-sugar determination; and (6) lumbar puncture.

The frequency of the various causes of coma in their frequency is given in Table 12 (Solomon and Aring).

Trauma and alcoholism outstrip all other conditions as causes of coma.

Cerebral hemorrhage is often associated with coma. The story indicates a sudden apoplectic onset often in a patient with a previous history of hypertension, with elevated blood pressure. florid facies, stertorous breathing, bounding pulse, and profuse perspiration. *Cerebral thrombosis* may be accompanied by coma provided the vessel occluded is large and the area of softening extensive, or if the occluded vessel is in a vital area. such as the medulla. In cerebral vascular lesions, onset with coma favors cerebral hemorrhage by far as compared with cerebral thrombosis. Coma is common also in *cerebral embolism*. Sudden onset with coma characterizes the onset in some forms of *brain tumor,* such as the glioblastoma multiforme, into which sudden hemorrhage may occur. Coma may supervene suddenly also in brain tumor associated with a sudden increase of intracranial pressure, as in straining at stool or following administration of an enema. Choked disc will be found in tumor cases. In the cases associated with

Table 12

Frequency of Causes of Coma

	No. of Cases	Per Cent
ALCOHOL	690	59.1
TRAUMA	152	13.0
CEREBRAL VASCULAR LESIONS	118	2.8
POISONING	33	2.4
EPILEPSY	28	1.7
DIABETES	20	1.7
MENINGITIS	20	1.7
PNEUMONIA	20	1.7
CARDIAC DECOMPENSATION	17	1.4
EXSANGUINATION	10	0.9
SYPHILIS OF CENTRAL NERVOUS SYSTEM	7	0.6
UREMIA	7	0.6
ECLAMPSIA	7	0.6
MISCELLANEOUS	38	3.2
	1167	100.0

onset after suddenly increased pressure, embarrassment of respiration is prominent due to herniation of the medulla through the foramen magnum. There may be Cheyne-Stokes respirations or slowed breathing. *Subarachnoid hemorrhage* may be ushered in by coma. The history of onset is characteristic, with sudden apoplectic headache and unconsciousness. Signs of meningeal irritation are present and lumbar puncture will reveal blood in the spinal fluid. *Convulsions* are often associated with coma, but by the time the patient is seen the convulsive attack is usually over; hence the history is all important. *Status epilepticus* is a particularly important cause of coma. Many conditions may be responsible for convulsions (*v.* Epilepsy). *Trauma* may be associated with coma under a variety of circumstances. It is not infrequently found in cortical laceration and contusion, and may persist under these circumstances for several hours or a few days. A particularly important consequence of trauma which is invaria- bly associated with coma is seen in mid- dle meningeal (extradural) hemorrhage. The coma in this condition is progres- sive, is sometimes delayed, and is asso- ciated with characteristic changes in blood pressure, pulse, etc. (*v.* Cranial Trauma). *Intoxications* of various sorts may be associated with coma. Excessive use of bromides or barbiturates may re- sult in coma, especially when used with suicidal intent. The history is usually clear in this condition. Alcohol is a com- mon cause. *Meningitis* of various sorts may be associated with coma. The coma is apt to be gradual in development, is accompanied by fever, signs of menin- geal irritation, and an increase of cells in the spinal fluid. It is readily detected as a cause of coma by the characteristic signs of meningitis. *Cardiac decompensa- tion* is a not uncommon cause of coma and is frequently overlooked. *Exsan- guination* is occasionally a cause of coma in esophageal varices due to cirrhosis of the liver, carcinomatous erosion of the gastrointestinal tract, rupture of aortic aneurysm, and hemoptysis. Among the *miscellaneous* causes are burns, encepha- litis, miliary tuberculosis, carcinomatosis, heart block, pernicious anemia, hysteria, leukemia, septicemia, and empyema.

IX. PAIN

Pain is such a frequent symptom that a consideration of its many causes is hardly feasible. More important than a review in detail of its causes is an analy- sis of the characteristic features of pain as it is encountered at various levels of the nervous system.

Peripheral nerve pain is an outstand- ing feature of peripheral nerve disease. such as neuritis, tumor, injury, etc. Its outstanding feature lies in its distribu- tion along the course of the affected nerve. Thus, in *ulnar nerve pain,* the distribution will be along the ulnar side of the arm and hand and in the fourth and fifth fingers; in *median nerve pain* along the median aspect of the hand and the thumb and first two fingers; in *sciatic pain,* along the back and side of the thigh and in the calf, etc. A history of pain will suffice to elicit its distribution and to make clear in most instances its periph- eral nature. Special types of peripheral nerve pain are seen in the pain of trigem- inal and glossopharyngeal neuralgia.

Peripheral nerve pain is constant or intermittent; hence no specific informa- tion is elicited from this aspect of its features. It is not infrequently asso- ciated with paresthesias. Increase of intraspinal pressure, as in coughing, sneezing, straining, etc., does not as a rule aggravate it, except in instances in which both the peripheral nerve and the posterior roots are affected as in triortho- cresyl phosphate (Jamaica ginger) neu- ritis or in neuronitis. It may be asso- ciated with sensory disturbances, but this is a variable feature dependent on the degree of involvement of the nerve, the degree of recovery from the lesion respon- sible for the nerve involvement, and the acuteness of the disease. Painful pares- thesias of a most disabling nature are characteristic of incomplete or irritative lesions of the peripheral nerve following injury. Sensory disturbances, both sub- jective and objective, occur in alcoholic neuritis, arsenic neuritis, etc., and are of- ten absent in acute infectious polyneuritis.

Radicular (posterior root) pain due to involvement of the posterior roots is found in a number of conditions: tabes dorsalis, spinal cord tumor, tuberculosis of the spine, pachymeningitis, herpes zos- ter, traumatic injuries of the spine, osteo- arthritis of the vertebrae, herniated nu- cleus pulposus, etc. It is characterized by distribution along the anatomical course of the root or roots which are affected. This can be determined by a glance at the root zone charts. The root pains most commonly misinterpreted are those of the middle and lower thoracic distributions, the pain in these areas being mistaken often for visceral disease. Thus pain in root zones T_4 to T_8 is mistaken often for gallbladder or stomach disease; pain in root zones T_8 to T_{10} for kidney disease, etc. Root pain is usually periodic, often paroxysmal, but may be constant. It is severe as a rule, reaching its greatest heights in the gastric crises of tabes. It is aggravated by any maneuvers which increase intraspinal pressure, such as coughing, sneezing, straining at stool, etc. Associated with the pain of root syndromes is evidence of superficial sensory changes, such as hyperesthesia in the skin in the involved root or roots, or decreased sensation to touch or pain (hypesthesia or hypalgesia). Because of the rich overlapping of adjacent root zones, sensory changes may not be detected in root disease unless more than a single root is affected. The diagnosis of root disease must often be established therefore on the characteristics of the root pain alone.

Central pain is a term used for pain originating within the central nervous system itself. Pain of central origin is possible at various levels: spinal cord, brain stem, thalamus, and cerebral cortex. Pain of *spinal cord* origin is seen in infiltrating tumors of the spinal cord and syringomyelia particularly. It is usually deep, ill-defined as to localization within a limb or limbs, and may be either constant or paroxysmal, more commonly the latter. It may be radicular in nature. It is often described as boring, cutting, etc. It is invariably associated with other evidences of spinal cord disease. It is due either to irritation of the pain fibers in the posterior horns of the spinal cord or to spinothalamic tract involvement.

Thalamic pain occurs particularly with the thalamic syndrome (*v.* Vascular diseases). It is characterized by a severe pain involving the arm and leg opposite to the lesion; it is deep, paroxysmal, or constant, and refractory to ordinary analgesics. With it are associated all the evidences of a thalamic syndrome, with hemisensory disturbances. Pain of *cortical* origin is rare, but it has been recorded in tumors involving the parietal lobe and in cysts of this area. It may involve any part of the opposite side of the body and has the same characteristics as other types of central pain. Intractable pain in the face or in the limbs may follow a thalamic syndrome. It is deep, often burning, and unyielding to treatment.

5

Neuritis and the Neuralgias

I. NEURITIS

1. General Features

Definition: Neuritis is a disease of the peripheral and cranial nerves, characterized by inflammation or degeneration of the nerves, with resulting impairment or loss of conduction along the nerve fibers, and by varying degrees of motor, sensory and reflex impairment. The term implies an inflammation, but in many instances no inflammation can be shown to be present. Hence the term "neuropathy" (Wechsler) has been suggested which simply substitutes one term for another without clarifying the problem. The term neuritis has the advantage of long usage. So long as one is aware of the fact that in many forms, as, for example, in parenchymatous neuritis, no inflammation is present, there is little danger of misunderstanding the term.

Classification: Many forms of neuritis are known, but in general they may be divided into the following main types: (a) *Mononeuritis,* involving a single nerve trunk; (b) *polyneuritis* or *multiple neuritis,* involving several nerve trunks.

Pathology: Neuritis may be divided from a pathological standpoint into the following groups:

1. *Interstitial Neuritis:* (a) Acute; (b) chronic (interstitial hypertrophic neuritis). 2. *Parenchymatous Neuritis.*

The normal peripheral nerve in cross section is composed of the epineurium surrounding the entire nerve, the perineurium surrounding the nerve bundles, and the endoneurium around individual fibers of small groups of fibers. These fibrous sheaths are spoken of as the interstitial portions of the nerves as contrasted with the parenchymatous portion composed of the axis cylinders and their myelin sheaths. No effort will be made to outline the histological features of normal nerve, save to point out the broad differentiation into these larger components.

The blood supply of nerves is received through the vasa vasorum and by means of nutrient arteries of adjacent vessels. The origin and number of the nutrient arteries supplying any given nerve are variable and there are long segments of nerve which do not receive a nutrient artery (Richards). The blood supply of a nerve is fundamentally segmental, with considerable overlap of supply between nutrient arteries entering the nerve at various levels. Thus a single vessel fails to dominate the circulation in a particular segment of nerve and collateral circulation is available on occlusion of one of the regional arteries.

A few general principles concerning the characteristics of nerves in health and disease appear to be pertinent. A cross section of any mixed nerve reveals the fact that it is composed of both myelinated and unmyelinated fibers with the former predominating. Furthermore, it is readily apparent that the size of the fibers varies greatly, some being thick and others thin. Conduction is fastest in the large fibers and slowest in the small. The myelinated fibers are thickest and conduct impulses faster than the small fibers.

147

By means of oscillograph recordings, it has been possible to classify nerve fibers into various groups and to correlate to some extent definite functions with specific types of fibers. There are three main types, classified according to their speed of conduction: A (fastest), B (intermediate), C (slowest). The A fibers are largest and mediate afferent impulses from proprioceptive receptors in skeletal muscles and tactile receptors in the skin. The B fibers are small myelinated fibers found chiefly in the preganglionic fibers of the autonomic nervous system. The C fibers are smallest and unmyelinated and mediate pain and temperature.

Ischemic changes in the nerve cause a falling out of sensations in the following sequence: Light touch, delay in appreciation of pin prick together with loss of cold, motor fibers, warmth, and finally pain. Local anesthesia causes a falling out in the following order: cold, warmth, pain, pressure. Spinal anesthesia produces a disappearance of sensation in the following sequence: pain, cold, warmth, pressure; and pressure causes disappearance as follows: pressure, cold, warmth, pain. From observations such as this and from the blocking of impulses by cocainization, it has been found that there exists a correlation between the types of fibers and the mediation of specific types of sensation. Pressure appears to be widely distributed in the fastest A fibers. Cold is chiefly mediated through the smallest A fibers; light touch through the larger A fibers; and pain through the B fibers.

Disease of a peripheral nerve by neuritis is capable of interrupting nerve conduction of all fibers, or it may involve some and leave others unharmed. In consequence, it is not surprising to find evidence of partial motor and/or sensory involvement in varying degrees. Nerve function, moreover, may be interrupted by neuritis at one point, at several points, or all along an entire nerve trunk, depending on the nature of the harmful agent.

1. Interstitial neuritis: This is found chiefly in the connective sheaths of the nerve, particularly in the perineurium and endoneurium, the changes in the nerve fibers probably following secondarily to these. The connective tissue sheaths are infiltrated with polynuclear cells or lymphocytes, depending on the nature of the infection. The blood vessels are dilated and at times small hemorrhages are visible. In mild cases there is a breaking up of myelin and a tendency on the part of the axis cylinders to swell and curl. In more severe cases, the myelin is completely broken up and the axis cylinders severely damaged.

Interstitial neuritis is found chiefly in infectious diseases. *Diphtheria* is commonly associated with this form of neuritis. In addition to infiltration of the interstitial tissue with polynuclear cells, hyperemia and hemorrhages are pronounced, and the myelin is damaged; the axis cylinders do not suffer severely.

Leprosy is associated with a severe interstitial neuritis which in many areas becomes nodular. The infiltration is lymphocytic and often perivascular. The myelin stains poorly and the axis cylinders are damaged, often severely. The interstitial reaction becomes so marked in the course of time as to cause a marked thickening of the connective tissue sheaths and an enlargement of the caliber of the nerves.

Syphilis is associated with a lymphocytic interstitial neuritis, seen particularly in the cranial nerves. *Malaria* and *periarteritis nodosa* are associated with this form of neuritis. In the latter it is characterized by a spotty myelin degeneration and by axonal degeneration. The blood vessels show the typical changes associated with the condition. A special form is seen in the *hypertrophic interstitial neuritis* (Dejerine-Sottas) characterized by marked hypertrophy of the sheaths of Schwann associated with proliferation of the Schwann cells and the formation of whorls. The myelin is degenerated and the axis cylinders destroyed. In some instances, an interstitial neuritis

in the interstitial tissue. Similar changes are found in lead neuritis.

Etiology: Neuritis is due to a wide variety of causes. These may be summarized best in Table 13.

It would be impossible to discuss all the causes of neuritis in detail. The causes of mononeuritis are discussed below under this heading. The causes of

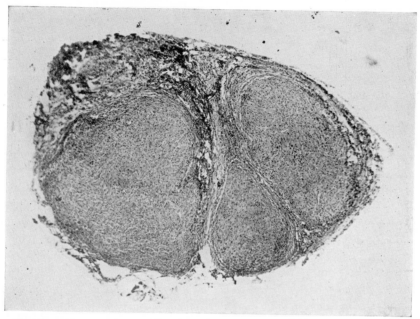

Fig. 53—*Interstitial neuritis.* Cross section of a peripheral nerve showing infiltration of the epineural and perineural sheaths.

develops as the result of infiltration of the nerve sheaths by hematogenous cells in *leukemia* and by carcinoma cells in *carcinoma.*

2. *Parenchymatous neuritis:* On the other hand, this form is unassociated with infiltrations of the nerve trunk but is characterized primarily by degeneration of the axis cylinders and myelin sheaths. It is found particularly in neuritis due to exogenous poisons, such as alcohol, lead, etc.; in avitaminoses; and in deficiency states. In alcoholic neuritis, the changes in the myelin and axis cylinders are often severe and proliferative changes are found

multiple neuritis are of a systemic or general nature as compared with the local causes of a mononeuritis.

Focal Infection: Infection in the teeth, tonsils, sinuses, prostate, bladder, kidney, or gastrointestinal tract is sometimes the cause, though there is great divergence of opinion about its importance. Its incidence is greatly exaggerated by its enthusiasts, but its denial as a factor in neuritis cannot be substantiated. The recovery from neuritis following removal of a bona fide focus of infection is strong evidence that this plays a part in the production of the

A

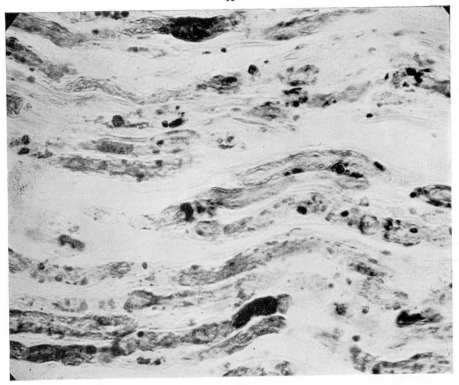

B

Fig. 54—*Parenchymatous neuritis* in a case of porphyria. A, Marchi degeneration of a peripheral nerve showing the destruction of the myelin sheaths. B, Demyelination in the anterior root, seen in myelin sheath stain, and showing areas of loss of staining corresponding to the demyelinated portions.

neuritis, though the mechanism is not well understood.

Fevers: Neuritis has been reported following or during the course of many fevers. Whether these cases should be regarded as cases of true multiple neuritis is open to discussion if this disease is confined to those instances in which a bilateral symmetrical neuritis is found. The fact remains, however, that neuritis has been recorded many times during such conditions as rheumatic fever, typhoid fever, influenza, pneumonia, malaria, and other fevers listed in Table 13. It occurs also during tuberculosis. There is nothing distinctive in the type of neuritis found in these disorders.

of beriberi, the response of alcoholic neuritis to thiamine injections, and the cure of such neuritis with thiamine despite continued ingestion of alcohol, all point to the importance of thiamine deficiency as the cause of alcoholic neuritis.

Table 13—Causes of Multiple Neuritis

Infection	Deficiency and Metabolism	Chemical and Drugs	Toxic
VIRUS BACTERIAL	Pellagra Beriberi Alcohol Pregnancy Carcinoma Diabetes Porphyrinuria Sprue Amyloid disease Polyarteritis nodosa	Lead Mercury Gold Antimony Arsenic Phosphorus Trichlorethylphosphate Aniline Carbon disulphide Carbon monoxide Dinitrobenzol	Sulfonamides Penicillin Isonicotinic acid hydrazide

Avitaminosis: This has been emphasized as the cause of the neuritis of alcoholism. It has also been shown to be the cause of neuritis in beriberi, pregnancy, and in many forms of gastrointestinal disorders, such as celiac disease, ulcerative colitis, stricture of the sigmoid, gastric carcinoma, gastric polyps, pyloric stenosis, and short-circuiting operations on the bowel. In alcoholism, the neuritis, as in beriberi, is due to a lack of thiamine (vitamin B_1). The similarity of the alcoholic symptomatology to that

Despite the evidence pointing to a thiamine deficiency in alcoholic neuritis, some doubt still exists with regard to thiamine deficiency as the sole factor in alcoholic neuritis.

In vitamin B_1 deficiency the chief biochemical abnormality within the nerve cells is a failure in the normal oxidative metabolism of the pyruvic acid formed during the breakdown of glucose. Pyruvate accumulates in the tissues and blood and nerve cells are deprived of their normal source of energy. A rise in the pyruvic acid level of the blood has been demonstrated in experimental vitamin B_1 deficiency and in humans vitamin B_1 deficiency even of mild degree have been detected by the blood pyruvate level.

Failure of some cases to respond to thiamine treatment has resulted in doubt concerning thiamine as the only causative factor. This objection is probably answered by the observation that neuritis resulting from thiamine deficiency

Table 14—Diagnosis of Cervical Rib Syndrome

Disease	Pain	Weakness	Vascular Symptoms	Sensory	Roentgen Ray	Miscellaneous
CERVICAL RIB	Shoulder (anterior), neck, arm and hand along peripheral nerve	In area of affected nerve, involving arm or hand muscles, or both	1. Weak or absent radial pulse 2. Low blood pressure on affected side	Present or absent in peripheral nerve distribution	Cervical rib; rudimentary rib; long transverse process	Horner's syndrome absent
SUPERIOR PULMONARY SULCUS TUMOR	Shoulder (posterior), axilla, arm, hand	In area of affected nerve, usually small hand muscles	None	Present	Shadow in apex of lung	Horner's syndrome constant and early
NEURITIS	Along peripheral nerves of arm	In area of affected nerve	None	Present in acute cases, Tenderness muscles & nerves	No findings	Horner's syndrome not present
BURSITIS	Local pain in shoulder	None; limitation of motion due to pain	None	None	Calcification of bursa in some cases	None
CERVICAL CORD TUMOR	Neck, shoulder, arm, radicular in distribution	Hands, shoulder girdle, arms (atrophy), later arms and legs	None	More or less well-defined sensory level	Changes in roentgen ray sometimes seen; erosion of bone	Horner's syndrome may or may not be present
ARTHRITIS	Shoulder and neck	None as a rule	None	None	Arthritis of spine	None
CERVICAL HERNIATED DISC	Root pain in shoulder and arm	Shoulder girdle muscles, arm also Atrophy may be present	None	In root areas of affected roots	Narrowed intervertebral discs	

is associated after a relatively short time with irreversible changes in the nerves, thus making correction of the deficiency ineffectual. Recent studies tend to show also that the period of hospitalization is frequently not decreased in cases of alcoholic multiple neuritis treated with thiamine. Similarly, in the neuritis developing during pregnancy, thiamine lack is assumed to be due to the persistent vomiting, and poor assimilation of foods. Factors giving rise to the neuritis are the persistent vomiting associated with the condition, nausea leading to decreased food intake, excessive intake of carbohydrate foods poor in thiamine, increased requirements of thiamine due to raised metabolism and increased fetal demands, and possibly poor assimilation due to low gastric acidity. The cause of the neuritis in the pernicious vomiting of pregnancy is probably a thiamine deficiency; the neuritis which develops in this fashion has no distinctive features. Pain and weakness are outstanding and the muscle and nerve tenderness, absence of reflexes, and sensory changes found in mixed nerve disease are all present. Atrophy of the muscles may be severe or mild. In most, if not all, of the cases of neuritis associated with the gastrointestinal conditions enumerated above, the thiamine lack is due to poor assimilation and absorption of proper vitamins. The neuritis of diabetes is said to be due also to thiamine deficiency but the evidence is not so clear as in the case of other disorders. The same may be said concerning thiamine deficiency in lead neuritis.

Virus Disorders: They are sometimes associated with neuritis. Certain cases of parotitis assumed to be due to a virus are sometimes associated with a multiple neuritis. Acute febrile polyneuritis is believed to be the result of virus in-fection. Anti-rabies vaccination has been associated with multiple neuritis.

Chemicals: Neuritis due to *chemicals* is sometimes important to recognize. In such instances, the neuritis results from direct action of the chemicals on the nerve tissue. Lead, arsenic, trichlorethylene, triorthocresyl phosphate, and carbon disulfide have a special affinity for peripheral nerves. Carbon disulfide neuritis occurs not infrequently in rayon workers. Carbon monoxide may at times cause a multiple neuritis in accidental or intentional exposures to the gas. In triorthocresyl phosphate neuritis due to Jamaica ginger ingestion or poisoning with apiol, there is extensive and severe neuritis with evidence of anterior horn involvement. Among rare causes are phosphorus, dinitrobenzene, and aniline. Phosphorus poisoning is found chiefly in matchmakers. The sulfonamides are at times associated with neuritis. Roentgen irradition has been complicated by flaccid paralysis without sensory loss.

There is some objection to the inclusion of so many widely divergent causes of neuritis. Walshe asserts that of the numerous causes usually listed, only about ten can be really incriminated. He would restrict multiple neuritis to those diseases producing a bilateral symmetrical affection of the nerve trunks. including both motor and sensory fibers. He divides neuritis into an acute infective type. a subacute variety of which diphtheritic neuritis is an example, and a chronic type of which the alcoholic variety is a paradigm.

Enough consideration has been given to the causes of neuritis to indicate that. in the problem of neuritis, the search for cause often supersedes the problem of diagnosis. In the consideration of the specific forms of neuritis, cause will be discussed further.

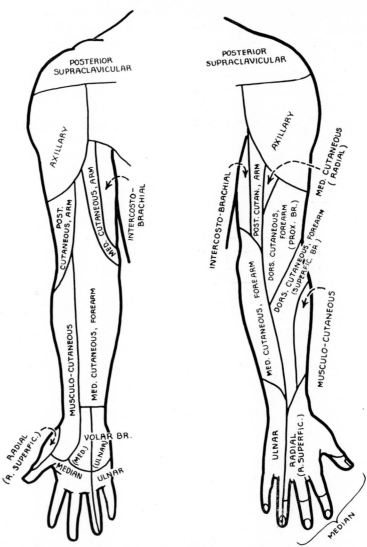

Fig. 55—*Peripheral nerve distribution* **of the upper limbs indicating the peripheral nerve innervation.**

General Symptoms: The symptoms of neuritis are similar in most respects for all cases of neuritis regardless of the cause, but they vary in their combinations. The symptoms of neuritis, whether multiple or mononeuritis, are due to a combination of factors. The pain is probably the result of irritation or stimulation of the peripheral nerve by the disease process. Break in the conduction of the nerve trunk accounts for the mus- cular weakness and the reflex changes, as well as the sensory disturbances. The degree of symptom deficiency varies with the many forms of neuritis and with the seriousness of injury of the nerve. In many forms of neuritis such as that due to alcohol, arsenic, porphyria, diabetes, vitamin deficiency, and virus infection (acute infectious polyneuritis) the nerve damage is severe, whereas in other forms it is mild or moderate. In some forms of neuritis the peripheral nerve injury may involve only focal parts of the nerve, as in ischemic neuritis, while in other forms it affects long stretches of the nerve trunk. As in the case of nerve injury, the closer the damage to the cell of origin, the more severe the effects. In some forms of neuritis the entire reflex arc is affected as in some forms of diabetic neuritis, acute infectious polyneuritis, alcoholic neuritis and arsenic neuritis. *Sensory* symptoms of one sort or another are present in most cases of neuritis. Chief among these is *pain,* which is usually the most distressing and urgent symptom. Its location varies with

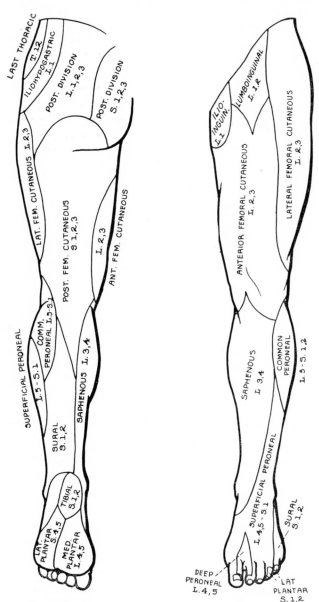

Fig. 56—*Peripheral nerve distribution* of the lower limbs indicating the cutaneous peripheral nerve innervation with their roots of origin.

the nerve or nerves affected, but a careful history will indicate clearly that it is distributed along the course of the affected nerve or nerves. It is variously described, is constant both day and night as a rule, but may be intermittent. Sometimes pain is absent in purely motor forms of neuritis. It is the one symptom demanding immediate relief. *Paresthesias* are found in some forms of neuritis. The hyperesthesias of alcoholic neuritis involving the feet are especially distressing. Hyperesthesias are also prominent in beriberi and in arsenical neuritis. *Tenderness of the muscles and nerve trunks* is always present in some degree in neuritis involving mixed nerves. It is absent in purely motor neuritis. It is sometimes extremely severe and at other times it is minimal. As a rule, it is well pronounced in most cases of neuritis. In acute infectious polyneuritis (Guillain-Barré) it is often minimal. Tenderness of the tendons, such as the *tendo achillis*, is often found. *Objective sensory changes* are commonly found. Their distribution depends on the nerves affected. They may be much less apparent than subjective sensory disturbances and may frequently be absent except in severe cases, or early in the course of the disease. In severe cases, there is loss or impairment of all forms of sensation (touch, pain, heat, cold, position, vibration). It is not uncommon, however, to find some forms of sensation intact while others are affected (pain or temperature). This may be due to recovery of some nerve fibers or to a different susceptibility of the fibers to damage.

Motor symptoms are, as a rule, present. There may be severe motor loss, or only minor decrease of motor power. Complete or almost complete paralysis may be found in some cases. There is frequently dissociation between the motor and sensory symptoms. Thus, there may be severe sensory symptoms and signs, and slight motor manifestations, or *vice versa*. It is obvious that the degree of motor weakness or paralysis will be a measure of the degree of interruption of the nerve. The specific types of motor loss will be found under diseases of the individual nerves. *Reflex changes* of some degree are always present. The tendon reflexes of the affected limb or limbs may be lost or decreased. Normal tendon reflexes are not found in neuritis. *Sphincter disturbances* are absent in the vast majority of cases, but may be found in forms of neuritis affecting the entire nerve to the posterior roots (neuronitis). *Electrical reactions* are of practical importance only if there is means of testing them. There is often decreased irritability of the muscles. Reaction of degeneration may be present if the entire nerve is destroyed. The electrical reactions are important in determining the prognosis. *Trophic disturbances* are common. They are seen in loss of subcutaneous fat tissue in the affected areas, smoothness and loss of corrugation of the skin, and brittle nails. *Vasomotor disturbances*, such as cyanosis or cold extremities, are commonly seen after neuritis.

2. *Mononeuritis*

Definition: Mononeuritis is a neuritis involving only a single nerve or nerve trunk.

Etiology: The causes of a mononeuritis are varied but not so numerous as those of polyneuritis. Mononeuritis usually results from some local condition. *Trauma* with bone fracture is a common cause, the nerve being involved as a result of compression by displaced bone fragments. Dislocations also may cause a mononeuritis, especially those of the head of the humerus, or dislocations of the elbow. *Tumor* of a peripheral nerve may cause a solitary nerve paralysis.

Other local causes are *stab* and *gunshot* wounds, pressure from *crutches,* pressure from tight plaster *casts* on the legs (peroneal paralysis), compression from tight *bandages, cervical rib,* and *infection. Callous formation* especially involving the humerus or the bones at the elbow may cause a mononeuritis involving especially the ulnar or median nerves.

Ischemia has been implicated as a significant factor in many types of mononeuritis. It is seen most clearly in (1) *arterial embolism,* the peripheral nerve involvement in such cases being accompanied by muscle necrosis and nutritional disturbances of the skin and subcutaneous tissue. In some cases the nerves alone may be damaged. It is also observed in (2) trauma. In some instances the associated injury to a blood vessel may be readily apparent, but in many the ischemic factor is not clear. Volkmann's contracture has been found to be the result of ischemic necrosis of the flexor muscles in the forearm. (3) Tourniquet paralysis, (4) occlusive vascular disease, (5) periarteritis nodosa. It is seen also in musculospiral paralysis (Saturday night paralysis), from lying on the arm against a hard edge, as with the arm hanging over the edge of the bed or a chair. It is seen sometimes in jobs requiring constant kneeling, as in cranberry pickers, resulting in peroneal paralysis and footdrop. Involvement of isolated nerve trunks is seen at times in *thromboangiitis obliterans.* Ischemic neuritis is found also in *embolism* and *arteriosclerosis.* Prolonged ischemia by a blood pressure cuff in local operations on the hand is sometimes a cause of mononeuritis. Paralysis of peripheral nerves sometimes follows application of a *tourniquet* for hemostasis in operation on the limbs. The radial nerve is most often affected. The median, ulnar, and femoral nerves are less often affected. The paraly-

sis of the muscles in such cases is the result of ischemia of the nerve trunk, but degeneration of the nerve fibers due to direct pressure may play a role. A tight *corset* or a military belt is sometimes responsible for isolated invovlement of the lateral femoral cutaneous nerve. *Serum injections,* especially tetanus, diphtheria and pneumonia serum, may cause neuritis of a single nerve or of multiple trunks. *Diphtheria, tetanus, and leprosy* are other causes. There are many special causes of mononeuritis involving the sciatic trunk which will be discussed in a consideration of this problem.

Ischemic neuritis poses problems of great clinical interest. The onset of paralysis in tourniquet paralysis follows after pressure of variable duration, twenty minutes to more than one hour. That which follows pressure cuff application to the arm follows constantly in twenty-five minutes. Nerve paralysis following a pressure cuff has a centripetal onset and affects touch before pain, and pain before motion. After paralysis has begun, the placement of a second cuff below the first, followed by removal of the first cuff, is succeeded by recovery from the paralysis and its reappearance after a further latency due to pressure from the second cuff. This suggests that the paralysis in such instances is due to ischemia of the compressed segment of nerve. There appears to be a great variation in the rate of extent of conduction impairment by compression of nerves. This variation is probably the result of uneven pressure on the nerve bundles (Denny-Brown and Brenner). Pressure on the nerve affects the motor function more than the sensory.

A special form of ischemic neuritis, though not a mononeuritis, is seen in *saddle thrombus* involving the lower portion of the aorta at its bifurcation. This is due to (1) embolism, most commonly associated with rheumatic heart disease, (2) arteriosclerosis of the aorta with thrombus formation, (3) abdominal aneurysm with mural thrombosis, and (4) infection. The condition is characterized by severe, sudden pains in the legs at times radiating into the lower back or inguinal regions; cold and clammy of the spinal cord, due to lessened blood flow in the regional vessels (lumbar, middle sacral and lateral sacral arteries).

Symptoms: The symptoms of mononeuritis vary with the cause. In most instances, the onset is rapid or sudden, as in the case of stab or gunshot wounds,

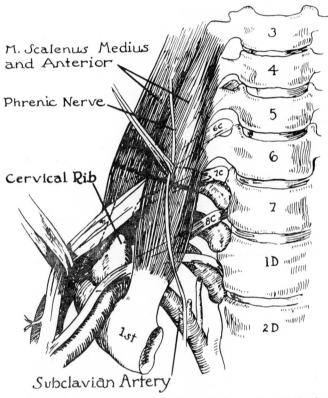

M. Scalenus Medius and Anterior

Phrenic Nerve

Cervical Rib

6C

7C

8C

1st

Subclavian Artery

3
4
5
6
7
1D
2D

Fig. 57—*Cervical rib*, showing the relationships of the nerves of the brachial plexus to the scalenus anticus muscle and the cervical rib, illustrating clearly the manner of compression of the nerves and the subclavian artery by the muscle and rib. (*Patterson: Amer. Surg. 111:531, 1940, J. B. Lippincott Co., Philadelphia.*)

limbs with color changes ranging from pallor to mottling and cyanosis; absence of pulsation in the vessels; weakness of the legs, ranging from slight to complete loss of power; loss of sensation; and absence of reflexes. In some instances evidence of spinal cord involvement is found. The clinical symptoms are the result of ischemia involving the cauda equina roots, peripheral nerves, and probably also the lumbosacral segments fractures, dislocations, and some ischemic conditions. In other instances, the onset is gradual, as in the case of cervical rib, callous formation, or toxic infectious causes. In the ischemic forms, paresthesias and pain are outstanding symptoms, whereas in those instances resulting from compression of the nerve, pain is not prominent. The painful paresthesias encountered in ischemic and in irritative lesions are extremely severe and difficult to cope with therapeutically. Pain is an important feature of cervical rib and the scalenus syndrome. Varying degrees of paralysis are seen, depending upon the nature of the cause, and the type of paralysis will depend naturally on the nerve which is affected. The same holds true of sensory disturbances. Trophic and vasomotor disturbances are seen in some forms, the latter quite prominently in cervical rib, the former in irritative nerve lesions associated with callous formation.

Since the specific disorders due to isolated involvement of nerve trunks depend upon the nerve which is compressed, these will be considered in a later section. Consideration must be given, however, to a special form of disorder causing a mononeuritis, namely, cervical rib.

Syndrome of the Thoracic Outlet: Pain in the arms is a common symptom, but frequently its cause is difficult to determine. Though its precise nature is often established accurately, there remain many cases for which no satisfactory explanation is available at present. Among the causes due to peripheral nerve involvement are cervical rib, scalenus anticus syndrome, thoracic rib, and costoclavicular compression. These may be grouped together for convenience into the *syndrome of the thoracic outlet*. The thoracic outlet is bounded by the first thoracic vertebra behind, the upper margin of the manubrium in front and the first rib laterally.

The symptoms produced by cervical rib, thoracic rib, the scalenus anticus syndrome and costoclavicular compression can be referred to an abnormality of the upper thoracic outlet (Walshe, Jackson & Wyburn-Mason), resulting in an asymmetry of the outlet. This tends to be narrower on one side, differs in outline on the two sides, is often higher on one side, the plane of the opening being abnormally tilted in the transverse and anteroposterior directions. Associated with this are abnormalities in insertion of the scalenus muscles. There may also be anomalies in the course of the subclavian artery. It may emerge from between two heads of abnormal scalenus insertions; it may lie higher than normal; and it commonly runs an abnormal S-shaped course in the presence of an anomalous rib. The space between rib and clavicle in which the third part of the artery runs may be altered in the presence of an abnormal rib. The space undergoes changes during movements of the arm and shoulder girdle and on elevation of the arm the clavicle may compress the third part of the subclavian artery. Stresses also occur on the lower components of the brachial plexus, the asymmetry of the thoracic outlet increasing the possibility of maladjustments between nerve roots and bone.

Cervical Rib Syndrome: In the case of the cervical rib, the clinical features are produced by compression of the subclavian artery and pressure on the nerve trunks of the brachial plexus by the cervical rib and the scalenus anticus muscle. Similar compression may be produced in the scalenus syndrome by the edge of a hypertrophied scalenus muscle, but the incidence of this condition is over-rated. The clinical symptoms of the syndrome may be of two main groups: one affecting primarily the upper cervical roots, causing symptoms chiefly in C_5 and C_6, and the other affecting mainly the lower cervical roots and involving chiefly the roots C_7 and C_8. In some instances, pain may be only slight in degree.

The cervical rib syndrome occurs chiefly in the fourth and fifth decades and is more common in women than in men. Direct trauma often precedes the onset, but just as frequently no such history is obtained and the symptoms appear gradually without apparent cause. There may be a history of occupation requiring repeated raising of the arms above the head. The outstanding symptom is pain, felt in the anterior portion of the shoulder, spreading to the supraclavicular area, and extending into the arm and hand. At times radiation into the arm is absent. The pain varies in

shoulders are brought forward, causing pressure of the neck structures against the scalenus muscle; (2) increased on turning the head to the unaffected side; and (3) increased on downward traction on the arm and shoulder. It is relieved by (1) sleeping with the arm above the head and (2) abduction of the arm. Pain and tenderness may be felt at the insertion

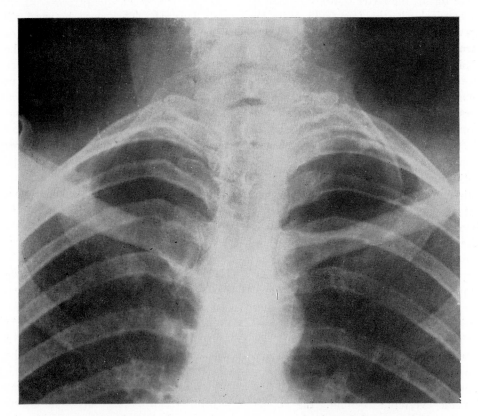

Fig. 58—*Cervical rib*. Photograph of x-ray showing bilateral cervical rib.

intensity from a tingling or numbness to a severe lancinating pain radiating along the specific nerve distribution. It is often felt along the ulnar side of the arm and hand, but it may be distributed along the median side or along both. The pain has helpful characteristic features. It is (1) worse at night, especially when sleeping on the back, due to pressure from behind as the

of the scalenus anticus muscle on pressure behind the clavicle. In some instances, a cervical rib may be palpated. Coldness, cramps, numbness, or blanching may be noted in parts of the hand or in the fingers.

The findings are of two kinds: Those referable to vascular and those due to nerve involvement. The *neurological* findings include weakness of the hand muscles, usually along the ulnar distribution, with atrophy of the interossei, and weakness of abduction and adduction of the fingers, etc. There may be similar weakness of the flexors of the fingers from median involvement or a combination of median and ulnar paralysis or weakness. Wrist-drop may be found. The degree of weakness varies with the compression of the nerve trunk or trunks. Sensory changes revealed as decreased sensation may be felt over the affected nerve area. Reflex changes are not as a rule present but decrease or loss of the biceps, radial or triceps reflexes may be found. Horner's syndrome has been described rarely in authentic cases. *Vascular* findings include decreased skin temperature of the affected fingers or hand, cyanosis, and sometimes edema of the hand. The radial pulse may be greatly diminished or obliterated, either spontaneously by turning the head to the unaffected side, by downward pressure on the arm, or by deep pressure over the scalenus anticus muscle. The blood pressure readings may be 15 to 20 mm. lower on the affected side. The hand and forearm are often colder on the affected side. *Roentgen studies* of the cervical vertebrae will reveal a typical cervical rib which is usually bilateral and attached to the thoracic cage; a rudimentary rib; or a long transverse process. In the last two types, the symptoms are produced by a fibrous band which compresses the involved structures.

The *diagnosis* of cervical rib is not difficult in typical cases. The history of anterior shoulder pain radiating into the arm and hand along one of the nerve trunks of the arm, the vasomotor changes in the hand, the difference in pulse and blood pressure on the affected side, the obliteration of the pulse by the maneuvers described all lead to a diagnosis of cervical rib which with such a history

and findings will be confirmed by roentgenologic examination. Unfortunately the entire spectrum of findings is not always demonstrable so that the neurological findings may be present without evidence of vasomotor disturbances. In some cases only the vascular disturbances are found, associated with pain. Pain is constant, but the findings may be variable.

The diagnosis of *cervical rib* can usually be established readily, but there may be difficulties in those cases with only a long transverse process or a rudimentary rib. In the presence of characteristic findings it may be assumed that these are responsible for the symptoms by means of the fibrous band attached to them.

The *treatment* of cervical rib is surgical. Section of the scalenus anticus muscle with release of compression of the nerves of the brachial plexus may cause complete remission of symptoms. Removal of the cervical rib may be necessary. Medical treatment is ineffective.

The diagnosis of *scalenus syndrome* offers great difficulty. The problem in such cases resolves itself into the symptoms and findings of cervical rib without its demonstration by the roentgenological examination. In definite cases, the diagnosis may be made with certainty, especially when real changes in the radial pulse are demonstrable. Such cases are few, so that the scalenus syndrome is more often suspected than established. In doubtful cases, with equivocal findings, the diagnosis is extremely difficult. Injection of the insertion of the scalenus anticus muscle with procaine may relieve the pain, but this in itself is not sufficient to confirm the diagnosis.

Shoulder Girdle Pain: The differential diagnosis concerns largely those conditions responsible for shoulder and arm pain.

The problem of pain in the shoulder girdle region lends itself to logical analysis. The complaint is common and the possibilities many, but a little scrutiny of the problem will result usually in proper segregation of cases.

The first and most important step in the orientation of shoulder girdle pain is an analysis of the pain itself; the next step is a determination of its cause. Pains in the shoulder girdle region may be grouped therefore into two large categories: (1) local and (2) radiating. In general, the *local pains* are produced by local causes, such as arthritis of the shoulder joint, bursitis, calcification of the supraspinatus tendon, and muscle disorders. In arthritis the pain is quite localized in the region of the joint, though there may be complaint of considerable soreness of surrounding structures. In bursitis the localized pain is most strikingly illustrated, for here the discomfort is produced by attempted abduction of the arm, is associated with spot tenderness over the diseased bursa, and with tenderness in no other portion of the shoulder girdle.

SHOULDER PAIN: It is claimed that lesions of the supraspinatus tendon and subacromial bursa are the commonest cause of pain in the shoulder (Armstrong). The mechanism is as follows: In the middle range of abduction of the humerus, the supraspinatus tendon with its covering bursa impinges against the overlying acromion so that, when a lesion of tendon or bursa exists, this pressure causes pain and muscle spasm accompanying any movement that tends to bring the lesion into contact with the acromion. The signs of the condition are as follows: (1) pain on abduction of the humerus in an arc of 60 to 120 degrees, (2) reversal of the normal scapulohumeral rhythm, and (3) tenderness on deep pressure over the supraspinatus tendon. Most patients recover spontaneously; others require acromionectomy.

It is also claimed that bicipital tendonitis is the commonest cause of shoulder and arm pain.

Pain localized to the shoulder region is found also in involvement of the *serratus magnus* muscle and in trapezius involvement. In these instances it is not so focal as in arthritis of the shoulder joint or in bursitis, but tends to be a more generalized pain involving the shoulder region. Sharp pain in the scapular region accompanies the onset of serratus paralysis, and appropriate maneuvers will demonstrate weakness of the muscle. It is essential of course to bear in mind the fact that focal pain may be felt in the shoulder girdle region in intraspinal disorders, but the incidence of such pain is not great.

In the case of *radiating pain* the problem is first that of determining whether the pain results from involvement of the peripheral nerves or spinal roots, a distinction which is not difficult to make in the majority of instances. Peripheral nerve pain spreads along one of the peripheral trunks in the shoulder and arm, is usually associated with muscle and nerve tenderness, and with muscle atrophy and reflex changes. A careful investigation of the location of the pain and its distribution will go a long way toward establishing its peripheral nature. Root pain on the other hand is distributed along the course of a posterior spinal root or roots. It is usually intermittent, radiating, and increased by any act which increases intraspinal pressure such as coughing, sneezing, or straining. It is unattended by motor manifestations.

Having determined whether the shoulder pain is of peripheral or radicular origin, the field of possibilities is thereby narrowed. In pain of peripheral origin the causes are apt to involve the nerves of the brachial plexus from their primary cords to the axilla. Among the common possibilities are cervical rib, the scalenus anticus syndrome, neuritis of the brachial plexus, and superior pulmonary sulcus tumor.

The cause of *superior pulmonary sulcus tumor* is still a matter of controversy, but the condition itself is a well-defined entity. It is due to tumors (carcinoma) found at the thoracic inlet and is characterized by severe pain around the shoulder, in the axilla, and down the arm; the early appearance of Horner's syndrome; atrophy of the hand muscles; roentgenological evidence of a homogenous shadow at the apex of the lung; destruction of the first, second, and third ribs; and often vertebral infiltration. The pain in superior pulmonary sulcus tumors is in the posterior part of the shoulder in contrast to that of cervical rib, which is in the anterior portion. It is worse at night and is usually increased by coughing. The tumor is presumed not to originate from lung, pleura, ribs, or mediastinum. While the syndrome is due to a special tumor, some regard the tumor as being of metastatic origin, since carcinoma from other parts of the body may metastasize to the apex of the lung or may originate within the lung and may produce a similar syndrome. Diagnosis is difficult in differentiating the tumor from a spinal cord neoplasm particularly, but the typical location of the pain (shoulder and axilla), the early appearance of the Horner syndrome, and the local rib destruction serve to characterize particularly the superior pulmonary sulcus tumor. Metastatic carcinoma should always be sought, especially if rib erosion is absent. Surgery and irradiation are of no avail. The pain must be controlled by cordotomy or root section.

In addition to the rare cause of superior pulmonary sulcus tumor, pain in the arm may be caused by thoracic conditions such as diffuse spasm of the esophagus and disturbances involving the diaphragm, such as esophageal hiatal hernia, diaphragmatic pleurisy, and subphrenic irritation.

ARM PAIN: *Neuralgic amyotrophy* (Parsonage and Turner) has been suggested as a term to cover a number of cases variously recorded as neuritis of the shoulder girdle (Spillane and associates). The condition is characterized by the sudden onset of pain without fever or systemic symptoms, the pain being severe, in the scapula, shoulder, outer arm, and sensations down the arm below the elbow; there is also the rapid development of muscle weakness and atrophy without fasciculations, usually maximal at the outset but in some instances progressing for two to seven days. Nerve root and spinal cord misplacement are sometimes found. In most instances, the weakness is confined to the muscles of the shoulder girdle and arm with occasional involvement of the forearm muscles, but a few instances are recorded with profound weakness of the thumb and index. Objective sensory changes are usually found, often over the outer arm in the circumflex area, and sometimes in root areas. Recurrent attacks are uncommon. Diagnosis requires distinction from anterior poliomyelitis, herniated cervical disc, brachial neuritis, and progressive muscular atrophy. The cause is unknown. Most of the cases have been observed in India, the Orient and the Middle East. It is doubtful whether this constitutes a special type of neuritis.

Brachial neuritis is easily distinguished by the tenderness of the nerve trunks and muscles which is not found in cases of cervical rib. The pain is likely to be more diffusely spread through the arm and to be more constant.

Pain in the hands and sometimes in the arms may be produced by what has been termed the *hyperabduction syndrome* which occurs with the arms in abduction in a sleeping or working position. The syndrome is characterized by paresthesias, numbness and pain in the hands and fingers. Gangrene may ensue. Pallor may be observed with the arms in abduction and normal color in adduction. The pulse is obliterated in various positions of abduction of the arms. The symptoms are produced by pressure on the subclavian artery and by ischemia of the brachial plexus trunks. Treatment consists of avoidance of over-abduction of the arms.

Among the causes of shoulder pain is the *shoulder-hand syndrome* occurring after myocardial infarction or long-standing angina pectoris. The condition is characterized by pain and stiffness of the shoulder, and swelling and pain of the fingers and hand. The pain in the shoulder may disappear and be followed by swelling of the hand and later by stiffness of the fingers and atrophy of the hand muscles.

Among the conditions causing arm pain, *thoracic rib* is relatively unknown and usually neglected. Malformations of the first rib consist of the following: (1) usually, a rudimentary structure terminating in a synosteosis or pseudarthrosis with the second rib near the scalene tubercle; (2) in a free termination of the soft tissues at the base of the neck, which may be connected by a ligamentous band with the manubrium sterni; or (3) rarely, by a distinct joint near its lateral angle before fusing with the second rib (White, Poppel, and Adams). It is usually associated with other skeletal abnormalities causing distortion of the thoracic outlet. These consist of deformities of the second rib, the upper end of the sternum, scoliosis of the cervicothoracic spine, and vertebral anomalies.

Symptoms of anomalies of the first thoracic rib consist of supraclaviclular bony prominence, pain in the arm and shoulder, weakness of the arm or hand muscles due to irritation of the nerves of the brachial plexus, and defect in the radial pulse due to compression of the subclavian vessels as they cross the thoracic rib. It is not possible to differentiate clinically thoracic rib malformations from a cervical rib. The differentiation can be made by an anteroposterior x-ray picture including all the cervical and upper thoracic vertebrae, provided the film is taken with a long exposure and with the mandible in motion. "Under these circumstances, the outline of the mandible will be blurred and the vertebra to which the uppermost rib is attached can be identified by counting downward from the base of the skull" (White). Treatment should first be along conservative lines. Scalenotomy alone is not sufficient to cause relief of the symptoms and must be accompanied by radical resection of the rib.

Pain in the arm and shoulder with evidence of delayed brachial plexus involvement has been found rarely as a result of compression of the subclavian vessels due to ununited fracture of the middle third of the clavicle.

Bursitis is readily distinguished by the local tenderness over the deltoid or acromial bursa. Limitation of arm movement is the result of pain associated with the bursitis and not to muscle weakness as in some of the associated conditions producing shoulder pain. Roentgen ray may reveal a calcified shadow. The diagnosis is usually easy. *Cervical cord tumor* may produce pain in the shoulder, the back of the neck and head, and down the arm. Early in its course only pain may be present, without evidences of cord compression. In this stage the diagnosis and the differentiation from other conditions is difficult. Growth of the tumor leads eventually to evidences of cord compression and may result in atrophy of the hand muscles, weakness of the arms and legs, and sensory disturbances. Subarachnoid block and increased protein content of the spinal fluid are helpful in establishing the diagnosis. *Arthritis of the cervical spine* may cause pain in the shoulder and arm and is easily established by a history of increased pain on movement of the head and by the demonstration of changes by x-ray examination.

A list of the conditions associated with pain in the shoulder includes the following, many of which need to be considered in the cervical rib-scalenus syndrome.

1. *Shoulder joint disorders*
   - (a) Arthritis
   - (b) Injury
   - (c) Tumor
2. *Bursa and tendon disease*
   - (a) Subdeltoid and subacromial bursitis
   - (b) Calcification of supraspinatous tendon
3. *Muscle disorders*
   - (a) Deltoid
   - (b) Serratus magnus
   - (c) Trapezius
   - (d) Other shoulder girdle muscles
4. *Peripheral-nerve disease*
   - (a) Cervical rib
   - (b) Scalenus anticus syndrome
   - (c) Brachial plexus neuritis
   - (d) Peripheral nerve disease of various shoulder girdle muscles
   - (e) Superior pulmonary sulcus tumor
   - (f) Tumors of peripheral nerves
5. *Intraspinal disorders*
   - (a) Extramedullary cervical cord tumors
   - (b) Herniated nucleus pulposus
   - (c) Pachymeningitis
   - (d) Syringomyelia
   - (e) Intramediary spinal cord tumor
   - (f) Radiculitis
   - (g) Metastatic carcinoma
6. *Vertebral disorders*
   - (a) Osteoarthritis of spine
   - (b) Fracture and fracture-dislocations of spine
7. *Visceral disease*

3. Polyneuritis, or Multiple Neuritis

There are many causes of polyneuritis (multiple neuritis) and numerous clinical manifestations. Unlike mononeuritis, which is usually the result of a local cause, polyneuritis results as a rule from systemic or general causes, of a bacterio-toxic, virus, deficiency, metabolic, or chemical nature. In its characteristic form, polyneuritis is usually symmetrical, involving both legs in most instances, but sometimes involving all the limbs. At times only the arms are affected. The cranial nerves escape in most forms, but in some forms of polyneuritis even these are affected. This is particularly true of acute infectious polyneuritis, but other forms of neuritis exist with cranial nerve involvement. The distal portions of the affected limbs suffer more than the proximal portions in acute infectious polyneuritis. Sphincter disturbances are not found in characteristic cases, but in some forms of polyneuritis even sphincter disturbances may be found.

The cause of multiple neuritis cannot always be determined. Among thirty-four cases of multiple neuritis the cause was established in fifteen cases (forty-four per cent), doubtful in six cases (eighteen per cent) and unknown in thirteen cases (thirty-eight per cent) in spite of careful investigation (Elkington). In another series of forty-six cases of multiple neuritis the cause was unknown in thirty-six cases (seventy per cent) (Mathews).

Diagnosis: That of polyneuritis is, as a rule, not difficult. Most, if not all, of the manifestations of nerve involvement discussed elsewhere are usually present—the pain, nerve trunk and muscle tenderness, reflex decrease or absence, and the motor and sensory weakness. The problem is one of establishment of cause rather than of diagnosis, which is, as a rule, easy. In not many instances is there difficulty in determining the diagnosis of polyneuritis, but problems arise in cases wherein there is relatively little muscle or nerve tenderness, or in which there is only slight motor or sensory involvement. In some instances, difficulty is offered by cases of purely motor neuritis. Specific problems of diagnosis will be discussed in a consideration of the various forms of neuritis.

Despite the characteristic features of neuritis already listed, the condition must be differentiated from other important neurological disorders. The pain and weakness of the limbs, usually of the legs, require distinction from *spinal cord tumor*. Apart from the absence of muscle and nerve tenderness and other signs of neuritis, cord tumors will, as a rule, give evidence of a history of progressive weakness or disability, evidence of weakness of the limbs, subarachnoid block (positive Queckenstedt test), sensory levels, increased spinal fluid protein, and sphincter disturbances. *Tabes dorsalis* enters the picture because of the leg pains, but is readily distinguished by Argyll Robertson pupils, posterior column signs (ataxia), and absence of reflexes.

Polymyositis may be hard to distinguish from neuritis. Dermatomyositis and acute polymyositis occur most often in children, but may be seen in persons of any age. Fever and leukocytosis may be present. The muscles are tender and weak. Erythema and other types of rash may be present.

Poliomyelitis is rarely confused with polyneuritis except in the occurrence of sporadic cases; fever, signs of meningeal irritation (neck stiffness, Kernig sign), and pleocytosis of the spinal fluid differentiate it; the pain and tenderness found in the early stages are muscular and not felt over the nerve trunks. The distinction may be difficult in early cases before the onset of paralysis, but the meningeal and spinal fluid findings will establish the diagnosis. In some instances, as in acute infectious polyneuritis, there may be difficulty in differentiating the disorder from poliomyelitis.

Acute ascending paralysis (Landry's paralysis) is often difficult to differentiate, especially since some forms of neuritis are characterized by an ascending picture. For such cases, the clinical picture is that of neuritis with an ascending picture. In most cases of Landry's paralysis, pain is not a feature, tenderness of the muscles and nerve trunks is absent, and fever is frequently present. Furthermore, it must be remembered that Landry's paralysis is a syndrome and that many causes are operative. *Myositis* must be ruled out in some cases. This can usually be done by means of the muscle tenderness without nerve tenderness or pain along the nerve trunks, the failure of reflex changes and sensory disturbances.

Arthritis offers few difficulties as a rule, the pain being confined to the joints with no radiation along the nerve trunks. The history of multiple joint involvement suffices to establish the diagnosis and roentgen ray changes are confirmatory.

These in general are the main diagnostic differentiations which appear in the course of a general diagnosis of neuritis. Special differentiations must be made in instances of neuritis involving special areas, as in sciatic neuritis or brachial neuritis. These will be considered in their separate sections.

Treatment: That of polyneuritis is similar in its essential details for most forms of the disease. For this reason it is advisable to consider the general features of treatment at this point. *Bed rest* is essential for all forms, both because of pain and weakness. *Diet* is important in all cases but especially in those instances associated with avitaminosis. A nutritious diet is sufficient for most cases. In the avitaminoses a high vitamin diet is indicated with special reference to the deficient factors. Dietary restrictions may be necessary in diabetic neuritis and insulin indicated. A high calcium diet is called for in acute lead neuritis and a low calcium intake in the chronic stages for purposes of deleading the tissues. Carbohydrate restrictions are necessary in sprue. *Hydrochloric acid* is valuable in alcoholic neuritis and in pellagra neuritis. *Iron* is important in many forms of neuritis, notably those due to alcohol, lead, pellagra, and in other forms associated with a secondary anemia. The control of pain is probably the most important and difficult problem. For this purpose drugs and physiotherapy are most helpful. *Salicylates* in large doses (45 to 60 grains daily) are helpful. Intravenous salicylates and iodides (15½ grains) are helpful in controlling pain in some cases. *Codeine* is often required to control the pain. *Meperidine (Demerol)* (50 to 100 mg.) three times daily by mouth helps to control pain. *Methadone* is a useful analgesic in doses of 5 to 10 mg. three to four times daily by mouth. It is not habit-forming, given orally. Morphine should not be given. Barbiturates may be necessary for sleep. Paraldehyde is helpful, especially in alcoholic patients. *BAL* (British antilewisite) has been found useful in some cases of polyneuritis, especially of the acute infectious type and in arsenic and diabetic neuritis. The drug is given intramuscularly in dosages of 2.5 mg. per kilogram of body weight daily for as long as seems necessary. *Heat* in the form of a lighted cradle over the legs often gives soothing but not complete relief. Short wave diathermy is soothing in the subacute and chronic stages but tends to aggravate the pain in the acute stages. Infra-red is helpful in the latter period and should be applied intensively two or three times daily. *Massage* is contra-indicated during the acute stages but is valuable after nerve and muscle tenderness subside. It should be given daily. *Splints* and sandbags are advisable to prevent deformities such as wrist-drop and foot-drop. *Vitamins* should be reserved for those patients in whom there appears to be a factor of avitaminosis. It is useless in other patients. Thiamine in patients in whom it is indicated may be given orally in small doses (10 to 30 mg. daily), or intravenously (100 mg. daily), or intramuscularly (50 mg. daily) in large doses. Other vitamins may be given as they seem indicated. *X-ray treatment* is often helpful in the acute stages of neuritis, and should be concentrated over the area of greatest nerve tenderness or the site of the neuritis.

4. Alcoholic Neuritis

Etiology: Alcoholic neuritis may occur at any age but it is more common in middle-aged drinkers. It may occur from twenty to seventy years of age, but has been found most frequently in subjects between forty and forty-five years old. It is more frequent in men than in women. It is more likely to occur in chronic drinkers than as the result of a single excess. The period of drinking necessary to bring on neuritis varies from a few days to weeks and depends on the general condition of the person. Alcohol in itself will not produce neuritis. This has been known for a long time, attention to this aspect of the problem being directed by the observation that many people drink excessively but relatively few develop neuritis. The neuritis of alcoholism is in large part due to avitaminosis, chiefly of the thiamine factor (B_1), but whether this explains the entire problem is still open to question. The observations on which this concept is based have been reviewed previously. Briefly they are: (1) the similarity between the neuritis of beriberi and that of alcoholism; (2) the known dietary insufficiency of alcoholics with emphasis largely on carbohydrates; (3) the occurrence of gastritis and achlorhydria in a large percentage of cases giving rise to difficulties in absorption; (4) the recovery of alcoholics from their neuritis despite the ingestion of alcohol, provided the diet and vitamin intake is normal; (5) the recovery of alcoholic neuritis with vitamin administration; and (6) the occurrence of neuritis with liver cirrhosis. Objections to this concept are based on the failure of recovery of many cases of alcoholic neuritis despite the administration of vitamins. This need not necessarily indicate absence of avitaminosis but rather the production of irreversible changes in the nerves before treatment is begun. In many cases of alcoholic neuritis, a history of an upper respiratory infection is obtained frequently preceding the onset of the neuritis. Whether this is a factor in the development of the condition is unclear. Gastric achlorhydria is found in 50 per cent of patients with alcoholic polyneuritis and hypochlorhydria in many more. Secondary anemia is found in a number of instances, sometimes of a severe degree.

Symptoms: The onset of alcoholic neuritis is acute as to attack, but gradual as to evidences of difficulty. There may be less disabling symptoms for days, weeks, or months before the serious attack of neuritis begins. Thus there may be paresthesias, cramps in the calves, or pains for some time before the onset. In other instances, the onset is quite acute, with rapid development of symptoms. The usual case develops over a period of a few days, before it reaches its full development of weakness.

The history is that of onset of pains in the legs and/or arms in a person who, by history from relatives or friends, is a confirmed alcoholic. Associated with the history of pains is almost always a complaint of painful paresthesias of the feet and/or hands, and usually weakness of some degree in the legs and arms. Foot-drop may be noticed by a complaint of a tendency to stumble, and weakness of the legs, arms, and hands may reach a severe degree so that by the time of examination the patient may be unable to walk. Numbness may be noted and in rare instances there may be complaints of disturbance of vision or of facial weakness. Sphincter difficulties are not, as a rule, present.

Pain is a prominent and usually the first symptom. It is usually in the legs, spreading out along the entire leg from the hip region to the foot, most common in the distribution of the sciatic nerve or one of its branches. It is constant and often intractable. Pain in the arms is almost as common as in the legs but is sometimes absent. Tenderness of the muscles and nerve trunks is usually pronounced, but need not parallel the degree of muscle weakness or the severity of the neuritis.

Paresthesias are severe in practically all cases, and are much more pronounced in the soles of the feet than in the hands; in severe cases, they are present in both. They are extremely painful and are usually experienced as sensations of heat or burning. Alcoholic patients are prone therefore to prefer keeping their feet uncovered or against the cold rungs of the bed. Stroking the soles is usually unpleasant and painful. The paresthesias constitute a striking feature of the disease and are often more difficult to control than the pain. In some cases they persist long after the pain has subsided and even after recovery has been complete in all other respects.

Paralysis is present in varying degrees. In severe cases, there may be complete or almost complete paralysis of the legs and arms in all segments of the limbs In less severe cases, the weakness is mild and may involve only selected muscle groups. Foot-drop is frequently observed, sometimes complete, at other times partial. Wrist-drop is common. The gait may be very ataxic and steppage in type. There is marked muscle atrophy in severe cases; in others, little or none may be present. In the majority of cases, atrophy of some degree is seen and is often rapid in development. The *cranial nerves* are not involved in the usual case. In rare instances, there may be impairment of vision due to optic neuritis or atrophy, or paralysis of the facial nerve. Multiple cranial nerve paralyses are rarely found. Retrobulbar neuritis with scotoma is sometimes seen. *Sensory disturbances* are present in the majority of cases, but it is surprising in how many they may be very slight or even lacking. In most cases in the acute stages, loss of pain, temperature, and deep sensation are lost in some degree in the legs, and less often in the arms and hands, particularly in the distal portions. Some forms of sensation may be affected and others normal, due to the difference in susceptibility of the nerve fibers to injury. The *reflexes* are lost or decreased in the affected areas. Under unusual circumstances, the reflexes may remain unchanged.

Trophic disturbances of the nails and skin are common in this form of neuritis. Brittle nails, dry scaly or red, shiny skin, and cold extremities are common. The trophic changes of skin and nails are quite characteristic. The skin of the legs becomes smooth, polished, and shiny, and the soles of the feet glossy. There are no sphincter disturbances in uncomplicated cases.

Excessive amounts of *arsenic* were found in the urine of patients with alcoholic polyneuritis, the amount of arsenic being greater in the more severe cases (Brown and Hastings).

Mental symptoms sometimes accompany cases of polyneuritis due to alcohol. These are characterized by confusion, disorientation, and confabulation, which, combined with polyneuritis, produce the so-called "Korsakoff syndrome." At other times, less definite confusional states are found (*v.* Alcoholic Encephalopathy).

Diagnosis: That of alcoholic polyneuritis offers no difficulties. A history of indulgence in alcohol is always available from one source or another. This together with the striking evidence of pain, nerve and muscle tenderness, the occurrence of muscle disability culminating in foot-drop and/or wrist-drop, the trophic changes in the skin and nails, and the severe paresthesias are characteristic. The neuritis associated with arsenic poisoning may give rise to a similar clinical picture but is not readily confused with alcoholic polyneuritis because of the history of arsenic poisoning.

Prognosis: As in all cases of neuritis, the outlook varies with the degree of damage to the nerve. In most cases, recovery is gradual and is complete in four weeks to two or three months. In severe cases, little recovery may ensue in spite of the most intense treatment. Contractures and trophic joint changes may develop in such cases and paralysis of the affected limbs persists. There may be very slow but incomplete improvement over a period of months. In some cases, paresthesias may persist in spite of good recovery of power and disappearance of pains. Mental symptoms recover in a large percentage of cases with proper treatment.

Treatment: *Rest in bed* is imperative. A *cradle* over the feet and legs to keep the covers off the limbs is often desirable and a lighted cradle helps for the soothing heat which it gives. Counterirritants, such as *methyl salicylate* or *chloroform liniment,* sometimes are helpful in relieving pain. *Salicylates* by mouth in large doses (45 grains or over a day) are helpful. In severe cases of pain, *codeine* affords relief. Intravenous salicylates sometimes help, given once or twice a day in 15½ grain doses. Morphine should never be given. *Thiamine chloride* is beneficial in many but not all cases despite the conception that alcoholic neuritis is due to avitaminosis. In the acute stages, it may be given intravenously in large doses (100 mg.). In other stages, 100 mg. intramuscularly may be given daily and continued for long periods. *Brewer's yeast* is often advisable. *Hydrochloric acid* is often helpful since many alcoholics have a decreased stomach acid content or even achlorhydria. *Iron* is sometimes necessary if secondary anemia is present. *Physiotherapy* in the form of *infrared* or *diathermy* should be given daily. Massage must not be given if the muscles are tender. *Splints* for wrist-drop and *sandbags* for foot-drop are necessary. *Massage* in the stage of recovery is essential to maintain good nutrition of the muscles. Treatment must often be continued for long periods of time.

5. Beriberi Neuritis

Etiology: This form of neuritis is the result of a deficiency of vitamin B_1 (thiamine). It is found chiefly in oriental countries and in hot climates, but it is frequent enough in other parts of the world. It is caused by the consumption of food lacking in the antineuritic vitamin, chiefly polished rice, or maize. There is some claim that vitamin A is in part responsible for the neuritis of beriberi.

Symptoms: The symptoms are those of polyneuritis associated with edema.

Two main types of beriberi may be differentiated. (1) wet beriberi, with predominant edema; and (2) dry or atrophic beriberi, with no edema but extensive atrophy of the muscles.

The neuritis is usually of a severe degree. *Paresthesias* are common in the legs and arms. Pains are frequent and cramps in the legs are common. Tenderness of the muscles and nerve trunks is pronounced. Objective *sensory disturbances* of varying degree are usually present. They may consist of patchy areas of loss or decrease of pain, touch, and temperature sensation, to large areas of a similar nature involving many nerve distributions. The *motor symptoms* are usually manifested as pareses of the arms and legs. They are more pronounced distally. In the legs, foot-drop, and in the arms, wrist-drop are usually found, but muscles in the more proximal portions of the limbs are not infrequently involved; the biceps and triceps in the arms, or the quadriceps and hamstrings in the legs. A steppage gait is common. The diaphragm is paralyzed at times in severe cases. The heart muscle is often affected and cardiac symptoms are common. *Edema* is an important feature of beriberi neuritis. It is usually seen about the ankles and over the tibiae, but it may spread up the thighs to the trunk and even involve the arms and face.

Treatment: This should consist of preventive measures consisting of a proper *diet* containing eggs, milk, fresh vegetables, and the avoidance of polished rice. Once the disease has developed, the administration of the antineuritic vitamin becomes specific. *Thiamine chlo-*

ride should be given in large doses either intravenously or intramuscularly (30 to 100 mg.) daily. Vitamin A may also be given. *Heat* and other physiotherapeutic measures are helpful in controlling pain.

6. Diabetic Neuritis

Etiology: The incidence of neuritis in diabetes is not easy to define because distinction must be made between unmistakable cases of neuritis and subclinical forms with only transient neuritic symptoms. Among one thousand consecutive cases of diabetes over a period of two and one-half years were twenty-five cases (2.5 per cent) of unmistakable neuritis (Jordan), but many more cases of a transitory type were seen. Others place the incidence much higher (10 to 50 per cent), but the criteria for the diagnosis of neuritis is so variable that comparable statistics are impossible. Diabetic neuritis occurs in about five per cent of all diabetics (Rundles).

Women seem to be more susceptible than men. Older patients with diabetes are more prone to develop the disease. In some cases, there is a direct connection between the hyperglycemia and the neuritis, but in the majority of instances no such connection can be demonstrated. In many cases hyperglycemia does not appear to be essential for the production of the neuritis, and the fact has often been noted that though there are many diabetics, very few develop neuritis. The more severe types of diabetic neuritis are seen almost entirely in patients whose diabetes has not been under adequate control for considerable periods of time (Root). Arteriosclerosis is present in a high percentage of cases, but its rôle in the neuritis is not clear. Deficient dietary intake has not been found responsible in most cases. A lack of thiamine (B_1) has been held responsible by some investigators because of the important rôle which vitamin B plays in the metabolism of carbohydrates. It is known that diabetic neuritis may develop despite adequate or even large intake of vitamins (Root). Foci of infection are found in many cases (38.5 per cent, Jordan).

As to the relationship with the diabetes, many discrepancies are found. Among them may be mentioned the following: (1) in many of the cases, the causative factor is probably not the diabetes itself; the neuritis is probably due to ischemia from arteriosclerotic vessels or other factors; (2) symptoms of neuritis occasionally precede the development of recognizable diabetes; hence uncontrolled diabetes is not the cause of all cases; (3) there is no close relationship between the occurrence of neuritis and the severity of the diabetes nor the control of the diabetes; diabetic neuritis is commonest in patients whose disease is unregulated and most frequently develops in patients whose treatment has been either neglected or poorly supervised (De Jong). It is not caused by hyperglycemia alone; it may occur in patients whose blood sugar level has never been excessive and in those who have never experienced either coma or acidosis (De Jong); (4) neuritis may first appear when a case of diabetes is brought under control with insulin; hence, in such cases, control rather than lack of control precipitates the neuritis; and (5) the diabetes may be mild or controlled, but the neurological changes may be severe.

Symptoms: Neuritis in diabetes may be divided into two main groups: (1) a group in which the evidences of neuritis are well pronounced and which conform to the general symptoms of neuritis; this group of cases is relatively infrequent in diabetes; and if the diagnosis of diabetic neuritis was made on these alone, the incidence would be very low; (2) a group in which the manifestations of neuritis are absent or few in number, the occurrence of the neuritis being established by changes in the tendon reflexes often on routine examination; the incidence of this group is high.

The clinical features of the first group are quite well defined. The onset of symptoms is, as a rule, gradual and often ill-defined, extending back for a period of weeks and months and characterized by vague pains and paresthesias. In other instances, pain is sudden in onset. The legs are much more often involved than the arms. *Pain* is common in the legs in some cases, especially at night. Pain was present in 83.3 per cent of a large group of patients reported by Jordan, with an intensification at night. In many of the cases, however, pain is either slight or not present. The pain may be continuous or intermittent. Paresthesias are often annoying in the feet. *Weakness* of the legs is present in at least two thirds of cases, is usually slight, but may be pronounced. Atrophy of the muscles is not usually present and is not often pronounced when it occurs. The pain is sharp in some cases and ill defined in others. Cramplike sensations are common. The pain is often referred along a specific nerve trunk, but in many cases no such distribution is described.

Decreased or absent patellar and Achilles *reflexes* are common. *Tenderness* of the nerve trunks is often found but it is not usually pronounced. *Sensory disturbances* are often present and are frequently poorly defined, both as to distribution and type of sensation affected. In some cases of diabetes, so-called "pseudotabes" is found, characterized by ataxic gait and incoördination of the legs, with loss of position and vibration sensations in the feet and toes. These are in reality cases of diabetic neuritis with secondary changes in the posterior columns of the cord. *Charcot joint* has been reported in cases of diabetic neuritis with extensive spinal cord involvement (Foster and Bennett).

Diagnosis: The diagnosis of this form of diabetic neuritis is not difficult. The occurrence of pains, usually of nerve tenderness, absent reflexes, and muscular weakness in a diabetic patient is sufficient to establish the diagnosis of neuritis and to indicate its cause.

Of even greater practical importance is the second group of cases of diabetic neuritis, the transient and subclinical group. This includes what may be termed the hyperglycemic group (Jordan), characterized by pains, usually in the legs, tenderness of the nerve trunks, and often, but not always, decreased tendon reflexes. The blood sugar in such patients is often, but not always, elevated, but the diabetes is always uncontrolled. Control of the diabetes is followed by a disappearance of the neuritis.

Probably the largest group of cases is that in which there is found absent patellar and/or Achilles reflexes during routine examination. No history of neuritis is obtainable in such cases, but there may be a vague account of muscle cramps or pains which were given no attention at the time of their occurrence. Cases of this sort are undoubtedly instances of neuritis, but must be regarded as asymptomatic.

Irregular, sluggish pupils are sometimes seen in diabetes. Retrobulbar neuritis is sometimes encountered. Paralysis of the third, fourth, or sixth cranial nerves may develop as a complication of diabetes, usually in mild diabetes of long standing, often associated with a diabetic retinopathy, and sometimes with peripheral neuritis. The third and sixth nerves are most commonly affected. The paralysis develops usually but not always with severe pain in and around the orbit, progresses rapidly, and clears up completely within a few weeks or months. The pupillary function is usually not affected. Pathological study of the condition has revealed fusiform enlargement of the retro-orbital portion of the nerve; destruction of some of the myelin sheaths and axis cylinders in the center of the nerve; increase in the connective tissue elements of the nerve and suggestive evidence of regeneration in the area of destruction (Dreyfus, Hakim, and Adams). The changes recorded have been attributed to incomplete ischemic neuropathy. Diabetes is responsible for so many changes in the peripheral and central nervous system that it is easy to attribute any complication arising in the course of the disease to the diabetes when in fact it may result from other causes. General paresis, brain tumor and spinal cord tumor have been seen in the course of patients with diabetes.

The spinal fluid protein may be increased in patients with minimal evidences of neuritis, but it is often normal in advanced cases (Rudy). On the other hand, increase of protein in the spinal fluid has been correlated roughly with the severity and duration of the neuritis (Root), as well as with difficulty of control of the diabetes.

Study of the electroencephalogram in patients having diabetes with frequent insulin reactions or seizures reveals no significant increase of abnormal reactions as compared with normals. Furthermore, long duration of diabetes fails to alter the incidence of cerebral dysrhythmia (Greenblatt, Murray, and Root).

The *prognosis* is usually good. Marked improvement occurs in a few weeks in many cases and within a few months in most cases. Severe cases may respond poorly. The prognosis in cases of diabetic neuritis is reported by some investigators to be worse in cases associated with arteriosclerosis of the limbs.

Treatment: This should consist of vigorous *diabetic measures. Vitamin B$_1$* should be given because of the as yet unproved contention that a vitamin B deficiency is present in cases of diabetic neuritis. Vitamin B$_{12}$ (1000 mcg./cc.) is said to be useful. BAL (2, 3 dimercaptopropanol) in doses of 100 mg. once or twice daily for seven to fourteen days is useful in some cases. *Physiotherapeutic measures* are valuable, as in all cases of neuritis.

7. Pellagra Neuritis

Etiology: The cause of pellagra is not yet definitely established. The preponderant evidence favors a dietary deficiency characterized by absence of thiamine and riboflavin from the diet and probably ascorbic acid as well. A lack of nicotinic acid does not account for all the symptoms; there seems to be also a concomitant riboflavin deficiency. Pellagra is the result of a qualitative and quantitative dietary deficiency. A survey of a large group of pellagrins with neuritis indicates a preponderance of women over men (thirty as compared with sixteen). The average age was forty-one, the age varying between eighteen and sixty-six years (Lewy, Spies, and Aring).

Symptoms: The neuritis of pellagra is usually of a mild or moderate degree. Some cases are severe. The arms and legs are about equally involved. Tenderness of the nerve trunks and muscles is usually present but is not invariably found. Spontaneous pains and cramps of the calf muscles are common. There appears to be about equal involvement of the motor and sensory nerves. Paresis is more common than complete paralysis, the arms and legs being about equally affected. Sensation (touch and pain) is often decreased in a glove-and-stocking type of distribution. The tendon reflexes are decreased or absent. In many cases the neuritis is associated with degeneration in the spinal cord, with resulting evidence of posterior and lateral column involvement (ataxia, loss of position and vibration senses, and Babinski sign). The pupillary reflexes are often sluggish and the corneal reflexes may be decreased. Mental symptoms are found in many cases with irritability, depression, and even hallucinations.

Treatment: A *high vitamin diet* is essential and should be fortified with *brewer's yeast*. Milk, vegetable, purees, eggs, and tomato juice are important. Powdered brewer's yeast (30 to 150 grains daily) in milk is important. *Liver* should be given either orally or by injection. *Nicotinic acid* (200 to 400 mg. daily) should be given. *Riboflavin* (1 to 3 mg. daily) is essential. *Iron* may be given to combat the secondary anemia, and *dilute hydrochloric acid* is usually prescribed. BAL (British anti-Lewisite) has been reported to give good results (*v.* treatment of multiple neuritis). Vitamin B_{12} concentrate (1000 mcg.) 1 cc. intramuscularly has been reported to be valuable.

8. Lead Neuritis

Etiology: Neuritis due to lead poisoning is said to occur in 5 per cent of cases with lead intoxication. Men are more commonly affected than women due to exposure to occupational hazards. The main sources of invasion of the lead are through the respiratory and gastrointestinal tracts. Little if any is absorbed through the skin. Lead poisoning is found in many industries and from many sources, among which are the mining of lead ore, spraying of fruit with lead, grinding or milling of lead, painting, the handling of gasoline containing lead, food

dyes, solder, water, lead glass, and the eating of lead by children. The burning of old storage batteries has produced lead poisoning.

The occurrence of lead neuritis bears no relationship to the length of exposure to lead poisoning. It may develop after short or long exposure. A vitamin (thiamine) deficiency has been assumed for cases of lead poisoning.

Symptoms: Lead may cause a mononeuritis or a multiple neuritis. One or both arms may be affected, more often the latter. The arms are more frequently involved than the legs, but neuritis involving the lower extremities is occasionally seen. The history is that of sudden onset of weakness of the wrists due to wrist-drop in the typical case, or there may be associated weakness of the feet as well. Pain is not a source of complaint in the typical instance. Apart from weakness the history contains little of significance.

A history of *lead colic* is often obtained, but it is surprising how frequently this is absent. The diagnosis must be suspected in the presence of typical findings, even though no history of lead poisoning is obtained. The usual history is that of *weakness* of the muscles, usually gradual in onset, associated at times with muscular pains. Acute, severe pain, such as characterizes other forms of neuritis, *e. g.,* alcoholic neuritis, is absent, since the neuritis of lead poisoning is chiefly of a motor type, but pain is sometimes a prominent complaint. The weakness is found first in the middle and ring fingers, which are found to fatigue early, and then spreads to the other hand and arm muscles. The typical case shows a weakness of the extensor muscles of the hand with a typical *wrist-drop.* The supinator longus is spared, a point of diagnostic significance for lead poisoning.

At times the triceps escapes also. Extension of the wrist and of the fingers is lost except by fixation of the wrist, when finger extension then becomes possible. When the legs are affected, the corresponding leg extensors are affected, with resultant *foot-drop*. There may be quite severe atrophy of the muscles if the paralysis persists. There is no tenderness of the nerve trunks or muscles since the neuritis is almost purely motor. *Sensory disturbances* are usually not found. Early in the paralysis there may be decrease of sensation over the radial nerve distribution. The triceps reflex is absent in cases of lead poisoning.

Cases of lead palsy may be divided into (1) an *arm* or *brachial* type, with predilection for the deltoid and biceps muscle groups; when the flexors of the arm are involved, the supinator longus, which is chiefly a flexor, escapes; this is a useful sign in cases of lead palsy; (2) *hand type,* simulating the findings of progressive muscular atrophy; in these cases there is progressive atrophy of the small hand muscles, the interossei, and the thenar and hypothenar eminences; and (3) *leg type* involving the foot extensors.

The cranial nerves may be affected in some cases of lead poisoning. *Optic neuritis* is encountered and in some cases retrobulbar neuritis is found. *Optic atrophy,* though rare, is reported. It is more often secondary in type, but primary atrophy has been described in lead poisoning.

In some cases of lead poisoning there is involvement also of the spinal cord, with or without evidences of peripheral nerve paralysis. In such instances, there may be evidence of a spastic paraplegia, with spasticity and weakness of the legs, amyotrophic lateral sclerosis with atrophy of small hand muscles, spasticity and weakness of the legs, overactive reflexes and Babinski signs, or syndromes simulating multiple sclerosis.

Secondary anemia, stippling of the red cells, and other features of lead poisoning in the blood smear are found in most but not all cases. Lead is also found in excessive amounts in the blood, urine, and feces in cases of lead palsy, but the degree of paralysis does not parallel the amount of lead found. Rarely, lead is found in the spinal fluid.

Prognosis: The outlook in cases of neuritis due to lead poisoning is not very good. There is little capacity for regeneration on the part of the nerves poisoned by lead (Villaverde). Recovery may occur if the source of poisoning is discovered and eliminated. Relapses are common, once there has been a neuritis due to lead.

Treatment: The indications for treatment of lead neuritis are different from those of chronic lead poisoning, since in such instances there is an excess of circulating lead and the object of treatment must therefore be to deposit lead in the bones. For this purpose, calcium is required and may best be given as *milk* (one to two quarts daily) together with *calcium lactate* (15 grains three or four times daily). After these measures, treatment may be directed carefully to the process of lead elimination by means of (1) *potassium iodide,* 5 grains three times daily, gradually increased to the point of tolerance; (2) a *low calcium diet,* with milk and eggs decreased in amount; and (3) *parathyroid extract* and *viosterol.*

Calcium Disodium Versenate has been used in lead poisoning with reportedly good results. One Gm. of the solution is added to 250-500 cc. of isotonic saline or 5 per cent glucose in water, and given intravenously over a one-hour period twice a day for five days. In children, the daily dosage is 30 mg. per kilogram of body weight.

Splints to hold the wrist and foot in normal position are indicated in order to prevent the development of deformities. *Massage* of the affected muscles is essential. *Electrical treatment* in the form of galvanism may help. Drugs have little effect on the neuritis.

9. Arsenic Neuritis

Etiology: Arsenic is used freely in commerce, industry, and medicine, so that cases of arsenic poisoning are not unusual. Neuritis may result from acute or chronic poisoning. Arsenic enters the body by the lungs through inhalation of dust, by the digestive tract, and possibly also by the skin. When absorbed through the gastrointestinal tract it induces stomatitis first, and eventually polyneuritis with melanosis and keratosis. Skin absorption is more likely to cause rashes, while medical arsenic compounds produce erythema, pigmentation, neuritis, conjunctivitis, and gastrointestinal disturbances.

Symptoms: Among the systemic symptoms of arsenic poisoning are headache, vertigo, insomnia, fatigue, epigastric pain, nausea, vomiting and diarrhea, melanosis and keratosis, and ridging, cracking, and transverse white lines of the fingernails.

Arsenic causes a polyneuritis characterized by severe pains and paresthesias. The latter are usually severe and exceed in intensity those of alcoholic neuritis. There is extreme tenderness of the muscles and nerve trunks, and often a severe degree of ataxia, producing the syndrome of pseudotabes arsenicosa. This is characterized by an extreme ataxia of the arms and legs. There is usually severe wasting of the muscles in which the small muscles of the hands and feet may suffer

most in some cases. The extensors of the fingers and toes suffer greatly. Optic atrophy is sometimes seen.

The diagnosis is not difficult if exposure to arsenic can be obtained by history. Arsenic should be suspected in cases of neuritis with severe ataxia, pains, and paresthesia, especially if these are associated with gastrointestinal symptoms, melanosis, keratosis, and changes in the nails.

In cases of chronic poisoning, the outlook is fair provided the source of the poisoning can be discovered and eliminated, but it may take months to produce a cure. A single large dose of arsenic taken with suicidal intent may produce more nerve damage than small doses taken over a long period.

British anti-lewisite (BAL) is valuable in arsenic neuritis. It is given in a dose of 2.5 mg. per kilogram of body weight The total dose so estimated is given twice the first two days, at twelve-hour intervals, and daily thereafter for one week. The course may be repeated after a lapse of a few days. The treatment must be stopped if respiratory embarrassment develops.

10. Neuritis Due to Other Chemicals, Poisons, and Drugs

The occurrence of polyneuritis on exposure to other poisons, chemicals, and drugs has already been referred to in the consideration of the causes of neuritis. Generally speaking, the neuritis which occurs with mercury, phosphorus, trichlorethylene, carbon monoxide, carbon disulfide, and the other causes listed under the heading of Chemical and Drugs in Table 13 is not in itself distinctive. A special and severe form of neuritis is found with *triorthocresyl phosphate* poisoning from the drinking of Jamaica ginger. The onset is sudden, and is sometimes associated with gastric symptoms but more often with a sense of coldness, heaviness, or soreness of the muscles. Pain may be present but it is not an outstanding symptom. The neuritis is chiefly motor in type. Foot-drop and wrist-drop are common. The weakness or paralysis may extend to the proximal muscles of the limbs, but as a rule the distal portions are most affected. Atrophy of the muscles develops and with it reaction of degeneration. Sensory changes are almost always absent (pain, touch, heat, cold), but loss of vibratory sensation is common. Tenderness on pressure over the calf muscles is often found. Paresthesias are not common. Mild trophic disturbances may be found. The Achilles reflexes are absent and the patellar reflexes often present. The arm reflexes may be affected. The cranial nerves are not affected. Recovery is said to occur in the muscles in inverse order of their involvement. In the upper limb, the forearm extensors are first improved, and then wrist extensors; in the leg the thigh, then the calf and foot muscles recover in the order named. Recovery occurs slowly even in mild cases, but severe cases may develop persistent paralysis.

In *carbon disulfide* poisoning, peripheral neuritis in varying degrees occurs very frequently, the neuritis in these cases being chiefly sensory in type and affecting largely the hands and feet. It has been reported in 76 per cent of cases (Lewy). Sensations of pins and needles, of crawling ants, a strange itching soreness, and dead fingers are early complaints. The arms and legs show a tendency to "fall asleep." Constant or paroxysmal pains in the muscles, especially in the calves, are frequent, as are pains along the peripheral nerve distributions. Shooting pains in the legs often become intolerable at night. Motor weakness may be present but is not very common. Sensory changes, however, are found frequently and tenderness

of the nerve trunk is usually present. The tendon reflexes are absent or decreased. The cranial nerves are affected in rare instances; among them are optic neuritis and peripheral facial paralysis. *Trichlorethylene* is an uncommon cause of neuritis, but has been found to cause sensory paralysis of the trigeminal nerve particularly, with numbness of the face. *Mercury* and *silver* are rare causes of neuritis.

Multiple neuritis has been reported following *gold* therapy for rheumatoid arthritis.

Neuritis has been reported as a complication of treatment with *sulfonamides* in a number of instances. *Sulfanilamide* has been responsible for foot-drop and for multiple neuritis, but it is less commonly the cause than other sulfonamides. Polyneuritis with increase of protein in the spinal fluid has been observed after the use of sulfanilamide. The neuritis seems to be typically that seen in mixed nerve affections, with pains, muscular weakness, nerve tenderness, reflex loss, and sensory disturbances. Most of the reported cases have recovered. Neuritis may develop with the use of *sulfathiazole* and *sulfamethylthiazole,* as well as with *sulfadiazine.* The onset of the neuritis after sulfonamides may be from one to fourteen days after treatment is started. Recovery occurs in two to five months. but symptoms persist as long as twelve to eighteen months in some cases. Optic neuritis, and trigeminal and vagus nerve involvement have been recorded with sulfonamide therapy.

Peripheral neuritis has been observed with *penicillin,* involving chiefly the sciatic, common peroneal, and cranial nerves. Recovery is slow.

A form of polyneuritis has been seen associated with multiple indolent ulcers, or jungle sore. Paralysis of accommodation is always present.

Table 15—Neurologic Complications of Serum Sickness
(After Doyle)

NUMBER OF CASES REVIEWED.........	49
SEX DISTRIBUTION:	
Males...........................	44
Females........................	5
AVERAGE AGE IN YEARS (46 patients)....	26.9
AVERAGE INTERVAL (in days between first injection and onset of serum sickness—39 cases)...................	6.8
AVERAGE INTERVAL (in days between onset of serum sickness and the neurological complications—35 cases)......	2.1

Serum Injected	No. of Cases
TETANUS ANTITOXIN.................	34
DIPHTHERIA ANTITOXIN..............	7
SCARLET-FEVER ANTITOXIN............	5
ANTIPNEUMOCOCCIC SERUM, Type I.....	2
ANTIMENINGOCOCCIC SERUM...........	1
	49

Table 16—Distribution of the Neurological Complication of Forty-nine Cases of Serum Sickness
(After Doyle)

Superior brachial plexus — unilateral motor......................	13
Mononeuritis (radial, 7; long thoracic, 1) .	8
Optic neuritis......................	6
Brachial plexus—bilateral motor.......	4
Brachial plexus—bilateral sensorimotor..	4
Superior brachial plexus—unilateral sensorimotor......................	4
Superior brachial plexus—bilateral motor......................	3
Superior brachial plexus—bilateral sensorimotor......................	3
Brachial plexus—unilateral motor......	1
Brachial plexus—unilateral sensorimotor......................	1
Central nervous system, meninges, brachial plexus—bilateral motor	1
Urticarial edema of the brain and meninges.......................	1

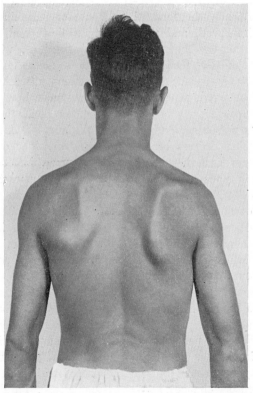

Fig. 59—*Serum neuritis.* Atrophy of the muscles of both shoulder girdles developing six days after an injection of tetanus antitoxin.

Isonicotinic acid hydrazide, used in the treatment of various forms of tuberculosis, may cause multiple neuritis, with prolonged use of the drug. Sensory symptoms (paresthesias) appear to predominate over motor, which tend to be mild. Glove-and-stocking anesthesia has been reported. Dupuytren-like contractures and Raynaud's phenomena have been observed. The symptoms disappear if the drug is discontinued, except in severe cases, where they may persist. This form of neuritis is associated with disturbance in pyridoxine metabolism. Increased urinary excretion of pyridoxine occurs in the disorder.

11. Serum Neuritis

Etiology: Neuritis develops in some instances of serum injection. The incidence is not high but no figures are available. The neuritis may involve a single nerve trunk or may manifest itself as a multiple neuritis. The complication has followed various forms of sera; tetanus antitoxin leads in the incidence of complications (fifty per cent); pneumonia, meningococcus, scarlet fever, streptococcus antitoxins, staphylococcus and paratyphoid-typhoid vaccines; and diphtheria sera or antitoxins have from time to time been complicated by the development of neuritis following injection.

The *pathogenesis* of the neuritis is not known. Early opinions regarded the neuritis as the result of a direct toxic reaction on the nerves. Recent investigators regard it as the result of a perineural urticaria and edema, with a resulting ischemic disease of the nerves.

Symptoms: Males have been more frequently affected than females. In the majority of cases recorded, the neurological complications have developed within two or three days of serum sickness and within four to eight days after injection, but occasional cases have developed within a matter of hours after the injection. The onset of symptoms is not uniform. Neuritic pains may develop within a few hours after the onset of serum sickness and generalized urticaria, flaccid paralysis developing within a few hours to days (Bennett). Serum sickness is usually present and develops four to eight days after the injection of serum. It is not always present, however, and serum neuritis may develop without the local itching, swelling, generalized urticaria, fever, and lymphadenopathy. There appears to be no relation between the site of injection and the nerve affected. Many cases show signs of palsies of the upper cord of the brachial plexus; others show radial, axillary, or bilateral brachial plexus involvement.

The median, suprascapular, axillary, and other nerves from the upper cord of the brachial plexus are especially susceptible. Motor symptoms are more common than sensory. Involvement of the long thoracic nerve with serratus magnus paralysis has been recorded. Table 16 (Doyle) indicates the main features of involvement after serum or antitoxin injections.

The findings depend naturally on the nerve involved. Among the manifestations which develop are *paralysis* of abduction of the arm (axillary nerve), weakness of wrist and finger flexors (median), paralysis of finger and wrist extensors (radial), or a combination of these and other nerves if the brachial plexus is affected. Muscle atrophy, sometimes of a severe degree, may develop. Optic neuritis and peripheral facial paralysis have been reported after injection of serum. *Pain* develops *pari passu* with the paralysis and may persist for some time after it is established; or it may precede the weakness by two or three days, being followed then by the development of paralysis. The pains may be widespread and involve the neck, shoulders, arms, and legs, and they may be confined to the nerve or nerves affected. *Muscle tenderness* is present and may persist for weeks. Fasciculations of the muscles have been observed in a few cases.

Prognosis: Generally, prognosis is good, even in patients with severe atrophy and absence of electrical reactions. About 20 per cent are left with residual weakness and atrophy (Bennett). Most patients recover within a period of six months but recovery may be delayed for as long as eighteen months.

12. *Acute Infectious Polyneuritis**

This disease has been variously described as infectious neuronitis, acute polyneuritis with facial diplegia, Guillan-Barré syndrome, acute febrile polyneuritis, polyneuronitis, motoneuronitis, myeloradiculitis, and neuritis with albumino-cytologic dissociation. These many forms represent one and the same disorder which is far from rare and constitutes an ever increasingly important form of neuritis.

Etiology: The cause of the disease is unknown. It has been attributed to

---

*The reigning confusion concerning the concept of acute infectious polyneuritis is nowhere more clearly exemplified than by a glance at the many synonyms used to describe one and the same disorder (after Pullen and Sodeman): acute febrile polyneuritis, infective polyneuritis, acute polyneuritis with facial diplegia, myeloradiculitis, polyradiculoneuritis, acute infectious neuronitis, radiculoneuritis, acute benign infectious myelitis, meningoradiculomyelitis, encephalomyeloradiculitis, Guillain-Barré syndrome, Guillain-Barré-Strohl syndrome, facial diplegia with polyneuritis, myeloradiculoneuritis, acute ascending paralysis, infective neuronitis, radiculoneuritis with acellular hyperalbuminosis of cerebrospinal fluid, acute infective polyneuritis, polyneuronitis, motoneuronitis, Landry's ascending paralysis, acute infective meningomyeloneuritis, acute toxic polyneuritis, and polyneuritis of unknown etiology.

either a bacterial or viral infectious agent, but the disorder is often not febrile or acute. Nutritional deficiency and allergy have been suggested as causes. Disturbance of the enzyme system of neurons has been proposed, due to toxic or allergic factors.

The disease is most common in the winter and autumn. No special incidence is found. Adults or children may be affected, but adults are more commonly afflicted.

The disease has been recorded with a number of conditions including influenza, infectious hepatitis, infectious mononucleosis, diphtheria, measles, mumps, scarlet fever, encephalitis, and chicken pox. The occurrence of the disease with so many diverse conditions raises the serious question of whether acute infectious polyneuritis is a disease *sui generis,* or whether it is not merely a form of neuritis which may occur in the course of many diseases. This appears to be a reasonable possibility.

Pathology: Changes are found in the peripheral nerves, but the findings have not been uniform. Acute neuritis (Bradford, Bashford, and Wilson) and degenerative changes in the nerves (Viets and Gilpin, and co-workers) have been recorded. Changes recorded by several investigators have been found in the spinal cord, involving posterior root ganglia, glial proliferation in the posterior roots and ganglia, degeneration of the posterior root ganglion cells, degeneration of the anterior horn cells, degeneration of the facial nuclei in the pons, and even infiltration about the nerve cells in the deep layers of the cortex. Recent studies (Roseman and Aring) reveal in the peripheral nerves and nerve roots: "(1) marked edema of the nerve bundles, (2) congestion, (3) moderate increase in cellularity with a tendency to focal accumulation of cells, (4) swelling and beading of the myelin sheaths, (5) swelling, beading, 'corkscrew' formation, and fragmentation and dissolution of the axis cylinders." The studies of Roseman and Aring showed further that the dorsal root ganglia were edematous and the nerve cells showed evidence of degeneration of varying degree; the axis cylinders were degenerated; phagocytes and lymphocytes were present in the tissue and the myelin was degenerated. The spinal cord showed a decrease in number and degeneration of the anterior horn cells in the cervical and thoracic cord particularly with some involvement of lower levels. There was a slight gliosis. The white matter showed mild changes in the myelin sheaths and axis cylinders. The brain stem showed changes somewhat similar to those of the cord, the process being diffuse with the greatest changes in the inferior olives. Changes were found in the vagus nuclei and in other nuclear groups. In the pons, the most severe degenerative changes were found in the facial nuclei. The cerebrum revealed a slight loss of nerve cells, shrinkage of ganglion cells, congestion, swelling of the oligoglia, and slight thickening and cellular infiltration of the meninges. Similar changes were found in the cerebellum.

It is apparent, therefore, that acute infectious polyneuritis is a disease which affects the peripheral nerves, the nerve roots, the anterior-horn cells, brain stem, cerebrum, and cerebellum. It often involves the entire reflex arc.

Symptoms: The onset is usually preceded by a history of recent infection, either a cold or grippe. Following this, there follows a latent period of days to months, with complete recovery often from the upper respiratory infection. The latent period between infection and the onset of neurological manifestations average one to three weeks. Fever is rarely present. *Pain* then develops in the legs and back but it is not constant. It may be so severe as to require heavy sedation and it may be preceded or accompanied by paresthesias of the feet and hands. Muscle and nerve tenderness is usually present but may be absent. *Weakness* of the hands and feet may develop gradually or suddenly after the onset of pain, within a matter of hours or days. It is symmetrical, often ascending in nature, being felt first in the distal portions of the limbs and ascending to involve the entire limb rapidly in a few hours or gradually over a period of several days. In some recorded instances, the motor weakness has progressed to its full development only after weeks. In most instances, the weakness is most severe in the proximal portions of the limbs but this is not an invariable characteristic. The weakness progresses as a rule to complete paralysis of the limbs, and sometimes of the thoracic and abdominal muscles. Despite the severe degree of paralysis, muscle *atrophy is not as a rule present early in the disease, and its absence constitutes one of the most striking features of the disease.* It may appear later. Muscle *fasciculations* are not present in the usual case but may be seen in some instances. The tendon *reflexes* are invariably absent, while the abdominal reflexes may be retained. The *sphincters are rarely involved. Sensory disturbances are usually absent,* but mild sensory deficit may be found so that hypalgesia or disturbance of position and vibration senses is sometimes found. Tenderness of the nerves and muscles is often present, but is not pronounced.

Peripheral *facial paralysis* is usually, but not always, present and is usually bilateral, causing facial diplegia. Unilateral involvement may be found. In the typical case there is loss of ability to wrinkle the forehead, close the eyes, blow out the cheeks, or to use the muscles of facial expression. The appearance of the face is blank; the voice is often nasal. Facial involvement may be severe or mild. Other cranial nerves may be affected. Optic neuritis, papilledema, oculomotor palsies, weakness of the masseters, palatal weakness, and hoarseness due to vocal-cord paralysis are present in some cases, either singly or in combination.

The spinal fluid reveals an increase of protein, which varies from 80 to 800 mg. (Roseman and Aring). The cells are not increased. Leukocytosis may be present.

The disease varies in duration. Recovery may occur in from three to four weeks, or may be delayed for a year or longer. Recovery usually is complete, but residual facial or limb weakness may remain. Death occurs in about 15 to 20 per cent of cases.

Diagnosis: This is usually not difficult. The onset of the disease after an upper respiratory infection, the ascending, progressive symmetrical paralysis, the facial diplegia, the absence of sensory findings, and the increase of protein in the spinal fluid are outstanding features. The increase of protein in the spinal fluid is an important factor in diagnosis, so much so that the diagnosis cannot be made without protein elevation. The spinal fluid protein is usually over 100 mg., but lower figures (75 to 80 mg.) have been recorded. The protein tends to return to normal with clinical recovery, but it may remain persistently high for some time after recovery begins. The problem is by no means simplified by the fact that increase of protein without increase of cells in the spinal fluid is found in other forms of neuritis (such as diphtheria or diabetes.)

On purely clinical grounds, this form of neuritis may be suspected in cases which develop with ascending paralysis, with predominant weakness in the proximial portions of the limbs, and with cranial nerve palsies, notably facial paralysis. None of these in itself suffices to establish the diagnosis, since the paralysis is not always ascending, the weakness pattern is not always predominantly proximal, and cranial nerve paralyses may be completely lacking. _Poliomyelitis_ is separated by the presence of fever, the the history of other cases in the community, the presence of cells in the spinal fluid in the acute stages, and the more rapid development. _Diphtheria_ is differentiated by the history of contact, the throat manifestations, and the more prominent sensory features of this form of neuritis. The disease may be indistinguishable from acute infectious polyneuritis.

13. Diphtheritic Neuritis

Etiology: This form of neuritis, once so common, has now become one of the rarities of neurological practice owing to the control of diphtheria. Both pharyngeal and cutaneous diphtheria were observed frequently in World War II. It is due to the diphtheria bacillus, occurs chiefly in children, but may be found in adults.

Symptoms: The symptoms appear two or three weeks after the appearance of the diphtheria, usually in outspoken cases; but in some instances the neuritis develops after a sore throat of diphtheritic origin, although usually it is not regarded as diphtheria. There appears to be no relation between the severity of the diphtheria and the neuritis; mild cases of diphtheria may develop neuritis, whereas severe cases of diphtheria frequently develop no neuritis. Cases are roughly of three categories: (1) those chiefly involving the cranial nerves, (2) those involving the extremities, and (3) those involving both.

In cases involving particularly the cranial nerves, the vagus is often affected with resulting palatal paralysis characterized by difficulty in swallowing and indistinctness of speech. The paralysis lasts a few weeks and then, as a rule, disappears. Accommodation paralysis is common after diphtheria. Oculomotor paralysis with ptosis, paralysis of movement of the eyeball, and strabismus may occur. Aphonia with paralysis of the larynx may occur; hoarseness is common. At times the facial muscles are paralyzed. Increase of spinal fluid protein is uniformly found.

Involvement of the extremities by diphtheria is due to a multiple neuritis. Pain and painful paresthesias are common. Apart from these distinguishing features, the neuritis is like that of other neuritides affecting the legs. The paralyses affecting the legs clear more slowly than those of the cranial nerves and may take months for full recovery to develop.

14. Other Forms of Infectious Neuritis

Neuritis may follow *influenza*. It is found also in *pneumonia*. *Malaria* is sometimes associated with neuritis. *Syphilis* is said to be a cause of neuritis. Undoubtedly it produces neuritis of the cranial nerves, but it is doubtful whether there is a syphilitic neuritis involving the nerves to the extremities. In any event, the diagnosis in such cases must be made with extreme caution. *Leprosy* is commonly associated with a neuritis. The nerves usually affected are the ulnar, median, and sciatic, singly, or as part of a multiple neuritis. The nerves are thickened and hypertrophic, and are felt as thick cords. Hyperesthesias are common and pain is a frequent symptom. Atrophy of the affected muscles and trophic changes in the skin (atrophy or pigmentation) and fingers (sloughing) may be found. Anesthesia of the skin is a common

finding and may be one of the first indications of involvement. It may be of the glove or stocking type or syringomyelic in nature. The outlook is not good. Progression of the neuritis is usual, with little evidence of improvement in most cases.

Polyarteritis nodosa is associated with multiple neuritis in about fifty-two per cent of cases (Lovshin & Kernohan). It has been attributed to two factors: (1) anoxemia and ischemia associated with the arteritis (2) a direct effect of the pathological agent of the periarteritis on the nerve trunks. The neuritis occurs early in the disease, either at the time of onset or within six months of the disorder. In general, it is widespread with severe, motor symptoms. The average duration of the disease is shorter in patients with neuritis, possibly because those cases with neuritis represent a more serious form of the disease.

Polyneuritis is an early symptom and an integral part of the disease. The neuritis is ischemic in origin and is secondary to the changes in the blood vessels. Extensive neuritis of the arms and legs is commonly found. Pain, tenderness of the nerve trunks and muscles, anesthesias, paralyses, loss of reflexes, and atrophies are found. Pain is often severe and is a prominent symptom. Transient attacks of diplopia may occur, and ophthalmoscopic examination may reveal papilledema and retinal hemorrhages, thrombosis of the central retinal artery, detachment of the retina, and albuminuric retinitis. Peripheral facial paralysis, and dysphagia may occur. Among the cerebral symptoms are headache, vertigo, focal and generalized convulsions, conjugate deviation of the eyes, chorea, myoclonus, tremor, hemiplegia, drowsiness, delirium, mental dullness, and coma (Woltman and Kernohan). The spinal fluid may be under increased pressure, may be yellow or cloudy, and may contain increase of cells and protein.

Infectious mononucleosis may be associated with neuritis indistinguishable from acute infectious polyneuritis. *Infectious hepatitis* is an occasional late complication by neuritis. At times multiple neuritis is found in association with *lupus erythematosus*. This latter disease needs consideration as an etiological factor in any patient in whom the cause of the neuritis is obscure.

Multiple neuritis is a frequent complication of *cutaneous diphtheria*. It was found to occur in 61 of 140 cases of cutaneous diphtheria (Gaskill & Korb). The neuritis develops relatively late after the appearance of the diphtheritic ulcers, at an average interval of 70.4 days, but it may develop during the acute stages of the ulcers. The neuritis begins with involvement of the cranial nerves or with paresthesias of the peripheral nerves. The former is characterized by loss of accommodation, loss of taste and numbness of the tongue, and weakness of the palate and pharynx. Motor peripheral nerve disease develops later. In severe cases, all stages may occur: cranial nerve involvement, paresthesias, and motor peripheral nerve disease. The neuritis runs a slow and insidious course. The spinal fluid protein is always elevated and gradually returns to normal with recovery. The early administration of *antitoxin* reduces significantly the incidence of neuritis. Apart from this, treatment is of no help.

15. Rare Forms of Neuritis

Sarcoidosis (Boeck's sarcoid) may sometimes involve the nervous system, but it is uncommon as a cause of nervous system disease. The cranial nerves are most frequently affected, particularly the facial nerves in association with uveitis and parotitis. There may be unilateral or bilateral facial nerve involve-

ment. In addition, there may be optic neuritis, optic atrophy, or choked disc due to either direct involvement of the optic nerve or involvement by pressure. There may be involvement of one or several other cranial nerves. There may be evidence of peripheral neuritis, either alone or in conjunction with cranial nerve involvement. Meningitis is sometimes seen, associated with mild cell increase (10 to 200 cells), chiefly lymphocytes. Encephalitis involving any part of the brain may develop in the course of the disease, embracing the cerebral hemisphere, brain stem, or cerebellum. The disease runs a slow and chronic course. There is usually slow recovery from the nervous system complications, but death may follow in patients with evidences of increased pressure.

Progressive, Hypertrophic, Interstitial Neuritis (Dejerine-Sotta): This form of neuritis is rare. It is the result of a true interstitial hypertrophy of the nerves and is often associated with degeneration of the spinal roots and spinal cord (posterior columns). The cause is not known. It occurs frequently in children but it also is found in adults and tends to occur in families. It is characterized by a multiple neuritis with particular involvement of the arms and legs, with claw-hand, talipes equinovarus, ataxia, sensory loss, loss of reflexes, and palpable nerves. The diagnosis of progressive, hypertrophic, interstitial neuritis is made on the basis of (1) family tendency, (2) palpable nerves, (3) glove-and-stocking type of anesthesia, (4) flat feet.

A special and rare form of *chronic progressive polyneuritis* has been described (Harris). The cases described have occurred in adults, the symptoms developing progressively over a period of many months or even years. The cause is not known, but a special endotoxin or neurotoxin of undisclosed type has been postulated. The common features consist of a slowly progressive paralysis, with muscle atrophy, decreased electrical excitability of the muscles, and few sensory symptoms. Hypertrophy of the nerves may be present but is not constant, and palpation of thickened nerves is not invariably present. Recurrent attacks following short periods of recovery may or may not occur.

Hematoporphyrinuric Polyneuritis: This occurs as a result of poisoning with Sulfonal, Trional, Veronal, and other barbiturates and also independently of these from the use of hematoporphyrin hydrochloride therapeutically. The neuritis develops acutely within a few days or weeks of taking the barbiturate, or it may develop gradually after years of barbital dosage. There is often no apparent relationship between the dosage of the drug and the symptoms, neuritis sometimes developing after trifling doses. The legs are usually affected, but all the limbs not infrequently. Pains in the limbs are common. Intestinal symptoms are common and include constipation, nausea, vomiting, and abdominal pains with distention. Fever, delirium, excitement, and moderate leukocytosis develop. The urine has a port-wine color due to the presence of hematoporphyrin (*v.* Porphyrinuria).

Hereditary Sensory Radicular Neuropathy (Hicks, Denny-Brown): This is a hereditary disorder, inherited as a simple mendelian dominant, occurring also in a sporadic and familial form. It is characterized by perforating ulcers about the feet, pains about the body and deafness. The pains are often felt as shooting or lightning pains in the legs. Pain and temperature sensations are lost in the lower limbs, involving the feet, in many instances extending to the middle of the leg and in some instances to the knees. The sensory disturbance is of a dissociated type, the loss of pain being greater than to touch and the loss of temperature greater than to pain. The deafness is slowly progressive and of a neurogenic type. The patellar and Achilles reflexes are lost; those in the arms retained. Postmortem study revealed a primary degeneration of dorsal root ganglia, deposits of amyloid being formed in the most severely affected ganglia. The disease is confused with tabes dorsalis, syringomyelia, pseudotabes diabetica and familial perforating ulcer.

Erythredema Polyneuritis (Pink Disease): This disease occurs in the young (three to fifteen months), involving either sex. The cause is not known. There is no familial incidence. The symptoms are fretfulness; irritability; loss of muscle tone with weak, flabby muscles; anorexia; gingivitis and stomatitis; constant sweats; erythema of the hands, face, cheeks, and nose, characterized by a bright pink over the face and pink or reddish blue over the extremities; swelling of the feet and hands with desquamation; falling off of fingernails and toenails; and in some cases gangrene. The onset in many instances seems to be correlated with some other acute illness. Photophobia, anorexia, hypotonia of the muscles, and the cutaneous rash are almost constant features. The entire bodily musculature becomes atonic, which may account for the sudden cardiac death seen in some cases. The reflexes are decreased or absent. Sensory disturbances cannot be evaluated, since the disease occurs in infants, but diminution of reaction to painful stimuli is reported. Irritability and photophobia are constant, and efforts to examine infants with the disease result in outbursts of crying and withdrawal. In some cases, extreme lethargy is found. Some of the subjects recover, others die.

The mortality in a group of fifteen patients was 13.3 per cent (Ratcliffe).

II. PERIPHERAL NERVE INJURIES

The problem of nerve injuries becomes of increasing importance because of increasing industrial hazards. Injuries to nerves, however, may result not only from industrial problems but from automobile accidents, gunshot wounds, stab wounds, prolonged pressure, fracture of the bones, dislocations, and other causes.

Incidence: There is hardly a nerve in the body which may not be subject to injury, but some nerves are more apt than others to be injured. The relative incidence of their involvement is given in Table 17.

Table 17—Incidence of Peripheral Nerve Injuries

	Foerster Cases	Frazier Cases	Pollock and Davis Cases
RADIAL	936	516	165
MEDIAN	800	269	93
ULNAR	742	492	136
SCIATIC	523	551	160
PERONEAL	183	395	120
TIBIAL	112	35	25
AXILLARY	82	. . .	7
MUSCULOCUTANEOUS	71	. . .	4
ANTERIOR CRURAL	30	. . .	19

It is apparent from this that the radial, median, ulnar, and sciatic are more commonly affected than other nerves in the body. The incidence of peripheral nerve injuries in World War II has been placed at 15 per cent (Spurling).

Syndromes: The clinical syndromes of nerve injury have been divided into a number of types. Though this grouping is in many ways artificial because of overlapping of features in each, it has some practical advantages, largely those of separation of complete and incomplete interruptions. For all practical purposes, however, it is sufficient to divide nerve injuries into complete and incomplete groups.

1. Syndrome of Complete Interruption: This is characterized by (1) immediate and complete paralysis of the muscles supplied by the interrupted nerve; (2) progressive and rapid development of hypotonia of the muscles; (3) atrophy which develops more slowly than hypotonia and eventually becomes pronounced; (4) loss of electrical reactions and the appearance of reaction of degeneration; (5) loss of sensation in the area supplied by the nerve; (6) absence of trophic changes; (7) absence of pain.

Distinction is often made in nerve injuries between *anatomical* and *physiological* interruption of function. The former refers to an interruption of function resulting from an actual section of the nerve and separation of its parts; the latter to interruption of function without actual section and separation of the nerve fibers. The distinction has been made in order to clarify indications for treatment, for the assumption is that in cases wherein recovery is developing after injury to a nerve, physiological and not anatomical interruption must be present. Consequently, conservative treatment is indicated. Actually the distinction between the two conditions is usually impossible on clinical grounds, for the symptoms and signs assigned to anatomical interruption hold equally as well for physiological interruption of function. It is safer, therefore, not to rely too strongly on the distinction between anatomical and physiological interruption and to confine oneself simply to determining whether complete interruption of nerve function is present.

It is possible from a single examination only to determine whether the nerve lesion is complete or incomplete. Upon subsequent recovery of function, it is possible to determine that there has been physiological interruption, but not until then. The criterion of return of function to indicate a physiological break is not safe, since it has been found that in cases in which this assumption has been made, operation has often revealed a complete anatomical separation. "Although many attempts have been made to discover a sign or group of signs which would justify at a single examination a differential diagnosis between a complete anatomical section of a nerve and one in which complete loss of function is not the result of discontinuity of the nerve but only a physiological interruption, none has been discovered." (Pollock.) Both conditions are characterized by complete paralysis, complete anesthesia, and complete reaction of degeneration of the muscles supplied by the nerve. Attempts to differentiate the condition by other criteria have failed.

2. Syndrome of Compression: This syndrome occurs because of compression of the nerve by callus, scar, ischemia (Saturday night palsy), etc., and is the result probably more of temporary than permanent interruption of the nerve. It is featured by (1) complete or incomplete paralysis, often the former; (2) partial muscular atrophy not as intense as in the syndrome of interruption; atrophy may be intense in the small hand muscles and slight in others; (3) relative preservation of muscle tone; this is extremely variable, however, and is not an absolute criterion; (4) only partial loss of electrical response; (5) sensory disturbances which are usually not as complete as in interruption of the nerve; (6) absence of pain, formication, or trophic lesions.

3. Syndrome of Irritation: This is an extremely important syndrome. Generally speaking, the injury to the nerves in this syndrome is incomplete, but it may vary from slight to severe degrees. Some degree of motion is usually retained and sensation is not completely interrupted. The general tendency is toward recovery. It is characterized by (1) pain which is absent in the first two syndromes; it is described as hot, burning and is often unbearable; (2) hyperesthesias of the skin in the area of the affected nerve; this is often of a severe degree, so that merely stroking the skin is very painful, causing a diffuse nonlocalizable painful sensation; (3) trophic disturbances, such as dryness of the skin, brittle nails, atrophy of the terminal digits, etc.; the skin is glossy, the nails brittle and yellowish, the muscles firm and fibrous; the changes are likely to persist; (4) muscle weakness of a variable degree.

NERVE CONCUSSION: It has been shown that the nerve is rapidly blown aside during expansion of a large temporary cavity that is formed by a high velocity missile, which passes near but does not strike the nerve directly. Functional damage can be done to nerves so displaced, and the loss of function can be attributed to a series of minor breaks in the myelin sheath of the nerve, due to compression and stretching of the nerve. Percussion of a peripheral nerve is followed in mild cases by myelin breakdown and rupture of the sheath of Schwann, without interruption of the axis cylinder, and in moderately severe cases by the same process, with complete interruption of impulses in motor fibers and intact sensation (Denny-Brown and Brenner).

III. DEGENERATION AND REGENERATION OF NERVES

In order to comprehend clearly the factors which govern recovery in nerves, as well as to understand the principles of treatment, consideration must be given to the histological features which accompany interruption of the nerve both as to degeneration and regeneration.

Section of a nerve by injury produces changes in the distal segment of the nerve, the proximal segment, and in the cells of origin of the nerve fibers within the spinal cord. In the central end changes are found for a short distance beyond the site of injury. These consist of degeneration of the myelin and axis cylinders for about 1 cm. beyond the site of section. Such changes appear about the third day and may proceed for some distance. These changes are of minor importance in the majority of instances, but in some cases the evidences of injury may extend for some distance along the central stump, especially in cases of evulsion and tearing of the nerves. Secondary changes are found in the anterior horn cells giving rise to the injured nerve. These consist of reversible changes within the ganglion cells, characterized by axonal chromatolysis, which are as a rule transitory and show a return to normal structure and function within a few days to several weeks. The changes in the ganglion cells begin as early as the first day after injury and reach their maximum development during the second and third weeks, after which recovery occurs. In some instances, the changes in the cells are more serious than in others, particularly in evulsions and in section of the nerve close to the cell of origin. The closer the injury to the cell of origin, the more serious is likely to be the damage to the nerve cells.

More important are the changes which develop in the distal stump. Changes in the axons are found in twelve hours after the section. Fragmentation and destruction of the axis cylinders begins within forty-eight hours and proceeds unabated until complete degeneration occurs by the end of the third to fourth week. Not all fibers are affected in the same fashion and it is probable that the fine fibers are more resistant than the larger ones and that some nonmedullated fibers are more resistant than the medullated axons. Degeneration takes place simultaneously along the entire axis cylinder and not by progression from one part to another. Similar degeneration affects the terminal endings of the nerve fibers within the muscles. The motor end plates degenerate, the process being complete in about six months. Reinnervation is carried out by penetration of nerve fibers into the old end plates and by accessory fibers. The muscle spindles also degenerate and again become reinnervated. The myelin breaks down simultaneously, the degeneration proceeding until all the myelin is removed and the nerve is bereft of both axis cylinders and myelin sheaths. Myelin degeneration begins on the first day and continues until all the myelin is removed by phagocytes.

The myelin destruction is seen in two stages, a Marchi stage from the eighth to about the twenty-first day, and a neutral fat stage thereafter. The Marchi stage reaches its maximum on the twelfth day. Removal of the disintegrated axis cylinders and myelin sheaths is carried out by fibroblasts and the cells of the Schwann neurilemmal sheaths which enlarge, become phagocytic, and remove the débris. The process is complex, but its essentials are as indicated. Complete demyelination occurs in about eight weeks. The result of the degenerative and phagocytic process is the removal of the broken down axones and myelin sheaths, leaving behind an empty tube composed of the neurilemmal sheath and the connective tissue septa of the nerve. The empty tube of the peripheral stump is made up of a number of Schwann tubes, each of perhaps half the diameter of the original fiber and filled with Schwann cells. Between this empty sheath and the vital central stump is a connective tissue scar which has developed as a result of the injury. It is this scar which the regenerating fibers from the central stump must traverse in order to fill in the empty sheath of the distal stump which offers the best route for the regenerating fibers.

Regeneration occurs from the central stump and begins in two or three days for medullated fibers. By the end of the second day fibers enter the scar proper. The power of regulation of fibers of the central stump is as good long after section as it is soon afterward. The rate of progression of the regeneration is variously estimated and no constant figures are available. The rate is usually estimated at 1 mm. a day. In cats, dogs, and rabbits, the growth of the axon has been found to be 3 to 4 mm. a day. It is believed by some that the rate of outgrowth of the axon tips declines with the distance from the lesion, but this has not been found to be universally true. In humans, the rate of regeneration for motor fibers is 1 to 2 mm. per day, and for sensory fibers 2.0 to 2.5 mm. per day (Sunderland).

Associated with the downgrowth of axis cylinders is the proliferation of the Schwann cells. These grow and expand markedly both from the central and distal stumps, chiefly from the latter. The outgrowth of the Schwann cells is of the greatest importance for the regeneration of nerves, "since it is the main agent by which physical continuity is restored between the intact axons of the central stump and the old pathways in the peripheral one" (Young). The outgrowing axons "are led into the peripheral stump along the Schwann bands which have grown out across the scar." They grow into the empty peripheral tubes alone and not in the Schwann bands. After downgrowth, the fibers thicken and medullate, their increase in diameter advancing progressively down the nerve. Medullation may develop *pari passu* with the growth of

the axis cylinder in some fibers, but is slower in others. It seems to be more rapid in the proximal portions and slower in the distal parts of the nerve, and is dependent on the central rather than the peripheral stump.

The rate of regeneration varies with different nerves. It appears to be influenced by (1) the level of section of the nerve, the greater the distance from the muscle innervated, the slower being the functional, not the anatomical, recovery; (2) the type of injury, recovery being materially slower in evulsion and suture than after crushing; (3) delay of suture; (4) infection; (5) age, recovery being slower in older subjects (Gutmann). In cases of secondary suture, regeneration is influenced by previous infection, the level of the injury, the presence of a scar, the type of suture operation, etc.

Clinical evidence of regeneration is manifested by improvement in the color of the skin, by change in muscle tone, return of sensation and motion, and disappearance of reaction of degeneration. The muscles become sensitive to pressure on pinching. The galvanic response on electrical examination begins to show evidence of return, while the faradic response is extremely slow to recover and often fails to reappear. Pin prick begins to be felt and with it deep pressure pain. Touch and appreciation of joint sense are slower to appear, while discriminatory sensations are slowest of all and may never return completely.

Changes also develop in muscle fibers after denervation. During one to three months after denervation, there is a loosening of the compact arrangement of the muscle fibers, an apparent increase of nuclei, and little change in the connective tissue. The blood vessels appear dilated. From three months on, there is progressive shrinkage of the muscle fibers, fading of the crossstriations, and thickening of the vessel walls. There is an increase of connective tissue, beginning around the vessels, spreading throughout the muscle, and finally obliterating the Schwann tubes. As the muscle fibers atrophy, they are replaced by fat and connective tissue. "Up to one year after denervation, it is possible to expect a fairly good degree of functional recovery; from then onward, the prognosis deteriorates; and as a rule from three years onward, the prospects are exceedingly poor" (Bowden).

Tinel's sign, which consists of a painful sensation referred to the periphery of a regenerating nerve on painful pressure, is of value in a sutured nerve where the ends are known to be in apposition; hence pressure over the nerve produces pain to a specific point which may be taken roughly as the point to which fibers have regenerated. In unsutured nerves, the sign is of less value, since the regenerating axons may be diverted and false-pain localization induced by pressure on the nerve.

Evidences of regeneration tend to appear in a more or less definite sequence: (1) sensory return, (2) arrest of atrophy and restoration of muscle tone, (3) return of faradic response in some cases, (4) disappearance of objective sensory disturbances, and (5) return of voluntary movements. Sensory regeneration is the first to reappear and is recognized by pain on pinching the skin, often, but by no means always, the first sign of regeneration; other sensory evidences consist of an aching of the muscles and formication on pressure of the nerve. Tinel's sign, already referred to, is generally regarded as unreliable as an indication of nerve regeneration. Sensory return precedes that of motor function in most cases. Two stages in the return of sensation are noted (Stopford): (1) a return of the ability to appreciate pin prick and extremes of temperature; and (2) the return of the

discriminative aspects of sensation, such as the localization of a sensory stimulus, the discrimination between strengths and types of stimulus, the recognition of position and passive movement, the recognition of fine differences of temperature, and the appreciation of very light touch. Recovery of the first group of sensations occurs early after nerve suture and is relatively good, while the recovery of the sensory impressions of the second group is later, and is less complete and perfect.

Return of sensory function begins between ten and fourteen weeks after nerve section. It is characterized by the following, based on the experiments of Trotter and Davies (Walshe): "(1) The progressive and simultaneous return of tactile, painful, and cold sensations, the return of actual heat being apparently delayed; (2) the development of two new phenomena not hitherto found in the area of sensory change, namely, peripheral reference and intensification. The returning sensory functions are hypoesthetic, and full acuity is not obtained for a further period of weeks." In peripheral reference, stimuli are referred minutely to the distal end of the area of sensory change. In intensification, an abnormally vivid quality is imparted to the returning sensations. The regenerating nerve trunk, moreover, is found to be abnormally sensitive to stimulation.

Motor recovery tends to recur in a definite order. Some nerves recover more rapidly than others, and some movements in the distribution of the affected nerves recover more rapidly than others. Thus in radial nerve lesions, the wrist and finger extensors tend to recover first, while in median nerve lesions the pronators, palmaris longus, and wrist flexor recover earliest, etc. Care must be exercised, however, in the return of motor function to differentiate carefully between true muscle movements and supplementary motility. This is often extremely difficult. The movements which cannot be supplemented in various nerve lesions are as follows: "In musculospinal lesions, extension of the proximal phalanx of the thumb and abduction of the thumb in the plane of the palm, and extension of the proximal phalanges of the fingers. In ulnar nerve lesions, flexion of the proximal phalanges of the ring and little fingers, with the distal phalanges extended, and lateral movements of the extended middle finger. In median nerve lesions, flexion of the distal phalanx of the index finger and thumb. In combined lesions of the ulnar and median nerves, all movements of the hand except flexion at the wrist and hollowing of the hand. In external popliteal lesions, eversion of the foot" (Pollock).

Radial nerve lesions show first a recovery of the wrist extensors, followed by the finger extensors, then the abductor and extensor of the thumb. In ulnar nerve lesions the intrinsic hand muscles are the last to recover. In median nerve lesions, the muscles of the thenar eminence and the flexor of the index finger recover last. In external popliteal lesions the extensors of the toes, and in sciatic nerve lesions the flexors and extensors of the toes, recover last. For spontaneous recovery of nerves the following order is found: tibialis, median, musculocutaneous, axillary, ulnar, radial, peroneal, and sciatic.

The time for expected evidence of regeneration is given in Table 18.

Management: The management of nerve injuries is a matter of some controversy. After it has been determined whether spontaneous recovery has developed to its fullest extent, it is necessary then to decide whether operative treatment is indicated. After this has been done, it becomes necessary to determine whether the nerve is recovering

Table 18—Approximate Time for Expectant Evidence of Regeneration

(*Stookey*)

Nerve and Level	Under Good Conditions, Months	Under Poor Conditions, Months
MUSCULOCUTANEOUS:		
Axilla............	5 to 6	8 to 10
MUSCULOSPIRAL:		
Middle third arm...	7 to 8	14
Lower third arm....	6 to 7	12
ULNAR:		
Wrist............	5 to 7	10
Elbow...........	10 to 12	16
Axilla............	15 to 16	22
MEDIAN:		
Wrist............	4 to 5	10
Elbow...........	8 to 9	15
Axilla............	12 to 14	18
SCIATICA:		
Middle third thigh.	10 to 12	18
Upper third thigh..	12 to 14	22
PERONEAL:		
Head of fibula......	8 to 9	14
Popliteal space.....	10 to 12	16
TIBIAL:		
Popliteal space.....	11 to 12	17

from operation and to evaluate the probability and degree of recovery. If this appears to be incomplete, accessory operations, such as muscle or tendon transplants and other procedures, may be considered. Generally speaking, treatment may be divided into operative and conservative measures.

Operative: Immediate suture of the severed nerve is always desirable wherever possible if it can be done under sterile conditions. Recovery is more prompt under such conditions. In the case of infected wounds, care must be taken to permit recovery from the infection before operation is undertaken. Experiences in World War II have made clear the following: "It has been established beyond all reasonable doubt that the optimum time to suture a divided peripheral nerve is within three to six weeks after wounding. . . . It has been clearly established that the time-honored custom of splinting an extremity because of damage to a major nerve trunk is, in the absence of an associated fracture, not only useless but actually harmful. It has been clearly demonstrated that by early application of competent physical therapy the fixed, ankylosed joint which had previously been the surgeon's bugbear in the management of all paralyzed extremities will almost never develop" (Spurling). It has been found also that "grafting of large nerve defects in the human subjects by either autogenous or homogenous grafts was as unsuccessful in practice as it was fallacious in concept" (Spurling). The time of repair of the nerve has been greatly shortened as a result of more rapid control of infection by means of the sulfonamide drugs.

Generally speaking, a radical attitude toward surgical exposure of the injured nerve seems best. "If this practice is followed, then it will happen, of course, that some who might have recovered without surgical treatment will undergo a needless operation. But even among a certain number of these patients regeneration may be hastened rather than jeopardized by liberating the nerve from scar tissue and by preparing a more suitable bed for the nerve. On the other hand, if loss of substance of a nerve is found at operation, the nerve may be sutured and the time lost in waiting for spontaneous regeneration saved" (Stookey).

Experience with peripheral nerve injuries in World War II has established beyond doubt that end-to-end suture should be carried out at the earliest possible moment. It has been demonstrated also that the harmful effects of infection upon the regeneration of nerve fibers is not so great as had been believed, and that nerve fibers are not so vulnerable to infection as had been presumed (Davis, Perret, and Carroll).

End-to-end suture in acute nerve injuries, whether in civil life or in war, offers few problems, since it seems clear that suture should be carried out at the first possible moment. In those patients, in whom suture has been delayed for some reason, operation appears to be indicated under the following circumstances: (1) the persistence of complete paralysis; (2) the palpation of a thickened mass, indicative of a neuroma; and (3) failure of progression of recovery in patients who have shown evidences of early recovery.

The types of operation available are matters of surgical treatment for which the student is referred to surgical texts.

Conservative: Conservative treatment should consist of *massage* of the affected limb daily, *electrical treatment, passive exercise* of muscles, and *splinting* to prevent contracture. These must be maintained over a long period and faithfully carried out. *Electrical examination* of muscle responses should be made from time to time in order to have a base by which to measure improvement. Electrical treatment may be given daily or on alternate days in the form of galvanism or faradism. Recent evidence indicates that muscle wasting can be controlled to a considerable extent by electrical stimulation. For this purpose, galvanism is best. To be effective, the treatment must be intensive and must be continued over a long period. It should be given at the rate of 90 stimuli daily, six days a week, and the stimuli should be strong enough to produce brisk contraction. The use of galvanism in the treatment of denervated muscle results in the decline of muscle wasting and in better return of function in the wasted muscles (Jackson). Massage and passive exercises should be given daily wherever possible. *Hydrotherapy* is often helpful and may be used in many forms, such as sprays, whirlpool baths, etc. *Heat* is useful, especially in the form of diathermy. Proper splints should be made in order to prevent deformities. The style of splint will depend upon the nature of the muscle deformity. Care must be taken to encourage the patient constantly, since recovery of a severed nerve is slow, and one must contend constantly with discouragement on the part of the patient.

In cases of recent nerve injury, it is extremely difficult to determine whether the signs of nerve injury are the result of an actual structural interruption of the nerve or of a physiological interruption due to loss of conduction of nerve impulses in an injured but not an interrupted nerve. Physiological interruption is present if recovery ensues. This may be complete or partial. It is true also that physiological recovery occurs sometimes before evidence of anatomical regeneration is found. Anatomical interruption is present if the signs of nerve injury develop: Atrophy of muscles, sensory loss, and loss of electrical reactions. Actually it is impossible to differentiate between the two conditions.

Nerve injuries associated with *closed fractures* of the limbs usually recover spontaneously, but in some instances incomplete recovery or complete lack of recovery occurs. Exploration in such cases should be carried out when it is apparent that recovery is overdue. Early exploration is desirable in ulnar nerve and peroneal nerve injuries, and in eight to ten weeks in radial palsy from fracture of the humerus if no return of function is apparent (Gurdjian and Smathers). It seems best to set no time limits, but to explore when it is apparent that recovery is lagging.

The *prognosis* of nerve injuries is much better than one would expect on theoretical grounds, and serves to illustrate the fact that if given an opportunity, injured nerves recover both spontaneously and after operation. The incidence of recovery has been variously reported from 50 to 86 per cent. It is estimated that after secondary suture, judged by rigid standards, complete regeneration occurs in 10 to 15 per cent of cases, marked but incomplete regeneration in 50 to 60 per cent, and total failure in 25 to 40 per cent. Following suture, recovery seems to be more complete in the radial nerve lesions, next best in the median nerve lesions, and poorest in ulnar nerve injuries. Brachial plexus injuries show a high incidence of spontaneous recovery.

IV. INVOLVEMENT OF INDIVIDUAL NERVES

1. Upper Extremity

Radial Nerve (C_5-C_8 and T_1): This is the main nerve of the posterior cord of the brachial plexus. It is chiefly a motor nerve, contributing only a small sensory innervation to the back of the hand and a small strip on the external surface of the forearm. It is frequently diseased both alone and in conjunction with other nerves. Neuritis of various sorts may single it out, as, for example, in jake paralysis, alcoholic neuritis, or acute infectious polyneuritis. It is frequently affected in lead poisoning. Fractures of the upper and middle portions of the humerus may injure it, since it lies in the arm on the lateral surface of the humerus. Tumors may occasionally be found along its course, either singly or as part of a generalized neurofibromatosis. Gunshot wounds in the axilla or arm may cause injury to the radial nerve and in war wounds it is the most frequently injured nerve in the body. Saturday night palsy causing paralysis of the radial nerve was formerly a common cause, the palsy resulting from compression of the nerve against the edge of a bed or chair during alcoholic stupor. Pressure on the nerve by

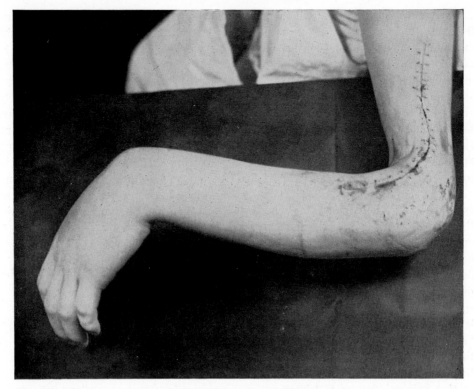

Fig. 60—*Radial nerve paralysis* resulting from injury of the nerve in the arm, illustrating the characteristic wrist-drop.

crutches may cause radial paralysis. Compression by a rifle sling may be a cause, the sling of the rifle being wound around the arm to steady it, resulting in ischemic compression of the nerve. In rare instances the radial nerve may be affected in the scalenus anticus syndrome.

The radial nerve is the main extensor nerve of the arm, wrist, and fingers. It supplies the triceps muscle and the anconeus, the supinator longus, the extensor carpi radialis longus, the extensor carpi radialis brevis, and the supinator brevis. It is, therefore, the most important extensor nerve of the arm and forearm, supplying as it does all the muscles on the extensor surface of the forearm. Its sensory component is unimportant, but it supplies a small branch to the posterointernal part of the arm, a narrow strip

on the posteroexternal surface of the forearm, and the dorsum of the hand to the proximal interphalangeal joint.

Injury of the nerve above the branch to the triceps muscle results in loss of extension of the forearm (triceps), loss of extension of the wrist with resulting wrist-drop (extensor carpi radialis longus and brevis), inability to extend the fingers (extensor communis digitorum), loss of extension of the thumb (extensor pollicis longus and brevis), weakness of the flexion of the elbow due to loss of action of the supinator longus, which is a powerful flexor of the forearm, and weakness of supination (supinator longus and brevis). The triceps reflex is absent and there is loss of sensation over the dorsum of the hand. Injury to the radial nerve above the origin of the triceps muscle is not common.

The most frequent site of injury is in the arm above the origin of the nerve to the supinator longus, resulting as a rule from fracture of the humerus. In such a case there will be wrist-drop with loss of extension of the wrist, loss of extension of the fingers and thumb, weakness of flexion of the forearm at the elbow, and weakness of supination. The picture is that of wrist-drop, with the action of the triceps muscle and the triceps reflex intact.

Injury of the nerve below the nerve to the supinator longus gives the same picture except that flexion of the forearm and supination are unaffected due to the intact supinator longus.

Isolated involvement of the deep *posterior interosseous branch* of the nerve in the forearm occurs at times. This is usually the result of injury, but instances of progressive paralysis of the nerve are recorded. The clinical picture is that of paralysis of extension of the fingers and

thumb with intact extension of the wrist, atrophy of the extensor forearm muscles, and intact sensation.

Median Nerve $(C_{6, 7, 8}$ and $T_1)$: The median is a mixed nerve, containing both motor and sensory fibers, forming part of the lateral and inner cords of the brachial plexus. It may be involved in any part of its course from the brachial plexus into the hand. It is subject to involvement by injuries, such as gunshot wounds, dislocations of the humerus or radius with compression of the nerve in the axilla or elbow, and cuts at the wrist and elbow, and by fractures of the humerus. It is involved frequently in multiple neuritis, as a mononeuritis in various types of infection, and in cervical rib compression at times. Isolated median nerve palsies have been reported in occupational hazards of many sorts—joiners, locksmiths, milkers, cigar makers, carpet beaters, and dentists. They have also

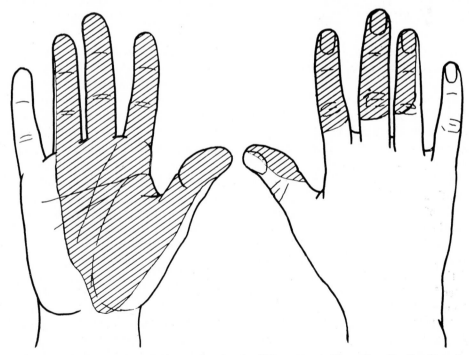

Fig. 61—*Median nerve paralysis*, showing in diagrammatic form the distribution of the sensory disturbance with involvement of the median nerve.

been found in fractures of the wrist. Unilateral palsy tends to occur in relatively young subjects, while bilateral palsy is more often seen in the middle-aged. In young subjects the condition is rare in the absence of injury; in the middle-aged group it may arise as a result of normal activity of the hands.

Neuritis of the median nerve may develop from compression of the nerve under the transverse carpal ligament in the wrist, in the carpal tunnel (Brain, Wright, and Wilkinson). The cases reported have occurred bilaterally in middle-aged or elderly women. The condition is characterized by pain, paresthesias and sensory loss within the area supplied by the sensory branches of the median nerve, and partial thenar atrophy limited to the abductor brevis and opponens pollicis muscles, or to the abductor brevis alone. Section of the transverse carpal ligament results in immediate relief of the pain and tingling, with gradual improvement in power of the affected muscles and the sensory loss. The development of symptoms is gradual. Occupation is probably the outstanding cause, as in rubbing and polishing.

The median nerve supplies all the muscles of the anterior surface of the forearm except the flexor carpi ulnaris and the ulnar portion of the flexor digitorum profundus. It supplies the pronator radii teres, flexor carpi radialis, palmaris longus, flexor digitorum sublimis, the outer heads of the flexor digitorum profundus, and the pronator quadratus. In the hand it supplies the abductor pollicis brevis, opponens pollicis, the superficial head of the flexor pollicis brevis, and the two outer lumbricals. The sensory supply of the nerve is on the palmar surface, to the radial half of the fourth finger, the middle and index fingers, the palmar surface of the thumb, and the corresponding areas of the palm; on the dorsum of the hand, to the distal two phalanges of the index, middle, and ring fingers. The median nerve is the chief flexor of the hand and fingers. It causes flexion of the hand on the forearm, flexion of the fingers, pronation of the forearm, and abduction, flexion, and opposition of the thumb.

Flexion of the fingers is not carried out exclusively by the median nerve. It is carried out as follows: at the metacarpophalangeal joints by the interossei, at the proximal interphalangeal joints by the flexor digitorum sublimis (median), and at the distal interphalangeal joints by the flexor digitorum profundus (median and ulnar), the innervation to the terminal phalangeal joints of the fourth and fifth fingers being through the ulnar nerve. Flexion is not entirely lost in median paralysis, therefore, but it is very greatly weakened.

The manifestations of paralysis due to involvement of the median nerve will depend on the level at which the nerve is injured by trauma or disease. Generally speaking, a lesion in the arm will cause the following: (1) paralysis of pronation of the forearm; (2) weakness of flexion of the hand at the wrist; this is not complete because of intactness of the flexor carpi ulnaris which permits some flexion of the wrist; (3) paralysis of flexion of all the fingers at the second joints and at the terminal joints of the thumb, index, and middle fingers; flexion is not absent at the metacarpophalangeal joints which are supplied by the ulnar nerve; the last two fingers flex by means of slips of the flexor digitorum profundus supplied by the ulnar nerve; (4) paralysis of flexion of the terminal phalanx of the thumb and of abduction and opposition of the thumb; (5) loss of sensation over the area of skin indicated above.

If the nerve is injured below the elbow, at the wrist or even in the palm, fragments of this syndrome will develop. If the injury lies below the point at which the nerves innervating the fingers are given off, only the muscles to the thenar eminence will be affected. This occurs in injuries at the wrist or in the lower part of the forearm.

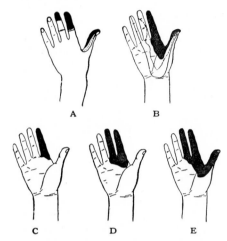

Fig. 62—*Median nerve. Sensory loss patterns in disease of the median nerve. (Stookey: Nelson Loose-Leaf Surgery, Vol. 2.)*

If paralysis is complete, atrophy of the thenar eminence is found, giving rise to the flat simian type of hand. Trophic changes may be found in the nails and skin.

Ulnar Nerve ($C_{7, 8}$ and T_1): This nerve is injured frequently as a result of stab or gunshot wounds, fractures at the lower end of the humerus, direct pressure at the elbow, cervical rib, scalenus anticus compression, and neuritis from various causes. Subluxation of the nerve from the ulnar groove or a progressive filling in of this groove are not infrequent causes of ulnar neuritis (Harris). These possibilities should be investigated in any obscure case of ulnar neuritis. The nerve supplies the ulnar flexor of the wrist, the terminal phalanges of the fourth and fifth fingers, the muscles of the hypothenar eminence, all the interossei and the

inner two lumbricals, the adductors of the thumb, and the short head of the flexor pollicis brevis. It supplies the skin on the ulnar side of the hand in the palm, and over the dorsum of the hand in a line passing through the middle of the ring finger.

Disease or injury of the ulnar nerve will cause (1) weakness of flexion of the hand on the forearm; this is never very great because of the intact flexors supplied by the median nerve; the hand deviates to the radial side in flexion; (2) diminished flexion of the last two fingers due to involvement of the two inner heads of the flexor profundus and paralysis of the terminal phalanges of the fourth and fifth fingers; (3) atrophy of the hypothenar eminence and weakness or paralysis of opposition of the little finger; (4) paralysis of flexion of the first phalanges on the metacarpals (metacarpophalangeal flexion) due to involvement of the interossei; (5) paralysis of adduction and abduction of the fingers due to involvement of the interossei, hence an inability to separate the fingers and to bring them together; (6) paralysis or weakness in adduction of the thumb; (7) sensory disturbances on the ulnar side of the hand in the region indicated.

Atrophy of some degree usually develops and is often pronounced. The interossei, lumbricals, and hypothenar eminence atrophy in the hand so that the dorsum and palm show deep indentations between the metacarpals, and the hypothenar eminence is flat and loses its rounded contour.

In ulnar neuritis there may occur focal paralysis of the small hand muscles without cutaneous sensory disturbances due to involvement of the deep palmar branch of the ulnar nerve. This is characterized by maintenance of the little finger in an abducted position, wasting of the interosseous muscles, and weakness of abduction and adduction of the

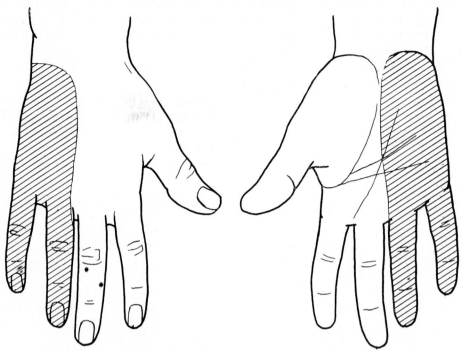

Fig. 63—*Ulnar nerve paralysis*, showing in diagrammatic form the distribution of the sensory disturbance with involvement of the median nerve.

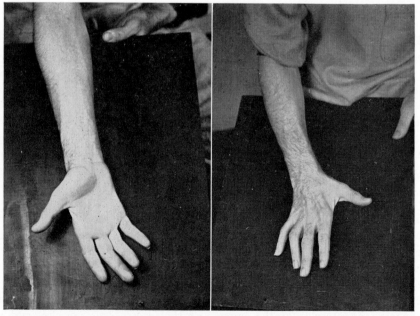

Fig. 64—*Ulnar nerve injury*, showing the atrophy of the interossei and of the hypothenar eminence and the characteristic flexion posture of the fourth and fifth fingers.

fingers. The difficulty has been found to be due to a callus overlying the ulnar nerve distal to the innervation of the hypothenar muscles.

Circumflex Nerve ($C_{5, 6}$) : This nerve is sometimes affected alone as a result of fractures of the shaft of the humerus, following serum injections, falls, or blows to the shoulder. The nerve supplies chiefly the deltoid muscle, but also the teres minor; hence disease or injury

causes atrophy of the deltoid muscle with a flattening of the shoulder and loss of its contour, with loss of abduction of the arm to the horizontal position. Sensation is lost over the shoulder to the upper arm.

Long Thoracic Nerve ($C_{5, 6, 7}$) : Isolated involvement of this nerve is seen occasionally. It occurs usually as a result of direct injury to the thorax, or indirectly through violent muscular contrac-

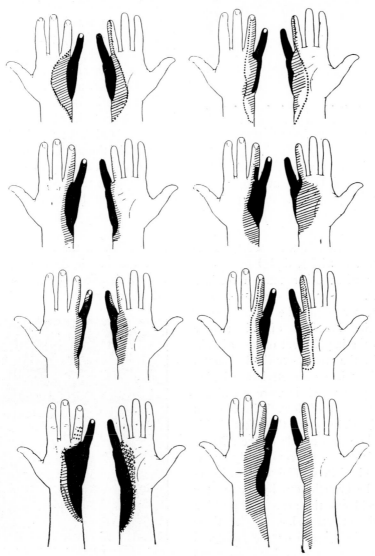

Fig. 65—*Ulnar nerve.* Sensory loss patterns in disease of the ulnar nerve. (*Pollock and Davis: Paul B. Hoeber, Inc., N. Y.*)

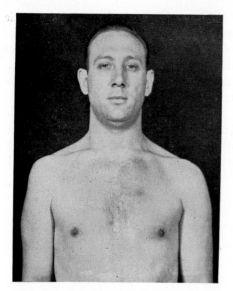

Fig. 66—*Deltoid paralysis* due to injury of the right axillary nerve, showing atrophy of the right deltoid muscle.

the hand can be inserted between it and the thoracic cage.

Onset of the paralysis is often acute. Pain is a prominent symptom and is usually felt along the base of the neck and downward over the scapula and deltoid regions. Pain may be felt under the scapula or in the axilla.

Suprascapular Nerve ($C_{5,6}$): The suprascapular nerve innervates the supra- and infraspinati, the function of which is outward rotation of the arm. The nerve is not usually involved alone. It is affected chiefly by trauma, particularly blows to the shoulder, but it may be involved also in neuritis. The shoulder is somewhat flattened due to involvement of the spinati, and there may be drooping of the arm, since one of the functions of the spinati is to fix the head of the humerus in the glenoid cavity.

Musculocutaneous Nerve ($C_{5,6}$): This nerve supplies the biceps, brachialis anticus, and coracobrachialis muscles. It is the chief flexor of the forearm on the arm. It supplies also the skin on the outer surface of the forearm to the base of the thumb. The nerve is rarely injured alone. It is affected chiefly by fractures of the humerus, stab or gunshot wounds.

tions of the arm with the arm raised above the head (swing at a golf ball, punching-bag practice). It may be injured also in carrying objects on the shoulder for a long period of time. It may be diseased following serum injection (serum neuritis), diphtheria, pneumonia, or after other toxic infectious conditions.

The nerve supplies the serratus magnus muscle. Paralysis of this muscle results in the impairment or loss of ability to raise the arm above the horizontal plane. There is a characteristic winging of the scapula which is more prominent and looser than its fellow. With the arm at rest, the shoulder of the affected side droops, while the scapula of the affected side stands out more prominently and is lower than its fellow. The scapular looseness can be brought out by having the patient hold out the arms and pushing against the affected side. Under these conditions the scapula on the paralyzed side stands out, its edge is pulled away from the thorax, and in marked cases

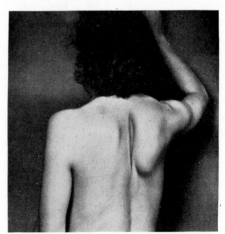

Fig. 67—*Serratus magnus paralysis*, showing the marked winging of the scapula.

Involvement of the musculocutaneous nerve causes atrophy of the biceps muscle, with loss of the biceps reflex, decreased flexion of the forearm on the arm, and loss or decrease of sensation over the outer aspect of the forearm. Flexion of the forearm on the arm is not lost completely in musculocutaneous involvement

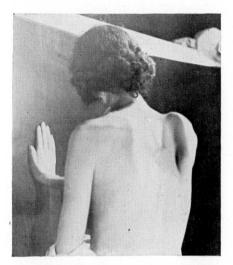

Fig. 68—*Serratus magnus paralysis* showing the winged scapula characteristic of involvement of the long thoracic nerve.

because powerful flexion is still possible by means of the supinator longus, which is supplied by the radial nerve.

Brachial Plexus: Injuries of the brachial plexus are not uncommon. They occur particularly in wartimes as a result of gunshot wounds, but their incidence is not high because missiles injuring the brachial plexus are likely at the same time to injure the great vessels of the neck and axilla, and to prove fatal. They represent only about 5 per cent of nerve injuries in war. Fractures, dislocations of the shoulder, operations on the thorax, forceps delivery, blows to the shoulder, infections of the neck, torsion of the upper arm, pressure by crutches, tumors, aneurysms, and neuritis may affect the brachial plexus.

Two types of syndrome develop: (1) the upper type (Erb), and (2) the lower type (Klumpke). The *upper type* results from involvement of roots of C_5 and C_6 and is particularly involved in birth injuries by traction on the hand and neck or pulling on the shoulders. It includes particularly the deltoid, biceps, brachialis, supinator, infraspinati and supraspinati muscles. There is inability to abduct the arm (deltoid), to flex the arm (biceps, brachialis, supinator longus), to rotate the arm outward (supra- and infraspinati), and to supinate the forearm. As a result, the arm is held in extension, internal rotation and pronation, and adduction. The lesion is usually combined with much atrophy and as a rule with no sensory disturbance. Marked deformities of the limb result from the severe atrophy and the long-standing nature of the process. The *lower type* of syndrome is characterized by a paralysis of flexion of the fingers (flexor digitorum), weakness of flexion of the wrist (flexor carpi ulnaris), paralysis of abduction and adduction of the fingers (interossei), and of abduction, adduction, and flexion of the thumb as well as opposition of the little finger due to involvement of the thenar and hypothenar eminences. The resulting paralysis and deformity is a combination of median and ulnar paralysis.

Lesions of the *secondary cords* of the brachial plexus occur at times and are characterized by distributions of paralysis similar to that of peripheral nerves. The *medial cord* involvement is characterized by paralysis of all the small muscles of the hands and of flexors of the wrist and fingers, especially the ulnar fingers. Sensation is lost along the inner arm and forearm. Lesions of the *lateral cord* cause paralysis of the biceps, coracobrachialis, and brachialis anticus muscles, and of the flexors of the fingers and wrist. The outer side of the forearm shows loss of sensation. Lesions of the *posterior cord* cause paralysis of the biceps, deltoid, and extensors of the wrist and fingers.

Generally speaking, brachial plexus lesions may be divided into those affect- ing primarily the roots, and those involv- ing particularly the cords. Root lesions are caused as a rule by supraclavicular injuries or disease, while cord injuries or disease are caused by infraclavicular le- sions. Supraclavicular disease rarely pro- duces cord involvement.

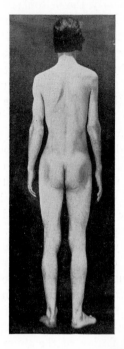
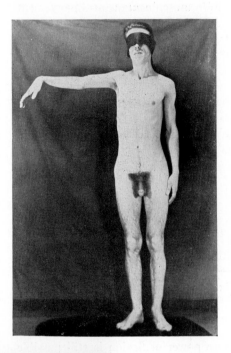
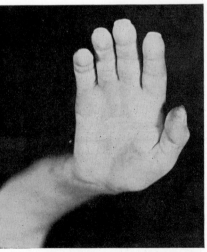

Fig. 69—*Brachial plexus injury* resulting from severe traction of the neck and arm, illustrating atrophy of the arm, forearm and hand muscles, and wrist-drop. The affected muscles revealed a moderate to severe degree of injury.

The upper and lower brachial plexus syndromes described are found in typical instances in many conditions, but the pattern of brachial plexus injuries in war conforms often to no definite plan and is characterized by many atypical forms, depending on the course of the missile, the introduction of infection, the occurrence of fibrosis, and the irregular injury of more than one part of the plexus in the neck or axilla.

2. Lower Extremity

Femoral Nerve $(L_{2,3,4})$: This nerve is not very commonly involved, but when it is, it is important that it be recognized. It is subject to injury by gunshot or stab wound in the groin, femoral aneurysm, tumor in the groin, inflammatory or tumor processes in the pelvis affecting the lumbosacral plexus, sudden contraction of the quadriceps muscle, and neuritis from various causes.

The femoral nerve supplies the quadriceps, sartorius, and pectineus muscles chiefly.

The symptoms are quite typical. Due to involvement of the quadriceps muscle which is supplied by the femoral nerve, there is loss of extension of the knee. Walking and standing are possible, but bouts of sudden falling because of the leg suddenly giving way beneath the patient are characteristic. There is atrophy of the quadriceps muscle, the entire front of the thigh being much smaller than the rest. The patella is very prominent on the affected side and a deep excavation can be seen above it. Decrease or loss of superficial sensation can be demonstrated at times over the front and inner side of the thigh, and along the inner aspect of the leg.

Sciatic Nerve $(L_{4,5}$ and $S_{1,2,3})$: The sciatic nerve is the largest nerve in the body. By means of its branches, it supplies most of the muscles of the thigh and leg. It supplies the main flexors of the leg on the thigh (hamstrings) by means of a special branch to the hamstring muscles and the biceps femoris. It divides into common peroneal and tibial branches anywhere between the sciatic notch and the popliteal space, the common peroneal dividing eventually into the superficial and deep peroneal nerves. By means of the peroneals, it is responsible for dorsiflexion of the foot; extension of the toes (extensor digitorum longus and extensor hallucis longus); abduction, eversion, and elevation of the foot (tibialis anticus and peroneus longus and brevis); adduction of the foot (tibialis anticus). Through the tibial nerve it is responsible for plantar flexion of the foot (gastrocnemius and soleus); flexion of the toes (flexor digitorum longus, flexor hal-

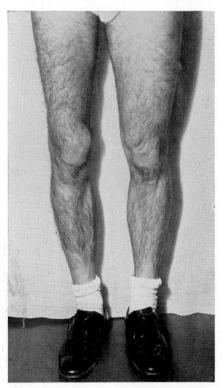

Fig. 70—*Femoral nerve* injury showing the characteristic atrophy of the right quadriceps muscle and the prominence of the patella on the affected side.

lucis longus, and flexor digitorum brevis) ; adduction of the foot (tibialis posterior). By means of its various sensory branches it is responsible for sensation over the leg and foot, the anteroexternal aspect of the leg and the dorsum of the foot by the peroneal nerve and the sole of the foot, the heel, and the outer surface of the foot by the tibial nerve.

The *diagnosis* of sciatica, regardless of its cause, may be determined by adherence to well-defined general criteria.

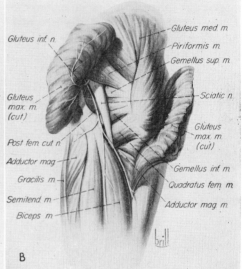

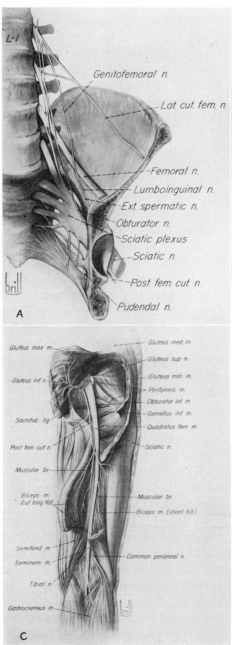

Fig. 71—A, Emergence of roots forming *sciatic nerve*; B, position of sciatic nerve in greater sciatic notch; C, sciatic nerve in thigh, showing its position and main branches.

These consist of (1) *Pain*. This is posterior thigh pain, which may be felt over buttock, posterior or posterior and lateral parts of the thigh into the calf and foot. Or it may, when due to root involvement, implicate only the buttock, the posterior part of the thigh or other parts of the leg. Anterior thigh pain and pain in the groin or genitals is not due to involvement of the sciatic roots or trunk. (2) *Weakness*. This is variable and may involve the thigh, leg and foot muscles supplied by the sciatic nerve, or only some may be affected. (3) *Tenderness of the sciatic trunk* in the greater sciatic notch is also variable and is not always present. (4) *Special signs* are present and are indicative of sciatica. Among these the most important are the *Lasègue* and *straight leg-raising sign*. The Lasègue sign is carried out by extension of the leg on the flexed hip. The straight leg-raising sign is executed by attempted raising of the entire leg with the leg in complete extension. Limitation of extension is found in sciatica, the degree of limitation being roughly proportional to the severity of the pain. The pain evoked by the tests mentioned is referred to the buttock and thigh region. It is due to stretching of the sciatic roots (L_5 and S_1) and eliminated by the application of local anesthetic to the sciatic roots and sciatic trunk. It is eliminated by section of the roots (L_5 and S_1) and by the application of local anesthetic to these roots. True sciatica is found very rarely without these signs. Many modifications of the signs have been described but they contribute little beyond the two signs described. Dorsiflexing the foot increases the pain (Bragard's sign). Flexion of the great toe also increases the pain (Sicard's sign). Flexion of the affected leg is noted on stooping (Neri's sign), and the pain is aggravated by passive dorsiflexion of the foot (Gowers' sign). Complete extension of the leg is impossible because of pain in the back and along the back of the thigh. Because of the pain which is generated by any movement which places the nerve on stretch, patients with sciatic pain, whether due to neuritis or other causes, avoid such stretch. Hence such patients stand with the affected leg flexed or with a compensatory scoliosis, they stoop feminine fashion in picking up an object with the affected leg flexed, they lie in bed with the affected leg flexed by a supporting pillow or bolster, and they avoid all activity such as climbing stairs. While most patients having sciatica are more comfortable lying down with the leg flexed, some prefer to sit up in a chair. (5) *Achilles reflex.* This is usually lost or decreased. (6) *Sensory changes.* These are variable and may not be present.

By means of these criteria a diagnosis of sciatica may be made. Thereafter the problem becomes one of determination of cause.

Disease of the sciatic nerve may be divided into two large groups: (1) *Sciatic neuritis*, and (2) *secondary sciatica* in which the symptoms are the result of secondary causes of many sorts.

1. *Sciatic Neuritis:* This is a true neuritis involving the sciatic nerve in all or part of its course. It is much less common than secondary sciatica, but there is no justification for the assertion that it is rare.

It usually follows infections of various sorts. Foci of infection in the teeth, tonsils, sinuses, or prostate are sometimes responsible, but are not so common as usually regarded. Exposure to cold and dampness, and other infections of various sorts, may be responsible for the neuritis.

The outstanding symptom of sciatic neuritis is pain in the leg. This is unilateral in almost all cases, but rarely may be bilateral. The left leg is more often involved than the right. The onset is usually acute and is sometimes but not often accompanied by pain in the back. Back pain, in fact, is not a common or striking feature of sciatic neuritis. The leg pain is, as a rule, constant, involving the region from the hip along the side and back of the thigh and calf of the leg, extending into the ankle or even the toes. In some instances, the pain may extend from the hip and back region only to the knee or be felt only in the hip. Pain is constant, but in some cases may be paroxysmal, radiating along the course of the nerve. The pain is severe, is usually increased on movement, and may sometimes be increased on straining, coughing, or sneezing. It is associated with tenderness over the nerve trunk in the sciatic notch and often in the popliteal space. This is usually pronounced in acute cases, but may be moderate in degree. Tenderness on pressure over the muscles and Achilles tendon is often present and is usually severe. Spasm of the back muscles may be present.

There is often great disproportion between the degree of pain and the amount of motor disability. Weakness of the leg may be great or slight and is usually not very pronounced. The evaluation of weakness is extremely difficult in the acute stages due to the severe pain which makes movement of the leg extremely unpleasant. Foot-drop may be present in some degree. Atrophy of the thigh and calf muscles (hamstrings, peroneal, tibials) may sometimes be seen, but is often lacking. The Achilles reflex is absent or decreased in most cases, but may be normal. The patellar reflex is retained. Sensory changes chiefly of superficial sensation may be noted.

DIAGNOSIS: The *diagnosis* of sciatic neuritis as against secondary sciatica is established largely on the basis of nerve and muscle tenderness along the course of the sciatic nerve in a patient who has had an acute onset of sciatic pain, and who may have in addition to the pain a loss or decrease of the Achilles reflex on the affected side, with or without muscle atrophy or sensory changes. Nerve tenderness may occasionally be found in cases of secondary sciatica due to nerve compression at a distance but it is uncommon, is usually not nearly so severe as is sciatic neuritis, and is as a rule not felt along the entire course of the nerve. In the last analysis, the differentiation between sciatic neuritis and secondary sciatica is made largely on the basis of tenderness of the muscles and nerve

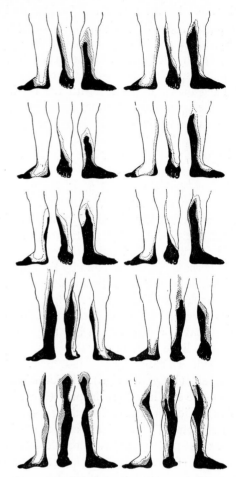

Fig. 72—*Sciatic nerve disease,* showing the sensory changes found in involvement of this nerve. *(Pollock and Davis: Paul B. Hoeber, Inc., N. Y.)*

trunks, particularly the latter, in the case of neuritis. The acute onset and the absence of back pain are additional helpful features. Atrophy of the muscles and sensory disturbances speak as a rule in favor of secondary causes. Back pain is more common in cases of secondary than in primary sciatica.

TREATMENT: This requires the use of many measures: (1) *Rest in bed* is essential. (2) *Boards* under the mattress to give a hard surface are helpful in supporting the back. (3) *Heat* in the form of infra-red applied several times a day along the nerve is valuable. Diathermy is likely to increase the pain in acute cases. A lighted cradle is often helpful. (4) *Salicylates* in large doses (15 grains) (three times a day) are helpful in controlling pain and often need to be used with *codeine* and *barbiturates* to relieve pain. Morphine and its derivatives should never be used. (5) *Salicylates intravenously* one or twice a day are sometimes helpful. (6) *Meperidine (Demerol)* (50 mg. [4/5 grain]) three times daily or *methadone* (5 mg. [1/12 grain]) by mouth three times daily helps to relieve the pain. (7) Injections around the nerve in the region of the sciatic notch should not be undertaken except under special circumstances and should never be practiced routinely.

Most cases of sciatic neuritis run a course of six to eight weeks. Some are terminated in three to four weeks; occasional cases may run for months with intermittent sciatic pain.

2. Secondary Sciatica. CAUSES: Pain along the course of the sciatic nerve due to secondary causes is more common than cases due to primary sciatica, or sciatic neuritis. Secondary causes of sciatica are much more common than primary sciatic neuritis. Table 19 gives a list, by no means complete, of the various causes of secondary sciatica.

Table 19—Causes of Secondary Sciatica

A. VERTEBRAE:
    (1) Sacralization of the 5th lumbar vertebra
    (2) Arthritis of the interarticular joints
    (3) Congenital abnormalities of the interarticular joints
    (4) Arthritis of the vertebrae
    (5) Long transverse process of 5th lumbar vertebra
    (6) Spondylitis:
        (a) Tuberculous
        (b) Pyogenic
    (7) Spondylolisthesis
    (8) Tumor:
        (a) Primary
        (b) Metastatic, especially from breast, prostate, and kidney

B. PELVIS:
    (1) Sacroiliac arthritis
    (2) Sacroiliac subluxation or strain
    (3) Hip disease:
        (a) Metastatic tumor
        (b) Infections
    (4) Infections:
        (a) Prostate
        (b) Female genital tract
        (c) Tuberculous abscess
    (5) Rectal impactions
    (6) Hernia:
        (a) Femoral
        (b) Inguinal
    (7) Tumors of lumbosacral plexus:
        (a) Carcinoma of ovary
        (b) Carcinoma of prostate
        (c) Carcinoma of uterus
        (d) Fibroids of uterus
        (e) Retroperitoneal sarcoma

C. MUSCLES AND FASCIA:
    (1) Tense fascia lata
    (2) Ischiogluteal bursitis
    (3) Myositis of gluteal muscles
    (4) Faulty posture producing faulty muscle balance
    (5) Irritation of pyriformis muscle
    (6) Herniation of fascial fat

D. SPINAL CORD:
    (1) Tumors, especially cauda equina, but thoracic and lumbar also:
        (a) Primary, intramedullary and extramedullary tumors
        (b) Metastatic
    (2) Herniation of nucleus pulposus or intervertebral disc
    (3) Hypertrophy of ligmentum flavum
    (4) Arachnoiditis
    (5) Pachymeningitis:
        (a) Syphilitic
        (b) Tuberculous
    (6) Herpes zoster
    (7) Tabes dorsalis
    (8) Hemorrhage around the cauda equina
    (9) Telangiectasis

E. MISCELLANEOUS:
    (1) Pes planus
    (2) Obesity and malnutrition
    (3) Hysterical

The causes of secondary or symptomatic sciatica are obviously numerous; hence this condition is more common than primary sciatic neuritis. Brief mention of the various causes is desirable. The *vertebral* causes listed are much more commonly responsible for low back pain without sciatic radiation than for sciatic pain. Under some conditions they may be responsible for pain along the sciatic nerve. Arthritis of the interarticular joints may cause sciatic pain if the proper roots are involved in the proper intervertebral foramina. Arthritis of the vertebrae may cause sciatic pain; but there is disagreement concerning its frequency, and its influence in causing sciatic pain is denied by some. In the presence of severe arthritis of the spine and the demonstration of no other cause for the sciatica, it may be assumed that the arthritis is the cause of the sciatic pain in a given instance. It should be understood also that arthritis of the vertebrae is common in advanced years and that it may be merely an incidental finding. The pain is probably produced by impingement of the arthritis on nerve roots in the intervertebral foramen. Severe arthritis of the spine is at times associated with arachnoiditis. Tumors of the vertebrae may cause sciatic pain by compression of the lumbosacral roots by either tumor or collapsed vertebrae, or by an extradural-tumor process as in metastatic carcinoma. Other vertebral causes are more often responsible for back pain than for pain along the sciatic nerve. *Spondylolisthesis* in itself is not responsible for sciatic pain; but when associated with a herniated disc, it is capable of causing sciatica.

Sacroiliac disease may cause sciatic pain in both arthritis of this joint and in acute sacroiliac strain. Sciatic pain in incidences as high as 36 per cent (Yeoman) has been attributed to sacroiliac arthritis. Anatomically, the lumbosacral trunk is separated from the sacroiliac joint in its lower third only by the thin joint capsule through which exudate breaks in disease of the sacroiliac joint. Hypertrophic arthritis may cause sciatic pain by pressure on the nerve trunk as it

passes over the sacroiliac joint in 25 per cent of cases (Hershey). In sacroiliac strain, sciatic pain probably results from the edema and exudate of the nerve as it lies adjacent to the joint. *Hip disease* may at times simulate sciatic pain, but the distinction between the two disorders is not difficult. The pain is not typically sciatic in distribution, is much more diffuse in its radiation, and is associated with definite evidences of hip disorder. Disease of the hip, once regarded as a very important cause of secondary sciatica (Bruce), is now looked upon as of only minor importance. *Pelvic tumors* are at times responsible for sciatic pain due to infiltration of the lumbosacral plexus by tumor cells or by compression. The former mechanism is seen in prostatic or uterine carcinomata, the latter in ovarian carcinoma. Fibroids of the uterus rarely cause sufficient compression to produce sciatic pain. Retroperitoneal sarcoma may cause sciatic pain by infiltration or compression of the lumbosacral plexus. A tense *fascia lata* may cause pain in the sciatic distribution (Ober) but the cause is not common. The diagnosis is made by demonstration of increased tension of the fascia lata by Ober's test.

Involvement of the entire sciatic nerve by *injury* is not uncommon. As a result of such section, all movements of the foot and toes are lost and flexion of the knee is almost entirely abolished, only slight flexion being possible as a result of the action of the gracilis muscle which is supplied by the obturator nerve. Sensation is lost below the knee, only the inner surface of the leg escaping by virtue of its supply by the internal saphenous nerve from the femoral.

A tense *pyriformis muscle* has been regarded as causing sciatic pain in many instances (Freiberg) due to irritation of the sciatic nerve by the muscle which lies between the lumbosacral trunk and the sacroiliac joint. Others have not found the muscle to be in this position in relation to the nerve. It is doubtful whether the pyriformis muscle is responsible for sciatic pain as frequently as it is regarded to be. Low back pain associated with sciatica has been found in some instances to be associated with *herniation of fascial fat*. The herniations occur at points where the fascia is weak, and are associated with areas of spot tenderness over the back. *Myositis* of the muscles of the back has been regarded as a not infrequent cause of sciatica. It is associated with tender points over one or more back muscles, injection of which with a local anesthetic relieves the sciatic pain. The sciatica in such instances is said to be "reflex" in nature, but the mechanism of production of the sciatic pain is not clear. *Intraspinal conditions* of many sorts may cause sciatic pain. Tumors, both primary and secondary, involving the cauda equina may cause sciatic pain and will be discussed later. Herniation of the nucleus pulposus is a common cause and will also be discussed later. Tumors of the thoracic region may at times cause pain in the sciatic distribution. Pachymeningitis is a rare cause.

SYMPTOMS: The symptoms of secondary sciatica vary with the cause, but in general the cases are characterized by pain in the back and along the sciatic nerve. The back pain is persistent, but may be intermittent. Back pain is much more common in these cases than in primary sciatic neuritis. The leg pain is felt along the course of the sciatic nerve as a constant severe pain, usually increased by movement or exercise, and by coughing, sneezing, or straining. It is felt in the region of the hip, along the side and back of the thigh and in the calf. It may extend into the ankle, foot or toes. It may in other instances be felt only to the knee or be lost in the calf. It may be associated with paresthesias in the foot or leg. There is no nerve or muscle tenderness in typical instances, but in some cases mild or moderate tenderness of the sciatic nerve may be felt on pressure in the sciatic notch. The muscles supplied by the sciatic nerve (hamstrings, peroneals, tibials, gastrocnemius) may show varying degrees of atrophy depending on the cause of the condition. This, however, is not constant. Similarly, sensory disturbances may or may not be found. The Achilles reflex may be absent, decreased, or normal. Lasègue's sign is usually present.

DIAGNOSIS: This is made when it is determined that a case with sciatic pain is not one of neuritis. This is true in cases with persistent pain, without tenderness of the muscles or nerve trunks, with evidence of involvement of a reflex, motor, or sensory nature in the area supplied by the sciatic nerve. The story and findings vary widely with the cause, but the general symptoms of back and leg pain are common to all causes except for variations in intensity and distribution of the pain. One feature distinguishes cases of secondary sciatica from sciatic neuritis: the absence of true nerve tenderness. The presence of tenderness of the nerve trunks does not in itself designate sciatica as due to neuritis, since spinal cord tumor and herniated disc may at times be associated with tenderness of the sciatic nerve in the sciatic notch. As a rule, it is not pronounced. Apart from this, the symptoms and signs are the same for the two conditions. The sciatic pain of secondary sciatica is more persistent than that of sciatic neuritis; but even this is variable, since many cases of secondary sciatica due to herniated nucleus pulposus give a history of intermittent and recurrent pain. On the other hand, the sciatic pain of caudal tumor, of Pott's disease, or of lumbosacral tumor is persistent and progressive. Secondary sciatica, moreover, is more often associated with muscle atrophy and sensory changes than is the case with sciatic neuritis. Generally speaking, cases of secondary sciatic pain are longer in duration than those of sciatic neuritis and have persisted longer when they appear for treatment.

All cases of suspected secondary sciatica should have routinely the following: (1) roentgenograms of the lumbosacral vertebrae, pelvis, and hip joints; (2) lumbar puncture, which should include, in addition to the routine, a total protein study; (3) orthopedic consultation.

Under some conditions, branches of the sciatic nerve may be affected. Chief among these are the two main branches—the peroneal and tibial nerves.

Peroneal Nerve: Peroneal palsy may result from crossing the legs. Woltman reported twenty-seven cases and stressed the importance of loss of weight, senility, and protracted convalescence. Its occurrence has been reported in healthy young soldiers, and the physical habitus was regarded as the most significant factor, the palsy occurring in tall, long-legged subjects where the nerve is more exposed (Nayler and Rangell). The nerve is probably compressed between the head and neck of the fibula of the uppermost leg, and the patella and external condyle of the femur of the lowermost leg.

This nerve is commonly affected by a variety of conditions. It may be involved in fracture of the leg, especially the fibula. Other causes include pressure from cast, ischemia from prolonged kneeling, as in floor cleaners or cranberry pickers, infections and toxic conditions of many sorts (alcohol, lead, diabetes), and gunshot wounds in war.

The peroneal nerve is the chief extensor nerve of the leg, hence symptoms of its involvement have reference to this function. The nerve dorsiflexes the foot, everts it, and extends the toes through the action of the peroneal muscles. Consequently, a common complaint is inability to lift the foot, stumbling, and dragging of the toes due to the foot-drop which is invariably present. Pain may be present, depending on the cause of the condition. Foot-drop is the outstanding sign. The patient walks with the foot hanging limply, the leg lifted high in a steppage gait in order to clear the ground with the paralyzed foot. There is inability to walk on the heel, whereas walking on the toes due to tibial action is intact. The outer aspect of the leg is atrophied due to loss of bulk of the peroneal muscles, and there is sensory loss over the outer aspect of the leg and the instep and dorsal surface of the four inner toes at their extremities.

Foot-drop and peroneal weakness are usually of peripheral origin. They may, however, be part of a lesion of the cauda equina and hence be of central origin. In such cases back pain and other manifestations of involvement of the affected limb are present.

Tibial Nerve: The tibial nerve is the main flexor nerve of the leg and foot supplying the tibial muscles on the inner aspect of the leg and the gastrocnemius group. It is involved in fractures, gunshot wounds, and neuritis. It is much less frequently involved than the peroneal nerve.

Because of the absence of plantar flexion of the foot, the presenting complaint is often one of loss of spring in the step. Plantar flexion of the foot and flexion of the toes are impossible. Atrophy of the inner side of the calf is seen. Sensation is lost over the sole of the foot, the lower third of the leg posteriorly, and the toes (plantar surface and dorsal aspect of terminal phalanges).

Lateral Femoral Cutaneous ($L_{2,3}$): This nerve is purely sensory in function, supplying the outer aspects of the thigh to the knee, spreading over the posterior aspect to the buttock. It is involved by trauma, or as the result of tight belts or corsets, due to its superficial position as it leaves the pelvic brim. It may be involved also by various toxic infectious conditions, such as typhoid, malaria, syphilis, diabetes, obesity, gout, and other conditions. Often the cause remains obscure. It has a long course in the abdomen and may be susceptible to compression or irritation by tumors or infection. It has been reported involved in appendicitis, cholecystectomy, and other abdominal conditions, as well as after abdominal surgery.

The syndrome (meralgia paresthetica) is characterized by pain and paresthesias along the outer aspect of the thigh, usually described as burning, tingling, or pricking sensations, usually associated with decreased pain and touch sensations over the lateral aspect of the thigh, but sometimes also with increased sensitivity to these sensations (hyperesthesia), making the wearing of clothes uncomfortable. There are no reflex changes and no muscle atrophies, since the nerve has no motor function.

The diagnosis of meralgia paresthetica is simple and quite characteristic. Care must be taken, however, to exclude femoral nerve involvement. Moreover, pain along the lateral and anterior aspects of the thigh may be due to lumbar root involvement centrally, and investigation must be made for such causes in proper cases which are associated with quadriceps atrophy and patellar reflex decrease or absence.

Gluteal: There are two gluteal nerves, the superior (L_4-S_1) and the inferior gluteal (L_5-S_2), their function being to supply the gluteal muscles. They may be involved by fracture of the pelvis, pelvic tumors or abscesses, or gunshot wounds. Involvement of the superior gluteal causes paralysis of abduction and internal rotation of the leg, the limb lying in external rotation. The gait is greatly disturbed owing to difficulty in fixing the pelvis. Inferior gluteal paralysis causes loss of movement of hip extension; hence stepping up and rising from a sitting posture are impossible. The glutei are atrophied.

The presenting symptom in cases of superior gluteal involvement is disturbance in gait, while in inferior gluteal paralysis there is difficulty in arising from sitting posture or in stepping. Cases of involvement of either nerve are rare. The complaint, together with the specific disability in movement of the limb with gluteal atrophy, gives the best clue to diagnosis. Once the diagnosis is made, vigorous search must be made for the cause, since involvement of these nerves is usually part of lumbosacral plexus involvement within the pelvis. Isolated involvement of the nerves by neuritis or other causes is rare.

Lumbosacral Plexus: The lumbosacral plexus is involved in processes of various sorts within the pelvis. Among these are infectious, tuberculous abscess, tumor (metastatic), fractures, and sometimes infections. The symptoms are due to a combination of involvement of the various nerves constituting the plexus. Pain in the leg and inability to move the limb normally are common complaints. Loss of power in the affected limb, usually associated with muscular atrophy, loss or decrease of Achilles and patellar reflexes, and sensory changes sometimes involving the entire leg, are found. The specific findings vary greatly with the nerves affected, different combinations of nerves being involved in many cases.

The diagnosis is difficult. The best clue probably is the involvement of more than one of the nerves passing to the leg. Differentiation from a lesion of the cauda equina is important and extremely difficult, the plexus representing merely a more peripheral extension of the caudal roots. Pelvic roentgenograms, as well as roentgenograms of the lower spine, pelvic examination, lumbar puncture, and even barium enema may be necessary to establish the diagnosis, a caudal tumor being more likely to be associated with an elevated spinal fluid protein, sometimes a xanthochromic fluid, and bladder and rectal disturbances (retention or incontinence) if the lowermost sacral roots or spinal segments are compressed.

V. CRANIAL NERVES

Under some circumstances the cranial nerves are involved in disease processes, either alone or in conjunction with the involvement of other parts of the nervous system. Hence some understanding of the disease processes which may affect them is essential.

Olfactory Nerve: This nerve is not important for most practical purposes, except for a few conditions. It may be affected in meningiomas of the olfactory groove, or fractures of the ethmoid plate with resulting loss of smell, which is usually not apparent to the patient.

Optic Nerve: The optic nerve is frequently diseased in neurological disorders. Knowledge of the conditions which may affect it is valuable in diagnosis. Examination of the optic nerve is readily accessible by means of the ophthalmoscope and should be routinely practiced.

1. Choked Disc: Among the disorders of the optic nerve of great importance is choked disc. This is characterized by an elevation of the optic nerve above the surrounding retina associated with hemorrhages and exudates in the latter. For details of the disorder, reference should be made to ophthalmology texts. Choked disc is practically always caused by brain tumor. Its incidence in tumor of the brain is discussed under that heading. It has also been found in tuberculous meningitis, multiple sclerosis, disseminated encephalomyelitis, Schilder's disease (encephalitis periaxialis diffusa), and syphilitic meningitis, but all these are rare causes. Choked disc when found must always be regarded as due to brain tumor until proved otherwise. Visual acuity in choked disc is not decreased until atrophy and organization of the swelling has taken place. It is, therefore, relatively slow in development, an important point of differentiation from optic neuritis. Enlargement of the blind spot is an early accompaniment of choked disc and serves to differentiate it from neuritis. Choked disc is usually but not always associated with headache and it is accompanied by increased intracranial pressure. Many ideas are extant concerning the origin of choked disc. Briefly stated, the following theories have been expressed: (1) *vasomotor,* maintaining that the choked disc is the result of changes in the caliber of the retinal vessels; choked disc is said to be produced by a low diastolic blood pressure in the retinal arteries with normal intraocular tension and simultaneous rise of retinal venous pressure; (2) *mechanical,* due to obstruction of flow in the cerebrospinal fluid, to lymph stasis due to congestion of the central retinal vein, or to venous stasis; (3) *edema of the brain* has been suggested as a cause of choked disc.

2. Optic Atrophy: The various types of optic atrophy (primary and consecutive) and their causes may be found discussed in detail in the proper texts. Their relationship to neurological disorders will be found referred to under their respective headings. Primary optic atrophy, characterized by a well-defined pallor of the optic nerve, is the result of any process (inflammatory, neoplastic, or degenerative) which interrupts the optic nerve between the retina and the optic chiasm by direct action on the optic nerve fibers. Secondary optic atrophy results from previous inflammation or edema of the nerve from whatever cause, with resulting organization and scar formation, producing a secondary atrophy of the nerve.

3. *Retrobulbar Neuritis:* This syndrome is frequently unrecognized and deserves special mention. The term is a poor one and refers to inflammation of the optic nerve behind the bulb. Actually the disease may involve the optic nerve anywhere along its course from nerve head (optic neuritis) to tract (retrobulbar neuritis) and the clinical manifestations of optic neuritis and retrobulbar neuritis are similar in all respects. The retrobulbar form is characterized by (1) acute loss of vision in one or both eyes; (2) sudden decreased visual acuity, usually of a moderately severe or severe degree; (3) a central scotoma in the visual field; (4) a nerve head of normal appearance.

The onset is usually sudden with pain in the eye or over the eye which may persist for days or be only transitory. The eyeball is painful on movement or palpation and there is tenderness at the inner wall of the orbit. Headache is sometimes present at the onset of the disorder and may persist for some time. It is usually unilateral, radiating out from the affected eye over the forehead and temple and becoming at times generalized. As a rule the pain is bearable, but in some cases may be extremely severe. In addition to the pain and headache, sudden loss or impairment of vision of one or both eyes completes the story of the patient with retrobulbar neuritis. This may remain unchanged, or it may improve or become worse by the time the patient presents himself for diagnosis and treatment.

The visual loss in retrobulbar neuritis is usually severe. While the usual field change is a central scotoma, paracentral scotomas are not uncommon. The optic nerve head is normal in appearance if the involvement is behind the optic nerve, but if the condition involves the nerve itself, optic neuritis develops. Visual acuity is greatly decreased as a rule. A late sequel of retrobulbar neuritis is pallor of the temporal side of the optic nerve, especially in multiple sclerosis, but this is by no means a constant sequel, since many cases run their course without visible effect on the nerve head even after more than one attack of retrobulbar neuritis. Optic atrophy may follow cases which manifest optic neuritis.

The outlook varies with the cause, some cases responding well to treatment if a specific cause is discovered, others showing no response at all.

The cause of retrobulbar neuritis is important. Sinus disease once held a hallowed place but is now known to be only a minor cause. Multiple sclerosis is the most common cause and an attack of retrobulbar neuritis may precede by some time other manifestations of the disease. A list of the more important causes of retrobulbar neuritis is shown in Table 20.

The diagnosis of retrobulbar neuritis is usually easy with the history of rapid loss of vision and the findings indicated above. Care must be taken to exclude brain tumor, especially tumor in the suprasellar region, which may simulate retrobulbar neuritis at times in its origin An extremely important study has been made of the subsequent course of cases of retrobulbar neuritis (Benedict). Of 400 cases of retrobulbar neuritis, a diagnosis of multiple sclerosis was made in 90.

Table 20—Causes of Retrobulbar Neuritis in 225 Cases

(Benedict)

Multiple sclerosis	155
Pernicious anemia and nicotine	14
Diabetes	14
Alcohol and tobacco	28
Syphilis	2
Congenital amblyopia	4
Familial	1
Sinus disease	1
Postpartum hemorrhage	1
Plumbism	2
Undetermined	3

The differentiation between optic neuritis and choked disc may be made on the following grounds:

	Optic Neuritis	*Choked Disc*
Optic nerve	1-2 D swelling	3-8 D swelling
Visual acuity	Affected early and severely	Affected late
Visual field	Scotoma present	Blind spot enlarged
Fundus	Swelling spreads out into retina and arteries sheathed	Swelling confined to optic nerve

Of these, 41 were later found to have developed other evidences of the disease, while in not a single instance in which further signs of multiple scerosis had not yet appeared was the retrobulbar neuritis found to be due to another cause. Of the various additional causes, a positive diagnosis of cause can usually be made at the first episode of blindness. The presence of overindulgence in alcohol or tobacco, sensitivity to tobacco, the presence of arteriosclerosis, diabetes, syphilis, or sinus disease, give positive evidence of the responsible cause. There may be a lapse of several years from the time of an attack of retrobulbar neuritis to that of further evidences of multiple sclerosis (*v.* Multiple Sclerosis).

The treatment in cases due to a specific cause consists of removal of the cause. There is a group for which no specific remedy is known and in which the cause cannot be determined. These patients should be given *typhoid-paratyphoid vaccine* intravenously in increasing doses from 25,000,000 to 450,000,000 bacteria, injections being given on alternate days. *Vasodilators* are also advocated. *Nicotinic acid,* 100 mg. (1½ grains) intravenously daily, or 100 mg. three to six times daily by mouth, is helpful. *Cortisone* has been used in treatment. Its value remains to be determined. Some patients respond dramatically; others not at all. It is given in doses of 10 to 25 mg. four times daily for one week or longer and is gradually reduced thereafter. ACTH is reported to be of value in optic neuritis due to multiple sclerosis.

Oculomotor, Trochlear, and Abducens Nerves: The oculomotor nerves (III, IV, VI) are frequently affected, either singly or in unison in neurological diseases. They may be affected (1) within the brain stem, by involvement of their nuclei; (2) peripherally in their course at the base of the brain; (3) within the orbit.

The ocular nerves are frequently diseased by a variety of processes. They may be affected within the brain stem by infiltrating tumors, multiple sclerosis, encephalitis of various sorts, hemorrhagic encephalitis (Wernick's polioencephalitis superior), hemorrhage, arteriosclerotic softenings, botulism, etc. At the base of the brain they may be involved in meningitis of various sorts, particularly syphilitic meningitis; subarachnoid hemorrhage; aneurysms of the internal carotid; posterior communicating or posterior cerebral arteries; meningiomas of the sphenoidal ridge; trauma; neuritis due to various causes (alcohol, lead, syphilis, etc.); sinus disease, especially ethmoid disease; and mastoid diseases affecting especially the abducens nerve (Gradenigo syndrome).

1. *Complete Paralysis of All Ocular Nerves:* This results in ptosis of the eyelids, complete immobility of the eyeballs, which cannot be moved in any direction (external ophthalmoplegia), and dilated pupils not reacting to light due to paralysis of the sphincter iridis and overreaction of the cervical sympathetic (internal ophthalmoplegia). Such paralysis may be unilateral or bilateral, more frequently the former. It is more likely to be the result of involvement of the nerves themselves than of their nuclei in the brain stem. Complete paralyses of all the ocular nerves are produced usually by lesions in the region of the cavernous sinus, where all the nerves are concentrated in one small area on their way to their respective muscles in the eyeball. The syndrome may be produced by meningitis, thrombosis of the cavernous sinus, or by tumors or aneurysms compressing the cavernous sinus. It may be produced also by lesions within the orbit itself or by myasthenia gravis. It is less often but by no means uncommonly the result of lesions within the brain stem, but encephalitis may produce complete ophthalmoplegia, as may also syphilitic meningoencephalitis, Wernick's polioencephalitis, poliomyelitis, and botulism. *Partial paralysis* of the ocular nerves may occur in various combinations either unilaterally or bilaterally and may be due to a variety of causes similar to those involving all the nerves. Partial paralyses are more likely to be due to lesions within the brain stem, particularly if other signs of involvement of cranial nerve or other systems are present.

2. *Isolated Paralysis of the Oculomotor (III) Nerve: Bilateral complete paralysis* of the oculomotor nerve is rare but may follow arteriosclerotic softening involving the nuclei in the midbrain, encephalitis, or multiple sclerosis. The eyes are held in divergent squint, the pupils are dilated, there is bilateral ptosis, and inability to move the eyeballs upward, inward, or downward. *Unilateral complete paralysis* is more common, and is usually due to compression of the nerve by aneurysm or tumor of the sphenoid ridge or by extension of a pituitary tumor, by meningitis, meningeal hemorrhage involving the nerve in the interpeduncular space, trauma, and penetrating wounds of the orbit. It is less likely to be the result of a brain stem affection, though such a lesion may at times cause complete oculomotor paralysis. The condition is characterized by dilatation of the pupil, ptosis of the eyelid with inability to open the lid, external strabismus because of the unopposed pull of the external rectus muscle, and inability to move the affected eyeball upward, inward, or downward. Reaction of the pupil to light is lost. *Incomplete paralyses* involving the oculomotor nerve are not uncommon either from brain-stem or nerve involvement. Loss or impairment of convergence is found without other evidence of oculomotor paralysis as a residual of epidemic encephalitis. Isolated muscles innervated by the oculomotor nerve may be involved in brain stem disease, since the various muscles innervated by the oculomotor nerve have specific localizations within the oculomotor nucleus. Isolated muscle paralyses may occur also from compression of the nerve itself by aneurysm, tumor, syphilitic meningitis, etc.

3. *Isolated Paralysis of the Trochlear (IV) Nerve:* This is not a common condition in neurological practice, but is frequently seen in ophthalmological practice. The nerve may be affected by lesions in the brain stem or by involvement of the nerve itself. The trochlear nerve innervates the superior-oblique muscle and moves the eyeball downward and out-

ward. This movement is lost in paralysis of the nerve. Torticollis is a constant accompanying sign with tilting of the head toward the shoulder. This is done in order to permit binocular vision without diplopia, the latter developing as soon as the head is held in the vertical position. Because of the tilting of the head, cases of trochlear paralysis are frequently mistaken for torticollis and are often treated as such for long periods of time before the correct diagnosis is made. There is inability to look downward and outward, but it is often difficult to pick out an isolated loss of movement of the superior oblique muscle which is supplied by the trochlear nerve. There is torsion outward in trochlear palsy. The condition may be confused with inferior rectus palsy, but in such instances there is torsion inward of the eye and difficulty in looking down.

4. *Isolated Paralysis of the Abducens (VI) Nerve:* The abducens nerve innervates the external rectus muscle. Paralysis of the nerve results in inability to rotate the eyeball outward. This is readily recognized by the internal squint due to the unopposed action of the internal rectus muscle. Diplopia is present, and the head is turned in the direction in which the eye muscle has been acting before it was paralyzed. Abducens paralysis is due to a variety of causes, most of which have already been discussed. It may be involved in lesions of the cavernous sinus, trauma, meningitis, meningeal hemorrhage, infection of the petrous bone in mastoid disease associated with pain in the face and eye (Gradenigo syndrome), and in increased pressure within the skull.

5. *Conjugate Paralyses:* Paralyses of the conjugate movement of the eyeballs occur under diverse circumstances and are helpful both in localizing and etiological diagnosis.

Examination of conjugate movements should include the following: (1) volitional movements; (2) attraction movements, consisting of quick movements of the eyes toward an object in the periphery which attracts the attention; (3) following movements.

1. *Paralysis of lateral gaze* is sometimes encountered. This syndrome is highly characteristic. It consists of inability voluntarily to move the eyeballs laterally in a horizontal plane. Despite this loss of voluntary movement of lateral gaze, the eyeballs can follow a directing finger readily to the paralyzed side in some forms of paralysis of lateral gaze. Paralysis of lateral gaze is indicative of a lesion in the pons, where a center is presumed to exist for such conjugate movement, separate from the nuclei of the oculomotor and abducens nerves. It results also from involvement of the supranuclear centers for conjugate gaze in the cerebrum. Conjugate, lateral gaze paralysis in cerebral lesions tends to be intermittent. These centers are located in the posterior portion of the opposite second frontal gyrus in the temporal lobe and in the gyrus angularis in the occipital lobe. Conjugate deviation of the eyes in cerebral lesions may result from irritative or destructive lesions. In irritative lesions, the eyes deviate to the opposite side, *i. e.,* they look away from the lesion. In destructive lesions, they gaze toward the side of the lesion due to the unopposed action of the centers in the opposite hemisphere. The distinction between a supranuclear and a pontine paralysis of lateral gaze is often difficult. The following points are helpful: (a) The presence of accessory signs may indicate whether a cerebral or brain-stem lesion is responsible for the paralysis of lateral gaze. Thus, the occurrence of an absent corneal reflex, motor paralysis of the trigeminal nerve, abducens paralysis,

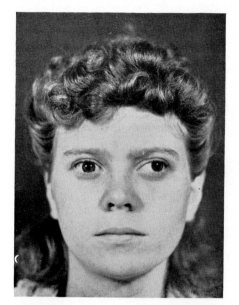
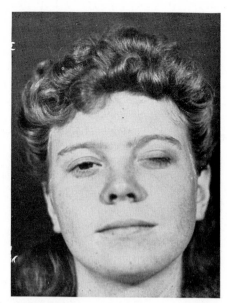

Fig. 73—*Partial ophthalmoplegia*, with involvement of the left oculomotor nerve, showing the ptosis of the eyelid and external strabismus in a case of cerebral aneurysm.

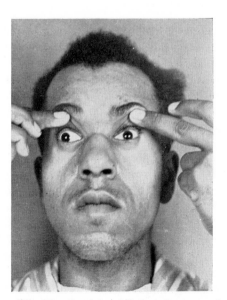
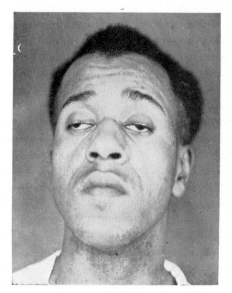

Fig. 74—*Partial ophthalmoplegia* involving the oculomotor nerve bilaterally and showing ptosis, paralysis of upward movement of the eyeballs, and bilateral external strabismus due to the unopposed action of both external rectus muscles.

or facial paralysis, point to a pontine lesion; (b) in pontine lesions, the eyes are unable to follow the directing finger; in cerebral lesions, this can be done but not in every instance; (c) the paralysis in a pontine lesion is permanent, while that of a cerebral lesion is transitory.

2. *Paralysis of upward convergence* (Parinaud syndrome) is characterized by

invasion of the superior colliculi; (b) involvement of the central gray matter around the aqueduct of Sylvius; (c) involvement of the nuclei of the eye elevators (superior rectus and inferior oblique muscles).

3. *Paralysis of divergence* is extremely difficult to determine. A center for divergence has not been demonstrated. Diver

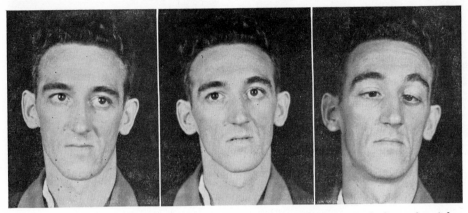

Fig. 75—*Paralysis of lateral gaze.* **Note the inability to look particularly to the right and the loss of near covergence with the right eye.**

an inability to move the eyeballs upward above the horizontal plane. It is usually associated with paralysis of downward gaze as well, but may not uncommonly exist with retention of the ability to look downward. It frequently exists without evidence of involvement of other ocular muscles, but it may be associated with changes in the pupillary reactions from the involvement of the adjacent pupillary fibers. It is rarely found as an isolated symptom, other evidences of involvement of the brain-stem being usually present. The syndrome is found in tumors of the pineal body, in infiltrating tumors of the collicular plate region (superior colliculus), in hemorrhagic encephalitis of Wernicke, and rarely as a distant symptom due to pressure in cerebellopontine angle tumor or in cerebellar tumor. Its exact cause is not known. It is thought to be due to (a) pressure or

gence paralysis is characterized by the following (Bielschowsky): (a) homonymous diplopia; (b) failure of increase of the angle of squint on looking to the right or left, but it increases or decreases on looking downward and upward; as a result, the head in some cases is held with the chin against the chest in order to promote convergence; (c) approach of the images closer to one another on bringing a test object close to the patient, and fusion at 10 to 15 inches from the patient; (d) the development of further diplopia when the test object is brought within this area because of the failure of convergence. There is much doubt on the part of some as to whether divergence paralysis is a true condition.

4. *Paralysis of convergence* is found in some conditions. It is characterized by loss of ability of the eyeballs to converge on near and far objects. Complete

loss is rare. It is found in encephalitis lethargica, which has a predilection for involving the oculomotor nerve complex and particularly the nucleus of convergence. Partial loss of paralysis of convergence is not uncommon in encephalitis lethargica, in old age, and in other conditions. Paralysis of movement of the internal rectus muscles with retention of convergence is designated as *internuclear ophthalmoplegia*. It is due to a lesion involving the medial longitudinal fasciculus (posterior longitudinal bundle) interrupting the fiber connections of the oculomotor nucleus. It is found almost exclusively in multiple sclerosis. Unilateral lesions have been described in association with vascular softenings.

Trigeminal Nerve: The trigeminal nerve is composed of a motor and sensory portion, the latter occupying most of the bulk of the nerve. The sensory division supplies the skin of the face, including the forehead and scalp, the cornea, orbit, eyeball, nose, lips, teeth, mouth, and anterior two-thirds of the tongue. The secretion of tears, saliva, and nasal secretion is carried out through trigeminal fibers. The motor root innervates the masseters and pterygoid muscles and is concerned with chewing and other jaw movements.

The trigeminal nerve is involved in a number of processes affecting it from gasserian ganglion to the periphery. The ganglion may be involved by tumors, both primary and metastatic, pachymeningitis, either syphilitic or tuberculous, or aneurysm. The nerve itself may be involved by a variety of processes, such as tumor (cerebellopontine angle), aneurysm, syphilitic meningitis, or neuritis from various causes. Infiltrating tumors of the pons sometimes involve the nucleus of the trigeminal nerve as do multiple sclerosis and various forms of encephalitis. Fractures of the base of the skull

rarely involve the nerve and meningeal hemorrhage is not a common cause of its involvement.

The *sensory portion* of the nerve is more frequently affected than the motor. Complete involvement is not so common as partial or fractional involvement. In cases of total paralysis of the sensory portion, there is loss of the corneal reflex

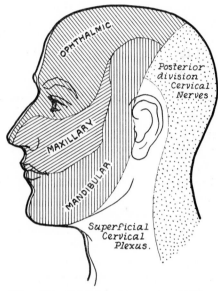

Fig. 76—*Trigeminal nerve*, showing the areas of supply of the three principal divisions. Interruption of one or all of the divisions results in corresponding loss of sensation of the affected areas.

on the side of the involvement, and a loss of superficial sensation over the area of distribution of the nerve (forehead, scalp, face, mucous membranes of nose, mouth, and the tongue). Such complete involvement is usually seen in disease affecting the gasserian ganglion; nuclear involvement in the pons results in less complete signs as a rule due to failure to destroy the nucleus in its entirety by the infiltrating process. The descending sensory root of the trigeminal nerve in the medulla produces loss of superficial sensation over the face on the side of the lesion, the distribution being of an onion-peel type.

Incomplete involvement of the sensory root is found more frequently than the complete paralysis. Loss of the corneal reflex may be the only evidence of sensory root involvement. It is found in cerebellopontine angle tumor, multiple sclerosis, encephalitis of various types, infiltrating tumor of the pons, syphilis, and other conditions. Isolated involvement of the first division of the trigeminus is found in cavernous sinus syndromes.

The *motor root* is less frequently affected than the sensory. Disease of this portion of the trigeminus is associated with atrophy of the ipsilateral masseter, pterygoid and temporal muscles, with weakness in opening the jaw, and deviation of the jaw to the paralyzed side by the healthy unopposed internal pterygoids.

The *trophic* and *vegetative* disturbances in trigeminal nerve disease are not common. Lachrymation is not affected as a rule. Taste is sometimes affected. *Paratrigeminal* involvement is seen in meningiomas, aneurysms, or pachymeningitis and is characterized by pain in the face, myosis, ptosis, and oculomotor paresis or paralysis.

Facial Nerve (VII): The facial nerve is frequently affected by disease of various sorts. It may be involved within (1) the pons, (2) the cranial cavity, (3) the fallopian canal, or (4) after its emergence from the base of the skull (stylomastoid foramen). In the *pons* it is affected by infiltrating tumors, hemorrhage, encephalitis, poliomyelitis, syphilis, tubercle, blood dyscrasias, and meningoencephalitis of various sorts. Within the *cranial cavity* it is affected by many processes. Tumors of the cerebellopontine angle frequently affect the nerve. It is often involved in trauma, especially in fractures of the base of the skull through the petrous portion of the temporal bone. Hemorrhage in the meninges sometimes involves the facial nerve. Meningitis of various sorts, but especially syphilitic meningitis, implicates it. Aneurysm of the posterior cerebral or basilar artery may compress it. In the *fallopian canal* within the temporal bone the facial nerve is often affected by mastoid infections, mastoid operations, trauma, tumor within the bone (cholesteatoma, sarcoma, or carcinoma), or by hemorrhage. It is injured also in the *neck* after its emergence from the stylomastoid foramen by gunshot wounds, stab wounds, cellulitis, parotitis, swollen glands, aneurysm. It may be involved anywhere along its course in many sorts of infection, in blood dyscrasias, in herpes (Hunt's syndrome), and in multiple neuritis with cranial nerve involvement, especially in acute infectious polyneuritis. *Tumor of the glomus jugulare* is a rare cause of peripheral facial paralysis. It is characterized by a history of aural polyps; progressive loss of hearing; chronic otorrhea; facial paralysis; pain; hemorrhage from the ear; and tinnitus with occasional episodes of dizziness.

There exists a large group of cases of facial nerve involvement for which no cause is definitely known. These constitute by far the largest group of cases. They are referred to usually as "rheumatic" in origin. They are probably of toxic-infectious origin, and frequently develop after exposure to draughts, cold, or extremes of temperature. In all probability these cases of facial paralysis are due to a neuritis of unknown origin, the cold acting merely as a precipitating agent. Ischemia of the nerve is said to be responsible for the cases of undetermined origin.

Peripheral Facial Paralysis (Bell's Palsy): Involvement of the facial nerve from its nucleus to the periphery produces a typical type of facial paralysis. The *symptoms* of this condition will be described only for the "rheumatic" type, since the onset and symptoms in cases due to other causes varies with the cause. The onset is, as a rule, abrupt, but it is not uncommonly rather gradual in onset even in the neuritic type. The usual account is of a feeling of numbness or stiffness in the face noticed on arising in the morning or while driving in an automobile, in typical examples. Upon examining the reason for this sensation in a mirror, the patient notices distortion of the face due to paralysis of the facial muscles, or the distortion is called to his attention by others. As the process develops he notices increased lachrymation and a painful sensation in the eye often described as a stabbing sensation, indistinctness in speech due to relaxation of the facial muscles, inability to eat on the affected side also due to relaxation of the facial musculature, and a loss of the food bolus on this side. In cases with a more gradual onset the numbness or stiffness is observed in one portion of the face and is found in the course of hours to involve the entire face. Frequently the onset is painless, but a history of pain behind the ear or in the face below the malar bone is not uncommon. Ringing in the ear may be present in some cases. In others the patient notices that taste is impaired, but this is not often noted even by perceptive patients.

Examination reveals a typical deformity which cannot be missed easily. There is inability to wrinkle the forehead on the affected side, to close the eyelid completely, to blow out the cheek, pucker the lips, retract the mouth, or whistle. The eye on the affected side waters freely and the sclera may be injected. The face is asymmetrical in repose, the corner of the mouth and the cheek on the affected side drooping. The palpebral fissure on the affected side is wider than its fellow. Laughing or voluntary movement of the face accentuates the deformity and reveals a distorted facial musculature, with pulling over of the facial muscles. Taste may be lost over the anterior two-thirds of the tongue as well as secretion of saliva. In some instances loss of tear secretion has been noted. Tenderness over the nerve in the face or in the parotid region is sometimes present. The eyelid closes incompletely, the eyeball rolling upward until the cornea is hidden (Bell's phenomenon). Hearing is affected in some cases.

In some cases the facial paralysis does not develop completely, only parts of the facial musculature being affected (forehead, eyelid), or all the muscles may be affected but slightly. In such cases it is difficult at one examination to determine whether or not greater paralysis will ensue.

In some instances bilateral peripheral facial paralysis is found, especially associated with bulbar paralysis, amyotrophic lateral sclerosis, or acute infectious polyneuritis. Some cases of facial paralysis have a tendency to recur. Multiple attacks of facial paralysis occur at times in the same patient, involving one or both sides of the face. Several attacks in each of three brothers has been reported. The syndrome of *crocodile tears*, consisting of lachrymation on chewing, is seen rarely. This is evoked by taking strongly flavored food into the mouth. It is due to faulty regeneration of the facial nerve fibers, the salivary fibers to the submaxillary and sublingual glands having grown along the path of the lachrymal nerve. The syndrome is associated with incomplete recovery, facial contracture and associated movements.

DIAGNOSIS: This is easy. It is readily distinguished from a *central facial weakness* by the fact that in the latter only the lower portion of the face is weakened and never to the same degree as in peripheral facial paralysis. In a central weakness there is a weakness in retraction of the corner of the mouth and asymmetry of the two corners of the mouth on opening the mouth. In fresh cases of central facial weakness there may be associated weakness of the muscles of the forehead and eyelid simulating a peripheral facial paralysis, but this is usually associated with a hemiplegia and passes off in the course of a few hours to a few days. In peripheral facial paralysis, the entire face is paralyzed—forehead, eyelid, and the muscles of facial expression.

The important problem in diagnosis is the determination of the site of the lesion in peripheral facial paralysis; whether it is in brain stem, cranial cavity, fallopian canal, or neck. This can be determined by the following: involvement in the brain stem is usually associated with involvement of other systems; along the peripheral course of the nerve, hyperacusis and loss of saliva and tears follow lesions between the internal auditory meatus and geniculate ganglion, while below the emergence of the chorda tympani only facial paralysis ensues.

PROGNOSIS: This is of greatest importance, since neither sex, but particularly women, choose to be marked by a permanent facial paralysis. Spontaneous recovery is said to occur in seventy-five to eighty per cent of cases; the incidence is given as only fifty per cent by some investigators. Most patients recover in two to five weeks. Some cases persist much longer and the patients may recover only in the course of two to three months, or longer. Patients with tenderness over the nerve recover more slowly. So long as the reaction to the electrical current persists and no reaction of degeneration is present, recovery can be looked for. Patients who develop contractures or involuntary spasms of the facial muscle will fail to recover completely.

TREATMENT: The treatment of peripheral facial paralysis will depend on the causes. In cases due to neuritis treatment is as follows:

The treatment of facial paralysis is largely mechanical; drug treatment is of secondary importance. In many cases spontaneous recovery will occur quickly. If there is no tenderness of the nerve or the facial muscles, *massage* may be started immediately. This is carried out by placing the thumb within the mouth against the inside of the affected cheek and the index finger against the outside of the cheek and gently stroking the cheek in an upward direction. This can be performed two to three times a day for five minutes at a time. Patients can be instructed in this maneuver and taught to carry it out readily. The *eye* should be washed frequently with boric solution and a drop of sterile oil instilled a few times a day in order to keep the cornea and sclera healthy.

Electrical treatments may be started after two weeks. Some prefer to begin such treatment almost from the start of the paralysis, but the better evidence appears to favor delay in the beginning of electrical treatments. The object is to maintain the nutrition of the facial muscles by their contraction by means of the electrical current. Galvanism or faradism may be used depending on which elicits the better response, but galvanism is the better current to use. Treatments may be given daily or every other day and should be continued until the facial paralysis has been cured. The rapid sinusoidal current is advocated by some. *Diathermy* is sometimes of help. *Infra-red* daily over the face, with the eye protected, is frequently soothing in patients with tenderness over the nerve trunk.

Acetylsalicylic acid, 5 grains three times a day, is frequently given. *Potassium iodide,* 10 drops three times a day, may be given. It has become the custom to give routinely *thiamine chloride,* 30 to 100 mg. intramuscularly daily, but there is no valid reason for so doing unless a vitamin deficiency can be demonstrated as the cause of the facial paralysis. *Neostigmine,* 15 mg. three times daily, is often helpful. Cortisone, 10 mg. three times daily, has been reported to be helpful.

In patients who fail to recover, *surgical operations* are indicated. These should be undertaken only when all chance of spontaneous recovery is gone, usually after six months. Various types of operations have been advocated, among them nerve grafts, end-to-end suture, neurolysis, and decompression of the nerve.

Auditory Nerve (VIII): The auditory nerve consists of two portions, the cochlear and vestibular parts, the former having to do with hearing, the latter with equilibration. The nerve may be affected in the brain stem, or anywhere in its peripheral portion. It gives rise to no perceptible symptoms when involved in the brain stem, either through its nuclei or the lateral fillets, unless it is involved bilaterally, since the pathways decussate in the brain stem and ascend both ipsilaterally and contralaterally. Hence only a bilateral lesion in the brain stem will destroy all the fibers of one nerve and cause deafness. Such lesions are rare but may follow infiltrating tumors, encephalitis, syphilitis, multiple sclerosis, syringomyelia, or other diseases. In its peripheral portion beyond the brain stem the auditory nerve is subject to disease by tumors (acoustic neuromas), syphilis (tabes, syphilitic meningitis), trauma, meningitis, neuritis, meningeal hemorrhages.

Disease of the cochlear portion of the auditory nerve gives rise to tinnitus and loss of hearing. The cochlear portion of the nerve may be affected without simultaneous involvement of the vestibular portion, and the opposite holds true. Frequently the two portions are affected together.

Disease of the vestibular portion of the auditory nerve gives rise to vertigo. Meniere's syndrome is a striking example of disease of the vestibular nerve. Its features are discussed under vertigo.

Glossopharyngeal Nerve (IX): The glossopharyngeal nerve is partly motor and partly sensory, the latter being its more important function. On the motor side it supplies the stylopharyngeus muscle, which elevates and widens the pharynx in swallowing. It supplies sensory fibers to the mucous membranes of the throat, tonsils, soft palate, and posterior part of the tongue, and taste fibers to the same portion of the tongue.

It is rarely diseased alone. It may be involved in syphilis, tumors, neuritis, fractures of the base of the skull, and local diseases of the pharynx. Symptoms of involvement of the nerve are few. Very little motor impairment is noticeable, since the stylopharyngeus plays such a minor rôle in swallowing. Most of the symptoms are sensory and consist of loss of sensation over the posterior part of the tongue, the throat, palate, and pharynx, and a loss of taste over the posterior third of the tongue. The latter is not constant.

The nerve is subject to the syndrome of glossopharyngeal neuralgia, a rare type of pain involving the glossopharyngeal nerve. This will be treated under the section of neuralgia.

Vagus Nerve (X): The vagus is a very long nerve which may be affected at the base of the brain, the jugular foramen, in the neck or thorax, or even in the abdomen. Its symptoms vary depending upon the point at which it is involved. Generally speaking, the vagus on the motor side supplies the musculature of the larynx, pharynx, and palate (external laryngeal, recurrent laryngeal, pharyngeal nerves). It supplies also visceromotor fibers to the heart, lungs, and alimentary tract. It carries sensory impressions from pharynx, larynx, epiglottis, trachea, esophagus, heart, lungs, stomach, and small intestine. It has two ganglia: superior, or jugular, and inferior, or nodosum.

The vagus nerve may be involved within the brain stem by a variety of processes, such as infiltrating tumors, multiple sclerosis, syringomyelia, encephalitis, syphilis, tubercle, poliomyelitis, vascular lesions such as thrombosis of the posterior inferior cerebellar artery, progressive bulbar paralysis, amyotrophic lateral sclerosis, and other disorders. Within the cranium it may be involved by tumors which compress it, by aneurysms of the vertebral or basilar arteries, fractures of the base of the skull, syphilitic meningitis, hemorrhage, gunshot wounds, and surgical operations. In the neck it is subject to injury by stab wounds, gunshot wounds, operations on the thyroid or other neck structures, tumors, aneurysms of the carotid or subclavian arteries, enlarged glands, tumors, aneurysms of the aorta, or other processes of the mediastinum.

1. *Lesions within the Medulla:* Those involving the vagus nuclei cause paralysis of the soft palate, pharynx, and larynx, resulting in difficulty in swallowing, aphonia, and hoarseness if the lesion is unilateral. About ten per cent of cases of laryngeal (vocal cord) paralysis are due to lesions of the central nervous system (Clerf). The patient may notice difficulty in swallowing and is aware of hoarseness in unilateral lesions. In bilateral lesions swallowing is impossible and the voice is lost. Examination reveals drooping of the palate on the affected side while at rest and pulling of the pharynx to the healthy side on phonation. On being asked to say "ah"

the palate is seen to move over to the sound side, while there is a so-called "curtain movement" of the posterior pharyngeal wall due to a pull by the constrictor of the sound side. The palatal and pharyngeal reflex is lost. The vocal cord on the affected side is abducted; this can be detected on direct laryngeal examination. Sensation is lost at the external auditory meatus and the pinna of the ear. Bilateral lesions result in complete aphonia, marked difficulty in swallowing, and respiratory and cardiac distress.

2. *Recurrent Laryngeal Paralysis:* This is not uncommon from neck wounds, tumors, or glands, compression by aneurysm, accidental section in neck operations, mediastinal tumors, and aneurysms. Paralysis of the recurrent laryngeal nerve has been reported in cardiac disease, especially in severe mitral stenosis and less commonly in congenital heart disease. It has been found rarely in patients with arteriosclerotic heart disease. The cause of the paralysis is not known, but it has been suggested that it is due to compression of the nerve against the arch of the aorta and the ligamentum arteriosum, due to dilatation of the pulmonary artery produced by engorgement of the lesser circulation. It is characterized by hoarseness, the vocal cord lying in the cadaveric position halfway between abduction and adduction. Complete aphonia follows bilateral recurrent laryngeal involvement. Cases of abductor paralysis of the vocal cords are found for which no cause is apparent. Adduction paralysis occurs in hysteria. In the case of bilateral, recurrent, laryngeal paralysis the vocal cords are immobile and there is aphonia, dyspnea, and laryngeal stridor on deep inspiration.

3. *Superior Laryngeal Nerve Lesions:* They are rare. They result from stab or gunshot wounds, or compression by tu-

mors or glands. The symptoms consist of hoarseness and easy fatigability of the voice from involvement of the cricothyroid muscle. There is anesthesia of the upper part of the larynx.

4. *Pharyngeal Nerve Involvement:* It is uncommon. It results in hoarseness and in bilateral cases in palatal paralysis and aphonia. There is also difficulty in swallowing and phonation. The palate fails to move at all on phonation and the voice is typically bulbar, having a distinct nasal quality. Attempts to swallow are characterized by regurgitation, especially of fluids, through the nose, due to inability to close off the pharynx by the palate.

Disease of the vagus nerve gives rise to a few syndromes which are sometimes important to recognize. The *syndrome of the jugular foramen* due to paralysis of the glossopharyngeal, vagus, and spinal accessory nerves is characterized by (1) difficulty in swallowing; (2) nasal regurgitation; (3) loss of sensation and taste over the posterior third of the tongue; (4) hoarseness; (5) paralysis of the sternomastoid and trapezius muscles.

The *syndrome of Avellis* is due to paralysis of the vagus and spinal accessory nerves. It is characterized by paralysis of the soft palate on one side, and abductor paralysis of the vocal cord. The *syndrome of Hughlings Jackson* is due to involvement of the vagus, spinal accessory, and hypoglossal nerves. It is characterized by (1) hoarseness due to paralysis of the vocal cord; (2) difficulty in swallowing from involvement of the palate; (3) weakness of the sternocleidomastoid and trapezius muscles; (4) hemiatrophy of the tongue. The *syndrome of the retropharyngeal space* is due to involvement of the glossopharyngeal, vagus, spinal, accessory, hypoglossal, and cervical sympathetic nerves and is characterized by (1) difficulty in

swallowing; (2) nasal regurgitation; (3) loss of sensation over the posterior third of the tongue; (4) hoarseness; (5) paralysis of the sternocleidomastoid and trapezius muscles; (6) hemiatrophy of the tongue; (7) myosis, enophthalmos, and ptosis (Horner syndrome). It is caused by tumor, adenopathies due to various causes, penetrating injuries, and aneurysms.

Spinal Accessory Nerve (XI): The spinal accessory nerve is not often involved alone. It may be affected by some of the syndromes already mentioned. It is injured in gunshot and stab wounds of the neck, operations in the neck, fracture dislocations of the cervical vertebrae, tumors of the foramen magnum or at the base of the brain, aneurysm, syringomyelia, poliomyelitis, amyotrophic lateral sclerosis, and neuritis. *Paralysis of the sternocleidomastoid muscle* is characterized by flatness of the neck on the affected side, and failure of the muscle to stand out on rotation of the neck. There is decrease of power in this movement. Peculiarly the loss of the muscle is little noticed and the resting posture of the head is unchanged. Paralysis of both sternocleidomastoid muscles causes weakness of flexion of the head on the neck. *Paralysis of the trapezius muscle* causes drooping and inability to raise the shoulder, weakness in shrugging the shoulder, difficulty in raising the arm above the horizontal plane, atrophy and flattening of the neck. The neck loses its normal contour. The scapula is slightly rotated downward and outward and in severe instances a slight winging of the scapula is seen.

Hypoglossal Nerve (XII): The hypoglossal is entirely a motor nerve supplying the muscles of the tongue. It may be involved in a variety of processes. Within the medulla it may be involved by such varied processes as progressive bulbar paralysis, amyotrophic lateral sclerosis, syringomyelia, infiltrating tumors, thrombosis of the anterior spinal artery, poliomyelitis, and syphilis. Outside the brain stem it may be compressed by aneurysm or tumor, severed by injury, or involved in meningitic or neuritic processes. It may be affected by processes involving its exit at the jugular foramen.

Disease of the hypoglossal nerve causes atrophy and weakness of one side of the tongue. In the mouth the tip tends to curl to the healthy side. The tongue on the atrophic side shows deep furrows, especially at its edges, fibrillary twitchings, and tends to be curved with the concavity on the side of the weakness. The tongue cannot be pushed firmly against the cheek. On protrusion it deviates to the healthy side. If the process is bilateral there is atrophy and fibrillations bilaterally with difficulty in phonation and swallowing, and inability to protrude the tongue. This type of peripheral paralysis of the tongue differs from a central weakness in the absence of atrophy and fibrillations in the latter and deviation of the tongue on protrusion to the weakened side, the tongue being pushed over by the healthy muscles.

Lingual spasm is seen rarely. It is characterized by attacks of spasm involving one side of the tongue. It has been reported to be relieved by section of the chorda tympani nerve (Cobb and Mixter).

VI. THE NEURALGIAS

The term "neuralgia" refers merely to pain along the course of a nerve. It is not in most cases a disease *per se* but must be regarded rather as a symptom complex or syndrome for which no assignable cause is known. In the case of such well-established entities as trigeminal or glossopharyngeal neuralgia,

on the other hand, the disease entity is well established beyond the syndrome stage. Save in the case of well-established processes, the diagnosis of a neuralgia should not be made except after careful search for specific causes has been made. Pain along a nerve trunk being merely a symptom, the conclusion that a neuralgia exists is tantamount to the assertion that no cause can be found. Before such a conclusion is reached, careful search for causes must be made.

1. Trigeminal Neuralgia (Trifacial Neuralgia, Tic Douloureux, Fothergill's Disease)

Trigeminal neuralgia is characterized by paroxysmal attacks of pain involving one or more branches of the trigeminal nerve.

Etiology: The precise cause of the disease is not known. Many conditions have been indicted as causing trigeminal neuralgia, but it is doubtful whether they can be regarded as more than inciting or precipitating causes. Arteriosclerosis is frequently found, but it is difficult to see how this can explain the pain. Trigeminal pain may be caused by affections of the ganglion, such as tumor, aneurysm, or pachymeningitis. It is found in intoxications, such as lead, alcohol, arsenic, etc., and in infections, such as grippe, syphilis, herpes zoster, tuberculosis, malaria, and other diseases. It is found also in gout, rheumatic diathesis, and diabetes. In many cases the disease occurs in the presence of diseased teeth, tonsils, or sinuses, but it is extremely doubtful whether these have any relationship to the disorder, since removal of the infected foci causes no relief of symptoms. So numerous are the cases for which no cause is found that the term "idiopathic" has been used for them. Exhaustion, overwork, and nervous strain have frequently been observed as predisposing causes. The bare fact is that after the many inciting conditions and predisposing factors are mentioned, it is still impossible to state the cause.

Symptoms: The sexes are about equally affected. Either side of the face may be involved, but there is a moderate preponderance of cases on the right side. Trigeminal neuralgia is a disease of middle life, most cases occurring at forty-five years or over. Cases in younger subjects are uncommon but they occur, while those in old people of sixty years or over are not uncommon.

The history in typical trigeminal neuralgia is quite characteristic and cannot be mistaken readily for other types of pain. The onset is sudden and the details as a rule are lost in obscurity. No precipitating cause is assigned as a rule by the patient and no antecedent twinges of pain have been experienced before the onset. The story is that of severe pain, so severe as to be unbearable, radiating from one portion of the face to another. It is often described as beginning at the ala of the nose and radiating along the maxilla toward the temporomandibular joint. Not infrequently it spreads along the side of the nose toward but not into the eye. It may begin at the corner of the mouth and spread along the lower jaw or start over the eye and radiate over the forehead. It is precipitated by movements of the face and often a spontaneous account of onset of pain by touching some part of the face is obtained. In most instances the pain is paroxysmal, the paroxysms occurring at irregular intervals, sometimes often, at other times infrequently. It may, however, give the appearance of a constant pain in those instances in which the paroxysms are repeated frequently. The pain may arouse the patient from his sleep. A history of previous bouts of pain with a free interval of varying periods of time is obtainable in many cases. If the patient is seen during a period of paroxysms there is often a history of failure to eat over a period of days for fear of precipitating attacks of pain.

The pain in most cases is in the second and third divisions. The first division is rarely affected (7 or 8 per cent). Second division pain is referred roughly along the upper jaw; third division pain, along the lower jaw. First division pain is referred over the forehead. Pain may begin in one division and spread later to another, but it may persist in one division for years. Bilateral pain occurs in rare cases. The pain itself is severe and variously described as "boring," "hot," "piercing," "tearing," and by many other names too numerous to mention. "Trigger zones" are frequently described. These are areas on the skin of the upper or lower lip, at the angle of the nose, or at the corner of the mouth, touching of which sets off a paroxysm of pain.

The pain is precipitated by talking, chewing, laughing, washing the face, brushing the teeth, or any voluntary movement of the facial muscles so that patients sit frozen with fear of movement of the face for any purpose, in order to avoid precipitating a pain paroxysm. Draughts of air or emotional upsets may set off a pain. During a paroxysm the patient suddenly holds the face, the eye waters, the nose runs, the face flushes, and the patient is in the throes of agony with the paroxysm for one to two minutes. Gradually he releases his hold on his face and emerges from the grip of the paroxysm, still fearful of another attack. The number of attacks varies from a few per day to pains every few minutes. In the typical case there is freedom from pain between paroxysms, but in some cases the paroxysms may be repeated so frequently as to give the impression of constant pain.

In the usual case also the pain lasts one to two minutes, but in some cases pains may last thirty to sixty minutes in typical cases of trigeminal neuralgia. Remissions from the pain are not uncommon and may last varying lengths of time from a few weeks or months to years.

Examination reveals nothing in the majority of cases. There is often evidence of retinal arteriosclerosis, but apart from this little else. The sensation over the face is unaffected and the corneal reflex is active. At the time of examination the patient is extremely apprehensive, is afraid to talk because of fear of precipitating pain, and prefers the history to be given by someone else. Manipulation of the face is resented and always there is a warning to avoid the areas of the trigger zones.

Diagnosis: The diagnosis of trigeminal neuralgia is not difficult in typical cases as described. The diagnosis is made in cases of face pain which develop in older subjects, with paroxysmal bouts of pain radiating along one or more divisions of the trigeminal nerve, with no neurological findings on examination. The paroxysmal nature of the pain is important, as is its distribution along one of the three divisions of the trigeminal nerve. This is a point of great importance, since cases of face pain with radiation beyond these areas of distribution must at once be suspected of not being trigeminal neuralgia. Not infrequently the pain radiates along areas not clearly those of the trigeminal branches, as, for example, along the side of the nose, but other features of the disease serve to make clear the nature of the disease. Trigger zones are extremely important and occur in no other type of facial neuralgia, though such zones are found in the throat and pharynx in glossopharyngeal neuralgia. Pain along the trigeminal nerve is found in *tumors of the gasserian*

ganglion. In such cases, signs of increased intracranial pressure are frequently absent, but they are characterized by the syndrome of anesthesia dolorosa, or anesthesia in the distribution of the trigeminal nerve, and absence of the corneal reflex; the pain in such cases is usually constant rather than paroxysmal, but this is not always true. Paroxysmal pain may be encountered in true gasserian ganglion tumors.

Herpetic neuralgia due to herpes zoster is much more common in the first division than in the second or third. It may be recognized by the vesicular eruption or scars, and by involvement as a rule of other cranial nerves due to the encephalitis which accompanies the herpes zoster. Absence of the corneal reflex and loss of sensation over the affected area are present.

Sphenopalatine neuralgia must be differentiated. Typical cases are characterized by pain of sudden onset behind the root of the nose, in the eyes, face, and often into the neck and shoulder. The pain is not referred along the branches of the trigeminal nerve but is much more diffuse and widespread. During paroxysms of pain relief may be obtained by cocainization of the sphenopalatine ganglion. If this is successful, alcohol injection of the ganglion can be performed for more permanent relief.

Atypical neuralgias must not be confused with trigeminal neuralgia. The term is applied to a wide variety of causes of facial pain not due to trigeminal neuralgia. These neuralgias occur at all ages and involve the face. They differ from true trigeminal neuralgia in the following respects: the pain extends beyond the confines of the trigeminal nerve, it is continuous and not paroxysmal, it is deep-seated rather than peripheral, is often bilateral, it differs in quality from that of trigeminal neuralgia, no trigger zones are present, and younger subjects are afflicted. Often the pain radiates into the neck or shoulder well beyond the anatomical distribution of the trigeminal nerve. Atypical neuralgias occur frequently in neurotic cases, but whether this has much to do with the pain is not known. The cause of the pain in the atypical neuralgias is not known, but efforts have been made to refer it to sympathetic impulses transmitted along the vessels of the neck and face.

Glossopharyngeal neuralgia may be distinguished by the occurrence of paroxysms of pain on swallowing, the pain being in the throat and not in the face.

Hysterical pain in the face, referred to as "psychalgia," is sometimes seen, but can be detected by a careful consideration of the personality and social background of the patient.

Arthritis of the temporomandibular joint produces face pain usually radiating into the face from the region of the joint. It may simulate trigeminal neuralgia, but the pain associated with it is not referred along the trigeminal branches. Tenderness of the temporomandibular joint is usually present and arthritis may be demonstrated by roentgenograms.

Malocclusion of the jaws may produce an indefinite type of face pain, but it is not readily confused with trigeminal neuralgia largely on the absence of paroxysms and atypical distribution of the pain.

Ciliary neuralgia is characterized by pain in the temple, eye, cheek, and jaws, usually unilateral, often associated with nausea, occurring in paroxysms lasting ten minutes to twenty-four hours, and regarded as a substitute form of migraine in which the pain is referred to the face and is unassociated with other manifestations of migraine (Harris). In many cases the pain is referred into the eye and around the eyeball. Injection of the

supraorbital or infraorbital nerve gives relief from the pain. Pain radiating into the face is found also in histamine headache (v. Headache).

The *auriculotemporal* syndrome is sometimes encountered and is characterized by flushing of the cheek and pinna, associated with profuse sweating, corresponding to the distribution of the auriculotemporal branch of the mandibular division of the trigeminal nerve. The syndrome is elicited on eating, usually something sour or acid, following which redness and sweating appear in the area indicated. Most cases have been associated with infection of the parotid gland.

Treatment: Permanent cure of the pain in trigeminal neuralgia is offered by *operation.* Section of the sensory root adjacent to the pons has many advocates and in skillful hands is extremely safe. Partial section of the root is performed. Other operations consist of tractotomy or section of the pain fibers passing to the face in the medulla; section of the trigeminal nerve through the posterior fossa is advocated by some. *Injection* (alcohol) treatment of the specific branch affected is advisable for those refusing operations, in old cases, or in doubtful instances. Relief lasts from six to twelve months. Injection of the gasserian ganglion is advised by some in preference to operation. *Medical treatment* is not as a rule effective. Trichlorethylene (fifteen to twenty drops) on a handkerchief, with the patient in a reclining position, helps soften paroxysms. It may be used several times a day in cases which are not hypertensive. Other medicaments are not effective. Morphine should never be given. Thiamine chloride in large doses is of little help.

Marcus-Gunn Phenomenon: In rare instances there develops in disease of the trigeminal nerve a peculiar reflex known as the "*jaw-winking reflex*" or the "*Mar-*

cus-Gunn phenomenon." This is character-ized by a slight ptosis of one eyelid and the production of an associated movement of the lid on opening or closing the jaw. Pro-trusion or lateral movements of the jaw, and mere opening or chewing movements result in elevation of the affected eyelid, causing great embarrassment to the pa-tient. Four varieties of the syndrome are reported: (1) when the mouth is opened and the mandible is moved to the opposite side, (2) when the mouth is opened but not upon lateral movement of the man-dible, (3) when the mandible is moved to the opposite side but not when the mouth is opened, and (4) associated movements of the eyelid and jaw without ptosis. In the majority of cases, the movement oc-curs on movement of the ipsilateral, external pterygoid muscle. The condition is usually congenital (ninety-three out of one hundred reported cases) but it may be acquired. In the latter case it may develop at any age and may fol-low trauma or infection. Males are more commonly afflicted than females and the left eyelid more commonly than the right. The eyeball is unaffected, and movement of both eyeballs is usually normal. The pupillary reflexes and the visual acuity are normal. The mechanism of the condition is poorly understood, but section of the motor supply to the exter-nal pterygoid muscle has cured the con-dition (Grant).

2. Glossopharyngeal Neuralgia

Etiology: Pain along the course of the glossopharyngeal nerve is rare, but it is important to recognize because of its confusion with trigeminal neuralgia. It may occur in the course of compression of the nerve by a cerebellopontine-angle tumor, by neuritis from syphilis, or by aneurysm. In most cases, the precise cause cannot be determined, and it has no relationship to infections of the throat, teeth, or sinuses.

Symptoms: The outstanding feature of the disease is pain of a paroxysmal nature. This pain is fully as severe as that of trigeminal neuralgia, occurring in paroxysms lasting only a few minutes. Between paroxysms the patient is per-fectly comfortable, though he lives in fear of occurrence of the pain. The dis-tribution of the pain is quite different from that of trigeminal neuralgia, an important feature which becomes appar-ent on taking a careful history. It is felt not in the face but in the throat, radiating to the ear of the affected side, and sometimes spreading out into the neck. It is precipitated by swallowing in particular, but it may be initiated by talking or yawning. Eating becomes impossible because of the paroxysms of pain initiated by swallowing, and loss of weight is a natural consequence. Trig-ger zones are frequently found in the pharynx. Nothing is found on examina-tion of most of these patients. In cases associated with cerebellopontine angle tumor or aneurysm, evidence of involve-ment of other cranial nerves and systems is found.

Diagnosis: The diagnosis of glosso-pharyngeal neuralgia is not difficult if one has seen a few cases or if one is on his guard against the entity. It is most often confused with *trigeminal neural-gia,* but a careful history will reveal the fact that the pain is not in the face but in the throat. *Otalgia* is often confused with it because pain is frequently felt chiefly in the ear in some cases and investigations are as a rule focused about the ear. The true nature of the disorder is revealed by the regular provocation of pain by a trigger zone in the tonsillar region or pharynx. Similar to glossophar-yngeal neuralgia are cases of *superior laryngeal neuralgia* which are said to comprise a true entity. In such cases paroxysms of pain lasting a few seconds to one minute are felt from the region of the thyroid cartilage to the angle of the jaw. The pain, like that of glossopharyngeal neuralgia, is precipitated by swallowing, but the trigger zone is in the pyriform sinus and a tender area can usually be elicited on the skin, just above and lateral to the thyroid cartilage.

Treatment: The only treatment of any value is *surgical*. Section of the glossopharyngeal nerve in the cranial cavity brings permanent relief from the pain. Medical treatment is without avail.

3. Tympanic Neuralgia (Neuralgia of Jacobsen's Nerve)

This type of neuralgia is rare, but occasional cases are confused with trigeminal neuralgia. It is due to involvement of Jacobsen's nerve, which is given off the glossopharyngeal nerve as a tympanic branch to join the tympanic plexus in the middle ear, thus innervating the mucous lining of the tympanum, eustachian tube, and mastoid cells. It is characterized by sudden short paroxysms of pain deep in the neck and ear. The trigger zone is probably located in the eustachian tube. Relief is afforded by section of the glossopharyngeal nerve.

4. Sphenopalatine Neuralgia (Lower Half Headache: Sluder's Neuralgia)

An unusual and not too common type of neuralgia is attributed to involvement of the sphenopalatine ganglion, which lies just beneath the maxillary division of the trigeminal nerve in the lateral bony wall of the nose. The pain of sphenopalatine neuralgia is said to be due to vasoconstriction of the vascular bed supplying the nasal mucous membrane, but there is doubt whether such vasoconstriction is accompained by pain. The ganglion gives nerve supply to the orbit, the sphenoidal and ethmoidal cells, the nose, the hard and soft palate, the tonsils, nasopharynx, and gums. From this diffuse nerve supply it can be seen that the pain in this type of neuralgia is diffuse and widespread. It is believed by some that sphenopalatine neuralgia is, in fact, due to a neuritis of the vidian nerve, caused in most instances by infection of the sphenoid sinus. According to this concept, sphenopalatine neuralgia is in fact a vidian neuralgia and is due to an irriation or inflammation of the vidian nerve (Vail).

The disease occurs preponderantly in patients between thirty and forty years but it may be found in younger or older subjects. Women are affected more frequently than men. The cause of the condition is not specifically known. Among the commonly attributed causes are infection of the sphenoid and ethmoid sinuses. Further causes are intumescence of the nasal membrane associated with intranasal deformities and systemic disorders including toxemia, anemia, and fatigue (Eagle). The intranasal deformities include deviation of the nasal septum, ledges, spurs, prominent turbinates, adhesions, and osteomas. Most patients with sphenopalatine neuralgia have an intranasal deformity involving contact with the middle turbinate. The pain is said to be due to irritation of branches of the sphenopalatine ganglion supplying the middle turbinate. In other instances, infection of the sphenoid or ethmoid sinuses appears to be responsible.

Pain, which is the outstanding symptom of sphenopalatine neuralgia, usually begins at the root of the nose, in and about the eye, the upper jaw and teeth, backward to the temple around the zygoma to the ear, frequently causing earache and tinnitus. It may spread at times to the region of the mastoid, down the neck and into the shoulder and arm. It may extend into the elbow and even the hand. The pain is unilateral and never extends above the level of the ear. It is lancinating and continuous, and may last for a few minutes to several days. Two main points of maximum pain are usually found, one in the region of the orbit and root of the nose, and the other in the region just posterior to the mastoid process in the temporal bone. Tinnitus and dizziness are occasionally described. Facial pain and burning, and a tingling and stinging sensation of the face are occasionally described.

Diagnosis: The condition is conclusively established if the symptoms are relieved within one to three minutes by cocainization of the sphenopalatine ganglion on the affected side. "When periods of cocainization of more than three minutes fail to alleviate the pain, the presence of sphenopalatine neuralgia is not likely" (Eagle). If cocainization is successful the ganglion may be injected with *alcohol* or removed *surgically*.

Among the conditions requiring differentiation are migraine, trigeminal neuralgia, dental abscesses and impactions, maxillary and ethmoid sinus disease, brain tumors, intracranial aneurysms, and temporomandibular disease. Migraine is readily distinguished by the history of unilateral headache associated with nausea and vomiting, often with scotomas, hemianopsias, or other transient phenomena, and relieved by ergotamine. Trigeminal neuralgia is easily distinguished by the typical paroxysmal pain distributed along the various branches of the trigeminal nerve. The pain is much less diffuse than that of sphenopalatine neuralgia and is never felt in the neck or shoulder. Dental abscesses or impactions are easily diagnosed by inspection and roentgenograms. Brain tumor rarely gives a history of diffuse pain such as is found in sphenopalatine neuralgia, is associated with bilateral headache, evidences of increased pressure, and signs of focal brain disease. Cerebral aneurysm may cause unilateral headache of a paroxysmal type, often behind the eye, but it is associated with cranial nerve palsies of varying sorts and often with signs of skull erosion by roentgenogram.

5. Geniculate Neuralgia (Hunt's Syndrome)

Geniculate neuralgia is due to herpes of the geniculate ganglion and is characterized by severe pain in the external auditory meatus and pinna, and sometimes in the throat. Evidence is at hand to indicate that the geniculate ganglion is not affected in herpes zoster oticus (Denny-Brown). Autopsy study of a case revealed damage to the facial nerve and 2nd cervical ganglion but none to the geniculate ganglion. Of twenty-two cases of herpes zoster with facial paralysis the geniculate was affected in only seven (Tschiassny). The pain usually appears before the skin eruption, which is seen in the external auditory canal, pinna, sometimes behind the ear, on the pillar of the fauces, and on the anterior two-thirds of the tongue. Swelling of the ear, often severe, is present. The pain is extremely severe and paroxysmal. Peripheral facial paralysis develops suddenly but is not present in every instance. It is found in the majority of cases. Tinnitus is almost invariably present and there may be loss or diminution of hearing.

The pain tends to disappear but may persist for some time. The deafness is persistent and the facial paralysis often fails to clear up. The condition is usually confused with middle ear disease due to the pain in the ear, the ear discharge from the erupted vesicles, and the development of facial paralysis. The diagnosis is readily made, however, by the recognition of the herpetic eruption in the ear. A small number of cases are found unassociated with herpes of the ear. The cause in these cases is unknown. Treatment should be directed toward eradication of infection in the nose and pharynx.

6. Occipital Neuralgia

Pain is fairly common in the region of the greater occipital nerve, radiating along the back of the head to the vertex. The group of occipital neuralgias is ill-defined and illustrates clearly the futility of the neuralgia concept. In most instances a diagnosis of occipital neuralgia is tantamount to a confession that there is unaccountable pain along the distribution of the occipital nerve.

In many cases pain along the occipital nerve may be traced to some specific cause, such as tuberculosis of the spine, spinal cord tumor, myositis, osteoarthritis, or pachymeningitis. In some instances, it is associated with infections of various sorts. In still another group, no cause save exposure to chill is found.

The pain is usually bilateral, usually constant, but may be paroxysmal, radiating over the back of the head to the vertex. It is severe, increased by moving and by coughing and sneezing. The scalp is often hyperesthetic. Tenderness over the points of emergence of the occipital nerves below the occipital protuberance is common.

The diagnosis is easy, but care must be taken to exclude secondary causes of occipital pain, such as tuberculosis of the spine, spinal cord tumors, tumors of the vertebrae, and osteoarthritis of the spine. Hysterical pain is frequently felt in the back of the head.

The treatment is usually satisfactory. *Salicylates, heat* (infra-red or diathermy), or *galvanism* give relief in many cases. *Alcohol injection* about the points of exit of the occipital nerves affords relief if other measures fail.

7. Phrenic Neuralgia

Phrenic neuralgia is extremely rare. It is characterized by pain in the shoulder or in the arm, associated with visceral disease, such as pericarditis, thoracic aneurysm, pleurisy, or suprarenal tumor. The pain is purely symptomatic and referred from the diseased viscera. If the diagnosis is made, it should be only as a preliminary to determining the precise underlying cause.

8. Intercostal Neuralgia

Pain in the distribution of the intercostal nerves is usually produced by specific causes, such as spinal-cord tumor, tuberculosis of the spine, metastatic carcinoma of the spine, osteoarthritis, pachymeningitis of syphilitic origin, aortic aneurysm, and other disorders. When due to neurological as opposed to systemic causes, intercostal neuralgia is usually root pain and should be investigated on this basis. In some instances, however, intercostal pain or neuralgia is due to no assignable cause. In such cases, the pain is felt along any of the intercostal nerves and is associated with tenderness along the spine. It is a safe rule to follow that the diagnosis of an intercostal neuralgia should be made with reluctance only after every effort has been made to exclude a structural cause. Intercostal neuralgia is frequently found in neurotic patients.

9. Brachial Plexus Neuralgia

Pain involving the nerves of the brachial plexus is usually the result of specific causes. Neuralgia of the brachial plexus may occur, however. It is more common in England than in this country, due probably to differences of climate. The usual causes include rheumatism, chills, exposure, or infection.

The symptoms are characterized by sharp pains in the neck and shoulder region extending into the arm and hand. The pain is usually constant, often dull and deep, but sometimes sharp and paroxysmal. There is usually no radiation along specific nerves; rather it is a diffuse pain spread throughout the arm. No changes can be detected in the muscles or reflexes. The pains tend to drag on indefinitely.

10. Lumbosacral Plexus Neuralgia

Pain along the various branches of the lumbar plexus is sometimes encountered. *Crural neuralgia* along the front of the thigh, *obturator neuralgia* along the inner aspect of the thigh, and other forms of neuralgia occur. In this as in all forms of neuralgia, it is important to exclude organic disease as a cause of the pain. Hasty conclusion that pain is the result of a neuralgia may lead to disaster.

11. Pudendal Plexus Neuralgia

This is felt along the nerves of the lower two or three sacral nerves ($S_{2 \text{ to } 5}$). Hence it is featured by pain in the perineum, scrotum, penis, and testes, to all of which regions a special type of neuralgic pain has been assigned. Pain involving the areas in question is quite sharp, paroxysmal, and excruciating. *Testicular neuralgia* is characterized by severe pain in the testis or testes, often of an excruciating nature, sometimes with symptoms of collapse, and associated with tenderness of the testicle. No cause is found as a rule. *Anoperineal neuralgia* is felt in the anus and perineum, and is more common in women than in men. *Coccygeal neuralgia* (coccygodynia) is usually found in women who give a history of a fall on the end of the spine. Pain of a severe, constant, or paroxysmal nature is felt in the end of the spine. but nothing is found to account for it. The symptom is frequent in neurotic women and resists treatment stubbornly.

12. Causalgia

Causalgia is a particular form of neuralgia found in injured nerves. It may follow immediately or soon after injury, or it may develop at a later period, some time after the injury. The nature of the injury varies. As a rule, the nerve is injured by gunshot or stab wounds, but causalgia may follow injury associated with fractures, or spinal anesthesia. It may involve any nerve in the body, but more particularly the median and sciatic. Its precise cause is not known, but it is presumably the result of activation of sensory fibers by sympathetic impulses. It is characterized by violent pains described usually as "burning" in nature but referred to variously as "like fire," "painful," "tingling," etc. Causalgic pain has the following characteristics (Medical Research Council, 1920) : "It is (1) spontaneous; (2) hot and burning in character, intense, diffuse, persistent but subject to exacerbations; (3) causalgic pain can be excited by stimulation which does not necessarily produce a physical effect on the limb; emotional excitement usually aggravates the pain and brings on a paroxysm; (4) it tends to lead to profound changes in the emotional state of the patient." The pain is superficial and usually localized at the termination of the nerve, in the palm of the hand (median), or on the sole of the foot (sciatic), but it may radiate over the entire distribution of the nerve. It is aggravated by movement, walking, or the slightest shock. It may be set off by the slightest touch of the skin, pin prick, heat, or cold. The skin is usually dry and the tendency is to keep moist the affected portions of the skin. Muscle wasting and weakness are usually slight or absent, as are reflex changes. Trophic changes are usually seen : the skin is dry, red, and glossy; the fingers thin; the nails friable and yellow; and the skin hyperesthetic. Treatment of the condition by drugs or local means is usually unsuccessful. *Alcohol injection* of the nerve has been reported as successful. The condition may resist treatment, but *sympathetic block* has been found to relieve the pain of causalgia in many instances. Many cases disappear spontaneously.

VII. PERIPHERAL NERVE TUMORS

Tumors of the peripheral nerve are of greater histological than clinical importance in the sense that their story in most instances is typical and their diagnosis readily made. Two main groups of tumors may be distinguished: (1) a benign group; (2) a malignant group. Classification of peripheral nerve tumors varies greatly and no two groups are similar.

In the benign group are included (1) tumors of the nerve sheath; these are variously grouped under several headings, such as "perineural fibroblastomas," "palisaded neurinomas," "myxoid neurinomas," or "neurilemoblastomas"; (2) tumors of nerve fibers, or true neuroma.

1. The Perineural Fibroblastomas

Palisaded neurinomas, or neurilemomas, arise from the sheath of subcutaneous nerves or the spinal or cranial nerves. They are covered by perineurium, are solitary, are palpable under the skin and painful on pressure, with pain referred along the distribution of the peripheral nerve affected. In the spinal canal they are attached to a nerve root producing root pain and pressure on the spinal cord (*v.* Spinal Cord Tumors). The peripheral nerve tumors of this type are characterized by pain, usually persistent, with typical radiation along the course of the peripheral trunk. Sensory changes are found in the region of the affected nerve.

2. Neurofibromas

These are found often associated with the sheaths of peripheral nerves. They are usually pedunculated and differ from the tumors of von Recklinghausen's disease in the absence of symptoms, their restricted numbers, their small size, and their failure to follow the entire cutaneous distribution of the nerve (Geschickter).

Tumors of the nerve sheath may be found involving the deeper nerves, especially the sciatic nerve in the thigh or popliteal space. They may also involve the femoral, median, and ulnar nerves, and the nerves of the sympathetic system. Tumors of this type occur more frequently in children, are not encapsulated, frequently extend along the nerve trunk without definite boundary, and tend to recur. They are characterized clinically by a history of persistent pain, but often there is relatively little pain, and simply evidence of rapid growth of the tumor by palpation. They must be *excised* widely. Recurrence occurred in 30 per cent of a large series of such tumors (Geschickter).

3. Neurofibromatosis, or von Recklinghausen's Disease

This is characterized by the congenital occurrence of nerve sheath tumors along the peripheral nerves, the spinal nerve and cranial nerve roots, and by areas of pigmentation. The disease is rare. Heredofamilial incidence occurs often but not constantly. The disease is congenital and its manifestations appear early in life, but in some instances are delayed. It is characterized by the presence of tumors under the skin, by pigmentary lesions, and in some instances by skeletal anomalies. The tumors are found in almost any location along the peripheral nerve trunks, their number varying greatly from a single or a few tumors to hundreds of neoplasms everywhere under the skin. The skin tumors are found under the skin of the scalp, limbs, and trunk, and are felt just under the skin. They vary in shape and size, they may be pedunculated, they may be extremely small or very large, and are usually soft. Plexiform neuromas are sometimes seen. The tumors may involve the roots of the spinal canal, the cranial nerves, the dura, and even the viscera. Microscopically, the tumors are neurofibromata, and in some instances meningiomas.

The symptoms vary widely. The age of onset of symptoms varies greatly from childhood to between thirty and fifty years. In many instances only the presence of subcutaneous nodules brings the patient to the physician. In other cases, pain along the distribution of a nerve or nerves affected by the tumor growth brings the patient. When the tumors involve the spinal canal, the symptoms are those of extramedullary spinal cord tumor (q.v.). In other instances, symptoms of brain tumor develop. Headache is often present in such cases and often signs of increased pressure are found. Examination reveals the tumor nodules under the skin and pigmentation of the skin. This consists of café-au-lait spots varying in size from small spots to very large areas of brownish pigmentation. In some cases, the pigmentation is scanty, in others very pronounced, and in still others absent. In spinal cord involvement, weakness of the limbs and a sensory level may be found. Many developmental anomalies have been described in the disorder. In some instances, the disease may involve the nerves of the spinal and cerebral cavities without implication of the peripheral nerves. Many variants of the disease are known and the disorder is not always found in its fully developed form. In addition to the central forms, there are pure nerve forms involving peripheral nerves alone, and cranial forms.

The diagnosis offers few difficulties in a typical case.

Malignant peripheral nerve tumors are characterized clinically chiefly by the tumor. This may be present for years and suddenly develop rapidly to a large size, or it may grow progressively and slowly for years. If the growth is rapid, a relatively large size is attained in a few months. Pain along the course of the affected nerve is usually present but it may be absent. If the growth is not removed, death ensues. Two classes of malignant tumors develop in the peripheral nerves (Stout): (1) those of mesoblastic origin, by far the most common; these are made up of the malignant neurofibroma and the much more common fibrosarcoma; metatasis occurs in 20 per cent of the fibrosarcomas; (2) those of neuroepithelial origin.

6

Diseases of the Spinal Cord

I. GENERAL CONSIDERATIONS

The spinal cord is subject to many forms of disease, most of which involve the cord primarily, others attacking it secondarily as part of a generalized involvement of the central nervous system. Infection in the spinal cord is in many instances only part of a generalized nervous system infection (meningitis, neurosyphilis, poliomyelitis), while in other instances it alone is involved (hypertrophic spinal pachymeningitis, epidural abscess, and herpes zoster). Tumors tend to affect it chiefly primarily, but metastatic tumors are common as well. Degenerative processes involve the spinal cord as part of general nervous system disease (amyotrophic lateral sclerosis, multiple sclerosis, Friedreich's ataxia) or in isolated form (syringomyelia, subacute combined degeneration, primary lateral sclerosis).

It is imperative, therefore, in the diagnosis of nervous disease involving the spinal cord to determine whether it alone is affected, or whether its involvement forms part of a generalized disease of the nervous system. Fortunately, this is within the means of the examiner to decide, since a thorough neurological examination will disclose the answer to this pertinent problem.

A few *anatomical considerations* appear pertinent. The spinal cord consists first of all of a number of segments (8 cervical, 12 thoracic, 5 lumbar, 5 sacral, 1 coccygeal). These are arranged metamerically so that specific segments are related to definite sensory dermatomes through the posterior roots, with definite muscle segments through the anterior horns and roots, and with specific reflex arcs (*v.* Chapter 2). The cord varies in size, being largest at the cervical and lumbar areas because of the innervation to the arms and legs derived from these areas, is thinner in the thoracic area, terminates in a tapering sacral portion, and is covered in its lowermost part by the fanning roots of the lower portion of the spinal cord, the cauda equina. The cord is surrounded by the meninges and is suspended in the vertebral canal, where it is attached loosely by the dentate ligaments. Despite the cervical and lumbar enlargements, it is less crowded in these areas than in the thoracic region because of the larger size of the vertebral canal in these regions. Consequently compression of the spinal cord in the cervical and lumbar areas is delayed in its detection frequently because of the greater room for expansion in these areas.

The spinal cord in its growth lags behind the growth of the vertebral column after the third embryonic month. As a result, the cord in the adult terminates at about the junction of the first and second lumbar vertebrae. The conus medullaris lies between the first and second lumbar vertebrae and the sacral segments of the cord beneath the twelfth thoracic and first lumbar vertebrae. Because of this difference in growth the cord segments fail to lie opposite their corresponding vertebrae, a factor which must be given consideration in laminectomies for tumors or other diseases of the spinal cord. Roughly speak-

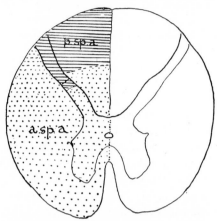

Fig. 77—*Spinal cord blood supply.* Schematic drawing of cord showing areas supplied by posterior spinal artery (lined area) and anterior spinal artery (dotted area). *(Bolton: Jnl. Neurol & Psychiat. 2:137, 1939.)*

ing, the spinal cord segment lags behind the vertebra by about one segment in the cervical area and two in the thoracic region. Thus, the sixth cervical segment lies opposite about the fifth cervical vertebra, and the sixth thoracic segment opposite the fourth thoracic vertebra.

The arrangement of the spinal roots is also important. The upper three cervical roots pass out horizontally, the first cervical emerging between the atlas and occiput. The lower three cervical roots are directed downward and outward, making their exit one vertebra below their segment of origin. Thoracic roots one to five make their exits two vertebrae below their origin, and thoracic roots six to eleven three vertebrae below. The roots of the cauda equina extend from the second lumbar vertebra to the sacral foramina.

Blood Supply of the Spinal Cord: This is provided by the anterior spinal and

posterior spinal arteries, for anatomical details of which the student is referred to anatomical texts. Three primary vascular chains are found supplying the spinal cord with blood. These are (1) an anterior spinal artery extending the entire length of the spinal cord and lying in the anterior fissure of the cord; (2) a pair of posterior spinal arteries situated near the entrance of the posterior roots on either side of the midline. These run the entire length of the spinal cord. They are formed by the radicular arteries which come to the spinal cord, divide

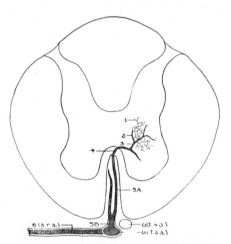

Fig. 78—*Spinal cord circulation.* Schematic diagram illustrating classification of the spinal vessels in man according to order of magnitude. *1* indicates capillary network (vessels of the first order); *2*, immediate precapillary (vessel of the second order); *3*, vessel of the third order; *4*, vessel of the fourth order, in this instance a paracentral vessel; *5A*, a sulcal vessel, for the right side; *5B*, a short common trunk of sulcal vessels; *6 (t.a.a.)*, a vessel of the sixth order, in this instance the truncus arteriosus anterior; *6 (t.v.a)*, the truncus venosus anterior; and *6 (a.r.a)*, the arteria radicularis anterior. *(Alexander.)*

into ascending and descending branches, and unite with the corresponding branches of the next higher or lower vessels. Generally speaking, the anterior spinal arteries which supply the anterior surface of the spinal cord derive their supply throughout the entire cervical and the upper two thoracic segments from the vertebral arteries, and below this level from the intercostal and lumbar arteries, and from the iliolumbar and lateral sacral arteries. The posterior surface of the cord is supplied by the posterior spinal arteries, deriving their supply in the cervical and upper thoracic segments from the vertebral or posterior inferior cerebellar arteries and below this from the terminal portion of the anterior spinal arteries. Within the substance of the spinal cord, the posterior spinal artery supplies the posterior portion of the posterior columns and the posterior horns, while the anterior spinal artery supplies the rest of the cord (Bolton). Within the spinal cord, the blood supply is provided by (1) the central arteries, which branch out peripherally; (2) the peripheral arteries around the circumference of the cord. The central arteries reach beyond the gray column into the surrounding white matter, but do not penetrate to the periphery. The peripheral vessels rarely reach the center of the gray column within the spinal cord. There is little or no anastomosis between the central and peripheral vessels of the cord. A rich capillary bed is found within the cord substance, different portions of the cord varying in richness of the capillary bed. The capillaries are larger and more numerous in the gray matter of the cord.

It is an interesting but little known fact that only one-fourth of the nerve roots in man are accompanied by segmental arteries which contribute to the circulation of the spinal cord. The blood supply of the spinal cord, in fact, depends upon from six to eight anterior radicular arteries and from five to eight posterior radicular arteries (Alexander and Suh). The entire cervical region receives three to five radicular arteries, which are more numerous here than in other portions of the spinal cord. From the eighth cervical to the ninth thoracic segments only two small anterior radicular arteries are usually seen. The lumbar radicular vessels are an important source of blood supply for the major part of the spinal cord.

The largest vessel to reach the cord, exclusive of the vertebral artery, is the anterior radicular artery of the lumbar area (ninth thoracic to third lumbar segments). The middle thoracic section of the spinal cord has the poorest local segmental circulation. This factor, in addition to the absence of anastomosis of any significance between the anterior and posterior spinal arteries, may explain the susceptibility of the midthoracic region to disease, as, for example, in subacute combined degeneration or even in tabes dorsalis, in which the lower portions of the cord are more susceptible to injury than the other portions.

From a physiological viewpoint, the spinal cord may be conceived as having two main systems of activity: one the system of reflex arcs mediated through the numerous spinal roots; the other the system of long ascending and descending tracts of the white matter whereby the cord is in close connection with all parts of the brain and brain stem.

From a pathological viewpoint, it is a matter of great interest that the cord seems to be susceptible to local vulnerability to a greater degree than the brain. Spinal cord diseases may be predominantly or exclusively in the gray matter (poliomyelitis, herpes zoster, progressive spinal muscular atrophy); in the white matter (multiple sclerosis, subacute combined degeneration, Friedreich's ataxia, tabes dorsalis); or in both the gray and white matter (amyotrophic lateral sclerosis, syringomyelia). The reason for this local vulnerability is not known. In some instances, it appears definite that in compression lesions of the cord, the motor fibers are more susceptible to injury than the sensory systems, but this is not invariably the case.

II. INFECTIONS

The meninges of the spinal cord may be affected by many sorts of infections. They may be involved secondarily by meningitis affecting both the brain and cord, as, for example, in pyogenic infections and syphilis, or they may be the seat of primary infection.

III. HYPERTROPHIC SPINAL PACHYMENINGITIS

Etiology: The most common causes are syphilis and tuberculosis. Syphilis is more commonly the cause than tuberculosis. Alcohol has been indicted in some cases, but this is without doubt only an incidental factor. Chronic pyogenic infections, trauma, and syringomyelia may be associated with pachymeningitis.

Pathology: Hypertrophic pachymeningitis consists primarily of a thickened dura. This is most commonly found in the cervical region, but it may involve also the lumbar and sacral regions of the spinal cord. The process may extend for two to several segments. The thickened dura shows much fibrous thickening and infiltration with lymphocytes, plasma cells, and even giant cells. The amount of infiltration varies, older processes showing more fibrous thickening, and more recent processes more infiltration. The underlying pia arachnoid also is thickened and infiltrated. The posterior and anterior roots of the spinal cord are compressed by the adherent meninges and are also infiltrated by lymphocytes and plasma cells. The spinal cord is invariably affected as a result of direct compression by the thickened dura acting essentially like a tumor, because of interference with blood supply due to diseased vessels. The spinal cord as a result shows areas of myelitis which may be scattered or may result in destruction of the entire cross section of the affected cord. In syphilis, evidences of involvement of other parts of the nervous system are often found. In such areas there is destruction of myelin and axis cylinders, infiltration of the white matter with lymphocytes and plasma cells, and perivascular infiltration with similar cells.

Symptoms: The symptoms of hypertrophic pachymeningitis may be divided into those of irritation and those of compression. The first and most prominent symptom is pain due to the involvement of the posterior roots in the disease process. In cervical pachymeningitis, the pain is usually along the outside of the arms and hands along the seventh and eighth cervical roots. It is usually bilateral and typically radicular in its distribution. In lumbar or sacral cases, the pain is felt in the legs and often is incorrectly regarded as sciatica. Atrophy and weakness of the muscles follow after the symptoms of pain due to anterior root and anterior horn involvement. There may be a relatively long latency between the occurrence of pain and the development of weakness and atrophy; or the latter may succeed pain quickly in the course of the disease. The small muscles of the hands are particularly affected, but the atrophy may involve the arm if the upper cervical regions are involved. Atrophy of the leg muscles is found in the lumbar and sacral cases. Associated with the atrophy and weakness is usually loss or decrease of the tendon reflexes. In the early stage sensory disturbances can be detected along the posterior roots affected.

After a varying period of time signs of compression of the spinal cord appear. In complete compression there develops the typical picture of a transverse syndrome with spastic paralysis of the legs or legs and arms, a complete sensory level, and sphincter disturbances. In cases of incomplete compression, the signs vary greatly. In such instances the clinical features may vary so widely as to defy classification. Ataxia of the arms and legs or of the legs alone is common and is associated with evidence of spastic weakness of the limbs. Weakness of the limbs associated with increased reflexes is common. An amyotrophic syndrome is sometimes encountered, just as in cases of cervical cord tumor, the outstanding features being atrophy of the hand and arm muscles, increased reflexes, and other pyramidal tract signs (spasticity, Babinski sign, etc.). Associated with the ataxia and weakness may be an incomplete sensory level involving only some modalities of sensation, a poorly defined sensory level, or in some cases a Brown-Séquard syndrome. Vesical incontinence occurs frequently.

Subarachnoid block can be demonstrated in some cases by the Queckenstedt test. In others, it is absent. Lipiodol injection may demonstrate a complete or a partial block, the latter characterized by streaking and breaking up of the lipiodol column. The Wassermann reaction of the blood and spinal fluid is usually positive in the syphilitic cases, but a negative reaction in one or the other is not uncommon. Abnormal colloidal gold curves are found in the syphilitic cases. The spinal fluid protein is increased as a rule.

The disease is slowly progressive with pain, loss of power, and signs of cord compression giving a picture like that of spinal cord tumor.

Diagnosis: The diagnosis is difficult to establish definitely. The disease is rare. It may be suspected in a patient with serological evidence of syphilis or in one having tuberculosis, with a history of slow progression characterized by pains, atrophy of the hands, weakness, and signs of spinal cord compression. The history is slowly progressive and is essentially that of spinal cord compression associated with root pains in the neck, shoulders, and arms in cervical hypertrophic pachymeningitis, and in the back and legs in lumbar pachymeningitis. In the presence of a positive spinal fluid, Wassermann reaction and other evidences of spinal fluid changes, the diagnosis may be made with some degree of certainty. In cases due to causes other than syphilis, the diagnosis is extremely difficult, so that one must be content merely with a diagnosis of spinal cord compression in many cases. The total impression is one of spinal cord tumor and cases of this sort are usually operated on for tumor, the diagnosis often being definitely established on exploration.

Spinal cord tumor is difficult to differentiate since the advance of the process is so much like tumor. The absence of positive serological reactions will tilt the balance in favor of tumor, but in most cases exploration is necessary to establish the diagnosis. Since the condition is more common in the cervical than in the lumbar region, particular difficulties are encountered in the differentiation from cervical cord tumor. The findings may be similar in the two conditions, only the evidence of syphilis in the spinal fluid findings giving a clue as to the condition in the syphilitic cases. *Syringomyelia* must be differentiated especially in the cervical cases. The absence of pain, the segmental disturbance of pain and temperature, the extremely slow advance of symptoms, and the greater incidence of trophic disturbances point to syringomyelia. *Cervical rib* and the *scalenus syndrome* may be suspected because of the pain, which is in the same distribu-

Table 21—Differential Diagnosis of Hypertrophic Spinal Pachymeningitis

	Pain	Motor Disturbances	Sensory Disturbances	Subarachnoid Block	Spinal Fluid Changes	Miscellaneous
HYPERTROPHIC SPINAL PACHYMENINGITIS	Always present. In neck, shoulder, arms in cervical cases. In back and legs in lumbar cases. Root pain	Complete paralysis or lesser degrees of weakness due to cord involvement	Usually ill-defined sensory level, but may be complete transverse syndrome	Usually present. May be absent early. Complete or incomplete	Usually shows evidence of syphilis	Pantopaque shows partial or complete block
SPINAL CORD TUMOR	Always or almost always present. Similar in type and distribution to pachymeningitis	Same as in pachymeningitis	Same as in pachymeningitis	Same as in pachymeningitis	No evidence of syphilis	
SYRINGOMYELIA	No pain, or severe pain of root or tract type	May be unilateral or bilateral or may be absent. Atrophy and weakness of arms and hands and at times weakness of arms and legs from pyramidal tract involvement	Segmental loss of pain and temperature	Absent as a rule. May be present	Absent. Protein may be increased	Myelogram shows greatly widened cord
CERVICAL RIB	Unilateral usually. Along arm and in shoulder	Weakness in a peripheral nerve area—ulnar, median or both	Often absent. Vascular disturbances usually present	Absent	None	Roentgenological evidence of cervical rib
NEURITIS	Unilateral or bilateral. Absent in purely motor neuritis. If bilateral, usually part of polyneuritis. Tenderness of muscles and nerves	In peripheral nerve areas	In peripheral distributions	Absent	None save for increased spinal fluid protein in acute febrile polyneuritis	
CERVICAL HERNIATED DISC	In shoulder and arm, unilateral	Weakness of shoulder and arm muscles possibly hand also	Radicular in type	Absent	Protein increased at times	Narrowed disc spaces in x-ray. Myelogram shows defect

tion as in these conditions, but the extreme atrophy and the signs of cord involvement help in the clarification of the issue. The pain of cervical rib is usually unilateral, that of pachymeningitis bilateral; cervical rib pain is aggravated by posture and is worse at night, spreads along peripheral nerves rather than roots, is associated with evidence of peripheral nerve disease and never with cord involvement, is accompanied by vascular changes such as a lower blood pressure and a feebler pulse on the affected side, and by evidence of cervical rib on roentgenologic examination.

Treatment: The outlook in cases of hypertrophic spinal pachymeningitis is not good as a rule. *Antisyphilitic treatment* does not dissolve the thickened dura, though it may help to relieve pain. *Operation* to remove the thickened dura is helpful, but since spinal cord damage is always present, full recovery cannot be anticipated.

Intensive antisyphilitic treatment should be given. Injections of bismuth, either soluble or insoluble, should be given (weekly or at five-day intervals for the insoluble and more frequently for the soluble preparations). Mercury and iodides may be useful. Arsenic is of little value. Penicillin should be given, but the results of treatment are not good.

Exploration may be necessary if there is no response to antisyphilitic treatment. Nonsyphilitic patients will be operated on for suspected tumors. In the syphilitic, specific treatment should be continued after operation.

IV. ACUTE EXTRADURAL ABSCESS

Etiology: The incidence of extradural abscess of the spinal cord is not definitely known. The condition is rare.

The infection may reach the extradural space by two paths: (1) By direct extension from infection in adjacent tissues by means of a retrograde thrombophlebitis. Furuncles, carbuncles, and cellulitis, are responsible for a large number of cases, especially furuncles. Furuncles are responsible in more than thirty per cent of cases (Gaul and Jaffe). The infected focus in such instances is usually in the same spinal cord dermatome as the extradural abscess. A furuncle in the skin at the eighth thoracic segment will be followed therefore by evidence of an extradural abscess at the eighth thoracic dermatome. (2) By metastasis from a distant focus of suppuration (lungs, septic abortion, extraction of infected teeth, mastoditis, trauma). This means of development of extradural abscess is not as well recognized as the first, but is fully as important, especially in the obscure cases.

Pathology: Extradural abscesses are most often located on the dorsal or posterior aspect of the spinal cord, since the extradural space is most pronounced in the dorsal and lateral portions and is only a potential space on the ventral surface. Abscesses have been found, however, on the ventral surface. The thoracic portion of the cord is most affected. The abscess is usually circumscribed, but in unusual instances the infection may involve the entire extradural space. The organism most commonly found is the staphylococcus, but streptococcus, pneumococcus, and Pseudomonas aeruginosa have been found.

The abscess lies on the outer surface of the dura, its structure being characteristically a collection of leukocytes, fibrin, and bacteria, usually grossly circumscribed. The dura is thickened, contains many leukocytes and usually bacteria. There is usually an accompanying meningitis of the underlying pia-arachnoid. Unfortunately, the process is not confined to the meninges. The spinal cord is softened and shows typical myelomalacia with gitter cells and scattered leukocytes. The spinal cord softening is usually confined to a few segments lying immediately beneath the abscess, but in some cases it may extend well beyond this. In cases in which the infection is subacute and involves large portions of the dura, the cord may be damaged in scattered areas along its entire length. Spinal cord destruction occurs invariably if the process has been sufficiently long. It is thought to be due to thrombosis of spinal or vertebral vessels, but evidence of this is often lacking. It is the spinal cord softening which demands early treatment of the condition. The infection is regarded by some as being primary in the extradural space, where it is said to begin as a thrombophlebitis. Others regard the primary process as an osteomyelitis of the vertebrae with subsequent extension to the extradural space (Browder).

Symptoms: A history of infection is always obtained, usually in the region of the cord involvement, but sometimes at a distance. There is as a rule a history of furuncle of the skin which has been treated, a cellulitis, or there may be a history of a septic abortion, bronchiectasis, or carbuncle. Some time after the onset of the infection (two or three weeks) the patient is seized with pain in one or more spinal root areas, usually constant in nature, increased by sneezing, coughing, and by other maneuvers increasing intraspinal pressure. The pain is persistent, and is usually in the back and thorax, since most cases are found involving the thoracic portion of the cord, but the location of the pain may be in the arms or legs if the abscess is cervical or lumbar in location. In a very short time, usually within a few days, complete paralysis of the legs develops suddenly, associated with sensory loss

and bladder disturbances. If the abscess is in the cervical area, the paralysis involves the arms and legs. In some cases the paralysis develops more slowly if the infection is subacute or chronic. Fever and chills are both common and striking early in the disease, associated with malaise and headache. Blood stream infection may be found. Examination reveals a severely ill patient with signs of meningeal irritation (neck stiffness, Kernig's sign), with leukocytosis, and with striking evidence of a complete transverse lesion of the spinal cord, with paralysis of the arms and/or legs, sensory paralysis to a definite level, and urinary retention or incontinence. Since the onset of paralysis is usually acute, the signs of spinal shock are usually present and as a result flaccid paralysis is found associated with absent reflexes and often with no pathological reflexes.

Lumbar puncture reveals an increase of cells in the spinal fluid, consisting of polymorphonuclear cells. If lumbar puncture is performed at the level of the lesion, it is possible to tap the abscess by careful withdrawal of the needle before entering the subarachnoid space. Roentgenological examination may show evidence of local osteomyelitis, but this is often difficult to demonstrate. Hydrodynamic studies of the spinal fluid show a complete block of the subarachnoid space. The spinal fluid protein is increased.

Diagnosis: The diagnosis is not difficult in the presence of a history of infection with the typical history described and signs of a transverse lesion with subarachnoid block. Some cases may develop slowly where the infection is subacute. The clinical features are those of a severe infection with acute and even apoplectic onset, severe prostration, usually a clear history of a local or distant infection, fever, leukocytosis, root pains, meningeal signs, evidences of spinal cord damage as indicated by a transverse spinal syndrome (complete motor paralysis, sensory level, etc.), and usually subarachnoid block. The history of an infection is important and the period of latency with pain, followed in several days or sometimes sooner by paralysis, is diagnostic, especially in the differentiation from a myelitis. The diagnosis must be made quickly in order to afford what relief surgery may offer, since once spinal cord damage occurs, little can be done to insure recovery. In the subacute forms of the disease, the development of symptoms is slower, frank pus is not usually found, there is a more diffuse dural and pia-arachnoid infiltration and thickening, and the process runs a longer course.

Myelitis of infectious origin usually must be considered, but here there is no evidence of subarachnoid block, and a history of local infection is lacking. The differentiation from infectious myelitis is sometimes extremely difficult, since both disorders occur with a preceding history of infection. In the case of extradural abscess, the infection is usually local, while in myelitis it is as a rule systemic and at times of an upper respiratory character. The onset of symptoms in myelitis is rapid, but may take place over several days, sometimes with an ascending paralysis. Pain is not a prominent symptom. A complete transverse syndrome is commonly seen in myelitis but subarachnoid block is not usually demonstrable. *Syphilitic meningomyelitis* differs in the absence of acute onset and the practically constantly positive Wassermann reactions of the spinal fluid. *Tumor* of the spinal cord can be excluded by the absence of the systemic symptoms (fever, headache, chills, etc.). The onset is gradual. Extramedullary

cord tumors are associated with pain, with a slowly developing syndrome of cord compression (paralysis, sensory level, urinary incontinence), and with subarachnoid block. *Metastatic carcinoma* may simulate the disorder chiefly by its rapid onset, but the systemic symptoms, the history of an infection, and the known presence of carcinoma help in the diagnosis. Carcinoma may be associated with a sudden development of paraplegia, but the cause is usually evident by virtue of the known presence of carcinoma elsewhere in the body. Where this is lacking, the absence of infection helps in the differentiation.

Treatment: Most of the cases have terminated fatally. Prompt diagnosis leading to immediate *laminectomy* is essential in order to aid recovery. In cases recognized early partial or complete recovery is possible before the destruction of the spinal cord substance has progressed too far. In delayed operation, the paralysis persists despite removal of the abscess, due to the underlying myelomalacia. Treatment with *sulfonamides* and *penicillin* has been helpful in cases which have been recognized early and operated on without delay.

V. ADHESIVE SPINAL ARACHNOIDITIS
(Meningitis Serosa Circumscripta Spinalis)

Etiology: The condition affects males more than females. There is no single cause of the disease, many different factors producing the condition. Among the conditions reported as producing spinal arachnoiditis are trauma to the spine, syphilis, spinal anesthesia, meningococcic meningitis, grippe, gonorrhea, typhoid fever, subarachnoid hemorrhage, lymphocytic choriomeningitis, tuberculosis, furunculosis, arthritis of the spine, influenza, and septic abortion. Tuberculosis of the spine has been found in some

cases. For some cases, no known etiology can be established. It is apparent, therefore, that spinal arachnoiditis
is found in association with many infections as well as with hemorrhage and
trauma, and that in this sense it may be
regarded as a secondary manifestation of
many generalized infections and other
systemic conditions. Spinal anesthesia
has become one of the most important
causes of archnoiditis of the spinal cord.
Its incidence is difficult, of course, to
estimate.

Pathology: Not much is known concerning the pathology of this condition,
since few cases have come to necropsy.
Any part of the spinal cord may be
affected, and the process may be localized in one area or involve the cord
diffusely. The posterior surface of the
cord is much more affected than the
anterior and some believe that it never
extends to the anterior surface. The thoracic cord is most often involved, the
cervical and lumbar areas suffering to a
much lesser degree. The arachnoid is
thickened and adherent to the dura and
the underlying pia. The adhesions are
associated with solitary or multiple cysts
which may compress the spinal cord.
Evidences of inflammation are absent,
the arachnoid showing fibrous thickening
without the presence of hematogenous
elements. The pia is also affected. The
adhesive arachnoiditis may vary in degree from single bundles of fibrous tissue
to dense adhesions obliterating the subarachnoid space and involving the spinal
roots. The adhesions themselves may
cause spinal cord changes by direct compression or interference with the blood
supply. These consist of demyelination,
usually of a spotty character and often
involving the marginal areas of the cord.
Cavitation of the cord, sometimes of a
severe degree, is found at times in cases
of arachnoiditis.

Symptoms: The clinical picture is
variable. The disease is one of middle
age. The onset may be rapid or gradual,
and frequently begins with pain which
involves the trunk in the distribution of
one or more thoracic segments. The pain
is radicular in type, usually unilateral
and later becoming bilateral. The pain
is intense and persistent. After a varying length of time there develop gradually as a rule, but sometimes rapidly,
symptoms of cord compression as in
tumor. These consist of weakness of the
legs and often of a noticeable ataxia.
Arm or hand weakness may develop in
cases involving the cervical area and leg
weakness in lumbar or cauda equina
cases. In many cases gradual cord compression develops without a history of
pain, but the compression is usually
incomplete. It is usually slow in development. There are almost never
signs of a complete transverse lesion
of the cord as seen in extramedullary
tumors.

In the thoracic cases, there is usually
weakness but not paralysis of the legs,
incomplete and indefinite sensory disturbances with an ill-defined sensory
level, no sphincter disturbances, and
overactive reflexes. Weakness but not
paralysis of the legs and partial sensory
loss usually to an ill-defined level are
found. In cases involving the cauda
equina roots sciatic pain, unilateral or
bilateral, is the outstanding symptom and
is associated with flaccid weakness of the
leg, atrophy of varying degrees, loss or
decrease of reflexes, and at times sensory
loss. Spinal puncture reveals an incomplete subarachnoid block in some cases
and rarely evidence of complete block.
The cells are not increased as a rule,
but in some instances may be elevated.
In some cases the protein content of the
spinal fluid is greatly increased. Pantopaque injection reveals usually an incom-

plete arrest of oil, with droplets spread diffusely about at the level of the lesion, giving the appearance of a guttering candle. Sometimes a complete arrest of oil can be seen.

Diagnosis: The clinical picture is that of a progressive lesion with incomplete signs of compression of the spinal cord with doubtful or incomplete evidence of subarachnoid block, and sometimes an increase of protein content of the spinal fluid. The development of the condition suggests spinal cord tumor, but the findings are more ill-defined than are usually found in tumor. The history of trauma or infection, particularly the latter, may lead to the diagnosis of arachnoiditis, which may be in part confirmed by the injection of iodized oil. The diagnosis can only be established by operation. It is almost impossible to make a definite diagnosis of arachnoiditis before operation, since the history and findings are those only of a slowly progressive lesion compressing the spinal cord. The appearance of pantopaque arrest may lead to the diagnosis, due to the guttered candle appearance by myelogram. A history of infection preceding the onset of symptoms or even in the dim past may help in establishing the diagnosis. *Spinal cord tumor* is most commonly confused with the condition. Extramedullary tumor may be separated by greater evidence of cord compression as seen in the more definite evidence of a transverse lesion, and by the presence of a complete subarachnoid block. Intramedullary tumor may be more difficult and even impossible to separate. *Spinal cord syphilis* offers no difficulties. Tabes may be readily differentiated by the Argyll Robertson pupils, the absence of reflexes, the evidences of posterior column disease and by the positive serological relations in most cases. *Pott's disease* may be

separated by the definite roentgenological findings.

Treatment: *Operation* affords the only good relief in order to destroy the adhesions between the meninges and cord and to empty the cyst often associated with the condition. In most cases, little can be accomplished, since the adhesions between the pia arachnoid and spinal cord are so firm that any attempt to remove them results in destruction of cord tissue.

VI. HERPES ZOSTER
(Zona, Shingles, Posterior Poliomyelitis)

Etiology: Herpes zoster is an infectious disease involving the dorsal spinal root, the spinal root ganglion, and the posterior horn of the spinal cord. It is sometimes referred to as posterior poliomyelitis.

The disease occurs at any age, but it is more common in middle-aged and older subjects. Men and women are about equally affected.

Cases of herpes zoster are divisible into two main groups: (1) a primary group in which the disease is caused by a virus; (2) a symptomatic group in which the herpes is an expression of root irritation associated with many types of disorders. It is not known whether the herpes in the latter group represents an expression of the primary disease process or whether the virus is activated in these instances by secondary causes. The primary form is due to a filterable virus which has been recovered in some cases from the nervous system and the spinal fluid. Herpes zoster virus can be isolated from the nervous system of animals and transmitted to other animals by intracerebral inoculation. Symptomatic herpes may occur after trauma, excessive anxiety, tuberculosis, syphilis, injections of bacterial vaccines and metals, metastatic carcinoma, cachexia, osteoarthritis of the vertebrae, Hodgkin's disease, syringomyelia, spinal cord tumor, and arsenic medication.

Pathology: The obvious lesions of herpes zoster are in the skin, but the important ones are in the nervous system. The condition is a myelitis involving the posterior root and its ganglion and the posterior horn of the spinal cord.

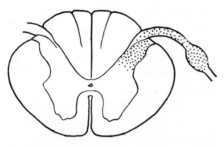

Fig. 79—*Herpes zoster,* showing diagrammatically the involvement of the posterior root and ganglion and the posterior horn of the spinal cord.

The posterior root and its ganglion are infiltrated by lymphocytes and sometimes plasma cells. Hemorrhage and necrosis may sometimes be found in the ganglion. The posterior root ganglion cells are severely damaged in many instances and proliferation of interstitial fibrous tissue cells occurs. The root and ganglion changes are responsible for the pain in herpes. Myelin destruction is found in the posterior root and to a lesser degree destruction of the axis cylinders. The posterior horn and posterior horn cells show similar evidences of infiltration and destruction. Areas of destruction have been found in a few cases in the white matter of the cord. The anterior horns or roots may be involved in rare cases. After the acute process runs its course, scar tissue is deposited in the involved areas, with compression and irritation of the nerve fibers in the posterior root. These are responsible for the persistent pain in herpes long after the skin eruption has disappeared.

Herpes zoster may affect the brain stem and produce encephalitis in conjunction with herpes about the face, especially in herpes ophthalmicus. The midbrain is most affected but any part of the brain stem may be involved. Infiltrations and cell destruction similar to those found in the cord are seen in the oculomotor nuclei, the trigeminal and facial nuclei particularly.

Symptoms: Herpes involves the trunk and limbs as a rule but may also involve the face. It is practically always unilateral but is rarely bilateral over the face, limbs, or trunk. The first symptom is fever and malaise, followed in three or four days by a vesicular eruption of the trunk, arm, or leg, distributed in the areas of a spinal root or roots with anatomical precision. The vesicles are found in the anatomical dermatomes of the affected nerve roots. Preceding or accompanying this may be paresthesias and pain. Indeed, pain may precede by several days the appearance of the vesicles. The pain is typically radicular, corresponding to the area of vesicular eruption. It is constant, but may be intermittent, is sharp, knifelike, and radiates along the root or roots affected. Hyperesthesia of the affected skin area is present in the acute stages. Decreased sensitivity to touch and pain may develop later. After several days (seven to ten as a rule) the eruption disappears, and often with it the pain. The latter, however, may outlast the eruption by days, weeks, or months, the persistent pain being the result of scar tissue formation in the posterior root and horn, relief from the pain representing a difficult therapeutic problem.

The symptoms are chiefly sensory in typical cases, but in some instances motor weakness is found. This is usually a peripheral or lower motor neuron weakness, the muscles involved corresponding to the root distribution of the sensory symptoms. It is usually associated with atrophy of the muscles and reflex loss. Herpes involving the arms is more likely to be associated with motor symptoms than that of the leg, where weakness is rare. Atrophy and weakness of hand or arm muscles, and atrophy and weakness of the thigh or leg, have been found in some cases. Paralysis of the oculomotor, trigeminal, or facial nerves may occur singly or in unison following herpes of the face. Upper motor neuron weakness in the form of hemiparesis has been reported.

Herpes may be associated at times with myelitis and varieties of the disease have been referred to as zoster myelitis. Brown-Séquard syndromes and other incomplete types of transverse myelitis have been observed in herpes.

Similarly, herpes may affect the brain stem and produce an encephalitis usually complicating ophthalmic herpes, herpes of the maxillary division, or herpes of the cervical roots. The midbrain is particularly affected, with resulting oculomotor paralyses. Facial paralysis and deafness sometimes are found.

Ophthalmic Herpes: This is due to involvement of the gasserian ganglion and its root. The vesicular eruption is over the forehead usually, but may involve the upper lid, the conjunctiva, and cornea. Pain is prominent and is found over the forehead along the supraorbital branch of the trigeminal nerve, radiating to the top of the scalp. Pain may be felt in the eye. Ophthalmic herpes may be associated with optic neuritis or atrophy, ophthalmoplegias varying from a single muscle involvement to complete oculomotor paralysis, and with exophthalmos in rare cases. Most patients with ophthalmic herpes recover without sequelae save for persistent pain in the forehead in some instances. In 5.7 per cent of the

patients, an encephalitis develops with the herpes ophthalmicus, producing infiltration and cell destruction in the brain stem, particularly in the mesencephalon, but involving also other parts of the brain stem. Associated with the herpetic encephalitis may be a variety of neurological conditions such as Argyll Robertson pupils, ophthalmoplegia, cerebellar disturbances, hemiplegia, and hemiparesis.

A cerebral form of herpes is known, due to encephalitic involvement of the cerebral hemispheres themselves. In such instances there may be signs of meningeal irritation (neck stiffness, Kernig's sign), a confusional psychosis, convulsions, and coma.

Diagnosis: The diagnosis is, as a rule, easy if there is a history of an eruption, evidence of scars of an old eruption, or if one is fortunate enough to see the skin manifestations in the acute stages. At times, patients are seen only with pain before the eruption has developed or after it has left without leaving traces of its presence. Careful inquiry should be made into cases of symptomatic herpes, in which the eruption is merely an indication of some irritating process such as Pott's disease, spinal cord tumor, osteoarthritis, syphilis, etc. Removal of the primary cause is indicated. Herpes encephalitis is readily recognized by the history of herpes ophthalmicus or herpes of the maxillary division of the trigeminal nerve, followed by signs of widespread brain stem involvement.

The outlook in most cases is good. In some instances, the pain may persist indefinitely after the skin eruption has disappeared, and in these cases the problem of control of the pain is extremely difficult. Herpes encephalitis is followed by incomplete recovery.

Treatment: *Irradiation* by roentgen ray is effective in the early stages but not later in the disease. Injections of *pituitary extract* (1 cc.) give symptomatic relief at times. *Codeine* or *morphine* may be necessary to relieve pain. *Aureomycin* (250 mg. every four to six hours) has been found to be helpful in controlling herpes zoster in the early stages. In persistent cases of pain lasting for months after the herpes, *section of the posterior roots or cordotomy* has been performed. Even by these means the control of postherpetic neuralgia may be impossible, since the pain often recurs after both ramisectomy and cordotomy. Subarachnoid alcohol injections should be avoided. Lobotomy has been performed for the relief of persistent pain.

VII. ACUTE ANTERIOR POLIOMYELITIS
(Infantile Paralysis)

Etiology: Poliomyelitis is an infectious disease caused by a filterable virus. This virus is small (10 millimicrons) and passes through very fine filters. It is pathogenic for certain monkeys, chimpanzees, and man; recent studies indicate that it is pathogenic for cotton rats and mice. It is strictly neurotropic and multiplies only in the nerve cells of susceptible hosts. It can be multiplied *in vitro* only in the brain and spinal cord of young human embryos but not in cultures of other organs (Olitsky and Sabin). There is no proof of the existence of a virus reservoir outside of man and no proof is available of an intermediary animate carrier in human cases. The evidence is now clear that poliomyelitis is caused by more than one virus. The *multiple* virus causation of the disease has demonstrated that poliomyelitis virus can be separated into three known antigenic groups: (1) Brunhilde or type 1, (2) Lansing or type 2, (3) Leon or type 3. It has been demonstrated further that more than one type of poliomyelitis virus may be present in a single

epidemic in a community. Studies show that second attacks in humans are due to reinfection with virus of an antigenic type different from that producing the first attack (Bodian). Poliomyelitis virus has been grown in tissue culture. Antibody is present in the serum of patients at the time of onset of paralysis. This raises the question of a viremia in the preparalytic period. Viremia appears to be an important part of the disease in animals (Bodian), virus appearing to multiply in the blood stream, initiated by escape of virus from the primary alimentary phase. Thus far, viremia in humans has been demonstrated rarely.

Though the evidence for the transmission of poliomyelitis by person-to-person contact is largely circumstantial (Howe), "there appears to be almost complete agreement that the virus of poliomyelitis usually is spread by person-to-person contact, and that it enters the body by the mouth. There is also general agreement that exit occurs by way of alimentary secretions or excretions, although it is not clear whether oropharyngeal secretion or fecal material is the principal vehicle of spread of infection" (Bodian). Modern laboratory studies have shown the virus of poliomyelitis to be present in stools during the acute stages of the paralytic disease in such a high percentage of cases that it seems justifiable to consider it a constant concomitant of central nervous system invasion. On the other hand, little is known about the incidence of virus in the stools or pharyngeal secretions *prior* to the onset of symptoms, though it has been described in the former twelve and nineteen days before onset (Howe). Within a week of the onset of symptoms the frequency with which virus can be demonstrated in the stools falls off, but virus has been shown to persist in some individuals for as long as eleven to twelve weeks. Virus has also been demonstrated in swabs taken from the throats of acute paralytic patients and in face masks worn by juvenile patients who had coughed and drooled into them. While virus has been isolated from the throat in nearly fifty per cent of the patients within three to five days of the acute onset of the disease, its incidence falls off very rapidly thereafter. Occasional isolations from abortive cases are recorded as late as the eleventh day. It is probable that the failure to detect virus in the oropharynx as long as in the stools reflects a real biologic difference since it is known that antibody may be present in the pharyngeal secretions, although it has not been demonstrated in the stools. It is therefore possible that the antibody response following infection clears the pharynx of virus in a relatively short time (Howe). It can be shown that humans become solidly immune to poliomyelitis virus (Howe). Monkeys paralyzed by inoculation of poliomyelitis virus do not become paralyzed again upon reinoculation of the same material.

Milk-borne infection has been traced in some cases and food infection in others. Flies appear to play no part in epidemicity. Elimination of flies has failed to affect the appearance or course of epidemics.

Air-borne infection of the virus has been demonstrated in monkeys, by the lower respiratory mucosa in rhesus monkeys and the oropharyngeal mucosa in cynomalgus monkeys. "The experiments open up the possibility that human poliomyelitis may, at least sometimes, be an air-borne infection and that the lungs may be a portal of entry" (Faber and Silverberg).

In other cases, the disease seems to have followed tonsillectomy. Instances of poliomyelitis (259 cases in the literature) have been found after removal of the tonsils up to within sixty days. Most of the cases of poliomyelitis have been of the bulbar type. The risk of development of severe poliomyelitis appears to be at least three times as great among persons who have undergone tonsillectomy within one month prior to exposure to the virus as among a comparable group not subjected to tonsillectomy (Anderson).

Multiple cases in a family have been observed in some instances. Multiple cases of poliomyelitis occurring in families were found in 9.2 per cent of 721 patients (Swartout and Frank). The diagnosis was confirmed by definite spinal fluid findings in 81.2 per cent and by questionably positive findings in 7.8 per cent. Two cases were found in 22 families; 3 cases in 5 families; and 4 cases in 2 families.

Intrauterine contraction of poliomyelitis has been reported and an instance described of the disease in a newborn infant whose mother contracted evidence of the disease after delivery (Bierman and Piscyek). Poliomyelitis has been reported in newborn infants $3\frac{1}{2}$ and 5 days after birth. In both instances the mother had poliomyelitis. The attack rate in poliomyelitis appears to be greater in pregnant than in nonpregnant women, but the severity of the disease appears not to be affected.

The evidence concerning the mode of infection in poliomyelitis may be summarized as follows: The most likely portal of entry in man is the mouth and pharynx. Virus is very common in the rhinopharyngeal secretions in the acute phase, but disappears rapidly from the upper respiratory tract. The risk of infection from virus elimination in the upper respiratory tract is of short duration. Virus elimination in the feces is constant in the acute phase; the quantity excreted in the feces is infinitely greater than from the upper respiratory tract; and the elimination of virus in the feces continues beyond the acute phase. Under certain conditions, the virus may be transmitted in contaminated water, milk, and food. Most workers believe at present that poliomyelitis is usually disseminated through contact (Rivers).

The virus has been recovered in nasal swabs from patients with poliomyelitis and in swabs from the throat and mouth (Ward and Walters). Only rarely has the virus been detected in the blood of human beings.

The relationship of the virus of human poliomyelitis to human sewage is at present under investigation. The presence of the virus in sewage raises the question whether it can then find its way into drinking water and swimming pools. Observations indicate that the virus can live in sewage for only a short time and that survival of passage through water purification plants is unlikely. There is no evidence that the virus can live or multiply in water. Furthermore, the disease does not behave like a water-borne disease (Maxcy and Howe). It has not been "correlated with poor water supplies nor have explosive outbreaks of widely scattered cases appeared in cities with municipal water systems" (Maxcy and Howe). Despite this evidence, it appears clear that the virus gains access to the body through the mouth and gastrointestinal tract.

The *incidence* of the disease varies in different climes. In temperate zones, it is most prevalent from August to October and falls off steadily in the winter and spring. In warm climates, the disease is less prevalent and is evenly distributed throughout the year. Though it is prevalent in the summer and fall, it may occur at any time of the year. Outbreaks have been recorded in cold climates.

The *age* distribution of poliomyelitis is quite uniform. The disease occurs chiefly in childhood. The age incidence varies in different epidemics and localities, the occurrence in childhood varying from 65 to 90 per cent. Adults are not infrequently afflicted, a tendency which appears to have increased in recent years. As the disease becomes established, the incidence of involvement of adolescents and adults becomes greater. The more frequent occurrence of the disease in adults in recent years has given rise to much speculation concerning the difference in age incidence. It has been suggested that the acquisition af specific immunity appears to be the most acceptable explanation of age selection. Furthermore, it appears true that when the disease is truly infantile in incidence most cases are of the paralytic type, whereas abortive cases become more numerous as it becomes established. It is a curious fact that the incidence of poliomyelitis is highest in countries with the highest standard of sanitation. The epidemicity of the disease grows steadily and seems to go hand in hand with advances in hygiene and living standards. Where the sanitation is primitive, facilities for spread of the virus are better and infants come earlier into contact with it. In countries with better sanitary arrangements, contact is delayed. The greater the density of population, the younger the age at which poliomyelitis develops, probably due to more frequent contact with adult carriers.

A *constitutional* factor is regarded by some as present in those developing poliomyelitis. The precise features of such a factor remain to be defined clearly, but it appears definite that healthy, robust children are most commonly afflicted. A familial tendency has been reported in some instances, but the incidence is rare. As predisposing factors, trauma and overexertion or strain deserve mention, since isolated cases of poliomyelitis have been found following these conditions. It has been suggested that genetic or endocrine factors may predispose to the disease. Operations have in some instances been followed by poliomyelitis, the paralysis corresponding to the seat of the trauma

reported in tropical countries. Poliomyelitis is apparently world-wide in distribution. Outbreaks have been recorded from the arctic regions to areas close to the equator. Though this is the case, it remains endemic in such places as Malta,

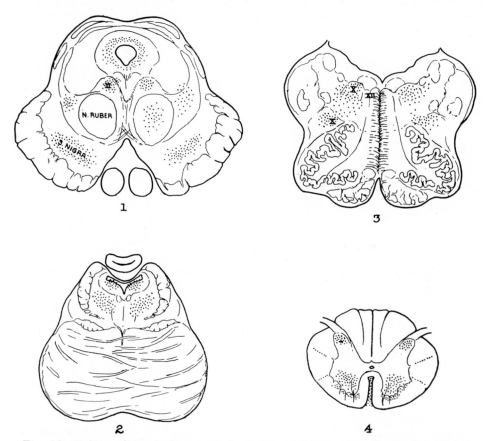

Fig. 80—*Poliomyelitis.* A diagrammatic sketch to indicate the distribution of the lesions in poliomyelitis showing the involvement of the gray matter in the mesencephalon (1), pons (2), medulla (3), spinal cord (4). Note the spread of the process beyond the anterior horns in the spinal cord and the involvement of the posterior horns. Similar involvement may be seen in the diencephalon and motor cortex, neither of which are shown here.

and the corresponding spinal segments. Muscle strain, such as overexertion during tennis or in other athletic contests, has resulted in reported cases of infantile paralysis.

As to *distribution,* poliomyelitis occurs chiefly in cool or temperate zones, though it may be found everywhere. It has been

El Salvador, Puerto Rico, Venezuela, Ecuador, and Palestine, where, with the exception of Malta, only small outbreaks have been noted. It is not yet known whether the preponderance of the disease in temperate climates is more apparent than real, but it seems possible that in tropical countries the disease is more uniformly present throughout the year and less apt to occur in outbreaks. It occurs in epidemics which may be small or very extensive. The disease is endemic, sporadic cases being found constantly throughout the year. Epidemics appear to occur when the endemic rate is highest. It has a tendency to confine its activities in a restricted area while adjacent cities or counties are free of the disease. It is more common in rural communities in recent epidemics, but it is not infrequently more prevalent in urban areas as well.

The epidemiological features of poliomyelitis are summarized by Maxcy as follows:

1. The disease is world-wide in distribution. "Wherever human populations have come under medical observation, sooner or later individuals showing typical paralysis have been found." Outbreaks have been found from Iceland and Greenland to New Guinea.

2. From no human community is the disease long absent.

3. Transmission can occur in any month of the year. It is misleading to refer to poliomyelitis as a summer disease. Epidemics usually occur during the summer and fall but may begin in the early spring and last into late winter.

4. The disease exhibits an irregular interannual periodicity. After a series of years in which the disease has fluctuated at a low level, a year may be expected during which it will attain an unusually rapid dissemination over a short period of time, involving a small locality but usually regional in character.

5. From an original focus, the spread is progressive in unpredictable directions.

6. It has no regular pattern as regards rural and urban distribution. It is not justifiable to say that poliomyelitis is a rural disease. "It has been conspicuously prevalent in epidemic form in rural areas during recent years, but there also have been epidemics in urban areas."

7. The total number of cases manifesting characteristic paralysis during an epidemic period rarely exceeds 2 per 1000 population of all ages. "More commonly the total attack rate based upon reported paralytic cases, when an epidemic has run its course, is in the neighborhood of 0.5 per 1000."

8. The number of individuals infected with the virus of poliomyelitis is far greater than is indicated by an attack rate based upon reported paralytic cases alone.

9. A considerable proportion of patients has had recent direct or indirect contact with a previous paralytic or nonparalytic, known or suspected, patient in the acute or convalescent stage.

Pathology: Poliomyelitis affects not only the spinal cord but the brain stem as well and in some cases also the cerebral cortex. In the majority of instances, the spinal cord is predominantly involved. In other cases, the brain stem is chiefly affected, producing the bulbar form of the disease. The incidence of involvement of the cortex is not precisely known, but it varies from epidemic to epidemic, some patients showing evidence of cortical involvement, others not. As in the clinical features of the disease, the pathological distribution of the lesions varies widely in different epidemics.

The disease is characterized by a patchy distribution in the involved areas. The gray matter is predominantly affected, but lesions may occur also in the white matter. The lumbar and cervical enlargements of the spinal cord are chiefly affected, but the thoracic cord is also often involved. The patchy nature of the disease is revealed by the uneven dissemination of the lesions. Thus, patches of involvement may be found in all levels of the spinal cord, while the cord between the affected areas is untouched. Or, there may be involvement of one anterior horn with escape of the opposite horn. Further, within an individual anterior horn some cells may be diseased while others escape, so that side by side may be seen diseased and healthy cells.

Poliomyelitis is a disease of the gray matter of the nervous system. It affects particularly the anterior horn cells of the spinal cord and their analogues, the motor nuclei of the brain stem, and the Betz cells of the motor cortex. It is predominantly a motor system affliction, therefore. Despite its exquisitely selective nature of motor gray matter, careful study of fresh cases reveals a spilling over of the process into the white matter around the anterior horns, into the posterior horns, and at times into the white matter of the spinal cord. Studies of bulbar poliomyelitis reveal the fact that changes in the medulla are frequent and involve chiefly the nucleus ambiguus, and the small and large reticular cells. In the pons the severest changes are in the dorsal half and most severe in the reticular formation. All the motor nuclei in the pons are about equally involved, but the abducens appears to be most severely affected. The hypothalamus is involved in most cases, especially in the region adjacent to the third ventricle, the supraoptic and periventricular nuclei being severely affected; the subthalamic area and the substantia nigra are also greatly involved. Lesions of maximum severity are encountered in the reticular substance, nucleus ambiguus, and supraspinal and spinal accessory nuclei. The motor cortex and the thalamus may be diseased. Cortical areas outside the motor cortex have been found in a few instances to be affected, but in the vast majority of cases the involvement is in the motor cortex (Area 4).

The histological features of the disease are constant in man. In the earliest stages, corresponding to the preclinical stage, the meninges are mildly infiltrated by lymphocytes which disappear within a few days to a week. In the paralytic stage, the anterior horn cells are destroyed or diseased and the anterior

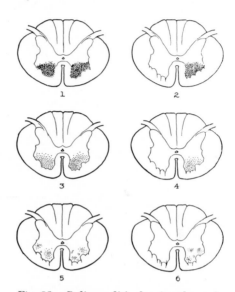

Fig. 81—*Poliomyelitis* showing the various possibilities in the ravaging of the anterior horns: 1, complete destruction of all anterior horn cells; 2, complete destruction of one anterior horn; 3, moderate destruction of both anterior horns; 4, moderate involvement of one anterior horn; 5, mild patchy involvement of both anterior horns; 6, similar involvement of one anterior horn.

horns infiltrated by lymphocytes which rapidly give way to microglia and later neuroglia. Congestion is marked in the acute cases. Perivascular infiltration by lymphocytes is common. The white matter of the cord, especially in its anterior and lateral portions, frequently reveals perivascular infiltration by lymphocytes but no destruction of myelin or axis cylinders. The changes in the brain stem are similar to those of the cord. The nerve cell damage may be complete or reversible and some cells may recover from the disease.

The primary point of attack of the virus of poliomyelitis is on the nerve cells themselves, the infiltrating process appearing secondary to this damage. The four to six weeks, or less. Statistical evidence from populations of motoneurons studied during acute and recovery periods indicates conclusively that a large proportion of motoneurons injured recover their normal appearance (Bodian). The view that poliomyelitis is a general infec-

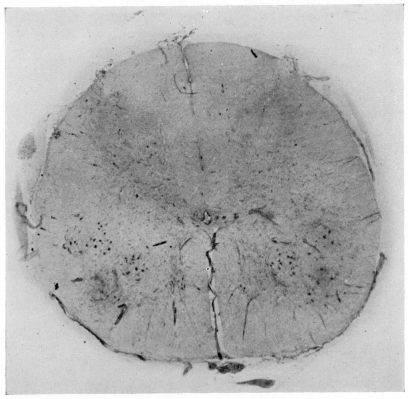

Fig. 82—*Poliomyelitis.* A low power view of the spinal cord in the acute stage showing the meningeal infiltration in the anterior fissure, the infiltration of the anterior horns and the perivascular infiltration of the vessels in white matter.

accumulating evidence indicates that the nervous lesions of the human disease are best explained on the assumption that the disease is neurocytotropic (Goodpasture). The process of nerve cell destruction rapidly reaches a peak within the first few days after onset. In paralytic animals, over 90 per cent of all the motoneurons in the limb populations are infected during the first few days. The cytopathological changes are reversed during the course of tion involving particularly the lymphatic tissue is not supported by present evidence, and doubt has also been cast by recent investigations on the assumption that the virus of poliomyelitis reaches the meninges first and proliferates in this region.

Pathogenesis: The portal of entry of poliomyelitis virus in the human is not definitely known. The most likely portal of entry is through the mouth and pharynx. Poliomyelitis can be produced in rhesus monkeys by injection into the peritoneal cavity, the tonsillopharyngeal region, or intracutaneously, subcutaneously, intravenously, into the brain, or into the intestines. Entry of the virus has been presumed to be through the nose and a large amount of evidence seems to support this contention. Intranasal inoculation of virus in monkeys is almost invariably followed by the production of the disease. Invasion of the nervous system by way of the olfactory bulbs takes place only after intranasal inoculation.

Experimental evidence is at hand to indicate that virus enters through the nasopharyngeal region, as attested by the occurrence of cases of bulbar poliomyelitis following tonsillectomy and by the production of bulbar poliomyelitis in monkeys after injection of virus into the tonsillopharyngeal region in amounts which were innocuous when given subcutaneously or intracutaneously, and by the recovery of the virus from swabs of the nose and throat. Entry of the virus through the tonsillopharyngeal region has been regarded as of special importance, and it has been found that in monkeys amounts of virus regularly innocuous when given intracutaneously or subcutaneously produced the disease in eighty per cent when injected into the tonsillopharyngeal region (Sabin). The relationship of tonsillectomy to bulbar poliomyelitis has attracted much attention in recent years because of the reportedly increased incidence of bulbar poliomyelitis following tonsillectomy during poliomyelitis epidemics. The evidence in favor of the higher incidence of bulbar cases cannot be disregarded. Of greater significance than the increased incidence of poliomyelitis following tonsillectomy is the fact that in those patients developing the disease, the poliomyelitis is always

of the bulbar variety, indicating a possible direct connection between the tonsillectomy and the occurrence of the bulbar poliomyelitis.

Regardless of the portal of entry of the virus, whether through the nose, pharynx, or gastrointestinal tract, it quickly reaches the nervous system by means not entirely clear. Several pathways may be utilized, the details of which cannot be considered here. "There is no acceptable evidence that the virus can enter the central nervous system except through neural channels. However, the exact site or sites of entrance in the human disease is not yet known" (Goodpasture). Within the nervous system it spreads by propagation along the axones, though some believe the spread is through the spinal fluid. The virus is presumed to multiply within the axones, but there is doubt as to the validity of this conception. Virus can be recovered in different parts of the brain stem and spinal cord after intranasal or intracerebral installation of the virus in monkeys. The virus has not been recovered in the spinal fluid in human cases. It is open to question how closely the events as observed in monkeys can be transferred to humans because of the artificial means of induction of infection.

Symptoms: The symptoms of poliomyelitis are usually divided into (1) the preparalytic stage; (2) the paralytic stage; and (3) the residual or chronic stage. The incubation period is not known but is probably from seven to fourteen days, with the seventh to the tenth days most vulnerable. The incubation period is difficult to calculate because there is difference of opinion about when poliomyelitis begins after exposure. A recent study indicates that the incubation period may vary from four to thirty-five

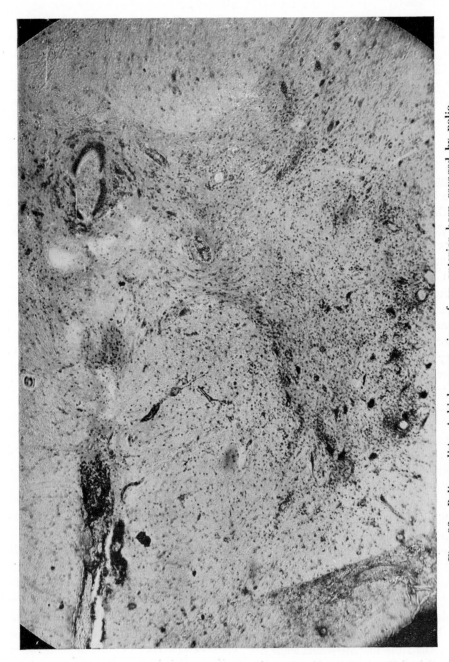

Fig. 83—*Poliomyelitis.* A high-power view of an anterior horn ravaged by poliomyelitis, showing the severe loss of ganglion cells and the heavy infiltration, as well as the meningeal infiltration in the anterior fissure.

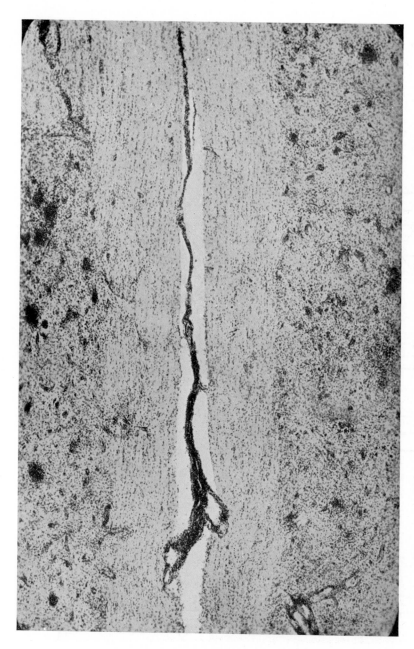

Fig. 84—*Poliomyelitis.* A longitudinal section of the spinal cord showing the heavy infiltration of the gray column and the absence of infiltration in the medially placed anterior white matter. Note the infiltration in the meninges of the anterior fissure.

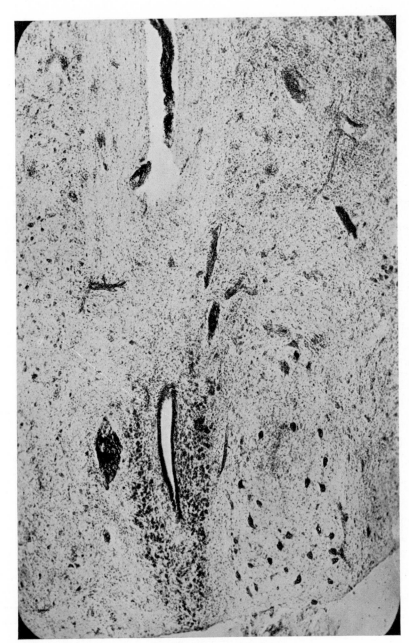

Fig. 85—*Poliomyelitis.* A longitudinal section of the spinal cord to show cell loss in many areas with well-preserved anterior horn cells in others.

days, with an average of 12.2 days (Casey).

In about 30 per cent of cases, the acute illness is ushered in with two febrile episodes, though the second is usually the only one recognized. In the first, the patient has an inconsequential illness with variable fever lasting twenty-four to thirty-six hours, followed by a normal temperature for one to eight days, usually two to three days, during which he feels well or relatively well; he then develops a more severe type of illness associated with involvement of the nervous system.

The *preparalytic stage* begins usually with a slight fever, malaise, upper respiratory symptoms such as coryza, and gastrointestinal symptoms, such as nausea, vomiting, diarrhea, or constipation. Leukocytosis is present at this stage, reaching as high as twenty thousand. The illness at this stage is not alarming and is not unlike many ordinary colds. It may last several days (four or five), but it is not uncommonly of only one or two days' duration or in some cases only fleeting or not present at all. Full recovery may occur at this stage, or the illness may progress with the development of headache, pain in the neck and back, and prostration which seems out of all proportion to the systemic condition. The patient at this stage is flushed and anxious; he is drowsy, much less alert than normal, and extremely irritable. He can be aroused, but on doing so is very irritable. He resents movement of any sort, has marked muscle sensitivity, and general hyperesthesia. Pinching of the muscles evokes marked pain. Signs of meningeal irritation are present as shown by neck stiffness and a positive Kernig's sign. The spine sign is positive; this consists of a spasm of the spine muscles with inability to flex the spine because of pain. Tremor may be seen in the preparalytic stage in the muscles which are destined to become paralyzed. It is not always found, but when present it indicates the seat of development of weakness.

Spinal puncture at this stage reveals an increase of cells in the spinal fluid (one hundred to two thousand). These are chiefly polymorphonuclear in the acute stage, but change quickly to lymphocytes, usually within a few days but in other instances in five to seven days. The spinal fluid protein is slightly increased at first, but later reaches a higher level (200 mg.). The spinal fluid sugar is normal. The colloidal gold curve may be abnormal but is not specific.

The disease may not develop beyond this stage and may be followed by complete recovery without progressing to the point of paralysis. At this time, the picture is that of a febrile disease with an increase of lymphocytes in the spinal fluid, and precise diagnosis is impossible. It may be correctly inferred in the presence of an epidemic but cannot be definitely established clinically at this stage.

Paralytic Stage: This develops after a varying length of time, anywhere from one to seven days after the onset of the illness. Systemic signs are not as prominent as in the preparalytic stage, but fever and malaise usually continue, though the muscle irritability and the neck and spine stiffness tend to disappear. They may persist for several days, or even weeks, even after the development of the paralysis. The cardinal symptom of this stage is paralysis, of which there may be some warning by the presence of tremors or loss of reflexes. The paralysis may develop gradually or rapidly, usually the latter. Paralysis may take two or three days in some cases to develop completely. It has all the features of a lower motor neuron paralysis: flaccidity, loss of reflexes, muscle fasciculations, and atrophy, with reaction of degeneration later. In some cases the paralysis is ascending, beginning in the feet and extending upward to the arms. The distribution of the paralysis varies; both legs are most commonly affected, then, in order of frequency, one leg, both legs and both arms, both legs and one arm, and one arm.

The presence of a Babinski sign is sometimes seen due to cerebral involvement, or to stimulation of the pyramidal pathways in the spinal cord by the perivascular cuffing seen in the disease during the acute stages. Paralysis of the respiratory muscles occurs not infrequently and may require the use of the respirator. Paralysis of swallowing or of the facial muscles may occur in the bulbar form of the disease. Paralysis of the bladder shown by inability to void is seen in some cases. Within two to three weeks after development of the paralysis, muscle atrophy is seen and sometimes is visible even earlier in rapidly developing cases.

There seems to be no parallel between the intensity of the preparalytic symptoms and those of the paralytic stage; mild preparalytic symptoms may be followed by severe paralysis and severe preparalytic symptoms may be followed by only mild evidences of paralysis. Paralysis is always possible as long as fever is present. Injections of pertussis vaccine and/or diphtheria toxoid one to three months prior to the onset of poliomyelitis have been reported to have some influence in the localization of the subsequent paralysis, but play no role whatever in the cause of the poliomyelitis.

Following the paralysis comes the *chronic* or *residual* stage, characterized by stability of the atrophies, and the development of contractures, etc. The muscles in this stage are atrophied and flaccid, muscular fasciculations are often but not always seen, and reaction of degeneration is demonstrable. Weakness is present in the affected muscles, varying with the degree of involvement. The affected limbs are cold and often somewhat cyanosed. Contractures are not infrequently seen in this stage.

Clinical Varieties: Various clinical or types of poliomyelitis have been described. The differentiation of types of poliomyelitis has some justification in the occurrence of epidemics of predominantly bulbar or spinal types. It is best to realize, however, that these represent merely patterns of the disease due to localization of the virus in specific areas. It is not known whether this localization is related to the type or virulence of the virus.

Bulbar Types: In some epidemics bulbar forms of poliomyelitis may predominate and may be the only evidence of involvement of the nervous system. Bulbar involvement may occur also in conjunction with paralysis of the extremities. Any of the motor nuclei of the brain stem may be involved (ocular, facial, vagus, hypoglossal). Facial paralysis is most common; difficulty in speech and swallowing, associated with palatal weakness or paralysis, ocular palsies, dysarthria, and tongue weakness also occur. In some instances, the only manifestation of poliomyelitis may be a facial paralysis, either unilateral or bilateral, following the systemic symptoms of the preparalytic stage. Isolated palatal paralysis may develop also. Abnormal electrocardiograms have been found in a high percentage of cases of poliomyelitis in children and adults, but are commoner in the latter and in patients with bulbar and high cervical paralysis. The EKG findings are nonspecific and appear to bear no relationship to the duration of the fever or the severity of the paralysis. They usually revert to normal within four weeks. Many of the bulbar cases recover completely, especially if there is only isolated cranial nerve involvement, such as palatal paralysis. Others terminate fatally, particularly the instances of multiple cranial nerve paralyses.

Cerebral Types: Cerebral forms occur during epidemics and are characterized by the presence of hemiparesis or hemiplegia. Focal convulsions have been recorded. The incidence of the cerebral form is disputed, but there seems to be no doubt that in some epidemics cerebral forms of the disease are found and correlate well with the pathological changes found in the brain.

Cerebellar Types: Some cases of poliomyelitis are characterized by extreme ataxia without evidence of other signs of poliomyelitis. It is doubtful whether such types are cases of poliomyelitis, but pure cerebellar forms have been reported in a few epidemics.

Meningeal Types: Not uncommon are cases of poliomyelitis with preparalytic symptoms, signs of meningeal irritation (stiff neck, Kernig's sign), and an increase of cells in the spinal fluid. These represent forms of the disease that have not progressed to the stage of paralysis. In epidemics such cases are not difficult to recognize, but when they occur in sporadic form it is extremely difficult to distinguish them from tuberculous meningitis, and lymphocytic choriomeningitis.

Abortive Types: These are probably the most important of all the variants of poliomyelitis. It is possible that most of the cases in an epidemic are of this type and that even endemic cases of an abortive nature are numerous but unrecognized. The difficulty lies, of course, in agreement on what constitutes abortive poliomyelitis; whether fever with gastrointestinal and upper respiratory symptoms, or cases with meningeal involvement, or others with mild febrile manifestations. No criteria for the determination of abortive types have been laid down. In epidemics the presumption that the types of case referred to are abortive cases of poliomyelitis is probably safe, but in nonepidemic years this assumption is not tenable. Most of the cases are manifested by fever, sore throat, headache, vomiting, or gastrointestinal symptoms.

As has been indicated, the assumption that such cases represent instances of abortive poliomyelitis is sound during epidemics for two reasons: (1) They are similar in their symptoms to cases which subsequently develop paralysis; (2) studies of such cases during epidemics have shown the isolation of poliomyelitis virus from nasopharyngeal washings in some cases (Paul, Salinger, Trask). In either case, the diagnosis cannot be confirmed save by neutralization tests and isolation of the virus from abortive cases, though the value of neutralization tests as indicators of resistance to the disease is open to question. The incidence of abortive cases of poliomyelitis has been found to be higher in families exposed to a fully developed case than in families not so exposed. In only a few instances has the virus been isolated from the nasopharyngeal washings in abortive cases very early in the disease. Many cases pass through the preparalytic stage with only febrile and upper respiratory symptoms or gastrointestinal symptoms. Others develop meningeal signs without subsequent paralysis. It is essential that such cases be recognized for what they are, but it is impossible in our present state of knowledge to do so save by neutralization tests of the serum, which have been found to be positive in the abortive cases. In the last analysis, the detection of abortive poliomyelitis depends upon laboratory investigations. Since these are not available for detection of poliomyelitis, the establishment of the diagnosis of abortive poliomyelitis is still difficult.

Diagnosis: The diagnosis of poliomyelitis in an epidemic is not difficult, particularly in the paralytic stages. Early diagnosis is essential. Fever, malaise, neck pain, muscle tenderness, and irritability associated with signs of meningeal irritation, leukocytosis, and stiff spine should lead one to suspect poliomyelitis. Lumbar puncture should be performed always in such cases in order to determine whether there is an excess of cells in the spinal fluid. The subsequent development of paralysis with atrophy and loss of reflexes will confirm the diagnosis of poliomyelitis. If the disease clears up without paralysis, the condition may be regarded as abortive poliomyelitis and safely diagnosed as such during epidemics, though final proof is lacking. Endemic cases cannot be diagnosed as abortive poliomyelitis with certainty save by laboratory controls.

Differentiation must be made from encephalitis, meningitis, neuritis, and myelitis. In the acute stage of the disease, before the onset of paralysis, the total picture is that of a febrile disease with an increase of lymphocytes in the spinal fluid. The diagnosis at this time involves, therefore, the differentiation of the disease from all conditions capable of causing a spinal fluid lymphocytosis. Many of these can be eliminated without difficulty, but the separation of poliomyelitis from others may never be successfully made if the disease fails to progress to the point of paralysis. The meningeal signs of the paralytic stage cause confusion with meningitis, especially when the spinal puncture reveals an increase of lymphocytes, which may cause confusion with *tuberculous meningitis,* but the demonstration of tubercle bacilli in the spinal fluid, and the low chloride and sugar content help in differentiation. The differentia-

tion from *lymphocytic choriomeningitis* is extremely difficult in endemic cases, since both disorders may simulate one another closely by their systemic symptoms. The absence of paralysis is of no help, since the problem still remains as to whether abortive poliomyelitis was present. The occurrence of headache, vomiting, and later paralysis in a child favors the diagnosis of poliomyelitis. The detection of the virus of lymphocytic choriomeningitis by neutralization test is diagnostic.

The bulbar forms may be confused with acute *encephalitis* and the differentiation may often be impossible. In some forms of encephalitis there will also be involvement of the white matter of the brain and cord, with indications of posterior column disease (loss of position and vibration sense), and disturbances of pain and temperature. Some forms of encephalitis may be differentiated by specific reactions (St. Louis encephalitis, Japanese encephalitis, etc.). *Neuritis* can be differentiated by the persistence of muscle and nerve tenderness long beyond the acute stage, the slower and less complete development of the paralysis, and the normal spinal fluid. The differentiation from acute infectious polyneuritis is more difficult, but the absence of cells and the elevated protein content of the spinal fluid is helpful. *Myelitis* due to various toxic-infective causes is differentiated by the presence of involvement of other systems outside the anterior horn cells.

"There is no rapid laboratory test to confirm a diagnosis. Demonstration of the virus in the feces is helpful, but the patient is either dead or on the road to recovery before this can be accomplished. Neutralization tests on specimens of acute-phase and convalescent serums are not particularly helpful because there are several immunological strains of poliomyelitis virus. There is no complement fixation test available at the present time" (Rivers).

Vaccine for the prevention of poliomyelitis (Salk vaccine) is recommended for all children and for adults under

done to make the patient comfortable in the acute stages and to prevent deformities in later stages. Transporation of patients in the acute stage of poliomyelitis may be harmful. During the acute febrile

Table 22—Differential Diagnosis of Poliomyelitis

	Onset	Fever	Meningeal Signs	Neurological Findings	Spinal Fluid	Miscellaneous
POLIOMYELITIS	Acute, with prepara-lytic stage	Present	In early stages	Paralysis, atrophy, reflex loss	Lymphocy-tosis in early stages Cultures negative	—
NEURITIS	Acute; no prodro-mal stage	Absent; present in some forms	Absent	Paralysis, reflex loss, atrophy but with pain, nerve tenderness and sensory disturbances	No changes, save in acute infectious polyneuritis —increase of protein but not of cells	
ENCEPHALITIS	Acute	Present	In early stages	Ocular paralysis and other brain stem palsies	Lymphocy-tosis in early stages Cultures negative	Requires separation from brain stem type of poliomyelitis. In latter, usually arms or legs affected
LYMPHOCYTIC FORMS OF MENINGITIS (V. MENINGITIS)	Acute	Usually, but not always	Present	None or scattered signs of cerebral involvement	Lymphocy-tosis	Tubercle bacillus in spinal fluid. Other causes may be demonstrated
PYOGENIC MENINGITIS	Acute	Always	Present	Only signs of meningeal irritation	Polynuclear cells in spinal fluid Cultures positive	

forty years of age. The vaccine has been in use long enough to indicate that the case rate of development in poliomyelitis is greater in unvaccinated than in vaccinated children.

Treatment: Though there is no specific treatment of poliomyelitis, much can be

stage of poliomyelitis, unusual physical exercise is associated with a significant increase in the incidence and severity of subsequent paralysis. *Before paralysis* develops, *bed rest* is essential in the febrile stage. Sedation may be given for restlessness and for relief of the irritability so commonly encountered in the disease. Small doses of phenobarbital, 0.008 to 0.016 Gm. (⅛ to ¼ grains), three or four times daily suffice in most cases, but more is required for adults. Sodium bromide, 0.648 to 0.972 Gm. (10 to 15 grains), three times daily may be used. A *footboard* should be used to keep the feet in good position and to keep the bed clothes off the painful limbs. If fluids cannot be retained by mouth, *intravenous glucose* may be given (1500 to 2000 cc. of 5 per cent solution). *Moist heat,* in the form of moist woolen packs, gives relief when applied to the spine or limbs if there is generalized muscle pain or spasm.

During the *paralytic stage, sedation* as in the preparalytic stage and the maintenance of fluid balance by *intravenous glucose* when needed are important. *Blood plasma* or *whole blood* may be used to restore plasma proteins, but convalescent or adult serum is of no value in the disease. *Footboards* or *plaster shells* may be used to maintain the feet in good dorsiflexion. *Heat* is important and is best used as warm moist packs, though radiant heat may also be used. Heat should be applied intermittently for not more than one to two hours daily. Most investigators and clinicians agree that the ritualized Kenny technic is not necessary and that intermittent, moist, warm packs are sufficient. If there is not too much muscle tenderness, *passive motions* may be used to prevent contractures and *active movement* encouraged in muscles that possess voluntary movement. Most contractures can be prevented by *proper positioning:* the knees slightly flexed, the feet in 90 degrees of dorsiflexion, the arms slightly abducted and externally rotated, and the back supported by a firm bed.

The bowels must be kept open, a problem which may become quite difficult in some cases of the disease. *Enemas* may be necessary. *Sodium chloride,* 0.486 Gm. (7½ grains), three times daily and 100 mg. (1½ grains) of vitamin C twice daily are important adjuncts in treatment because of the profuse loss of fluid. *Thiamine chloride,* 100 mg. intramuscularly daily, and *neostigmine bromide,* 15 mg. three times daily by mouth, should also be given.

The *respirator* becomes important in some cases of poliomyelitis. The respirator is most useful for patients with thoracic-cage and diaphragmatic paralysis, but it should also be used in those with bulbar paralysis, though its use in the latter is condemned by many clinicians. Since, however, some patients with bulbar paralysis may be given an opportunity for recovery if life can be maintained during the acute stages of the disease, the use of the respirator becomes justified. The respirator should be used in patients with respiratory distress, fatigue, or cyanosis. It has been demonstrated that in bulbar poliomyelitis, anoxia and CO_2 accumulation due to difficulty in swallowing, with secretional obstruction, are responsible for most severe central effects. Treatment should be designed to clear the airways. Potassium deficiency has been found to be present in bulbar poliomyelitis.

Massage and *exercises* become important in the convalescent stage when muscle tenderness has subsided. Passive and active exercises may be used, and massage must be light and soothing. *Muscle reeducation* is important in this stage, and there should be frequent check of the muscles to serve as a guide to treatment and to stimulate the morale of the patient. *Underwater exercises* in tub or pool are useful at this time. Braces may be necessary and should be ordered by an orthopedist. Attention must be given to the prevention of deformities in the ambulatory stage just as in the acute phases of the disease. Later, *orthopedic operations* of various sorts may be necessary to provide correction of deformities.

The sulfonamides are of no value in poliomyelitis, but they may be used with or without penicillin in patients requiring respirator treatment, in order to prevent pulmonary infection.

VIII. ACUTE ASCENDING PARALYSIS
(Landry's Paralysis)

Etiology: Acute ascending paralysis, or Landry's paralysis, is a syndrome resulting from many causes and is caused by no single agent. It occurs in either sex at any age.

In at least one-third of the cases, the specific cause is unknown. In these instances a virus has been presumed to be the cause, but has not been demonstrated. Ascending paralysis may develop also in poliomyelitis, tick bite, sting of the weaver fish, vaccine therapy, antitetanus injections, typhoid fever, herpes zoster, lymphogranuloma, malaria, leukemia, rabies and antirabic vaccine therapy, neuritis, spinal cord syphilis, disseminated encephalomyelitis, and other conditions (Thorner, Alpers, and Yaskin). It is obvious, therefore, that the groups of symptoms known as Landry's paralysis may be produced by a variety of conditions.

Pathology: No uniform pathologic findings are demonstrable in the nervous system as might be expected with the varied etiology. Many of the patients, almost a third (thirty per cent), show no nervous system lesions. In others, anterior horn cell damage, mild or severe, is found. The anterior horn cell changes vary in type and degree. Axonal chromatolysis, acute degenerative changes, and chronic cell disease are found in the course of the disorder. In some patients, inflammatory changes are found, with lymphocytic infiltration in the anterior horns. This is not frequent. Severe cases clinically may show few or no changes in the anterior horn cells. This is the most constant finding. In some patients, not many, degenerative and inflammatory changes are found in the peripheral nerves and anterior roots. The changes in the peripheral nerves and/or anterior roots may be associated with those in the anterior horns or they may be independent of them.

It is believed by some that Landry's paralysis is a form of peripheral neuritis, but a survey of all reported cases reveals the fact that the peripheral nerves are affected in 15 per cent of the cases characterized by degenerative changes and in 25 per cent of those with inflammatory lesions. Peripheral nerve changes are seldom present without changes in other parts of the nervous system. The nuclei in the brain stem show changes similar to those of the anterior horns. Some authors assert that Landry's paralysis is the result of a polyneuritis of the Guillain-Barré type. The Guillian-Barré syndrome, acute infective polyneuritis and Landry's paralysis are said to fall into a single category (Haymaker and Kernohan). "Taken as a whole, the disorder is characterized by a polyradiculoneuropathy which may begin in any peripheral neurons, spinal or cranial, circumscribed or widespread, may affect predominantly the motor or the sensory neurons or both to the same degree; it may remain essentially a radicular disorder, or . . . it may extend into the central nervous system at any point, and either ascend or descend, the outcome usually being dependent on the degree of involvement of respiratory or cardiac nerves." (Haymaker and Kernohan). The muscles have been inadequately studied in Landry's paralysis, but the claim is made for some cases that the primary change is at the myoneural junction. Degeneration of the tracts in the white matter of the cord has been found. Generally speaking, there is no uniformity in the type, degree, or distribution of the lesions in Landry's paralysis.

Symptoms: The clinical features of acute ascending paralysis are variable and often atypical, hence the numerous problems which arise in the diagnosis of this seemingly easily recognized entity. The typical form is readily diagnosed. It begins abruptly in a person who has had a nasopharyngeal infection shortly before the onset, or with no prodromal symptoms whatever. The onset is often with fever, but the disease may be entirely afebrile in its onset, and even in its entire course. Fever of some degree is usually present but is not always found. Systemic symptoms are usually present and consist of malaise, vomiting, a feeling of profound fatigue, or aching of the muscles. Within a short time there is weakness of the feet and legs, leading quickly to complete paralysis. Then follows gradually or rapidly ascending paralysis, involving the abdominal and thoracic muscles and finally the arms. The paralysis may develop in the course of hours or days, the ascension being rapid or slow. The unfolding of the ascending paralysis has taken as long as seven to ten days in some instances. Descending paralysis is seen in very rare instances. The large muscle groups are affected first in the development of weakness and paralysis. The vesical and rectal sphincters are involved in fifty per cent of cases. The illness may progress no farther than the arms. It usually advances to affect the muscles of deglutition and respiration, as a result of involvement of the centers in the medulla. Ocular paralyses, paralysis of the muscles of chewing, and aphonia may develop. In most cases (eighty per cent), the course terminates in death, but in some instances there is partial or complete recovery.

Examination reveals flaccid, atonic muscles which are usually completely paralyzed. The tendon reflexes are absent as a rule. Sensory disturbances are not usually present. There is no tenderness of the muscles or nerve trunks in most cases. Laboratory studies are not of much help in the diagnosis. There is usually no leukocytosis, and the findings in the spinal fluid are generally normal.

Diagnosis: The diagnosis of acute ascending paralysis is easy in a case in which there are fever, a history of ascending paralysis, and signs of flaccid paralysis of the limbs. When one is confronted with a case in which there is no fever, the diagnosis may be difficult to accept. It should be recognized, however, that in some cases of acute ascending paralysis fever and systemic reactions are not present. For this reason, the diagnosis of hysteria is not uncommonly made in such cases, and great care should be exercised to avoid this error. In every instance, careful search should be made for a cause, since the syndrome is, in most cases, a symptom of one of its many causes.

The problem of Landry's paralysis is greatly complicated by a tendency to regard all cases with a history of ascending paralysis as Landry's paralysis. This is obviously not the case, since a history of this nature is found in many disorders —poliomyelitis, acute infectious polyneuritis, syphilis, rabies, and disseminated myelitis. The ascending history, therefore, has no absolute significance and does not in itself indicate Landry's paralysis. The chief features of this disease are: an onset of bilateral symmetrical paralysis of the legs; rapid or gradual extension to involve muscles of the arms and trunk, sometimes the muscles of swallowing, occasionally those of mastication and phonation, and rarely ocular movements; loss or diminution of tendon reflexes, and usually, but not always, the presence of sphincter disturbances and the absence of sensory findings.

Poliomyelitis offers a difficult problem in differentiation. In a typical case, the preparalytic symptoms and the spinal

Most cases are fatal. Cases with bulbar symptoms are almost always fatal. In other cases, complete or partial recovery may take place, despite the development of severe paralysis.

Treatment: Little can be done in the cases with unknown cause, save *symptomatic treatment,* such as rest, fluids, elimination, sedation, etc. In cases secondary to some specific cause, such as

Table 23—Causes of Myelitis

Infections	Toxic	Degenerative	Vascular	Trauma	Compression
Syphilis	Carbon monoxide	Multiple sclerosis	Arteriosclerosis	Concussion of spinal cord	Extramedullary tumor
Gonorrhea	Lead	Friedreich's ataxia	Embolus from coronary or	Compression of cord by dislo-	Metastatic carcinoma
Measles	Arsenic	Syringomyelia	valvular disease	cated vertebra	Hodgkins disease
Mumps	Alcohol	Subacute combined	Syphilitic vascular disease	Laceration	Tuberculosis of vertebrae
Chickenpox	Spinal anesthesia	degeneration			
Influenza	Triorthocresyl phosphate	Neuromyelitis optica	Acute and Subacute necrotic myelitis		Osteitis deformans
Malaria	Carbon bisulfide		Hematomyelia		
Tuberculosis					
Diphtheria					
Endocarditis					
Undulant fever					
Extradural abscess					

fluid findings are helpful. The distinction is often academic in so far as treatment goes, but of great importance from the standpoint of infection and management. Neuritis can be recognized by the muscle and nerve tenderness, the sensory findings, and the absence of sphincter disturbances. Syphilis can be detected by the positive blood and spinal fluid reactions. In cases of development of the syndrome following vaccine therapy a history of injections is obtainable.

syphilis, poliomyelitis, etc., the treatment is that of the primary disease. The respirator may be required in some patients.

IX. MYELITIS

Myelitis refers merely to an inflammatory or degenerative condition of the spinal cord. It is due to a wide variety of conditions and may therefore be regarded as the central nervous system involvement of some other primary state. It is not in itself a diagnosis unless the specific cause of the myelitis can be designated. To refer to a condition as "myelitis" or "transverse myelitis" indicates nothing; the specific cause must be indicated such as syphilitic myelitis, arteriosclerotic myelitis, etc. The term myelopathy is preferred by some because of the absence of inflammatory changes in some forms of the syndrome, and it is urged that the designation myelitis be reserved only for instances in which infection or inflammation is present. Since the term myelitis, however, is in common usage, it is employed here for all forms of spinal cord involvement.

Etiology: Myelitis is practically always secondary to a variety of causes and may result from: (1) Infections of many sorts, such as syphilis, gonorrhea. measles, mumps, chickenpox, influenza, malaria, tuberculosis, diphtheria, spinal cord abscess, endocarditis, undulant fever, and still other infections. Syphilis is probably the commonest cause of myelitis. (2) Poisons such as carbon monoxide, lead, arsenic, anesthetics for spinal anesthesia, intraspinal serum in the treatment of syphilis (Swift-Ellis). (3) Degenerative conditions such as multiple sclerosis, Friedreich's ataxia, syringomyelia, etc. (4) Vascular conditions such as arteriosclerosis, syphilis, embolic vessel occlusions, coronary thrombosis. (5) Trauma. (6) Tumors, both primary and secondary. (7) Miscellaneous or ill-defined causes. Infectious forms of myelitis referred to as neuromyelitis have been reported in epidemic form in South America. Their precise etiology is not known.

In the various causes listed, the myelitis or cord involvement is secondary to some other systemic illness. In other instances, the disease is associated with an infection of unknown origin. Cases of this sort are uncommon (disseminated myelitis or encephalomyelitis), but they occur and the term infectious myelitis should be reserved for them. Whether they represent primary infectious types of myelitis is not known at present. They are regarded as of virus origin by some, but their virus causation has not been proved.

Pathology: Due to the variety of causes of myelitis, its pathological background varies widely. A description of the various forms of myelitis would lead to infinite detail; hence only the more general features of spinal cord involvement in myelitis is possible. The many forms associated with separate disease entities will be considered under their various headings. Myelitis usually involves the spinal cord alone, but may be part of a generalized cerebrospinal involvement of the nervous system. Any part of the spinal cord may be affected. It may destroy the entire circumference of the spinal cord at any level (transverse myelitis), it may produce only partial destruction of a segment, or it may produce scattered lesions at many levels of the cord, causing a diffuse myelitis.

The cord is usually swollen in the acute state and may show hemorrhages on section. The fundamental point in common in all causes of myelitis is cord degeneration characterized by destruction of myelin and loss of axis cylinders. In some cases, inflammatory elements, such as lymphocytes and plasma cells, are found free in the tissue and around blood vessels, with infiltration of the meninges as well. Complete necrosis of the cord substances may be found in some forms, with extensive phagocytic response and mesodermal proliferation. The nerve cells within the gray matter of the cord may be severely degenerated. Mesodermal reaction is usually prolific, with dilated, proliferated, or infiltrated vessels. Scar formation by glial cells is found in some forms and not in others.

Symptoms: A variety of clinical forms may develop. Chief among these is *transverse myelitis*. This may develop suddenly or come on gradually in the course of hours or a few days. The onset is often febrile with severe systemic symptoms. There may be pain in the trunk or extremities, and usually paresthesias of the limbs and retention of urine. The patient with the fully developed disease shows complete motor, sensory, and sphincter paralysis. The legs usually, but also at times the arms and legs, are completely paralyzed. These are at first flaccid, later becoming spastic after a few days to a few weeks, but in some cases persisting as a flaccid paralysis. The legs are almost always in extension but may at times develop a flexion posture. The reflexes are lost at first, but later become overactive, and pathological reflexes develop. Complete sensory loss is present to the level of the lesion. This involves all forms of sensation uniformly. Bladder and rectal incontinence are present. Bedsores commonly develop. *Incomplete transverse myelitis* may develop. The picture may be that of a Brown-Séquard syndrome, or of disseminated lesions spread throughout the cord, the clinical features varying, of course, with the areas diseased. Paralysis, ataxia, isolated Babinski signs, and disturbances of vesical function are among the signs encountered. Ascending forms of myelitis due to many causes are well known.

Leukocytosis may be found in some of the acute forms of myelitis. Spinal fluid studies may show an increase of cells; the Wassermann reaction and colloidal gold curve are positive in syphilis. Subarachnoid block, either incomplete or complete, may be demonstrated in acute cases, the swollen cord compressing and obliterating the subarachnoid space.

Scattered cases of a special form of myelitis have been recorded under the terms *acute* and *subacute necrotic myelitis*. The cause of the disease is not known. Pathologically, the condition is characterized by degeneration of the white matter, which may involve portions of the cord or its entire cross section, and by loss of myelin and axis cylinders. The areas of destruction in their advanced stages are necrotic; in their early stages they are patchy, with swollen and destroyed myelin and axis cylinders, and with large numbers of phagocytic cells. The gray matter is not as severely affected, but changes are found in the anterior horn cells. The patches of necrosis are associated with disease of the vessels, characterized by hyaline thickening of the small arteries and veins, but an occasional larger vessel may be affected. Thickening of the vessels both inside and outside the spinal cord occurs. It is probable that this form of myelitis is primarily vascular in origin.

Clinically, the *acute form* of subacute necrotic myelitis is characterized by a rapid development of symptoms affecting particularly the lumbar and sacral segments of the spinal cord, with a resulting rapidly developing flaccid paraplegia which fails to recover. The reflexes are absent. The symptoms unfold with a varying degree of rapidity, covering a period of two days to two weeks, in which time the legs become completely paralyzed. Pain and other subjective sensory disturbances such as paresthesias are not prominent, but objective sensory disturbances appear early with rapid development of a sensory level which may reach to the midthoracic or lower thoracic segments. Sphincter disturbances appear within a few weeks of the onset of weakness. The spinal fluid reveals no evidence of subarachnoid block, but the protein is greatly increased (500 to 1000 mg.) in the cases recorded, and the cells are increased.

The *subacute form* is gradual in onset and progressive without remissions. The presenting symptom is weakness of the legs, but pains in the legs are common. The past record in the reported cases has revealed a history of albuminuria, gout, cardiovascular disease with auricular fibrillation, and hypertension. The motor weakness is characterized by a spastic paraplegia with atrophy of the muscles and overactive reflexes, but flaccid paraplegia with areflexia may develop. The sensory disturbances develop some time, usually months, after the motor disturbances, and are characterized by the progressive ascending development of a sensory level with involvement of all forms of sensation. Sphincter disturbances appear early. The spinal fluid shows no evidence of subarachnoid block despite the history of progression of symptoms. The protein is increased and the cells may be normal in amount or there may be a moderate lymphocytosis.

Spinal cord tumor must be differentiated because of the progressive history, an almost impossible task because of the history, the sensory level, and paralysis. The absence of subarachnoid block and of root pains will exclude extramedullary tumor, and the ascending type of sensory loss will favor subacute necrotic myelitis. Pott's disease may be excluded by the absence of root pain and by roentgenologic studies, and metastatic carcinoma by the same studies. Syphilitic meningomyelitis will be associated with evidences of syphilis in the spinal fluid.

Amyotrophic lateral sclerosis, which must be considered because of the atrophy, is excluded by the presence of the sensory findings. Subacute combined degeneration is excluded by the absence of paresthesias and the sensory level, which does not occur in this disease; the normal blood findings and gastric analysis are important in excluding this disorder as well.

Diagnosis: The problem in myelitis is usually that of a complete or incomplete transverse spinal cord lesion, which has developed gradually or suddenly, for which a cause is sought. The problem resolves itself further into a search for infectious, toxic, vascular, traumatic, or compression factors which could cause the syndrome. It is beyond the province of this section to consider the differential features of all the possible causes of myelitis, but some comment on a few is essential. Many of the infectious cases are febrile in onset. In cases following exanthemata there is a history of a recent exanthem, such as chickenpox, measles, mumps, etc., with subsequent signs of involvement of the spinal cord.

Gonorrheal cases follow closely on the acute infection. The onset is sudden, with pain, incontinence, and evidences of myelitis occurring two to three weeks after a severe attack of gonorrhea. Recovery is slow and may be incomplete. Syphilis is detected by positive serological reactions of the spinal fluid and by other signs of syphilitic disease, such as Argyll Robertson pupils. The various forms of syphilitic myelitis are described subsequently. Some infectious cases have no demonstrable cause. Rarely, myelitis is associated with coronary disease, due to embolus of one or more spinal vessels. It has also been described in rheumatic heart disease. A history of exposure to lead, treatment with arsenicals for syphilis, exposure to carbon monoxide, etc., are helpful in other cases. Vascular cases are not so easy to detect. Those due to arteriosclerosis give evidence of peripheral arteriosclerosis. Anterior spinal artery occlusions often give a history of exertion preceding the onset of symptoms. Traumatic cases give a clear history of injury. In all cases of myelitis it is essential to exclude spinal cord tumor first in order to proceed to operation if necessary. This is usually possible by means of a history of pain and progression of symptoms, and positive evidence of subarachnoid block by lumbar puncture. Metastatic lesions can be detected by a history of carcinoma elsewhere in the body. Neuritis may simulate myelitis but is detected by the muscle and nerve tenderness, the absence of sensory level, and of sphincter disturbances.

Dissecting aneurysm of the aorta must be considered in the causation of obscure spinal and cerebral vascular disorders and unexplained cases of myelitis. The symptoms of this condition may be either cerebral or spinal, and appear to be more frequently the former. Neurological symptoms occur in eleven to twenty-nine per cent sometime during the cause of the disorder. The condition occurs about once in every 400 to 500 postmortem examinations. It is more frequent in men, 2 or 3:1, and is commonest in the 5th or 6th decades, though no age is entirely exempt. It is on the whole an acute affliction, eighty per cent of the patients dying within a few days, and from eighty to eighty-five per cent within the first two weeks. Death (eighty to ninety per cent) is due to rupture into the pericardial, thoracic, or abdominal cavities.

The onset is usually dramatic, with sudden violent pain in the chest, back or abdomen with a feeling of impending death. The pains tend to be migratory, spreading from one region to another. Hypertension is almost always present and is maintained in the face of a serious vascular disturbance, but it is not always found, especially in the younger group of patients. The leukocyte count is elevated in the presence of a normal temperature. The heart may give little helpful information, but the presence of a cardiac murmur and the appearance of a precordial rub during the course of the illness are of diagnostic importance. There is no characteristic electrocardiogram, but there may be evidence of ventricular strain. Roentgenograms reveal an enlarged heart with a tortuous aorta which may be dilated and calcified.

Neurological findings are important in establishing the diagnosis. These may involve brain, spinal cord or peripheral nerves, and though nervous system involvement is usually cerebral or spinal in its predominant location, it is at times diffuse. The cerebral symptoms may consist of hemiplegia, complete or partial; seizures; episodes of unconsciousness, and attacks of vertigo. The spinal cord symptoms are evidenced usually by manifestations of a partial or complete transverse myelitis.

The diagnosis of dissecting aneurysm of the aorta is based on the following features (Moersch): (1) The sudden onset of symptoms with prostration and collapse, (2) the presence of severe and usually prolonged and migrating pains, (3) the presence of hypertension, (4) the presence of neurological symptoms, (5) normal to only slightly elevated temperature, (6) an enlarged heart with a cardiac murmur and transitory pericardial rub, (7) an electrocardiogram that is not diagnostic, (8) roentgenographic findings of enlarged heart with tortuous aorta which may be dilated and calcified,

(9) increased leukocyte count, (10) albumin in the urine and at times red cells.

Prognosis: The outlook in cases of myelitis depends to a large extent on the cause. In cases following exanthemata, recovery usually takes place. Patients with infectious cases of unknown cause do poorly as a rule, while those with disease due to necrosis of the cord fail to recover much if any function. Syphilitic myelitis responds poorly to treatment, as does gonorrheal myelitis. Patients with persistent flaccid paralysis do less well than those with shorter duration of flaccidity, and high cervical cord involvement is more serious than when involvement is lower down, owing to interference with respiratory function.

Treatment: All the patients require *general measures* of a similar nature. These include an air or soft rubber mattress to prevent pressure sores. Great care must be taken to keep the skin clean. The patient must be moved from side to side several times a day to prevent prolonged pressure on any one area. The skin must be cleansed and powdered frequently and contact with incontinent urine and feces avoided. A urinal should be kept in place for male patients and a large pad for females. A daily enema takes care of the rectal incontinence adequately. The problem of catheterization will be encountered early in patients having retention. Catheterization may be carried out followed by bladder washing, or a permanent catheter inserted with tidal drainage to prevent bladder infection. Bedsores are difficult to treat, but zinc oxide powder, gentian violet, and ultraviolet lamp are helpful. The sores must be covered with heavy gauze pads. Massage of the paralyzed limbs is helpful in maintaining nutrition and should be given daily if possible. Care should be taken to prevent contractures.

X. NEUROMYELITIS OPTICA
(Neuropticomyelitis, Diffuse Myelitis with Optic Neuritis, Devic's Syndrome)

This disease is not clearly defined as to etiology or classification. It has come to the fore in recent years and claims made for it as a disease *sui generis*. It is as yet impossible to support this contention, and its inclusion as a separate entity is doubtful.

Etiology: The disease may occur at any age, in young or old, and in either sex. It is more common in the middle-aged or in older people. The exact cause is not known, but those who regard it as a distinct entity believe it to be of virus origin. This opinion has not been substantiated. The prevailing opinions are that it is either a separate entity of the demyelinating group of diseases or that it is a subgroup of multiple sclerosis.

Pathology: Any part of the cord may be attacked, but thoracic involvement is more common than others. The cord destruction often involves a complete transverse section. The disease is characterized by patchy demyelination of the brain stem, spinal cord, optic nerves, and tracts. The diseased areas show myelin loss in greater or lesser degree, axis cylinder destruction and disease, proliferation of blood vessels, and perivascular infiltration with lymphocytes or plasma cells with evidence of neurological repair in older lesions. The optic nerves and tracts show areas of destruction similar to those of the cord and brain stem.

Symptoms: Neuromyelitis optica, as the name implies, is characterized by symptoms involving the optic nerves and the spinal cord. The onset is usually abrupt with either signs of optic nerve or cord involvement. Either set of symptoms may occur first, with an interval varying from days to one year before the appearance of the remaining signs, or, less frequently, the double symptomatology may be simultaneous in onset. The optic nerve symptoms consist of impairment of visual acuity varying from mild blurring to amaurosis, field defects, especially paracentral scotomata and orbital or retroörbital pain. The optic nerve involvement may be unilateral or bilateral, and if bilateral may be simultaneous in onset or separated by a period of days to months. In some instances, examination of the optic discs reveals papilledema. This occurs in optic neuritis when the lesion is at or near the disc. Examination of the fundus may reveal little or no change in patients with retrobulbar neuritis when the lesion is behind the optic disc. The spinal cord symptoms are usually those of a complete transection with bilateral paralysis, complete sensory loss, and loss of sphincter control. They may appear simultaneously with the eye symptoms or after an interval of weeks or months. This may be preceded by pain in the back or legs. The cord lesion is not complete in all instances.

The most common causes of death are urinary infection and decubitus ulcers. Accurate prognostic statistics are not available, since newer methods have been employed to combat these complications. Indications are that the mortality rate is in the neighborhood of ten per cent.

Some patients recover entirely from both the optic nerve and cord lesions. These patients constitute a minority. The sequelae which result from the optic nerve involvement range from a small scotoma, usually paracentral, to complete amaurosis. Permanent sensory impairment, partial to complete paralysis or sphincter disturbances may remain either alone or in combination as sequelae to the cord lesions. In addition, recent follow-up studies have shown that these patients frequently develop other neurologic manifestations as diplopia, cerebellar signs, and hemiparesis.

Laboratory studies are negative. The spinal fluid shows no subarachnoid block. An increase of cells in the spinal fluid is found in some cases.

Diagnosis: The diagnosis of neuromyelitis optica is made on the basis of simultaneous or near simultaneous involvement of the eyes and spinal cord, with loss of vision and indications of a complete or incomplete myelitis resulting in remission or failure of recovery.

There is no *bona fide* evidence that the disease constitutes an entity. On the contrary, there is much to indicate that it is merely a form of multiple sclerosis. The pathology, the remissions, and the signs are so similar as to make differentiation impossible, and follow-up studies show that those patients who recover frequently develop other attacks involving other systems as do patients having multiple sclerosis.

Remissions occur in some cases (ten to fifty per cent). Others remain stationary and still others proceed to a fatal outcome.

Treatment: The treatment of the loss of vision is often without avail. *Vasodilators* may be tried as in the treatment of retrobulbar neuritis. *Thiamine chloride* intramuscularly may be helpful. The disease should be treated like multiple sclerosis (*q.v.*).

XI. SYPHILIS OF THE SPINAL CORD

Syphilis occurs in many forms in the spinal cord. No classification of spinal cord syphilis is entirely satisfactory, but the following represents a combined clinical and pathologic grouping which covers most of the forms encountered:

1. *Meningeal:*
   Hypertrophic pachymeningitis
   Meningomyelitis
2. *Parenchymatous:*
   Tabes dorsalis
   Syphilitic amyotrophies
   Gumma of spinal cord
3. *Vascular:*
   Thrombosis of the anterior spinal artery

Of these, tabes dorsalis is by far the most common, the other forms of spinal

months or as late as twenty-five to thirty years after infection. The average latency is given in some series as twenty years.

Pathology: Tabes dorsalis is a disease predominantly of the spinal cord and its roots, but it affects also the cranial nerves, the brain stem, and in some cases the brain itself.

The thoracic, lumbar, and sacral seg-

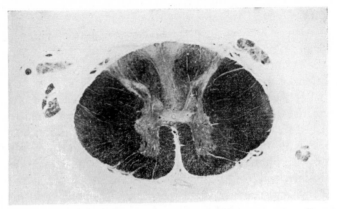

Fig. 86—*Tabes dorsalis.* Myelin sheath stain showing the demyelination of the posterior columns and the posterior roots.

cord syphilis lagging far behind in incidence.

1. Tabes Dorsalis (Locomotor Ataxia)

Etiology: The syphilitic nature of tabes is beyond question and needs no elucidation. There is some evidence to indicate that there may be a superimposed factor of dietary deficiency accounting for some of the cord damage in the disease. The disease occurs in about seven to ten per cent of patients with neurosyphilis. It is much more common in men than in women.

It is most frequent between thirty and fifty years of age, but it may occur in both younger and older age groups. The disease makes its appearance from five to fifteen years after the initial infection, but instances are known of its occurrence as early as twelve to eighteen

ments of the spinal cord are affected much more commonly than the cervical region. In the affected areas, meningeal infiltration by lymphocytes and plasma cells is found in the pia arachnoid. The meninges become fibrosed and adherent as the disease progresses. The posterior roots and their ganglia are diseased, forming the basis for the pains, girdle sensations, and paresthesias so common in the process. Infiltration of these areas by lymphocytes and plasma cells is followed later by destruction of myelin and axis cylinders and scar formation. Within the cord itself the changes are confined to the posterior or dorsal columns, where loss of the myelin sheaths and axis cylinders is found associated with heavy scar formation. The cord changes are responsible for the ataxia which is so prominent in the disease.

The various cranial nerves affected give the picture of a typical interstitial neuritis, with infiltration of the nerves by lymphocytes and plasma cells and destruction of myelin and axones. Among those affected are the optic, oculomotor, trigeminal, and auditory nerves.

The pathologic basis for the trophic changes in tabes (ulcers, arthropathies) is not agreed upon, but the bare roots lying between pia and cord are presumed to be particularly vulnerable to a toxin or to a localized meningitis. Still others regard the primary damage in the radicular nerve, which is the point at which posterior and anterior roots come together before reaching the ganglion, the primary process being a neuritis of this

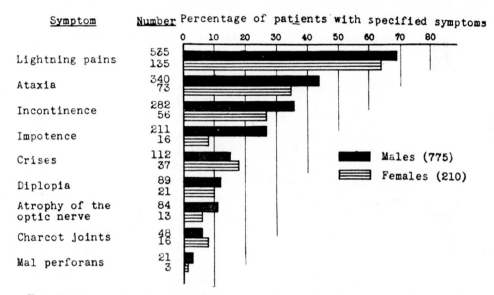

Fig. 87—*Tabes dorsalis.* Frequency of symptoms in patients with tabes dorsalis under treatment. (*O'Leary, et al.*)

not clear. Impairment of sensation contributes to their development, but disease of a special set of trophic fibers is postulated by some, and for the arthropathies (Charcot's joints) the factor of trauma is regarded as important.

The mode of development of tabes has fascinated pathologists for many years. It is regarded by some as due to the direct involvement of the posterior column fibers primarily, the root changes following secondarily. Cases supporting this view are rare. Others regard tabes as being due primarily to disease of the posterior roots, with secondary degeneration of the posterior columns. The precise locus of involvement of the roots is nerve or the formation of syphilitic granulation tissue induced by the settlement of spirochetes in this area.

Symptoms: A characteristic word picture of the symptoms of tabes is difficult because of their variability, depending on the stage of development of the disease. A history of a primary infection is almost never volunteered, and is obtained only on direct examination. The history is longstanding. The presenting symptom may be acute, but a retrospective study will reveal that unrecognized or mild symptoms have been disregarded. As a rule, the presenting complaint is pains in the legs, which are usually severe enough to require attention, but pain in the arms or trunk, girdle sensations, dimness of vision, incontinence of urine, difficulty in walking, or loss of sexual potency may bring the patient to the physician for the first time. Following a varying length of time in the usual case the leg pains are succeeded by difficulty in starting the stream of urine or by occasional incontinence, and later by sexual impotence and ataxia, with inability to walk, particularly noticeable in the dark, and with loss of balance on closing the eyes. In other instances, the presenting complaint may be loss or dimness of vision because of the optic atrophy not infrequently found in tabes. In still others, ataxia may be the first symptom and may or may not be followed by pains; it is usually associated with a history of incontinence.

Pains and *paresthesias* occur very commonly in tabes (ninety per cent), as may be surmised from the involvement of the posterior roots in the disease. They occur early as a rule, often as the first symptom of the disorders, but late development is sometimes seen and they may be present for a long time before other symptoms appear. They are most frequent in the legs but may occur in the arms or trunk. Their frequency varies, but once established they appear often and do not disappear spontaneously. They are described usually as lightning pains shooting down the legs from hip region to knee, ankle, or foot, or as boring, tearing pains usually felt deep in the tissues. They are increased by coughing, sneezing, etc., and often by movement. Arm pains may radiate and shoot down the arms into the fingers. Sometimes the pains are felt first in the ankles or knees and remain localized but severe. Often associated with the pains are *paresthesias* of various sorts. These are felt usually in the feet as sensations of the feet falling asleep, tingling, or numbness. Paresthesias along the ulnar nerve are common. The sensation of walking on cotton or air is frequently described. This is due to loss of proprioceptive sensation associated with the disease in the posterior columns, the patient failing to recognize when the feet are on the ground or feeling in the usual case as if the feet are treading on cotton, air, springs, etc.

Girdle sensations may appear early and are experienced as tight sensations around the abdomen or waist as if a tight belt were being drawn around the affected part. Similar sensations may be felt around the ankles or thighs. They are often extremely painful. They may be experienced as sharp pains or as band-like constrictions.

Associated with the pains may be objective sensory disturbances, usually ill-defined, patchy areas of decreased pain or touch sensation over the inner aspect of the legs, the trunk, and in some cases the arm. The loss of pain sensation on squeezing the testes is regarded as an early sign of tabes. Squeezing the tendo achillis elicits no pain and no pain is elicited on compression of the ulnar nerve in the elbow.

Ataxia is a prominent symptom but is not present in all cases About one-fourth of all patients with tabes fail to develop the symptom. When present, it is usually well marked. It develops gradually but in some cases may appear acutely. It is increased by loss of vision and may first be noticed on closing the eyes to wash, the patient falling into the wash bowl. The gait is extremely unstable, the base wide, the legs lifted high, the feet slapped down vigorously, and the eyes glued to the ground or on the feet. The patient is unable to stand with the feet together and falls with the eyes closed (Romberg's sign); nor can he walk heel to toe in a straight line. So aware are most tabetic persons of their disability that the mere request to stand with the feet together throws them into a panic. The ataxia of tabes is always associated with evidences of loss of posterior column sensation and is directly proportional to such loss. Loss of position and vibration senses are found in severe cases in the affected limbs, and impairment of these sensations in milder cases.

In patients in whom the cervical cord is involved, there is marked ataxia of the arms, with inability to make coördinated movements, and with much clumsiness.

Reflex disturbances appear early in the disease and are constant features of tabes dorsalis. Absence or decrease of the Achilles reflexes may be one of the earliest signs of the disorder. Similarly, absence or decrease of the patellar reflexes may precede all other evidences of the disease. Both may exist without any evidence of ataxia. The Achilles reflexes may disappear before the patellars, and absent Achilles with retained patellar reflexes may be found early in tabes dorsalis. In patients with cervical cord involvement, absence of biceps, triceps, and supinator reflexes is found.

Among the reflex disturbances of cardinal importance in tabes are those involving the pupils. Most important is the *Argyll Robertson* pupil, which is found in seventy to eighty-five per cent of patients with tabes. It is not pathognomonic of tabes, since it is found in other forms of neurosyphilis, but it is found most commonly in the tabetic form of neurosyphilis. The Argyll Robertson pupil has the following characteristics: (1) It is a contracted, small, irregular pupil, but it may be dilated; in its characteristic form, it is contracted. (2) It does not respond to direct light but responds in accommodation movements. This is not always true, since failure of

reaction to light and in accommodation occurs in advanced stages. (3) It dilates very imperfectly with mydriatics. (4) It fails to dilate on painful stimuli.

Irregular, sluggishly reacting pupils are found in patients with tabes who fail to show Argyll Robertson pupils. A normal pupil is rare in tabes dorsalis.

Visceral crises of many sorts are found. The commonest form is the gastric crisis, which is characterized by attacks of severe abdominal pain associated with vomiting, sweating, tachycardia, and extreme shock. The pain has no relation to food intake. During attacks, no food, either liquid or solid, can be taken by mouth. The attacks vary in intensity and character. Some are much more severe than others. In some instances, pain is unassociated with vomiting. Relief is obtained only by morphine in large doses and then not constantly. It may persist for hours or days. Many other forms of crises occur (rectal, bladder, laryngeal, testicular, uterine, etc.). Rectal crises are featured by paroxysms of rectal pain and tenesmus; bladder and testis crises by pain in these regions, and laryngeal crises by stridor and severe dyspnea.

The cause of visceral crises in tabes is obscure. It is thought to be due to (1) inflammation of the autonomic ganglia, (2) irritation of visceral afferent fibers in the posterior roots, or (3) irritation of the sympathetic fibers that emerge from the spinal cord through the posterior roots.

Sphincter disturbances develop in many patients with tabes (seventy-five per cent). They may develop early, but are usually found in later stages of the disease. The bladder wall is atonic, and difficulty in passing urine due to an atonic detrusor muscle as well as incontinence due to a relaxed atonic sphincter are common complaints.

Sexual impotence is likewise common, and often an early symptom. It is manifested by inability to develop and maintain an erection. Sexual libido usually remains unimpaired. A form of *sacral tabes* occurs with only sexual and sphincter disturbances, loss of reflexes, and pupillary disturbances.

taining the leg fibers, but cases of tabes may run their course without evidence of disturbance of deep sensation, particularly cases of so-called optic tabes. The ataxia of tabes is dependent on the loss of deep sensation and is always proportional to the degree of deep sensory involvement. Position sense is lost in the

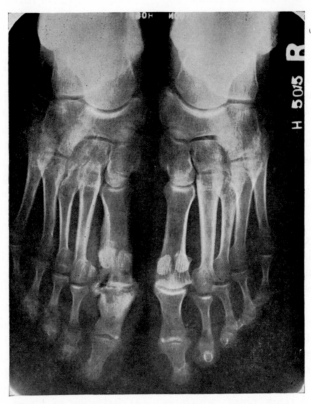

Fig. 88—*Tabes dorsalis.* Charcot joint involving the great toe in an early case of tabes without posterior column signs.

Trophic disturbances of many sorts may be found in tabes. Indolent painless ulcers on the heel or sole of the foot are characteristic. Joint changes, the typical Charcot's joints involving the knee most commonly, but also the elbow, spine, and ankle, are encountered.

Sensory disturbances appear commonly but not constantly. Deep sensation is most affected due to involvement of the posterior columns, especially those con-

great toes, or greatly impaired. In severe cases it may be lost in the large joints (knee, ankle) as well. If the cervical cord is affected, position sense may be lost in the thumbs. Vibration sense is lost over the feet and legs, usually in the same degree as position sense, but a disproportion between the two is not unusual, one being affected more than the other. Vibration sense may be lost and position sense retained. Loss of vibration sense over the sacrum may be an early sign in tabes.

Other forms of sensory involvement are less common, though the patchy areas of decreased pain and touch over the legs and arms have already been mentioned.

Motor Disturbances: Hypotonia of the muscles is common and is most pronounced in advanced cases with resulting hyperextension of the joints. Atrophy of the muscles occurs in four to eight per cent of cases and may involve the arms or legs as well as the tongue, jaw muscles, etc. Marked muscle wasting is sometimes seen in the marasmic form of tabes. Loss of muscle power is not usual, though occasional cases of tabes with later development of hemiplegia have been seen.

Cranial Nerve Involvement: This is quite usual in the disease. The *optic nerve* is frequently affected. Optic atrophy of the primary type is found in twenty to twenty-five per cent of cases. It is sometimes an early symptom. Some cases of tabetic optic atrophy proceed without the development of ataxia. The *oculomotor nerves* may be affected, ptosis and strabismus occurring quite frequently. *Trigeminal symptoms,* such as facial pains of a ticlike character, loss of corneal reflex, ulcers of the mouth, and loss of teeth without pain are found. *Auditory nerve* involvement is common and impairment or loss of hearing is frequently found. Other cranial nerves may also be affected. *Vagus* involvement is sometimes found, associated with swallowing difficulties.

Mental symptoms are found occasionally. These are found most often in cases of taboparesis in which cases of tabes develop signs of cerebral involvement such as are found in paresis. These include evidence of mental deterioration (loss of memory and concentration powers, emotional instability, personality changes, etc.). In other instances, *tabetic*

psychoses have been described (Jakob), quite apart from those found in taboparesis. Their existence as an entity is rare, but it is true that cases of tabes are found with psychosis apart from the mental symptoms of taboparesis. Paranoid types of reaction predominate.

Laboratory Findings: Apart from the serologic changes in the blood and spinal fluid, there are no laboratory findings of significance. It is essential to recognize that negative serologic reactions in blood and/or spinal fluid may occur in tabes. The Wassermann reaction of the blood has been found negative in thirty to thirty-five per cent of the patients, hence the blood Wassermann test cannot be relied upon to confirm a diagnosis of tabes in at least one-third of the cases. In a fresh, untreated case, the cell count of the spinal fluid is elevated (fifteen to one hundred lymphocytes), the globulin and protein increased, and the colloidal gold curve abnormal in fifty to sixty-five per cent of cases, showing no characteristic form. The Wassermann reaction of the spinal fluid is negative in ten to twenty per cent of cases. This percentage is even higher if small amounts of fluid (0.1 cc.) are used in the test. Large amounts of fluid may be necessary to obtain a positive reaction. In some cases the Wassermann reaction of both blood and spinal fluid may be negative. In such patients there are usually other abnormal spinal fluid changes, but this is not always true.

The incidence of negative spinal fluid findings in tabes in variously estimated and is not a matter of agreement among all clinicians. No good statistics are as yet available, and the discrepancies in the estimates of negative spinal fluid findings may be attributed to the following factors: (1) many of the negative reports were made by older laboratory methods; with newer and more sensitive methods,

Table 24—Differential Diagnosis of Tabes Dorsalis

	Onset	Pupils	Reflexes	Posterior Column	Incontinence	Spinal Fluid	Miscellaneous
TABES DORSALIS	Chronic. Pains in legs; ataxia as a rule	Argyll Robertson as a rule; or irregular and poorly reactive to light	Absent: usually patellar and/or Achilles	Loss of position and vibration senses	Usually; late or early	Wassermann usually positive. Gold sol often abnormal. Cells, globulin increased	Optic atrophy some cases. Auditory and other cranial nerves affected
MULTIPLE SCLEROSIS	Chronic with history of remissions	Not abnormal	Overactive	Loss of position and vibration senses often, with other spinal cord signs	Not present	Colloidal gold abnormal often; Wassermann negative	Temporal pallor often, signs of pyramidal tract involvement (Babinski's sign) often
SUBACUTE COMBINED DEGENERATION	Chronic	Not abnormal	Absent or decreased; or overactive	Loss of position and/or vibration senses. May predominate or be exclusively present. Usually associated with Babinski sign or spasticity	Not present	Not abnormal	Pernicious anemia usually present. Other causes also found
NEURITIS	Acute	Not abnormal	Absent	Not affected	Not present	Not abnormal save in acute infectious form with elevated spinal fluid protein	Tenderness of muscle and nerve trunks

it is quite probable that the incidence would be found to be lower. Thus, among 100 patients with tabes tested by newer methods, only 2 had normal blood and spinal fluid findings, and only 12 per cent had negative blood Wassermanns (Merritt, Adams, and Solomon). (2) The reports of blood and spinal fluid Wassermanns are not always comparable in and vibration senses), absence of reflexes, Argyll Robertson pupils, and abnormal reactions in the blood and spinal fluid.

Early diagnosis is essential in order to give treatment its best chance. The diagnosis is tenable in patients with a history of leg pains and paresthesias, or with a history of bladder disturbances

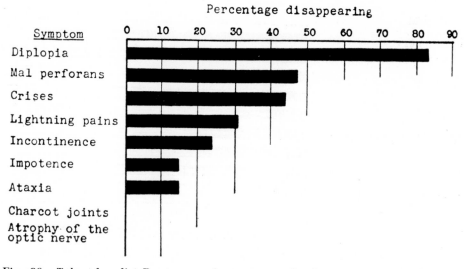

Fig. 89—*Tabes dorsalis.* Percentage of symptoms of tabes dorsalis disappearing under treatment. (*O'Leary, et al.*)

many cases because of differences of method and technic.

Despite more refined methods of laboratory diagnosis, the fact remains that there are patients with tabes, having all the clinical features of the disease, with negative spinal fluid findings. These patients usually are those with long-standing disease, having the so-called burned out cases.

Diagnosis: The diagnosis of tabes in an advanced case is easy, but the prospects of treatment in such instances are poor. The history of leg pains or girdle sensations, bladder and sexual disturbances, and difficulty in walking is supported by the finding of ataxia, disturbances of deep sensation (loss of position and leg pains, with Argyll Robertson pupils, absent Achilles reflexes and/or absent patellar reflexes, and positive blood and spinal fluid Wassermann reactions. In all patients with suspected tabes, examination of both blood and spinal fluid is imperative. The diagnosis of early tabes is sound in such a patient, even with negative blood and/or spinal fluid reactions, provided the syndrome of *tonic pupil* (Adie's syndrome) can be excluded (*v.* Pupils).

Tabes may be found with optic atrophy and absent reflexes, without ataxia. This form, known as optic tabes, usually fails to develop ataxia and is diagnosed on the basis of Argyll Robertson pupils, primary optic atrophy, absent Achilles and patellar reflexes, and abnormal serological reactions. Signs of posterior column disease are absent.

Gastric crises may simulate gastric and gallbladder disorders, but the pupillary and tendon reflex responses will make their nature clear. Many a patient having tabes with gastric crises has been operated on needlessly for some abdom-

ical reactions, absence of Argyll Robertson pupils, and the blood and gastric findings of primary anemia. *Pseudotabetic syndromes* with severe ataxia occurs in diabetes, arsenic poisoning, and alcoholism, but are readily distinguished *Spinal cord tumor* is a remote diagnosis because of pains, but is distinguished by the presence of subarachnoid block,

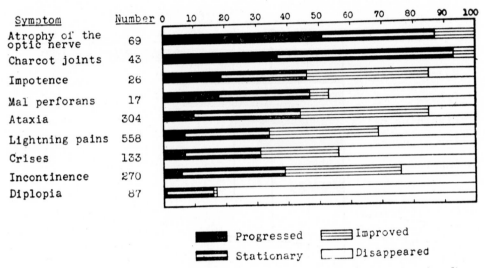

Fig. 90—*Tabes dorsalis.* **Final result of treatment in patients with tabes dorsalis.**
(O'Leary, et al.)

inal condition. There is little need for the failure to recognize gastric crises or the other visceral crises found with tabes, for by the time these develop other evidences of the disease are well pronounced and examination will not fail to reveal them.

The pains make a differentiation from *neuritis* necessary, but the muscle and nerve tenderness, the absence of Argyll Robertson pupils, and the negative serological reactions are helpful. Some cases of tabes are wrongly diagnosed sciatica because of the leg pains. *Subacute combined degeneration* of the anemic type is differentiated by the presence of signs of pyramidal tract involvement (Babinski, overactive reflexes), negative serolog-

the absence of a sensory level, and the negative serological reactions.

Prognosis: Tabes is, on the whole, a disappointing form of neurosyphilis to treat. The disease progresses slowly and runs a course of ten to twenty years. Ataxia, incontinence, and impotence are difficult to influence. It is impossible, however, to speak of the prognosis of tabes as a whole, since the various symptoms of the disease respond variously to treatment. The leg pains respond better than the ataxia, but pains may be extremely resistive to all forms of treatment and may defy relief. Gastric crises respond poorly as a rule, and the ataxia of tabes is most discouraging of all to handle, since treatment can hardly replace destroyed axis cylinders or myelin sheaths. Optic atrophy responds poorly as a rule.

Tabes has a tendency to spontaneous arrest in a respectable percentage of cases (10 per cent). In other instances, the disease may become arrested, though signs of the disease persist. Ataxia, incontinence, optic atrophy, and other symptoms may continue owing to irreversible damage of the respective parts, but the disease may not progress and may remain stationary for years.

Treatment: The treatment of tabes dorsalis is discouraging in a large number of cases from the standpoint of disappearance or even improvement of symptoms, but it is satisfactory from the standpoint of arrest of the disease, since a good number of cases become arrested either spontaneously or as a result of treatment, with persistence of symptoms. It is essential to keep in mind in the treatment of tabes as well as in other forms of neurosyphilis that the response to treatment must be evaluated on the basis of both clinical and serological improvement. Clinical improvement with reversal of blood and spinal fluid findings is the goal of all treatment, but not infrequently it occurs without reversal of either the blood or spinal fluid reactions or with reversal of one or the other. In such instances, the possibility of recurrence or advance of symptoms is always possible and treatment must be continued constantly. Of the serological reactions, the spinal fluid findings are a more valuable index to treatment than is the blood Wassermann reaction. Evaluation of improvement must include all the categories of the spinal fluid tests and not the Wassermann reaction alone. Here, too, it must be clearly understood that reversal of the serological reactions does not indicate cessation of activity, since progression of symptoms can and

does occur in tabes and in other forms of neurosyphilis with negative reactions This serves but to emphasize the necessity for close correlation of clinical and laboratory studies in the treatment, not only of tabes, but of all forms of neurosyphilis.

The treatment of tabes is outstandingly a treatment of individual symptoms. It is not possible to compare the treatment results in patients with severe ataxia with those in patients with symptoms due to root involvement such as pains or girdle sensations, or with the responses of the cranial nerve to treatment. Hence an analysis of the treatment results of tabes becomes invariably an analysis of the response of individual symptoms.

The treatment of tabes dorsalis is unsatisfactory as to cure in many cases but encouraging in the possibility of arrest of the disease and in the treatment of symptoms by specific therapy. In this sense, it is often a treatment directed against the improvement of symptoms. As in all other types of neurosyphilis, the treatment of tabes is an *individual problem;* and for this reason, the handling of tabetic neurosyphilis by uniform courses of treatment is to be discouraged. Each case must be handled on its own merits. Thus, a patient with cachectic type of tabes with pronounced ataxia cannot be treated in the same fashion as one having early disease with no ataxia but with incontinence and lancinating pains.

By the time a patient with tabes reaches the physician, he has usually had some type of treatment, but this is not always the case. In those patients in whom the disease is in an early stage, with pains in the legs, absent reflexes, and slight evidence of posterior column damage, treatment with *penicillin* (10,000,000 to 14,000,000 units) is advisable. For most patients with tabes, *penicillin* therapy is sufficient. Root pains and other symptoms usually respond well to this form of treatment. Incontinence of urine may be improved, as well as ataxia if it is not too far advanced. Dosages of ten to fourteen million units are used, the total dosage being given over a period of ten to fourteen days. The penicillin may be given in a single daily dosage of one million units until the total is completed. The penicillin may be repeated as often as seems necessary to control the symptoms. Some prefer administering the penicillin over a twenty-four-hour period at intervals of six hours. The root pains may be aggravated during the course of the treatment, but subside later. Under rare circumstances malarial therapy needs to be used in addition to penicillin. This form of treatment should be used (1) in patients with early disease, who have had a trial of treatment by arsenicals and bismuth and whose disease has advanced in spite of such treatment; (2) in patients with well-established tabes, who are not cachectic and can tolerate fever therapy; and (3) in patients with optic atrophy. Treatment in the last group is unsatisfactory, since no method is yet available which can assure arrest or recession of optic atrophy. The best possibilities are offered, however, by malaria and penicillin. Malarial fever should be maintained for 150 hours at over 100°F. (37.7°C.) if possible, and for at least 100 hours. Penicillin should be given in doses of 7,000,000 to 10,000,000 units over a 14-day period, preferably in aqueous solution every three hours throughout the twenty-four-hour period but also in 300,000 unit doses in peanut oil every twelve hours if three hour doses are not possible.

In tabes as in other forms of neurosyphilis, the cell count and protein content revert to normal (two to three months) before the Wassermann reaction and the colloidal gold.

Despite specific treatment directed against the disease, symptoms persist or even reappear after patients have been successfully treated, judging by clinical and/or laboratory criteria. *Symptomatic treatment* is often necessary, therefore, during the course of tabes.

Root pains offer a perplexing problem. They may be controlled at times by large doses of *salicylates* (0.972 Gm. [15 grains] four times daily) if they are not too severe or by *salicylates* and *codeine* (0.0324 Gm. [½ grain] three to four times daily). *Meperidine (Demerol)* (50 mg. [¾ grain] three to four times daily) may be used. Given by mouth, addiction is not a serious problem. Morphine must never be used in tabetic root pains for fear of addiction. The same holds true of Dilaudid and other opiates.

The gastric crises of tabes are extremely difficult to control and often defy treatment. *Morphine* is necessary in crises, even large doses often failing to control the pain. *Barbiturates* in large doses may help, preferably *amobarbital sodium* (Amytal Sodium) (.486 Gm. [½ grain]) intravenously, repeated as often as necessary to maintain narcosis. *Paraldehyde* intravenously (2 cc.) may be of help. *Atropine* in large doses may be helpful. Gastric lavage is sometimes helpful. Malarial treatment gives relief in some cases. Operation consisting of section of the posterior roots of the spinal cord (rhizotomy) has been resorted to in some cases and in others cordotomy has been performed. Cordotomy to be effective must be bilateral and above the third thoracic segment. The *bladder incontinence* and *sexual* symptoms respond poorly to treatment.

Since the treatment of tabes is often outstandingly a treatment of symptoms, a consideration of the response of individual symptoms to treatment seems advisable.

The *ataxia* of tabes, if well established, cannot be influenced by treatment or can be influenced only to a minimal degree. It is dependent on destruction of the posterior columns which no amount of treatment can correct.

The *optic atrophy* of tabes and other forms of neurosyphilis responds poorly to treatment. The best therapy by far consists of intensive treatment early in the development of eye symptoms in an effort to prevent further advance of blindness. Tryparsamide should never be used. Drug therapy is of very questionable value. Penicillin in large doses and in repeated courses should be used. Malarial therapy or typhoid vaccine therapy are successful in checking the advance in some cases and, generally speaking, offer the best means of treatment in most instances combined with penicillin. While nothing can be done to restore sight, strong efforts should be made to salvage what remains of eyesight. Most patients with tabetic optic atrophy develop rapid blindness in a short time without treatment; hence proper treatment is essential.

2. Syphilitic Meningomyelitis

Etiology: Syphilitic meningomyelitis is a form of syphilis involving the meninges and cord with a varying clinical picture. Little is known concerning its latency and its age incidence, except that it tends to occur in the middle-aged.

Pathology: Any part of the spinal cord may be affected, but the thoracic and lumbar cords are predominantly involved. The meninges are fibrosed and adherent and contain lymphocytes and plasma cells. The spinal cord damage is variable. There may be a complete transverse syndrome, only involvement of the pyramidal tracts, posterolateral damage, or diffuse areas of involvement of the cord. The posterior roots and ganglia are infiltrated and diseased. The diseased areas are characterized by destruction of myelin and axis cylinders and perivascular infiltration with lymphocytes and plasma cells in both the gray and white matter.

Symptoms: The disease in its most frequent form is seen as a complete transverse myelitis. This usually begins with pains and paresthesias in the trunk and legs. After a variable period of time weakness of the legs develops progressing to complete paralysis, with incontinence of urine, and sensory loss. The picture is one of a complete transverse syndrome (Chapter 2) with motor, sensory, sphincter, and reflex changes.

In other cases, spastic paraplegia develops with incontinence and few sensory changes (Erb's syphilitic paraplegia). Still other patients develop a typical posterolateral sclerosis syndrome with combined ataxia and weakness of the legs.

The serology of the blood and spinal fluid in patients with syphilitic meningomyelitis is almost always strongly positive. The cells are increased, the globulin is elevated, the Wassermann reaction is positive, and the colloidal gold curve abnormal.

Prognosis: The outlook in most cases is poor. The transverse syndromes fail to respond to treatment, while the spastic paraplegias fail to respond or advance, their course being normally slow.

Treatment: Not much is to be gained by treatment. *Mercury* and *bismuth* are to be preferred to arsenic. *Iodides* are also useful. Fever treatment has no value. *Penicillin* has been of little value but should always be used in that same dosage as in tabes.

3. Syphilitic Amyotrophies

Rarely, syphilis may be responsible for one of the amyotrophies such as progressive muscular atrophy or amyotrophic lateral sclerosis. These are in reality forms of syphilitic myelitis or meningomyelitis. The pathology of progressive muscular atrophy of syphilitic origin consists of loss of cells in the anterior horns, with lymphocytic and plasma cell infiltration in the tissues and around the vessels. In amyotrophic lateral sclerosis, the pyramidal tracts are involved in addition to the anterior horn cells and infiltrative changes are found.

The symptoms of the syphilitic type of progressive muscular atrophy and amyotrophic lateral sclerosis are similar to those of the more common degenerative type (*q.v.*) with the minor differences that in the syphilitic type they are likely to develop in younger subjects and somewhat more rapidly.

The symptoms consist mainly of loss of power of the arms and legs, and weakness and clumsiness of the hands. These develop gradually, over a period of months, and are associated with considerable weakness at the time of presentation of the patient for relief. Atrophy of the small hand muscles, atrophy of the arms and shoulder girdles, weakness and spasticity of the legs, and at times atrophy of the leg muscles, muscle fasciculations, and overactive reflexes are present. Bulbar symptoms which are characteristic of the degenerative form of amyotrophic lateral sclerosis are not found in the syphilitic form, and the disease in the syphilitic type is more often asymmetrical than in the degenerative form.

The Wassermann reactions of the blood and spinal fluid are usually positive. The cells may be increased and the colloidal gold abnormal.

The outlook is poor and *antisyphilitic treatment* is of little avail in the disappearance of symptoms. It is valuable in causing arrest of the disease. *Mercury, bismuth,* and *iodides* are preferred to arsenic. *Penicillin* should be given, but its use is of doubtful value.

4. Syphilitic Vascular Disease

Syphilis may at times be responsible for vascular disease of the spinal cord, particularly thrombosis of the anterior spinal artery. The pathology and symptoms are the same as in anterior spinal artery occlusion from other causes (*q.v.*). The serology is positive as a rule in both blood and spinal fluid. Relatively little can be expected from treatment, since the vessel occlusion results in cord softening from which there is no restitution.

XII. TUMORS OF THE SPINAL CORD

Types: Spinal cord tumors may be extramedullary or intramedullary. Extramedullary tumors may be extradural, lying on the outer surface of the dura, or subdural, lying beneath the dura. The subdural location is more common than those in the extradural area.

Extramedullary tumors include new growths of many sorts arising from many sources. Among them are tumors of vertebral origin (sarcoma, osteoma, hemangioma, herniated nucleus pulposus), meningeal origin (fibroblastomas), blood vessel tumors (hemangioma, telangiectasis), congenital and parasitic cysts, etc. Their varied structure and nature are seen in the following list:

EXTRAMEDULLARY TUMORS OF SPINAL CORD

Meningioma	Lipoma
Perineural fibro-	Tuberculoma
blastoma	Arachnoid cysts
Neurofibroma	Herniated nucleus
Hemangioma	pulposus
Chondroma	Hypertrophied liga-
Osteoma and osteo-	mentum flavum
sarcoma	Echinococcus cyst
Sarcoma	Teratoma
Metastatic carcinoma	Dermoid cyst
Lymphosarcoma	Cholesteatoma
Giant cell tumor	Extradural cyst

A perusal of the list of possible extramedullary spinal cord tumors reveals how diverse is their nature and therefore how varied their manifestations and outlook.

Intramedullary tumors include fewer varieties of lesions than those outside the cord substance. Most of them are gliomas, but tuberculoma, hemangioma, sarcoma, and lipoma are found within the cord substance. Of the gliomas, different types are found, chiefly of a slowly growing variety.

Incidence: The actual incidence of spinal cord tumors has never been accurately computed, but they probably form one or two per cent of all neurological lesions. They are, therefore, not common. They are much less common than brain tumors, which outnumber those of the spinal cord eight or nine to one.

Extramedullary benign tumors outnumber intramedullary growths in a ratio of three to one. The chances favor a removable type of lesion much more frequently than in cerebral tumors.

Either sex may be affected, with no predominance in one or the other.

The *age* incidence of spinal cord tumors is spread over a number of decades. Their greatest incidence is between the ages of twenty and sixty, with probably most of them occurring from thirty to fifty or thirty to sixty. Rarely, spinal cord tumors have been reported in children under ten, but their occurrence at this age is most unusual. They occur somewhat more frequently in the second decade (ten to twenty).

Pathology: A knowledge of the pathological features of the many types of spinal cord tumor goes far toward an appreciation of their clinical characteristics; hence they will be considered here in some detail.

1. Extramedullary Types

(a) Fibroblastomas: The fibroblastomas are of meningeal (meningioma) or nerve sheath (perineural fibroblastomas) origin. The meningioma is attached to the dura and is usually subarachnoid in location, while the perineural type is not adherent to the dura. Both types are attached to one or more nerve roots, accounting for the pain so common in these tumors. The spinal cord is compressed, pushed to one side, and may even be flattened by the encroaching neoplasm, giving rise to the symptoms of cord compression characteristic of tumor.

Not all the symptoms of fibroblastomas are caused by root or cord compression. Some are caused by interference with the venous circulation, with resultant spinal cord changes, and others may result from interference with the spinal fluid circulation. The tumors often measure 1 to 2 cm. in length and about half this in diameter, but they may extend for three or four segments in a long sausagelike mass measuring 5 to 6 cm. in rare cases. The meningiomas are associated with increased vascularity of the adjacent bone. Some fibroblastomas may be of the hourglass or dumbbell-shaped variety, part of them being subdural or intradural and another part extradural, the two being connected by a small isthmus of tissue.

Most fibroblastomas are found within the thoracic portion of the vertebral canal. Next in frequency come cervical fibroblastomas, then lumbar, and finally caudal. Their relative occurrence may be seen at a glance at the accompanying chart. Most fibroblastomas are found on the lateral surface of the spinal cord or in anterolateral or posterolateral positions. Relatively few are found entirely posteriorly and still fewer entirely on the anterior surface of the cord.

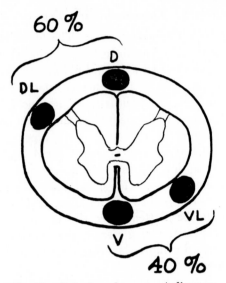

Fig. 91—*Spinal cord tumors*. A diagram illustrating the common locations of extramedullary spinal cord tumors.

(b) Metastatic Carcinoma: These tumors are always extramedullary and practically never within the cord substance. Only a few cases are on record of metastatic carcinoma invading the spinal cord itself. The breast and prostate are the most prolific sources, but carcinoma anywhere in the body may involve the cord. As a rule, the vertebrae show evidence of invasion by carcinoma, but it is not unusual to find it without evidence of bone metastasis. Carcinoma may involve any part of the vertebral column. It is chiefly extradural but may be subdural, and spreads in a sheetlike mass over the dura, sometimes covering several segments. It is adherent to the dura and invades the nerve roots. The spinal cord is softened and shows extensive destruction beneath the mass, due at times to occlusion of extradural blood vessels by the carcinoma or to compression of the cord by an extensively invaded vertebra which has buckled and compressed the cord. In the latter type of case, no intraspinal carcinoma is found, the compression syndrome resulting from the invaded and buckled vertebra. Intramedullary invasion of the spinal cord by carcinoma practically never occurs.

Metastatic carcinoma is not always associated with evidence of cord compression. Symptoms resulting only from compression and/or root infiltration with carcinoma may follow metastasis to the cauda equina. Similar metastasis may involve one or more roots in the vertebral canal without cord compression. In many such instances, compression eventually follows if the condition is not detected.

(c) Hemangioma: Blood vessel tumors of the spinal cord are rare. They may be primary within the spinal canal, or they may develop as extensions of a vertebral hemangioma which is primary within the body of the vertebra, the soft tissue protruding into the canal. Rarely, acute cord compression may be due to hemorrhage within such a tumor. Hemangioma of the vertebrae may be detected by their characteristic roentgenographic findings featured by longitudinal striations within the affected vertebra or vertebrae. Hemangioblastomas are found in rare instances, similar in histologic structure to those found in the posterior fossa. Telangiectases are also encountered within the spinal canal. They are usually venous and may extend for several segments over the surface of the cord. In rare instances they may run the entire length of the cord. The varices may follow along spinal roots and cause root pains. Telangiectases are often associated with vessel abnormalities within the cord proper.

(d) Sarcoma: Sarcomas of the spinal cord are rare. They include the following types: Lymphosarcoma, osteosarcoma, reticulum cell sarcoma, spindle cell and giant cell sarcoma. They arise often within the vertebrae (osteosarcomas), extending into the spinal canal from this primary focus. Roentgenologic evidence of their presence is usually found. Melanotic sarcoma may involve the spine. Lymphosarcomas are almost always extradural and are usually found on the posterior surface of the cord.

(e) Lipoma: These tumors are rare. They involve any part of the cord, they may be extradural or intradural, they are encapsulated, and they not infrequently are composed of an intramedullary portion with an extramedullary extension. They have no characteristic clinical features. They are often associated with a spina bifida.

(f) Herniated Intervertebral Disc: This may be regarded as a tumor in the sense that it gives evidence of its presence on protrusion into the spinal canal. Actually, it is not a new growth. It consists of a herniation through the lacerated annulus fibrosus of the nucleus pulposus which protrudes into the spinal canal or, probably more often, of the annulus itself. Hence the term herniated intervertebral disc is more accurate than herniated nucleus pulposus. The protrusion is usually posterior through a small tear in the annulus fibrosus. Posterolateral herniations occur. These are most often seen in the lumbar and cervical regions but are found also rarely in the thoracic region. The protruded tissue is seen as a fibrous cartilaginous mass measuring 0.5 to 1 or 2 cm. lying extradurally on the posterior surface of the canal and often compressing spinal roots. It may be multiple, and it may be found not infrequently at necropsy without having given symptoms during life. Associated with the protrusion of the nucleus pulposus is narrowing of the intervertebral disc, but this occurs also in decalcifying disease of the bone and herniation of the nucleus pulposus upward into the spongiosa of the vertebral body. Rarely, calcification of the intervertebral disc is found in association with herniation of the nucleus pulposus.

(g) Miscellaneous: Osteomas of the spinal canal are rare, as are osteochondromas. Giant cell tumors of bone may at times affect the vertebrae, causing symptoms of cord compression. Tumors of this type usually appear in the young. There is roentgen ray evidence of their pressure, in addition to signs of spinal cord compression. The same may be said of parasitic cysts (echinococcus), and teratomas. The teratomas may be intramedullary, subarachnoid, or subdural. They may be found usually in the cervical, lumbosacral, or sacrococcygeal regions, are chiefly cystic, and are at times associated with syringomyelia. Dermoids, epidermoids, and chordomas are rare. Granulomas have been referred to (pachymeningitis). Neurological symptoms are common in myeloma, paraplegia being one of the earliest to appear. The vertebrae are commonly involved. The myeloma is usually in the epidural space. Hodgkin's disease occasionally is characterized by the development of an extradural mass of tissue, usually in the thoracic region. The same is true of leukemia. Most of the cases of spinal cord involvement associated with Hodgkins disease are the result of extension of the disease to the extradural space without bone involvement. In other instances there may be (1) invasion of the vertebrae with destruction of the bone and compression of the spinal cord by collapse of the vertebra, (2) extension into the subdural space from the extradural space, (3) invasion of the nerve roots in the intervertebral foramina, (4) degeneration of tracts within the spinal cord itself, without evidence of infiltration. Achondroplasia is not infrequently associated with involvement of the spinal cord, due to narrowing of the spinal canal. Partial or complete transverse syndromes may develop. Decompression may afford relief. Encroachment on the spinal cord may occur in Paget's disease.

Spinal extradural cyst is a rare condition occurring in adolescents, with a history of progressive paraplegia without pain or with very little pain. Objective sensory disturbances are slight, and their upper level is usually in the midthoracic region. Spontaneous remissions occur in the disease. There is usually erosion of the interpedicular spaces of the vertebrae. The condition is sometimes associated with kyphosis dorsalis juvenilis and vertebral epiphysitis (Scheuerman's disease). Improvement of symptoms may follow diagnostic removal of spinal fluid (Turner). The cysts are regarded as the result either of (1) congenital diverticula of the dura mater, or (2) herniations of the arachnoid through a dural defect. The available evidence seems to favor the latter concept. Compression of the spinal cord may develop rarely from *aneurysm of the aorta,* resulting in spastic paraplegia and pain. The process is gradual and progressive. The symptoms may be produced by (1) erosion of the vertebrae with direct compression of the spinal cord, (2) epidural hemorrhage due to rupture of the aneurysm, (3) kyphosis, with pinching off of the spinal cord. The reported cases have all been due to syphilis.

2. Intramedullary Tumors

(a) Gliomas: By far the largest number of intramedullary spinal cord tumors are gliomas. Most of these are thoracic or cervical in location. They may extend for two or three to seven or eight or even more segments. Gliomas extending the entire length of the spinal cord have been described. They may involve any portion of the spinal cord, but some, such as the ependymomas, have a distinct predilection for the lumbosacral portion of the cord. The cord diameter is enlarged in the invaded areas and may fill or almost fill the vertebral canal. In this fashion they tend to block the subarachnoid space, in many instances giving evidence of partial or complete subarachnoid obstruction. The manner of invasion of the cord varies from case to case. In some instances, the tumor may destroy almost the entire cord substance, leaving only a rim of cord tissue around it. In others, it may invade only a small part of the cord diameter; or it may destroy much in one area and relatively less in another. Infiltrating tumors may be sharply demarcated from the surrounding tissue and have been removed *in toto* in a few instances. In the usual case, they are diffusely infiltrating and hardly discernible from the rest of the tissue. The degree of destruction in an infiltrating spinal cord tumor is not proportional to the degree of invasion. In other words, a glioma may invade widely, but may not give rise to evidence of extensive cord destruction, since many intact functioning nerve fibers may pass through the invaded tumor area. Some gliomas of the spinal cord are in part or wholly cystic. Syringomyelic cavities associated with infiltrating tumors are not uncommon. The types of glioma found in the spinal cord vary to include ependymomas, astrocytomas, glioblastoma multiforme, polar spongioblastoma, astroblastoma, oligodendroglioma, medulloblastoma. Of these, the relatively benign ependymomas outnumber all others (sixty to seventy per cent). Astrocytomas occur next in frequency. Other glioma types are rare. The medulloblastomas involve the spinal cord by secondary extension from tumors of this type in the posterior fossa. They usually extend into the spinal subarachnoid space, but may penetrate into the central canal of the cord. They may form a thin film of cells or a very thick layer extending the entire length of the spinal subarachnoid space, chiefly along the posterior surface. Similarly, they may

entire literature) to invade the spinal cord. It has no specific features.

(d) Hemangioma: It may be intra-medullary and widely invasive. It is sometimes cystic.

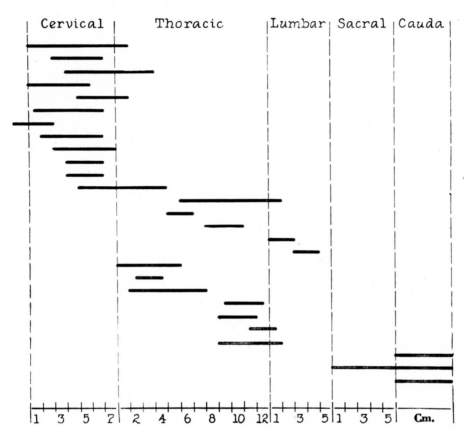

Fig. 92—*Intramedullary spinal cord tumor,* illustrating the longitudinal extent of 27 tumors involving the spinal cord. (*Shenkin & Alpers.*)

form a small plug in the central canal or such a large one as to destroy a good deal of the surrounding spinal cord.

(b) Tuberculomas: They may at times invade the spinal cord. They are usually solitary, well-defined, only locally destructive, and differ in no way in their structure from tuberculomas elsewhere in the body.

(c) Carcinoma: It has been reported on very rare occasions (nine cases in the

3. *Symptoms of Extramedullary Tumors*

The symptoms of spinal cord tumor vary according to whether the tumor is extra- or intramedullary. In either instance, the course of the disease is slow, chronic, and progressive, all of these important diagnostic factors. The story as a rule covers a period of many months or years and is characterized by a steady progression of symptoms, usually without letup. In rare instances the onset is acute, with sudden evidence of cord compression after straining or even after lumbar puncture. In such instances symptoms have usually been present prior to the onset of the acute compression of the cord.

Pain is an important symptom of extramedullary tumors, but is not as prominent in the intramedullary group. It is frequently the first symptom (eighty to ninety per cent), and in those instances in which it is not, it makes its appearance sooner or later during the course of the illness. In unusual instances, extramedullary tumors run their course without pain, especially in the case of tumors situated on the anterior surface of the cord. Pain may be the only symptom for a long period in rare cases. The pain is variously described as sharp, tearing, boring, lancinating, etc., and is felt usually on one side around the thorax and abdomen, in the leg or arm, depending on the location of the tumor. Since the majority of extramedullary fibroblastomas are in the thoracic region, the pain is most often in the thorax or abdomen and is often referred to the axilla or scapula. It is distributed along the course of a spinal root or roots, a careful description of the pain making this clear. It is increased by movement, coughing, sneezing, jarring, etc., and is often relieved by change of posture. The pain usually remains persistent in the area in which it is felt. On the other hand, it may persist for months, then disappear completely or recur after a long interval. Intervals of freedom from pain are not uncommon and may in some instances cover a long period of time. The pain in the thorax or abdomen is not infrequently regarded as due to intercostal neuralgia or to visceral disease (gallbladder, appendix, stomach, pelvis) and operations are sometimes needlessly performed in such cases. Cervical tumors frequently produce pain in the back of the neck, in the shoulder or arm; thoracic tumors in the back, under the scapula, shoulders, in the region of the kidney, or under the costal margin; lumbar tumors in the back or leg along the distribution of the sciatic nerve or along other nerve roots in the leg. Pain is often not present in tumors situated on the anterior aspect of the cord.

Accompanying the pain or following it, *paresthesias* make their appearance in a large percentage of cases. They appear very frequently (seventy-five to eighty-five per cent) in both extramedullary and intramedullary tumors, and are referred to as sensations of numbness, tingling, formication, burning, dryness, coldness, stinging, pins and needles, etc. They are probably more constant in intramedullary growths. They may be felt at the level of the tumor or well below it and in the latter instance are the result of irritation of sensory tracts within the spinal cord. Heaviness of the limbs or a sensation of walking on cotton or air may be encountered.

Pain and paresthesias or pain alone may exist for some time before the onset of *motor symptoms*. These appear as a later symptom, following pain and paresthesias as a rule, but they may be the very first symptom of an extramedullary tumor in a small group of cases (ten to fifteen per cent). The duration of the latent period between the onset of pains and the development of motor signs is not constant. It varies widely, but in most cases covers a period of months. In the case of cervical and cauda equina tumors, where there is much room for the tumor to expand, motor symptoms are, as a rule, slower to develop than in the case of tumors in the thoracic canal. They are manifested first as a subjective feeling of numbness or weakness, usually felt in both legs but sometimes in only one. The weakness varies, depending upon the level of the cord compression, whether cervical, thoracic, or lumbar, and on the site of the tumor, whether lateral, posterior, or anterior.

In cervical tumors, weakness of an arm may be the first evidence of motor involvement, or a spinal hemiplegia is at times seen. Leg weakness is usually the first sign of motor involvement due to the predominance of tumors in the thoracic region below the cervical cord level. The weakness of the legs progresses slowly but definitely and the gait, at first described as clumsy, later becomes shuffling and spastic. Examination reveals a typical extensor spastic weakness of the legs, with dragging of the feet in walking, overactive reflexes, and Babinski's signs. Flaccid weakness or paralysis is found in some tumors, especially in cauda equina tumors and in tumors compressing the anterior surface of the cord. Flexion paraplegia is found in some cases of long-standing paralysis of the legs. Some extramedullary tumors may run their course with only motor weakness, without the involvement of sensory disturbances. While the development of weakness of the legs is slow in most cases, covering a period of months to years, it is rapid in others. Sudden paraplegia may develop in a fibroblastoma after straining at stool or following diagnostic spinal puncture due to the removal of the pad of spinal fluid between the tumor and the spinal cord. In metastatic carcinoma, sudden onset of paraplegia is usual, due to the cord destruction which accompanies carcinoma. Sudden paraplegia may develop also in sarcoma, leukemia, Hodgkin's disease, etc. Remissions from the weakness, complete or almost complete, are occasionally seen in cord tumors. During these periods the limbs may regain much of their power, only to lapse again later.

After the cord has been subjected to compression for a time, *sensory symptoms* appear. These are manifested by the occurrence of a sensory level which is often one or two segments lower than the level of the cord compression by the tumor. Above this level is a zone of hyperesthesia one or two segments in width and often an area of only slightly disturbed sensation. The sensory level develops slowly as a rule and is associated in severe cases with an interruption of all forms of sensation (pain, touch, heat, cold, position, and vibration). In some instances, only one or two sensory modalities may be affected or the sensory impairment may be slight and sensory level difficult to determine. Involvement of the sacral dermatomes is found in extramedullary growths due to the fact that the fibers from these dermatomes lie externally in the spinothalamic tract and are compressed first by tumors on the outside of the spinal cord. The sacral dermatomes, on the other hand, are often spared in the case of intramedullary tumors. A Brown-Séquard type of sensory involvement is not infrequently found in extramedullary tumors. *Tenderness of the spinous processes* is found often in both extra- and intramedullary tumors, the tender spine or spines being as a rule a little below the level of the tumor. A vasomotor level is often present and may be an early sign of extramedullary cord tumors. *Sphincter disturbances* are present in almost all cases, usually manifested as incontinence of urine or difficulty in starting the stream. In severe cases, rectal incontinence is present. Sphincter disturbances usually develop late.

4. Symptoms of Intramedullary Tumors

The history of complaints is usually long, for it seems to be well demonstrated that gliomas may grow within the cord for a considerable period without giving rise to symptoms. The length of the clinical course has been found to een to twenty months) to several years (four to five years). In this respect the intramedullary tumors cannot be differentiated from the extramedullary group.

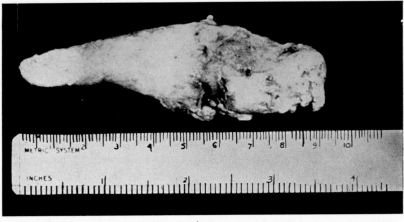

A

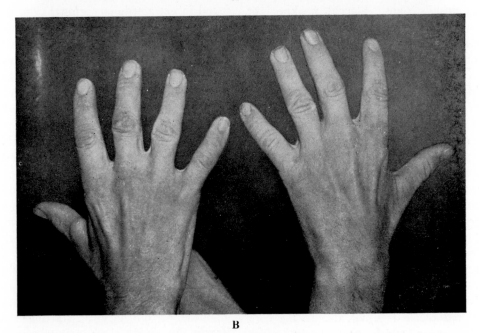

B

Fig. 93—*Cervical cord tumor*, showing the atrophy of the interossei due to compression of the lower cervical roots, and the tumor removed at the level of C5-C8.

vary widely between limits of six weeks to seventeen years. It is difficult to give an accurate estimate of the average duration of symptoms except to say that they usually vary from several months (eight-

The onset of symptoms conforms to no uniform pattern. In a surprising number of patients the onset is with pain; in others, paresthesias appear first; in still others, motor weakness, and, in rare instances, the onset has been with sphincter disturbance. Once symptoms have developed they are likely to progress steadily, but remission of symptoms is not unknown and may be seen not infrequently in a large series of tumors.

The pain encountered in intramedul-

often referred to areas distant from the level of the tumors, and is described as a burning or boring sensation conforming neither to root nor to peripheral nerve distribution. In some instances, an anesthesia dolorosa is found. In many cases, spinal pain is encountered. This is usu-

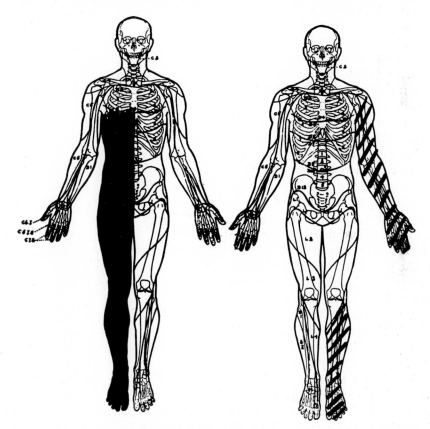

Fig. 94—*Spinal cord tumor*. An infiltrating tumor of the spinal cord showing a Brown-Séquard type of sensory dissociation with loss of pain and temperature in the left figure (black) and loss of position and vibration in the right figure (cross hatch).

lary gliomas may be of several varieties. Typical root pain is not unusual and may be indistinguishable from that of extramedullary tumors. It may usher in the disease, appear within one or two months after the onset of symptoms, or develop later in the course of the illness. On the other hand, it may conform to the features of so-called tract pain, in which case it is likely to be diffuse, is

ally a dull, aching soreness of the back muscles, usually influenced by posture. Associated with the history of pain is that of paresthesias, though the latter may precede the pain and in some instances usher in the disease. Once they appear they are likely to be both persistent and progressive, and they are so variously described as to merit no accounting of their many manifestations.

They are found in segments of the body corresponding to the level of the tumor, but it is not unusual to encounter them at levels well below the tumor location.

Motor symptoms may usher in the picture in many instances. Once the motor symptoms appear, they tend to be progressive. The motor findings depend naturally upon the level of the infiltrating tumor, its longitudinal and horizontal extent through the spinal cord, the degree of blockage of the subarachnoid space, and the rapidity of growth of the tumor on the motor side. Cervical cord tumors are prone to develop an amyotrophic syndrome with a combination of anterior horn and pyramidal pathway involvement; thoracic and lumbar gliomas on the other hand usually develop a spastic limb weakness. Sensory examination discloses usually a well-defined sensory level, though it is claimed by some that this is not as a rule present. This is more likely to involve superficial than deep sensation, though all forms of sensation may be affected. The sensory level is, as a rule, sharp, though it may be ill-defined. Since the tumor grows within the spinal cord, the observation that the lowermost segments are spared or are less affected than those at the level of the tumor is a very important feature. A Brown-Séquard syndrome is encountered at times, and anogenital sparing is common.

Sphincter disturbances are apt to be late in intramedullary tumors, and by no means appear in every case (sixty per cent). Early incidence is well known, however, and in rare instances sphincter trouble has ushered in the clinical picture.

Tenderness of the spine may be present. Cranial nerve signs are sometimes encountered, especially in tumors of the cervical cord.

Manometric studies show a high frequency of subarachnoid block which may be complete or partial, but in some instances the manometric studies are normal. The total protein may be increased or normal in value. When increased it appears to be highest in infiltrating tumors of the cervical cord. It is often increased without a corresponding pleocytosis.

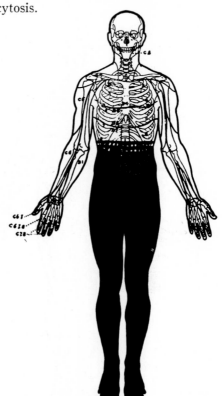

Fig. 95—*Spinal cord tumor* showing a typical complete sensory level at T8 with loss of touch, pain, and temperature sensations.

The outstanding feature is the progressive development of *motor weakness* involving usually the legs, but in some instances all the extremities, painless in many instances, but not infrequently accompanied by paresthesias or pains of the type described. Paresthesias occur very frequently, often at a distance below the level of the tumor. The motor weakness develops gradually over a period of months or years to complete paralysis of

Table 25—Upper Vertebral Levels of 296 Tumors of the Spinal Cord
(Elsberg)

Vertebral Level	Extradural	Intradural	Extradural and Intradural	Intramedullary	Totals
CERVICAL 1 TO 3......	4	12			16
CERVICAL 4 TO 8......	17	28	2	5	52
THORACIC 1 TO 3......	10	24	1	5	40
THORACIC 4 TO 8......	2	48		1	74
THORACIC 9 TO 12.....	12	6	1	3	52
LUMBAR 1 TO 3........	6	20		15	41
LUMBAR 4 TO 5........	8	12			20
SACRAL..............	1				1
TOTALS..........	83	180	4	29	296

Table 26—Relative Frequency of Histological Types
(Elsberg)

Types of Tumors	Extradural	Intradural	Extradural and Intradural	Intramedullary	Totals
PERINEURIAL FIBROMA..	5	5	..	..	59
MENINGEAL FIBRO-BLASTOMA..........	4	69	..	.	73
SARCOMA.............	22	9	..		31
ANGIOMA } HEMANGIOBLASTOMA	4	5	..	..	9
FIBROMA.............	4	2	..	..	6
NEUROFIBROMA (von Recklinghausen)..	1	3	1	..	5
DERMOID.............	0	4	..	..	4
LIPOMA..............	1		..	3	6
EPENDYMOMA.........	0	0	..	11	11
CYST................	2	1	..	..	3
GANGLIONEUROMA......	2	..	..	..	2
CHONDROMA HERNIATION OF NUCLEUS PULPOSUS	27	..	..	..	27
GRANULOMA..........	2	..	..	..	2
METASTATIC AND SECONDARY..........	11	2	1	..	14
UNCLASSIFIED........	..	8*	..	..	8
GLIOMA.............	..	..	..	14	14
TUBERCULOMA........	..	..	..	1	1
TOTALS..........	85	159	2	29	275

*Mostly tumors of the conus and cauda equina, many of which, perhaps, should be classified as intramedullary growths.

the affected limbs, usually of a spastic nature. In rare instances, the paraplegia may be flexion in type instead of the typical extension posture of the limbs. *Sensory disturbances* develop *pari passu* with the motor weakness usually, but may lag behind. They are characterized by transverse sensory loss to the level of the lesion, or by a Brown-Séquard type of sensory disturbance. *Sphincter disturbances* are common, particularly incontinence of urine.

5. *Spinal Fluid in Spinal Cord Tumors*

Much dependence is placed upon the spinal fluid findings in tumors affecting the spinal cord, since the history of pain and progressive motor impairment is by no means pathognomonic.

Manometric (Queckenstedt) tests are extremely important (*v.* Spinal Fluid, Chapter 2). In extramedullary tumors, subarachnoid block is present in almost all cases. Subarachnoid block is tested by means of an ordinary lumbar puncture. With the needle in place and a water manometer attached, the jugular veins are compressed lightly and then firmly for ten seconds. Under normal conditions there will result a rapid rise and fall of the fluid column in the manometer, the pressure returning to normal within ten to fifteen seconds. This is a negative Queckenstedt test. If a complete block is present due to obliteration of the subarachnoid space by tumor, there will be no rise of the fluid column whatever (positive Queckenstedt). If partial block is present, the rise will be slow and slight, and the fall will likewise be slow with failure to return to the normal level. Straining and coughing will produce a rise in the fluid level even if complete block is present. When present, it is an extremely important finding in support of the diagnosis of extramedullary tumor. In some in-

stances, extramedullary tumor may be present without any evidence of block whatever, while in others only partial block is found. In intramedullary tumors the block is partial or absent, but in other circumstances may be complete.

Next to manometric tests, the *total protein* content of the spinal fluid gives the most information in spinal cord tumor. It is increased (100 mg. or more) in many (sixty-five to seventy per cent) cases, the level depending on the site of the tumor, and the degree of block of the spinal fluid pathways. Generally speaking, the lower the level of block in the spinal subarachnoid space, the higher the total protein level in the spinal fluid. In some cases the spinal fluid protein reaches as high as 3000 to 4000 mg., but this is not common. The spinal fluid is yellow (xanthochromic) in some cases, a valuable finding in a suspected instance of spinal cord tumor. In rare instances the *Froin Syndrome* is found. This is characterized by xanthrochromia, high protein content of the spinal fluid (3000 to 4000 mg.), and coagulation of the fluid on standing.

In some instances, the cell count in the spinal fluid is increased, but in most cases it is normal.

6. *The Roentgenogram in Cord Tumors*

Roentgenograms may be helpful in some cases by disclosing bone destruction, as in carcinoma and sarcoma. Erosion of the pedicles of the vertebrae may be found in some encapsulated tumors. Calcification of a tumor may be seen on rare occasions. Pantopaque studies to diagnose tumor are helpful and in many instances are necessary in order to establish the diagnosis. The contrast medium is injected into the spinal canal and followed by fluoroscopy. Complete arrest is seen in many extramedullary tumors, incomplete arrest in arachnoiditis, intra-medullary and some extramedullary tumors.

7. *Varieties of Cord Tumors*

(a) **Cervical Cord Tumors:** Tumors of the cervical cord region possess features peculiar to their location. Some cervical cord tumors are situated high in the cervical region and penetrate through the foramen magnum. The *foramen magnum* and *high cervical cord tumors* are of several sorts. They may be primary fibroblastomas involving the foramen magnum and upper cervical cord region, or they may be posterior fossa tumors which have penetrated through the foramen magnum (ependymomas). Their specific features are ill-defined. Pain in the back of the neck and head is common, as is also pain in the shoulder. The pain often radiates over the back of the head to the vertex. Weakness of one or both arms, astereognosis, and in some cases choked disc are found. Due to the penetration of the tumors into the posterior fossa, symptoms referable to this area are not uncommon. Vertigo, difficulties in swallowing and articulation, and ataxia are sometimes found. Atrophy of the sternomastoid muscles, unilateral atrophy of the tongue, and atrophy and weakness of the shoulder girdle muscles are seen. Particularly frequent is the shoulder girdle atrophy due to compression of the upper cervical roots. Evidences of compression of the cord and of a transverse lesion are very late in appearing due to the roominess of the cervical canal, which permits considerable growth of the tumor before cord compression symptoms develop.

The diagnosis of a high cervical cord tumor penetrating into the foramen magnum is difficult. It is made on the basis of a history of long-standing, persistent pains involving the back of the head and neck, and often involving shoulder girdle; on the history of weakness of an arm or shoulder, or of both arms and shoulders; on accessory symptoms such as vertigo, and difficulties in articulation and swallowing; on the demonstration of atrophy of the shoulder girdle muscles, sometimes unilateral tongue and sternomastoid atrophy, and few sensory disturbances. Signs of cord compression appear late, subarachnoid block is usually difficult to demonstrate, and the total protein of the spinal fluid may or may not be elevated. The symptoms and signs are those only of root irritation (pain) for a long period of time and tumors in this region are therefore often regarded as cases of neuralgia for long periods of time.

Cervical cord tumors below the third cervical segment give a story and findings different from those of the high cervical tumors. Here, too, because of the roominess of the cervical canal, root symptoms are long persistent before evidences of cord compression develop. Pain in the shoulder, between the shoulder blades, or along the arm is frequent. It is constant or intermittent, increased by coughing, sneezing, etc., and is present for months or years before cord compression symptoms develop. The pain may be felt along the outer side of the forearm and hand if the lower cervical roots are involved ($C_{7,\,8}$) or along the medial aspect if the midcervical roots ($C_{5,\,6}$) are affected. Paresthesias of the little and ring fingers may develop in tumors affecting the roots of the seventh or eighth cervical segments, or of the thumb and first two fingers in the case of the fifth and sixth cervical roots. These may be present without pain. Weakness of the fingers or arm, unilateral or bilateral, follows symptoms of pain. There may be a loss of dexterity in the use of the fingers, or clumsiness may be noted in many movements. After a long period of time, weakness of the legs develops with stiffness and sometimes ataxia. Paresthesias of the feet and legs may occur early, before arm symptoms develop. Weakness of the legs may also be an early symptom. Incontinence is late in appearing.

Examination reveals very little in the early stages of root irritation. Later there appears atrophy of the small hand muscles or of the arm or shoulder girdle muscles, unilateral or bilateral, associated with muscle fasciculations, and loss or decrease of the biceps or triceps reflexes. At this stage, the picture is that of amyotrophic lateral sclerosis with arm or shoulder pains, usually without lateral column findings (spasticity, increased reflexes, Babinski's sign), giving rise to an impression of an amyotrophic syndrome. A unilateral Horner's syndrome may be found at this stage. In the advanced stages, there is in addition evidence of cord compression with a complete or incomplete transverse syndrome, characterized by weakness of the legs, spasticity, overactive reflexes, Babinski's signs, and a sensory level involving all or a few forms of sensation. In this fully advanced stage, therefore, there is pain in the arms or shoulders, atrophy of the hand, arm, or shoulder girdle muscles, evidences of a transverse lesion, and, as a rule, indications of subarachnoid block with a high protein content of the spinal fluid. The diagnosis in this stage offers no difficulties.

(b) Thoracic Cord Tumors: Apart from the location of the pain, there is very little of localizing significance in thoracic tumors. In high thoracic tumors, the pain is felt frequently under one shoulder blade and is often mistaken for gallbladder colic. The pain may also be felt around the chest or abdomen on one or both sides. Thoracic tumors may at times give rise to pain in the leg, mistakenly regarded as typical sciatica. Gir-

dle sensations around thorax or abdomen are common. Pressure symptoms produce motor and later sensory paralysis, with paralysis of the legs and a sensory level which is usually well defined. The abdominal reflexes may be lost early in some tumors and testicular pain may be lost early in low thoracic tumors. Choked disc has been associated at times with tumors in the upper cervical region of the spinal canals, especially with those encroaching on the foramen magnum. Very rare instances of choked disc has been reported associated with spinal cord tumors of the lower thoracic cord.

(c) Lumbosacral Cord Tumors: The pain in lumbar cord tumors is in the leg or

Table 27

Frequency of Tumors Compared to Number of Vertebrae and to Relative Lengths of the Cervical, Thoracic, and Lumbar Cord

(Elsberg)

Vertebrae	Length of Spinal Cord (Ravenel)	Tumors
Cervical 7 = 29%	10 cm. = 23%	68 = 23%
Thoracic 12 = 50%	26 cm. = 58%	166 = 56%
Lumbar 5 = 21%	8.5 cm. = 19%	62 = 21%

legs. It may be felt along the sciatic distribution or in one of its branches. Sphincter disturbances appear early. Weakness of the legs appears early and changes affecting the patellar and Achilles reflexes are found.

(d) Cauda Equina Tumors: The features of caudal tumors are relatively easy to define on paper but are difficult to combine in the diagnosis of tumor. *Back pain* is a frequent early symptom and may persist for a long time before other features develop. *Pain* in one or both legs is common (eighty-five per cent), and is more often unilateral than bilateral. It is frequently dismissed as sciatica, since the radiation is often typically along the sciatic nerve. Nerve tenderness is usually not present, but may be present in moderate degree at the sciatic notch. It is wise to remember that in some cases local compression may cause typical tenderness along the entire nerve trunk sufficient to resemble neuritis very closely. Lasègue's sign is usually positive. Pain in the perineum or in the bladder or rectum occurs at times. Pain may be completely absent throughout the life cycle of a cauda equina tumor.

Accompanying the pain or following it by some time is *motor weakness*. This may develop as weakness in one or both legs, and is more often unilateral than bilateral. The weakness in severe cases may develop into complete or almost complete paralysis, which is flaccid in type. More often the weakness remains partial and may involve only some muscle groups. Atrophy of the affected muscles is usually present, but is by no means constant and is not necessarily severe. It may be quite slight —a little flattening of a muscle or a mild decrease in bulk. The distribution of the weakness and muscle atrophy varies greatly. In severe cases, the quadriceps, hamstrings, and the calf muscles may all be involved. In other instances, only the quadriceps or hamstring groups may be affected, or only the gastrocnemius group, or there may be varying combinations of weakness and atrophy. Foot-drop may be noted by the patient, who may complain of an inability to clear his foot of the ground or a propensity to stumble frequently. In cases of quadriceps weakness, the leg will be found to give way under the patient due to inability to lock the leg in extension. In other cases, inability to plantar flex the foot may be noted. *Sensory disturbances* when present are radicular in type. They are frequently absent. Saddle types of sensory disturbances may be found. *Bladder dis-*

turbances, such as difficulty in starting the stream, may occur. Loss of sexual libido and potentia may be present. Both bladder and sexual disturbances are said to be more common involvements of the sacral portion of the cord (conus medullaris), but the distinction is often academic because the conus may be compressed by a tumor in the cauda equina, and because also sphincter and sexual disturbances may be produced by involvement of the sacral roots.

The Achilles tendon reflex is absent or decreased and the patellar reflexes are similarly affected if the lumbar roots are involved.

The manometric tests in cauda equina tumor are often of no help because the spinal canal in its lowermost portion is so roomy that only a very large tumor could cause a complete subarachnoid block. The spinal fluid may be yellow and the protein is often increased. Pantopaque injection may often be necessary in order to establish the diagnosis of tumor.

The diagnosis of a cauda equina syndrome is quite difficult, but may be suspected in the presence of a long history of unremitting pain in the back and leg or legs, atrophy of the leg or legs with weakness of varying degree, reflex changes, and/or sensory disturbances. The diagnosis becomes extremely difficult if nerve tenderness is present, since the very same picture may be produced by cauda equina or peripheral neuritis. As between the two, an increase of spinal fluid protein will favor tumor, but may be associated with some forms of neuritis. Sphincter disturbances will favor tumor. Only the subsequent course may settle the issue. Cauda equina syndromes vary widely in their manifestations from full-blown types to syndromes which resemble sciatica, with little or no muscle atrophy or weakness and only mild reflex changes, to others with no pain but with definite motor, sensory, and reflex disturbances.

Cauda equina syndromes result from a variety of causes, such as encapsulated tumors of various sorts, herniated nucleus pulposus, arachnoiditis, metastatic carcinoma, sarcoma, pachymeningitis.

general practitioner; the second is the task of the neurologist or neurosurgeon.

The decision as to whether a spinal cord tumor is present will be determined by a chronic, progressive history with root pain for long periods in the chest, abdomen, arms, or legs, often with pares-

Table 28—Differential Diagnosis of Spinal Cord Tumor

	Onset	Motor Symptoms	Sensory Symptoms	Spinal Fluid
SPINAL CORD TUMOR	Slow; pain usually prominent. Progressive	Weakness of limbs; spasticity as rule. Flaccid some types	Sensory level usually	Protein increased. Subarachnoid block
SYPHILITIC MYELITIS	Chronic	Spastic weakness	Sensory level, usually ill defined but may be complete	Positive reactions of Wassermann test, colloidal gold, etc.
MULTIPLE SCLEROSIS	Chronic; often with remissions	Spastic weakness	Posterior column signs. Sensory level rare	Colloidal gold curve abnormal in many cases
ARACHNOIDITIS	Chronic; progressive; often after history of infection or trauma	Not very severe	Ill-defined sensory level	Subarachnoid block incomplete. Protein elevated
PACHYMENINGITIS	Chronic; pains prominent	Often not very severe	Ill-defined sensory level as a rule	Subarachnoid block incomplete. Protein elevated
SYRINGOMYELIA	Very slow	Atrophy in hands and arms; spasticity of legs may develop	Segmental loss of pain and temperature. Later, sensory level if cavity expands	Not abnormal as a rule. Protein may be increased
TUBERCULOSIS OF SPINE	Relatively fast	Spasticity develops slowly	Sensory level found	Subarachnoid block often

8. Diagnosis and Treatment of Spinal Cord Tumors

Diagnosis: The diagnosis of spinal cord tumor resolves itself into (1) the determination of whether tumor is present; (2) the localization of the tumor. The first lies well within the province of the

thesias, with progressive weakness of legs or/and arms, and with sensory disturbances. The suspicion may be confirmed by manometric tests and by other spinal fluid studies, such as increase of spinal fluid protein. In infiltrating tumors, and sometimes in extramedullary tumors, pain may be absent and only the progressive weakness, sensory and sphincter disturbances may be found. All these lead only to the decision that tumor may be present. Attention is again called to the fact that root pains may persist under the shoulder, or in the abdomen, down the legs, etc., and be mistaken often for disease of the gallbladder or appendix, and sciatica. A similar history and findings may be given by infectious myelitis or by other forms of myelitis, but the progressive nature of the disorder extending over a period of months or years is the outstanding feature, particularly of the meningiomas and perineural fibroblastomas compressing the spinal cord. In contrast to this is the onset in the case of metastatic carcinoma involving the spinal canal. Here the symptoms frequently develop suddenly or with only a short period of pain. In some instances pain may be present for long periods before evidences of cord compression such as paralysis and sensory disturbances develop. Spinal cord tumors are sometimes characterized by a minimum of signs. In such instances their outstanding feature is pain, their primary complaint, characterized by radicular features, occurring often at night and increased by coughing and straining. The neurological examination is usually normal in such instances. The spinal fluid protein is usually increased, but the hydrodynamics are usually normal. The diagnosis in such instances is made by myelogram. The problem of diagnosis is made doubly hard by the fact that under some circumstances no evidence of involvement of the vertebrae is found. The diagnosis of metastatic carcinoma offers no difficulties where carcinoma has been known to be present, but where it has not been previously established the diagnosis may be difficult. Acute onsets are found also in acute extradural ab-

scess and at times in Pott's disease and lymphosarcoma.

Having determined that a spinal cord syndrome exists due to root pain and signs of cord compression, the next step consists in establishment of tumor as the cause. Manometric tests are here of great value, but an extramedullary tumor may run its course without pain and Lipiodol or Pantopaque injection may be necessary in some cases.

Any transverse *myelitis* may resemble tumor. Those of infectious origin are usually more rapid in onset, but this is not a rigid differentiation, since tumor may at times develop rapidly as in carcinoma, sarcoma, etc. *Syphilis* can be determined by a positive serology. *Multiple sclerosis* may at times resemble cord tumor, especially in those types with a progressive course without evidence of remissions, with or without a sensory level. In such cases, no block can be demonstrated, the colloidal gold curve is often abnormal, and other signs of nervous system involvement may help. *Arachnoiditis* may be impossible to differentiate from tumor except in the presence of a previous history of infection and by Lipiodol studies. *Pachymeningitis* may also be impossible to differentiate except by exploration or by serological studies when due to syphilis. *Syringomyelia* is usually distinguishable from tumor by its relatively early onset, extremely slow progression, and by the segmental dissociation of sensation. *Cervical rib* and *scalenus anticus* syndrome are differentiated by the unilateral pain, the difference in pulse on the two sides, and the confinement of the syndrome to the lower cervical and upper thoracic segments without involvement of other limbs. Roentgenologic studies may help greatly in the diagnosis of cervical rib. *Superior pulmonary sulcus tumor* may be confusing, but can be diagnosed readily by unilateral shoulder and arm pain, Horner's syndrome, and by roentgenograms of the chest. *Pott's disease* may offer difficulties, but can be diagnosed by the typical roentgenologic findings. In early cases, these may not be present. *Dislocation* of the spine as a result of fracture offers no problems if found in acute trauma, but may be overlooked in old cases of trauma. Roentgenograms of the vertebrae will reveal the deformity. Spondylitis of the Marie-Strümpell type may involve the upper cervical vertebrae and compression of the cervical cord has been observed in the extreme flexion of the head observed in such instances. Rarely, compression of the medulla has been observed due to dislocation of the atlanto-axial joint and the odontoid process. Progressive disability similar to that produced by spinal cord tumor is seen at times in *achondroplastic dwarfs.* It may be the result of tumor or of herniation of an intervertebral disc into the congenitally narrowed spinal cord.

The *level* of the spinal cord lesion offers real problems in diagnosis. This can usually be determined by the sensory level and the zone of hyperesthesia above it. It is well to remember, however, that the sensory level is often one or two segments below the zone of compression. In the absence of sensory disturbances, the reflex disturbances and the muscle weakness may help to establish the tumor level. Vasomotor and pilomotor reactions may help. In doubtful cases, contrast media, such as iodized oil or air myelography, may be required to establish the level.

Treatment: Generally speaking, the outlook in benign extramedullary tumors is good if the tumor is *removed* in time. Rapid progression of symptoms and the rapid development of cord compression offers less chance of recovery than more slowly developing disability. The paralysis resulting from carcinoma responds poorly because of destruction of the underlying cord. Flexion paraplegia offers poor chances of recovery. Flaccid paralysis responds poorly, when due to complete cord interruption.

Intramedullary tumors offer less chance of recovery than extramedullary tumors. Some are cystic and *emptying the cyst* may bring improvement. Others respond to *irradiation* but not with complete recovery. In some instances of well-defined intramedullary tumors, *complete removal* of the tumor has been effected with relief, but not cure, of disabilities.

Massage, splints, and *other mechanical measures* may be necessary in the aftercare of tumor patients.

XIII. HERNIATED INTERVERTEBRAL DISC *(Herniated Nucleus Pulposus)*

This condition has assumed increasing importance as a cause of low back and leg pain. Since the symptoms result from a protrusion of the intervertebral disc into the spinal canal, with resulting root and in some instances cord compression, it may be considered in the discussion of spinal cord tumors. Though it acts like a spinal cord tumor as to course and symptomatology, it is not a new growth. Herniation of the annulus fibrosus may occur without evidence of herniation of the nucleus pulposus.

Herniated intervertebral disc is associated with low back and leg pain (sciatica). It is claimed by some to be the most common cause of sciatica, but this is an extravagant claim (*v.* Sciatica. Chap. 5). The incidence of herniated disc as a cause of sciatica is difficult to determine. Some state it to as high as ninety per cent. In a series of 354 cases it was found to be the cause of leg pain in forty-two per cent (Alpers).

The *location* of herniation of the intervertebral disc is well established. Most cases occur in the lumbar region, involving particularly the discs of the fourth and fifth lumbar vertebrae. About ninety to ninety-five per cent of lumbar herniations occur at the fourth lumbar and lumbosacral discs. These far outnumber the herniations elsewhere in the spine. Cervical herniations account for a smaller percentage, but herniations in the cervical region are more common than usually appreciated. Thoracic herniations

cated—slipping without falling, a missed golf swing, stepping off a curb unexpectedly. Falling on the buttocks or back has been found responsible in some cases. There are many instances of herniated disc in which no history of trauma is available. The disorder occurs in laborers, but it is equally as frequent in those who do not engage in strenuous exertion. Lumbar puncture has been reported as causing herniation of the nucleus pul-

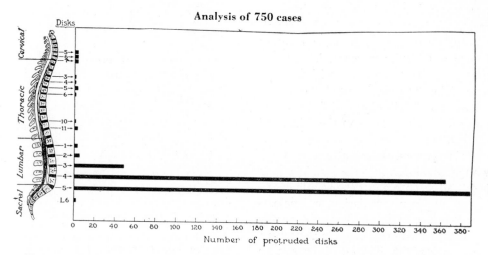

Fig. 96—*Herniation of nucleus pulposus,* illustrating the great preponderance of the disorder at L4 and L5 discs in a series of 750 cases. (*Love & Walsh: Surg. Gyn. & Obst., 77:497, 1943.*)

are uncommon. The herniations are usually single, but are found to be multiple in about twelve per cent of cases. Males far outnumber females so affected, figures varying from seventy-one per cent (Bradford and Spurling) to eighty-five per cent (Barr). More than seventy-five per cent of cases are found in or beyond the fourth decade; a few instances are reported in the second decade of life.

The *cause* of the herniation is, in most instances, trauma (fifty per cent). The most common type of trauma is that of lifting a heavy object with the body in the flexed position. Other forms of trauma of a less significant nature have been impli-

posus. The condition may occur also in degenerative conditions involving the spine — osteoarthritis, and osteitis deformans. Because of the absence of a history of injury in about half the cases, it is believed that the herniation is preceded by a degeneration of the intervertebral disc.

Symptoms: *Symptoms of Lumbar Herniations of Intervertebral Disc:* These are ushered in by pain in the low back, usually following an attempt to lift a heavy object with the body flexed. There may be an account of a "snap" in the back at the time of injury, followed by severe back pain often described as "lumbago." The pain remains localized in the lower portions of the back for varying periods of time; months, or years. It is usually constant, but may be intermittent, and periods of remission are common. It is relieved often by posture, patients preferring standing to sitting or lying down; it is aggravated by bending over and straightening up and occasionally by coughing, sneezing, etc. After a varying period of time, pain appears usually in one leg or in some instances (fifteen per cent) in both legs. In some cases, the leg pain may develop simultaneously with the back pain; in other instances (thirty per cent), it may appear as the first symptom, without back pain. The leg pain is usually typically sciatic in distribution, with radiation along the back and side of the thigh, and the back of the leg. Not infrequently it may involve only the buttock or thigh without extension into the leg. The pain is felt all at once along the sciatic distribution and is not radiating or lancinating; it is usually severe, is aggravated by posture, and often by coughing, sneezing, and moving the bowels. It varies in severity. It is usually bearable, but it may be excruciating from the onset. It may be increased by compression of the jugular veins, thus increasing intraspinal pressure which is transmitted along the subarachnoid space and into the subarachnoid coverings of the nerve roots (Naffziger test).

The pain in herniated disc is usually recurrent, the typical case giving a history of more than one episode of back and leg pain varying in duration and number. Several such attacks may have been experienced or only a few. There may be complete relief from pain between episodes or the pain may be inconstant and bearable.

Examination reveals a loss of the lumbar lordosis in most cases (sixty per cent) with spasm of the paravertebral muscles and in some cases lumbar scoliosis. Manipulation of the leg is painful, and Lasègue's test is almost always positive (v. Sciatica). Movements of the lumbar spine are limited; extension of the spine is painful; lateral flexion of the spine is restricted, especially to the pain-

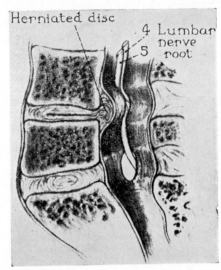

Fig. 97—*Herniated intervertebral disc* showing the protrusion of the intervertebral disc with compression of roots L4 and L5. *(Courtesy of Dr. R. A. Groff.)*

ful side; hyperextension of the lumbar spine usually increases the back and leg pain. Pain is elicited also on the straight leg raising test. Tenderness along the sciatic nerve is not usually present, but has been reported by some authors in a high incidence of cases. Weakness of the leg is difficult to evaluate in most cases, due to the defensive reaction produced by the pain. Weakness of plantar flexion of the foot, weakness of dorsiflexion and foot-drop, and at times weakness of the thigh muscles is seen, associated with varying degrees of atrophy of the affected muscles. Atrophy is not a common feature, however. Diminution or absence of the Achilles reflex is found in most cases, at least eighty to eighty-five per cent of lumbosacral herniations and fifty per cent of all lumbar herniations, and decreased or absent patellar reflex is found in herniations at times (ten per cent). Decreased pain sensation is found at times on the outer aspect of the leg and foot (S_1 and S_2), but is often absent.

In some instances, the herniation may be so extensive as to produce evidence of complete compression of the spinal roots, as in spinal cord tumor, causing a complete motor paralysis of the legs, a sensory level, and subarachnoid block.

Symptoms of Cervical Herniation: Though herniated disc is commonest by far in the lumbar region, protrusions occur also in the cervical canal. As elsewhere, trauma is not always found in such cases. The protrusions are lateral and are most common at C_5 and C_6 vertebrae but occur also at C_7 and C_8. The history is always that of pain in the shoulder radiating over the convexity of the shoulder and into the arm. The pain is usually intractable, fails to respond to rest, drugs, and physiotherapy, and is of a characteristic root nature, being increased on coughing, sneezing, and straining. Atrophy of the shoulder girdle muscles is always found and at times those of the arm. Muscle fasciculations also are found occasionally. Reflex and sensory changes may be found, with loss either of the biceps or triceps reflexes.

Under some circumstances, a herniated disc in the cervical region may cause only compression of a single root (Murphy and Semmes; Bucy and Chenault). The seventh cervical root is usually affected. The syndrome is characterized by (1) precordial pain, (2) pain at the upper angle of the scapula, and (3) pain along the lateral and medial surfaces of the arm. Hypalgesia and hypesthesia are found along the index and middle fingers. The history of pain in the arm is often preceded by an account of "crick" in the neck recurring for months or even years before the severe attack ensues.

Herniated disc in the cervical region is said to be common (Brain), but it is doubtful whether it can account for the majority of cases of arm pain. As in the case of herniated disc in the lumbar region, trauma may play a prominent rôle, but in many cases develop without trauma or with insignificant trauma. Arthritis of the cervical vertebrae appears to play a significant rôle in some cases.

Because of the firm anchorage of the cervical spinal cord by the ligamenta denticulata and the crowding of the spinal canal by the cervical cord, disc protrusions in the cervical region may cause not only root compression but compression of the spinal cord as well. The lower cervical discs are more commonly affected than the upper, especially C_5 and C_6, and C_6 and C_7 discs. In such instances the herniation is central rather than lateral.

The symptoms may be ushered in by (1) acute pain involving the neck and arm, (2) insidious and intermittent pain in the neck and arm, and (3) acute or gradual onset of symptoms of compression of the spinal cord. Pain is almost always present and is radicular in nature, involving roots C_5, C_6, and C_7 most commonly. Pain is commonly felt in the root of the neck to the tip of the shoulder, the supraclavicular fossa, and the lateral aspect of the arm. Muscle weakness and fasciculations are common.

Herniated cervical disc may simulate progressive spinal cord disease such as amyotrophic lateral sclerosis, multiple sclerosis, posterolateral sclerosis and syringomyelia. The clinical picture in such instances is that of progressive spinal cord disease, but with features not typical of the conditions simulated by the disc. Most important are the absence of signs above the spinal cord level and the presence of pain in the neck, shoulders, or arms. Roentgen examination reveals normal vertebrae, a narrow disc or discs, or arthritis.

Symptoms of Thoracic Herniation of the Intervertebral Disc: These are less well defined than those of the cervical region, since herniations in this portion of the vertebral column are less common than elsewhere. Pain of a radicular type in the chest or abdomen is the only symptom for some time, and may remain the only symptom. Compression symptoms, such as weakness of the leg and sensory paralysis, may develop just as in the case of thoracic tumors if the herniation is large enough to obstruct the spinal canal. Herniations of intervertebral discs in the thoracic region occur in the ratio of 2 to 3 to 100 in the lumbar and cervical regions combined (Love & Kiefer). The protrusion appears to be more often midline than lateral, giving rise usually to a picture of an incomplete transverse lesion.

Diagnosis: The *diagnosis* of a herniated intervertebral disc is often difficult on clinical grounds alone despite advances which have been made in the recognition of the condition. In lumbar herniations, the history is that of low back pain following exertion or of low back pain appearing without adequate cause, in both instances with persistence of the pain, often with remissions. After a varying period of time or at times simultaneously with the back pain there develops pain in the leg along the sciatic distribution. This is associated with pain on stretching the sciatic nerve by various manoeuvers, at times with tenderness along the sciatic nerve, and is increased on movement of the trunk, and at times on sneezing and coughing. Weakness and atrophy of the leg muscles may be present but is usually not found. The Achilles reflex is usually absent or decreased, the patellar reflex is similarly af-

fected in a small percentage of cases, and sensory disturbances will usually be absent.

The history and findings to this point suggest a disturbance involving the spinal roots within the vertebral canal. They are not pathognomonic, however, and they may be produced by other conditions. Lumbar puncture is usually unnecessary with a history of this nature unless spinal cord tumor or some other cause is suspected. The *spinal fluid* findings reveal a clear fluid in most instances, and a xanthochromic fluid in a small percentage of cases. The total protein is reported to be increased in eighty per cent of cases, the level of the protein varying from 45 to 250 mg. Subarachnoid block is found rarely, in only five per cent of cases, and then only in the case of massive herniations. The spinal fluid, therefore, is likely to reveal only an increase of protein, usually moderate in degree, a finding which may be produced by a number of conditions. The spinal fluid examination is not as a rule helpful and routine spinal fluid examination is not necessary in herniated disc.

Roentgenologic examination reveals nothing specific in most instances, but should always be carried out. Narrowing of the intervertebral disc is often found, a finding of value in cases of herniation of the intervertebral disc, but often present without it. Hypertrophic osteoarthritis may be found.

Despite the very suggestive history of low back pain, sciatic pain, and the findings which have been described, it is difficult to make the diagnosis of herniation of the intervertebral disc with certainty, even in the presence of an increased protein in the spinal fluid. Many authors, however, believe that no more than these findings are required for a diagnosis. For absolute certainty, a myelogram is necessary in order to establish the diagnosis. This may fail to reveal a herniation when present. The diagnosis by myelogram is not always dependable, since both false positives and negatives may be found. Pantopaque myelograms are positive in ninety to ninety-six per cent of cases. In order to avoid unnecessary explorations, myelogram should be performed. Exploration is justified in the presence of a negative myelogram if all other features indicate a herniated disc. False positive myelograms usually offer little difficulty, since careful analysis of the entire problem reveals features not characteristic of herniated disc, such as atypical distribution of the pain, absent Lasègue or straight leg-raising signs, etc.

In the last analysis, the clinical diagnosis of herniated disc can be made with certainty in a case with sciatic pain if (1) a history of trauma is obtained; (2) a narrowed intervertebral disc is found by roentgenologic examination; (3) the myelogram is positive.

It may be presumed to be present in a patient with recurrent sciatic pain, without evidence of sciatic neuritis, if a history of trauma is obtained and if no other cause is demonstrable. In such instances, the diagnosis may be confirmed only by exploration.

Low back pain alone, without radiation into the leg, is said to be caused most frequently by herniated disc. The evidence for this is lacking in important respects. While herniated lumbar disc often begins with low back pain, the diagnosis cannot be made on this feature alone.

The *differential diagnosis* of herniated disc involves, as a rule, consideration of the many causes of sciatica (*v.* Sciatica). Primarily, distinction must be made from those conditions which involve the spinal canal. Spinal cord tumor is usually readily separated by the greater incidence of motor and sensory findings in the limbs, by a longer history, the absence of a history of injury, and by more characteristic spinal fluid changes. Sacroiliac disease becomes important to differentiate because of the history of acute onset with pain in the back, but the differentiation is not difficult. The differentiation from conditions involving the lumbosacral plexus may be hard at times, but the greater extent of involvement of the limb, the more profound sensory disturbances, and the recognition of pelvic disease sufficient to account for the process will help.

It is sometimes difficult to differentiate a vascular lesion with leg pain from one of neurological origin. The pain in arterial occlusive disease is more diffuse and does not follow nerve channels. It appears and increases rapidly in proportion to the amount of exercise and it subsides quickly after exercise is completed. The peripheral pulses are absent, the foot is pale and cool, and oscillometric studies reveal reduced amplitudes.

Arthritis with encroachment on the intervertebral foramen may produce a root syndrome similar in all respects to that of a herniated disc.

Treatment: The treatment of herniated disc is not necessarily surgical. Since there is a frequent history of remission of the pain, it may be assumed that under these circumstances the herniation is relieved. That this is probably the case is evidenced by the fact that in many instances the pain will disappear completely with (1) *rest* in bed; (2) *salicylates* in large doses (gr. 15 four times daily); (3) *diathermy* to the back and leg daily; (4) *massage;* (5) infra-red to the back and area of the sciatic foramen twice daily; (6) hot tub soaks daily; and (7) if salicylates and heat fail to control pain, *codeine, meperidine (Demerol)* (50 mg. [¾ grain] three times daily), or *methadone* (5 mg. [½₂ grain] three times daily) may be used. Seventy-five per cent of the patients will recover with medical treatment and will therefore not require surgery.

Surgical removal of the herniated disc should be reserved for (1) those patients in whom the pain is so severe either in the first or subsequent attacks as to defy relief; (2) those patients with repeated recurrences of sciatic pain, leading to loss of work and income; (3) those patients who choose surgical relief rather than medical methods. Ten per cent of laminectomies for herniated disc result in negative explorations. The cause of the pain in these patients has not been disclosed. In properly selected patients the leg pain disappears dramatically after operation. The back pain may persist.

The possibility of recurrence of the herniation is always present whether the treatment has been medical or surgical. Recurrences have been reported in five to ten per cent of patients operated upon. Cramps involving the leg and thigh muscles sometimes develop after operations for herniated disc. They disappear spontaneously in two or three weeks but may persist longer at times. Similarly, sciatic pain may at times persist following operation, despite the successful removal of a protruded disc.

XIV. INJURIES OF THE SPINE AND SPINAL CORD

1. Fractures of the Spine

The problem of spine fractures may be divided into three aspects: (1) simple fracture of the body, transverse processes, etc.; (2) fracture dislocations without injury of the cord; (3) fracture dislocations with spinal cord injury.

Etiology: The actual incidence of spine fractures is not specifically known. Men are more commonly affected than women, probably because of greater ex-

posure to industrial hazards, such as mining, automobile accidents, etc. Most spine fractures occur in adults, though their incidence in children is by no means unknown.

Spine fractures may occur as the result of direct or indirect injury, such as direct blows to the spine or by falls on the head, buttocks, or feet, by the fall of a heavy weight on the head or shoulder, by diving into shallow water, by gunshot wounds, muscular violence, convulsion therapy, etc. Direct blows are probably more prone to produce fracture of the spinous or transverse process, while indirect violence is more commonly responsible for crush fractures.

Acute flexion is the most important factor in the production of compression fractures. Cervical fractures are usually the result of acute forward flexion of the head, as in diving accidents. Similarly, thoracic and lumbar fractures result from acute flexion of the trunk at the point of fracture. Relatively slight accidents may at times cause compression fractures, as, for example, a fall down a few steps on the buttocks.

Nature and Location of Fracture: Many fractures of the spine involve relatively unimportant parts such as transverse or spinous processes. These are frequently asymptomatic. In war, spinal cord injuries occur in less than one per cent of battle casualties (Everts and Woodhall). About forty to fifty per cent of spine fractures are compression fractures. In seventy per cent of these subjects the spinal roots and spinal cord are uninjured, leaving relatively fewer patients with cord damage.

In the majority of cases only one vertebra is crushed, but multiple crushes may occur. The vertebrae most commonly involved are the fourth, fifth, and sixth cervical, and the eleventh or twelfth thoracic, the first or second lumbar (seventy to eighty per cent). Of these, the twelfth thoracic and the first lumbar are most commonly involved (fifty to sixty per cent), and the first lumbar is much more commonly injured than any other single vertebra. Compression fractures of the cervical vertebrae are not as common as fractures of the thoracic and lumbar vertebrae.

Pathology: Injuries to the spinal cord by vertebral dislocations or fracture-dislocations or by gunshot wounds may give rise to one or to a combination of changes. Probably the most common type of lesion in such instances is *contusion* of the spinal cord, produced by a direct blow of the displaced vertebra or of a fractured portion of it. Edema is severe in the early stages and may be associated with hemorrhage in the subarachnoid space in severe cases. The cord immediately after injury appears bluish, contused, and swollen. Microscopic study of such spinal cords reveals that the greatest degree of damage is at the level of the injury with some extension for a very short distance above it, approximately one segment in extent. Damage may be produced for some distance, both above and below the level of the lesion. Fresh hemorrhages are seen in the acute stages scattered everywhere through the cord. The myelin is destroyed, there are many phagocytic cells (compound granular corpuscles), and as the condition becomes more chronic, astrocytes are found. Polymorphonuclears, lymphocytes, and plasma cells are seen in the tissue and around the blood vessels may be red cells, lymphocytes, or polymorphonuclear cells. The ganglion cells show varying degrees of change, depending on the stage of the process; many are lost at the level of the injury. Within the pia-arachnoid are many red blood cells, and at times lymphocytes. Similar changes are seen in *laceration* of the spinal cord due to penetrating missiles or pieces of fractured bone. The difference is largely one of degree, but if the laceration is extensive the damage may be as severe as that which is seen in contusion.

Hemorrhage into the spinal canal occurs in some cases and may be extradural, subdural, or subarachnoid. (1) *Extradural hemorrhage* is rare. It may attain sufficient size to compress the spinal cord, to give signs of progressive paralysis, and subarachnoid block by the Queckenstedt test. The spinal cord changes may be reversible despite the compression, but if the condition is unrecognized and the compression persistent, loss of myelin and axis cylinders develop with reactive glial formation and compound granular corpuscles. (2) *Subdural hemorrhage* is also rare and gives rise to findings similar to those of extradural hemorrhage. (3) *Subarachnoid hemorrhage* is found in all cases of contusion and laceration and at times in cases with no cord damage. Microscopically, red cells are found in the subarachnoid space. *Hematomyelia* or hemorrhage into the substance of the spinal cord may develop as the result of direct injury to the cord or without such injury, the trauma being sustained in the vertebral column alone. The spinal cord in such instances is swollen and edematous. The hemorrhage may be single or multiple, large or small, and involves gray matter more commonly than white substance. It may at times extend for as many as six to ten segments. Around the hemorrhage within the spinal cord are areas of perivascular infiltration by red cells, lymphocytes, and polymorphonuclear cells. The hemorrhage in hematomyelia tends to spread longitudinally in the gray matter, while in the white matter are punctate hemorrhages and leukocytic infiltrations. Thrombus formation, congestion, and areas of necrosis are seen. Destruction of myelin and axis cylinders and of the anterior horn cells occurs. Cavity formation develops later as the hemorrhage becomes older.

General Symptoms of Spinal Fractures: The features of simple fractures or of compression fractures without cord injury are not primarily neurological in the sense that they do not cause evidences of root or cord damage. The features of compression fractures of the vertebrae or of fracture dislocations are variable. In many cases only pain is experienced, usually in a single root area in the lower part of the trunk or chest. In fracture dislocations, crush of the underlying cord usually occurs. It is not invariable, however, so that in many instances there may be fracture-dislocation without injury to the spinal cord. This may be complete or partial. Complete crush results in the picture of *complete cord transection,* with immediate paralysis of the legs, or arms and legs, depending on the location of the crush. Paralysis may develop slowly and may be progressive. The paralysis is flaccid as in all cases of spinal shock, is associated with absent reflexes, and may later become spastic if the patient survives. Sensory paralysis to the level of the crush is present, with sphincter disturbances, at first retention then incontinence of urine, and incontinence of feces. In all severe spinal lesions retention develops first. This is followed in cervical and thoracic lesions by automatic emptying after days or weeks. In conus and cauda equina injuries detrusor action is feeble and the bladder is incompletely emptied with great straining. In *partial injuries* many combinations of symptoms develop depending on the areas injured. Spinal hemiplegias, paraplegias, or monoplegias are seen, together with various combinations of sensory symptoms. Root pains are not uncommon in partial injuries or in fractures of the spine without disloca-

tion. They may be extremely severe and their traumatic origin may not be suspected in the presence of a minor degree of injury.

Topical Features of Spinal Fractures: The characteristics of fracture of the spine associated with underlying damage of the spinal cord varies with the level of the injury, and it is essential, therefore, that some knowledge be had of the specific features encountered with injuries at different levels, together with the specific problems which they create.

Cervical Fractures and Dislocations: Fractures of the cervical vertebrae are less common than those of the lumbar and thoracic vertebrae but are by no means rare. Of the cervical vertebrae involved, the fifth and sixth are most commonly affected. Cervical dislocations are most likely to occur between the first and second, and the fourth, fifth, and sixth vertebrae. "Nearly all cervical spine injuries occur as the result of indirect violence which causes excessive flexion" (Munro and Wegner). The commonest causes of cervical cord injury by fracture are (1) automobile accidents, (2) diving into shallow water, and (3) falling down stairs. The severity of the neural and skeletal damage does not run parallel one to another; there may be severe cord damage with little evidence of vertebral injury, or there may be little or no cord damage with severe compression fracture. The flexion produced by the blow causes a shearing stress on the facets, which become dislocated as a result of the blow.

FRACTURES AND DISLOCATIONS OF THE ATLAS: Fractures of the atlas are rare. Dislocation or fracture-dislocations are more common than fractures alone. The latter are likely to be associated with skull and/or axis fractures. Of the injuries which involve the atlas and axis, dislocation without fracture is most common, followed by fracture of the odontoid in frequency, and least frequent is fracture of the lateral masses of the atlas or axis, with or without dislocation or fracture of the odontoid. When involved the posterior arch, or both the anterior and posterior arches, is most commonly involved. Direct violence seems to be of little importance in the production of atlas fractures. The common cause is a fall upon the head, the force of the blow being transmitted from the vertex to the occipital condyles and the underlying atlas. In rare instances the atlas may be fractured by a fall with the head in extension, the posterior arch being crushed between the occiput and the arch of the axis; or the anterior arch may be fractured by means of the odontoid with the head in full extension.

The outstanding clinical signs of fracture of the first vertebra consist of rigidity of the neck muscles and limitation of movement. Nodding is most limited, but rotation of the head is also restricted. The head is held stiffly as if balancing a weight, or the head may be supported with the hands, particularly in making a change from the upright posture. In cases of fracture of the anterior arch a lump may be felt in the pharynx at the level of the palate. Dysphagia and dysarthria may be found. Pain along the back of the head in the area of the greater occipital nerve may be present and if found is of great diagnostic value. Spinal cord injury is found often but not invariably.

Dislocations of the *atlas on the axis* result from trauma such as automobile accidents, falls, sudden turns of the head, traumatic dislocations being associated frequently with fracture of the odontoid process. Dislocation may occur also from (1) infections (pyogenic, syphilitic, tuberculous osteomyelitis) with relaxation of the ligaments supporting the atlas; (2) bone decalcification

and joint involvement associated with cervical infection as sinusitis, pharyngitis, tonsillitis, mastoiditis; (3) congenital absence of the odontoid process. The symptoms are similar in many respects to those of fracture alone and consist of a torticollar position of the head, the head being bent forward and tilted to one side. Thus in a dislocation on the right the head will be turned to the left and tilted to the right. In bilateral dislocations the head is tilted forward. The chin is often held tightly against the larynx, it is difficult to open the mouth, and dysphagia and dysphonia may be present. Pain is present in the occipital area. Extension of the head is painful and the chin is supported in the hands on arising. Lateral flexion of the head is only slightly possible from the side to which it is tilted, and rotation of the head past the midline is impossible, so that the entire body must be turned in order to see over the opposite shoulder. A mass can be felt in the pharynx on the side to which the head is tilted. Paralysis is infrequent in cases which survive, but involves the arms more than the legs when present. Quadriplegia may be present in other cases of cord compression. In still others pain in the neck and back of the head may be the only symptoms. Roentgenograms confirm the clinical findings and show the anterior arch of the atlas anterior to the odontoid, with lordosis of the lower cervical spine. Death occurs instantly in those cases in which injury of the medulla is produced by the compression.

The *axis* is fractured most commonly at the base of the odontoid process and this is caused by pressure of the head on the rigid spine, the head being in hyperextension. It may be fractured alone or be the seat of dislocation or of fracture-dislocation. Involvement of the axis by one of these processes is usually associated with injury of the atlas. The symptoms of dislocation of the axis are similar to those described for dislocation or fracture-dislocation of the atlas. An associated fracture of the odontoid process is usually present and may or may not be accompanied by evidences of compression of the spinal cord just as in the case of involvement of the atlas.

Fractures of the *odontoid* process are rare. They occur often with anterior or forward dislocation of the atlas and in such instances there is usually displacement of the loose fragment of the odontoid with resulting root and cord compression, often resulting in death. The outstanding symptoms are pain in the neck and spasmodic limitation of motion (Osgood and Lund). The pain is exaggerated by motion and relieved by immobilization. Pain over the back of the head is common, due to pinching of the greater occipital nerve. There is often a complaint of a lump in the back of the throat and difficulty in swallowing, and palpation reveals in such cases a bulging of the posterior pharyngeal wall on one side. Associated with the odontoid fracture may be only the neck pain and the limitation of motion of the neck; or there may be evidences of compression of the spinal cord with quadriplegia, sensory and vesical paralysis, either complete or incomplete; or there may be delayed signs of involvement of the spinal cord and its roots. It is important to recognize the significance of pain in the back of the head and neck following cervical injury and to determine the presence of odontoid fracture by careful roentgen studies, in order to avoid delayed compression of the spinal cord in unrecognized instances which have survived the odontoid fracture. Such cases may, by a sudden turn of the head or by sneezing or sudden exertion, bring on fatal paralysis by compression of the spinal cord by a loose fragment of odontoid which has not been recognized.

In some instances delayed signs in fractures and dislocations of the atlanto axial region are found. In such instances symptoms may appear days, months, or years after the trauma, the manifestations at the time of the accident being absent, insignificant, or rapidly disappearing. The onset of symptoms following a latent period of freedom from difficulties after the trauma may be rapid or slow. The cause of the delayed development of symptoms has been ascribed to redislocation, progressive dislocation, excessive callous formation, pachymeningitis with resulting pressure on the spinal cord, irritation or abnormal mobility, arachnoiditis, and the late development of an osteomyelitis. The signs vary, but evidence of involvement of the spinal cord is present and is manifested by spastic paraplegia or quadriplegia; at times associated with a sensory level and evidence of subarachnoid block. While the condition is rare, it should be considered in all cases of obscure and progressive cord involvement in the cervical region. In rare instances choked disc and internal hydrocephalus may follow fracture of the odontoid process with subsequent arachnoiditis and the development of internal hydrocephalus due to obstruction of the subarachnoid space at the entrance to the spinal cord.

FRACTURE AND DISLOCATION BELOW THE ATLAS-AXIS LEVEL: The findings in cases of cervical fracture-dislocations below the level of the axis vary with the level involved. They may be grouped for the sake of convenience into two groups: (1) Those above the fourth cervical segment and therefore involving the phrenic nerve innervation; (2) those developing below the fourth cervical segment. In all such instances pain is present at the site of the fracture and evidences of the fracture-dislocation are readily demonstrable by roentgenograms. Most of the dislocations are anterior; only rarely are they posterior.

Fracture-dislocations above the fourth cervical segment are usually associated with cord damage. Quadriplegia is present, with paralysis of all the limbs, sensory paralysis is present, and vesical and rectal disturbances are found. Fever is often present. Death follows because of the respiratory paralysis ensuing from involvement of the innervation to the phrenic nerves.

Fracture-dislocations below the fourth cervical segment are characterized also by evidences of cord compression, with motor and sensory paralysis and sphincter disturbances, but with variations in the clinical features depending on the level of the cord compression. Injury above the fifth cervical segment involves the arms and the motor paralysis will therefore be a quadriplegia. Injury between the fifth and sixth cervical segments results in a lesion which produces a characteristic posture (Thorburn position) of abduction of the arms, flexion of the forearms and external rotation. Injury below the sixth cervical segment permits movements of the arms, but with partial paralysis of the hands. The motor paralysis in such instances will, therefore, involve chiefly the legs, with only partial paralysis of the upper extremities and with a sensory level to the lower cervical segments.

Owing to evidences of injury to the cord in compressions below the fourth cervical segment the outlook for such patients is poor and permanent paralysis is followed eventually by retention of urine, pyelitis, decubitus ulcers, sepsis, and death.

The mortality in dislocations of the cervical vertebrae was 16 per cent in World War II (Ellis).

Minor injuries to the cervical portion of the spinal cord sometimes occur as the result of dislocation between the fourth and fifth, or fifth and sixth vertebrae, with momentary nipping of the cord on displacement (Walshe). Such cases are characterized by (1) limitation of movement of the head and neck with pain and stiffness on movement; (2) some generalized weakness of the upper limbs, sometimes associated with weakness and wasting of the small muscles of the hand; (3) changes in the tendon reflexes of the arms—some are increased, some abolished or decreased and the supinator reflex may be inverted; (4) slight hypertonus of the extensor muscles of the legs; (5) absence of sensory loss at the time of examination; (6) absence of defects of sphincter control: (7) slow and incomplete recovery. Cases of this sort are mistaken for progressive muscular atrophy or amyotrophic lateral sclerosis.

Thoracic and Lumbar Fractures: These may be considered conveniently together, since most fractures of the vertebrae are found in this portion of the spinal column, and since also they have many clinical features in common.

Fractures involving the thoracic and lumbar vertebrae are compression fractures. Of the forty per cent of compression fractures which comprise all spinal fractures, only one third are associated with cord injury, leaving a large number in which no cord damage occurs. Most of the compression fractures of the vertebrae are found in the thoracic and lumbar areas, involving particularly the twelfth thoracic and first lumbar vertebrae. It is clear that the lower thoracic vertebrae are more liable to fracture than the upper and that the lower the fracture the greater is the likelihood of dislocation (Munro).

The *cause* of thoracic and lumbar fractures is direct violence, fall from a height being the most common cause. Automobile accidents, stab wounds, gunshot wounds, and other forms of violence form other causes of the disturbance. In all cases there is acute flexion at the site of the fracture. The mechanism is similar to that of a nut crushed between the jaws of a nutcracker, the jaws being represented by the vertebrae above and below the one broken. "The posterior part of the body is protected by the strength and rigidity of the articular processes, and hence the spinal body after the injury becomes wedge-shaped with the narrow part in front. The extent of wedging depends on the amount of violence" (Irwin).

SYMPTOMS: Those of fracture-dislocations of the thoracic or upper lumbar vertebrae consist of complete paralysis of the legs with sensory paralysis and loss of all forms of sensation to the segmental level involved, together with sphincter paralysis. These are the symptoms in complete transection of the cord. In less severe instances the degree of paralysis varies. There may be weakness but not paralysis of the legs, weakness or paralysis of one leg, and varying types of sensory syndrome, such as the Brown-Sequard sensory syndrome, or a partial transverse sensory syndrome involving all forms of sensation in minor degree or only some forms of sensation. Pain in the back is present in all forms.

Injuries of the lower lumbar vertebrae cause lesions involving the cauda equina and conus medullaris, causing incontinence of urine and feces, impotence, loss of sensation in the perianal region, and paralysis of the legs with atrophy and absence of reflexes due to involvement of the cauda equina roots.

Diagnosis: The diagnosis of a spinal fracture must resolve itself into a con-

sideration of (1) the location of the injury; (2) the nature of the injury, whether fracture, dislocation or fracture-dislocation, and if fracture whether it involves the spinous processes, the transverse processes, the body or other parts of the vertebra; (3) the determination of the presence of injury to the spinal cord. The first two problems are usually readily determined by the nature of the symptoms, the location and type of injury, and by the aid of roentgen and physical examinations. The problem of injury to the spinal cord is one which is of paramount importance and requires careful clinical study. Injury may result in complete compression or transection of the spinal cord, resulting in a transverse syndrome, or in partial injury with the features which have already been mentioned. It is extremely important to determine whether the paralysis resulting from cord injury has been instantaneous, or whether it has developed in the course of hours or days. In the former case, laceration and destruction of the cord tissue by the displaced vertebra may be assumed; in the latter case, meningeal hemorrhage, either extradural or subdural, is probably present. The extent of the injury may be determined at the time of the accident or shortly thereafter. At such time it is possible to determine whether there is a partial or a complete cord transection and to map out the level of the injury. The degree of displacement of the injured vertebra is of no value in this connection, since there is usually some recoil of the displaced vertebra after injury. Hence the degree of damage to the spinal cord as indicated by the degree of paralysis, both motor and sensory, is the only safe guide to the degree of injury. Beyond this nothing can be settled in the acute stages. The upper level of the damage is determined by the sensory level and gives a clue also as to the location of the injured vertebra. Following this it is important to decide whether the cord injury is associated with subarachnoid block due to edema, meningeal hemorrhage, dislocation of the vertebra, or displacement of a fragment of fractured bone. This is determined by the Queckenstedt test. If subarachnoid block is found to be present, operation will probably be decided upon ; if it is not present, operation is not indicated.

After the determination of the level and extent of the spinal cord injury and the presence or absence of subarachnoid block, it is then possible to decide upon the nature and type of the bone injury by roentgen and other examinations. Under ordinary circumstances, in the case of complete or even of incomplete cord transection, there is no difficulty in determining the location of the injury. This may be difficult under the following circumstances: (1) in the case of fractures which are not readily demonstrable by roentgenologic studies; (2) in the case of partial injury to the spinal cord; (3) in the case of spinal cord concussion in which lesions may be found at a level some distance above or below the point of impact of a missile (v. Spinal Cord Concussion).

The specific features of fractures and fracture - dislocations involving various portions of the spinal cord have already been described and need no restatement. Special attention is called to the difficulties of diagnosis in the case of odontoid fractures. The presence of neck pain, pain over the back of the head in cases of cervical fracture without injury to the cord should lead to careful roentgenologic studies of the odontoid process for evidences of fracture. Elsewhere, the actual demonstration of fracture or fracture-dislocation offers no difficulties.

It is essential to recall, however, that complete transection of the spinal cord may be found without evidence of vertebral dislocation under two circumstances: (1) in spinal cord concussion; (2) in complete spontaneous replacement of the dislocated vertebra.

The outlook in most cases of fracture-dislocation depends upon the site of injury and the degree of injury to the spinal cord. In evaluating prognosis, it is well to remember that not all patients with cord crush succumb, and that what appears to be a complete destruction of the cord at a definite level is due, not to cord damage, but to a functional interruption of pathways from which complete or incomplete recovery may ensue. Bedsores with subsequent infection and urinary tract infection are the commonest causes of death after spinal injury. Patients with extensive and complete cord damage usually succumb early or late, while those with partial damage may recover. Patients with severe motor and sensory damage usually do poorly, while those with pure motor or predominantly motor damage have a better prognosis. Cervical cord injuries are fatal in a high percentage of cases (fifty per cent). In high cervical cord crush the outlook is particularly poor because of damage to respiratory mechanisms. Thoracic and lumbar cord injuries are fatal in many patients having complete cord crush.

Treatment: A patient with a fracture-dislocation with injury to the spinal cord presents three immediate problems: (1) the treatment of shock; (2) the determination of the extent of the injury by neurological and roentgenological examinations, and (3) care of the bladder and skin. Other factors can be dealt with later. The immediate treatment depends upon the neurological signs disclosed and the roentgenological findings.

All patients having cord injury are in some degree of spinal *shock*. External heat should be applied. The head should be lowered. Patients should be placed between blankets, hot water bags placed at the feet, and fluids given freely. Care must be taken to avoid pneumonia by protecting the patient against unnecessary exposure. The bowels must be kept open and fecal impactions avoided. Patients should be moved off their backs to one or the other side every two hours and should never be allowed to lie in a wet bed. Lumbar puncture is usually not necessary, but may be required to determine whether subarachnoid block is present. Fluid may be necessary by hypodermoclysis or veniclysis if intake by mouth is limited, and intravenous plasma or serum may be necessary. Sufficient protein must be given by diet or transfusions to maintain the serum protein at 6.0 mg. or better (Munro).

All patients should have *roentgenograms* of the spine, since exact information is required in order to determine treatment, but this can be postponed if subarachnoid block is not present. Generally speaking, it is best to make roentgenologic study routine on admission. Fracture-dislocation is usually seen by roentgenograms, but in some cases with evidence of complete crush of the cord no dislocation is found, the deformity having been reduced spontaneously. A crush fracture without dislocation can be treated with immobilization and traction alone, whereas a fracture-dislocation with evidence of cord damage must be handled differently.

Cervical dislocations are treated by slow traction, in order to reduce the dislocation. This is done by a collar, fixing the head to the top of the bed, using the inclined body as the reduction force. A halter may be used with pull under the chin and occiput, led over a pulley at the head of the bed and attached to a weight. The weight necessary may vary from 20 pounds or more. In other cases, traction is made by a loop of rustless steel passed through two adjacent holes in the skull on either side of the midsagittal plane. Other reduction methods are advocated. *Thoracic* and *lumbar injuries* are treated by the general measures mentioned and by plaster cast.

Treatment of the patient with paraplegia resulting from injury to the spinal cord requires attention to the following details (Freeman): (1) unnecessary movement such as rotation or flexion of the spine; (2) frequent movement of the patient, at least every two hours; (3) care of the bladder, including avoidance of distention or continuous contraction; encouragement in the development of an automatic bladder; avoidance of urinary sepsis; and prevention of urinary calculi by exercising upper extremities in bed and by early ambulation; (4) care of the skin, including avoidance of prolonged pressure by frequent turning; a clean, dry, smooth, and flat bed; maintenance of adequate protein intake; and surgical repair of large decubitus ulcer; (5) care of the bowels by use of Prostigmin, enemas, and rectal tube; removal of fecal impactions; and development of proper bowel habits; (6) prevention and treatment of anemia, hypoproteinemia, and vitamin deficiencies; (7) proper attention to the psychological attitude of the sufferer. Much can be accomplished by muscle training and rehabilitation and by the proper use of braces. Training should be started as soon as there is any movement in the limbs.

Prevention of *bladder infection* is of extreme importance, and control of the bladder function essential in all cases. The problem of treatment of the bladder is controversial. Many are loath to empty the paralyzed bladder, but careful catheterization causes little real trouble. A permanent catheter with tidal drainage is safe and is the method to be preferred. The development of an automatic bladder is not as common as one would wish. Some degree of infection is to be expected from every catheter installation, but careful use of an indwelling catheter causes a minimum of difficulty. Complete transverse lesions of the spinal cord with retention of urine have had treatment of the latter by transurethral resection of the vesical neck (Emmett) with encouraging results. In acute injuries the problem of emptying the bladder is one of the most acute one has to handle, and the assumption that an automatic bladder will develop within hours or days is often erroneous for the good reason that it fails to occur, especially in the presence of sepsis. While the development of an automatic bladder is to be wished for, it occurs too infrequently and too late; in the meantime a sick patient requires emptying of a distended bladder, for which an indwelling catheter with tidal drainage is a wholly safe procedure despite assertions that such a maneuver increases the mortality in these patients. If balanced bladder function fails to return within three to six months, cause must be sought for the failure. Increased physical activity and ambulation should be encouraged. In patients with upper motor neuron lesions and conus activity, pudendal nerve anesthesia, pudendal neurectomy, or transurethral resection may be indicated. Patients with lower neuron lesions and inactivity of the conus are best suited for transurethral resection. Routine use of penicillin and/or sulfonamides is advisable in order to avoid infection.

Decubital ulcers constitute an important problem and must be avoided by careful attention to care of the skin, every effort being made to keep it dry and powdered, and to turn the patient frequently. Air or soft rubber mattresses are desirable. Pressure sores precede bedsores, which may be avoided by keeping the patient constantly dry, by maintaining serum protein at 6.0 or better and blood chlorides at a normal level (Munro). The skin should be rubbed with a mixture of alcohol and camphor. If sores develop, luminous heat and infrared are helpful.

The *bowels* should be treated by mineral oil or high cleansing enemas daily. Abdominal distention may be treated by means of a rectal tube. Prostigmine (1.0 cc. initial dose and 0.5 cc. every four hours subsequently) is helpful in stubborn cases.

Sedatives may be necessary in order to relieve pain. Morphine should be used cautiously in acute cases, since shock is present. Barbiturates may be used for restlessness.

The problem of operation upon the spinal cord always requires consideration and disposal. Nothing is to be gained by routine operation in patients with complete transverse lesions. The cord has been damaged by the dislocated vertebra and operation cannot restore its function. *Operation* is indicated if (1) there is roentgenologic evidence of impingement of a missile or bone in the spinal canal; (2) subarachnoid block is present; (3) progressive paralysis develops due to extradural hemorrhage. Laminectomy is performed by some if subarachnoid block persists in spite of efforts at reduction of the dislocation. In patients with partial cord injury, operation may be performed if there is evidence of pressure on the cord by bony fragments. Operation on patients with complete cord injury months after trauma is never justified. Late operations may be performed on patients with progressive symptoms with subarachnoid block, and on patients with adhesive arachnoiditis following trauma.

2. Concussion of the Spinal Cord
(Contusion of the Spinal Cord)

Etiology: Spinal cord concussion is an entity too often overlooked in spinal cord trauma. It is caused by blows of many sorts to the spinal cord; by falls on the end of the spine, gunshot wounds which ricochet off the spine, stab wounds, and external blows against the spine. It is a manifestation, therefore, of many sorts of injury, both indirect and direct, to the spine transmitted from vertex or sacral region, or from lateral blows. Concussion of the spinal cord is in reality diffuse contusion of the cord, and the term "spinal cord contusion" is preferred by some.

Pathology: Unlike concussion of the brain, spinal cord concussion is characterized by numerous areas of destruction in the cord. These involve most particularly the thoracic portion of the cord, the cervical being next in frequency and the lumbar least of all. They involve both gray and white matter, and vary in size and distribution. They may be spread throughout the entire length of the cord, or they may be confined to only a few areas. They may be minute or there may be destruction of the entire cord at one or more segments. In gunshot wounds, the areas of destruction may be spread diffusely above and below the level of the blow to the vertebra. In some instances of gunshot wound, the cord may be completely transected by the bullet which has ricocheted off a vertebra without penetrating either the vertebra or dura.

The changes produced in the spinal cord by missiles striking the vertebrae are determined in part by the mobility of the vertebrae in various parts of the vertebral column. In cats, shots passing the cephalic edge of thoracic spinous processes produced severe cord damage, while those striking the middle of the thoracic spines caused none.

The areas of destruction are seen as foci of hemorrhage or softening in both gray and white matter, with destruction of myelin and axis cylinders, with scar formation in the older foci.

Symptoms: There is no characteristic set of symptoms due to the fact that the lesions are frequently widespread and consist of minute hemorrhages or softenings scattered about either diffusely throughout the cord or confined to a few areas. The onset of symptoms follows directly on the trauma but may be delayed for days or weeks. Weakness of one limb or part of a limb, scattered sensory disturbances, ataxia, atrophy of a limb or part of a limb, reflex disturbances, and abnormal reflexes are seen in varying combinations. Many groups of symptoms in spinal cord concussion are transient in character, but many are not, and serious permanent disability may occur. Transverse lesions with motor and sensory paralysis, urinary and fecal retention, abdominal distention, hematuria, etc., occur in both cervical and thoracic concussion. Spastic quadriplegia, spastic hemiplegia, brachial monoplegia, and spastic cerebellar types have been described in cervical concussion. Bulbar symptoms, such as difficulty in swallowing, have been seen in some subjects.

Diagnosis: This depends in large part on a history of injury to the spine. Following this, there develop diffuse symptoms and signs which are difficult to classify and are therefore usually regarded as psychogenic. Careful examination will disclose true evidence of neurological disease characterized by scattered cord involvement. This is sufficient to establish the diagnosis.

The outlook is poor for recovery due to the destruction of the cord substance. Treatment is purely symptomatic.

XV. VASCULAR DISORDERS OF THE SPINAL CORD

1. Meningeal Hemorrhage

Etiology: Meningeal hemorrhage affecting the spinal cord may be either extradural or subdural. The condition is rare. The causes are the same as those of meningeal origin elsewhere. Trauma of all sorts is the most important cause. Other causes include embolus, blood dyscrasias, birth injury, scurvy, typhoid fever, arteriosclerosis.

Pathology: Extradural hemorrhage is the result of arterial bleeding. It is seen as an accumulation of fresh blood on the outside of the dura, usually confined to a few segments. Subdural hemorrhage is seen beneath the dura as an accumulation of fresh blood. It is more widely dispersed than extradural hemorrhage.

Symptoms: Following trauma there develops progressive weakness in the legs or in all the limbs until a complete transverse syndrome develops with flaccid paraplegia, loss of reflexes, sensory disturbances, and bladder and rectal disturbances. Pain is a striking complaint early in the disease, due to root irritation. The paralysis in patients having meningeal hemorrhage is seldom complete, since the extradural space is roomy and the hemorrhage finds plenty of room in which to expand.

Diagnosis: Both extradural and subdural hemorrhage in the spinal canal are rare, and are more often suspected than proved. The history of a progressive weakness and development of a transverse syndrome following trauma by no means indicates hemorrhage, since this may at times occur in crush of the cord. Hemorrhage should be suspected, however with such a history, particularly if subarachnoid block can be demonstrated,

and it can be seen by roentgenograms that no dislocation is present to account for the block. Under such conditions, exploratory laminectomy is justified.

Treatment: *Operation* with removal of the clot is the only treatment for either extradural or subdural hemorrhage.

2. Anterior Spinal Artery Thrombosis

Etiology: The condition is rare. Syphilis is the most important cause in many cases. Arteriosclerosis occurs in some cases. Trauma or a history of trauma occurs in most cases, but it is doubtful whether trauma alone can cause thrombosis of the anterior spinal artery. It is probable that it acts as a precipitating factor rather than a cause.

Pathology: Occlusion of the vessel results in softening of the spinal cord. Since there is some dispute as to the distribution of the anterior spinal artery, the extent of the softening is a matter of debate. The anterior spinal artery in the cord supplies the anterior horns, the anterior half of the cord, and the pyramidal tracts. The anterior horns and anterior surface of the spinal cord are softened, including the spinothalamic tracts. The pyramidal tracts are probably also softened in anterior spinal artery occlusion, since injection experiments demonstrate that these are supplied by the anterior spinal artery. The softened areas show typical myelomalacia, with gitter cell formation and little glial replacement. Occlusion is more common in the cervical region.

Symptoms: The anterior spinal arteries may be occluded in the medulla, where they supply the pyramids, the medial lemniscus, and the hypoglossal nerve. Occlusion of the vessel in the medulla results, therefore, in quadriplegia, loss of position and vibration senses in the legs and to a lesser degree in the arms, and atrophy of the tongue.

Most frequent seats of occlusion are in the cervical and thoracic regions. The onset of symptoms in the cord is frequently with pain, sometimes severe. Paresthesias often occur and may precede the onset of pain and paralysis. Trauma may precede the onset of symptoms (stretching and yawning, lifting a heavy weight, etc.). The onset is sudden and apoplectiform in typical cases. The symptoms (paralysis, sensory disturbances, etc.) usually develop rapidly in the course of one-half hour or they may take a few days to reach their peak, the weakness of the limbs, the sensory loss and the the sphincter disturbances developing gradually over the course of a few days. Paraplegia develops as a result of pyramidal tract involvement. Atrophy, fibrillation, and weakness of the muscles is seen at the level of the lesion due to anterior horn cell destruction. Loss of pain and temperature sense is found due to spinothalamic tract involvement. Complete transverse syndromes have been observed in the disease, but it is doubtful whether they are the result of pure anterior spinal artery occlusion, since the artery supplies only the anterior portion of the spinal cord. The picture is that of an incomplete transverse lesion.

Diagnosis: The diagnosis is tenable in the presence of a history of indirect trauma with an anatomical syndrome (paralysis, segmental atrophy, pain and temperature loss). *Hematomyelia* is usually associated with direct trauma and with segmental sensory loss as in syringomyelia if the hemorrhage is confined to the central gray matter of the spinal cord. *Fracture - dislocation* offers the greatest difficulty, but can be differentiated by roentgenological studies. *Cord tumor* may develop rapidly, but subarachnoid block and a complete transverse syndrome serve to separate it.

Intermittent claudication of the spinal cord has been described in a number of instances but it is doubtful whether it is in itself an entity. It is essentially a vascular spasm involving the spinal arteries, but since anastomosis is quite rich in the spinal cord it is doubtful whether symptoms can be assigned to the arterial spasm. Transitory weakness of one or both legs, transitory Babinski's signs, pain in the legs, and increasing weakness of the legs in walking occur. Examination reveals no weakness with the limbs at rest, but the tendon reflexes are exaggerated and a Babinski sign appears after walking.

Treatment: If syphilis is the cause. *antisyphilitic treatment* is indicated. Otherwise the treatment is purely *symptomatic* as in transverse myelitis syndromes. The outlook in most cases is poor.

3. Hematomyelia

Etiology: The condition is rare. Hemorrhage into the spinal cord may occur with trauma, which is by far the most common cause. The trauma may be of various sorts of both direct and indirect type—a fall on the back or buttocks, a blow to the back, severe strain as in lifting a heavy weight, coitus, emotional excitement, etc. Spontaneous hematomyelia may develop in tumors of the spinal cord, purpura, scurvy, salvarsan treatments, typhoid fever, myelitis, or for no demonstrable reason.

The hemorrhage in cases of hematomyelia is usually massive and may extend through several segments or almost the entire length of the cord. Smaller hemorrhages are also found, confined to a few segments. Most of the hemorrhage is within the gray matter in the region of the central canal, but it often extends into the entire cord circumference. The tissue surrounding the hemorrhage is edematous, the myelin is swollen and fragmented, the axis cylinders swollen and gitter cells are seen in the tissue.

Symptoms: The onset is almost always sudden in both the spontaneous and traumatic varieties. In the former there is a history of sudden weakness due to no obvious cause; in the latter, the sudden onset follows trauma. Slow development is seen in some cases. Within a very short time paralysis develops, associated with sensory disturbances such as loss of pain and temperature, or a ensuing paraplegia or quadriplegia, and a sensory level or a segmental type of sensory disturbance. The decision to operate is not easily settled. The problem is that of an apoplectic cord disturbance, sometimes progressive in nature, with motor and sensory paralysis. *Myelitis* in some form is most often considered. The history of trauma is helpful, but often the condition cannot be recognized save

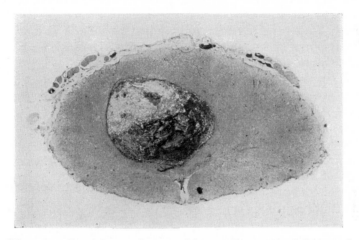

Fig. 98—*Hematomyelia.* A hemorrhage in the central portion of the spinal cord in a case of injury of the cord.

complete transverse sensory syndrome. Sphincter troubles are common. The findings vary in accordance with the level of the spinal cord affected. In cervical lesions quadriplegia results; in thoracic and lumbar lesions paraplegia. After a varying length of time, usually a few weeks, recession of symptoms occurs, and sequelae of various sorts are found, depending on the degree of involvement of the nervous tissue.

The diagnosis is not difficult in cases of trauma. The symptoms are likely to be progressive. In spontaneous cases, the diagnosis is not clear; only an intramedullary cord involvement is diagnosable in such cases, the true nature of the disorder being disclosed by operation. The symptoms are those of a rapidly developing paralysis in most cases, with by *exploration.* *Tumor* can be ruled out by spinal fluid studies, but partial block may be found in hematomyelia due to the cord swelling.

XVI. CAISSON DISEASE

Etiology: Caisson disease occurs in individuals working under high atmospheric pressures in deep sea diving, or in diving bells in the building of bridges, tunnels, or skyscrapers. It affects, therefore, adult males who are so employed. It is caused by nitrogen gas emboli which form on too rapid decompression after prolonged compression. Under such conditions, nitrogen gas bubbles are set free in the circulation due to oversaturation of the blood and tissues with nitrogen which has failed to be absorbed under the conditions of increased atmospheric pressure. Under conditions of compression, the circulating blood is exposed to a partial pressure of nitrogen and oxygen proportional to the air pressure. The oxygen is absorbed by the tissues, but the nitrogen is not and accumulates in the body until the tissues are charged with nitrogen. If decompression is slow, nitrogen is excreted by the lungs until the normal equilibrium is established with the atmospheric pressure. If decompression is too rapid, the blood and tissues are left with a partial pressure far above atmospheric pressure, and the nitrogen which saturates the tissues leaves the blood and tissues in bubble form and lodges as nitrogen emboli in many parts of the body.

Pathology: Free gas is found in the circulation and in the lungs, liver, and other organs. Fat tissue contains an unusual amount of nitrogen bubbles. The brain and spinal cord are often severely damaged and show softenings and hemorrhages. The softenings are similar to those found in vessel occlusion from other causes, and are composed of gitter cells and dissolution of the tissues. Their extent is dependent on the size of the occluded vessel. Bubbles of nitrogen are found in the brain and cord.

Symptoms: The symptoms develop quickly after decompression and specific symptoms found depend upon the site of the emboli. Muscle and joint pains are extremely common (bends) and usually usher in the illness. The pains are usually in the legs, but may often involve the abdomen and the arms. Vertigo, staggering, loss of equilibrium, nausea and vomiting, are almost as common as pain. Dyspnea is very common. Pruritis and erythema are frequently found. Air emboli involving one of the branches of the cerebral vessels may cause hemiplegia, hemianopsia, monoplegia, aphasia, or other symptoms referable to cerebral

disease. Tinnitus, deafness, strabismus, or diplopia may occur.

The spinal cord is not infrequently affected, with pictures characterized by paraplegia, sensory and sphincter disturbances. A complete transverse myelitis may sometimes be produced. The symptoms may be delayed in some cases for several days.

Some patients recover completely with recompression, but in some instances the occlusion of a cerebral vessel with resulting hemiplegia results in permanent disability. The same holds true for most spinal cases.

Treatment: *Immediate recompression* is imperative in patients with the bends, followed by *gradual decompression.* Even hemiplegias and paraplegias may recover under these circumstances. Recompression should be started as soon as possible after acute symptoms develop. Long delay may result in permanent injury to the brain or spinal cord. Symptoms are usually relieved by compression to the same level of pressure as that which the patient left, but pressures of 5 to 15 pounds higher are sometimes necessary.

XVII. DISEASES OF THE VERTEBRAE

Involvement of the vertebrae becomes important under some circumstances because of accompanying evidences of root and spinal cord involvement. Relief is therefore sought for pain, and the opinion of the neurologist requested.

1. Spondylarthritis Ankylopoietica
(*Spondylitis Deformans, Spondylose Rhizomelique, Marie-Strümpell Disease*)

Etiology: The disease involves chiefly young males during the third and fourth decades. The exact cause is not known, but the process is probably an infectious disease of the vertebral column and adjacent structures, usually described as a nonspecific infectious arthritis. Trauma is said to play a part in about 15 per cent of cases, but its part is doubtful in causing the disease. Heredity is probably a factor, since the disease has been found in several members of one family and in one instance has been followed through three generations. Syphilis has been indicted in some cases. Endocrine imbalance, notably parathyroid deficiency, has been blamed. Pulmonary tuberculosis is a fairly frequent complication. A previous history of rheumatic arthritis is sometimes found and in a few instances the disease has developed in patients with atrophic arthritis.

Pathology: The disease is a destructive arthritis which begins in the vertebrae as an infectious process, which leads to a destruction of the joint cartilage, followed by connective tissue repair and finally by calcification, and ankylosis of the joints. The small intervertebral articulations are affected first. The vertebrae show high grade atrophy without tendency to collapse. The intervertebral discs escape. Calcification of the longitudinal ligaments of the spine, ossification of the ligamenta flava, and calcification of the costochondral junctions occur. In the hip and shoulder joints the process resembles a severe atrophic arthritis. Changes may be found early in the sacroiliac joints. The intervertebral foramina are narrowed by the arthritis, thus pinching the posterior spinal roots and accounting for the pain.

Symptoms: The process is a chronic progressive condition characterized by pain and stiffness in the back, sometimes with exacerbations and remissions, and with involvement of the shoulder and hip joints in some types (Marie-Strümpell). As a rule, the shoulder and hip joints are not involved. Two forms have been described: that of Bechterew with root pains and that of Marie-Strümpell. Though there are minor variations in the

radiological appearance of the two, the weight of evidence favors the view that they are merely variants of the same disease.

The onset is usually gradual, with a slowly developing stiffness of the spine which becomes apparent to the patient over a period of months. A low grade fever and leukocytosis are usually present. An acute onset is sometimes seen, often following an injury or infection. The disease involves primarily the vertebrae and the adjacent structures in all the cases. The progressive spine stiffness develops gradually at first without pain, but pain appears in almost all subjects sooner or later. It is typical root pain which may appear anywhere, depending upon the roots pinched. Pain in the thorax, neck, and lower back is common. Careful inquiry will reveal one or more roots to be affected on one or both sides. The root pain which is paroxysmal is not continual but has exacerbations. Against the root pain is often a background of dull constant pain.

Examination reveals a stiff, rigid, "poker" spine usually in the thoracic and lumbar regions, but often affecting the entire spine. The normal lumbar lordosis is lost. The head is thrust forward and the trunk held rigidly in walking. Kyphosis develops, but not in all cases. The spine muscles are held in spasm and become atrophic later in the disease. No signs of spinal cord involvement can be demonstrated, but hyperesthesia in the pain zones corresponding to the root irritation may be found.

Roentgenologic studies in advanced cases show decalcification about the joints, blurring of the joint surfaces, narrowing and obliteration of the affected intervertebral discs in some cases.

Diagnosis: The diagnosis is made without difficulty, the stiff spine and back pain being quite distinctive in the early stages and the root pains later. Roentgenologic evidence of the condition may not be present early in the disease and may lag far behind clinical features by months or years. There is little value in distinguishing types of the disease, as for example, the Marie-Strümpell type with stiff spine, involvement of hip and shoulder joints, no kyphosis, relative absence of root pains, and atrophy of the muscles, as against the Bechterew type with kyphosis, root pain, and no involvement of the larger joints. The two types are part and parcel of the same disease. From the standpoint of diagnosis, the distinction between the two forms is not important; but from the prognostic standpoint, the distinction is of some value since one form is associated with severe root pain (Bechterew), while the other is not (Marie-Strümpell).

Hypertrophic arthritis of the spine may be confused with spondylitis. It occurs usually after the fourth decade, and fever and leukocytosis are uncommon. The roentgenograms show degeneration of the intervertebral disc, narrowing of the intervertebral spaces, exostoses, and bony bridging.

Prognosis: The disease is usually slowly progressive, though it may cease to progress at any stage. Bony ankylosis develops after 10 to 20 years and pains cease.

Treatment: Adequate *physical* and *mental rest* and a *high vitamin diet* are important. *Warm climates* are better than cold. *Salicylates* help keep the patient comfortable and if used should be employed generously. Anemia is sometimes present and should be treated with *iron*. Vaccines are of doubtful value. *Infected foci should be removed. Local heat* is extremely important, as *infra-red*, and gives great comfort. *Paravertebral injections* or rhizotomy may be necessary for the relief of pain. *X-ray treatment* offers real help and should always be used.

2. Kümmel's Disease

This is a rare disease of the vertebrae which follows trauma, sometimes severe but most often of a minor nature. The trauma may be direct or indirect, is soon recovered from, and months later is followed by rarefaction of the vertebra with gibbus formation and kyphosis. The process is noninflammatory.

The condition is at times associated with neurological symptoms such as root pains and paralysis of the legs, bladder, and bowels due to compression of the spinal cord by the buckled vertebra.

3. Hypertrophic Osteoarthritis

Osteoarthritis of the spine may at times be associated with neurological symptoms. The causes are those of arthritis elsewhere, and the condition is found most frequently (eighty-five per cent) after the fourth decade. It is characterized by calcium deposits on the vertebrae, with spur formations and bridging. In advanced cases, the intervertebral discs are degenerated and may become calcified.

Root pains appear most commonly in arthritis of the spine. They may be felt in the neck, trunk, arms, back, or legs, depending on the root or roots compressed. Not uncommonly, cases of sciatica are suspected of being due to osteoarthritis, and it is sometimes responsible for leg pains. The pains are due to compression of the posterior root in the intervertebral foramen by the hypertrophic arthritic process. In rare instances, compression of the spinal cord has been observed due to impingement of the hypertrophic arthritis upon the spinal canal. There may be no evidence of arthritis elsewhere in the body.

The *diagnosis* of root pain due to osteoarthritis of the spine is usually difficult to establish because osteoarthritis may not be demonstrable by roentgenogram in early cases, while in advanced cases the relation between the pain and the arthritis is hard to establish because of the frequent occurrence of arthritis of the spine without symptoms. If the root pain corresponds to the involved vertebra, the assumption may safely be made that it is due to the arthritis. Osteoarthritis of the spine is too often diagnosed by exclusion in cases of leg pain.

Treatment: This consists of the treatment of arthritis elsewhere: *general hygiene, proper diet, salicylates,* and *physiotherapy,* particularly *heat.*

4. Neurological Complications of Scoliosis

Scoliosis may rarely be associated with neurological symptoms in structural scoliosis, poliomyelitis, or rickets. The scoliosis of syringomyelia and Friedreich's ataxia is not considered in this group, since the spinal cord symptoms are not caused by the bony deformity. Rarely, cases appear with evidences of root pains, the location of which varies due to the region of scoliosis. Trunk pains are most common. Still more rare are cases of spinal cord compression secondary to severe scoliosis. Paraplegia, transverse syndromes, and syringomyelic syndromes have been reported. Subarachnoid block is not present as a rule. The reason for the cord symptoms has been variously ascribed to narrowing of the vertebral canal, pressure of the cord against the inner wall of the spinal canal by the angle of the scoliosis, or torsion of the spinal cord by an abnormally stretched dura.

In early cases, *orthopedic measures* such as plaster cast have been found to be successful. In advanced cases, *laminectomy* has been performed on the region of pressure on the cord with reported relief in some patients.

5. Tuberculosis of the Spine
(Pott's Disease, Tuberculous Spondylitis)

Etiology: Tuberculosis of the spine occurs usually in children or in young adults. It is caused by invasion of the vertebrae by the tubercle bacillus. Neurological complications, notably the paraplegias, occur in eight per cent of cases of Pott's disease.

Pathology: Pott's disease affects particularly the second dorsal to third lumbar vertebrae. The vertebrae most commonly affected are the tenth, eleventh, and twelfth thoracic and first lumbar vertebrae. The reason for this special predilection is not known.

The process begins as a tuberculous infection of the vertebra. More than one vertebra may be involved. With extension of the process comes destruction of the vertebra, collapse, and the development of kyphosis. With this the process spreads into the surrounding tissue and cold abscess develops. This may remain confined beneath the anterior ligament of the spine or spread out into the tissues and invade the spinal canal.

Beneath the collapsed tuberculous vertebra there develops an extradural abscess with a pachymeningitis. The epidural infection extends to form an extradural abscess, and later extension of the process directly into the spinal cord. Inflammatory foci are present in the posterior and anterior roots. The cord becomes compressed by the process. Degeneration is found in various parts of the cord, with demyelination and loss of axis cylinders. Inflammatory foci are numerous and perivascular infiltration with lymphocytes and plasma cells is seen. In some cases the destruction in the cord is the result of mechanical compression only, without invasion by the tuberculous process. Complete demyelination of the cord segment or segments may be found.

The pathological process is thought to be due to a blood stream infection, but lymphatic extension from a neighboring focus is proposed by some. In very rare instances, direct extension has been found from pulmonary tuberculosis.

Symptoms: The neurological complications of Pott's disease may appear rapidly (six to ten months) or may develop slowly after the tuberculous disease of the vertebra. Rarely, the onset may be sudden with compression of the spinal cord in the cervical region, due to rapid subluxation or sudden collapse of the atlas or axis with sudden death. A similar onset may develop in the thoracic region. One of the earliest signs is pain, which is usually found to be a typical root pain, sometimes appearing in a child or young adult without previous evidence of disturbance. It is important to recall that root pain may be the only symptom of Pott's disease for some time and that so far as treatment is concerned it is desirable to recognize the condition at this time. The pain may persist for some time and may be followed by paraplegia within the course of weeks or months. This may develop suddenly in apoplectic fashion or the paraplegia may be slow in development. The late paraplegias developing after the bony deformity has been present for some time are usually the result of reactivation of a small tuberculous mass inside the spinal canal (Butler). The paraplegia is usually associated with extension of the legs, spasticity, increase of reflexes and Babinski's sign. Flexion paraplegia may be seen occasionally.

Spinal cord involvement in Pott's disease may be manifested only by root pains, by root pains and spastic paraplegia, or by spastic paraplegia and sphincter disturbances, with or without sensory disturbances. The paraplegia in some cases may be associated with objective sensory disturbances as in complete transverse cord syndromes. Sphincter disturbances are frequent. A kyphosis is usually present, sometimes developing suddenly.

Lumbar puncture reveals evidence of a complete subarachnoid block (positive Queckenstedt test) and increased spinal fluid protein. Xanthochromic fluid is sometimes seen.

Roentgenologic study of the spine in well-developed cases reveals the typical deformity of tuberculosis of the vertebra, with destruction, kyphosis, destruction of the intervertebral disc, and abscess in the surrounding tissues. In early cases with pain only there may be no changes visible in the roentgenograms.

Diagnosis: The diagnosis of Pott's disease in a well-developed case is easy, the kyphosis, roentgenological changes, the spastic paraplegia, and the subarachnoid block being quite characteristic. In early cases with only root pain, without roentgenological changes, the diagnosis is more difficult and can only be suspected. *Metastatic carcinoma* may simulate the condition, particularly in view of the rapid onset of the paraplegia in such patients, but its occurrence in older people, the previous history of carcinoma in most cases, the evidences of cachexia, and the roentgenologic findings of carcinoma in the bone are usually sufficient to distinguish the condition. *Spinal cord tumor* is differentiated by the history of pains, the evidence of a transverse lesion, and subarachnoid block in the absence of a destructive process in the vertebrae. *Syphilitic meningomyelitis* is easily differentiated by the positive serological findings in the spinal fluid.

Treatment: It is generally agreed that *hygienic measures,* a *nourishing diet, fresh air, heliotherapy,* and continuous and prolonged *dorsal recumbency* are to be employed. The possibilities of bladder and bowel dysfunction and the danger of trophic ulceration require critical nursing supervision. An effort to secure complete *immobilization of the spine in hyperextension* is to be made by the use of a Bradford or Herzmark or Rogers frame, a plaster bed or circular body cast, or an accurately fitting brace.

The *surgical management* in cases of tuberculous spondylitis *with* cord compression will depend, in great part, on the attitude of the attending physician as to the surgical treatment of tuberculous spondylitis *without* cord compression, and, indeed, of bone and joint tuberculosis in general. While there is considerable agreement that fusion of the spine by any one of several technics is an invaluable measure in adults for securing the absolute immobilization so necessary in effecting a local cure, there is some disagreement as to the indications for this procedure in children and young adults. Most patients with early nerve root or cord involvement will demonstrate clinical improvement or recovery by simple prolonged dorsal recumbency. Recurrence or even exaggeration of the neurologic features, however, must be anticipated if the tuberculous spondylitis continues to be active, and, indeed, has been known to occur several years after an apparent cure. It is probable that fusion or arthrodesis of the spine should be utilized in the treatment of tuberculous spondylitis with neurologic complications, if and when the patient's general condition permits, irrespective of the age of the patient, or of the site, duration, or extent of the lesion.

The results following the use of laminectomy in the treatment of these patients have been generally unsatisfactory, except in a very few in whom this procedure may have prevented an irremediable lesion of the spinal cord from pressure of a pachymeningitis, or from a sequestrum or a cold abscess within the spinal canal. It might be stated broadly, that decompressive laminectomy is indicated if, in spite of adequate external spinal fixation, symptoms of cord compression continue without sufficient evidence that the progression is due to changes in the position or degree of destruction of the involved bony elements. In these patients, a minimal amount of bone is to be sacrificed, since this serves further to weaken the spinal column, and this procedure should be fortified, immediately or later, by an arthrodesis of the spine.

Recumbency, following fusion of the spine, must be continued, despite complete ankylosis of the spinous processes and laminae of the involved vertebrae and healthy vertebrae above and below, until the clinical and roentgenographic pictures indicate sufficient healing of the spinal lesion itself. Residual paralysis of the limbs may require the use of external appliances to assist the ambulatory patient.

Associated paravertebral abscesses usually tend to diminish in size and to calcify or disappear following the successful treatment of the bony focus. Therapy directed to the abscess itself appears to be indicated when the abscess is contributing to the nerve root or cord compression. Such mechanical effects may be alleviated by repeated aspiration. Successful approach to a mediastinal abscess may require a costotransversectomy.

XVIII. SYRINGOMYELIA

Etiology: Syringomyelia is a chronic, slowly progressive disease, characterized by cavity formation in the spinal cord. Its exact cause is not known. It occurs most frequently in individuals between 20 and 40 years of age, but it has been known to occur in childhood and in persons as old as 60 to 65 years. Males are more commonly affected than females.

Though the cause of the disease is not known in the majority of cases, contributory causes of many sorts have been recorded in the disease. *Spinal cord tumors* have been found to be associated with syringomyelic cavities. It is doubtful, however, whether the cavities are the

recorded also following *hematomyelia*. Cavity formation may follow *spinal cord concussion* and other forms of *trauma* of the spinal cord, especially in persons with severe indirect injury to the vertebral column. The cavities in such patients have developed in the areas of softening produced by the concussion. Multiple sclerosis and Pott's disease have been observed with cavity forma-

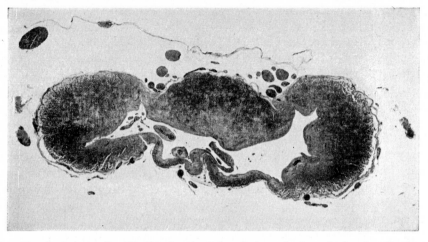

Fig. 99—*Syringomyelia*. Myelin sheath stain of the spinal cord showing the large cavity and the destruction of the central, dorsal and lateral parts of the cord.

same as in syringomyelia, though they resemble them closely. The reason for the association of intramedullary tumors at times with cavity formation is not known. Similar cavity formation may be seen in infiltrating tumors of the brain stem. *Emboli* of the spinal cord have been found to produce cavities. *Thrombosis* of *spinal arteries* is not infrequently associated with cavity formation. This appears to be particularly true of anterior spinal artery thrombosis. *Syphilis* is sometimes found to produce cavity formation of a syringomyelic type. This is true of syphilitic meningomyelitis and pachymeningitis especially, but it has been seen also in tabes. Rare cases have been recorded in congenital syphilis. Syringomyelic cavities have been

tion. *Familial* forms of lumbosacral syringomyelia have been recorded.

Pathology: The outstanding feature of syringomyelia is the cavity within the spinal cord. The cord is enlarged and fluctuant, and may fill the dura. The cavity may extend for only a few segments or it may extend the entire length of the spinal cord and even into the medulla and brain stem. In one recorded case, the cavity extended through the entire brain stem to the lateral ventricle. It occupies the central portion of the cord, and may extend into the posterior and anterior horns, the posterior columns, or may destroy the entire cord circumference, leaving only a thin rim of tissue. The form of the cavity varies greatly from case to case and even from segment to segment. It may be slitlike or a round or oval cavity. Cavities may be single or multiple, may be extensive in one segment and small in another, their form and size varying from one level to another. They frequently follow along the nerve root entrance into the cord, and as slitlike cavities along the nerve entrance zones in the medulla. Slitlike cavities may develop in a single posterior horn without involving the central gray matter.

The cavity is filled with thick yellow fluid which causes distention of the cord. Microscopic study shows a dense glial network around the cavity, composed chiefly of glial fibers and few cells. The degree of cord destruction depends on the extent of the cavity. Posterior column degeneration is common. Anterior horn cell destruction is practically constant. Pyramidal tract involvement is also common. The entire substance of the cord may be destroyed, leaving only a thin layer at the circumference.

Syringomyelia is regarded by some as being of congenital origin due to arrested development of the spinal cord, the syringomyelic cavity resulting from failure of closure of the ectodermal tube. Others look upon it as an acquired disorder resulting from vascular softening with resulting cyst formation trauma, or lymph stasis. By still others the disease is regarded as primarily neoplastic (blastomatosis), the glial formation being regarded as primary and tumorous in nature.

Symptoms: Syringomyelia affects young people in particular, the typical subject showing a combination of motor and sensory disturbances, usually with trophic disturbances. The cervical cord is much more commonly affected than other portions, hence the predominance of symptoms in the hands and arms. Involvement of the thoracic and lumbar cord is not altogether uncommon, however.

Motor symptoms are constant and together with the sensory features usher in the disease. Weakness is a common complaint and is associated with atrophy of the hand muscles usually, but in some instances of the leg or foot muscles. The small muscles of the hand undergo atrophy, weakness, and show fibrillations. The thenar and hypothenar eminences atrophy together with the interossei and lumbricals, giving rise to the flat simian hand.

Sensory symptoms also are common. Paresthesias occur frequently and are experienced as feelings of numbness, prickling, formication, cold sensations, etc. Girdle sensations and even severe pains may be felt. Pain may be a persistent and disabling symptom of syringomyelia. It is usually felt in the shoulders and arms, and may resemble root pain due to other conditions such as herniated cervical disc and spinal cord tumor. The most common objective sensory disturbance consists of a segmental loss of pain and temperature sensations, the extent depending naturally on the extent of the cord damage. Less common are unilateral segmental sensory loss of pain and temperature due to involvement of the fibers in the posterior horn before crossing over to join the spinothalamic tract. Disturbances of deep sensation (loss of position and vibration senses) are almost always found, either singly or together. The legs or arms may be involved.

Vegetative disturbances are found frequently. Hyper- or hypohidrosis may be seen in the involved segments or may extend beyond them. Horner's syndrome may be present from involvement of the spinal cord or medullary fibers. Vasomotor disturbances are found in almost every case in the form of cyanosis of the hands and feet. Bladder symptoms are not found in the early stages of the disease but may be found in later stages. Sexual and rectal disturbances are not common.

Trophic disturbances are seen constantly in syringomyelia. These are of many sorts. Scoliosis or kyphoscoliosis is seen constantly and involves the thoracic vertebrae chiefly. The vertebrae themselves may be denser or may show rarefaction. Trophic skin changes are extremely common and are seen as callous formations, brittle and hypertrophied nails, atrophy of terminal phalanges, edema, enlargement of hand or foot, pigmentations, skin ulcer, etc. Charcot joints are sometimes found. Cervical ribs have been observed in the disease. Spontaneous fractures are often found. Exostoses are common. Arthropathies are common, affecting chiefly the shoulder and elbow joints, and the small joints of the hands. Ankylosis may develop in the affected joints, causing great limitation of motion.

Unusual accompaniments are sometimes seen. Choked disc is seen in rare cases, associated with internal hydrocephalus. Spina bifida, spina bifida occulata, duplication of the spinal cord, and meningocele are sometimes seen. Deformities of the skull such as oxycephaly are rare occurrences. Epileptic attacks have been observed in cases with hydrocephalus.

Clinical Varieties: The symptoms described may be found in various combinations, depending upon the area of cord which is diseased.

Cervicodorsal Type: Since the syringomyelic cavity affects the cervical region most commonly, the cervical syndrome is seen often in the disease. It is characterized by onset with paresthesias of the hands or sometimes with pain in the arms. Atrophy of the small hand muscles appears early and may extend to the arm and shoulder. Loss of pain and temperature sensations is found over the arms and upper part of the trunk, usually bilaterally, sometimes unilaterally. Horner's syndrome may be present. Spasticity of the legs or of all the limbs often develops as the cavity extends, and ataxia from posterior column involvement may be found. Trophic and vegetative disturbances appear constantly.

Lumbosacral Type: Cavity formation in the lower cord is manifested by atrophy of the thigh and foot muscles, which may develop later into severe contractures. Loss of pain and temperature is found to involve the lower limbs, perineum, and genitalia. The reflexes are overactive and a Babinski sign is present in lumbar involvement if the pyramidal tract is affected. Absence of the Achilles reflex is found in predominant sacral involvement.

Bulbar Type (Syringobulbia): Syringomyelia may affect the brain stem, giving rise to syringobulbia. This is rare as an isolated manifestation of the disease. Bulbar symptoms are more commonly seen as part of syringomyelia involving the cord. Atrophy and fibrillations of the tongue, usually unilateral, are common. Facial paralysis may be seen. Sensory involvement of the face is common due to involvement of the descending root of the trigeminal nerve. The loss affects pain and temperature on the side of the lesion and is of the concentric variety, the sensory impairment not being found in the peripheral nerve distribution of the trigeminal but rather as concentric areas of sensory loss over the face. The corneal reflex is lost. Paresthesias involving the face are common. Vertigo may be one of the first symptoms of syringobulbia. Pupillary disturbances have been observed. Argyll Robertson pupils have been reported.

Diagnosis: The diagnosis of syringomyelia is not difficult in a typical case.

The onset in early life, the very slow progression, the combination of motor symptoms, segmental loss of pain and temperature, vegetative, and trophic disturbances usually involving the upper limbs is sufficient to establish the diagnosis. Progress of the disease is very slow and there may be long periods of months or years in which no visible progression is made.

Intramedullary and extramedullary spinal cord tumor offer the greatest difficulties. The former, since it grows within the cord, may simulate syringomyelia closely. The progress of tumor is faster than syringomyelia. Though some tumors may progress slowly, they rarely progress as slowly as syringomyelia. The dissociation of sensation is not likely to be found in tumor unless it remains confined to the central canal region. More often tumors spread out and cause a transverse sensory syndrome. Bladder incontinence is more common in tumor. Spinal fluid studies are helpful; protein increase is more constant in tumor, as is subarachnoid block, but both may be observed in syringomyelia. Myelogram may offer the only means of differentiation. If syringomyelia is present, a greatly enlarged spinal cord may be seen. *Hypertrophic pachymeningitis* progresses more rapidly than syringomyelia, is characterized by pains and by evidence of compression of the cord. Dissociated loss of pain and temperature is not found. *Syphilitic meningomyelitis* may simulate syringomyelia very closely in cases with involvement of the central gray matter. The serological findings in the spinal fluid are positive and sufficient to establish the diagnosis. The onset is more abrupt and the course more rapid than syringomyelia. *Cervical rib* or *scalenus anticus syndrome* may resemble syringomyelia largely because of the atrophy of the hand muscles, but the absence of the typical dissociated sensory loss is enough to distinguish it, while the roentgenological evidence of cervical rib and the vasomotor changes establish the true diagnosis.

Syringomyelia may simulate herniated cervical disc. In patients with severe pain the differentiation from a laterally displaced herniated disc may be very difficult, and similar difficulties may be present in centrally displaced discs, in these patients without pain. As in spinal cord tumor, myelogram may be necessary to establish the diagnosis.

The *nuclear amyotrophies,* such as progressive muscular atrophy and amyotrophic lateral sclerosis, are characterized by the absence of sensory findings. They require differentiation from the bulbar form of syringomyelia. *Leprosy neuritis* needs to be considered largely because of its resemblance to *Morvan's disease,* which is a form of syringomyelia characterized by weakness of the arms with ulcers of the fingertips.

Prognosis: The disease is slowly progressive and usually continues for years. Rare cases have been reported with an acute course, with death in a few years. Death ensues from some intercurrent disease, such as pneumonia, tuberculosis, etc.

Treatment: Syringomyelia cannot be treated by medical means. Early cases of the disease should be given a trial with *irradiation,* since good results have been found with such treatment. Advanced cases are unaffected by irradiation. *Operation* to open the syringomyelic cyst and relieve pressure within the cord sometimes gives good results. and may halt the advance of the disease.

XIX. FRIEDREICH'S ATAXIA
(Hereditary Spinal Ataxia)

Etiology: Friedreich's ataxia is a disease which begins early, from five to twenty years of age, the greatest incidence being at puberty. Cases are known which have had their onset late in life (fifty to sixty years). It is a heredo-familial disease which can often be followed through several generations, but sporadic cases are not uncommon. Blood relationship can often be demonstrated in the affected families. Atypical forms of the disease and other types of neurological disorder (myopathies, epilepsy, multiple sclerosis) are often found in the affected families. Direct etiological factors are not known.

Pathology: The disease affects primarily the spinal cord, which is small and atrophic. The posterior columns, spinocerebellar, and pyramidal tracts are chiefly affected. Degeneration is found in the posterior columns, particularly affecting the column of Goll and, to a lesser extent, the column of Burdach; in the spinocerebellar pathways and Clarke column cells, and the pyramidal tracts. The posterior column degeneration is primary and not dependent on posterior root or ganglion disease. While the degeneration of the spinocerebellar tracts is chiefly spinal, it may be followed into the cerebellum, and degenerative cerebellar changes are found in the disease. The cerebellum is smaller than normal, the Purkinje cells are degenerated and decreased in number, and secondary changes are found in the fibers of the cerebellum. Degenerative changes are sometimes found in the cerebrum, basal ganglia, the dentate nucleus, and thalamus.

Symptoms: Typical cases are characterized by the fully developed symptom complex, but many atypical forms are known. The disease begins gradually in late childhood as a rule, with difficulty in walking and with other evidences of incoördination in a child who appears up to this time to have developed normally. *Ataxia* develops as the first symp-

tom, almost always in the legs. The gait is extremely ataxic, with high lifting of the feet and much lurching, representing a combination of tabetic and posterior column incoördination. Walking becomes totally impossible eventually. Even sitting and standing become impossible. Romberg's sign is often but not always present. *Muscle irritability* and restlessness are common, often giving the impression of chorea. The motor restlessness involves the hands and arms particularly. Speech disturbances are seen constantly. The speech is hesitating, slow, and indistinct even in early stages, and becomes more pronouncedly disturbed in later stages. The patellar and Achilles *reflexes* are lost or decreased. Reflex loss is one of the earliest and most characteristic symptoms of the disease. In rare cases, however, the reflexes may remain intact for years during the course of the disease or throughout the disease. The reflexes, once lost, may return after disease of the pyramidal tracts appears. With the latter comes weakness of the legs and Babinski signs. The abdominal reflexes are retained almost always but may be lost. *Sensory disturbances* are constant in the form of loss or impairment of position and vibration senses in the great toes and less constantly in the thumbs. Pain and temperature disturbances are not affected. *Nystagmus* is a constant symptom, though exceptions to this have been noted. It is usually a horizontal nystagmus, but rotary and vertical nystagmus is seen at times. Optic atrophy is seen, though it is more frequent in the cerebellar form (Marie's disease). Ocular palsies occur in the form often of internal and external rectus weakness, and diplopia is a common symptom. Muscle atrophies are seen not infrequently in Friedreich families, in the form of spinal muscle atrophy, or myopathies. *Friedreich's foot* is constantly seen. The typical deformity is a pes cavus with talipes varus or equinovarus. The metatarsophalangeal joints are dorsiflexed and the terminal phalanges plantar flexed. This position becomes fixed eventually. The *mentality* may be unimpaired or mental deficiency of varying degree may exist. *Kyphoscoliosis* is an almost constant feature (eighty-five per cent). Skeletal anomalies of various sorts are found.

Other features of involvement of other systems are seen in Friedreich's disease. Among them are spina bifida, retinitis pigmentosa, syndactylism, supernumerary digits, blue sclerae, cataract, albinism, deafness, alopecia, ichthyosis, and other manifestations, indicating a rather diffuse ectodermal involvement apart from the nervous system. Diabetes mellitus has been found in some cases.

Atypical forms or formes frustes are common and many varieties have been described. These include atypical cases seen in families of Friedreich's ataxia or families of atypical cases may be seen without clear-cut development of the disease. Among them are patients with Friedreich's foot, absent reflexes, and nystagmus. Or subjects exist with mild ataxia, absent reflexes, Babinski's sign, and Friedreich's foot.

Diagnosis: The diagnosis in a typical case is clear. The disease occurs in families, but may be found sporadically, comes on usually in puberty with a normal developmental history, is characterized by ataxia, speech disturbances, scoliosis, nystagmus, absence of reflexes with intact abdominal reflexes, disturbances of deep sensation, Babinski signs, and Friedreich's foot. It may be confused with Marie's *hereditary cerebellar ataxia*, which is probably a similar disease. It is characterized by a later onset than Friedreich's ataxia (twenty to forty-five years), by outstanding cerebellar signs, and by direct inheritance. Among its features are optic atrophy, cerebellar incoördination of arms, legs, and trunk, severe speech disturbances, oculomotor palsies, and often mental deterioration. Sensory disturbances, scoliosis, and Friedreich's foot are not found and the reflexes are increased rather than lost as in Friedreich's disease.

Friedreich's ataxia is one of a group of heredodegenerative diseases in which transitions between one and another group are frequently seen. Among these are Friedreich's ataxia, cerebellar ataxia, and myopathies. Myopathic disturbances may be found in Friedreich's ataxia itself or may be seen in pure form in Friedreich's families. The distinction between Friedreich's ataxia and Marie's hereditary cerebellar ataxia is not distinct and definite. The ordinary distinctions of age of onset, ocular involvement and hereditary features merge into the two forms in many instances. Families are on record in which both forms appeared in a study of 6 generations with hereditary ataxia (Schut).

Prognosis: The disease runs a very chronic slow course with long periods of lack of progression of symptoms. Death usually occurs from some intercurrent disease.

XX. NEURAL MUSCLE ATROPHY
(Charcot-Marie-Tooth Atrophy)

Etiology: The disease affects males much more frequently than females and occurs most often in the first two decades of life. It is a heredofamilial disease, occurring in the second to sixth generations of families. Incidental factors of many sorts have been accused, among them alcohol, lead poisoning, syphilis, tuberculosis, and endocrine factors, especially pituitary and thyroid deficiencies.

Pathology: The peripheral nerves and spinal roots show degenerative changes in myelin sheaths and axis cylinders as well as proliferative changes in the Schwann cells. The peripheral nerve changes are much more pronounced than those of the spinal roots, which are slight. Changes are found also in the spinal ganglia. Degeneration of the posterior columns of the spinal cord is constant but varies in intensity. Both posterior columns are affected diffusely in the lower portions of the cord, but only the column of Goll in the cervical region. The anterior horn cells of the spinal cord are also diseased; many cells are lost in the lumbar region of the cord and are degenerated in other cord levels. The affected muscles show atrophic changes.

Histological study of the muscles in progressive neuromuscular atrophy suggests that the muscular changes in the disease are due to a disorder of the peripheral motor nerves. In the early stages, the muscles show increase in the hypolemmal nuclei and some increase in connective tissue. In later stages, there is a greater increase in connective tissue and hypolemmal nuclei; degenerative changes in the nuclei and sarcoplasm; and degeneration of myofibrils.

Symptoms: The onset of symptoms is gradual and may be ushered in following an acute infection. The disease does not affect all afflicted members of a family in the same way. Some may be more severely affected than others. *Motor symptoms* are outstanding, particularly atrophy and weakness of the leg and especially the foot muscles. The peronei and extensors of the toes are most affected and may be the only muscles involved for some time, the disease spreading later to other leg muscles. Because of the muscle atrophy, the foot assumes a hollowed position and may even resemble

clubfoot. The foot deformity may be the only sign of the disease early in the illness. The foot is held in foot-drop, with typical dropping of the toes and steppage gait. The process extends to the upper limbs after years, involving the small hand muscles chiefly. The shoulder girdle muscles may be affected. Fibrillations of the affected muscles are often seen. The reflexes are absent and the electrical reactions decreased. Scoliosis is often present.

Sensory disturbances are common. Spontaneous pains are found early in the disease. Objective sensory disturbances are found but are not constant. Superficial sensation is most affected. Hypalgesia and hypesthesia are found most marked in the distal portions of the limbs, especially the legs.

Vasomotor changes are found in the feet (cyanosis). Trophic changes are found in the skin and nails. *Mental* symptoms have been reported.

Diagnosis: The disease is not difficult to recognize as a rule. The familial history, combined with onset in childhood or adolescence of symmetrical weakness of the feet and legs, with progressive development of foot-drop, weakness and atrophy of the legs, reflex loss, and sensory disturbances forms a characteristic picture which offers no difficulties as a rule. In some instances, it is necessary to separate the disorder from *hypertrophic interstitial neuritis,* which also has a familial incidence, occurs in childhood, and is associated with similar leg weakness. In patients with this disorder, however, the nerve trunks are thickened and easily palpable, pains are more pronounced, sensory loss is more definite, there is often evidence of spinal cord involvement and of involvement of the arms. *Friedreich's ataxia* also has a familial incidence, but the distinction from neuritic muscular atrophy is not difficult in view of the presence of nystagmus, dysarthria, ataxia, loss of reflexes with positive Babinski's signs, and evidence of posterior column disease. *Peripheral neuritis* with foot-drop and weakness of the leg is easily differentiated by the presence of muscle and nerve trunk tenderness, usually a history of an acute onset, pain, and sensory disturbances. The tenderness of the muscles and nerve trunks is sufficient to indicate the diagnosis. In some instances, *progressive muscular atrophy* may involve primarily the lumbar cord, with resulting weakness of the legs, foot-drop, and reflex loss. The age of onset is later than in neuritic muscular atrophy, and familial features are lacking. Except for these, the distinction may in some cases be quite difficult. The distal type of *myopathy* is rare, but may simulate the condition in question. Fasciculations are absent, the patellar and Achilles reflexes are retained as a rule, sensory disturbances are absent, and there is no familial incidence. Other forms of myopathy are associated with evidences of atrophy without fasciculations elsewhere in the body, in some instances with hypertrophy, and with no sensory changes.

Treatment: No medical treatment is of value. *Orthopedic measures* may be applied to correct the foot-drop. The disease is slowly progressive, but is characterized by remissions, sometimes of long duration.

XXI. FAMILIAL SPASTIC PARALYSIS

Spastic paralysis of a familial form is a rare affliction. It is characterized by a progressive spastic paralysis occurring usually in the third to sixth generations, with onset as a rule at the same age in the afflicted subjects, and with similar clinical pictures in all cases. There is often blood relationship among the various members of the afflicted families.

The age of onset varies; sometimes the disease appears early (three to six years), later (twenty to thirty years), or even in older persons. The outstanding symptom is spasticity of the legs with attendant increase of reflexes and Babinski's sign without sensory signs. Most of the cases are purely spastic, but in some instances muscle atrophies, speech disturbances, visual defects, nystagmus, athetosis, ataxia, chorea, and other disturbances have been recorded. The disease is manifested by demyelination of the pyramidal tracts in the spinal cord, but degenerative changes in the Betz cells of the motor cortex are also found.

XXII. SUBACUTE COMBINED DEGENERATION (*Posterolateral Sclerosis; Combined Degeneration; Subacute Combined Sclerosis; Funicular Myelitis*)

Etiology: Subacute combined degeneration is a progressive process involving the posterior and lateral columns of the spinal cord. The cause of the condition is a matter of controversy. Some regard pernicious anemia as the only cause and speak therefore of the neuroanemic syndrome. Such a conception seems to be too narrow. While pernicious anemia is undoubtedly the most important and most frequent cause, the syndrome has been observed in other conditions. Among these are chronic alcoholism, gastric carcinoma, obstructions and fistulae of the intestinal tract, and sprue. Many other diseases (sixty in all) have been reported with findings similar to those of subacute combined degeneration as seen in pernicious anemia, but pathological verification of other causes is unusual.

The syndrome of involvement of both posterior and lateral columns is symptomatic of involvement of many neurological disorders, a matter which will be discussed subsequently.

The condition occurs equally in males and females. It is most common about forty to forty-five years of age, but it may at times occur earlier and sometimes is found late in life (sixty to sixty-five years). It occurs at times in families.

Pathology: Subacute combined degeneration associated with pernicious anemia affects particularly the thoracic and lumbar portions of the cord but

syndrome. The posterior columns vary in involvement; the column of Goll is more affected than that of Burdach as a rule. There may be severe involvement of the posterior columns and little of the lateral, or *vice versa*. The peripheral nerves have been found to show degeneration in some cases. Microscopically, the areas of degeneration show loss of

Table 29—Conditions Associated with or Frequently Considered to Be the Cause of Subacute Degeneration of the Spinal Cord "Like That Seen in Pernicious Anemia"

(Woltman and Heck)

Endocrine Dysfunction	Infectious Diseases	Nutritional Disorders	Poisoning	Miscellaneous Diseases
Acromegaly	Respiratory diseases	Alcoholism	Absinth	Anemia, splenic
Addison's Disease	Chorea	Beriberi	Arsenic	Anemia, secondary
Diabetes mellitus	Diphtheria	Dysentery	Barium	Amyotrophic lateral
Exophthalmic	Erysipelas	Gastric carci-	Chloral	sclerosis
goiter	Influenza	noma	Ergot	Anclyostomiasis
Myxedema	Malaria	Obstruction of	Lathyrus	Arteriosclerosis
	Measles	bowel	Lead	Infestation with bo-
	Leprosy	Carcinoma of	Morphine	thriocephalus
	Rabies	pancreas	Phosphorus	Caisson disease
	Scarlet fever	Pancreatitis	Phosphin	Icterus, hemolytic
	Sepsis	P e r n i c i o u s	Strychnine	Jaundice
	Smallpox	anemia	Tea	Leukemia
	Syphilis	"Prepernicious"		Nephritis
	Tetanus	anemia		Pregnancy
	Typhoid	Pellagra		Primary degeneration
	Typhus	Scurvy		Senility
	Tuberculosis	Sprue		Shock
				Unclassified disease

may involve the entire length of the spinal cord. It never extends beyond the cord into the brain stem. The spinal cord shows degeneration in the posterior columns, the pyramidal tracts, the spinocerebellar tracts, and even in the anterior portions of the cord. The designation posterolateral sclerosis is therefore a misnomer, the process extending beyond these areas. Under rare circumstances, the entire circumference of the cord may be demyelinated, giving a transverse

myelin and axis cylinders with only a mild tendency to gliosis in the affected regions. There is a tendency to repair, as shown by gliosis in pernicious anemia patients treated by liver injections. The degenerated areas have a lacelike, spongy appearance which is quite characteristic of the disorder. The anterior horns of the spinal cord usually escape, but hemorrhages are occasionally found within them. The cerebral cortex shows evidence of damage in some cases as seen by scattered ischemic areas, areas of coagulation necrosis, and infarcts.

Symptoms: The clinical features of subacute combined degeneration are characterized by great variability. Since the disease occurs most frequently in pernicious anemia, the symptoms found in connection with this disorder will be considered. The onset is usually sub-disease. They are probably not dependent on the anemia. _Ataxia_ is an early symptom and usually persistent. Difficulty is noted in walking, from slight lurching to extreme incoördination. The degree depends upon the degree of destruction of the posterior columns and cerebellar pathways which is greater in some cases than in others. In some in-

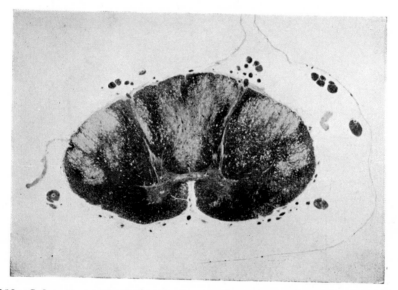

Fig. 100—*Subacute combined degeneration*, associated with pernicious anemia, showing in a myelin sheath stain the demyelination of the posterior and lateral columns of the spinal cord.

acute or chronic, symptoms developing gradually and slowly.

Paresthesias are constant. They may vary in intensity from case to case, being more pronounced in some cases than in others, but they are always found. They occur most commonly in the feet, but may spread to involve both hands and feet, and they are variously described as prickling, sticking, tickling, numbness, etc. They cannot be rubbed away. They seem to be aggravated by cold and relieved by heat. Paresthesias of the tongue are sometimes seen. The paresthesias have been ascribed to the anemia, to posterior column, and to peripheral nerve stances, the ataxia is slight. Position and vibration senses are usually lost, but one may be lost without the other. _Motor symptoms_ of some degree accompany the ataxia. Weakness and easy fatigue are early symptoms.

As in ataxia, the weakness and other pyramidal tract signs may vary greatly. One of the early manifestations is a positive Babinski's sign, which may be the only evidence of pyramidal tract disease. Spasticity may develop in varying degree. In some cases flaccid paralysis is present. The reflexes of the lower limbs may be increased at first, but later disappear. Sphincter disturbances of the bladder are always present in some degree. Sensory disturbances apart from those of deep sensation occur rarely, but may be found in some cases. Transverse sensory syndromes may be seen in rare instances with typical motor and sensory paralysis of a complete transverse syndrome. not uncommon (sixty to sixty-five per cent). No specific type of mental reaction is found. Organic reaction types are common, with intellectual deficit, memory loss, and confusional episodes. Paranoid and affective reactions (depressions) are common; these are probably

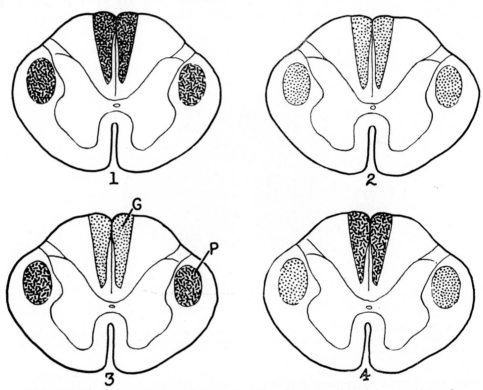

Fig. 101—*Subacute combined degeneration* showing the possible patterns of involvement. The columns of Goll are shaded because symptoms are more common in the legs. (1) Severe involvement of posterior and lateral columns, (2) mild involvement of the posterior and lateral columns, (3) mild involvement of posterior and severe involvement of lateral columns, (4) severe involvement of posterior and mild involvement of lateral columns.

drome. *Ocular symptoms* are not infrequently encountered. Retinal hemorrhages, optic neuritis, and primary optic atrophy have all been observed. Optic atrophy has been recorded rarely in subacute combined degeneration. Changes in the visual fields are rare, scotomas of the cecocentral type with varying degrees of peripheral contraction having been recorded. *Mental symptoms* are related less to the disease than to the specific personality of the patient.

Diagnosis: The clinical features of subacute combined degeneration of the anemic type are characterized by gradual onset with paresthesia, associated with ataxia and paraplegia, both well marked, with paraplegia and slight ataxia, or with ataxia and slight pyramidal tract involvement (Babinski's sign). The number of possible combinations is great, the signs depending on the fortuitous degree of involvement of the posterior and lateral columns. Similar types of syndromes with involvement of posterior and lateral columns may be found in multiple sclerosis, syphilis, Friedreich's ataxia, lead poisoning, amyotrophic lateral sclerosis, arteriosclerosis, leukemia, caisson disease, spinal cord injuries, and other disorders. In these disorders the posterolateral sclerosis forms but part of the clinical condition in which it is found, other features of multiple sclerosis or whatever other condition may be present indicating the nature of the disorder.

The disease, when due to pernicious anemia, is associated usually with the typical *blood picture* of the disease. Central nervous system disease is found in eighty to ninety per cent of patients with pernicious anemia. In many instances (forty to fifty per cent), the spinal cord disease is already present when the anemia is discovered. In others it develops during the course of the disease. Most important of all the patients, however, are those in whom the cord manifestations antedate the blood findings of pernicious anemia. That the spinal cord manifestations are not dependent on the blood findings is shown by the fact that the nervous symptoms and signs may precede development of the blood findings sometimes by several years. Hence cord manifestations may be found without anemia. Conversely, intense anemia may be found without cord manifestations. The involvement of the spinal cord early in pernicious anemia as a first manifestation of the disease has been variously estimated from twenty-five to thirty-five per cent, the discrepancy being due to inclusion of symptoms such as paresthesias as evidence of central nervous system involvement. The occurrence of nervous symptoms as the first sign of the disease requires emphasis, despite the fact that it is a well-known clinical fact.

Achlorhydria or *achylia gastrica* is found constantly, though some believe that in a small percentage of cases of pernicious anemia free hydrochloric acid is found. The diagnosis of subacute combined degeneration of the anemic type in the absence of anemia will depend on the finding of achlorhydria or achylia gastrica. A spastic paraplegia or a posterolateral sclerosis with gastric anacidity may be suspected rightfully as being due to pernicious anemia provided gastric carcinoma can be excluded. Cord symptoms have preceded the development of the blood findings by as long as thirteen years.

Neuritis may be difficult to differentiate in the early stages with paresthesia and reflex loss, but the occurrence of nerve and muscle tenderness and the sensory findings of neuritis usually suffice, as well as the absence of sphincter involvement. *Tabes* can be differentiated by the Argyll Robertson pupils, the pains, and the positive serological reactions. *Multiple sclerosis* may be confused with the condition, but the occurrence of history of remissions, temporal pallor, and absence of abdominal reflexes is helpful. *Spinal cord tumor* may be associated at times only with posterolateral sclerosis, without evidence of superficial sensory loss. This may be found in both intramedullary and extramedullary tumors. Pain is usually present, but it may be absent in intramedullary tumors. Evidence of subarachnoid block, either partial or complete, and increase of the total protein in the spinal fluid are extremely helpful in establishing tumor as a cause.

Because pyramidal tract signs may predominate or may be exclusively present. *primary lateral sclerosis* must be considered. There is serious doubt concerning the existence of this entity, and the probabilities favor the fact that patients with pure pyramidal tract disease involving the legs, or arms and legs, develop eventually other signs of nervous system disease and become subjects of multiple sclerosis, amyotrophic lateral sclerosis, or some other form of disease in which the pyramidal tracts are regularly affected.

Among the many other conditions which may cause a posterolateral syndrome, the differentiation is not as a rule difficult, since the cause is usually clear and pernicious anemia is readily excluded by blood and gastric studies. *Nutritional disorders* as a cause of the syndromes must be sought after carefully in all cases with an obscure cause. Despite the most careful survey, there still remains a group of cases for which no cause seems to be found. Some of these cases prove subsequently to be due to pernicious anemia, and others to multiple sclerosis; still others remain unsolved.

Treatment: The treatment is that of pernicious anemia or of whatever condition is associated with the process. *Thiamine chloride* (100 mg. [1½ grains]) intramuscularly daily may be helpful *Curare* (50 units) intramuscularly daily may aid in relieving spasm. *Neostigmine bromide* (15 mg. [¼ grain]) three times daily may be helpful. *Vitamin B₁₂* offers real help in the improvement of the spinal-cord signs associated with pernicious anemia. Given in doses of 100 to 1000 micrograms for extended periods, it has been found to produce definite improvement in the subacute degeneration of the spinal cord associated with the disease. It should always be used and continued over long periods.

7

Diseases of the Meninges

The meninges may be the seat of infection, hemorrhage, or tumor formation. The first two conditions will be dealt with in this chapter, the last will be considered under tumors of the brain.

I. MENINGITIS

Classification: Infection of the meninges is spoken of as meningitis. It may involve the dura (pachymeningitis) or the pia-arachnoid (leptomeningitis). Following is a general working classification of meningitis: Pachymeningitis externa, pachymeningitis interna, leptomeningitis.

Under the group leptomeningitis are included all the forms of meningitis involving the pia-arachnoid.

Mode of Infection: The meninges may become infected in several ways: (1) By the blood stream. This is probably the pathway for meningococcus infection, and for some forms of pneumococcic meningitis and for septicemias due to other organisms. (2) By direct extension. This mechanism is portrayed by the introduction of infection through head injury with skull fracture and the direct introduction of infection through the nose or ear, or by compound fracture. It is seen also in bullet wounds and in the direct extension of infection into the meninges by osteomyelitis developing from disease of the sinuses or mastoids. (3) By retrograde thrombophlebitis, seen in meningitis secondary to infections of the face with thrombophlebitis, cavernous sinus thrombosis, and meningeal infection. A similar mechanism is seen in spinal cord extradural abscess (pachymeningitis externa) which follow infection of the skin, or in extradural or brain abscess subsequent to mastoid or sinus infection. (4) By spinal fluid pathways. This is a hypothetical possibility as yet unproved as a means of introduction of infection except by direct inoculation as through lumbar puncture.

General Clinical Features: Regardless of cause, all cases of meningitis have features in common which are readily recognized. These are true of all cases of meningitis and are indicative only of the presence of foreign substances in the meninges. It is essential, therefore, that the general features of meningeal infection be recognized.

Headache is present in some degree in every case. Often it is intense; in some cases it is mild. It has no specific features except that it is generalized, is often though not always accompanied by vomiting, and is increased by coughing or sneezing.

Meningeal signs are likewise present in practically every case. In exceptional instances, in patients with profound stupor, they may be totally lacking throughout the course of the meningitis. They may all be present in a particular patient, or some may be found and others not. (1) *Neck stiffness* is a constant finding. This is characterized by a resistance of the neck to flexion, varying in degree from total rigidity with absolute inability to flex the neck muscles

345

and with the head held in hyperextension, to a slight resistance to complete flexion. The neck muscles are usually sore to the touch. (2) *Brudzinski's sign* is found in many cases but is not constant. This consists of flexion of the legs at the knees on attempted flexion of the head. More constant is (3) the *Kernig sign,* which is taken by extending the leg on the flexed thigh. A positive test

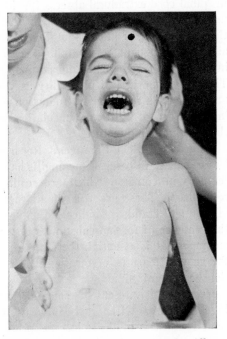

Fig. 102—*Meningitis,* showing neck stiffness in a child with tuberculous meningitis. The neck stiffness is so great that the patient is being lifted bodily from the bed.

is shown by the inability to extend the leg completely due to pain in the back: a negative sign is shown by complete extension of the leg. Kernig's sign, when present, is bilateral. It may, however, be unilateral, or it may be lacking altogether in cases of frank meningitis. (4) *Spine stiffness* and soreness is found in many cases.

Mental confusion occurs commonly. It may vary from slight evidence of disorientation to complete delirium. Apathy,

stupor, and coma are found commonly. It has no specific features and is probably indicative of a toxic-infectious process, and has nothing to do specifically with the meningeal involvement itself.

Fever is almost always present in some degree, the nature and extent varying with the type of meningitis. In meningococcic, pneumococcic, streptococcic, and staphylococcic meningitis, the temperature is high (over 102° F.) and often of a septic variety. In tuberculous meningitis, it is often not over 100° to 101° F.; in syphilitic meningitis, fever is usually absent, and in lymphocytic choriomeningitis the temperature may be normal or slightly elevated. The point of importance is that fever is present in all forms of meningitis with few exceptions. It constitutes, therefore, one of the cardinal features of meningeal infection, associated with it being other evidences of a systemic infection, such as chills, rapid pulse and respirations.

Headache, meningeal signs, fever, and mental confusion are the outstanding clinical signs of meningeal infection. On these findings alone it is possible to infer that meningeal infection is present. Additional signs are sometimes but not always found, and are dependent on the occurrence of spread of the infection beyond the meninges into the brain, on brain edema, or other processes such as the nature of the meningeal and cerebral reaction evoked by the offending organism. Some infections, such as tuberculosis, are associated with infiltration of both the brain and the meninges. *Convulsions* may develop; they are usually generalized, but may be focal. *Hemiplegias* or *monoplegias* may be found, and even aphasia may develop. Loss of pupillary reflexes is seen in severe cases of meningitis and cranial nerve signs may develop, especially in basilar forms of meningitis. Choked disc, oculomotor paralyses of varying degree, facial paralysis, deafness, and other cranial nerve involvements may be found. It is to be emphasized, however, that these are not common to all forms of meningitis and that the diagnosis of meningitis is made without them.

The tendon reflexes are absent in meningitis due to the overwhelming toxic found in the spinal fluid; they will be considered under the specific forms to be discussed, but in general both sugar and chlorides are affected, usually decreasing in amount in most forms of meningitis.

Diagnosis: The *diagnosis* of meningitis depends on a history of headache, the presence of meningeal signs, and the

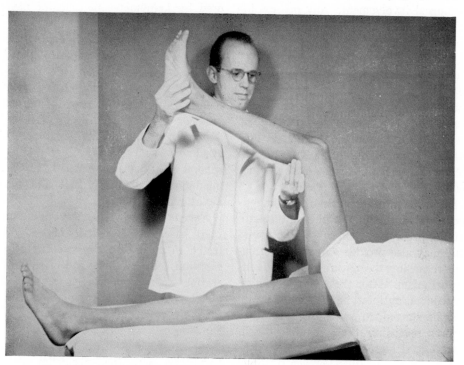

Fig. 103—*Meningitis,* illustrating the Kernig's sign found in cases with meningeal irritation.

reaction, except in those instances in which hemiplegia or monoplegia develops, in which case they are increased.

In every case of meningitis, there is an increase of cells in the *spinal fluid.* The number and nature of the cells will depend on the cause of the meningitis. Lymphocytes predominate in some forms, and polymorphonuclear cells in others. Bacteria are not found in every form and cultures are not always positive in meningitis. Syphilitic and virus meningitis, for example, show no organisms by smear or growth. Chemical changes are

findings of an excess of cells in the spinal fluid, with or without organisms by smear or culture. With these findings it is possible only to make a diagnosis of meningitis. Establishment of the cause constitutes the next step in the analysis and can only be determined by laboratory studies such as direct smear examination, blood and spinal fluid cultures, animal inoculations, etc.

The occurrence of headache and meningeal signs and even fever does not indicate specifically a meningitis or inflammatory involvement of the meninges; it indicates only disease of the meninges. Headache and signs of meningeal irritation may be produced by blood in the spinal fluid (subarachnoid hemorrhage), which may be accompanied at times by fever. Similarly, meningeal carcinomatosis, extension of tumors into the meninges, etc., may give rise to evidences of meningeal involvement. Any process involving the meninges, whether it be infection, hemorrhage, neoplastic involvement of the meninges, or even an excess of fluid (meningismus), will give rise to headache and signs of meningeal irritation. The occurrence of fever and evidences of systemic involvement favor meningitis, an impression which is confirmed by an excess of polymorphonuclear cells or lymphocytes in the spinal fluid.

Following the diagnosis of a meningitis, blood and spinal fluid culture are routine procedures. Smear of the spinal fluid may also provide valuable information regarding the nature of the offending organism. After these simple routine procedures, antibiotic and chemotherapy may be started, to await the laboratory reports regarding the offending organism. The studies include the identification of the organism wherever possible, and its sensitivity to the various antibiotic and chemotherapeutic agents.

General Pathological Features: All forms of meningitis have features in common, an understanding of which is helpful in treatment and prognosis. Some degree of *hyperemia* is present in all forms. This is seen in dilatation of the pial vessels, both large and small, more marked in some forms than in others. It is particularly pronounced in the pneumococcic and influenzal types of meningitis, but it is found also in severe degrees in other forms as well. The hyperemia involves the vessels within the brain substance, the smaller vessels of the brain tissue being dilated and filled with red cells. *Edema* of the brain is found in some degree in all cases. The gyri are swollen and bulging in severe cases, with crowding of the sulci; in other instances, the gyri are less swollen but are puffed and edematous. The swollen and edematous brain is largely responsible for the increased intracranial pressure as measured by manometer in cases of meningitis. Internal hydrocephalus due to blockage of the spinal fluid circulation contributes in some cases to the increased intracranial pressure. The perivascular spaces are dilated and edematous in practically all parts of the cerebral cortex. Excessive accumulations of fluid may be found at times in the subarachnoid space over the cerebral hemispheres or in the basal cisterns. In serous meningitis particularly, such fluid accumulations are striking.

Encephalopathy in some form is found in all cases of meningitis. This is manifested in most cases by swelling of the ganglion cells, swelling and often proliferation of the endothelial cells of the blood vessels, perivascular and perineuronal edema, and hyperemia. The ganglion cell changes are not permanent. They are reversible, the cells reverting to normal with the subsidence of the infection. The changes thus far described constitute evidences of reaction to the infection on the part of the cerebral cortex as well as other parts of the brain and may be best regarded as an encephalopathy. The point of importance is that changes are found always in the brain as well as in the meninges in cases of meningitis. In some instances, an actual encephalitis is found associated with the meningitis. This is true particularly in tuberculous and syphilitic meningitis, in which types perivascular infiltrations and hematogenous elements are found in the brain substance. Encephalitis is found also in association with lymphocytic choriomeningitis; at times it is found also in streptococcic meningitis.

Meningitis may be predominantly basilar, predominantly hemispherical, or both. The tuberculous and syphilitic forms of meningitis are chiefly basilar, but spread over the convexities as well. Pneumococcic and influenzal meningitis swathe the hemispheres and the base of the brain in a heavy exudate. The streptoccic form of meningitis involves all parts of the brain but tends to be heavier over the hemispheres. In some instances, the exudate is found within the ventricles.

Recovery from meningitis may result in complete absorption of the exudate without after effects. In some instances, the exudate becomes organized, with a resulting arachnoiditis which may cause late symptoms after the meningitis has receded. This may result in internal hydrocephalus if the arachnoiditis is in the posterior fossa and obstructs the flow of cerebrospinal fluid; it may produce focal symptoms such as hemiplegia, aphasia, etc., depending on the location of the arachnoiditis; or it may cause mental deficiency if it is widespread and associated with extensive cortical damage.

II. PACHYMENINGITIS EXTERNA
(Extradural Abscess)

Etiology: Pachymeningitis externa, or extradural abscess, is a collection of pus outside the dura, between this membrane and the skull. It may be frontal or temporal in location, and develops secondarily to disease of the sinuses or mastoids. It may occur with disease of any sinus but is more common in frontal sinus disease. A cerebellar location is at times encountered secondary to mastoid infection or lateral sinus thrombosis. Infection is by direct extension, with osteomyelitis of the frontal bone or of the petrous portion of the temporal bone, or by retrograde thrombophlebitis from the infected mastoid or sinus.

The dura in such cases is usually covered by a moderately thick layer of pus which is adherent to the membrane. In some instances, no free pus is seen, but the dura is greatly thickened and is infiltrated by inflammatory elements. The dura is adherent to the underlying brain tissue in greater or lesser degree and the underlying brain itself may be the seat of inflammation in the form of scattered foci of polymorphonuclear infiltration.

The organisms most commonly associated with the disease are the streptococcus and pneumococcus.

Symptoms: The onset of the disease is acute, following acute frontal sinus or mastoid disease. *Headache* is the outstanding symptom. It appears acutely and may be frontal, behind the eye, or occipital. It is usually accompanied by a slight or high *fever*. Neck stiffness or Kernig's sign may be present, but signs of meningeal irritation are unfortunately often absent Vertigo and nystagmus may be present in cases secondary to mastoid disease.

The spinal fluid reveals no changes in uncomplicated cases, but in cases associated with a leptomeningitis, there is an increase of cells (polymorphonuclears) in the spinal fluid.

Osteomyelitis of the frontal bone or bones is seen in some cases, and in such instances there is pitting edema of the soft tissues of the forehead to the hairline.

Diagnosis: The detection of an extradural abscess is notoriously difficult. Indeed, it is safe to assert that except in unusual instances the diagnosis cannot be made with certainty before operation. It may be suspected, but can only be established by direct exploration. The first step in diagnosis is the establishment of a focus of infection in the sinuses or mastoids, which is not difficult, since the condition follows acute disease of either of these areas. If with such a history, headache and fever persist or recur after recovery appears to have set in, one is justified in suspecting an extradural abscess. The persistence of headache and fever after the sinus or ear infection seems to have come under control is *a priori* evidence that the condition may be present. Similarly, their persistence after sinus or mastoid operation with good drainage is indicative of probable extradural infection. If, in addition, osteomyelitis of the frontal or temporal bone is detected by roentgenograms, the assumption becomes a certainty. Mild meningeal signs such as neck stiffness and Kernig's sign are helpful but are not diagnostic, since they may result from a serous meningitis or from a localized or sympathetic meningitis associated with the sinus or ear infection. The presence of evidences of lateral sinus thrombosis aids in the assumption that an extradural abscess may be present in the temporal area, since this condition is at times associated with an extradural collection of pus. The presence of leukocytosis is of no help, since it is part of the sinus or ear infection.

Meningitis may be eliminated by the more pronounced fever, the increase of cells in the spinal fluid, and the frank evidence of meningeal irritation. *Brain abscess* is often difficult to differentiate. Choked disc and focal signs are helpful.

Treatment: The treatment is *surgical.* Cleaning out the abscess, with removal of the thickened dura, is necessary. Use of the *sulfonamides* and *penicillin* is mandatory and should be carried out as soon as the diagnosis is established.

III. PACHYMENINGITIS INTERNA
(Subdural Abscess)

This condition, as the name implies, consists of a collection of pus beneath the dura, the latter being thickened, infiltrated by polymorphonuclear cells, and covered on its undersurface by pus which is quite adherent to it. The infection extends from an extradural abscess usually by direct fistula, but sometimes without.

Subdural abscess follows infection of the paranasal sinuses in the majority of instances, but it may be secondary to ear infection, and may even be metastatic from lung infection. There is no specific age incidence. The disease usually follows an acute episode of a chronic infection, and is especially prone to occur in chronic frontal sinusitis. The onset is with local pain followed by generalized, severe, persistent headache often associated with nausea or vomiting and with a pronounced rise in temperature. Confusion and somnolence follow, and are succeeded often by stupor. Neck stiffness is common. Jacksonian seizures are common (fifty per cent); hemiplegia or hemiparesis, and aphasia occur. Roentgenograms reveal frontal sinusitis as a rule and sometimes osteomyelitis of the frontal bones. The cerebrospinal fluid is under moderately increased pressure. There is a moderate increase of cells in the spinal fluid but bacteria are not demonstrable by smear or culture. Death ensues in most cases.

The treatment is *surgical.*

IV. LEPTOMENINGITIS

By far the greatest number of cases of meningitis involve the pia-arachnoid (leptomeningitis). Most of the various forms of meningitis are secondary to other foci within the body. The chief primary forms of meningitis are the menigococcic, pneumococcic, and virus forms. While pneumococcic meningitis is primary at times, it is as a rule secondary to foci elsewhere in the body in the majority of instances. All other forms are secondary.

The chief forms of meningitis are shown in the following table (Neal, Jackson, Applebaum) :

Meningococcic meningitis .... 1216 cases
Tuberculous meningitis .... 961 cases
Pneumococcic meningitis .... 209 cases
Streptococcic meningitis .... 203 cases
Influenzal meningitis .... 111 cases
Staphylococcic meningitis .... 27 cases

Causes: Meningitis may be caused by a wide variety of organisms. It may be caused by the Meningococus, Streptococcus, Pneumococcus, Staphylococcus, Hemophilus influenzae, Friedlander's bacillus, Mycobacterium tuberculosis, Gonococcus, Treponema pallidum, Cryptococcus neoformans, Gaffkya tetragena, Streptothrix, virus infections, Actinomyces, B. anthracis, Leptothrix, Brucella melitensis, and other organisms.

Frequency of Occurrence: The more frequent forms of meningitis are indicated in a group of 642 cases (Lindsay, et al.):

	Cases	Per cent
Meningococcus	205	31.9
Influenza	180	28
Pneumococcus	100	15.6
Streptococcus	73	11.4
Staphylococcus	50	7.8
Friedlander's bacillus	5	1.6
Morgan's bacillus	1	0.8
Undetermined	27	4.2

The relative figures may vary in different groups, but it seems true that meningitis is most commonly caused by the meningococcus, pneumococcus, streptococcus, and H. influenzae organisms, with staphylococcus not as common a cause as in the other groups.

Types: Most cases of meningitis are secondary to foci of infection elsewhere in the body. Relatively few are primary in origin.

V. MENINGOCOCCIC MENINGITIS
(Cerebrospinal Fever, Epidemic Cerebrospinal Meningitis)

Etiology: Meningococcic meningitis is caused by the meningococcus, which is a Gram-negative diplococcus. It grows readily in culture and is easily identified.

Table 30—Primary Forms of Meningitis

Type	Source of Infection
MENINGOCOCCUS...	Nasopharynx—blood stream
PNEUMOCOCCUS....	Lungs
VIRUS...........	Unknown
INFLUENZAL......	Lungs. nasopharynx

Secondary Forms of Meningitis

Type	Source of Infection
TUBERCULOUS.....	Lungs, glands, epididymis, kidney, etc.
PNEUMOCOCCUS....	Sinuses, mastoids
STREPTOCOCCUS....	Mastoids, sinuses, septicemia
H. INFLUENZAE....	Lungs, nasopharynx
GONOCOCCUS......	Gonorrheal urethritis, epididymitis, etc.
STAPHYLOCOCCUS..	Infections in general, septicemia
B. TYPHOSUS......	Intestinal tract
B. COLI..........	Intestinal and urinary tracts, middle ear
B. PESTIS........ (Plague)	Skin inoculation (flea), or lungs
B. MALLEI........ (Glanders)	Skin infection from horses, and other animals
CRYPTOCOCCUS....	Unknown
B PROTEUS.......	Chronic ear disease; contaminated wounds, urinary and intestinal tracts, lateral sinus thrombosis
B. PYOCANEUS.....	Lateral sinus thrombosis
SPOROTHRIX......	Lungs, bones, periarticular tissues, kidneys, eyes and ears
PASTEURELLA TULARENSIS.....	Skin; digestive tract; respiratory pathway
B. ANTHRACIS.....	Skin—face, neck, ear, arm, nose, mouth
ACTINOMYCES.....	Skin, chiefly after jaw infection
TRICHINELLA......	Alimentary tract
SALMONELLA......	Alimentary tract
LEPTOTHRIX......	Mouth, pharynx, lungs, throat, ear, bones, gastro-intestinal tract
M. CATARRHALIS...	Respiratory tract, throat, ears
B. MELITENSIS	Alimentary tract, skin
GAFFKYA TETRAGENA.....	Sinuses, lungs, pleura, pericardium, endocardium

There are several strains of meningococcus, four different groups being identified.

The disease affects people of all ages. It affects the young most commonly, but is also found commonly in adults. It occurs most often at one to ten years, but is frequent to sixteen years of age. It is found at times in epidemic form, but it is always endemic. Cases are spread by carriers of the meningococcus usually and to a lesser degree by close contact with a case of the disease. Direct contact seems not to be important, since multiple cases are not common, and the occurrence among doctors and others in close contact with cases is very low. Similarly, epidemics in schools are not frequent. The transmission seems to be from adults to children. The meningococci are found in the secretions of affected cases and in carriers. The latter may be temporary or chronic. The chronic, healthy passive carriers are the main source of transmission and outnumber cases of menigococcic meningitis ten to thirty to one. Individual predilection is presumed to play a part, since some persons may come in contact with meningococcic meningitis for days without developing the disease, while others succumb. It is found most often in the late autumn and winter months. Constitutional factors have been accused in the development of the disease. Spread of the disease is favored by crowding.

Pathology: The meningitis covers both the cerebral and cerebellar hemispheres, and the base of the brain. Predominantly basilar or cerebral hemisphere exudates may be found, the meningitis being more pronounced in one or the other area. In a typical case the cerebral hemispheres are covered with a creamy exudate which tends to be heaviest along the vessels and spreads thinly over the gyri. The exudate is usually heaviest over the anterior portions of the brain. The brain stem and cerebellum are also heavily covered with exudate, the degree of involvement of these parts as well as the cerebrum varying from case to case. The meninges in the acute stages contain numerous polymorphonuclear cells among which are macrophages of various sorts. These increase in number as the disease becomes more chronic. The meningococ-

cus can be found in and among the cells by special staining. The underlying cortex is as a rule free of exudate, but the ganglion cells show evidence of cloudy swelling or of more severe toxic changes.

Recovery from the meningitis may result in complete resolution of the exudate, but in some instances firm adherence of the thickened meninges to the underlying cerebral cortex or to other structures (cranial nerves) results, with subsequent impairment of function.

Pathogenesis: Meningococcic meningitis is regarded as but one manifestation of a disease which may involve and localize in many parts of the body, producing endocarditis, arthritis, nasopharyngitis, and meningococcemia.

Two concepts prevail concerning the development of meningococcic meningitis: (1) that of direct extension; (2) that of a blood stream infection. The evidence at present favors the conception that meningococcic meningitis begins as a blood stream infection and that invasion is probably by way of the blood stream. Herrick was able to recognize about forty-five per cent in the premeningeal stage, and about four per cent of these failed ultimately to show signs of meningitis. There are many other reports, furthermore, of the recovery of meningococcus from the blood stream before meningitis develops; many of the subjects never developed meningitis. In rabbits, meningitis can be produced by the intravenous injection of meningococci following the production of hyperemia of the meninges and after spinal drainage.

The direct extension concept is based on the fact that the meningocous can be found in the nasopharynx and also at the base of the brain, the assumption being that it must reach the latter locus by direct extension along the perineural pathways.

Symptoms: The incubation period is most commonly three to five days, but extremes of one to ten days are found at times. Sudden onset, often within a matter of hours in a previously healthy person, is common, especially in epidemic cases. The disease often appears first as a mild nasopharyngitis; in the course of a few days severe chills, drowsiness, vomiting, and fever may develop. Following the mild nasopharyngitic stage comes the phase of *meningococcic septicemia,* which lasts usually about two days, but may be fulminating. Apathy and great prostration are found in this phase. Fever is present (102° F. or more) and petechiae are found over the face, neck, and trunk and to a lesser extent over the limbs. They may be very numerous in severe cases and may coalesce to leave almost no normal skin visible. Hemorrhages into the skin, mucous or serous membranes are characteristic of meningococcal sepsis (Strong). *Petechial hemorrhages* are found in the skin in from fifty to eighty-two per cent of cases and are more commonly seen in epidemic forms of the disease. The specific rash is always hemorrhagic, cannot be obliterated by pressure, and invariably becomes manifest before the end of the first twenty-four hours of infection, if it is to appear. It is usually sparse and requires search. Any part of the skin or mucosa may be affected. The rash reaches full development within a few hours and fades rapidly, leaving only a faint brownish skin discoloration. The lesions are about 1 to 3 mm. in diameter and vary in shade from a rose color to a deep red. Purpuric spots or ecchymoses may accompany the rash in severe cases. Widespread rash occurs in severe cases, but the absence of a rash does not indicate a mild case.

Following this phase comes the development of *meningitis* with headache, neck stiffness, positive Kernig's and Brudzinski's signs. During the septicemic stage, there may be minimal evidences of meningeal irritation. The septicemic phase may not be very striking in many endemic cases. The earliest sign of meningeal involvement is severe, intractable headache which is found in ninety-nine per cent of cases. It is generalized, but is more severe in the frontal and occipital regions. It is unrelieved by any form of treatment. When the meningitis is fully developed, the patient has high fever (102° F. or more), flushed face, dilated pupils, severe prostration, herpes labialis, headache, vomiting, and marked neck stiffness often resulting in opisthotonos. The respirations are irregular and rapid. Confusion, irritability, and delirium are conspicuous. Drowsiness is common and unconsciousness may develop. The tendon reflexes are almost always absent.

The total picture is that of extreme prostration, with fever, meningeal signs, confusion, delirium, and deepening unconsciousness if the infection persists without letup. As recovery develops, the meningeal signs recede and the mental clouding fades gradually until the patient is clear, is without headache, confusion, and fever.

In some cases, *fulminating forms* are seen. These appear suddenly, with severe prostration, the onset being of a septicemic nature with chills, severe headache, and vomiting. Fever is present and delirium is common. Purpuric eruptions of the skin are constant in this form of the disease. The blood culture is positive. The spinal fluid may show nothing or may contain many polymorphonuclear cells, with organisms seen in the smear. The fulminating form of the disease is usually fatal, terminating often within forty-eight hours. In some instances, the fulminating form is associated with the

Waterhouse-Friderichsen syndrome in which there is found adrenal hemorrhage, purpuric eruptions, and collapse. Patients with this syndrome often die before meningitis develops.

Chronic forms of the disease occur in children, especially in the form known as *posterior basic meningitis*. The onset is like that of an upper respiratory infection, with gradually developing lethargy, fever, meningeal signs, opisthotonos, and extensor spasticity of the limbs. Hydrocephalus develops and emaciation becomes marked, with death occurring in six to eight weeks.

Other chronic forms are found in adults in the chronic septicemic form characterized by fever, purpura, headache, leukocytosis, without the presence of signs of meningeal irritation.

Spinal Fluid Findings: *Lumbar puncture* should be performed for diagnostic purposes only. Repeated lumbar puncture is not necessary and may be hazardous, since the associated brain edema and increased pressure may produce foraminal herniation and death with frequent lumbar taps. The Queckenstedt test should never be performed because of the danger of causing herniation of the medulla into the foramen magnum. After diagnostic lumbar puncture, the procedure should be reserved for (1) a check of the findings before discharge, (2) study of the spinal fluid findings which have failed to respond properly to treatment, and (3) study of the spinal fluid findings in malignant types of meningitis, such as tuberculous meningitis, in order to determine the effect of treatment.

The spinal fluid findings are of great importance in the diagnosis. The cells are increased, varying in number from one to ten thousand in most cases, but numbering less than one thousand or as high as twenty thousand or more in others. Poly-

nuclear cells predominate, but macrophages are also found. The *protein* is increased always, varying in amounts from 45 mg. to 1000 mg. The *sugar* content is decreased as in bacterial meningitis in general. The sugar content often falls below 40 mg. and is often absent. *Chlorides* are not as a rule diagnostically decreased in meningococcic meningitis. They often fall, but usually are not abnormally low. They average 650 to 700 mg., but may fall below 650 mg. There is nothing significant in the colloidal gold curve.

Sequelae: The disease when recovered from may be followed by sequelae of one sort or another due to adhesive meningitis which follows the acute infection. Internal hydrocephalus may follow blockage of ventricular flow by the adherent meninges.

The ill-effects of the present-day treatment of any form of meningitis must be recognized clearly. Apart from the toxic effects of the various sulfonamides and antibiotics, the physician treating meningitis must be prepared for the development of cortical damage as a delayed or late sequel of treatment. Eradication of the infection is followed at times, in severe cases of the various types of meningitis, by adhesive arachnoiditis, followed by ischemic-anoxic ganglion cell disease, and resulting in mental retardation or deficiency, convulsions, hemiplegia, paraplegia, and other distressing symptoms. Abducens paralysis occurs in 4 to 20 per cent of cases. There has been no decline with the use of sulfonamides, a recent survey showing 15 per cent involvement. Facial paralysis occurs in 1 to 5 per cent and is usually unilateral. Auditory nerve deafness is common and is due to meningitis rather than to otitis media. The incidence is 2 to 25 per cent, with an average of 5 per cent. It has not decreased with the use of sulfonamides and is usually bilateral. Optic nerve involvement with resulting atrophy and decrease of vision or blindness occurs in 12 per cent (Farmer).

Diagnosis: Meningococcic meningitis in its general clinical manifestations is similar to other forms of purulent meningitis. The signs of meningeal irritation, the headache, and the presence of polynuclear cells in the spinal fluid lead tentatively to a diagnosis of purulent meningitis. The demonstration of purpura is extremely important, however, and should lead to a tentative diagnosis of meningococcic meningitis, but the best confirmatory finding is, of course, a positive blood and/or spinal fluid culture. Meningococci may be demonstrated in the purpuric spots. In those cases having a characteristic onset with a nasopharyngitis, followed by fever, chills, severe headache, purpuric spots, and signs of meningeal irritation, the diagnosis of meningococcic meningitis may be made with safety before confirmatory laboratory studies are available.

In instances in which purpuric spots are not found, the diagnosis can only be that of purulent meningitis, until the laboratory studies identify the causative organism. In such instances, the meningitis may be the result of any of the organisms responsible for a purulent meningitis. Pneumococcic meningitis may be suspected if a focus of infection is disclosed, by history or examination, in the sinuses or in the mastoid region. The same may be said of streptococcic meningitis. Staphylococcic forms may be suspected in the demonstration of a focus of infection, such as furuncles, osteomyelitis, etc. The organism may be found at times in the cells of the spinal fluid exudate by direct smear and they have been seen at times in the blood stream by the same method.

The most cogent reason for differentiation of meningococcic meningitis from other forms of meningitis lies in the treatment, since the outlook is more hopeful in the meningococcus forms.

In some cases, the meningococcic infection may assume a chronic form. *Chronic* meningococcemia is characterized by a more or less protracted febrile illness, arthralgia, and cutaneous eruptions. The fever may be extremely irregular, with peaks occurring daily, on alternate days, or on every third day. Symptoms referable to the joints are the principal source of the patients' complaints. The cutaneous lesions include petechial eruptions, maculopapular lesions, or small, widely scattered, tender nodules resembling those of erythema nodosum. The spleen may or may not be palpable. Meningeal symptoms may appear at varying intervals. The cases resemble rheumatic fever. Sulfadiazine is ordinarily curative (Martin and Snell).

Treatment and Prognosis: It is assumed, of course, that the *usual routine care* of a febrile patient is used in all cases. Feeding may be difficult in confused cases, and nasal tube feeding may be necessary. Fluids may be given by hypodermoclysis or by vein despite the brain edema associated with the condition, in order to maintain nourishment. Sedation may be necessary in confused cases and for this purpose paraldehyde by mouth or rectum is a useful drug. Tepid sponge baths or alcohol rubs are indicated with high fevers. The patients having acute septicemia may be given *adrenal cortex extract* (desoxycorticosterone acetate) intramuscularly.

The treatment of meningitis is subject to such frequent changes and modifications owing to the discovery of new drugs that it is hardly possible to keep its discussion current.

In *meningococcic meningitis*, the first and most important factor in the treatment is early diagnosis. Experiences during World War II indicate unqualifiedly that the mortality of meningococcic meningitis can be reduced to as low as 1 per cent if the diagnosis is established early and treatment begun immediately. If a diagnostic lumbar puncture reveals a high cell count of polynuclear cells, the assumption must be made that the meningitis is due to the meningococcus, provided no focus of infection is found in the ear, mastoid, or sinuses, and the possibility of influenzal meningitis can be eliminated in a child. If the meningococcus is demonstrable in smears of the spinal fluid, the assumption is definitely supported. Blood culture should be taken, but treatment must be started before it is reported, lest valuable time be lost.

The drugs of choice in meningococcic meningitis are *penicillin,* and *sulfadiazine.* *Penicillin* is given in doses of one million or more units daily. In many instances it is sufficient in the treatment of meningococcic meningitis. In those instances of sensitivity to penicillin or inability to use it for other reasons it must be supplanted by other drugs. It is given in single large doses or in smaller doses (300,000 units) at intervals of three to six hours. The *sulfonamides* are extremely effectual in meningococcal meningitis and are regarded by many as the drugs of choice. In some instances both penicillin and sulfonamides are necessary. In many instances either drug may be used. In the average case, with a conscious, not desperately ill subject, sulfadiazine may be given intravenously as sodium sulfadiazine, 3 to 5 Gm. (45 to 75 grains). The dosage is then maintained at 1 Gm. (15 grains) of sulfadiazine every three hours until clinical improvement sets in, when it can be reduced to 1 Gm. every four hours. If vomiting develops, the drug must be given intravenously. In stuporous, se-

verely ill patients the drug must be given intravenously, 3 to 5 Gm. (45 to 75 grains) of the sodium salt being given as an initial dose and 1 to 2 Gm. (15 to 30 grains) every three hours thereafter. Oral administration may be used when the patient regains consciousness and there is no vomiting. After the temperature has returned to normal, the drug may be withdrawn, but only if the clinical signs have cleared and a diagnostic lumbar puncture reveals no excess of cells in the spinal fluid. Children from one to three years receive 3 to 4 Gm. (45 to 60 grains) of the drug on the first day; and those from three to seven years, 4 to 7 Gm. (60 to 105 grains). Aureomycin is reported to be an effective agent in the treatment of meningococcic meningitis. It is given in doses of 0.25 Gm. orally at four hour intervals (1.5 Gm. daily) for children and for adults 1 Gm. every eight hours (3 Gm. daily) after an initial dose of 50 mg. per kilogram of body weight. Terramycin may also be used. Intrathecal medication is not necessary in meningococcic meningitis.

The treatment of *fulminating meningococcic infection* (Waterhouse-Friderichsen syndrome) is difficult even under the most favorable circumstances, since the infection, virulent and swift, strikes with overwhelming force. Treatment must be started with *sodium sulfadiazine* intravenously (3 to 5 Gm.), repeated in a few hours, and with a large initial dose of *penicillin* (100,000 units). Thereafter, it can be maintained at 1 to 2 Gm. of sulfadiazine and 75,000 units of penicillin every three hours. Since most of the patients with this type of infection are prostrated, the sulfadiazine must be given either intravenously as the sodium salt, or by nasal tube. In addition, the following should be given: (1) *glucose* (5 per cent) in saline intravenously, 1500 cc; (2) *adrenal cortex extract.*

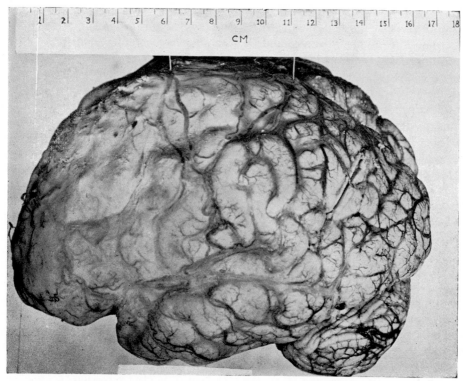

Fig. 104—*Pneumococcic meningitis*, showing the thick, dense exudate covering the brain and completely obscuring the frontal lobes.

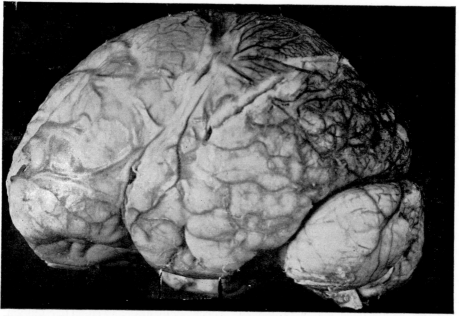

Fig. 105—*Pneumococcic meningitis*, showing the characteristic heavy purulent exudate obliterating the landmarks in the underlying brain.

VI. PURULENT MENINGITIS

Definition: By purulent meningitis is meant any form of meningitis caused by pus-forming organisms with a purulent exudate composed chiefly of polynuclear cells. Strictly speaking, the meningococcic form is a purulent meningitis, but it has so many problems peculiar to itself that it is treated separately. Purulent meningitis includes, therefore, most of the forms of acute meningitis exclusive of tuberculous, syphilitic, and virus forms.

Pathology: Regardless of the specific organism causing the disorder, the brain and spinal cord findings have many similarities. The brain is swollen and edematous. The pia-arachnoid contains exudate. In streptococcic forms this exudate tends to follow along the course of the blood vessels, leaving the intervening gyri more or less uncovered. In the pneumococcic and influenzal varieties, the brain, both at the base and over the cerebral hemispheres, is swathed in a heavy exudate which obscures the underlying brain and in severe cases obliterates it completely. Cranial nerves and vessels are caught in the mesh of exudate. The ventricles are often distended and contain pus. Thrombi may be found in the veins or sinuses. The choroid plexus is often distended and covered with exudate. Histologically, the meninges are filled with polynuclear cells among which may be many macrophages. Fibrin deposit is seen in some forms, especially in the streptococcic varieties. For the most part, the inflammatory process is confined to the meninges, but in some types (streptococcic, influenzal) changes may be seen in the cortex in the form of encephalitic areas of perivascular infiltrations with polynuclear cells, and minute hemorrhages.

In cases which have had a prolonged course, a tendency to organization of the exudate may be seen with the development of fibrous tissue and the formation of an adherent arachnoiditis.

Etiology: The forms due to streptococci follow infections of the mastoid most commonly, but develop also following sinus disease. Pneumococcic forms appear secondary to sinus and mastoid disease, but occur also, though less commonly, after pulmonary infections. Type III pneumococcus infection is most often secondary to otitic infection. Pneumococcic meningitis may follow operations of the nose and throat, head injuries, and upper respiratory infections exclusive of pneumonia. Influenzal meningitis occurs after upper respiratory infections or from foci in the lungs, otitis media, etc. Rarer forms include staphylococcic and gonococcal meningitis. The former develops secondarily to foci of infection elsewhere, such as furuncles on the skin and osteomyelitis. Gonococcic meningitis is secondary to genital infection in almost all instances, but rare cases occur in which the source of the infection is not clear. Colon bacillus infection develops after otitis media, genitourinary infections, gastrointestinal infection, trauma, or as part of a general infection; anthrax is found developing after cutaneous anthrax; actinomycosis follows jaw infection with the fungus or from other sources. Meningitis is found not uncommonly as a complication of fevers of various sorts, such as typhoid and paratyphoid fever, typhus, mumps, scarlet fever, etc. It occurs also as a manifestation of brain abscess, and may be found in pulmonary infections, subacute bacterial endocarditis, and many other diseases.

Meningitis may occur at any age. Many forms occur commonly in adults, but some forms, such as the meningococcic, influenzal, and colon bacillus varieties, are more common in children.

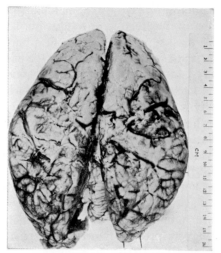

Fig. 106 (see Fig. 107).

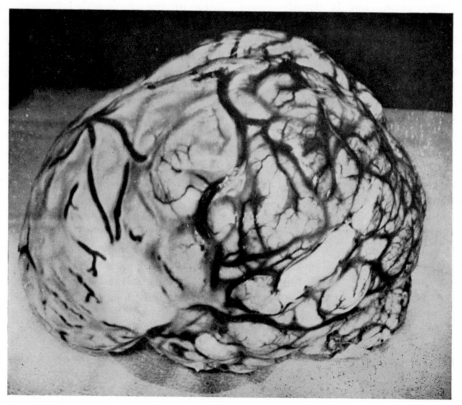

Fig. 107—*Influenzal meningitis*, showing clearly the thick exudate covering the frontal areas, obscuring the cortex completely.

Symptoms: The symptoms in general are similar to those of meningococcic meningitis, but are masked often by the symptoms of the primary infection. The onset is usually abrupt with headache, malaise, and fever, but it varies greatly in severity. The early symptoms may be somewhat mild, consisting of headache, vomiting, moderate fever, chills, and slight evidences of meningeal signs. The spinal fluid in such cases shows cell increase but organisms may be hard to recover. In severe cases, the symptoms are more pronounced. Within a short time complete prostration develops and stupor sets in. Restlessness is commonly seen, and with it confusion and delirium. Convulsions may develop, especially in children. The temperature varies, but is usually found around 102° to 104° F., the pulse is rapid, the respirations increased and sometimes of the Cheyne-Stokes type. Headache is a common complaint if the patient is conscious, and vomiting is often present. Examination reveals all the signs of meningeal irritation. Neck stiffness is always present and may be so severe as to cause marked neck retraction. Tenderness of the neck muscles is often seen. Kernig's sign is usually found and the Brudzinski sign is often seen. In some cases with encephalitic foci, evidences of brain involvement may be found in the form of monoplegias or cranial nerve paralyses. Remissions may occur during the course of the illness, the temperature at these times approaching normal, the mentality becoming clear, and the spinal fluid findings receding but not reaching normal.

Leukocytosis is found invariably. A positive blood culture is present in practically all the forms, and organisms can be demonstrated on smear of the spinal fluid. Positive spinal fluid cultures are usually obtained.

Spinal fluid examination reveals cloudy or frankly purulent fluid, and an increase of cells of a polynuclear variety (ninety to ninety-six per cent), ranging usually from a few hundred to 10,000 cm³., but sometimes reaching 20,000 cm³. The pressure is increased in over ninety per cent and varies usually from 200 to 500 mm. of water. The protein content is elevated. The sugar content is usually decreased, often below 40 mg. The chlorides are often decreased below 700 mg. Examination by smear often fails to show the offending organism. Only cultures of the spinal fluid establish the cause in many cases.

Diagnosis: The diagnosis of the various forms of purulent meningitis raises special problems, each related to the specific cause of the meningeal infection. In general, the symptoms as outlined are characteristic of all forms of meningitis due to pyogenic organisms. *Pneumococcic meningitis* gives rise to no characteristic clinical picture and is associated with no signs or symptoms which can be regarded as pathognomonic. It may be presumed to be present if meningitis develops during an acute pneumonia; or it may be regarded as a possibility in patients with known sinus or mastoid disease. It is practically always secondary to infection elsewhere in the body. Among the sources of infection are otitis media, pneumonia, sinuses, head injuries, endocarditis, and eye disease. In some instances (twenty-five per cent), the infection is primary with no known source of the meningitis. Middle ear infection and mastoiditis are the most common sources, and head injuries also account for many cases. The head injury may be trivial or there may be a long period of latency between skull fracture and the development of meningitis. Influenza and upper respiratory infections account for five per cent of cases. Cellulitis of the ear, pituitary tumor, lung abscess, and pneumococcic peritonitis have been found to be sources in rare cases. The disease may develop at any age, but seems to be more common in the first and fifth decades; more than one-half the cases occur before the age of twenty-one, the next high peak being in the fifth to sixth decades. It has been found in the newborn.

The diagnosis in the last analysis is made by examination of the spinal fluid in a patient with signs of meningitis developing during acute pneumonia or secondarily to mastoid, sinus disease, or other infections elsewhere in the body. In such a patient the spinal fluid pressure is increased, is hazy in appearance or frankly purulent, contains large numbers of polynuclear cells, and has decreased sugar and increased protein contents. In more than half the cases, the organism can be demonstrated in the spinal fluid with the aid of typing sera. If this fails, culture will permit identification of the organism. Any of the various types of pneumococcus may cause meningitis, and no definite pattern of type distribution is found in pneumococcic meningitis. The higher types of pneumococci are less likely to cause meningitis. The only exception seems to be Type III pneumococcus, which has a specially high incidence in the causation of pneumococcic meningitis, due probably to its high incidence in ear and sinus infections. Multiple infections of the meninges by pneumococci are extremely rare. Rare instances also are found of mixed pneumococcus and H. influenzae infection and of pneumococcus and Staphylococcus aureus infection.

Streptococcic meningitis is secondary usually to infections in the sinuses and to otitis. With rare exceptions, the meningitis is caused by Streptococcus hemolyticus. The clinical features of streptococcic meningitis are as already described and have no characteristics which might be regarded as diagnostic. Meningitis due to *Streptococcus viridans* is rare, occurring in an incidence of 0.3 to 2.4 per cent of all types of purulent meningitis. It develops in the course of subacute bacterial endocarditis, in ear, nose and throat infections, and in a large group of cases (thirty-five per cent) the source is unknown and the meningitis is assumed to be primary. The treatment of choice appears to be large doses of penicillin and a sulfonamide.

Influenzal meningitis, like the other forms of purulent meningitis, has no characteristic symptomatology. It is essentially a disease of infancy and early childhood, most cases occurring in the first two years of life. A seasonal incidence seems to be demonstrable, most cases occurring in the last quarter of the year. The disease is primary in a high percentage of cases (sixty-one per cent, Neal, et al.). In adults, influenzal meningitis is ordinarily secondary to acute sinusitis, otitis media, head injuries, or operations on the skull. In infants and children, the earliest signs are those of a gastrointestinal disturbance, irregular fever, irritability and a bulging fontanel. In adults, the symptoms are those of a systemic infection as outlined above. Leukocytosis is always present. The spinal fluid shows a marked increase in polynuclear cells. The diagnosis can only be inferred in an infant who develops signs of meningitis, since the disease is largely one of infancy and early childhood. It can be established with certainty only by laboratory examinations. The organism can be demonstrated often in the blood stream early in the disease. It can be seen in direct smear in the spinal fluid as a Gram-negative bacillus. Six types of influenza bacillus are known (a to f), of which type b produces the majority of infections in infants and children.

Staphylococcic meningitis is much less frequent than the other forms of purulent meningitis. There is usually a history of a staphylococcic infection elsewhere in the body—a furuncle on the face, osteomyelitis, a carbuncle, etc. It has no distinctive clinical features.

Colon bacillus meningitis is most common in infants under three months of age, but there is wide discrepancy with regard to the incidence of colon bacillus as a cause of meningitis in infancy, estimates varying from three out of fifteen hundred cases of meningitis to thirty per cent of cases of meningitis in infants. The portal of entry of the organism is unknown in many cases, but in those cases in which it has been determined the middle ear, the genitourinary and gastrointestinal tracts are the most common source. The diagnosis in adults is based on evidences of meningitis, usually with indications of a generalized infection. In children and infants, the first symptom may be a failure to nurse properly, irritability, and later vomiting and convulsions. The temperature is not high, rarely rising above 101° F., occasionally normal temperatures being recorded. Hydrocephalus may develop. The diagnosis in both infants and adults must await identification of the organism in the spinal fluid. The spinal fluid is turbid, there is an increase of cells (three to ten thousand) with a mixture of polynuclears and mononuclears, the former predominating. The organisms may be seen in the direct smear in many cases or may be demonstrated in cultures. The spinal fluid may be infected for several weeks. Without chemotherapy the fatality rate is eighty per cent.

Gonococcic meningitis is secondary to gonococcic infection elsewhere in the body, resulting either from an acute gonococcic infection or from exacerbation of a chronic infection. Very few cases are recorded in the literature, but gonococcic meningitis is said to be more common than it seems to be. It is often overlooked because of the close resemblance morphologically of the gonococcus and meningococcus. In most cases, in addition to a urethritis there are other gonococcal complications occurring before, during, or after the meningitis. These are prostatitis, cystitis, arthritis, endocarditis, and purpura. In a few instances, the meningeal infection has followed the urethritis directly, without intervening complications of other sorts. The meningeal infection follows a gonococcemia.

In addition, there are many unusual forms of meningitis which deserve only brief mention. Meningitis due to *Friedlander's bacillus* is rare, occurring about once in one hundred cases of meningitis (Sicard and Pluvinage). It develops in the course of septicemias or complicates an infection of the nose, throat, or ear. It has been reported following sinus infection and mild angina. The onset of the meningitis may be slow or sudden. Cutaneous hyperesthesia and sphincter disturbances are comparatively frequent. The meningeal signs vary greatly in intensity. The fever is often moderate in degree. The blood culture is nearly always positive. The pneumobacillus can be demonstrated in smear and culture of the spinal fluid, which contains large numbers of polynuclear cells. In very rare instances, meningitis may result from infection with *Gaffkya tetragena*. The clinical features are similar to those of meningococcic meningitis. The diagnosis must depend on the identification of the organism by smear and culture. It is often mistaken for the meningococcus or the staphylococcus. *Enterococcic meningitis* is rare and has no characteristics which may be regarded as diagnostic. The enterococcus can be demonstrated in the spinal fluid. Meningitis due to *salmonella infection* has been reported, due to S. suipestifer and panama. The meningitis in such cases has no specific features, the diagnosis depending on the identification of the organism in the spinal fluid. In the case of S. suipestifer infection, a history of contact with pork is obtained.

Treatment: *General care* is important. The patient must be kept in good general condition. Restlessness should be treated with sedation such as paralyde-hyde, chloral hydrate, or some similar remedy if the restlessness becomes harmful to the patient. Nasal feeding should be used if the patient cannot take food spontaneously, and the diet in any case should consist of liquids and semisoft foods enforced with vitamins. Fluids should be given in accordance with the condition of the tissues and, despite the brain swelling, should be given freely if needed. Much harm can be done by indiscriminate dehydration. *Transfusions* should be given as often as necessary in all forms of meningitis and constitute an important feature of the treatment.

Simultaneous double meningitis may develop rarely, most commonly in children. The offending organisms have been found to be *H. influenzae*, associated with *Neisseria intracellularis, Streptococcus* and *Diplococcus pneumoniae.*

Pneumococcic meningitis: The treatment of pneumococcic meningitis is concerned with two major and allied problems: (1) the treatment of the meningeal infection, and (2) the treatment of the focus of infection from which the meningeal infection developed.

The mortality of pneumococcic meningitis, though significantly less than in the days before the sulfonamides and antibiotics, is still high (35 per cent). Treatment of the meningeal infection requires the use of all possible means of combating it. *Sodium sulfadiazine* should be given intravenously (3 to 5 Gm. [45 to 75 grains]) as soon as the diagnosis is made and should be continued by this route as long as the patient is stuporous (2 Gm. [30 grains] every eight to twelve hours). If a nasal tube is used for feeding, sulfadiazine may be given by tube, 1 to 2 Gm. (15 to 30 grains) every three hours. In patients who are conscious, the drug may be given by mouth in doses of 1 Gm. every three hours until improvement develops, when it should be continued every four hours. *Penicillin* must be given with the sulfadiazine in doses of 300,000 units intramuscularly every six hours.

In view of the resistance of pneumococcic meningitis to treatment, *combined sulfadiazine and penicillin* treatment is essential. Penicillin should be continued as long as there is clinical indication of its need. Penicillin should be given in doses of one million units every two hours (500,000 units for children). This should be continued until the patient is afebrile for four days, and the dosage resumed at the former level if the temperature rises after withdrawal of the drug. *Intrathecal penicillin* is justified in those cases in which the situation is desperate, though there is controversy concerning its value so given, and it has distinct hazards. It may be given in doses of 25,000 units, diluted in 10 cc. of saline, after an equivalent volume of spinal fluid has been withdrawn. *Streptomycin* has been reported to be efficacious in the treatment of pneumococcic meningitis.

Elimination of the focus of infection in the sinuses or mastoids is fully as important as the conquest of the meningeal infection. Of one thing there is no doubt: the focus must be eradicated whether by drugs or surgery. In some instances, drug treatment will dispose of both areas of infection, but in many the focus must be dealt with individually. When to operate on an offending mastoid or sinus infection is a problem which cannot be answered dogmatically. If the meningeal infection is brought under control, the mastoids or sinuses can be dealt with after the meningitis is cured. If, on the other hand, despite adequate treatment, the battle with the meningitis fails to be favorable and temperature persists, it is necessary to operate on the focus of infection while meningitis still is present. A measure as extreme as this is essential only because the situation in such instances is desperate, and the meningitis will not respond so long as the original focus of infection remains active.

Streptococcic meningitis: This should be treated in the same fashion as pneumococcic meningitis, except that intrathecal penicillin is not necessary. The same rules apply for elimination of the focus of infection responsible for the meningitis.

Influenzal meningitis: This form of meningitis responds well to *streptomycin, sulfadiazine* and *specific serum.* Sulfadiazine is given intravenously (1 to 3 Gm. [15 to 45 grains]) in stuporous or severely ill patients and maintained by this method until the drug can be given by mouth. Since the disease occurs chiefly in children, the dosages are lower than those for adults. The drug is given in doses of 1 to 2 Gm. (15 to 30 grains) intravenously and repeated every eight to twelve hours until it can be maintained by mouth in doses of 1 Gm. every four hours. For adults, it is given intravenously (3 to 5 Gm. [45 to 75 grains]) in severe cases and continued at doses of 1 Gm. every three hours either intravenously or by mouth as the occasion demands.

Hemophilus influenzae anti-serum, type B, is given in an initial dose of 100 mg.

of antibody in 200 cc. of saline, and allowed to drip into a vein over a two- to four-hour period. This should be repeated. The serum may be given intramuscularly. The serum should be given with one of the other agents used, though there is difference of opinion regarding its value.

Streptomycin has been found to be effective in influenzal meningitis. Though the mortality of this form of meningitis has been reduced to as low as 20 per cent by sulfonamides and specific serum, the routine use of streptomycin is advisable in addition to these remedies because of (1) failure of some patients to respond to sulfonamides and serum alone, and (2) mounting evidence that streptomycin alone is effective in some cases. The dosage varies. For infants, 0.5 to 1.0 Gm. (7½ to 15 grains) daily in divided doses is given; and for older children, 2.0 Gm. (30 grains) daily intramuscularly in divided doses. The intramuscular administration may be fortified by giving 0.1 to 0.5 Gm. (1½ to 7½ grains) of streptomycin in 5 to 10 cc. of saline intrathecally once in twenty-four to forty-eight hours. *Aureomycin* and *terramycin* are said by some to be the agents of choice in influenzal meningitis. *Chloramphenicol* is equally effective. Aureomycin is given as the hydrochloride, intravenously during the acutely ill period on the basis of 10 mg. per. kg. of body weight, administered every eight hours until the patient is conscious. It is then continued orally in divided doses, 2 to 3 grams per day for adults. This should be continued until the patient is afebrile for one week. Terramycin is given in the same dosage.

Prognosis: The sulfonamides and antibiotics have placed in the hands of the physician potent means of combating the many forms of meningitis. Diseases, which in many of their forms seemed hopeless, have now been brought under control, and future outlooks are brighter as newer compounds are discovered. *Meningococcic meningitis* mortality has been reduced to 1 per cent under controlled conditions, as in the Army during World War II. In civil life, the general mortality has been reduced to 10 per cent and in some instances lower. The outlook in the *fulminating form* of meningococcic meningitis is still grave, but the possibilities of help are increased if the diagnosis is made early and intensive treatment begun without delay. *Pneumococcic meningitis* still carries a high mortality despite combined sulfonamide and penicillin treatment. Recovery rates of 45 per cent are reported. *Influenzal meningitis* has been rescued from almost certain death in every instance to reported recovery rates of 75 per cent and higher with combined sulfonamide, serum, and streptomycin treatment. Prior to streptomycin, the mortality rate was higher, but with the latter added to other means of treatment, the majority of the patients can be expected to recover.

VII. TUBERCULOUS MENINGITIS

Etiology: Tuberculous meningitis occurs most commonly in children, but may develop at any age. It is the most frequent form of meningitis in childhood. It appears most commonly in children under six years of age. It does not occur in infants below three months and is rare in infants of three to twelve months. It is more frequent in the summer months. It is more common in males. It is always secondary to tuberculosis elsewhere in the body, as, for example, pulmonary tuberculosis, tuberculous epididymitis, tuberculosis of the kidney, mediastinal or abdominal glands, or tuberculosis of the bones or other parts of the body. It may develop as part of a miliary tuberculosis. The source of the tuberculosis is not

always apparent, but in most instances the source of the meningeal infection is apparent either in the lungs or elsewhere. In not a few cases the source remains hidden in tuberculous glands in the mediastinum or abdomen. The most frequent source is thoracic (73.9 per cent); other sources are abdominal (22.8 per cent), cervical glands (2.1 per cent), unknown (1.2 per cent) (Blalock and Griffin).

Pathology: The process is a meningoencephalitis. The brain is usually swollen and edematous, and is moderately congested. The meningeal exudate is heaviest over the base of the brain, over the chiasm, cerebral peduncles, and pons. In its fresh state it appears as a fibrinous exudate in which minute tubercles may be seen. Tubercles can be found also over the cerebral hemispheres, usually extending along the blood vessels. They are especially numerous in the Sylvian fissures. They may be seen also over the superior surface of the cerebellum. Tubercles may sometimes be seen in the brain substance, either as a small solitary tubercle or as scattered tubercles about 1 cm. in diameter throughout the brain.

The meninges contain many lymphocytic cells. The blood vessels are heavily infiltrated with lymphocytes. Giant cells are occasionally seen. The underlying brain substance shows perivascular infiltration with lymphocytes and lymphocytic infiltration in the parenchyma of the brain.

The means by which tuberculous meningitis develops is not clear. Blood stream extension seems improbable in most cases. Lymphatic extension may explain the process in some cases. Extension of the infection into the meninges from a cortical tuberculoma has been suggested as the causative mechanism.

Symptoms: The onset of the disease is apt to be insidious with apathy, irritability, listlessness, fretfulness, and loss of

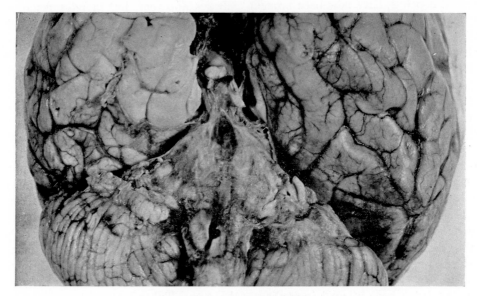

Fig. 108—*(See: Fig. 109)*

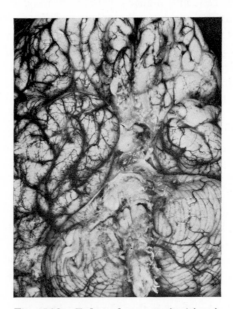

Fig. 109—*Tuberculous meningitis.* A
view of the base of the brain from a
case of tuberculous meningitis showing
the fibrinous exudate closely adherent
to the structures of the pons, mesencephalon and diencephalon. Upon high
magnification, the fibrinous and adherent nature of the exudate in tuberculous meningitis is clearly seen.

interest. These prodromal symptoms may last for a few days or may persist for several days or a few weeks. During this period signs of meningeal irritation are lacking and examination of the spinal fluid reveals nothing. The onset may in other instances be acute with headache, stupor, and fever. Headache appears early and may be a prominent symptom. A slight fever is noted early in the disease and with the listlessness and fretfulness may be the only symptom at this stage. The disease may pursue this course for several days. The patient presents a characteristic picture as the disease develops to more advanced stages. He lies in bed, usually resenting examination and fretting over being moved. Somnolence is a very striking feature, patients drowsing constantly and appearing apathetic. Convulsions may develop and stupor may in some instances supervene, deepening rapidly into coma. Hemiplegia or monoplegia is found in some cases. Meningeal signs are present, with stiffness of the neck, Kernig's sign, and often Brudzinski's sign. Fever is usually of a low grade (99° to 101° F.) and is irregular. The pulse and respirations are increased in rate.

The spinal fluid is under pressure. It is usually clear, but may be misty or yellow, and a clot often develops on standing. The cells vary from fifty to five hundred and are predominantly lymphocytes. In occasional cases polynuclear cells predominate early in the disease and sometimes throughout its course. The sugar is decreased (45 mg. or below). The chlorides are moderately or greatly reduced, usually below 650 mg. and constitute an important feature of the disease. The decrease in chlorides is greater than in other forms of meningitis, but it is not pathognomonic, since other forms of meningitis may be associated with a low chloride content of the spinal fluid.

The tubercle bacillus is found sometimes on direct smear of the spinal fluid sediment, but is more often not found. In rare instances the spinal fluid may contain blood.

The usual case runs a course of two to four weeks, but chronic and more prolonged cases are not uncommon.

Diagnosis: The diagnosis is usually not difficult. The disease should always be suspected in a child with slight up and down fever, with listlessness, somnolence, and signs of meningeal irritation, which may be very mild. If the spinal fluid reveals an increase of lymphocytes, the diagnosis is probable even if no tubercle bacilli are found. If the spinal fluid chlorides are below 650 mg. further confirmation is added, but the diagnosis is not established, by the low chloride content of the spinal fluid. If a known source of tuberculosis is present in the body, the evidence indicates at this stage that a meningeal infection is present, with fever, and an excess of lymphocytes in the spinal fluid. Under such circumstances, a presumptive diagnosis of tuberculous meningitis may be made and will probably be sustained later by the demonstration of tubercle bacilli in the spinal fluid.

In many cases the problem is that of a child or adult with slight fever, with a history of listlessness, somnolence, possibly with convulsions, with signs of meningeal irritation and with an excess of lymphocytes in the spinal fluid. No tubercle bacilli are found in the spinal fluid and no evidence of tuberculosis can be found in the body. The problem in such a case is that of a lymphocytic form of meningitis of undetermined origin. If such a meningitis is found to be tuberculous in origin it will be established by the demonstration of tubercle bacilli in the spinal fluid or by a webbed clot in the spinal fluid. Until such evidence can be found, the problem resolves itself into a consideration of those conditions which are capable of causing meningitis with an excess of lymphocytes in the spinal fluid.

The differential diagnosis of the lymphocytic type of meningitis must include consideration of the following forms:

1. *Acute lymphocytic meningitis:*
   Lymphocytic choriomeningitis
   Lymphocytic meningitis due to other viruses

2. *Meningoencephalitis varia:*

Mumps	Herpes zoster
Poliomyelitis	Herpes simplex
Rabies	Vaccinia
Lymphogranu-	Infectious mononucleosis
loma venere-	
um	

3. *Bacterial infections:*
   Tuberculosis
   Syphilis
   Tetanus
   Pyogenic organisms (brain abscess)

4. *Fungus and Parasitic infections:*
   Cryptococcus
   Cysticercosis
   Coccidiomycosis

5. *Meningitis Sympathica:*
   Serum
   Spinal anesthesia
   Pantopaque
   Ear or mastoid infection
   Brain abscess

Acute lymphocytic choriomeningitis is associated with less pronounced systemic signs than in tuberculous meningitis. No tubercle bacilli are found in the spinal fluid and the general tendency is toward recovery. A prodromal illness resembling a grippal attack is found in over seventy-five per cent of cases. Following this there develop headache and other symptoms of meningeal involvement. There may be a history of contact with mice, and the lymphocytes in the spinal fluid usually exceed 600 per mm³. No organisms are found by smear or culture, but the diagnosis can be made by the demonstration of virus or of neutralizing antibodies to the virus. The condition is benign and fatal cases rare.

Acute syphilitic meningitis is characterized by severe headache of sudden or gradual onset, associated with varying cranial nerve signs, such as deafness, optic neuritis, facial paralysis, difficulty in swallowing, etc., usually without fever but rarely with fever, sometimes with convulsions or hemiplegia, and with positive Wassermann reactions of the blood and spinal fluid and abnormal colloidal gold reactions. The sugar and chloride contents of the spinal fluid are normal. Unless there is a clear-cut history of recent infection or of antisyphilitic treatment, the diagnosis in the last analysis is made upon the abnormal serological reactions unless such diagnostic findings such as Argyll Robertson pupils are demonstrable, when a tentative diagnosis of syphilitic meningitis is tenable.

Poliomyelitis begins acutely with prodromal signs, fever, and evidences of meningeal irritation. In the preparalytic stage, it may resemble tuberculous meningitis very closely, the patient showing the listlessness, nausea, vomiting, and other signs which develop in tuberculous meningitis. The spinal fluid in this stage shows an excess of lymphocytes without significant changes in sugar or chlorides. The diagnosis is made readily if the disease is epidemic; otherwise it is first established definitely upon the development of paralysis. If paralysis fails to develop, recovery ensues, in which case tuberculous meningitis is excluded by virtue of the recovery as well as by the failure to demonstrate tubercle bacilli on repeated examination of the spinal fluid.

Encephalitis may offer difficulties in the early stages when a meningeal reaction is present. The encephalitis following measles, varicella, vaccinia, etc., is readily detected because of the history

Table 31—Differential Diagnosis of Tuberculous Meningitis

Disease	Age	Symptoms	Signs	Spinal Fluid	Diagnosis
TUBERCULOUS MENINGITIS	Children predominantly	Gradual onset, somnolence, listlessness, fever, diplopia, facial weakness	Meningeal signs. Ocular palsies, or facial paralysis, or other cranial nerve palsies	50-500 lymphocytes, chlorides 650 mg. or less. Sugar reduced. Tubercle bacilli present	Diagnosis definitely established by demonstration of tubercle bacilli. Death almost invariable. Rare recoveries
LYMPHOCYTIC CHORIO-MENINGITIS	Adults chiefly	Grippal onset, fever, followed after a latency by headache, and in some instances diplopia and other signs of encephalitis	Meningeal signs all cases. Ocular palsies much more unusual than in tuberculous meningitis	50-3000 lymphocytes. Sugar and chlorides normal. Protein increased	Complement fixing antibodies for soluble antigen about 4 weeks after onset. Neutralizing antibodies to virus 2 to 3 months after onset. Recovery usual
SYPHILITIC MENINGITIS	Adults chiefly	Gradual onset with severe headache, no fever, plus cranial nerve palsies—deafness, diplopia, facial paralysis, etc. Convulsions, hemiplegia, aphasia at times	Meningeal signs. Irregular pupils, ocular palsies, facial paralysis, nerve deafness, palatal weakness. Hemiplegia, aphasia at times	50-500 lymphocytes, sometimes more. Wassermann of spinal fluid usually positive. Colloidal gold usually abnormal. Chlorides and sugar normal	Diagnosis in the last analysis depends on abnormal Wassermann reaction in spinal fluid and other evidences of syphilis
POLIOMYELITIS	Children usually	Acute onset with fever, gastrointestinal symptoms, headache. Later, weakness of one or more limbs	Meningeal signs in prodromal stage. Muscle tenderness, irritability	25-200 lymphocytes. Chlorides and sugar normal	Prodromal poliomyelitis detectable in epidemics; otherwise difficult. Development of paralysis indicates diagnosis. Chlorides and sugar normal and help to differentiate from tuberculous meningitis
ENCEPHALITIS	Children and Adults	Vary with type of encephalitis. Fever, headache, somnolence, diplopia, in some forms convulsions	Meningeal signs in very acute stages. Ocular palsies prominent	15-100 lymphocytes. Sugar and chlorides normal	Meningeal signs transitory and disappear rapidly. Encephalitic signs predominate
ASEPTIC MENINGITIS	Any age	Acute, following focus in mastoids, sinuses, sinus thrombosis, abscess, etc.	Meningeal irritation and almost nothing else save fever	Excess of cells, 50% lymphocytes, and 50% polynuclears	Dependent on focus of infection and sterile spinal fluid. Disappears with removal of focus
INFECTIOUS MONONUCLEOSIS	Adults chiefly	Acute, with fever, headache	Lymphadenopathy, splenomegaly, lymphocytosis	Excess of lymphocytes. Otherwise negative	Enlargement of lymph glands, splenomegaly and demonstration of agglutinins in blood

of development during the course of the illness in question. All these may show an excess of lymphocytes in the spinal fluid. Meningeal signs, however, are not pronounced and tend to disappear within a short time. Lethargic encephalitis and St. Louis encephalitis can be differentiated by their acute onset with fever, somnolence, ocular paralyses, and by the predominance of encephalitic over meningeal signs. The latter are present early but are not persistent. The spinal fluid reveals an excess of lymphocytes but no tubercle bacilli are found.

Acute aseptic meningitis (meningitis sympathica) develops as a result of infections adjacent to the meninges, as, for example, in sinusitis, otitis media, petrositis, brain abscess, and venous sinus thrombosis. In such cases the presence of a focus of infection is usually known either by history or symptoms. The signs of meningeal irritation in such cases are those common to all cases of meningitis—headache, vomiting, neck stiffness. There is an excess of cells in the spinal fluid, about fifty per cent of which are polynuclears and the rest lymphocytes. The sugar content is normal. No organisms are demonstrable by smear or culture. The diagnosis is made by the demonstration of a focus of infection and by the presence of a sterile spinal

Infectious mononucleosis rarely may produce a meningeal reaction with an excess of lymphocytes in the spinal fluid. The condition is detected readily by the development during the course of the illness of lymphadenopathy, splenomegaly, lymphocytosis, and the development of agglutinins in the blood.

In some instances, *tuberculous meningitis* may develop slowly and chronically. The symptoms in such instances may persist for weeks with signs of meningeal irritation and all the other evidences of tuberculous meningitis.

Treatment: Until the advent of *streptomycin*, the treatment of tuberculous meningitis was looked upon as almost hopeless. Streptomycin for the first time offers hope of a potent means of coping with tuberculous infection of the meninges. For infants it should be given intramuscularly in divided doses of 0.5 to 1.0 Gm. (7½ to 15 grains) daily; and for older children, in doses of 2.0 Gm. (30 grains) daily in divided doses. For adults, it may be given in doses of 2.0 to 3.0 Gm. (30 to 45 grains) daily intramuscularly in divided doses. Recovery in fifty to sixty per cent of patients is reported with combined intramuscular and intrathecal streptomycin. Recovery is slow, requiring a year or more, and the drug must be given over a long period. The majority of deaths occur in the first three months, and the relapse rate after a full course of treatment is low (Cairns, Smith, and Vollum). Precise rules about stopping treatment are difficult to define. Intramuscular streptomycin is recommended for at least 180 days, regardless of the patient's progress and should not be stopped until the patient is gaining weight and the protein and cells of the spinal fluid have been steadily falling for at least two months.

Other drugs are available for treatment besides streptomycin. These include isoniazid and para-aminosalicylic acid (PAS). In the acute phases, isoniazid is given orally in doses of 8 to 10 mg. per kilogram of body weight, in two or three divided doses. This treatment should be continued until there is definite improvement, when the dosage can be reduced to 5 mg. per kilogram of body weight. After recovery has occurred, isoniazid should be continued in doses of 100 to 200 mg. given three or four times daily. Care must be taken to avoid neuritis which sometimes results from isoniazid.

Para-aminosalicylic acid (PAS) is given in doses of 3 Gm. four or five times daily.

Treatment should be continued for a year or longer in order to avoid recurrence. Streptomycin can be discontinued after the recovered phase and treatment continued with isoniazid and PAS, because of the tendency of streptomycin to neurotoxicity.

In the moribund patients, or those severely ill, cortisone or hydrocortisone has been suggested as an accessory form of treatment.

Reports of recovery from tuberculous meningitis are already available, but dosage technics remain to be standardized. Increased cell counts in the spinal fluid may persist after clinical improvement has been attained. The probabilities are that the infection is merely suppressed in these patients and that relapse will occur where the cell count fails to return to normal.

VIII. ACUTE LYMPHOCYTIC CHORIO-MENINGITIS (Benign Lymphocytic Meningitis, Acute Aseptic Meningitis)

Acute lymphocytic choriomeningitis is a term used to designate a specific group of cases of benign meningitis of virus origin. The disease has been observed in epidemics as well as in sporadic cases and seems to be more common now than formerly. Most of the cases occur during the fall months.

Etiology: The disease is caused by a virus, but as already stated, by no means all of the cases of this disorder are found to neutralize the known virus which has been discovered for the disease. It is also probable that all the cases grouped in this heading are not identical. Several viruses may perhaps be responsible. The virus responsible for the disease has been isolated in widely separated portions of the United States, in England, France,

and Japan, suggesting that it is worldwide in distribution.

A virus causing lymphocytic choriomeningitis has been isolated in monkeys, rats, mice, and guinea pigs. A similar virus has been isolated from the spinal fluid in some human cases in this country and found to be identical with the virus found in lower animals. The virus is obtained easily from the spinal fluid and blood. "Wild mice caught in nature have been shown to be infected by the virus, and the epidemiology of the disease in some way is associated with this rodent host" (Rivers). Specific neutralizing antibodies have been found in the blood in many cases. Virus has been reported to be isolated from the nasopharynx.

All ages are susceptible. Most cases occur between fifteen and forty years of age; the disease is not common in the first decade.

Pathology: The pathology is that of a generalized infection, with visceral as well as nervous system lesions. The changes in the nervous system have been studied best in animals, but fatal human cases also have been described, though they are not numerous. The meninges are infiltrated with lymphocytes. The underlying brain tissue is usually not involved, but in some fatal cases encephalitic foci have been found in the brain and brain stem (cerebral cortex, pons, mesencephalon, and medulla). The ganglion cells of the midbrain may show evidence of damage (Viets). Inflammatory changes are found in the walls of the ventricles, with lymphocytic infiltration and glial proliferation under the ependyma. The choroid plexus may be thickened and scarred (Machella, et al.). Arachnoiditis involving the spinal cord has been reported (Barker and Ford).

Studies of mice reveal that the infiltration is greatest on the sixth to the ninth day after intracerebral inoculation. It is greatest at the base and in the major cerebral fissures. The choroid plexuses are infiltrated, particularly those of the third and fourth ventricles. Ventricular infiltration appears about the seventh day. The infiltration is chiefly lymphocytic with scattering of macrophages and polynuclear cells. Perivascular infiltrations are seen in the period of greatest meningeal, plexal, and ventricular infiltration, around the vessels under the meninges and ependyma. The infiltrations diminish after the ninth day. The meningeal and plexal infiltration is less in guinea pigs. Monkeys show a variable picture, from slight to moderate focal or diffuse infiltrations. The meninges of the spinal cord are sometimes affected. Visceral infiltrations are common. They consist of polyserositis with serous exudate of the pleura and peritoneum, fatty degeneration of the liver, and to a lesser extent of the kidneys; focal necrosis in the liver, and rarely in the adrenal cortex and corpora lutea; diffuse and sometimes focal necrosis in the thymus, spleen, lymph nodes, and bone marrow; and generalized lymphocytic infiltrations in the pleura and peritoneum, renal cortex and pelvis, liver, salivary glands, pancreas, lungs, heart, adrenal glands, and less frequently the tissues of the gastrointestinal and genitourinary tracts (Lillie and Armstrong).

The disease in humans develops in some cases from virus-carrying gray mice and it is well established that there is a reservoir of infection in gray mice. The evidence suggests that in a number of cases of lymphocytic choriomeningitis the virus was transmitted from mice to humans (Farmer and Janeway).

Symptoms: The clinical picture is quite typical. General systemic symptoms develop first and may be followed by evidences of central nervous system involvement or may disappear without the latter. Prodromal symptoms develop five to ten days after exposure to the virus and vary in duration from seven to twenty days. Fever (100° to 103° F.) usually is present, and often returns to normal before meningeal symptoms develop. Symptoms of grippe, such as malaise, backache, and muscle aches, develop, associated with fatigue, weakness, and somnolence. There is often an upper respiratory infection before the disease sets in, characterized by cold, cough, sore throat, or bronchitis. Virus is present in the blood at this stage and a leukopenia is present. The disease may progress no farther than this stage or go on to the development of meningitis.

Evidences of central nervous system involvement are indicated by the development of headache, fever, and vomiting, which appear after an incubation period of twelve to twenty-three days. The headache is generalized and quite severe; the fever varies from 101° to 104° F., and is associated with chilly feelings. Lumbar backache is common. Drowsiness, disorientation, and memory defects are noted occasionally. Abdominal and thoracic pain have been reported. The pulse may be normal or only slightly accelerated with the increased temperature. Neck stiffness is always present; Kernig's sign is usually present (fifty per cent), and Brudzinski's sign much less frequent. Photophobia may be marked. Choked disc may be found occasionally. The leukocyte count is usually normal (six to eleven thousand) but may reach as high as twenty thousand. The sedimentation rate is normal or slower than normal.

The developing picture is therefore that of a meningeal infection with fever, photophobia. headache, backache, muscular pains, and abdominal cramps. Examination reveals, outstandingly, evidences of meningeal irritation with neck stiffness and Kernig's sign but usually no evidence of involvement of the brain tissue itself. Encephalitic signs are sometimes seen. In a few instances, reports of encephalitic or encephalomyelitic forms of lymphocytic choriomeningitis have been recorded. In such cases, fever and headache develop, associated with which may be mental confusion and hallucinations, drowsiness, diplopia, aphasia, hemiplegia, or other focal signs. Choked disc may be found, as well as hemiplegia and paraplegia.

The spinal fluid is under normal or increased pressure and contains an increase of lymphocytes (fifty to three thousand or over), ninety-five to one hundred per cent of the cells being lymphocytes. Verified cases are on record without increase of cells in the spinal fluid. These are probably abortive cases. The sugar content is normal but may be reduced to 35 to 40 mg. The chloride content is normal. The protein is increased (50 to 200 mg.) Virus can be isolated from the spinal fluid during the first seven to ten days of meningitis, but after this is no longer detectable. Stained smears show no organisms and cultures are negative

Diagnosis: The detection of the condition is not difficult as a rule. The picture is usually that of an acute meningitis with a lymphocytic increase in the spinal fluid. This usually begins with prodromal symptoms which often resembles a grippal attack, following which evidences of headache, backache, vomiting, and other symptoms develop; fever and meningeal signs are demonstrable and an excess of lymphocytes is found in the spinal fluid with otherwise normal chemistry of the fluid. In some instances, evidences of encephalitis may develop, associated with signs of focal brain in. volvement, such as ocular palsies, hemiplegia, aphasia, or other focal signs. In most instances, probably, the disease

stops at the prodromal stage, does not go on to the development of meningeal signs, and is often disposed of as a grippal attack.

The problem in most instances is that of a febrile illness with a lymphocytic meningitis, without organisms demonstrable by smear or culture.

In the last analysis, the diagnosis must be made by the demonstration of virus in the patient's spinal fluid or by the development of antibodies in the convalescent serum. For this, special laboratory studies are necessary. Complement fixing antibodies for the soluble antigen and not the virus appear about four weeks after onset and can be detected for several months. Neutralizing antibodies to the virus itself do not appear until two to three months after onset, but usually persist for several years. The diagnosis may be suspected clinically under the following circumstances (Farmer and Janeway): (1) in the presence of a history of handling dead mice or where there has been contact with mice excreta; (2) the presence of a definite prodromal illness, since in over seventy-five per cent of the cases a febrile systemic infection has been reported; (3) the cell count of lymphocytes is higher in cases of lymphocytic choriomeningitis than in acute aseptic meningitis. It is apt to exceed six hundred cells per cc.

Aseptic meningitis of virus origin may be due to lymphocytic choriomeningitis, mumps, herpes simplex, leptospirosis, and other virus infections such as poliomyelitis. Meningitis may result from involvement of the meninges by the Coxsackie virus, which has been recovered from the spinal fluid of such patients. The differentiation depends for the most part on laboratory identification of the offending virus. Often this is unsuccessful in our present state of identification of viruses, and the diagnosis frequently remains virus meningitis of undetermined origin or aseptic meningitis. In instances of aseptic meningitis due to virus infection, it is essential to separate such cases from the start from those cases of aseptic meningitis associated with a focus of infection or to other causes (v. Acute Aseptic Meningitis).

Treatment and Prognosis: Treatment of the condition is purely *symptomatic*. Headache is the most prominent complaint and is best relieved by lumbar puncture. Large doses of salicylates are also helpful. Barbiturates may be necessary to relieve restlessness and quiet anxiety. Sulfonamides have not been found to be useful.

The outlook is almost uniformly good. Occasional fatal cases have been reported, but they are unusual. Convalescence is gradual. The fever persists in slight degree for one or two weeks, the meningeal signs disappear gradually, and the excess of cells in the spinal fluid disappears. Recovery is usually complete, but personality changes, prolonged fatigue, headache, impairment of memory, depression, dizziness and strabismus have been reported as after effects. Spastic paraplegia due to spinal arachnoiditis complicating the disease has been recorded in one instance.

IX. ACUTE ASEPTIC MENINGITIS
(Meningitis Sympathica, Protective or Reactive Meningitis, Serous Meningitis)

Definition: The term "acute aseptic meningitis" is nondescript and refers to a sterile meningitis occurring secondary to a focus of infection outside the meninges. It has several forms. It may be mainly cerebral or basilar. Its nature is not clear since good pathological studies are not available.

Etiology: The most common cause is probably otitis media or mastoiditis, both of which are at times associated with a sterile meningitis or meningitis sympathetica. Other causes include venous sinus thrombosis, pneumonia, typhoid fever, influenza, malaria, cervical adenitis, brain abscess, lead poisoning, alcoholism, and fevers of various sorts. Trauma is a not uncommon cause. The condition may develop after a mastoid operation. Often no specific cause can be determined.

Symptoms: The symptoms vary widely. The onset may be acute as in any meningitis or it may be gradual. Headache is a prominent feature and fever may or may not be present. Neck stiffness is found. There may be optic neuritis or even choked disc. Other cranial nerve palsies may be found. The spinal fluid is sterile and contains an increase of cells, usually polynuclear cells, an increased amount of protein, and normal sugar and chlorides.

Diagnosis: It is difficult to prove definitely. It may be suspected in otitic cases in the presence of a focus of infection in the ear and a sterile spinal fluid, but these criteria are not absolute because (1) a spinal fluid may be sterile and subsequently show evidence of infection, (2) a brain abscess or sinus thrombosis may be accompanied by a sterile fluid and an increase of lymphocytes in the spinal fluid, but may be detected by the presence of localizing signs in the first, and chills and fever in the second.

In acute cases occurring during ear disease, fevers, or exanthemas, the clinical features are those of an acute meningitis with a sterile spinal fluid. If the spinal fluid shows an increase of cells consisting chiefly of polynuclear cells, the assumption must be that the meningitis is of the acute aseptic type if the spinal fluid is persistently sterile. The diagnosis therefore depends upon (1) the demonstration of a focus of infection; (2) the presence of a sterile spinal fluid.

It must be remembered, however, that sterile fluids may often show organisms on repeated study, so that the diagnosis of a sterile fluid must not be made on the basis of a single examination.

Treatment: *General care* should be given as in any meningitis. Lumbar puncture repeated as often as indicated gives great relief and often cures, even resulting in a disappearance of choked disc. Care must be exercised lest lumbar puncture be performed too often in the presence of increased pressure. Hypertonic solutions (fifty per cent sucrose) are helpful in reducing the fluid collection. *Operation* is necessary for the chronic subtentorial forms.

X. RARE FORMS OF MENINGITIS

Among the rare forms of meningitis is that due to torula infection, which is but one form of infection of the nervous system by higher fungi. Among those invading the nervous system are actinomyces, endomyces, streptothrix, sporathrix, blastomyces, saccharomyces, and coccidioides. *Cryptococcus meningitis* is characterized by meningeal thickening due to fibroblasts and endothelial cells and by infiltration of the meninges by giant cells and yeast cells. The brain is penetrated along the course of the blood vessels. The brain lesions are of three general types: a diffuse or granulomatous meningitis; small granulomas or cysts in the cortex, and deeply placed lesions, solid or cystic, lying chiefly in the basal ganglia but sometimes in the white matter of the cerebrum and cerebellum (Freeman).

The *symptoms* are characterized in some cases by prodromal complaints with respiratory infection predominating, and in rare instances by symptoms of several weeks' duration. The onset is at times acute with severe headache, vomiting, and vertigo, but more often insidiously with headache, which may be the only manifestation for some time. The headache becomes progressively more persistent and severe, is associated with stiffness and pain in the neck, and with nausea and vomiting. Disturbances in sleep, amblyopia, and diplopia are common, and mental phenomena follow. The temperature is normal at the outset, but fever develops later. There is evidence of a chronic upper respiratory infection, and enlargement of the lymph nodes is often found. The pulse is increased; there is neck stiffness and a positive Kernig's sign; neuroretinitis, choked disc, or optic neuritis occurs in two out of three cases; strabismus, stiff pupils, nystagmus, and ptosis occur; the patellar and Achilles reflexes are often lost; a positive Babinski's sign may be found. There may be a slight leukocytosis. The spinal fluid pressure is increased; the fluid is usually slightly hazy, occasionally cloudy or yellow, in most cases a pellicle forms; the cells vary from ten to thousands, 300 to 700 per cc. being average; the cells are lymphocytes but polymorphonuclears are found, at times as high as thirty per cent.

The condition is confused with brain tumor, especially in the early stages before the diagnosis is evident. It may resemble tuberculous meningitis and encephalitis. The diagnosis is often accidental and is made on the finding of the peculiar bodies in routine examination of the spinal fluid. These bodies are readily identified by India ink stain. The treatment is not as a rule successful, but a few recoveries have been reported following therapy with Amphotericin.

Coccidioidal meningitis develops from a focal lesion in the skin or lungs. Infection by coccidioides may be generalized, with the nervous system involved as part of the infection, or the nervous system may be chiefly affected. Meningitis is the chief manifestation, characterized by headache and meningeal signs, the process being chronic. There is slight fever and leukocytosis. The spinal fluid pressure is increased; the cells vary in number from fifty to two thousand, chiefly lymphocytes (seventy-five per cent) and organisms are usually found. Paraplegia due to involvement of the meninges of the cord is not uncommon and gives rise to motor and sensory paraplegia resembling spinal cord tumor.

Chronic meningitis may also be produced rarely by the *sporothrix*. Sporotrichosis produces skin lesions which are gummatous and may be mistaken for syphilis or tuberculosis. The infection may become systemic, involving the lungs, bones, periarticular tissues, kidneys, eyes, and rarely the brain. Fever is present in the meningeal form and the meningeal disease runs a chronic remitting course. Mental confusion, tetanoid attacks, and microptic hallucinations have been reported in the disorder. The spinal fluid pressure is increased and there is an excess of lymphocytes; red cells may be found in the fluid. The diagnosis is made by the demonstration of sporothrix spores in the spinal fluid.

Meningitis may develop in epidemic jaundice or *Weil's disease* (Spirochaeta icterohemorrhagiae). The symptoms are those of meningitis in general, headache being most prominent. Neck stiffness and Kernig's sign are found. The cell content of the spinal fluid may reach one thousand or more with polynuclear cells predominating early and lymphocytes later. Meningismus may be found without associated increase in the cell content of the spinal fluid.

Actinomycosis is at times associated with cerebral complications such as meningitis, cerebral abscess, and cerebellar abscess. The infection develops from contact with infected hay or grain. The meningeal infection almost always develops following a primary infection elsewhere in the body which spreads to the meninges by direct extension. In the pure meningitic form, headache predominates and is associated with neck stiffness and Kernig's sign. All cases terminate fatally.

Infection of the brain by *Blastomyces* (Oidiomycetes) is characterized by the presence of lesions resembling tubercles or gummas, usually multiple and sometimes large. In some instances, meningitis may result. Infection of the brain is always secondary to infection of the skin or lungs. The essential lesion consists of a miliary abscess tending to heal with the production of large amounts of fibrous tissue and a central zone of necrosis. Organisms can be demonstrated in the miliary abscesses, and lymphocytes and endothelial cells are abundant. Cutaneous lesions are abundant. Fever develops in generalized oidiomycosis, leukocytosis is mild. Hemiplegia is not uncommon.

Endomyces infection of the meninges is rare. One instance of meningeal infection has been recorded in a furrier, and lasted for six months. Signs of chronic meningitis were present. The process involved only the cerebral meninges. Infection of the meninges by *saccharomyces* is not proved though instances have been recorded.

Aspergillus infection of the orbit is not uncommon, but invasion of the brain is rare (Freeman). The characteristic lesion appears to be a miliary abscess. Headache, meningeal signs, hemiplegia, and pleocytosis of the spinal fluid may be found.

Infection of the nervous system by molds is extremely rare. Aspergillus infection has been mentioned. Infection due to the Mucoraceae has been recorded and has been associated with meningeal involvement and brain necrosis. In the recorded cases of mucromycosis, entrance was by way of the orbit. Headache, neck stiffness, confusion, and evidences of focal brain damage are found.

A benign form of meningitis has been described in young swineherds and has been designated *benign meningitis of swineherds* (Leptospira pomona). The etiology is unknown. Bacterial, serological, and animal experiments have produced negative results. A filterable virus has been isolated from the blood of a patient with disease of young swineherds. This form of meningitis has been found to attack mainly young laborers occupied in the making of cheese, the byproducts of which are fed to pigs. The pig is probably the transmitting agent. The intermediary host is not known. The disease begins suddenly with chills and high temperature, coated tongue, vomiting, and obstipation or diarrhea, after a prodromal stage that may last several days and is characterized by listlessness and general indisposition. The feces have the odor of pigs. Violent headaches and dull sensorium suggest typhoid or paratyphoid infection. Meningeal signs are marked. Restlessness is pronounced but somnolence and delirium are lacking. Perspiration, cyanosis, and a slight eruption on the skin are additional features. The spinal fluid is usually clear; in rare cases is opalescent and reveals an excess of lymphocytes, sometimes extremely high. Lumbar puncture eases the headaches and seems to shorten the duration of the illness. Venesection has been found to be beneficial.

Meningeal symptoms characterized by headache, by neck stiffness, and Kernig's sign may develop during the course of fevers such as pneumonia, typhoid fever, typhus fever, malaria, and other febrile diseases. The manifestations are precisely those of meningitis from which the condition cannot be differentiated clinically. Neck stiffness and Kernig's sign are found. Choked disc may be seen in some instances. Lumbar puncture reveals increased pressure but without evidence of cellular increase in the spinal fluid. Such cases are regarded as instances of *meningismus*, are benign, and recovery takes place with subsidence of the febrile illness with which the meningeal symptoms were associated. The meningeal signs result from an excess of fluid in the subarachnoid space without increase of cells: hence the term serous meningitis, which is often applied to instances of this sort. Lumbar puncture relieves the headache and often cures the condition.

In rare cases meningitis may be caused by *lymphogranuloma venereum,* the diagnosis of which on purely clinical grounds is extremely difficult. The diagnosis is made by the Frei test, which is specific for the disease. Weil's disease, with or without jaundice, may also be associated with meningitis. The disease is characterized by chills, fever, headache, muscular pains and weakness, jaundice in most cases, tenderness of the muscles, hemorrhagic manifestations, enlargement of the liver, and skin eruptions. In some instances there may be meningitis with increase of cells in the spinal fluid; in others, only a meningismus. The spinal fluid is clear or yellow and the cells which are polynuclear in type may reach as high as one thousand.

Bacteroides infection of the central nervous system arises most commonly from chronic otitis media. It occurs in both males and females, more commonly in adults than children, and its symptomatology is that of other meningeal infections. Bacteroides infection should be suspected when meningitis or brain abscess develops in the presence of chronic otitis media. In meningitis, the cell count varies from 2000 to 45,000 cells per cc. The diagnosis depends on cultivation of the organisms, and anaerobic cultures should be made repeatedly in cases in which gram-negative bacilli are seen in smears or in which aerobic cultures are sterile (Smith, McCall, and Blake). The course may be acute, with death in four to nine days, or recovery may be prompt or prolonged. Bacteroides meningitis is most extensive over the base of the brain, the exudate being composed chiefly of polymorphonuclear cells.

XI. MENINGEAL HEMORRHAGE

Hemorrhage into the meninges occurs most frequently as the result of causes which are not primarily infectious, but a discussion of this problem appears to be logical at this point. There are three types of meningeal hemorrhage: (1) extradural, or epidural; (2) subdural; and (3) subarachnoid. Under certain conditions there may be a combination of these various forms. At times one meets with all three forms in a single case. Not infrequently subdural and subarachnoid hemorrhage is found in the same case.

1. *Extradural Hemorrhage*

Extradural hemorrhage, as the name implies, is characterized by bleeding which occurs on the dura, between the dura and skull.

Etiology: In almost all instances, extradural hemorrhage is traumatic in origin. It occurs in three per cent of all head injuries. The trauma may be trivial or severe. In most instances, it is a very severe injury caused by the impact of a moving object, developing very frequently after a blow from a stone, a baseball bat, a baseball, etc. Very often, too, the hemorrhage develops after a blow to the head when the latter comes in contact with some stationary object; hence a moving missile is not a *sine qua non* for the development of this form of hemorrhage. The blow is more frequently delivered in the temporal region, but a blow to any

part of the skull may cause extradural bleeding.

Very rarely bleeding on the dura may occur as the result of a mycotic aneurysm or in blood dyscrasias, but these causes are rare.

Pathology: Extradural hemorrhage is almost always arterial in origin due to traumatic rupture of the middle meningeal artery. In rare instances, the bleeding may be of venous origin arising from the lateral sinus or the longitudinal sinus. Venous bleeding extradurally is comparatively rare, however; so that for all practical purposes it is safe to say that extradural hemorrhage is arterial in origin in practically all instances. Extradural hemorrhage in the posterior fossa is of venous origin, the bleeding occurring from one of the dural sinuses.

The cause of the hemorrhage is usually rupture of the middle meningeal artery, except in those cases in which the bleeding is venous in origin. Rupture of the vessel is caused by a shearing or clipping effect on the middle meningeal artery by the fractured skull, the fracture line passing through the middle meningeal groove. The hemorrhage is usually located in the frontotemporal region, covering more of the temporal than frontal area. If it is very extensive it may spread over the entire lateral surface of the hemisphere, but as a rule it does not do so. Not infrequently the hemorrhage may be entirely frontal, due to bleeding from a branch of the middle meningeal artery. Rarely it may lie entirely posteriorly over the occipital lobe. The location of the hemorrhage bears a vague and poorly understood relationship to the site of the trauma, but is not always under the seat of the trauma. Almost always the hemorrhage is unilateral and on the same side as the trauma. Sometimes it is on the side opposite the trauma. Very rarely it is bilateral.

The hemorrhage resulting from extradural bleeding varies in size and extent. It may cover a small portion of a lobe or it may extend over a large part of the lateral surface. More often it tends to confine itself to one area and to grow by thickness rather than by spreading out laterally. Grossly, the hemorrhage is usu-

tients with extradural hemorrhage in which the blow has been so severe as to cause hemorrhage elsewhere. The extent of this subarachnoid hemorrhage varies; sometimes it is thick over both hemispheres and sometimes mild.

Microscopically, one sees a clot firmly adherent to the underlying dura. If a

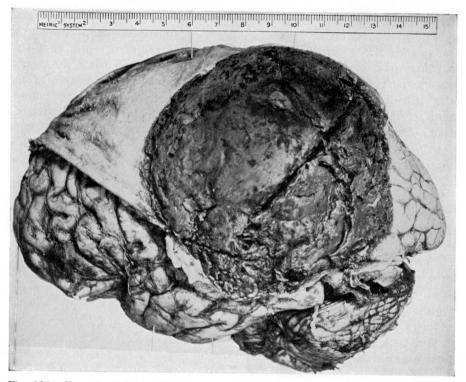

Fig. 110—*Extradural hemorrhage.* An extensive extradural middle meningeal hemorrhage in the fronto-parieto-temporal area. The hemorrhage is clearly seen lying on the dura and is firmly adherent to it.

ally a firm clot at necropsy, lying on the external surface of the dura. It is firmly adherent to the dura. The brain beneath the hemorrhage is indented and depressed, due to pressure from the overlying clot. It may be softened if the pressure from the clot is great enough to interfere with venous drainage into the pial veins. It also contains hemorrhages of varying size within its substance in some instances but not invariably. There may also be blood in the subarachnoid space in pa-

few days have elapsed between the trauma and death, there may be signs of fibrous penetration into the superficial layers of the clot. The vessel spaces under the clot in the dura are greatly dilated and filled with blood.

In almost all cases of extradural hemorrhage, there is a fracture of the skull, which may be linear or depressed, but is usually linear. In rare instances, fracture of the skull is not present. The fracture line is seen in the temporal bone, or in the frontotemporal or parietotemporal areas.

Symptoms: The symptoms of extradural hemorrhage are quite dramatic. There is first of all a *history of trauma,* either severe or trivial. After this comes what is known as the *lucid interval,* which may last a few minutes to a few hours. This lucid interval is extremely characteristic of extradural hemorrhage and has the following features: After the trauma, the patient gets up and goes about his work apparently free from symptoms for a varying length of time, lasting from a few minutes or half an hour to several days. As a rule, it is minutes to a few hours in length. It is probable that the patient is not entirely clear during this period, but compared with what follows he is certainly lucid and clear. The reason for the lucid interval is not well known. It is probable that this represents the time from the onset of the hemorrhage to such a time when the hemorrhage has reached a sufficiently large size to compress the brain and to interfere with consciousness.

Following the lucid interval, the patient lapses into *unconsciousness.* At first his loss of consciousness is not very deep, but as time goes on it becomes more and more profound, the patient finally lapsing into a very deep stupor. This increasing loss of consciousness is very characteristic of extradural hemorrhage and is one of its most outstanding symptoms. The story of trauma, lucid interval, and ever-deepening stupor when obtainable is striking.

Unfortunately the history of a lucid interval is often not obtained and in large series of cases has been found to be absent in fifty per cent of cases (Munro and Maltby). In such instances, the injury is followed immediately by loss of consciousness from which the patient never recovers. Careful observation, however, will reveal in such instances a deepening stupor, the patient becoming more profoundly unconscious with the lapse of time. Absence of the lucid interval is due to associated brain injury or to some complicating factor such as alcoholism.

There may be focal cerebral signs, but as a rule these are difficult to obtain because of the fact that one deals often with a stuporous patient. Hemiparesis or hemiplegia is present in about fifty per cent of cases. In some instances, the hemiplegia is on the same side as the clot. These may be evident before the development of stupor. Jacksonian convulsions are sometimes found, but are usually absent. A unilateral fixed pupil is regarded by some as being of distinct diagnostic value, but it is often absent. When present it is apt to be on the same side as the clot. The patient is in shock and stupor and cannot be aroused. The breathing is stertorous and deep. The weakened limbs are usually flaccid, but hypertonus may be present. Sometimes there is more evidence of involvement of one side than the other. The spinal fluid pressure is high in about two-thirds of the cases. Roentgenologic study of the skull reveals a fracture in all cases, with rare exceptions. The demonstration of a fracture line is therefore important in diagnosis.

In patients with extradural hemorrhage, there is an evermounting temperature, a fall of the pulse, with a rise in blood pressure. The temperature mounts rapidly and continues to rise until it reaches 106° or 107° F. (41.1° or 41.7° C.). The pulse also falls very rapidly and the blood pressure rises. These signs are more likely to appear late in the course of the bleeding. The temperature, pulse, and blood pressure charts are of great help in the diagnosis of extradural hemorrhage. In cases of extradural hemorrhage in the posterior fossa, there is a history of injury to the back of the head, headache, increasing stupor, hyporeflexia, hypotonia, and neck stiffness. Fracture of the skull is always present. The development of extradural hematoma in infants and children is not as commonly recognized as in adults. Though the over-all clinical picture resembles that of adults there are important differences. A history of head injury is always present. Of great importance in the diagnosis is the progression of drowsiness to stupor or coma, associated with evidence of medullary compression or localizing signs. Hemiparesis is common, as is dilatation of the pupil on the side of the lesion. Profound anemia may follow the extravasation of blood; hence anemia and shock following head injury in an infant may point to intracranial bleeding. Fracture of the skull can usually, but not always, be demonstrated.

Diagnosis: The diagnosis of extradural hemorrhage is at once one of the most baffling and simple in neurological practice. A careful history is of the utmost importance, but it is often very difficult to obtain. One is confronted in a typical case with a patient in profound stupor, breathing stertorously, with rising temperature, and with a history of trauma, lucid interval, and constantly deepening stupor. Under such circumstances the diagnosis is not difficult.

In the absence of a lucid interval or in the presence of a lucid interval which has lasted only a few minutes and has therefore passed unnoticed, the diagnosis is profoundly difficult. The problem in such instances concerns a patient who has suffered a blow to the head, has never recovered consciousness, and who appears to be in profound shock. Careful study reveals the fact that the stupor has become more profound than on admission to the hospital; that the limbs which could move on painful stimulation, develop evidences of weakness of one side; that the temperature may be rising and the pulse falling; and that the spinal fluid pressure may be high. This picture will show no change except for increasing stupor, rising temperature and blood pressure, and falling pulse. In such cases it may be impossible to differentiate the condition from a very severe cerebral concussion or from subdural bleeding. Confirmation of the possibility of extradural hemorrhage is obtained by the demonstration of a fracture line, but it does not establish the diagnosis. It is helpful only in clinching one's impression of extradural hemorrhage. This condition, incidentally, is one in which it is justifiable to move a patient with an acute head injury for roentgenograms of the skull, since the latter are so helpful in diagnosis. The only definite way to establish the diagnosis is by the making of bilateral trephine openings over the temporal or frontal areas in the hope of disclosing a hemorrhage. Such a procedure is justified whenever there is a grave suspicion that an extradural hemorrhage may exist. Extradural hemorrhage is an acute condition and one in which temporizing is fatal. Consequently, if there is a healthy suspicion of its existence in a stuporous patient with head trauma, where there is a rising temperature, signs of profound shock, and a linear fracture of the skull, trephining to establish the diagnosis and hence to effect a cure is justified. While the symptoms of extradural hemorrhage fulminate in the course of twenty-four to seventy-two hours as a rule, cases lasting a week or longer are sometimes observed.

Treatment: There is only one treatment for extradural hemorrhage: *ligation of the bleeding middle meningeal* *artery.* This is usually not difficult to find, but when the tear is low down and the bleeding from the artery in its passage through the foramen spinosum, the problem is much more difficult. If the vessel is tied off quickly, the outlook is good. If delay in operation has been too long, the outcome is not so hopeful and death is frequently seen. In patients who recover, the emergence after operation from a profound stupor to relative clarity is a most dramatic experience and one not easily forgotten.

2. Subdural Hemorrhage

Etiology: Chief among the causes is trauma. This is without doubt the most important cause of the condition. The incidence of subdural hematoma in patients with head injury varies from 1 per cent (Browder) to 10 per cent (Munro), the lower incidence probably being more accurate. The trauma is usually a direct injury to the head, but in rare instances an indirect injury such as a prat fall may be the cause of the subdural bleeding. Trauma acts by the tearing of a vein or veins traversing the subdural space, with subsequent bleeding. The trauma may be very slight and hardly noticeable in the chronic cases, or it may be very severe in the acute cases. Most often, however, in the chronic cases the violence is great (Putnam). A history of trauma is not always available and spontaneous non-traumatic subdural hemorrhage has been found in acute and chronic forms (Scott), the acute forms simulating a cerebrovascular accident. The cause of such cases is not clear.

Among other causes of subdural hemorrhage may be mentioned blood diseases such as pernicious anemia, leukemia, and purpura hemorrhagica. The incidence in pernicious anemia has been emphasized by Huguenin. Scurvy is sometimes a cause of subdural hemorrhage. Subdural hemorrhage has been found in the region of a metastatic tumor involving the pia-arachnoid, in the vicinity of cerebral abscess, in cerebral aneurysm, and in arteriovenous aneurysm on the surface of the brain (Landig, *et al.*). It occurs also in infectious diseases such as measles, scarlet fever, variola, typhus fever, pertussis, anthrax, and syphilis. Of these, pertussis has been emphasized as a cause of the conditions because of the association of severe straining and increased intracranial pressure. The same has been felt to be true of tuberculosis. Subdural hemorrhage is seen in syphilis. It may be large in these cases but is more often slight in degree. The association of chronic alcoholism with subdural hemorrhage has been emphasized by a number of authors. There is no question that subdural hemorrhage is frequently found in chronic alcoholics, either with or without a history of trauma, but the incidence of alcoholism is by no means universal, and alcoholism, like syphilis, must be regarded as a frequent concomitant of subdural hemorhage but by no means the most important cause.

The incidence of subdural hemorrhage in children has been found to be great, according to recent studies. The cause in almost all these cases is birth trauma. It has also been found in other conditions in children, as, for example, in rickets, scurvy, measles, scarlet fever, syphilis, tuberculosis, diphtheria, pertussis, hemorrhagic diatheses, pernicious anemia, tuberculosis, otitis media, and sepsis.

Spontaneous fractures of the long bones have been found in children with subdural hematoma in the posterior fossa. Occurrence of such fractures, without adequate cause, must always lead to a search for subdural hematoma.

Pathology: The lesions are bilateral in from one-third to one-half of all the cases due to trauma. On the other hand, in forty-two cases of acute subdural hematoma, thirty-eight were unilateral. The size may vary from that of a microscopic ecchymosis to a large collection of blood or fluid covering almost an entire cerebral hemisphere. Small hemorrhages are more common than large ones occurring from veins traversing the subdural space, or from laceration and contusion of the brain with associated tear of the overlying membranes. In rare instances, it has been found to be arterial in origin from underlying cerebral hemorrhage.

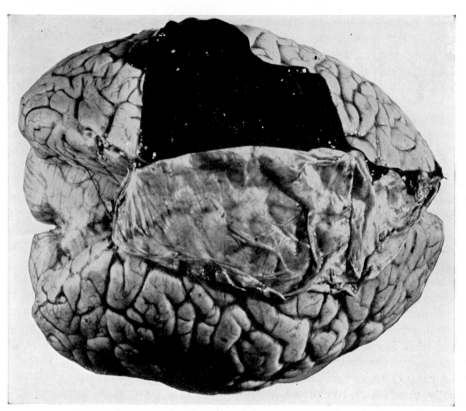

Fig. 111—*Acute subdural hemorrhage,* shown with the dura reflected back and the fresh hemorrhage covering the left fronto-parietal region.

rhages are more common than large ones and Putnam points out that the hemorrhage reaches a thickness of possible clinical significance in only a small percentage of cases. Most of the hemorrhages are located in the frontoparietal region, but extend to the temporal and occipital areas when they are unusually large. They are less frequently more marked in either the temporal or occipital areas.

The hemorrhage in subdural hematoma is venous in origin, the bleeding

In acute hemorrhage there is a collection of blood beneath the dura adherent to its undersurface. Associated with the acute hemorrhage are often subarachnoid hemorrhages and even extradural hemorrhage. In chronic subdural hematomas, there is a collection of fluid in a cyst which has formed after the subdural hemorrhage. This cyst is encapsulated. It has a thin, translucent, or, at times, transparent membrane called the neomembrane which encloses the clot. The dura in such cases is definitely altered, but not to a very serious degree. On the undersurface of the dura one usually sees dilated vascular spaces, sometimes very numerous, most of which are filled with blood. Among these spaces are numerous, large, round cells containing hemosiderin, depending on the duration of the process. Hemosiderin may be found free in the tissue. On the undersurface, also, there is frequently an increased number of fibroblasts, but this is not always present. There is as a rule no increase in thickness of the dura in these patients. Occasionally the vessels in the dura are atheromatous.

The dura and neomembrane in the nontraumatic cases show changes similar to those in the traumatic group. In the former, however, the hemorrhage may be very small and may consist of only a thin layer of blood on the undersurface of the dura with reactive changes on its undersurface. Solid clots are found in a considerable number of cases, especially in those associated with birth injury, or in nontraumatic cases due to scurvy, purpura, etc. (Munro).

The brain in cases of subdural hemorrhage shows a variety of pictures. In the acute cases due to trauma there are frequently punctate and confluent hemorrhages scattered throughout the brain. There may also be lacerations of the cortex. Subarachnoid hemorrhage is usually present. In the chronic cases where there has been cyst formation, the brain is compressed on the side of the lesion and there is an area of excavation due to pressure from the cyst, varying in size according to the size of the cyst. In such patients the underlying cortex may show secondary changes in the ganglion cells.

Pathogenesis: There are several problems in the pathogenesis of subdural hemorrhage which are important. Among these are: (1) the source of the hemorrhage; (2) the source of membrane, and (3) the mode of formation of cyst. These problems will be considered serially.

Source of Hemorrhage: The hemorrhage is the result of tearing of a cortical vein which runs through the subdural space in the pia. This rupture occurs from trauma to the head.

Source of Membrane: This has been a source of mystery for a long time, but recent studies have thrown much light on the source of the neomembrane which encloses the subdural clot and later the cyst. During the second week after the hemorrhage there are usually manifested the first efforts at granulation and encapsulation. There is formed a thin layer of fibroblasts along the dura in contact with the blood and prolongations of these are sent out into the clot. From these is formed a layer on the outside of the clot, composed of fibroblasts, eventually enclosing the clot after a number of weeks (O'Leary).

This is still a moot point. Some believe that the origin of the membrane is due to an inflammatory process on the inner side of the dura; hence the term "pachymeningitis hemorrhagica interna," which is used to describe this condition (Virchow). According to Virchow, the dura first becomes inflamed and a thin film of fibrin forms over it. Capillaries grow into this and more fibrin is deposited. The vessels may rupture and give rise to ecchymoses or to massive hemorrhage. Others maintain that the membrane develops by means of a hyperplastic process involving the fibroblasts in the subendothelial layer of the dura (Wohlwill). Another concept is that of Ford Robertson, who found in early cases minute granulations growing from the undersurface of the dura, and also proliferation and degeneration of the endothelial lining of the perivascular channels. At the same time the capillaries proliferated. Small hemorrhages form and are organized from the undersurface of the dura. Robertson therefore believes that the granulations come first and the hemorrhage after this.

Source of Cyst: The origin of the fluid in the cyst is not clear. First of all, the contents of the cyst vary widely and seem to have relatively little relation to the time factor. The cyst contents may be a reddish brown gelatinous clot or a colorless fluid. When seen fresh at operation, the color is often a mixture of red and green. The condition of the clot has little relation to the length of the interval between trauma and onset of symptoms, operation or necropsy (Putnam). Partly solid clots have been found after forty-five days or longer. In no instance has complete organization of a clot been reported. It has been suggested that the membrane enclosing the blood acts as a semipermeable membrane and that, by a process of osmosis, fluid is absorbed into the cyst until finally the entire contents are cystic (Gardner).

Symptoms: Subdural hemorrhage occurs more frequently in males. It may occur at any age from infancy to senescence. The chronic subdural hematoma occurs most frequently in middle age. The symptoms vary in the acute and chronic forms. In the *acute* form there is usually profound loss of consciousness. There is usually severe injury of the brain in association with acute subdural hemorrhage. In a group of 194 acute mixed subdural hematomas, there was an associated major brain injury in 184 cases; fracture of the skull in fifty-five; extradural hemorrhage in eleven; subcortical hemorrhage in seven, and ventricular hemorrhage in one case (Munro). Detection of acute forms is difficult but is possible in sixty-two per cent of cases (Munro). This is probably too generous an estimate. Unfortunately the majority of patients suffer severe head injury, are in surgical shock, and manifest profound loss of consciousness during the early stages of the disorders when correct diagnosis is vital. The problem of diagnosis in such patients is therefore that of a patient with prolonged and persistent loss of consciousness, probably associated with slight temperature elevation, and with increased spinal fluid pressure. The spinal fluid contains blood. Munro refers to hematomas of this type as acute mixed subdural hematomas because of the presence of spinal fluid and blood in the subdural space due to a tear in the arachnoid. "Since these patients have, as a rule, severe brain injuries in addition to their hematomas, since many of them are in surgical shock for a varying period after the receipt of the injury, and since these hematomas are expanding lesions, there is an associated compression of the brain that is beyond that which may be produced by uncomplicated cerebral injury" (Munro). There may be very few signs, but a dilated pupil on one side and a hemiparesis or hemiplegia are important signs when present. The *chronic* form is better defined. This is practically always due to trauma, which may at times be so slight as to pass unnoticed. It may be a single severe trauma or repeated insignificant injuries such as the constant bumping of the head against a stationary object in the performance of work. On the other hand, it may be a single slight blow such as a slap on the face, a blow on the chin, or a minor football injury. Unconsciousness follows the trauma in the majority of cases, but in some cases no history of unconsciousness can be obtained. Following the trauma there develops a lucid interval as observed in extradural hemorrhage. The period following the head injury may be followed by an interval in which no symptoms are present or by one in which there may be dull headache associated with mild vertigo. This is again followed by more severe headache. The free interval may vary from one day to several weeks, or even to several years. Instances are recorded in which the symptoms did not occur until two to five years after the trauma.

Subjective symptoms of a minor degree may be noted for some time before they become serious enough to require attention. These consist of attacks of dizziness, headache, and sometimes of vomiting. They may persist for a long period before more severe symptoms develop. The recurrence of headache is probably the most striking feature of subdural hematoma. This develops some time after the trauma, weeks, months, or longer. It is not invariably present. The free or lucid interval may be followed by drowsiness, lack of concentration, abnormalities in the state of consciousness or even convulsions.

The development of symptoms in cases of subdural hemorrhage is slow, progressive and irregular, and variability in signs constitutes one of the outstanding features of the disease. Symptoms and signs may be present one day, only to disappear sometimes for long periods. Trotter has explained this variability in symptoms by the fact that after the hemorrhage reaches a size sufficient to produce symptoms, a physiologic diminution in the size of the brain may dispel them again, only to have them reappear later. The diagnosis of subdural hemorrhage, therefore, requires observation in many instances and is not made by a single examination.

Signs of increased pressure are found in many cases, but they may be entirely absent. In addition to subjective signs, such as headache and vomiting, choked disc is frequently but not always found. Among the signs sometimes of value is that of a dilated pupil on the side of the hemorrhage. This has been observed in many cases, but is not always present, and when observed cannot always be relied upon as a localizing sign. A variety of cranial nerve signs has been recorded, including strabismus, nystagmus, myosis, deafness, and loss of convergence.

Hemiparesis or hemiplegia is sometimes found but is not common. Sometimes the hemiplegia is homolateral to the clot. Generalized convulsions occur infrequently. Jacksonian convulsions are encountered in some cases, but are surprisingly uncommon in view of the cortical pressure exacted by the subdural hemorrhage. Mental signs are quite frequently seen and may be the only indication of disturbance in addition to vague signs of increased pressure. They vary widely, from confusional episodes separated by periods of clarity to severe signs of mental deterioration and personality changes. These mental signs may be present for a long period.

Among 245 cases of subdural hematoma the following incidence of signs was encountered: headache, sixty-five per cent; vomiting, forty per cent; choked disc, forty per cent; coma, thirty-five per cent; slowed pulse, seventeen per cent; bilateral plantar extensor response, fourteen per cent; impaired respiration, eleven per cent; stupor, nine per cent; relative intracranial hypertension, 8.3 per cent; diplopia, 6.2 per cent; absence of abdominal reflexes, 6.2 per cent (Klemme & Stuck). In another series (Bergman, Nathanson & Friedman), seventy-six per cent were admitted to the hospital because of changes in behavior or disturbances in the state of consciousness. Seizures occurred in thirty per cent and choked disc in twenty-one per cent.

The temperature is usually normal but may be subnormal. The pulse is frequently slow and may be valuable as a diagnostic sign. The spinal fluid pressure is usually elevated, the degree of elevation varying with the amount of increased pressure. Not infrequently the spinal fluid is xanthochromic. In acute subdural hemorrhage it may be bloody from rupture of the hemorrhage into the subarachnoid space.

Diagnosis: The diagnosis of subdural hemorrhage is often extremely difficult and is frequently missed. The spontaneous variety may be impossible to diagnose when it is acute. The diagnosis of an acute subdural hematoma is an extremely difficult problem, since the clinical picture is that of a patient who has suffered severe head injury, is unconscious, has blood in the spinal fluid in most instances, and has a spinal fluid pressure which may be high or normal. There are no features in the total picture which differ from those of severe brain laceration and contusion, and herein lies the difficulty in making a diagnosis. The problem resolves itself, therefore, into a decision as to whether a patient such as the one described, with persistent loss of consciousness, harbors a subdural hemorrhage. There are no clinical features which permit sound conclusions. If a hemiparesis or hemiplegia develops during the period of observation, or if a unilateral fixed and dilated pupil persists, there may be supporting evidence for the conclusion that a subdural hemorrhage is present. Both these signs, however, may be associated with laceration and cerebral hemorrhage and are not specific. In the last analysis, the diagnosis of acute subdural hemorrhage can be made only by trephining or by air injection. Since these patients are in shock, trephining is on the whole a simpler procedure. The decision as to whether trephining is necessary cannot be reduced to a formula. It is only possible to state that in patients with severe head injury

with persistent loss of consciousness, with evidence of increasing stupor, or with signs of focal brain damage, trephining of the skull is justified in order to determine whether a subdural hemorrhage is present.

In the chronic type, the history of trauma, a careful history with a lucid period, followed by headache, impairment of mental function, possibly with unilateral weakness, and with signs of increased pressure help to establish the diagnosis. Abnormalities in the state of consciousness occurring in combination with a history of head injury constitute the most valuable and probably the most consistent evidence of subdural hematoma. All other signs are variable. The general course is that of a posttraumatic patient who develops progressive symptoms after a varying period of time which may be weeks, months, or years after the trauma. The difficulties are multiplied when one considers that chronic cases may run a completely asymptomatic course without signs of increased pressure. Such cases may exist for years without evidence of difficulty. It has been frequently said that subdural hematoma is often diagnosed when it does not exist, and that it often exists when it is not diagnosed. This still remains true. It is probably better, however, to err in the first direction than in the second.

In patients suspected of having a subdural hematoma, the diagnosis, in asymptomatic patients, may be established by means of an encephalogram. This will show in all instances a shift of the ventricular system to the side opposite the hematoma, and a compression of the ipsolateral ventricle. More recently, it has been pointed out that there may be in some patients a subdural collection of air under the hematoma. Arteriography is also a helpful diagnostic aid.

In acute cases, where encephalography is not feasible because of the patient's stupor, trephining is justified in order to determine whether subdural hemorrhage is present.

Subdural hematomas may become calcified or ossified in rare instances. The reported cases appear to be equally divided among those in which hemorrhage occurred in infancy and those in which it occurred in adult life. In children, thickening of the skull is usually found on the side of the hematoma, but this is not seen in adult cases. The reason for the deposit of calcium in some subdural hematomas is not known, but it does not seem to be related to the duration of the lesion or to its contents. The clinical symptoms differ in no way from those of subdural hematoma without calcification, except that there may be a greater susceptibility to convulsive seizures. Roentgenologically, the outstanding feature is a large mass of calcification or ossification in the roentgenograms of the skull.

Relapsing juvenile subdural hematoma has been described as an entity separate from the chronic subdural hematoma of adults (Davidoff and Dyke). The assumption is that the hematoma in cases of this nature develops as the result of an early trauma at birth or in infancy, that the effects of this trauma pass unnoticed or are disregarded, and that the occurrence of another trauma causes further bleeding into the already established hematoma and accounts for the development of recent symptoms. In some instances, there may be evidences of changes following the original injury, as seen in enlargement of the skull, mental retardation, headache, and vomiting. It occurs in young subjects with a history of an early trauma occurring years before admission to the hospital, with a super-imposed recent trauma of a few to several months' duration. Intracranial pressure is moderately increased and there are minimal localizing signs. Roentgenograms of the skull reveal, on the side of the hematoma, elevation of the sphenoid ridge, superior orbital plate and superior orbital ridge; deepening, widening, and lengthening of the middle fossa; atrophy of the inferior and lateral wall of the superior orbital fissure; hypertrophy of the frontal and ethmoid sinuses, and thickening of the skull. Pneumograms reveal slight to moderate displacement of the ventricular system.

A special form of subdural hematoma has been found following high explosive blast injuries resulting from bomb and shell blast, from torpedoes exploding in compartments, and from concussion blasts of depth bombs which are transmitted through the water. Death follows immediately in many of the subjects; others are unconscious and show evidence of injury to the abdominal and thoracic viscera. The clinical picture in the surviving patients is not clean-cut. Vague neurotic complaints, headache, and memory disturbance are common, with few signs of brain damage. Many of the cases are regarded as neurotic. Pneumogram in suspected cases reveals the nature of the lesion.

Since the over-all picture of a chronic subdural hematoma is that of an expanding lesion, one of the chief conditions from which it must be differentiated is *brain tumor*. The differentiation may be impossible, since both conditions give rise to signs of increased intracranial pressure. The point of distinction is the history of head injury. This is not always reliable, however, since the onset of symptoms in some cases of brain tumor may be related to a history of trauma which is followed by a free interval, simulating closely the history of a subdural hematoma. A similar story may at times be encountered in *brain abscess,* though this is unusual. The problem here, too, is that of an expanding lesion, but the history of a previous ear or sinus infection will help make the proper diagnosis.

Among the rare conditions simulating subdural hematoma, that of *subdural hydroma* is of practical importance. Subdural hydroma is an accumulation of fluid between the dura and arachnoid. It has been variously reported as posttraumatic subdural cyst, circumscribed hydrocephalus, meningitis serosa traumatica, and traumatic arachnoiditis. The condition follows injury to the head and is probably due to a tear in the arachnoid, which permits escape of cerebrospinal fluid into the overlying subdural space. Accumulation of fluid takes place with little or no absorption. Locking of the fluid has been ascribed to the attendant brain edema, which forces the brain into the arachnoid opening and blocks the return of the fluid into the subarachnoid space. The locked fluid acts by pressure on the brain, thus producing neurological symptoms.

It is believed by some (Munro and Merritt) that subdural hydroma represents only a phase of subdural hematoma, the hydroma representing a fluid form of subdural hematoma in which the original blood clots had completely dissolved. The fluid in the subdural space may remain free, or it may become encapsulated with a thin membrane. The protein content of the fluid may be very high, and fluid in subdural hydromas has been known to coagulate. The condition is usually unilateral and invariably extends upward over the hemisphere from the Sylvian fissure. The amount of fluid varies from a few ounces, which is usual, to 500 cc., which is rare. The fluid is usually under tension and may be clear, yellowish, or tinged with blood. The protein is usually increased. The symptoms are similar to those of subdural hematoma. The outstanding symptom is headache, which is severe and persistent. The mental state found in subdural hematoma is usually found; and focal signs, such as hemiparesis, hemiplegia, aphasia, and focal convulsions, may be present. The differentiation from subdural hematoma is impossible except at operation.

Treatment: The treatment of subdural hematoma is entirely *operative.* The type of operation depends on the desires of the neurosurgeon. Two methods are at present in wide use: (1) the reflection of an osteoplastic flap with complete removal of the subdural hematoma and its contents; (2) the drilling of two or more trephine openings, splitting the dura and washing the contents of the clot through, leaving the membrane *in situ.* Thus far no recurrences or other ill effects have been recorded following this procedure.

The outcome after operation on a subdural hematoma is not as good as might be expected, possibly because operation is too long delayed in many cases. Despite this, the results are good. Operation offers the only hope for recovery. There is no other method of treatment.

3. Subarachnoid Hemorrhage

The disorder comprises seven per cent of all cerebral vascular disease and approaches in frequency parenchymatous cerebral hemorrhage (Stevenson). Subarachnoid hemorrhage is responsible for two per cent of sudden deaths (Ayer).

Subarachnoid hemorrhage is in reality a syndrome rather than a disease *sui generis.* It is a group of symptoms resulting from bleeding from a meningeal vessel and may be due, therefore, to a wide variety of causes. Two main groups of cases are recognized—a spontaneous group and a secondary group. In the spontaneous variety, the subarachnoid hemorrhage results from a defect in the vessel wall, resulting in bleeding into the subarachnoid space. The term sponta-

mon cause of the bleeding is a miliary *aneurysm* of one of the basilar or cerebral vessels. This is congenital in origin, due to a defect in the media of one of the vessels, resulting in a thinning out of the vessel wall at the point of bifurcation of a vessel. This congenitally weakened vessel gives rise to an

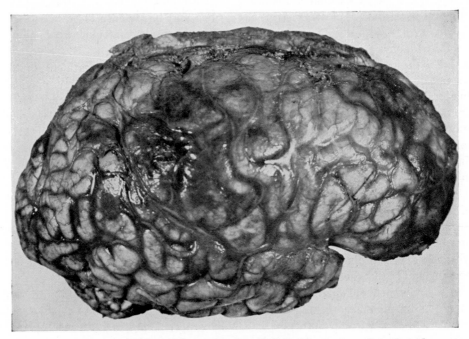

Fig. 112—*Subarachnoid hemorrhage*, showing the bleeding in the subarachnoid space over the cerebral hemisphere.

neous in such instances is used to designate cases in which the bleeding has occurred due to a spontaneous rupture of a cerebral vessel. The secondary variety represents a group of cases in which the bleeding into the subarachnoid space constitutes only an incidental part of a general disease process, as, for example, blood dyscrasias, pertussis, etc. The distinction between the spontaneous and secondary varieties of subarachnoid hemorrhage serves a useful purpose clinically.

Etiology: Subarachnoid hemorrhage results from a large variety of causes. In the spontaneous cases the most com-

aneurysm and ruptures when subjected to the strain of increased pressure. Congenital aneurysms of this type are not found in every patient having spontaneous subarachnoid hemorrhage owing either to a lack of careful search or to obliteration of evidences of the aneurysm in the meningeal bleeding. Their incidence has not been accurately determined. Arteriography has demonstrated that some of the cases previously attributed to miliary aneurysm are in reality due to vascular anomalies of various sorts, such as arteriovenous communications, hemangiomas, and telangiectases.

The many other conditions which may give rise to the condition include (1) trauma, (2) arteriosclerosis, (3) septic or infectious emboli, (4) ruptured intracranial aneurysms, (5) massive cerebral hemorrhage invading the subarachnoid space, (6) intraventricular hemorrhage, (7) blood dyscrasias, (8) ruptured vascular neoplasm (Sand). Trauma is probably one of the most important causes of all. Subarachnoid hemorrhage is also found in syphilis, cerebral hemorrhage, cardiorenal disease, tuberculosis, blood dyscrasias, such as hemophilia and purpura, leukemia, Hodgkin's disease, pernicious anemia, scarlet fever, measles diphtheria, diabetes, epilepsy, pertussis, acute meningitis, brain tumor, and sepsis. It may be the only cerebral manifestation of an embolic process from a subacute bacterial endocarditis. The condition is due, therefore, to a large variety of causes.

Since subarachnoid hemorrhage may occur in a large number of conditions, the age incidence varies greatly. It may occur in young subjects (fifteen to twenty years of age). It is common in men with cardiovascular disease. It is most common between twenty and forty years of age. It is more common in men than women. The specific cause of the onset of the subarachnoid hemorrhage is not always possible to define, but in some instances is found to be physical exertion, emotional excitement, and sexual excitement during intercourse. In the majority of cases, however, physical exertion cannot be implicated as a cause of the onset. In a series of 150 of these patients, there was no history of exertion in ninety per cent (Magee).

Pathology: The pathology of subarachnoid hemorrhage is very simple. There is bleeding of varying degree in the subarachnoid space. It may be chiefly over the cerebral hemispheres or chiefly at the base of the brain. Or it may be found both over the vertex and the base of the brain. The brain shows a film of hemorrhage varying from a few to several millimeters in thickness. It may cover the entire brain or be found chiefly in focal brain areas. Sometimes there may be evidence of repeated hemorrhages in the subarachnoid space; in such patients

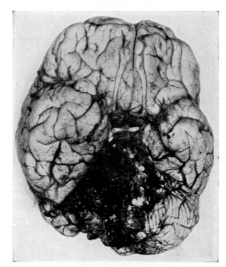

Fig. 113—*Subarachnoid hemorrhage; an extensive subarachnoid hemorrhage covering the entire brain stem, due presumably to a miliary aneurysm.*

a clot of two, three, or more layers may be found, usually over the base of the brain. In cases due to trauma, there is frequently also laceration of the brain. In other cases there may or may not be damage to the brain itself. As a rule, there are punctate hemorrhages in one or more areas; in some cases, they may be generally spread throughout the brain. In still others, there may be massive cerebral hemorrhage, ventricular hemorrhage, or subdural bleeding.

The fate of hemorrhage into the subarachnoid space is of great practical interest. Histological studies reveal that in most instances the blood disappears from the subarachnoid space spontaneously. In some instances, particularly if the bleeding is extensive, organization may take place and adhesions form between the thickened pia-arachnoid and the brain substance (Forster and Alpers).

Pathogenesis: The pathogenesis of subarachnoid hemorrhage contains some points which are not generally agreed upon. It is generally believed that suba-

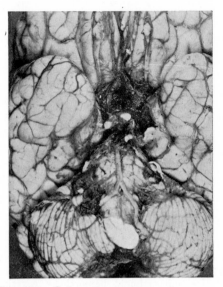

Fig. 114—*Subarachnoid hemorrhage*, over the base of the brain, involving particularly the chiasmal and interpeduncular areas.

rachnoid hemorrhage in many cases results from the development of a minute cerebral aneurysm resulting from a muscular defect in the media located at the point of bifurcation of the vessel and that this defect dates from intrauterine life. Degeneration of the internal elastic membrane is presumed to occur in the final production of the aneurysmal sac. Opposed to this view is the contention that defects in the muscular coat are common at the points of bifurcation of vessels but that aneurysms form at these sites only in the cerebral vessels. A study of a group of aneurysms reveals that the medial defect is constant and the elastica inconstantly deficient (Forster and Alpers). Aneu-

rysms are not always found at the bifurcation of vessels and in some instances the internal elastic membrane is found intact in aneurysmal sacs. Many spontaneous subarachnoid hemorrhages, especially those associated with focal lesions, are the result of vascular malformations rather than aneurysms (Wechsler).

Symptoms: The onset of *spontaneous subarachnoid hemorrhage* is dramatic. In most cases the onset is with intense headache which is followed quickly by loss of consciousness. At times vomiting accompanies the headache. The onset is apoplectic, often without prodromal symptoms, but the latter may be present over a varying period of time. These consist of tinnitus, giddiness, and sometimes mild fleeting headaches. A history of prodromal symptoms is usually lacking, however. Fifteen percent of patients have had previous attacks of hemorrhage within three months (Hyland). A history of migraine is found in a respectable number of sufferers from subarachnoid hemorrhage (15 per cent, Wolff), and periodic headache occurs even more frequently (26 per cent). It is not possible to predict which of the patients with recurrent headache will eventually develop subarachnoid hemorrhage.

Usually the immediate result after the onset with headache is some impairment of consciousness. This may be very profound, from which the patient cannot be roused; or it may be less profound and result only in an impairment of consciousness from which the patient is readily aroused. Headache persists and may be so severe as to be felt through the impairment of consciousness. The headaches are usually frontal and occipital, and the pain often radiates into the back of the neck. The headache of subarachnoid hemorrhage develops with apoplectic abruptness, is severe and memorable.

It is the most frequent and most striking symptom.

Mental symptoms are not uncommon early in the disease. They may appear almost simultaneously with the onset of symptoms and persist long after all other evidences of the disease have gone. Cases with mental symptoms persisting for weeks or months after subarachnoid hemorrhage are not uncommon. The usual mental picture consists of a confusional psychosis with clouding of the sensorium and marked delirium. Restraints are often necessary so severe is the confusion.

Hemiparesis may accompany the subarachnoid hemorrhage. This is not a very frequent complication, but sometimes may be an outstanding feature of the disease.

Outstanding among the signs of the disease are signs of meningeal irritation. In practically all cases, there is neck stiffness, a Brudzinski, and Kernig sign. These may be the only signs present and in most cases this is true. Patients have been observed, however, in whom there was known bleeding in the subarachnoid space without signs of meningeal irritation. Kernig's sign is not always present and only neck stiffness may be found. These meningeal signs persist for several days, but usually disappear before complete recovery has taken place.

In isolated cases there may be evidences of cortical irritation as seen in the rare occurrence of generalized or jacksonian convulsions. Weakness of the face and tongue, or monoplegias of the arm or leg have been observed. It must be emphasized, however, that these are not common and that they are usually absent.

Cranial nerve palsies are common in hemorrhage over the base of the brain. If there is hemorrhage into the sheath of the optic nerve, various degrees of swelling of the nerve may be present from neuritis to marked choked disc. Oculomotor paralyses are not common. but there are in some instances difficulties in convergence or internal rectus paralyses. External rectus palsies are more frequently encountered. Peripheral facial paralysis from hemorrhage into the sheath of the facial nerve is common, especially in fracture at the base of the skull. Sometimes deafness or hypoacusis, tinnitus, and vertigo are present due to hemorrhage into the sheath of the auditory nerve. The lower cranial nerves are not very often injured. The pupils are usually normal, but myosis and anisocoria have been observed. Hemianopia has been reported occasionally. Loss of visual acuity with optic atrophy may develop after the hemorrhage. Sciatic pain in one or both legs may result from subarachnoid hemorrhage which fills the spinal subarachnoid space and penetrates around the spinal nerve roots.

The blood pressure is normal in the vast majority of cases. In some instances, vascular hypertension is found, especially in the cardiorenal cases.

The spinal fluid findings are of the greatest importance. The pressure is increased in many cases but normal in others. The fluid is bloody. The amount of blood varies greatly, but in general the fluid contains many red cells. Its gross appearance is like blood in most cases; in others, it is spinal fluid with a gross admixture of red cells. The bloody fluid may be differentiated from a bloody fluid due to a technical error by the fact that it is bloody no matter how much fluid is withdrawn and by the fact that the supernatant fluid after centrifuging is xanthochromic. After four or five days to a week the fluid is no longer grossly bloody but becomes xanthochromic. It finally becomes entirely clear.

In about one-third of the cases recurrence of the subarachnoid hemorrhage develops. These may often develop while the patient is still in bed, suffering from the original attack (Magee), within three or four weeks of onset.

Diagnosis: The diagnosis of subarachnoid hemorrhage is, as a rule, very simple. The apoplectic onset with severe headache and signs of meningeal irritation, usually in a young person who has

The differentiation from *cerebral hemorrhage* is made on the basis of age, the presence usually of hypertension and diseased vessels, and the more definite evidence of hemiplegia.

Subdural hematoma is more difficult to differentiate because it may exist with the subarachnoid hemorrhage. Usually the spinal fluid is not bloody in subdural hematoma, but in cases where the bleeding has ruptured into the subarach-

Table 32—Prognosis of Spontaneous Subarachnoid Hemorrhage

Author	No. of Cases	Mortality	Mortality with First Attack	Mortality with Recurrent Attacks	Recurrent Attacks
Strauss, Globus & Ginsberg (1932)..	36	39%			
Ohler & Hurwitz (1932)............	24	50%			
Strauss and Tarachaw (1937).......	105	37%	37%		
Sands (1941)....................	120	34%			
Sahs and Keil (1943).............	64	28%			
Magee (1943)...................	150	56%	35%	21%	33%
Wolf, Goodell & Wolff (1945).......	46	33%	11%	22%	52%
Hamby (1948)...................	130	51.5%	34%	17.5%	35.4%
Hyland (1950)..................	191	52%	39%	13%	
Mount (1951)...................	130	40%			
Dekaban & McEachern (1952)......	87	37%	18.4%	18.6%	20%

no hypertension and no previous history of difficulty, plus the presence of blood in the spinal fluid, establishes the diagnosis definitely. The condition is differentiated from various forms of *meningitis* by the absence of a septic temperature and the differential spinal fluid cell count. In subarachnoid hemorrhage, the fluid contains free red blood cells, thousands to two or three million, while in purulent meningitis leukocytes of various types prevail. Smears and cultures will also help to establish the differentiation.

noid space the differentiation may be impossible immediately and can be made only on prolonged observation. Under these conditions, signs of increased pressure and localizing signs will more often develop in patients with subdural hematoma.

Brain tumor may begin suddenly and can be differentiated by the prodromal history of headache over a long period and by the presence of choked disc.

Since rupture of an arterial aneurysm with subsequent subarachnoid hemorrhage is a common cause of death in *coarctation of the aorta,* this must be considered in the presence of the cardinal features of this condition: hypertension of the upper limbs, lower blood pressure of the legs, collateral arterial anastomoses with rib erosion by x-rays, a systolic murmur over the upper precordium and in the left interscapular region, and cardiac hypertrophy.

Prognosis: In subarachnoid hemorrhage, it varies with the cause. In young people recovery from a single attack is usually the rule, but fatal cases are by no means uncommon. A mortality rate of fifty-eight per cent in the first attack in a series of 150 cases is recorded by Magee. It is responsible for two per cent of sudden deaths. Mortality rates have been reported as follows: thirty-nine per cent (Wolff), forty-one per cent (Sands), and twenty-eight per cent (Sahs). The prognosis tends to be worse in the presence of generalized vascular disease. In the spontaneous variety, a history of proved or presumptive previous attacks makes the prognosis better. This history is usually found in young persons with congenital aneurysms or aneurysms with cerebral arteriosclerosis in young persons (Strauss). Unconsciousness at the onset, advanced age, the existence of preexisting hypertension and papilledema all render the prognosis worse.

A relatively large number of patients (twenty-nine per cent) have been found to die during the first episode of bleeding (Wolf, Goodell, and Wolff). Most patients who die in the first attack die within twenty-four hours. Survival of seven to ten days is usually a good prognostic sign. The survival of the first attack of bleeding is not assurance that no further episodes will develop. Recurrences may develop one to twenty-seven years after the initial hemorrhage, with resulting death from the subsequent bleeding episode. Other patients develop no recurrences.

Treatment: The treatment of subarachnoid hemorrhage varies with the cause. Patients having traumatic subarachnoid bleeding should have daily lumbar punctures until the fluid is clear. Since the spinal fluid pressure is usually high in the first days of the disease, it is best to remove enough fluid only to reduce the pressure by half until the pressure becomes normal. After this the fluid may be drained.

In patients with spontaneous hemorrhage, especially in those having hypertension, it is wiser not to perform daily lumbar tap for fear of inducing more bleeding. Some tap all patients having subarachnoid hemorrhage, but it is wiser not to tap the spontaneous type except for diagnosis. Lumbar puncture may be repeated apart from a diagnostic tap under two circumstances: (1) to relieve intractable headache, when this cannot be controlled by other means, and (2) in stuporous or comatose subjects in order to influence this symptom by decreasing intracranial pressure. Since the blood in the subarachnoid space is absorbed without harmful after effects in the majority of cases, there is no sound reason for daily lumbar punctures (Alpers and Forster).

In the acute stages, the patient must be treated for shock with hot water bottles, hypertonic solutions, and sedatives in case of motor restlessness. The nasal tube is advisable in stuporous patients. In patients with vomiting, intravenous glucose (five per cent) is necessary to maintain fluid balance. Because of the associated brain edema in the acute stages, hypertonic solutions are advisable, especially when headache is intractable and stupor persistent. Magnesium sulfate (twenty-five per cent) by rectal drip is best if the patient is conscious and can retain the solution. In other instances, fifty per cent sucrose, 50 cc. intravenously, is useful once or twice in twenty-four hours.

Based on the high mortality in the first episode of subarachnoid hemorrhage, surgical treatment has been advocated. Angiography must be performed if the patient survives the hemorrhage. Often this must be bilateral in patients without localizing signs. The value of surgery in treatment of aneurysm with subarachnoid hemorrhage has not yet been clearly demonstrated.

8

Encephalitis

I. GENERAL FEATURES

The problem of encephalitis is complex and difficult. Many forms of encephalitis exist, but the specific cause is known for only a few of them. To add to the confusion, new forms are still being discovered; hence it is almost impossible in our present state of knowledge to offer more than a working classification of the encephalitic group of diseases.

The term encephalitis, strictly speaking, implies an inflammation of the brain, with infiltration of the brain tissue by hematogenous elements, usually lymphocytes and plasma cells, sometimes punctate hemorrhages, perivascular infiltration by the same elements, nonspecific degenerative changes in the affected areas, and glial response, in the acute stages microglial and astrocytic, and in the later stages astrocytic with glial scar formation. The term, however, has come to be used for many other diffuse conditions of the brain and brain stem without inflammatory reactions, as in lead encephalitis or encephalopathy and hemorrhagic encephalitis. Whether the inclusion of the latter is justified cannot be determined here, since it would involve an academic discussion of the nature of inflammation.

The following is a tenable working classification of encephalitis in its various forms:

Table 33—The Various Forms of Encephalitis

1. POLIOENCEPHALITIS
   (Polioclastic Encephalitis):

   Encephalitis lethargica
   St. Louis encephalitis
   Japanese B encephalitis
   Louping ill
   Australian X disease
   Rabies
   Herpes zoster
   Herpes simplex

2. DISSEMINATED ENCEPHALOMYELITIS
   (Myeloclastic Encephalitis):

Influenza	Equine encephalomyelitis
Typhus fever	Tick bite encephalitis
Toxoplasmosis	Vaccinia
Typhoid fever	Gonorrhea
	Antirabic inoculations

3. SUBACUTE SPORADIC ENCEPHALITIS:

   Subacute inclusion body encephalitis
   (Dawson)
   Subacute sclerosing leukoencephalitis (van
   Bogoert)
   Nodular panencephalitis (Pette-Döring)

4. ENCEPHALITIS OF TOXINS AND METALS:

Lead	Manganese
Arsenic	Carbon monoxide
Carbon disulfide	Pneumoconiosis
Botulism	Mushroom poisoning
Alcohol	Ergotism
Mercury	Lathyrism

5. "HEMORRHAGIC" ENCEPHALITIS:

Trauma	Blood dyscrasias
Avitaminosis, chiefly B deficiency	Lead
Arsphenamine poisoning	Phosphorus
Acute hemorrhagic necrotizing encephalitis	

397

**Table 33—The Various Forms
of Encephalitis—Continued**

6. EMBOLIC OR METASTATIC ENCEPHALITIS:

Heart disease:
Subacute bacterial endocarditis
Mitral stenosis
Vegetative endocarditis
Pulmonary disease:
Lung abscess
Bronchiectasis
Septicemia
Thrombophlebitis
Osteomyelitis

7. POSTINFECTIOUS ENCEPHALITIS:

Measles   German measles
Chickenpox   Scarlet fever
Smallpox
Pertussis
Mumps

In only a few of the many forms of encephalitis described has the specific cause been established. A number of forms of encephalitis are arthropod-borne, and are transmitted either by mosquitoes or ticks. Among these are Japanese B encephalitis, St. Louis encephalitis, Western equine encephalomyelitis, Eastern equine encephalomyelitis, Venezuelan equine encephalomyelitis, Russian tick-borne encephalitis, and probably West Nile encephalitis. These are included in Table 34.

Diagnosis: The *diagnosis* of encephalitis in itself offers difficulties in many instances. Two steps can be determined in the attainment of a diagnosis; the first is the recognition that an encephalitis exists, and the second is the determination of the cause. Each step offers difficulties, some of which are great, because of the similarity of many of the forms.

Table 34—Encephalitis of Known Virus Etiology

Epidemic Type, Usually Seasonal		*Sporadic Type*	
Name	*Mode of Transmission*	*Name*	*Mode of Transmission*
POLIOMYELITIS..........	Probable contact infection	Mumps Lymphogranuloma venereum	Contact
JAPANESE "B" ST. LOUIS WESTERN EQUINE VENEZUELAN EQUINE RUSSIAN SPRING- SUMMER AUSTRALIAN X EASTERN EQUINE	Arthropod-borne	Rabies...............	Bite
		Virus B...............	Monkey
		Lymphocytic chorio-meningitis	Mice
WEST NILE SEMLIKI FOREST	Probably arthropod-borne	Pseudo choriomeningitis Herpes simplex	Unknown
FOCAL HEMORRHAGIC MENINGO EN- CEPHALITIS	Unknown	Measles Influenza Infectious Mononucleosis	? ?

Encephalitides of Questionable Virus Etiology

Epidemic Type		*Sporadic Type*	
Name	*Mode of Transmission*	*Name*	*Mode of Transmission*
VON ECONOMO TYPE.....	Unknown	Postinfection Postvaccinal	Unknown

The recognition of encephalitis is sometimes easy and at others extremely difficult. In many instances, there is a history of onset with fever, following which are obvious evidences of brain involvement, usually with signs of brain stem disease predominating (ocular palsies, peripheral facial weakness, difficulties in swallowing), but in some forms with disease involving the cerebral hemispheres as the outstanding feature (convulsions, hemiplegia, aphasia). In other instances, as in the cases associated with intoxications, the development is not that of a febrile illness, but is more gradual or may be afebrile, associated with indications of brain damage. In many of the encephalitides of this group there is evidence of an organic mental syndrome, associated with other evidences of brain involvement. This is often true of lead encephalitis, carbon disulfide poisoning, manganese, and alcohol. The onset in avitaminosis encephalitis and in carbon monoxide is abrupt. Embolic encephalitis develops abruptly with or without fever and with evidences of brain damage as shown by focal signs involving the cerebral hemispheres or brain stem.

It is obvious that the first approach to a diagnosis of encephalitis must be the demonstration that brain damage is present, whether this affects the cerebrum or the brain stem. Following this demonstration, it then becomes necessary to establish the cause of the encephalitis. This is obvious in many instances and obscure in others. In the case of the exanthems (chickenpox, smallpox, measles, scarlet fever, German measles), the occurrence of brain symptoms during the course of the illness indicates clearly the reason for the encephalitis. The same holds true of vaccinia, gonorrhea, influenza, and other infections. Similarly, the occurrence of cerebral symptoms during the course of valvular disease of the heart or of pulmonary infections is sufficient to point to the source of the embolic encephalitis developing during the course of cardiac and pulmonary disease. The source of the cerebral involvement in intoxications is clear in alcoholism and in the case of industrial hazards such as manganese, lead, and carbon disulfide, in which the history of exposure to the chemical in question is obvious. The problem becomes more difficult, however, in those cases in which exposure to an offending chemical is not obvious and may require a good deal of search in order to determine the cause of the cerebral symptoms. The problem of cause in hemorrhagic encephalitis is likewise not difficult to trace.

It is in the group of epidemic encephalitis that the greatest difficulties are encountered in the establishment of precise cause, since many of these forms of encephalitis resemble one another in being epidemic and in giving rise to similar clinical manifestations. In the last analysis, it is only possible clinically to arrive at a diagnosis of encephalitis. The specific type can be determined in most cases only by means of intricate laboratory tests, either neutralization or complement fixation tests. Only by the latter means can it be specifically determined that a case of encephalitis is due to the St. Louis or to some other specific virus. By careful attention to epidemiological data, however, a clue as to the specific cause may be obtained, a history of dog-bite in rabies, contact with horses in equine encephalomyelitis, etc. The clinical symptoms of lethargic encephalitis, St. Louis and Japanese encephalitis are similar in many ways and only laboratory tests can determine the precise cause. The specific virus causing St. Louis encephalitis and Japanese B encephalitis can be detected only by neutralization or complement fixation tests, using a mouse as the test animal. The same is true of louping ill and equine encephalomyelitis. The viruses of the various forms of encephalitis bear a family relationship to one another, the precise nature of which is still unknown. Thus, West Nile encephalitis which is due to a virus, is antigenically related to the viruses of St. Louis and Japanese B encephalitis, yet distinct from both of them. A similar relationship has been found to exist between the Russian tick-borne virus of spring-summer encephalitis and the tick-borne virus of louping ill encephalitis found in sheep in Scotland. Studies reveal more and more that the viruses of the various encephalitides are geographically widespread. Thus an epidemiological survey revealed the presence of West Nile virus and the virus of St. Louis and Japanese B encephalitis over broad expanses in Central Africa.

The diagnosis of encephalitis is too frequently a matter of exclusion, and is reached because no other diagnosis seems to fit the picture. This is a dangerous clinical habit which frequently results in backfiring and the disclosure of some process other than encephalitis, often a brain tumor. With so many etiological possibilities it should be possible in almost all cases to designate the type of encephalitis responsible for the clinical picture. Despite the many causes, however, there will still remain cases of obscure or unknown etiology for which no grouping can be found.

"Exclusive of Russian spring-summer encephalitis, lymphocytic choriomeningitis, mumps meningoencephalitis, Venezuelan equine encephalitis, herpes simplex encephalitis, and lymphogranuloma venereum, the viruses that attack the nervous system are so rarely found in the blood or spinal fluid that to seek them in these materials is not worthwhile for clinical purposes" (Rivers).

The electroencephalogram has been reported to be of diagnostic value in encephalitis. Changes in the electroencephalogram were found in cases of encephalitis (Gibbs & Gibbs). The acute phase is characterized by slow waves of very high voltage, the clinical severity correlating with the EEG changes. Periodic slow waves are frequently encountered in the subacute stages. Subacute cases showed less abnormality, characterized by scattered slow waves. The EEG records tend to return to normal after the acute phase. The EEG cannot make a diagnosis of encephalitis, but in a suspected case it may help support the diagnosis (Radermecker).

II. EPIDEMIC ENCEPHALITIS

Included in this category is a group of cases which contains many features in common both clinically and pathologically, but is characterized by separate and distinct causes in those types on which the cause has been determined. Pathologically, all the diseases listed as epidemic encephalitis involve almost exclusively the gray matter of the brain and to a very large degree the gray matter of the brain stem in particular. In encephalitis lethargica the involvement is especially in the mesencephalon, with particular involvement of the periaqueductal gray matter, the oculomotor nuclei, and the substantia nigra. The diencephalon is also involved, especially the hypothalamus and to a lesser degree the basal ganglia (pallidum, putamen, caudate). The medulla and pons are less affected. In the St. Louis type of encephalitis, the lesions are found chiefly in the gray matter of the mesencephalon, thalamus and pons, but are present as well in the cerebral hemispheres. The same holds true for Japanese B encephalitis.

Etiologically, the various members of the group are related but distinct. The viruses of St. Louis and Japanese B encephalitis are distinct from one another. That of encephalitis lethargica has not been identified. Clinically, the various forms may resemble one another so closely that their causal identification will depend on neutralization tests or other laboratory means of identification.

1. Encephalitis Lethargica
(Epidemic Encephalitis, Sleeping Sickness, Economo's Disease)

Epidemic lethargic encephalitis, as the name implies, tends to occur in epidemics, but is also found sporadically. The disease is characterized by (1) its epidemic tendencies; (2) its polymorphous clinical features; (3) the occurrence of sequelae which are more disabling than the disease. There is good reason to believe that there is more than one disease which is referred to as encephalitis lethargica, and that several forms of the disease may exist.

Etiology: The disease affects all ages with no special predilection for one or the other sex. The precise cause is not known. The present tendency regards a virus as the cause of epidemic encephalitis, but the virus has never been isolated. Efforts to identify it with herpes febrilis virus have not succeeded and the occurrence of herpes virus appears to be coincidental. Similarly, attempts to demonstrate that the cause of the disease is identical with that of influenza have not succeeded; nor has the streptococcus etiology of the disease borne fruit. Bacteria appear not to be related etiologically to epidemic encephalitis. Inclusions have been found in the ganglion cells of some subjects and are thought to represent virus activity.

The disease tends to occur in the colder months, but the method of transmission is not known. Direct contagion is improbable. The incubation period is from nine to twenty-one days.

Pathology: The changes in acute epidemic lethargic encephalitis are predominantly in the brain stem (mesencephalon, pons), basal ganglia and to a lesser degree in the cerebral cortex and cerebellum. The meninges over the brain stem particularly are infiltrated slightly with lymphocytes. Within the brain stem the changes are of two types: degenera-

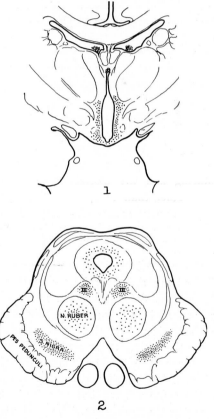

Fig. 115 — *Encephalitis lethargica* (Economo). A diagrammatic sketch illustrating the main site of the pathological process in lethargic encephalitis. Note the particular involvement of the gray matter of the mesencephalon, especially the substantia nigra and the periaqueductal gray matter.

tive and infiltrative, consisting of destruction or disease of ganglion cells and infiltration of the tissue with lymphocytes and plasma cells as well as perivascular infiltration of the vessels in the affected regions. Hemorrhages may be found early in the process. Glial proliferation is found in the affected areas after subsidence of the process (Fig. 115).

nia, etc., or it may recede and leave no immediate residuals, but may be followed years later by sequelae. These are assumed to be the result of old inflammatory foci which have persisted and become reactivated later to produce the many clinical sequelae characteristic of the disorder. For this reason the term chronic encephalitis has been given to

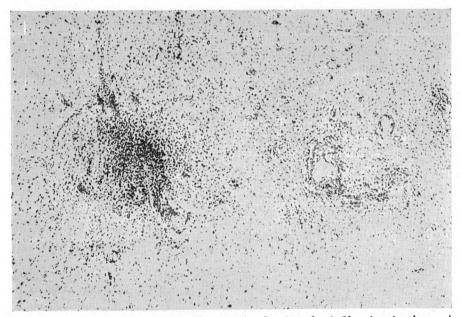

Fig. 116—*Epidemic encephalitis* (Economo), showing the infiltration in the periaqueductal gray matter, involving particularly the region of the oculomotor nuclei, destroying the ganglion cells.

The areas of the brain most commonly affected are the central gray matter of the midbrain (oculomotor and convergence nuclei), the substantia nigra, the subthalamic region, the gray matter between the nucleus ruber, and the reticular substance. The basal ganglia are likewise affected. The cerebral cortex is involved in the acute process, but to a lesser degree than the brain stem. The cerebellum is sometimes affected and in rare instances the spinal cord (Fig. 116).

The acute pathological process recedes and leaves behind immediate residuals, such as oculomotor paralyses, hypersom-

the cases with sequelae. Whether such chronic encephalitic foci exist in every case with sequelae has not been demonstrated beyond question.

Symptoms: The *onset* of the disease varies and differs often from case to case and from epidemic to epidemic.

The symptoms of encephalitis lethargica are so numerous and so varied that a mere recital of them would in itself be formidable. Not all of them are found in a single case and combinations of them vary greatly, depending upon the degree of invasion of the nervous system. Usually the onset is with fever, headache, and vertigo, and often with upper respiratory symptoms (rhinitis, cough). The fever is persistent and variable. The initial symptoms last for several days and lead eventually to full expression of the disease. In other cases, the onset may follow what seems to be a "grippal" infection, with slight fever, exhaustion, and symptoms of a common cold. In

have disappeared. It may be slight, characterized by a tendency to nod at odd moments, or it may be so profound as to produce a stupor from which the patient can be aroused but into which he lapses quickly when left alone. In some cases, *insomnia* is found instead of sleepiness, and in such instances reversal of the sleep rhythm is common, patients sleep-

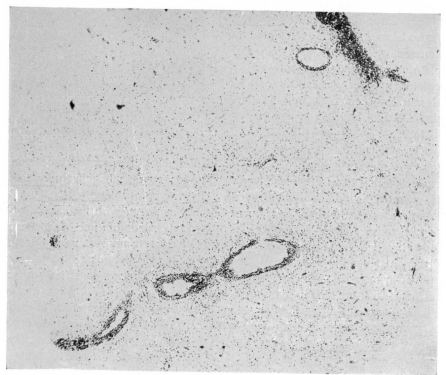

Fig. 117—*Epidemic encephalitis* (Economo), showing the perivascular infiltration with lymphocytes, characteristic of the process.

still other cases, the onset is sudden with high fever and oculomotor paralyses, while in others a psychosis may usher in the disease (Fig. 117).

Lethargy, sleepiness, or *hypersomnia* is a prominent symptom, the term sleeping sickness being derived from this feature of the disease. It is possible that this symptom is related to damage of the anterior reticular formation. It usually appears early and sometimes persists when all other evidences of the disease

ing in the daytime and finding it impossible to sleep at night. *Neck stiffness* and other signs of meningeal irritation may be found very early but are never very striking. *Delirium* and mental states of many other sorts are common.

Ocular paralyses are a common feature of the disease, as one might gather from the predilection of the disorder for the central gray matter of the midbrain. Together with lethargy, they are probably the most constant features of the disease.

Pupillary disturbances of many sorts occur; irregular, contracted, dilated, or fixed pupils are seen and even Argyll Robertson pupils have been described. A paradoxical pupillary reaction is not uncommon (dilatation of the pupil on stimulation by light). *Impairment* or *loss of convergence* is an early sign and persists in practically all cases as the only evidence of the disease after all other signs have disappeared. *Ophthalmoplegias* of various sorts are commonly encountered, with ptosis, diplopia, and complete or incomplete paralyses of the oculomotor muscles. Paralysis of the facial muscles occurs, as well as dysphagia. Vertigo is often a feature of the disease.

Paralyses of various sorts may be encountered in the acute stages of the disease, among which may be included hemiplegia or monoplegia. *Parkinsonism* is seen rarely as an acute manifestation of the disease rather than as a sequel. *Epileptic attacks,* both focal and generalized, have been described but are rare. *Hyperkinesias* of various sorts—chorea, torticollis, tics, athetosis—are seen in some cases. *Myoclonic twitchings* may sometimes be the outstanding feature and may involve all parts of the body. *Hiccough* is a distressing symptom of the disease at times and may persist for long periods. Some forms are characterized only by this symptom. *Mental symptoms* of one form or another may dominate the picture. Delirium is common; manic states, catatonia, depression, and other mental reactions may be found and are usually associated with other features of the disease (Fig. 118).

The *spinal fluid* findings are of no value except in the acute stages and here, too, are of little value unless studied in the very acute phases. The cells are increased in the early stages and number 20 to 100 or more, chiefly lymphocytes.

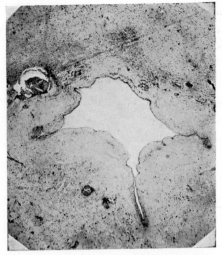

Fig. 118—*Epidemic encephalitis* (Economo). A high power view of the aqueductal region showing the heavy infiltration in this region.

The spinal fluid sugar may be increased but has no diagnostic value. The protein may be increased.

The acute stage of the disease lasts for varying periods of time. It persists for weeks or even months and may result in complete recovery, death, or in sequelae which may develop some time after the disease.

Sequelae: The after effects of epidemic encephalitis are more distressing than the disease itself. They may appear shortly after the disease or some time later, and they may develop in patients with a clear-cut history of encephalitis, in those with a history of "grippe" or "influenza," or without a history of an acute illness of any sort (Fig. 119).

Postencephalitic parkinsonism or paralysis agitans is one of the most distressing of the after effects of encephalitis and undoubtedly its most common sequel. It will be considered in detail in extrapyramidal disorders. *Oculogyric crises* are not uncommon. They are characterized by sudden forceful upward spasm of the eyeballs, lasting for several seconds to several minutes. They may occur infrequently or may develop several times a day. No effort on the part of the patient relieves them; they subside spontaneously. They are usually found associated with parkinsonism. *Palpebral* spasm is a rare sequel and is characterized by a spasm of the palpebral muscles of the eyelids, resulting in their forceful closure, which is relieved spontaneously. *Respiratory disorders* such as tachypnea, bradypnea, tics, etc., are sometimes seen and are usually regarded as hysterical in the absence of a history of encephalitis. The occurrence of other sequelae (parkinsonism, etc.) stamps their origin clearly. *Tics* of various kinds occur, among them diaphragmatic tics, facial tics, etc. *Paralysis or impairment of convergence* of the ocular muscles is an almost constant sequel, and constitutes an important sign of the disease. *Myoclonus* is a rare sequel. *Myasthenic syndromes* giving rise to a picture of myasthenia gravis are occasionally seen. *Amyotrophies* sometimes follow the disease and amyotrophic lateral sclerosis syndromes have been described. *Behavior disorders* are seen, especially in children. They are characterized by reversal of behavior, stealing, vagrancy, truancy, and other forms of behavior problems.

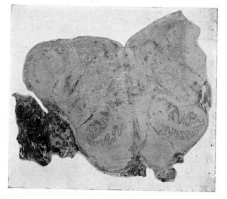

Fig. 119—*Epidemic encephalitis.* **A survey section of the medulla showing the infiltration in the gray matter, indicated by the dark areas around the vessels.**

Diagnosis: The diagnosis of lethargic encephalitis is both easy and difficult. In epidemics, as in the case of poliomyelitis, the diagnosis is easier when the physician is on guard against the disease than in sporadic cases. Sporadic cases occur sometimes with great frequency. The diagnosis of the disease is based chiefly on an onset with fever, malaise, and grippal symptoms, associated with lethargy and oculomotor paralyses. This, however, is merely one means of arriving at the diagnosis, since the manifestations of the disease are so numerous that many combinations of symptoms are possible. In some cases, mental symptoms may predominate; in others, hyperkinetic phenomena (tics, chorea, etc.), and, in others, ocular phenomena.

In the last analysis, the diagnosis is reached in two ways: first, the determination that an encephalitis is present, and secondly, the determination that it is of the type known as lethargic encephalitis. The diagnosis of an encephalitis can be made by the demonstration of scattered lesions in the nervous system, giving rise to diffuse scattered signs, developing acutely with fever. The specific determination of an epidemic type of encephalitis cannot be made with absolute certainty since the precise cause is not known, but it may be inferred safely by the combination of symptoms mentioned.

It must be remembered that insofar as sequelae are concerned many forms of postencephalitis sequelae occur with no previous history of encephalitis. Many of the patients give a history of mild "grippe" or influenza which has probably been an unrecognized attack of encephalitis of a mild nature.

Brain tumor is often confused with encephalitis, especially tumor involving the brain stem. The differentiation is sometimes difficult, since tumor may exist without choked disc, and since encephalitis may develop with choked disc, and may give a history of progression of symptoms. In general, evidences of increased pressure favor tumor by far and a progressive history is greatly in favor of tumor, though it may exist with encephalitis. The onset of symptoms in infiltrating tumor of the brain stem is usually gradual and afebrile in contrast to that of encephalitis, but it may in unusual cases be abrupt in appearance. The differentiation must be made chiefly on the basis of the more gradual onset in tumor, the progressive nature of the process, and evidences of increased intracranial pressure. The signs of involvement of the brain stem may be quite similar in the two conditions.

Meningitis may be difficult to separate in the early stages when signs of meningeal irritation are present. Meningoencephalitis of tuberculosis or lymphocytic choriomeningitis may be confused, but the former may be differentiated by the discovery of tubercle bacilli, low spinal fluid chlorides, a pellicle in the spinal fluid, and persistent and pronounced meningeal signs, which are fleeting in encephalitis. Lymphocytic choriomeningitis is characterized by severe meningeal signs which are persistent without, as a rule, evidence of encephalitic involvement of the brain or brain stem. The signs are purely meningeal. A history of prodromal symptoms is usually present.

Poliomyelitis is readily separated by the development of the paralyses which are typical of the disease. In the preparalytic stages, it may be impossible to differentiate from encephalitis except by specific injection tests into animals. Clinically, the differentiation of preparalytic poliomyelitis and encephalitis may be impossible.

Syphilitic meningitis may be confused temporarily but serologic studies soon make the differentiation clear. Severe headache is striking in syphilitic meningitis. Cranial nerve palsies such as those encountered in encephalitis are common. Fever is unusual, meningeal signs are marked, and the serological studies of the spinal fluid reveal the presence of syphilis.

Botulism may give a picture simulating encephalitis very closely. Oculomotor palsies are common and may simulate those of encephalitis. The afebrile course, the history of onset after food ingestion with gastrointestinal disorders, the occurrence often in several members in a group, all of whom have eaten the same food, tend to balance the diagnosis in favor of botulism. In the absence of a specific history of food poisoning, the differentiation may be very difficult.

Hysteria was often diagnosed in previous times when the relation of the tics, respiratory disorders, etc., to encephalitis was not recognized. There should be no difficulty in making the diagnosis as against hysteria, the latter resulting usually from a hasty impression. Convergence paralysis, signs of parkinsonism should be of help in the differentiation.

Prognosis: The mortality of the acute disease is about twenty-five to thirty per cent. Probably thirty-five to forty per cent of the patients will develop sequelae. The severity of the acute attack bears no relation to the sequelae. A severe attack may be followed by no sequelae, while the latter may develop after a very mild attack or in the complete absence of a previous history of encephalitis. Patients with bulbar symptoms have a grave outlook. The outlook in parkinsonism will be discussed later. The prognosis in other sequelae such as oculogyric crises, respiratory disorders, tics, etc., is not good in so far as relief is concerned. They persist indefinitely and are relieved only temporarily by treatment.

Treatment: The acute stages must be treated like any febrile disease. Specific remedies are not known. The sulfonamides are of no value. Of the sequelae, oculogyric crises and palpebral spasm may be treated with some relief by atropine (0.5 per cent solution) given in ascending doses beginning with one drop daily and increased gradually until five to ten drops are taken three times a day. Other drugs, such as hyoscine hydrobromide, bulgarian belladonna, and stramonium, may be used. Hyoscine may be given in dosages of gr. $\frac{1}{200}$ to gr. $\frac{1}{100}$ three or four times a day. Stramonium may be given as the tincture (gr. 15 to 60 three times a day), or as the leaf (gr. $2\frac{1}{2}$ three or four times a day). Respiratory disorders respond poorly to treatment, but may be decreased by sedatives such as bromides or barbiturates (phenobarbital). The tics and myoclonic twitchings are difficult to control by medication. Section of the phrenic nerves for diaphragmatic tic, respiratory disorders, and hiccough have given only temporary relief. Conduct disorders in children respond poorly to ordinary psychotherapeutic measures and often require institutional care.

2. Additional Forms of Epidemic Encephalitis

Among other forms of epidemic encephalitis is that described as *St. Louis encephalitis* due to outbreaks of the disease in that city. Sporadic cases have occurred in the St. Louis area since 1937. The term is an unfortunate one, since St. Louis encephalitis has been found in other areas as well, in one instance as far afield as Central Africa (Smithburn). A specific virus has been isolated for the St. Louis type, distinct from that of epidemic encephalitis lethargica. St. Louis encephalitis resembles Japanese B encephalitis clinically, but the two disorders have been found to be due to two distinct viruses. Virus has never been demonstrated in nasopharyngeal washings. The disease in transmitted by a mosquito vector, the mosquito Culex tarsalis appearing to be the main means of transmission in some groups (Hammon). The virus is passed by the infected female tick through her eggs. Domestic fowl have been found to be the main reservoir for the infection of mosquitoes. Other forms of mosquito may also spread the disease (Culex pipiens). Virus was transmitted to susceptible animals by bite of the dog tick. Virus has been demonstrated in bodies of chick mites.

Pathologically, there are diffuse lesions of the brain and cord, featured by hemorrhages, cellular infiltration, perivascular cuffing, and ganglion cell disease. The disease resembles Japanese B encephalitis in its clinical manifestations. It has no respect for sex or color and seems to be more serious and more common in older subjects. The incubation period varies, but averages between nine and fourteen days. The spread is by human contagion, but individual susceptibility, in which age plays a part, is more important than contagion.

The clinical picture is characterized generally by sudden onset with headache, fever, stiff neck, mental confusion, tremors, and only occasional transient ocular manifestations (Hempelmann). Complete recovery occurs rapidly in most cases after two to three weeks, following a stormy course.

Three types of the disease were observed in the St. Louis epidemic of 1933: (1) an *encephalitic form* in which evidences of involvement of the nervous system were present from the onset; (2) a *systemic form* with signs of a general infection for several days before nervous system involvement; (3) mild and *abortive forms.*

The average subject has first symptoms of a general nature, such as extreme lassitude, malaise, chills, or chilly sensations, grippelike pains in the back and limbs, nausea or vomiting, and abdominal pains. Photophobia, conjunctivitis, and sore throat may be found rarely. Following these general manifestations, there appear signs of involvement of the nervous system, either quickly or after several days. These are manifested by fever, severe headache, stiff neck, somnolence, mental confusion, and tremors. Mild transient vertigo, tinnitus and deafness, retention or incontinence of urine and feces are sometimes encountered. Signs of meningeal irritation (neck stiffness, Kernig's sign) are present; the abdominal reflexes are absent and the tendon reflexes often increased; pathological reflexes (Babinski's sign, etc.) are sometimes found; ocular palsies are very rare. Mild blurring of vision, transient diplopia, and strabismus may be observed. Fever persists for the first two or three days, then falls rapidly, reaching normal seven to ten days after onset. Occasionally it persists four to six weeks. Moderate leukocytosis (twelve to twenty thousand) is usually present. The spinal fluid reveals an increase of cells (fifty to 250), most of which are lymphocytes. Cell counts of five or six hundred to eleven hundred may be found. The spinal fluid sugar is normal.

The diagnosis is made by the demonstration of neutralizing or complement fixing antibodies. A single convalescent serum is of no value and specimens must be taken at the onset, after two and six weeks and the titers compared.

St. Louis encephalitis is indistinguishable clinically from lethargic encephalitis, except that in the latter ocular paralyses are common, while they are rare in St. Louis encephalitis. Convalescent and recovered patients possess neutralizing antibodies in their blood (eighty to eighty-five per cent), while patients with lethargic encephalitis fail to show them. Neutralization tests establish the identity of St. Louis encephalitis. Early in the disease, cases are often regarded as *grippe,* but this is excluded by the subsequent course with the evidence of encephalitic involvement. *Tuberculous meningitis* may resemble St. Louis encephalitis, but in the former the course is more insidious and terminates fatally, there are often cranial nerve palsies, and the spinal fluid reveals pellicle formation, tubercle bacilli, and decreased sugar and chlorides. *Poliomyelitis* offers no difficulties in the paralytic stage, but in the pre-paralytic stages may resemble St. Louis encephalitis. The subsequent course with the development of flaccid paralyses makes the distinction clear and later neutralization tests confirm the diagnosis.

Japanese B encephalitis is caused by a virus which differs from that of St. Louis encephalitis and is transmitted by mosquitoes. It is considered to be identical with Russian autumnal encephalitis. The natural reservoir is probably in horses and possibly in man. Its clinical features are similar to those of St. Louis encephalitis. It occurs in both endemic and epidemic forms, the more severe epidemics appearing to occur at intervals of five to six years. The maximal morbidity occurs during the summer months, especially in August and September. Men are more often affected than women. The mortality is greater in the higher age groups. The mortality rate is sixty-five per cent. The diagnosis depends on the isolation of the virus from the blood; it is rarely found in the spinal fluid.

In a group of American military patients in whom a positive diagnosis of Japanese B encephalitis was established by serological methods, it was found that drowsiness, lethargy, mental confusion and disorientation, and semicoma and coma in the more severe cases, occurring in association with high fever, nuchal and spinal rigidity, leukocytosis, and pleocytosis, constituted the most important diagnostic criteria. "The onset was usually sudden with fever and extremely severe headache, although the mental confusion and lethargy, and even the stiffness of the neck and spine, . . . frequently did not appear until several days later." Convulsions were seen in two fatal cases. The pupils were usually contracted, diplopia was not observed, and dissociated eye movements were found in only one case, though common in native children with the disease.

"Athetosis, incoordination, and tremor of the hands were not uncommon, and difficulty in writing could be easily demonstrated. Difficulties in speech varied from slurring to complete aphasia. The reflexes were variable. The abdominal reflexes were usually absent, while the tendon reflexes were most often exaggerated, although occasionally they might become diminished or disappear. Positive great toe reflexes were uncommon." The fever was high and lasted seven to eleven days. A relative bradycardia was invariably present. A leukocytosis of 10,000 to 25,000 was present with a definite increase in the number of mature and immature neutrophiles. The spinal fluid was clear, under normal or slightly increased pressure, and contained 22 to 660 leukocytes per cc. The cells were chiefly mononuclear (Sabin).

Sequelae have been reported in Japanese B encephalitis. Hemiplegia, aphasia, dementia, convulsive attacks, character reversals, neuroses. and psychoses have been found in patients who have suffered from the disease.

Louping ill is a disease found in sheep, which can be transmitted experimentally to monkeys and man. In the few instances found in man, the disease developed in laboratory workers handling the virus. The onset is apparently acute, with an influenzalike group of symptoms — fever, headache, malaise, backache, and prostration. Recovery develops following this group of symptoms, only to be followed by evidences of encephalitis after several days. With this there is again fever, headache, diplopia, sometimes dizziness, and at times evidences of meningeal irritation. Ocular palsies and optic neuritis may be demonstrable. Leukocytosis is present. The spinal fluid is sterile and reveals mononuclear pleocytosis and, in some instances, red cells. The virus was not recovered in the blood or spinal fluid of the reported human cases, but the cases are regarded as being due to louping ill because of exposure of affected patients to the virus and because all the subjects were found to have neutralizing antibodies for the virus of louping ill.

West Nile fever is due to a virus which is related to that of the St. Louis and Japanese encephalitis. It is widespread in Central Africa, but no good account is available of its clinical manifestations

III. RABIES (*Hydrophobia, Lyssa*)

Rabies is a form of encephalitis produced by a specific virus injected by the bite of a rabid animal. The disease occurs in all countries, and while many animals are capable of propagating the disease, the dog is mainly responsible. Cats, wolves, skunks, foxes, and other wild animals are capable of transmitting the disease.

Etiology: The *cause* of the disease is a filterable virus which enters the body, usually through a bite. In exceptional instances, it may be introduced through a cut in the skin if it comes in contact with the saliva of a rabid animal, or through the mucosa of the mouth or nose.

Pathology: The *pathology* is that of an acute encephalitis most pronounced in the brain stem (mesencephalon, diencephalon, pons, and medulla), but with extensive involvement also of the spinal cord. The cerebrum is affected to a lesser degree. Histological examination reveals a predominant involvement of the grav matter involving the brain stem and spinal cord. In the affected areas there is a severe loss of ganglion cells and a heavy infiltration of lymphocytes in the tissue and around the vessels. Microglial cells are prominent soon after the infection develops. Negri bodies are found in the cytoplasm of the ganglion cells invariably in rabies in animals but inconstantly in the human. There is a distinct relationship between the site of the bite and the development of symptoms. Bites around the face and neck are followed by shorter incubation periods than those at a distance from the brain stem.

Symptoms: The *symptoms* of rabies develop after an incubation period varying from twenty to ninety days, but cases are known to develop months after infection. The end of the incubation period is characterized by slight fever, malaise, restlessness, and apprehension. This is followed in two or three days by the characteristic period of excitement characterized by at first a slight sense of fullness of the throat and eventually by violent spasms of swallowing and respiration until swallowing becomes difficult and then impossible. Even drinking becomes impossible. The slightest stimulus brings on attacks of spasms of difficulties in swallowing and breathing. Even swallowing saliva becomes impossible;

hence the accumulation of the saliva around the mouth. Generalized convulsions are common. Delirium may develop in this stage. Anxiety and apprehension are intense. Death may occur at this time or the period of excitement may be followed by paralysis and coma. High fever develops, paralysis becomes complete, respiration and deglutition are impossible, and death follows by the seventh day of the disease.

Diagnosis and Treatment: The *diagnosis* is not difficult. The history of a bite by a rabid dog is enough to make the diagnosis. If the animal responsible for the bite is known to be rabid, it should be killed and its brain examined for Negri bodies. *Treatment* should be instituted at once. This consists of immediate cauterization of the wound with phenol or fuming nitric acid. Vaccine may be given after a delay of a few days to determine whether the biting animal is rabid. Daily injections of ascending doses are given for two to four weeks, active immunity developing before the disease develops. Antirabies vaccines may sometimes produce encephalitis and other neurological conditions such as myelitis or neuritis. The incidence of such complications is low—about 1 in 1,000 to 1 in 4,000 treated. Myelitis is probably the most frequent sequela. Multiple neuritis may develop and involve the facial nerve. Encephalitis is rare. Because of the seriousness of the sequelae, it is essential that the diagnosis of rabies be certain before the vaccine is administered.

In persons in whom the disease has already developed, sedatives to quiet apprehension and restlessness are strongly indicated. Their choice depends largely on what seems to give best relief. Morphine is often the only sedative capable of quieting the convulsions.

IV. SUBACUTE SPORADIC ENCEPHALITIS

Among the sporadic encephalitides there has evolved in the past few years a group of subacute infections which have a similar clinical and pathological picture. On the European continent these are called "subacute sclerosing leukoencephalitis" (Van Bogaert); they are related to the nodular panencephalitis of Pette and Doring. There is a tendency in Great Britain and America to isolate a group of encephalitis cases under the term "subacute inclusion body encephalitis of the Dawson type," since, in many of the subjects, type A intranuclear inclusion bodies can be found in the neurons and oligodendroglia. Careful studies have demonstrated these inclusion bodies in the Van Bogaert type of subacute sclerosing leukoencephalitis. In like manner a characteristic astroglial response in the white matter can be seen in many, if not all, of the patients having inclusion body encephalitis or the nodular panencephalitis described by Pette and Doring—panencephalitis—because the white and gray matter are involved often with a sclerosing astroglial response. Glial nodules are prominent especially in the cortex and brain stem as in Japanese "B" encephalitis. An etiological factor has not been identified, but the virus origin of these closely related sporadic encephalitides is assumed by most authors. The pathology is closely similar to that in some patients with diffuse sclerosis, as in Schilder's third patient. In addition, a necrotizing type of encephalitis of shorter clinical course, but associated with intranuclear eosinophilic inclusion bodies and localized predominantly in the rhinencephalon, has been identified. In many of these patients, herpes simplex has been isolated as the causative agent. In other subjects with identical pathological conditions, search for a virus has not been attempted, or none has been isolated.

The clinical pictures of subacute inclusion body encephalitis and of subacute sclerosing leukoencephalitis are identical. There is first a gradual onset of a somewhat ill-defined psychiatric picture with such symptoms as apathy, confusion, and memory disturbances. This progresses over a period of weeks or months to dementia. It is often mistaken for a schizophrenic reaction pattern in the early stages. Prominent, as time goes on, are symptoms of hyperkinesia or dyskinesia, most frequently described as tic-like movements, tremors, or abnormal myoclonus. Parksonian features and other manifestations of rigidity are common. Decerebrate rigidity and complete dementia are terminal events. More or less characteristic periodic slow wave bursts are common in the EEG. Frequently the colloidal gold test shows a first zone reaction.

The pathological picture in these subacute encephalitides is essentially that of a panencephalitis with involvement of cortex and subjacent white matter principally in the anterior half of the brain and decreasing in intensity caudally. There is a moth-eaten, variable demyelination with corresponding astrogliosis. The "U" fibers are not spared. Damage to axons and myelin varies to the stage of neutral fat. There are signs of subacute inflammation with lymphocytes and plasma cells perivascularly and in the parenchyma, with meningeal inflammation primarily over the more involved cortex. Type A intranuclear inclusion bodies are frequently observed in cortical neurons and in the oligodendroglia of the cortex and white matter. In the involved cortex, microglia proliferate to prominent rod cells and fibrous glia are diffusely present.

In the acute necrotizing encephalitis of herpes simplex origin, frank softening is found usually in the inferior temporal cortex and white matter, hippocampus, and fornicate gyrus with signs of inflammation and eosinophilic intranuclear inclusions.

V. DISSEMINATED ENCEPHALO-MYELITIS

Definition: The term "disseminated encephalomyelitis" refers to a condition or conditions with widespread involvement of the brain, brain stem, and spinal cord. This form of encephalitis, unlike the preceding group of epidemic encephalitis, involves both the gray and white matter, the lesions predominating by far in the white substance. On the other hand, the lesions in the epidemic encephalitis group of patients are almost exclusively in the gray matter, involving the brain stem in particular. Disseminated encephalomyelitis is found in its best-defined form following infections of various sorts, such as measles, chickenpox, smallpox, German measles, and other infections. In this form it is a clearly delineated and well-established clinical and pathological type.

Whether there exists in addition to this a group of cases commonly referred to as encephalomyelitis disseminata is not yet clearly established. That there is such a group in which the cause is not known is probable. The cases in question develop acutely, usually without known cause, and with evidences of disseminated involvement of the nervous system. Some of the cases in question undoubtedly represent examples of acute multiple sclerosis. Their pathological features are no more definite unfortunately than their clinical forms and final judgment concerning the group in question must be withheld for the time being. The group of cases in ques-

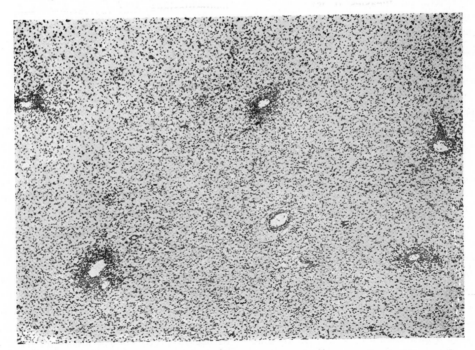

Fig. 120—*Disseminated encephalomyelitis* (perivenous) in a patient with measles showing the accumulation of mononuclear cells around the venules in the white matter of the brain.

tion is most commonly considered in differentiation from acute multiple sclerosis (q.v.) and neuromyelitis optica. Their existence as a specific entity must be conceded, but their exact cause is very much a matter of doubt at the present time. The term "disseminated encephalomyelitis" is at present widely employed clinically, but without very much knowledge as to its precise definition.

1. Postinfectious Encephalitis

Etiology: One of the chief forms of disseminated encephalomyelitis is that which follows infections of various sorts. These are of many forms such as measles, mumps, vaccinia, influenza, scarlet fever, chickenpox, smallpox, German measles, pertussis, typhus fever, and still other fevers. Most of these have clinical features in common. The incidence of encephalitic complications in these various diseases has not been determined with accuracy. In measles it is said to be 0.4 to 0.5 per cent; in vaccinia one case in one hundred thousand vaccinations. The incidence in other cases has not been worked out. It is still not known whether the encephalitis complicating these various diseases is caused by the organism responsible for the original infection, whether it is due to a secondary invader, whether it is caused by an organism activated by the infection, or whether it is an allergic or hyperergic response.

Pathology: The only feature which many of the diseases have in common is the dissemination of the lesion; the basic pathology varies widely. In some forms (measles, vaccinia), the pathological features are similar. They consist of disseminated areas of demyelination affecting gray and white matter, but predominating in the latter. In the gray matter, they are found in the cortex, basal ganglia, and brain stem; in the white matter,

they are found in the cerebrum, the internal capsule, and the long tracts of the brain stem and spinal cord. The essential lesion consists of demyelination and destruction of the axis cylinders in the areas around the veins, associated with perivascular cuffing by glial cells and often of lymphocytes, plasma cells, and leukocytes. The close relationship to the vessels has given rise to the term "perivenous encephalitis." In measles the lesions have a predilection for the edge of the cord, the marginal zones of the cerebral cortex, and the subependymal white matter. (Fig. 120).

In other forms (influenza, acute disseminated encephalomyelitis), the lesions are characterized by scattered patches of tissue destruction occurring in both the gray and white matter, but chiefly in the cerebral white matter, in the optic tracts, and in the long tracts of the brain stem and spinal cord, with demyelination, destruction of axis cylinders, gitter cell accumulations, and perivascular cuffing with lymphocytes and plasma cells. The disease resembles so closely acute multiple sclerosis that it is impossible under the microscope to differentiate the two diseases with accuracy (Fig. 121).

The eventual outcome of the lesions in the perivenous forms has not been studied extensively for want of material, but

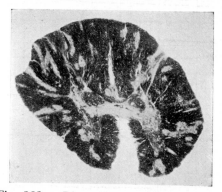

Fig. 121 — *Disseminated encephalomyelitis* **(perivenous) in a case of measles showing areas of demyelination in the spinal cord. (Courtesy of Dr. Charles Davison.)**

Table 35—Features of Postinfectious Encephalitis

Disease	Appearance	Onset	Symptoms	Spinal Fluid	Residuals	Mortality
MEASLES	3 to 5 days after rash	Acute, with or without fever, usually with fever	Lethargy, confusion; convulsions. Cranial nerve palsies, hemiplegia	No characteristic findings	Common; ca. 4 out of 10 cases	10 to 25 per cent
GERMAN MEASLES	2 to 6 days after rash	Acute, with normal or slightly elevated temperature	Mild as rule. Meningeal signs. Hemiplegia, convulsions and other symptoms	Lymphocytes increased (10 to 200)	None	Low. Benign as a rule
CHICKENPOX	9 to 13 days after onset of illness	Acute	Hemiplegia, chorea, ocular palsies		None	Recovery invariable
VACCINIA	7 to 14 days after vaccination	Acute with fever	Headache, drowsiness, ocular palsies, convulsions, hemiplegia, etc.		None as a rule but some are reported	35 to 50 per cent
SMALLPOX	8 to 16 days after eruption	Acute	Similar to vaccinia		None as a rule	
MUMPS	On subsidence of parotitis	Acute	Meningeal signs prominent. Ocular palsies. Facial paralysis, hemiplegia, etc.	Lymphocytes increased	None	Recovery in most cases
PERTUSSIS	No constancy	Acute	Convulsions, hemiplegia, etc.	No changes as a rule. Blood pressure some cases	Not uncommon	75 per cent mortality in cases with convulsions

Table 36—Features of Acute Epidemic Encephalitis

Disease	Onset	Clinical Features	Spinal Fluid	Laboratory Identification	Sequelae
ENCEPHALITIS LETHARGICA (von Economo)	Acute with fever; grippal symptoms	Ocular palsies prominent. Lethargy, delirium, loss of convergence	Lymphocytes increased (20 to 100) in acute stages; none later	None	Common—parkinsonism, behavior disorders, etc.
ST. LOUIS	Acute with fever; grippal symptoms	Meningeal signs. Confusion; somnolence. Ocular palsies rare	Lymphocytes increased (50 to 250)	Neutralizing antibodies in blood. Transmitted by mosquitoes	Few. Much less frequent than in lethargic encephalitis
JAPANESE B		Similar to those of St. Louis type		Neutralizing antibodies in blood	Sequelae common
LOUPING ILL	Acute with grippal symptoms	Headache, diplopia, meningeal signs	Lymphocytes increased	Neutralizing antibodies in blood	

it is probable that the demyelinated areas develop scars (astrocytes, glial fibers), or they may disappear completely and leave no trace of their presence.

Punctate hemorrhages are seen in some forms (mumps, pertussis).

Symptoms: The manner of onset is quite similar for many of the diseases which may be complicated by an encephalitis. Usually the onset is abrupt, with headache, vomiting, often convulsions, and sometimes mental confusion. In other instances, there is a more gradual development of symptoms with irritability for a few days prior to the development of headache, etc. Fever is frequently on the down grade when encephalitic complications develop and may even be normal. With their appearance, a secondary rise of fever occurs as a rule, but need not always be present.

Nervous-system complications are of two types: (1) cerebral, (2) spinal. Both cerebral and spinal complications occur in practically all the diseases affected. Cerebral manifestations predominate in all forms; in some diseases, such as pertussis, the spinal cord syndromes are unusual. Peripheral nerve involvement is found in most of the diseases. The spinal fluid shows an increase of cells in most of the forms, especially early in the disease.

Measles Encephalitis: This form of measles develops usually in children two to eight years of age, but no age at which measles occurs is spared. The encephalitis may precede the measles rash; it may occur with the rash, or appear at varying periods after it. Onset before the appearance of the rash is rare. In typical cases, the encephalitis occurs three to five days after the appearance of the rash, but a shorter or longer latency is not uncommon. The onset may be gradual or abrupt, is usually but not always with fever which may sometimes be very high and may de-

velop in a patient previously afebrile for several days. The symptoms vary greatly and baffle concise description, depending as they do on the distribution of the lesions. *Lethargy* and *mental symptoms* (delirium, confusion, catatonic states, excitement) are usually present. The mental state varies from that of mild irritability or apathy to profound stupor or delirium. *Convulsions,* either tonic or clonic, generalized or focal, are common and occur in about half the cases. They occur most often at the onset of the encephalitis, but are not uncommon as a terminal manifestation. *Cranial nerve manifestations* appear in varying numbers and include aphonia, ocular palsies, deafness, blindness, facial and bulbar paralysis, optic neuritis, pupillary changes (inequality, fixation of pupils), and choked disc. *Hemiplegia* or paraplegia may develop, the former being much more common than the latter.

The reflexes may be decreased, absent, or overactive and Babinski's sign may be found. Signs of meningeal irritation are commonly present. The *spinal fluid* shows an increase of cells (up to three hundred lymphocytes), the chloride and sugar content being normal, and the protein increased. No organisms are found. There is usually a mild leukocytosis. The mortality has been variously recorded as between ten and twenty-five per cent. The outlook is poor in very young patients. Fever of rapid onset and constant increase and bulbar symptoms have a poor prognosis. Residual symptoms are common. Any of the neurological symptoms may become permanent or may persist for a long time before recovery ensues. In general, of ten patients, four will recover completely, two will die, and four will have one or more major or minor debilitating residual symptoms (Hamilton and Hanna).

Residual symptoms were found in thirty-nine per cent of the subjects and consisted of changes in personality, mental deficiency, choreiform movements, tremor, cord bladder, and foot-drop (Fox, Kuzma and Stuhler). A study of patients with measles encephalitis, followed fourteen months to six years, reveals that there is a close correlation between the length of the illness and the psychological outcome, those with short illnesses having a better outcome. The observed changes consisted of personality difficulties, difficulties in perception and attention, and impulsive behavior (Meyer and Byers).

German Measles (Rubella) Encephalitis: This is a rare form of measles encephalitis. The reported cases have been found in subjects varying in age from five to thirty-five years. It develops in a manner similar to ordinary measles and occurs two to six days after the rash with a normal or slightly elevated temperature. The onset occurs abruptly as a rule, usually with headache as the presenting symptom. Convulsions and mental confusion are frequent. Meningeal syndromes, ocular palsies with diplopia and strabismus, hemiplegia, delirium, stupor, convulsions, and transverse cord syndromes have been recorded. The disease is short as a rule. Mild cases show only headache, vomiting, and neck stiffness. Convulsions are found usually in fatal cases. The spinal fluid shows an increase of cells (ten to two hundred lymphocytes), with an increase of protein and no organisms. The diagnosis is not difficult, since the symptoms occur in obvious relationship to the rubella.

2. *Vaccinia and Other Forms of Encephalitis*

Vaccinia is at times associated with an encephalitis, but the frequency of this complication is difficult to estimate.

There seems to be a direct relationship between the number of vaccinations performed and the incidence of vaccinal encephalitis in those countries in which the complication has been a problem. In patients so affected, focal areas of damage are found throughout the nervous system, with extensive involvement of both the gray and white matter. The meninges show a mild infiltration with small round cells early in the disorder. Scattered throughout the nervous system are areas of perivascular demyelination, chiefly around the veins. Associated with this is an increase of cells around the affected vessels. These are chiefly glial in nature. Degeneration of the nerve cells is seen in the affected regions. Symptoms of encephalitis develop seven to fourteen days after vaccination in the average case (eighty-two per cent) and in the majority between the tenth and thirteenth day (sixty-five per cent). Onsets as early as the second day and as late as the sixteenth to twentieth days have been recorded. The clinical picture is variable, since, as in the other forms of encephalomyelitis, the symptoms are dependent upon the number and distribution of the lesions. The onset in most cases is rapid and the course acute. Fever, headache, vomiting, and drowsiness are the predominant symptoms in the majority of cases. Strabismus, mental confusion, and hemiplegias or hemiparesis may develop. Convulsions develop in some cases. Rare cases of myelitis develop after vaccinia (Dixon). The mortality rate is high (thirty-five to fifty per cent), the actual rate varying from year to year. Death may occur in two to four days in acute cases or in less severe cases in seven to fourteen days. Recovered subjects seem to show no residuals as a rule, but sequelae have been reported.

Central nervous system symptoms occur in *brucellosis* with surprising frequency and are manifested by evidences of meningitis, encephalitis, or meningoencephalitis. Spinal cord manifestations occur also, producing signs of incomplete or complete transverse myelitis. Focal signs of various sorts may develop, such as hemiplegia, hemianopsia, and aphasia. The differentiation between brucellosis and psychoneurosis may be extremely difficult. Postencephalitic paralysis agitans has been noted in brucellosis (Harris). Neuritis has been reported on several occasions. Psychoses have been observed during the acute stages of the disease, and neuroses are common.

The importance of the disorder is illustrated by the facts that (1) central nervous system manifestations may be the only expression of the disease and (2) vague encephalitic, meningoencephalitic, and neurotic disorders may be found to result from brucellosis. The spinal fluid shows increased pressure, cell increase, increased protein, and decreased glucose and chloride content.

Varicella encephalitis is probably more common than reports indicate. Very few instances have been recorded. The complication develops usually on the ninth to the thirteenth day of the illness. The pathology is similar to that of vaccinia and measles encephalitis. The neurological manifestations develop rapidly, with muscular weakness or paralysis the outstanding feature. The legs are most often affected by paraplegia, but the process may extend to the arms as well. Irritability or delirium is quite constant; stupor and mental dullness may be found. The temperature is usually slightly elevated, rarely rising above 100° F. Vertigo, vomiting, tremors, and choreiform movements have been recorded in some cases. A bulbar form of the disease has been reported and is characteristic by dysarthria, dysphagia, ocular palsies, and other symptoms referable to the brain stem. The spinal fluid findings are not characteristic; the cell count may be normal or increased. Many complications have been reported, among which are hemiplegias, chorea, ocular paralyses, athetosis, and transverse myelitis. Recovery always occurs.

Mumps encephalitis may occur without symptoms (latent encephalitis), but with an increase of cells in the spinal fluid, or with evidence of a frank meningitis or meningoencephalitis. Meningitis is common as a complication of mumps. In a small percentage of cases true encephalitis develops. *Mumps* is a systemic disease with special predilection for the salivary glands, mature gonads, pancreas, and breasts, and also for the central nervous system. The most frequent nervous system manifestation of mumps is a meningoencephalitis with an increase of lymphocytes in the spinal fluid usually below 200 cells. Many other varieties of nervous system involvement occur. The meningoencephalitis of mumps may occur prior to or in the absence of the usual manifestations of mumps, particularly parotitis, or it may develop during the typical mumps picture. The incubation period has been found to be twelve to twenty-six days, most commonly eighteen to twenty-one days. There appears to be no correlation between central nervous system involvement in mumps and the severity of the parotid gland or gonadal involvement. In an obscure case of lymphocytic meningitis or meningoencephalitis, mumps must always be suspected, particularly in the absence of parotid gland swelling. The diagnosis can be established by specific serological tests. Virus has been found in the saliva, spinal fluid, and blood of humans. Meningeal signs are prominent and there is an increase of cells in the spinal fluid. Ocular palsies may develop. Peripheral facial paralysis, optic atrophy and neuritis, deafness, hemiplegias, and aphasia have been found in the course of the disease. The outlook in mumps encephalitis is usually good. Fatal cases of mumps meningoencephalitis have been reported on rare occasions. The disease has been associated with perivascular demyelination, as have other types of postinfectious encephalitis.

Smallpox is associated with nervous system complications at times. The relative incidence is shown in the occurrence of twenty-five cases with nervous system complications among ten thousand cases of smallpox (Ralleston). The cases resemble closely those seen after vaccinia. The symptoms develop at varying periods of time after the rash, eight to sixteen days usually, but sometimes longer. Encephalitic, meningitic, and myelitic pictures predominate. The picture for the encephalitic forms varies, depending upon the region of the brain stem affected. Hence no characteristic picture is possible. The symptoms may be entirely bulbar, with dysarthria and dysphagia predominating, or these may be associated with spastic paralysis of the limbs, ataxia, and sometimes mental changes, suggesting a diffuse involvement of the nervous system resembling multiple sclerosis. Drowsiness, coma, loss of sphincter control, disturbances of speech, and paralysis of the limbs with or without sphincter disturbances are found. The onset in some cases is that of a transverse myelitis with paralysis of the legs, sensory paralysis, and sphincter disturbances. There may later be extension of the process to the upper limbs. The outlook is often good. There may be fleeting, transitory symptoms, or severe cases leaving evidence of permanent damage.

Pertussis encephalitis is not uncommon. The pathological findings in cases of pertussis complicated by cerebral disorders are not uniform and there is considerable variation in the findings at post-mortem. Punctate hemorrhages, meningeal hemorrhage, or congestion of the brain are found in some cases. Extensive degeneration of the nerve cells has been reported in some instances. The most common type of cerebral involvement is characterized by the sudden onset of convulsions, a complication occurring in about eight per cent of pertussis cases. Somnolence often precedes the convulsive attack. The convulsions are usually generalized, but may be focal, and are unassociated with objective neurological findings. The mortality rate is high (seventy-five per cent), death ensuing after a single convulsion or after a series. The spinal fluid is usually normal, but may contain blood. Hemiplegias, paraplegia, cranial nerve palsies, mental retardation, meningitis, and bulbar syndromes have been described as encephalitic complications of the disease. They may occur at any time during the course of the whooping cough. It is important to realize that the occurrence of cerebral symptoms in pertussis need not be due invariably to encephalitis. Tetany may develop in those patients in whom severe alkalosis has developed as a result of vomiting. Severe injury to the nervous system may follow the administration of pertussis vaccine given in usual dosage. Symptoms appear acutely within twenty minutes to seventy-two hours following injection. The onset is usually abrupt with high fever, restlessness, irritability or drowsiness, followed quickly by generalized or occasionally unilateral convulsions and coma. Hemiplegia or hemiparesis is common and symptoms of bulbar palsy have been reported. Sequelae are common and recurrent convulsions have been recorded in many instances. Among the sequelae have been recorded "cerebral palsies" and mental retardation. Complete recovery may occur. Autopsy studies reveal that the changes are degenerative in character. The pathogenesis is unknown, but it is not due apparently to contaminated or faulty vaccine.

Virus has been isolated from human brains infected with *herpes simplex*. The virus of herpes simplex is capable of causing encephalitis in man.

Toxoplasmic encephalitis occurs in children. It has been reported in identical twins. It is caused by an encephalitozoon. Its clinical features are not too well-defined. In *adults* it is characterized by malaise and weakness for several days followed by chills and fever, the latter sustained throughout the illness. A maculopapular eruption is present, covering the entire body but sparing the hands, soles of the feet, and scalp. Pulmonary infection is usually present. The *infantile form* is featured by chorioretinitis, hydrocephalus, and meningoencephalitis characterized by generalized convulsions, disorientation, neck rigidity, and increase of cells in the spinal fluid. The brain shows necrotic and granulomatous foci. The diagnosis is made by laboratory identification of the toxoplasma after death or in infants with chorioretinitis and cerebral symptoms.

Equine encephalomyelitis has come to the fore in recent years in two forms, an eastern and a western form of the disease. It occurs in horses and mules and has been described frequently in man. The disease in man is caused by a virus which is different for the eastern and western forms. It has a seasonal incidence, occurring during the summer and early autumn, is transmitted by mosquitoes and ticks, and there is evidence to indicate that birds may harbor the virus.

The virus can be isolated from the brains of human cases, and neutralizing antibodies can be demonstrated in the convalescent serum.

The disease is a meningoencephalitis with focal areas of destruction of nerve cells, and infiltration with polymorphonuclears, lymphocytes, and microglial cells. Perivascular cuffing is common. Vascular thrombi are found scattered about in the tissues.

The clinical features of the eastern and western types are not identical. *Eastern equine encephalomyelitis* occurs chiefly in children, has a mortality of sixty per cent, and is often followed by residuals. The disease has been transmitted experimentally by mosquitoes, but virus has not been isolated in mosquitoes caught in nature.

In most cases the onset is sudden with high fever (102° to 105° F.), irritability or drowsiness, vomiting, cyanosis, and convulsions. Cyanosis is marked in all the cases. Neck rigidity is constant and muscular twitchings and rigidity are common. In older children, the onset is more gradual, over a period of four to ten days, and is usually associated with headache and dizziness. All the patients become comatose or semicomatose rapidly. The temperature continues to rise in the fatal cases and falls by lysis in those which recover, reaching normal in four to five days. Leukocytosis is common. The cells in the spinal fluid are increased (200 to 2000 cm^3) and are mostly polymorphonuclears, but later change to lymphocytes after two or three days. Sequelae are not uncommon after the acute attack (hemiparesis, hemiplegia, aphasia, mental retardation and emotional instability). The residuals appear to be permanent and may even be progressive.

The frequency of the disease in man parallels closely that in horses, but most patients have no contact with horses, the transmission of the disease taking place probably through mosquitoes.

The diagnosis is suspected in communities where the disease is present among horses. The symptoms resemble those of other forms of encephalitis, but the high fever and the frequent onset with stupor are important features. The diagnosis is made with certainty only by the demonstration of neutralizing and complement-fixing antibodies in the blood.

Western equine encephalomyelitis is epidemic in the late summer, is found chiefly in adults, has a mortality rate of five per cent, and is not followed by the severe residuals of the eastern type. Culex tarsalis is the most important vector, and birds, including domestic fowl, are an important source of virus infection for the mosquitoes (Hammon, Reaves, and Galindo). The virus has been transmitted experimentally by mosquitoes and chicken mites, and has been found in mosquitoes caught in nature. The disease in *infants* resembles closely that of St. Louis encephalitis. The onset is sudden with fever, refusal to eat, vomiting, neck rigidity, twitching, and occasionally convulsions. The temperature climbs rapidly to 103° to 105° F. within twenty-four to forty-eight hours and falls to normal in the next three or four days. Cyanosis is conspicuous in the acute stages. After several days of quite severe prostration, recovery occurs completely in four to seven days. The disease in *adults* is similar to that of the eastern form, but is milder and is followed by recovery in two or three weeks. In fatal cases, the onset is abrupt, beginning usually with severe frontal headache, followed promptly by dizziness and prostration. When first examined, the patient appears very ill, is disoriented or partly stuporous, and has high fever. The neck is tender and stiff

and sometimes retracted. The limbs show tremor and may be spastic. There is a moderate leukocytosis. The cells of the spinal fluid rarely rise above one hundred but may be as high as five hundred, of which about two-thirds are lymphocytes.

Venezuelan equine encephalomyelitis is immunologically distinct from the Eastern and Western forms of equine encephalomyelitis. The virus is easily obtained from the blood and throat washings of human beings, and the diagnosis is confirmed by neutralization and complement fixation tests. The disease is highly pathogenic for horses, but there is an absence of infection in man in Venezuela. It has been found to be the cause of encephalitis in a group of laboratory workers handling the virus and is therefore known to be capable of causing encephalitis in man (Lennette and Koprowski).

Embolic or metastatic encephalitis is a convenient term given to encephalitis developing from foci of infection in the heart and lungs especially, but occurring also in blood stream infections, after the extraction of teeth, and from thrombophlebitis. In heart involvement, the disorder develops especially as a complication of subacute bacterial endocarditis, but it occurs also in vegetative endocarditis, and in mitral stenosis in which mural thrombi have developed. In pulmonary diseases, metastatic encephalitis is found in association with pulmonary abscess and bronchiectasis. The encephalitis in such cases develops from minute emboli discharged into the brain. Cerebral complications have been recorded in acute rheumatic fever, presumably due to rheumatic involvement of the brain. Psychoses have been attributed to rheumatic brain infection due to endarteritis of a chronic type with associated brain erosions (Bruetsch). Though changes of this type doubtless occur, it is doubtful whether they account for very many instances of psychosis.

The pathology consists of foci of cell accumulations composed of polymorphonuclear leukocytes. Perivascular cuffing by leukocytes is found in their vicinity. Scattered leukocytes are found in the surrounding tissue and endothelial swelling and proliferation are found in the vessels near the embolic foci. Punctate hemorrhages are not uncommon. Softening of the tissue due to plugging of vessels by emboli is sometimes seen.

The onset of symptoms is usually sudden and abrupt as in any embolic brain process. Fever may be present, but is not constant. Headache and neck rigidity are common. Convulsions may develop. Signs of many sorts may be found, including hemiplegia, monoplegia, aphasia, convulsions, stupor, brain stem syndromes, and ocular palsies. The signs vary with the distribution of the lesions. The spinal fluid shows an increase of cells in cases with meningeal symptoms, but as a rule no cell increase is found.

The significance of metastatic encephalitis varies. In most cases it is a serious symptom In heart disorders, especially in subacute bacterial endocarditis, the encephalitis may be terminal or may be followed by recovery. In blood stream infections, it is usually of serious import. In pulmonary infections, its significance is similar to that of heart disease.

Encephalitis is associated rarely with *gonococcal* infections. *Cryptococcus neoformans* (torula) infections are sometimes associated with encephalitis, but are much more often the cause of a meningitis. The clinical features of these cases are similar to those of a meningoencephalitis from other causes (headache, neck stiffness, drowsiness, etc.). The spinal fluid shows an increase of

cells (three hundred to seven hundred lymphocytes) ; the torulae may be seen in the smear. They are easily demonstrated by India ink preparations. They resemble red cells in the unstained specimen. *Trichiniasis* likewise is complicated by nervous system complications at times, among which are meningitis, encephalitis, neuroretinitis, optic neuritis, and diplopia. Absence of reflexes is common. Generalized weakness is also commonly present. The main differentiation in cases of trichiniasis is from polyneuritis, poliomyelitis, encephalitis, meningitis, dermatomyositis, and periarteritis nodosa. Larvae are sometimes found in the spinal fluid, together with an increase of cells.

In some cases, *infectious mononucleosis* causes an encephalitis. There is no constant order of appearance of the neurological symptoms in infectious mononucleosis. They may appear early or late. In instances in which the involvement of the nervous system is severe, the changes in the blood picture tend to be delayed, and symptoms of involvement of the nervous system may be the first manifestation of the disease. They are characterized by headache, dulling of the sensorium, irritability, facial nerve paralysis, oculomotor nerve palsies, optic neuritis, ataxia, and signs of meningeal irritation. Neurological complications of various types may develop during the course of infectious mononucleosis. The most frequent manifestation of nervous system involvement is *meningitis*, which may develop at any time during the course of the disease. Signs of meningeal irritation—headache, neck stiffness, and Kernig's sign—are usually present. The spinal fluid contains an excess of lymphocytes, with normal sugar and chloride values, and sterile culture. Encephalitis may develop, with cranial nerve paralyses of various types, such as ocular palsies, facial paralysis, and palatal paralysis. Cerebellar symptoms may be noted. Convulsive seizures may develop in the course of infectious mononucleosis. Optic neuritis has been reported. The disease is often confused with poliomyelitis, lymphocytic choriomeningitis, and epidemic encephalitis before the lymphadenopathy, the blood picture, and the splenic enlargement develop. Recovery from the neurological symptoms in cases of infectious mononucleosis is stated to be complete in eighty-five per cent of cases (Bernstein & Wolff).

Neurological symptoms due to central nervous system involvement occur frequently in systemic *lupus erythematosus*. Symptoms of many sorts have been described. These include generalized and focal convulsions, subarachnoid hemorrhage, aphasia, paralyses of various types (monoplegias, hemiplegias, quadriplegias, and paraplegia), choked disc, and diplopia. Psychiatric manifestations occur such as anxiety, depressions, paranoid reactions, and hallucinations. Isolated involvement of the spinal cord has been reported. It has been suggested that nervous system manifestations may precede evidences of systemic infection. The pathological changes consist of vasculitis characterized by fibrinoid changes in the walls of small blood vessels with proliferative changes leading to narrowing or occlusion of the lumen and the production of infarcts.

Relapsing fever (treponema recurrentis) may be responsible for encephalitis or meningoencephalitis. They may appear at any time during the course of the illness, but are more common after the third week. The most common nervous complications consist of meningitis, encephalitis, or meningoencephalitis. The spinal fluid usually shows a cell increase, sometimes as high as 2000 cells per cc. The majority

of subjects recover completely without residuals. Meningitis may exist alone; there may be evidence of encephalitis without meningitis; or meningoencephalitis may be found. Ocular palsies develop in the encephalitic group; facial paralysis of the peripheral type may develop. The organism is often found in blood smears.

The *Rickettsial diseases*, such as typhus fever and Rocky Mountain spotted fever, are associated with encephalitis at times. Typhus fever is borne by the louse and Rocky Mountain spotted fever is transmitted by the wood tick. Nervous symptoms are common in both diseases (headache, delirium). The essential lesion is a disease of the smaller blood vessels with numerous thromboses, and with necroses in the spotted fever type. Encephalitis associated with the acute state of Rocky Mountain spotted fever usually clears up, but prolonged residuals have been recorded. These include hemiplegia, impaired vision and photophobia, seizures, mental retardation, and disturbances in behavior. These usually recede, but residuals such as hemiplegia of more than one year in duration have been recorded. In typhus fever encephalitis, deep stupor develops and results in death. A form of lymphocytic encephalitis has been described in association with *pleurodynia*. Fever and severe pain in the upper abdomen or lower thorax usher in the disease. Pharyngitis, headache, apathy, vertigo, photophobia, and nuchal rigidity are found. The spinal fluid shows an excess of lymphocytes. Recovery is the rule and no sequelae have been noted.

Otogenous encephalitis is not infrequently seen in association with mastoid disease. The encephalitis involves the temporal cortex as a rule and resembles closely brain abscess from which it can be distinguished by absence of signs of increased intracranial pressure. The distinction between otogenous encephalitis and brain abscess is not as a rule easy. Both conditions develop in association with middle ear or mastoid disease and both are accompanied by signs of focal involvement, usually of the temporal lobe —hemianopsia, central facial weakness, hemiparesis. It is quite possible that in many cases of otogenous encephalitis the condition represents the early stages in the development of a brain abscess which has not progressed to fruition of the abscess. In some instances, operation has been performed without disclosure of an abscess, but with evidence of encephalitis. In the last analysis, the distinction is made on the basis of recovery in the case of encephalitis and the development of signs of abscess in those cases in which the latter is present.

Infective hepatitis is associated with brain changes in fatal cases, the changes being probably in the nature of an encephalitis. In this group, coma, delirium, and convulsions are present. Other more fatal groups are associated with symptom complexes, such as (1) generalized muscular rigidity with increased reflexes and sometimes Babinski's sign, (2) choreiform movements, and (3) peripheral neuritis.

Cerebral malaria results largely from infection with P. falciparum (aestivo-autumnal, malignant tertian). The symptoms result from plugging of the capillaries by plasmodia, pigment-laden leukocytes and erythrocytes. The onset varies, some cases developing with coma, some with somnolence, and others with fever. Severe headache is common and photophobia and vertigo are frequent. Convulsions may develop and confusion and disorientation are almost constant. Aphasia is sometimes found. Neck stiffness, transient paralyses (monoplegias, hemiplegias, and quadriplegias), dys-

arthria, athetoid movements, and trismus have all been observed. The blood count is low or normal and the fever usually high. The spinal fluid pressure is usually normal (Fitz-Hugh, Pepper, and Hopkins), and the fluid is usually clear but may be xanthochromic or hemorrhagic. The mortality rate is high; twenty-five per cent for all cases (Fitz-Hugh *et al.*). The occurrence of coma and convulsions is associated with a mortality rate of eighty per cent.

Rare instances of encephalitis have been reported with *cat scratch fever*.

World War II has brought to the United States instances of encephalitis resulting from infection with *Schistosoma japonicum*. The cerebral complications associated with this disease are of two types: (1) those due to a diffuse encephalitis and (2) those associated with a large granuloma, causing symptoms and signs of brain tumor. In the group due to encephalitis, the manifestations vary, depending upon the areas of the brain affected—convulsions, hemiplegia, aphasia, or cranial nerve palsies. In the group due to granuloma, the signs are focal and resemble those of brain tumor.

VI. ENCEPHALITIS DUE TO TOXINS AND METALS

Encephalitis is not rarely found as the result of toxins and metal poisonings. Botulism, mushroom poisoning, ergotism, lead, arsenic, and other metals may be associated with evidence of nervous system involvement.

Lead encephalopathy is found in both children and adults, the lead poisoning resulting from the same causes as in lead neuritis. The brain in affected cases shows diffuse ganglion cell damage, vessel disease, and in some instances foci of encephalitis, though the last are rare. In *children* the signs of lead encephalopathy frequently simulate those of brain tumor, especially cerebellar tumor. Headache, vomiting, choked disc, convulsions, and cerebellar dyssynergia are found. The total picture resembles tumor so closely that the diagnosis of the latter is often made. In *adults* many sorts of manifestations are found. These develop gradually as a rule, but may appear suddenly. Convulsions appear not infrequently. Psychoses are not uncommon, and are characterized by confusion, evidence of deterioration, and other psychotic trends. Hemiplegia or aphasia may be seen during the course of the disease. Mental deterioration may be marked and may resemble general paresis very closely. Optic atrophy and choked disc are seen rarely. A meningitic form of the disease is known, the meningitis being of the serous type.

Lead encephalopathy may simulate brain tumor, central nervous system syphilis, epilepsy, chronic alcoholism, and neuroses. It is diagnosed by the presence of a lead line, basophilic stippling and anemia, and lead in the urine, feces, and blood (*v.* chapter on Intoxications).

Botulism is often associated with encephalitic symptoms. Poisoning occurs from spoiled food containing B. botulinus. The clinical features resemble closely those of encephalitis. The onset is sudden and usually preceded by gastrointestinal disturbances. Diplopia, ocular palsies of many sorts, ptosis, dysphonia, dysphagia, facial paralysis, drowsiness, and other bulbar symptoms are found. Generalized weakness and eventual paralysis, with decrease or loss of reflexes, are present.

The condition resembles epidemic encephalitis very closely. If a history of onset after eating tainted food is obtained, the diagnosis is facilitated, but the connection is not recognized frequently by the patient and can only be brought out by direct questioning. Obscure cases should always be investigated from the standpoint of their relation to food ingestion.

Despite the evidence of severe brain stem involvement, there is often nothing to be seen on examination of the nervous system. In some cases, nerve cell degeneration and endothelial swelling are found.

Encephalitis may develop following exposure to carbon disulfide, mercury, manganese, alcohol, carbon monoxide, and other chemicals. These are considered in detail in the chapter on Intoxications.

VII. HEMORRHAGIC ENCEPHALITIS

The term "hemorrhagic encephalitis" refers to a pathological rather than a clinical entity, the outstanding feature of which is scattered hemorrhages variously distributed in the nervous system. The condition is, therefore, not in reality an encephalitis, since no inflammatory or infectious processes accompany it. The term, however, has the advantage of established usage and the group is therefore considered in the encephalitis category. A clinical diagnosis of hemorrhagic encephalitis has no standing in most instances, the term being merely a descriptive one to indicate the type of lesion occurring in a wide variety of diseases.

Many different conditions may be associated with a hemorrhagic encephalitis. Among them are alcoholism, avitaminoses, phosgene and carbon monoxide poisoning, methyl chloride poisoning, influenza, diphtheria, pneumonia, malaria, dysentery, typhoid and typhus fever, pernicious anemia, head injuries, scurvy, erythema multiforme, purpura hemorrhagica, sulfonamide compound and arsenical poisoning. The large number of clinical conditions in which hemorrhagic encephalitis is found makes it impossible to consider in detail the various clinical manifestations which may develop as a result of the condition. It is clear that the disorder constitutes in many instances a complication of the disorders in which it is found and will be discussed in the consideration of these various entities. In a few instances, the condition is of sufficient significance to require brief but separate discussion.

The essential features of the disease are scattered punctate hemorrhages. These are distributed in both gray and white matter, but are more numerous in the latter. All parts of the nervous system are susceptible. The cerebral cortex, basal ganglia, the gray matter of the brain stem, the cerebral white matter, and the long tracts of the brain stem are particularly susceptible. The hemorrhages are perivascular. They are replaced eventually by glial cells.

One of the special forms of hemorrhagic encephalitis is that of Wernicke, *polioencephalitis hemorrhagica superior*. This disease occurs frequently in alcoholics, but is found also in nonalcoholic conditions, such as carcinoma of the gastrointestinal tract, carcinoma of the stomach, atrophic gastritis, and following cholecystectomy. Alcohol *per se* is probably not responsible for the condition. Recent views indicate that a nutritional deficiency is responsible, particularly a deficiency in thiamine hydrochloride, but multiple deficiencies are probably a factor in most cases. The disease can be produced quite regularly in pigeons deprived of thiamine when large supplies of vitamins A_1, B_2, C, and D are fed. It cannot be produced in pigeons receiving thiamine, though they are deprived of all other vitamins.

A review of the literature makes clear the following points (Jolliffe, Wortis, and Fein): (1) The clinical syndrome is not clear cut, but in general consists of clouding of consciousness, varying ophthalmoplegias, and ataxia. Furthermore, the syndrome is frequently preceded or accompanied by a delirious episode, and in those patients who recover a residual Korsakoff syndrome is frequently seen. (2) The spinal cord and peripheral nerves are probably involved in the process in addition to the brain. (3) The syndrome is usually associated with chronic alcoholism, but the evidence is fairly good that it is not due primarily to alcoholism. A nutritional deficiency, especially of thiamine, seems to be the most obvious common factor.

The pathology of Wernicke's syndrome is found in the periventricular gray matter, the hypothalamus, mammillary bodies, oculomotor nuclei (third, fourth, and sixth), the vestibular nuclei, and the thalamus. Lesions are seen constantly in the mammillary bodies, less constantly in the other hypothalamic nuclei and thalamus, frequently in the gray matter around the aqueduct, in the posterior colliculi and the junction of gray matter of diencephalon and mesencephalon, and in the gray matter of the fourth ventricle. The cerebral cortex and cerebellum are sometimes affected. The lesions consist of small hemorrhages, vascular proliferation, glial proliferation, foci of degeneration, absence of inflammatory infiltration, and varicose deformities of the blood vessels.

The *clinical features* are not clear cut. The *onset* is usually abrupt. The duration of symptoms varies from a few days to several weeks. Disturbances of consciousness are seen in every case; in some patients drowsiness developing into coma dominates the picture, while in others drowsiness, apathy, excitement, and delirium are present. Confusion and delirium in varying degrees are seen constantly, with slight or severe degrees of confusion and disorientation. A clear mentality is never seen in patients with Wernicke's encephalopathy. The delirium and stupor may develop very rapidly. Ocular disturbances are common. There may be irregularity and inequality of the pupils, diplopia, strabismus, and ophthalmoplegias varying from slight disturbance of ocular movements to complete ophthalmoplegia. Impairment or loss of upward gaze is common. Ataxia is a common feature. It is often extreme in the limbs. Dysarthria is usually present. Peripheral neuritis is present in almost every case. Many cases terminate fatally.

There is good evidence to indicate that in patients who recover, the ophthalmoplegia responds to thiamine chloride, but since multiple vitamin deficiencies are present it is best to give vitamins A, C, and D in high doses in addition to the thiamine.

Arsphenamine given intravenously sometimes gives rise to a hemorrhagic encephalitis or myelitis. The condition develops following intravenous arsphenamine usually in syphilitic cases, and occurs most often after the second injection (fifty per cent). The size of the dosage appears to bear no relation to the development of the condition. The reaction may develop immediately or within the first three days after injection. It develops once in every sixty-five hundred cases and once in every thirty-six thousand injections. The cases of hemorrhagic encephalitis are characterized by onset with headache, chills, vomiting, nervousness, and dizziness. Fever often is present. Convulsions (eighty per cent) and unconsciousness (seventy-five per cent) occur in most cases. Cyanosis, icterus, skin rash, and respiratory changes are common. The oculomotor nerves are frequently affected. Mental confusion

and delirium are found in about half of the subjects. Other scattered signs of various sorts develop, depending upon the areas destroyed by the hemorrhage, hence a detailed analysis of the symptoms is impossible. The condition is fatal in seventy-six per cent of the patients, death occurring in two to thirty-five days. Some die within twenty-four hours.

Transverse myelitis is a rare complication of intravenous arsphenamine injection and is the result of hematomyelia. The outlook for recovery in such cases is poor. There is usually complete loss of power in the limbs, sensory, bladder, and rectal paralysis.

In other diseases associated with hemorrhagic encephalitis, the condition is incidental and has no specific features. The encephalitis associated with these various conditions will be discussed subsequently.

In some instances, hemorrhagic encephalitis is presumed to be at the basis of a condition known in boxers as "*punch drunk*." The condition is said to be found in at least fifty per cent of mediocre fighters and not commonly found among agile boxers who know how to guard themselves against punishment. Chiefly affected are less expert but courageous fighters who take considerable punishment in a fight or those used for training who are knocked down several times a day. The early symptoms are represented by occasional clumsiness of one foot, slight ataxia, and periods of confusion. In the more severe cases, the legs drag in walking, and tremors, dysarthria, deafness, physical slowing, and even mental deterioration requiring commitment to an institution may supervene. In some instances, a progressive neurological disorder develops leading to mental or physical helplessness.

9

Syphilis of the Brain

I. INTRODUCTORY

Neurosyphilis constitutes an important and frequent cause of nervous disorder. The spinal cord types have already been considered. Classification of the various forms of neurosyphilis is unsatisfactory because of many transitions and ill-defined forms. No single classification covers all the possibilities, but the following grouping constitutes a useful working basis:

1. *Meningeal syphilis:*
   Latent syphilitic meningitis
   Acute syphilitic meningitis
   Chronic syphilitic meningitis
2. *Vascular syphilis:*
   Cerebral vascular syphilis (Heubner)
   Syphilitic endarteritis
3. *Meningovascular syphilis (cerebrospinal syphilis)*
4. *Parenchymatous syphilis:*
   General paresis
   Taboparesis
   Juvenile paresis
   Syphilitic optic atrophy
5. *Asymptomatic neurosyphilis*

Invasion of the nervous system generally takes place during the first two years of the disease or not at all (Ford and Stokes).

II. MENINGEAL SYPHILIS

Syphilis involving the meninges may assume the following forms: (1) Latent, (2) acute, (3) chronic.

1. Latent

Latent syphilitic meningitis is found in many cases of syphilis during the secondary stages (twenty-five to forty per cent), but may be found also during the primary stage of the disease. It is, as a rule, asymptomatic, but may be disclosed by lumbar puncture, which reveals an increase of cells in the spinal fluid, always lymphocytes, without evidence of a positive Wassermann reaction of the fluid. In some instances there may be headache and neck stiffness. This form of syphilitic meningitis has no clinical significance save to indicate that syphilis attacks the nervous system early in the course of the disease.

2. Chronic

The *chronic form* of syphilitic meningitis is seen as part of general paresis or tabes. It is found also in localized form as an arachnoiditis, at times involving the optic chiasm in syphilitic optic atrophy.

3. Acute

Etiology: This is an important form of meningeal syphilis, but it is comparatively rare, its incidence being estimated at about 1.6 to 2.4 per cent of cases of neurosyphilis. It occurs with greatest frequency in the early stages of syphilis when it is found in the latent form usually without symptoms. The well-pronounced type to be described below is found chiefly in the later stages. It may occur at any age. Females are affected a little less than males, and races of all sorts may be afflicted. It is difficult to estimate carefully the time of occurrence of the meningitis after the primary infection. It may occur at any time after in-

427

fection, but the majority of cases occur within one year of the initial infection (Merritt and Moore). Cases may develop several years after the initial infection, they may be found in congenital syphilis, and they may develop as a complication of tabes dorsalis and general paresis.

Pathology: The meningeal infiltration is largely basilar in distribution, but it may spread over the convexities as well, or be confined to the convexities alone. In a typical instance, the pia-arachnoid over the midbrain, pons, and medulla is thickened, has a whitish gray appearance and is adherent to the underlying brain stem structure. In the meshes of the meninges are numerous lymphocytes and plasma cells which usually infiltrate the blood vessel walls as well. The exudate is often not confined to the meninges, but extends into the brain tissue, where it is seen as collections of lymphocytes and plasma cells in both the gray and white matter of the brain stem or cerebrum. Syphilitic meningitis is therefore a meningoencephalitis. The cranial nerves at the base of the brain are often infiltrated and are the seat of an interstitial neuritis. Of these, the optic, oculomotor, trigeminal, auditory, and hypoglossal nerves may be involved. Associated with the basilar meningitis is often an acute external hydrocephalus due to the involvement of the lateral recesses by the syphilitic process and the failure of spinal fluid to escape by the foramina of Luschka and Magendie.

Symptoms: The symptoms of the disorder are striking. The onset is usually acute or subacute. *Headache* is constant and usually very severe, due both to the meningitis and its accompanying hydrocephalus. It is often more severe than the headache of brain tumor. The development of symptoms is characterized in the majority of cases by a sudden

or relatively sudden onset of headache which may be present for a varying period of time before relief is sought. As a rule, the severity of the headache is such that relief is sought within a relatively short time after its appearance. The headache is felt in the back of the head or it may be frontal. *Nausea* and *vomiting* accompany the headache in almost every case. In some forms, headache, nausea, vomiting, and vertigo are the only symptoms of the disorder. In others there may be in addition a history of convulsions, of sudden loss of power on one side of the body, of disturbance in speech, and of mental symptoms such as confusion, delirium, or psychosis of other forms. In still other instances in which *cranial nerve involvement* is outstanding, the history, in addition to headache, will consist of complaints of sudden onset of ringing in the ears, deafness, paralysis of one side of the face, difficulty in swallowing, difficulty in protrusion of the tongue, all of which may be found in various combinations or all together in a single case. The onset in such cases may be with cranial nerve palsies and little if any headache.

Fever is not a prominent feature of syphilitic meningitis. A low-grade fever is found in most cases during the first part of the illness. High fevers over 101° F. are uncommon, but they occur. *Neck stiffness* is constant and with it may be found other signs of meningeal irritation, such as Kernig's sign. Cranial nerve paralyses are found in many combinations and forms. They may be bilateral or unilateral (fifty per cent) and they may involve a single nerve, two, three, or more nerves. The facial and auditory nerves are most frequently affected, followed next by the optic and oculomotor nerves, after which in order of frequency come the abducens, trigeminal, glossopharyngeal and vagus, hypoglossal, trochlear, olfactory, and spinal accessory nerves. The pupillary reactions are usually normal but Argyll Robertson pupils may be found. Choked disc is found in some cases, usually associated with considerable loss of visual acuity. In some series, the incidence of choked disc has been found to be as high as fifty-nine per cent (Merritt and Moore). Pto-

may be encountered in the form involving the convexities. These may be generalized or focal or of the petit mal variety. Mental dullness is usually present and psychoses may even be encountered.

The blood Wassermann reaction is positive in sixty per cent of cases. The spinal fluid shows an increase of cells

Table 37—Blood and Spinal Fluid Findings in Syphilis of Brain

Disorder	Blood Wassermann	SPINAL FLUID					
		Cells	Protein	Sugar	Chlorides	Wassermann	Colloidal Gold
ACUTE SYPHILITIC MENINGITIS	Positive in 60%	25-200 lymphocytes, usually over 100 (75%)	Increased	Normal or decreased	Normal or decreased	Positive in 90%	Any type but commonest forms 5555432100 1123321000
VASCULAR NEUROSYPHILIS	Positive in about 50%	0-100 lymphocytes	Increased or normal	Normal	Normal	Positive but may be negative even with 1 cc. of fluid	Variable
GENERAL PARESIS	Positive in 90%	0-200 lymphocytes; average 25-50 cells	Increased	Normal	Normal	Positive with 0.05-0.2 c.c. of fluid in 95% and with larger amounts in remainder	5555432100 5432100000 5555555555 4444321000

sis of one or both eyelids, and paresis or paralysis of one or several ocular nerves may be seen, resulting in strabismus or ophthalmoplegias of varying degree. The corneal reflex may be absent. Tinnitus, deafness, and vertigo are often found. Peripheral facial paralysis may be present, as well as dysphagia, dysarthria, and lingual weakness. Hemiparesis or hemiplegia and aphasia are sometimes found, as well as other evidences of invasion of the brain or brain stem. Convulsions

(twenty-five to two hundred, all lymphocytes); the Wassermann reaction of the spinal fluid is positive in about ninety per cent of cases; the globulin and protein are increased, and the colloidal gold curve is often abnormal though it has no specific features (5555432100 in fifty per cent; midzone and other curves, fifty per cent). The sugar content is normal or slightly reduced and the same is true of the chlorides. In those cases in which the Wassermann reaction of the spinal fluid is normal, other features of the spinal fluid are abnormal. The spinal fluid Wassermann may be positive with 0.1 cc. of spinal fluid, but is often negative in dilutions of less than 0.5 cc. Entirely normal spinal fluids are extremely rare.

Diagnosis: The diagnosis of acute syphilitic meningitis is not difficult in the majority of instances. The presenting symptom is severe headache, with which are combined nausea and vomiting in most cases, and in many others a combination of complaints referable to involvement of the cranial nerves—facial paralysis, tinnitus, deafness, and vertigo, loss of vision, diplopia, and a number of other difficulties. Examination in such instances reveals evidence of meningeal irritation (neck stiffness, Kernig's sign) in all instances. Save for the meningeal findings, and choked discs, nothing more may be found in one group of cases of acute syphilitic meningitis, referred to as *acute syphilitic hydrocephalus*, characterized by severe progressive headache, nausea, vomiting, and choked disc. Cases of this sort may be difficult to separate from *brain tumor*, but the spinal fluid findings will be conclusive. The remaining cases may be divided into two large groups: those in which the signs are largely *cerebral* (convulsions, hemiplegia, aphasia), and those in which there are cranial nerve paralyses due to predominant *basilar* involvement of the brain. The cases characterized by cerebral symptoms are in reality instances of meningovascular syphilis with syphilitic endarteritis of the cerebral vessels associated with the meningitis. The cranial nerves may be unilaterally or bilaterally affected; and may be affected in varying combinations.

Though any conceivable combination is possible, studies of large groups of cases

of the *basilar form* of syphilitic meningitis reveal a tendency to fall into three main groups: (1) interpeduncular (optic and oculomotor nerves); (2) cerebellopontine angle (facial and auditory); (3) bulbar (vagus, spinal accessory, and hypoglossal).

Regardless of the type of presenting clinical picture, lumbar puncture will usually be performed because of the meningeal signs and will disclose evidence of syphilis. The blood Wassermann is unreliable as an index of diagnosis, since it is negative in 40 per cent of cases.

Not all cases of acute syphilitic meningitis present the same type of problem in differential diagnosis. In those patients with meningeal signs and cranial nerve paralyses, the problem is that of differentiation of those conditions which may produce a basilar lymphocytic meningitis — tuberculous meningitis, lymphocytic choriomeningitis, poliomyelitis, infectious mononucleosis, etc. These have been considered in the discussion of tuberculous meningitis.

The problem of diagnosis of acute syphilitic meningitis involving the cerebral hemispheres presents more difficulties than the basilar form. The diagnosis of syphilitic meningitis may not be so easily reached, but since spinal fluid studies will be indicated by the persistent headache, the convulsions which may be focal, and the meningeal signs, the diagnosis will often be established by this means. The progressive course with headache, convulsions, and focal brain symptoms, such as hemiplegia and aphasia, resembles closely *brain tumor*, especially if choked disc is present. Tumor may be differentiated by the persistently elevated spinal fluid pressure, by the evidence of syphilis in the spinal fluid findings, and by the response of the symptoms to antisyphilitic treatment.

Syphilis and tumor may, however, co-exist in rare instances. The possibility of solitary *cerebral gumma* must be considered seriously in the cerebral cases with focal symptoms. Gumma is rare and in any event is essentially a neoplasm requiring operative removal; hence the problem is in reality that of a brain tumor with positive serological reactions.

Those cases with a *cerebellopontine angle syndrome* consisting of headache, tinnitus, deafness, facial paralysis, present special problems and require differentiation from angle tumor. This can be accomplished by the absence of characteristic Barany findings, by the absence of signs of increased intracranial pressure, and by the presence of the evidences of syphilis in the spinal fluid.

Treatment: Syphilitic meningitis is one form of neurosyphilis which responds well to *penicillin*. For this form of central nervous system syphilis, it is safe to use penicillin alone unless there is danger of loss of vision or unless the symptoms of acute syphilitic hydrocephalus fail to improve. Penicillin (crystalline penicillin G) should be given in doses of 10,000,000 to 14,000,000 units over a period of ten to fourteen days. In most instances, the symptoms will clear up satisfactorily, and the spinal fluid findings will be reversed.

The results of treatment are often dramatic, both symptoms and signs responding well within a few treatments with sudden clearing of headache and cranial nerve paralyses. In other cases, the symptoms clear more slowly but completely and in still others they fail to recede by routine treatment with trivalent arsenic, requiring fever therapy for their complete removal. Serological reversal occurs in sixty to eighty per cent of cases. Adequate treatment arrests the disease; patients inadequately treated frequently develop later evidence of neurosyphilis.

III. VASCULAR SYPHILIS

Several forms of vascular neurosyphilis are known. Most of these are of greater pathological than clinical interest. The form of greatest practical importance is that of syphilitic endarteritis of the larger cerebral vessels (Heubner). Other types, such as syphilitic endarteritis of the small cerebral vessels, chronic syphilitic vascular disease, and syphilitic arteriosclerosis, are only of interest from a pathological viewpoint and are associated with no distinctive clinical features. Syphilis involving the cerebral blood vessels may develop in association with meningitis (meningovascular syphilis) or in a chronic form without meningeal reaction. The former has already been considered in the cerebral form of acute syphilitic meningitis.

Etiology: Vascular neurosyphilis develops chiefly in young subjects with an average age of thirty to thirty-five years, well outside the age incidence of arteriosclerosis. The incidence of this form of neurosyphilis is difficult to ascertain, but it probably constitutes about three to five per cent of all forms of neurosyphilis. Moore gives the incidence of vascular neurosyphilis as 1.3 per cent among white males, 0.3 per cent in white females, 2.4 per cent among colored males, and 0.6 per cent among colored females. Males appear to be more susceptible than females, but in a proportion much less than that found in parenchymatous neurosyphilis such as general paresis. It may develop at any time during the course of the disease, both early and late, but it is preponderant during the first five to seven years after infection.

The larger arteries of the brain and pia are usually affected by the process which when fully developed occludes the vessel lumen. It is characterized by infiltration of the vessel adventitia by lymphocytes, fibrous proliferation of the intima with splitting of the elastica, and endothelial proliferation. The media usually escapes, but in some cases may show atrophy and even infiltration. Meningeal

set varying from thirty or thirty-five years to fifty-five years. Vascular hypertension is usually present, and syphilitic vascular disease is found in the majority of cases in the form of syphilitic aortitis and an enlarged heart (thirty-five per cent). The symptoms are those of vascu-

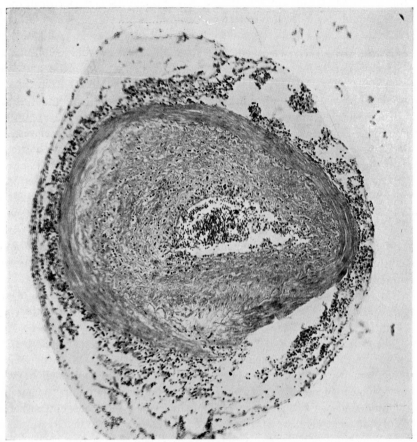

Fig. 122—*Syphilitic vascular disease,* showing the Heubner form of syphilitic endarteritis involving the middle cerebral artery. Note the infiltration of the adventitia and the almost complete occlusion of the vessel lumen.

infiltration is often present in the acute stages, but is not found in the chronic forms. Foci of lymphocytic and plasma cell infiltration in the brain may be found in some cases. Softening of the brain tissue is found in the area supplied by the occluded vessel.

Symptoms: Young male adults are most commonly affected, the age of on-

lar occlusion. The onset is usually gradual, extending over a period of days, weeks, or months, with complaints of light-headedness, dizziness, or headache extending over long periods. These prodromal symptoms are succeeded by those due to actual occlusion of the affected vessel. There is, therefore, a history of either sudden loss of power affecting one side of the body, of a gradual loss of power involving first one part and extending to others over a period of hours until an entire side is paralyzed, or of sudden or gradual loss of speech or vision depending upon the areas involved.

The evidence of occlusion of a cerebral vessel by cerebral vascular syphilis is shown by the gradual or sudden loss of consciousness, the actual onset depending on the rapidity of vessel occlusion. In cases with gradual onset mental confusion or transitory loss of consciousness may develop and the symptoms progress over several hours. In rapidly developing cases the onset is sudden and apoplectic, the patient falling into unconsciousness wherever he may be. The signs depend upon the specific vessel which is occluded. Hemiplegia is the most common manifestation, due to occlusion of a branch of the middle cerebral artery in the internal capsule. Aphasia, convulsions, hemianopsia, and other evidences of focal damage may be found. The pupillary reactions usually show no deviation from the normal, but irregular, sluggishly reacting pupils and Argyll Robertson pupils may be found.

Any of the syndromes found in vascular disease from other causes may be encountered in cerebral vascular syphilis (v. Vascular Disease).

The blood serology is positive in fifty per cent of cases. The spinal fluid pressure is increased in the acute stages, but is normal later. The cell count is usually normal, but may be increased (fifty to one hundred lymphocytes). The globulin content is increased. The Wassermann reaction of the spinal fluid is positive in nearly all cases with large amounts of spinal fluid. The colloidal gold reaction is often negative, but may show nonspecific variations from the normal in the form of a paretic curve or other abnormalities. There is considerable difference of opinion concerning the incidence of negative spinal fluid reactions in vascular neurosyphilis, but there is no doubt that this form of central nervous system syphilis may be encountered with a negative special fluid Wassermann.

Diagnosis: The *diagnosis* is not difficult. The picture is usually that of a young adult who has developed a vascular accident often with hypertension, sometimes without it, with a history of syphilis, evidences of syphilitic cardiovascular disease, signs of focal brain damage, and changes in the blood and spinal fluid indicative of syphilis. The serological reactions, however, are not dependable, since they are frequently negative. It is important to recognize the fact that this form of syphilis may be associated with a negative Wassermann reaction of both the blood and spinal fluid, in which case the diagnosis must depend on other evidences of syphilis such as irregular, sluggish pupils, syphilitic vascular disease, etc.

The condition must be differentiated from hypertensive disease; this can usually be done on the basis of the serological reactions and the absence of evidences of syphilis.

Treatment: *Penicillin* should be used in all cases in doses of 10,000,000 to 14,000,000 units over a period of 10 to 14 days. This may be repeated as indicated. The results of treatment with penicillin are not as satisfactory as in other forms of neurosyphilis. Some of the older forms of treatment may be necessary for this reason. *Heavy metals* such as mercury, bismuth, and iodides may be used. Large doses of iodides (50 to 75 grains three times daily) by mouth are desirable. Mercury may be given as daily inunctions until signs of mercury intoxication appear (tenderness of gums, etc.), as injections of soluble mercury (succinimide, $\frac{1}{6}$ grain to ¼ grain) given three to five times a week, or as mercury salicylate in weekly injections. Bismuth may be given weekly in the form of the insoluble salt, or it may be given as aqueous soluble bismuth two or three times a week. All treatments should be continued for long periods as long as there is clinical indication for their use.

age of cases. Its incidence has been variously estimated; it occurs in about ten per cent of cases of syphilis. About two per cent of cases of general paresis are instances of juvenile paresis. It is possible that the incidence of general paresis and of other forms of neurosyphilis may become decreased as a result of the penicillin treatment of primary syphilis.

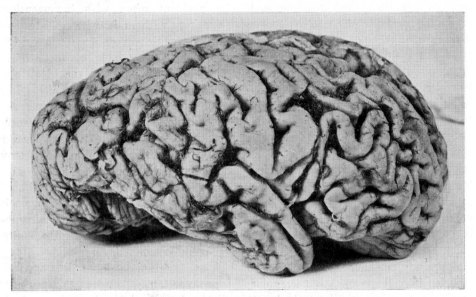

Fig. 123—*General paresis. (See: Fig. 124.)*

The outlook in cases of syphilitis endarteritis (Heubner) is good as to outcome from the acute episode. It is poor as a rule as to recovery from the hemiplegia or other evidence of focal brain damage. Treatment does little to reopen the occluded vessels. Some patients, however, recover wholly or in part. Generally speaking, however, the outlook for recovery of function is not good.

IV. GENERAL PARESIS (*General Paralysis of the Insane; Dementia Paralytica; Paresis*)

Etiology: General paresis is the most important of the cerebral forms of neurosyphilis. It is caused by the Treponema pallidum, which can be demonstrated in the brain of paretics in a large percent-

It is too early to state definitely whether this is the case. The *sex* distribution favors men by far in a ratio of about three to five to one. The reason for the preponderance of general paresis in men is not known. It has been suggested that pregnancy protects against the development of paresis in women. Whether the difference in glandular construction is a factor of importance is not yet known. It has been found that the excess of males over females is much less marked when general paresis develops before the childbearing period. The ratio of primary syphilitic infection favors males in a ratio of about two to one, a proportion far below that of the incidence of general paresis.

The *age* of onset of the disease varies, its greatest incidence being from thirty to fifty years (sixty-five per cent), the age of greatest activity and productivity in man. Cases may develop in younger subjects, but instances of development of paresis before twenty-five years of age must be regarded as juvenile paresis unless proved otherwise. Onsets between sixty and seventy years are uncommon but are known. Acquired cases have been found in subjects as young as twenty-two and as old as seventy-nine years of age. The onset is much earlier in cases of juvenile paresis, the average age being thirteen years, but rare instances of juvenile paresis have been reported at twenty-five years of age or slightly older. The *latent period* between the original infection and the onset of general paresis varies from ten to twenty years and averages about fifteen years. Cases are known in which latencies under five years were present despite

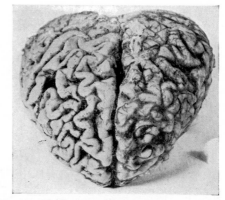

Fig. 124—*General paresis.* The meninges have been stripped away from the cortex, showing the cortical atrophy and the wide separation of the gyri.

vigorous treatment, and others have been reported of less than one year, though these are rare. Latencies of thirty years or more have also been described.

The reason for the *susceptibility* of some cases to general paresis while others escape is not known. Various ideas have been advanced, among them being

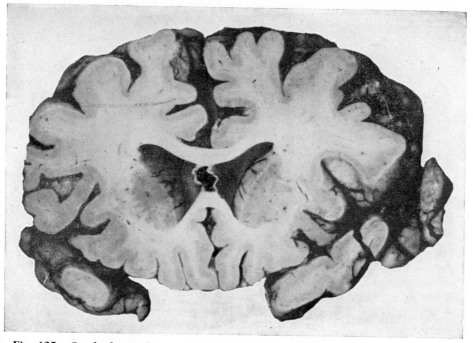

Fig. 125—*Cerebral atrophy* in general paresis, demonstrated by the wide separation of the gyri.

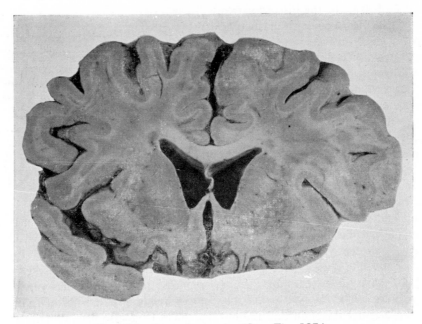

Fig. 126—*General paresis.* *(See: Fig. 127.)*

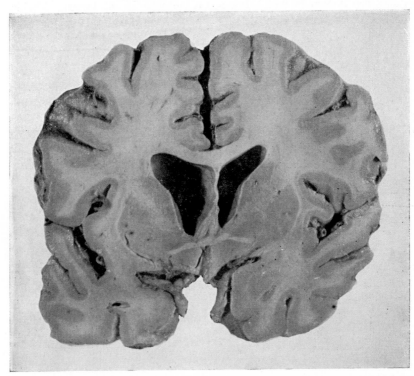

Fig. 127—*General paresis,* showing a cross section of the brain with atrophy of the gyri as shown by their separation and atrophy of the white matter revealed by the dilatation of the ventricles.

a constitutional susceptibility, the nature of which cannot be defined; a neurotropic tendency on the part of the spirochete, or a special neurotropic form of the organism which attacks the nervous system in cases infected by this form. There is evidence to support this hypothesis, but there is also much evidence opposed to it. Thus, pure neurotrope forms are hard to find, since other

rence of general paresis to occupation have been unsuccessful, as have efforts to demonstrate that it is more prone to occur in those who use their minds rather than their hands, or in those of unstable emotional construction, particularly neurotics.

General paresis may attack any *race*. It is common in the white race and for a long time was thought to be unusual

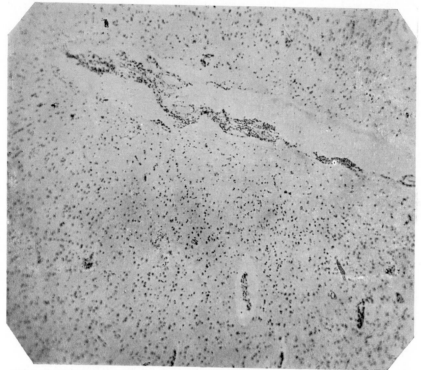

Fig. 128—*General paresis.* The infiltration of the meninges, the loss of the orderly lamination of the frontal cortex, and the perivascular infiltration are clearly shown.

parts of the body are attacked by this form, while the dermatrope form invades the nervous system in a large percentage of cases early in the secondary stages. Instances are on record of the development of paretic neurosyphilis or of tabes in cases which were infected from the same source. While these and other findings are suggestive they do not prove conclusively that general paresis results from a special neurotropic strain of treponema. Attempts to link the occur-

among the dark races. It has been shown to occur commonly, however, among Negroes, Chinese, Hawaiians, Arabs, and others. Contrary to the usual belief, neurosyphilis is not rare in the tropics. The application of modern clinical and laboratory methods indicates a neurosyphilis rate of 20 per cent among unselected cases (Cook).

Pathology: General paresis is a meningoencephalitis of syphilitic origin. It involves all parts of the brain and even attacks the spinal cord. While the cerebrum is most affected by the disease, the subcortical structures do not escape. The frontal and temporal lobes are most involved and within these, specific areas are more affected than others, but other parts of the cortex are also affected. Subcortical structures are commonly affected, usual, however, for no weight loss to be found. The dura is thickened and adherent to the inner table of the skull. The pia-arachnoid is thickened and often adherent to the underlying brain tissue. It is more involved over the frontal areas than elsewhere, but may be thickened over the entire brain. The cortex is

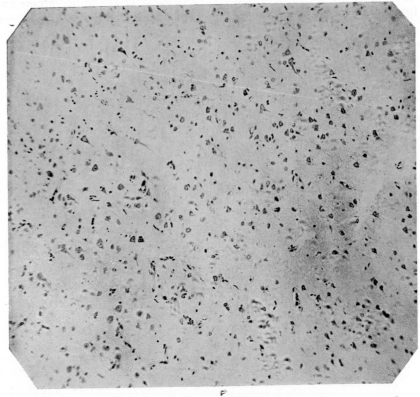

Fig. 129 — *General paresis.* High power view of the frontal cortex to show the disorderly arrangement of the ganglion cells.

among them being the striatum, pallidum, and hypothalamic region. The brain stem structures, such as midbrain, pons, and medulla, are not much involved in the typical case. The cerebellum is not often affected except in juvenile paresis. The optic nerves are involved in a small percentage of cases.

The brain of general paresis is decreased in size, weighing 100 to 1000 grams less than normal. It is not unatrophied, especially in the frontal lobes, but no atrophy may be present in some cases. There is also atrophy of the subcortical white matter, with a concomitant internal hydrocephalus of mild degree. Granular ependymitis is found in all cases, especially in the floor of the fourth ventricle. Syphilitic aortitis is found in at least thirty-five per cent of cases.

The cerebral cortex shows typically an

infiltration of the pia-arachnoid with lymphocytes and plasma cells, varying in degree from case to case. The cortical architecture is greatly disturbed and wind-blown in severe cases and moderately disordered in others, the ganglion cells being disarranged, and often diseased and reduced in number. The microglial cells are hypertrophied in the form of rod cells and the astrocytes increased, producing a definite gliosis. The cortical capillaries are increased in number. Perivascular infiltration with lymphocytes and plasma cells is found in varying degrees, being marked in some cases and mild in others. Granules of iron are found in the microglial cells. The white matter shows perivascular infiltration in varying degree, gliosis, and small areas of demyelination, giving it a moth-eaten appearance. Spirochetes may be demonstrated in many cases in the cortex. Vascular changes, such as the endarteritis of Heubner, are found rarely in paresis and are not part of the characteristic picture of the disease. The spinal cord may show demyelination, especially in the posterior and lateral columns.

Symptoms: The onset of symptoms in general paresis is usually gradual. A history of primary infection is often not obtained. The so-called prodromal symptoms consist of the gradual and insidious development of nonspecific complaints, which are difficult to connect with paresis unless the physician is on his guard against them. Neurotic symptoms of various sorts may develop slowly in a person not prone to such complaints. Easy fatigue, excessive anxiety, apprehension, somatic complaints of various sorts, may appear without awareness on the patient's part that they occur. Slight difficulties in concentration and memory may develop and be dismissed as inconsequential until they become more pronounced. Loss of memory for names, the location of familiar objects, and difficulties in simple arithmetical problems may be found. The memory for recent experiences is more impaired than that for remote events. Mild changes in personality develop, consisting among other things of irritability, impairment of judgment in personal and business problems, depression, or a sense of well-being. The number of symptoms referable to the changes in personality noted in general paresis may be multiplied greatly. The essential kernel is that the symptoms which develop are abnormal for the personality of the patient; hence the particular manifestations vary greatly. Reversal of character, such as pilfering or lying, philandering, and other traits, may appear. These are often unnoticed even by those close to the patient, so slight may they be.

The *onset* in not a few cases is sudden. Convulsions in an adult with no previous history of epilepsy may usher in the disease. An acute psychotic episode may be the first overt manifestation of the disorder. In other cases, the disease may be ushered in by a sudden loss of power on one side of the body, with disappearance of the hemiparesis or hemiplegia in the course of a few days. In some instances, the onset is associated with an injury to the head. The probabilities are that in such cases general paresis was present, was either asymptomatic or produced only mild symptoms to which no attention was paid, and that the process was activated by the head injury.

In the well-established phases of the disease, the symptoms are easily recognized. *Mental symptoms* of various sorts and degrees are found. In some cases, these are severe and dominate the picture; in others, they are slight. Many sorts of mental pictures may develop so that general paresis may be associated with any form of psychosis. The *deterio-*

rated form is common and is characterized by mental confusion and disorientation, loss of memory, loss of mathematical capacity even for simple problems, impairment of judgment, and loss of ability to concentrate. Patients with this form are careless and slovenly in appearance and habits. Delusional formations are common. Other types of mental reactions consist of *agitated, depressed, euphoric,* and *excited* types. These are self-explanatory for the most part. Euphoria is found in many paretics, but is not always present. It may consist of a sense of well-being out of all proportion to the patient's condition, or may be associated with delusions of grandeur often of a very flowery nature. Facetiousness is often present to a severe degree.

In some cases, the evidences of psychosis are few, but signs of mental impairment can be seen in the presence of euphoria, memory disturbances, and other features of decreased mental function.

The *neurological findings* in general paresis are not many, but when taken with the symptoms and the mental picture are quite characteristic. Pupillary changes are often found. The Argyll Robertson pupil is found in thirty-five to forty per cent of cases. Irregular and sluggishly reacting pupils are common, and normal reacting pupils are not uncommon (ten per cent). Tremors of the eyelids, lips, tongue, face, and fingers appear constantly. The speech is poorly enunciated and is referred to as slurred. In early cases, the difficulty in enunciation may be so slight as to escape the attention of intelligent patients; in advanced cases, there is severe slurring both on spontaneous speech and test phrases. Many types of test phrases may be used to bring out the slurring: "Truly rural; Massachusetts artillery; third riding artillery brigade; Methodist Episcopal;

particular statistics," etc. The tendon reflexes are generally hyperactive. The handwriting is tremulous. Optic atrophy is found in a small group of cases (five per cent). Ocular palsies are found at times. Evidences of spinal cord involvement, especially of the posterior and lateral columns, are encountered. Convulsions are found in a small percentage of cases and may be the first symptom of the disease which the patient recognizes. They are usually generalized and indistinguishable from ordinary epileptic attacks. Transient attacks of hemiplegia, hemiparesis, monoplegia, or monoparesis are not uncommon. The attacks of weakness or paralysis last a few hours to a few days and invariably clear up. Attacks of aphasia of a transitory character are also seen at times.

General paresis is characterized by the occurrence of remissions (two to ten per cent) which appear suddenly either with or without treatment and disappear as suddenly as they develop. They may last six months to a year or for several years, are often terminated by a convulsion, and are followed as a rule by rapid deterioration.

Atypical Forms of Paresis: General paresis appears not only as typical paresis but in atypical forms as well. Of these, *Lissauer's paresis* is best known. This is a form of the disease with focal manifestations, such as aphasia, focal convulsions, hemiplegia, hemianopsia, etc. These are the result of a greater confinement of the disease to a single area of the brain in contrast to the more widespread character of typical paresis. The onset is at any age and is likely to be abrupt.

Juvenile paresis is a congenital form of general paresis with similar pathological and clinical features as the adult form of the disease save that it has a tendency to affect the cerebellum more severely than the adult form. The onset is usually at an average age of thirteen years but it may develop from twelve to nineteen years of age. The symptoms and signs of the disease are those of adult paresis, but mental symptoms, such as rapid deterioration or failure to develop mentally, are outstanding. The blood Wassermann reaction is positive in ninety per cent of cases, and the spinal fluid findings are as follows: cells, ten to 250 lymphocytes; globulin increased in amount; Wassermann reaction, one hundred per cent positive; colloidal gold curve almost always paretic in type. The outlook both with and without treatment is poor, probably because the condition develops insidiously and much damage has been done before treatment is undertaken.

Senile paresis occurs rarely and is found in persons of sixty to seventy years, thirty or more years after the initial infection. It tends to react poorly to treatment. *Stationary paresis* is a form of the disease which has burned itself out and has developed a complete remission. This form of the disease is uncommon. Pathologically, it shows a relatively normal cerebral cortex or a mild, burned-out meningoencephalitis. The blood and spinal fluid reactions are those of typical paresis. *Galloping paresis* is a very malignant, rapidly developing form of paresis.

Blood, Spinal Fluid, and Other Laboratory Findings: The Wassermann reaction of the blood is positive in ninety per cent of untreated subjects. The spinal fluid examination shows consistent abnormalities. The cells are increased in number (twenty-five to two hundred or more lymphocytes); the globulin is increased and the total protein high; the Wassermann reaction is positive in one hundred per cent of patients, even with small amounts of spinal fluid; the colloidal gold reaction is the typical first zone or paretic curve (5555543210). Variations in the spinal fluid findings occur; the cells may be normal in number or only slightly increased, and the colloidal gold reaction may not show a strong paretic type of reaction. It is important to recognize the fact that the paretic type of curve is not pathognomonic of general paresis. It is found in other forms of neurosyphilis (tabes, cerebral vascular syphilis, syphilitic meningitis, asymptomatic neurosyphilis), and in unrelated conditions, such as multiple sclerosis, tuberculous meningitis, and brain tumor.

The spinal fluid is said to show a negative Wassermann reaction and to be normal in rare cases of general paresis. The diagnosis under such conditions is hazardous, and the contention has not been supported by post-mortem studies.

The electroencephalogram (EEG) has been found to be abnormal in many but not in all instances of general paresis. No typical EEG has been found in cases of paresis. The EEG may show improvement in treated cases or may remain unchanged.

Changes in the spinal fluid formula are found after treatment with penicillin alone or combined with malaria. These consist of an early decrease in the number of cells and protein to normal in most cases. This is followed by a gradual flattening of the colloidal gold curve, the slowest response being the reduction of positivity of the complement fixation reaction. Persistence of the positive Wassermann reaction does not indicate impending relapse, but its persistence after eighteen to twenty-four months of treatment indicates persistent activity. Reversal of the Wassermann reaction occurs in malarial and penicillin treatment and in tryparsamide therapy. The colloidal gold curve is changed from the paretic to other types, but is reversed to complete normal in a smaller number of instances.

Table 38—Differential Diagnosis of General Paresis

Disease	Age	Sex	Onset	Physical Signs	Spinal Fluid	Course
GENERAL PARESIS	30 to 50	Males 3 to 5:1	Gradual usually, with memory impairment, personality changes, impairment of intellectual function. Later psychosis. Acute at times with convulsions, paresis, paralysis	Pupils irregular, sluggish or at times Argyll Robertson. Tremors eyelids, face, lips, tongue, fingers. Speech slurred. Overactive reflexes. Psychosis or organic deterioration	Cells 10 to 200 Wassermann positive Colloidal gold 5555432100	Progressive deterioration, psychosis; death in average case in 2 to 3 years
ALCOHOLIC ENCEPHALOPATHY	Adults	Males more than females	Gradual, with memory loss, difficulties in concentration, personality changes and intellectual deterioration. History of alcoholic excess of long standing	Pupils may be irregular and react sluggishly. Tremors face, tongue, hands. Speech slurred. Reflexes decreased, overactive or absent	No changes of significance	Gradual deterioration
CEREBRAL ARTERIOSCLEROSIS	60 or more	No preponderance in either sex	Gradual with evidences of intellectual impairment; memory loss, disturbance of concentration. Delusional formations	Retinal arteriosclerosis. Evidences of intellectual loss	No changes of significance	Gradual, progressive deterioration
BRAIN TUMOR FRONTAL	Any age	No preponderance	Gradual with difficulties in concentration and memory. At times personality change. Headache	Choked disc. Often nothing else. Hemiparesis or aphasia at times	Spinal fluid pressure elevated	Progressive with headache, increasing pressure and death
IDIOPATHIC EPILEPSY	Childhood puberty as a rule. Adults not infrequently	No significant preponderance	Usually long standing history of convulsions with no reference to significant physical factor or activities	No significant signs. Abnormal electroencephalogram	No changes of significance	Continuance of convulsions over years
LEAD ENCEPHALOPATHY	Children and Adults	No significant preponderance	Sudden with convulsions, headache. Gradual with intellectual deterioration	Evidences of lead poisoning clinically and by laboratory tests. Choked disc at times. Signs of organic deterioration. Cerebellar signs at times	No changes of significance	Gradual progression
MULTIPLE SCLEROSIS	19 to 30	No preponderance	Varied, with blurred vision, weakness of legs, incoördination, etc. Convulsions in small percentage of cases. Remissions in many cases	Pallor of discs, intention tremor, slowed speed, pyramidal tract, cerebellar, and posterior column signs in varying degree	5555432100 not infrequently	Gradual progression, with remissions, but not in early instances
BROMIDISM	Adults	No preponderance	Gradual, with symptoms of intellectual impairment and confusion	Sluggish pupils, dysarthria, confusion, decreased reflexes	Often an increase of protein	Improvement on withdrawal of drug

It is believed by some that the cell count and protein content of the spinal fluid are the best index of arrest of the disease process (Dattner), while others look on the Wassermann response as the best guide.

Diagnosis: The problem of general paresis is presented to the physician in many guises. Patients may appear with a well-pronounced psychosis as the first indication of difficulties, a psychosis which may assume many forms and is associated with evidences of organic mental deterioration of varying degree. They may present themselves also with symptoms of neurosis or of mild personality deviations; or they may appear first with a history of convulsions or transient pareses in a previously healthy person. The point of greatest significance is the appearance of symptoms of emotional, personality, and intellectual deviations associated with evidence of organic brain disease, and with specific changes in the spinal fluid formula.

The diagnosis of general paresis in a well-developed case is not difficult. The history of memory loss, difficulties in intellectual function, changes in personality and character, and evidence of psychosis, together with the pupillary changes, the tremor, the slurred speech, the hyperreflexia, and the objective evidences of mental impairment or psychosis make the diagnosis possible even without blood and spinal fluid studies. With confirmation by these studies, the condition is clearly established. The majority of patients entering mental institutions have a well-defined syndrome, for the most part easily recognizable. Such patients are hospitalized because of the psychosis which is usually well advanced at the time of confinement, but which can be found to have developed gradually before hospitalization became necessary. Cases seen first in office practice, how-

ever, are more difficult to recognize because of the early symptoms which are never as definite as those of the advanced case.

Early diagnosis is essential in order to offer the best possibilities for treatment. It is important, therefore, to recognize the disease in its prodromal or less advanced stages. The occurrence of neurotic traits without exciting cause in a previously well-adjusted person, slight change in judgment, deviations from the ordinary social amenities, the development of coarse traits, excessive fatigue, disturbance of concentration or memory, must all excite suspicion. They are often so slight as to be dismissed without serious consideration and are likely to be discarded as manifestations of neurosis. A social history obtained from other members of the family or from friends may be helpful in suspicious cases. Unexplained deviations from normal behavior and character must always lead to the suspicion that general paresis may be present. The occurrence of the symptoms mentioned should lead to investigation for evidences of organic brain disease. In those patients in whom the history reveals clearly that there has been a deviation from the normal in emotional and social adjustments and intellectual functions, studies of the blood and spinal fluid are indicated for evidence of syphilis. It is far better to err on the side of safety than to overlook a single instance of early general paresis during a period in which treatment is hopeful.

General paresis must be suspected in adults who develop convulsions without a previous history of fits; in instances in which transient hemiplegia or hemiparesis develops; and in persons with rapidly developing psychosis of an organic type. A social history will support the possibility of paresis in such cases, and further confirmation will be derived from the presence of tremors, overactive reflexes, slurred speech, and spinal fluid studies.

Alcoholic encephalopathy may not only simulate the mental features of general paresis but may show all the physical features as well. A history of alcoholism is always obtainable and the negative Wassermann reactions of blood and spinal fluid in an untreated patient will settle the diagnosis.

Cerebral arteriosclerosis may simulate paresis closely and may be confused with senile paresis. The presence of retinal arteriosclerosis, the age of onset, and the negative serological reactions are helpful in differentiation.

Frontal lobe tumor may simulate paresis due to the evidences of organic deterioration found in some cases, but the history of headaches and the signs of increased intracranial pressure will establish the diagnosis of tumor. Because of the occurrence of convulsions in some cases of paresis and its onset with convulsive attacks in some cases, it may be confused with *epilepsy* or with a number of other conditions which produce convulsions. Among these are *lead encephalopathy,* which will usually show evidence of lead poisoning in the blood smear, serum, or urine, and give a history of exposure to lead. *Uremia* is differentiated readily by the presence of nitrogen retention and evidences of kidney damage.

Multiple sclerosis has been confused at times with paresis because of the euphoria, the slurred speech, the remissions, and the presence of a paretic type of colloidal gold curve. The onset in a relatively young person, the signs of scattered involvement of the brain and spinal cord (ataxia, cerebellar signs, pyramidal tract disease) and the negative Wassermann reactions serve to establish the diagnosis of multiple sclerosis.

Bromidism may simulate general paresis in all details. The symptoms may be very similar and examination may reveal sluggishly reacting pupils, intellectual impairment, confusion, dysarthria and decreased reflexes. A history of the use of bromides is usually obtainable.

Presenile dementia such as Alzheimer's disease may simulate general paresis.

Prognosis: The outlook in general paresis is poor without treatment. Death occurs in two to three years after the disease is manifested in the average case, but some patients may live for five or six years. With treatment, the figures vary with different series. After malarial treatment, complete remissions are obtainable in sixty to eighty per cent of patients if treated within the first year (Freeman, Pfeiffer). These figures, however, are probably too generous; complete remissions develop in thirty to forty per cent of cases after early treatment, and incomplete remissions with residual deterioration in an additional twenty to thirty per cent. The percentage of remissions in combined malaria and penicillin treatment is better than for either of these forms of treatment alone. The results of treatment with penicillin are on the whole good. Improvement by penicillin treatment alone has been recorded in over seventy per cent of the patients, and with combined penicillin and fever therapy in eighty per cent. Affective types appear to have a better prognosis, while demented forms do not respond as well. Remissions drop to ten to twenty per cent or less if the disease has been present ten years or longer. The outlook is better in the manic and euphoric types of paresis and less good, though not bad, in the depressed, simple demented, and paranoid forms. Galloping paresis has a poor outlook.

Treatment: General paresis may be treated by means of (1) drugs or (2) artificial fever. The drug of choice is *penicillin. Artificial fever* may be given as (1) tertian malaria, (2) quartan malaria, (3) heat cabinets of various sorts, and (4) typhoid-paratyphoid vaccine injections.

It is important for good treatment, not only of general paresis but of all forms of neurosyphilis, that the following general principles be recognized: (1) Each case must be handled on its individual merits. General principles of treatment can apply only within broad limits. The duration and type of treatment must be decided upon as an individual problem. (2) It is best to treat the clinical problem as a whole rather than to treat only the serology. There are numerous instances in which the serology has become negative while many clinical symptoms persist; there are other instances in which the clinical symptoms improve or disappear completely in the presence of persistently positive blood and spinal fluid reactions. The laboratory findings must be regarded as only a part of the clinical picture, all aspects of which must be given their proper evaluation. While it is true that in the majority of instances clinical improvement parallels laboratory improvement, this is not always the case. It is true further that in the face of clinical improvement, a persistently positive blood or spinal fluid Wassermann reaction indicates the probability of recurrence of symptoms and further trouble. To this extent, therefore, one must be guided by the laboratory findings in the handling of treatment. One must not be lulled into the false security of believing, however, that reversal of laboratory findings to normal means a disappearance of symptoms. After five years it is generally

believed that a negative spinal fluid will not become positive. Nevertheless, the clinical features are of most importance, since neurosyphilis may be present with a completely negative spinal fluid. (3) Courses of treatment should be dispensed with. The patient should receive treatment as long as he appears to need it. Interrupted course of therapy may do more harm than good.

Penicillin is the most important of the present treatments for general paresis. Opinions at present are divided concerning the question whether penicillin alone is sufficient in the treatment of paresis, whether it should be combined with malarial therapy, and what represent the indications for one form of treatment as opposed to the other. Most investigators agree that penicillin alone should be used in the treatment of general paresis, and some believe that this is the only drug necessary. It should be given in dosages of 20,000,000 to 30,000,000 units, administered by injection of 1 million units in a single dose daily. If penicillin fails to control the symptoms in such cases, fever therapy should be used.

Despite the favorable results obtained with penicillin, fever therapy is necessary in some patients. These include the following: (1) those who fail to react to penicillin, (2) those who are sensitive to penicillin, (3) patients with optic atrophy. The fever of choice is malaria, but typhoid-paratyphoid vaccine may be used. The penicillin and malaria treatments may be carried out simultaneously. The malaria is given as tertian malaria, 10 cc. being injected intravenously or intramuscularly from another paretic patient undergoing treatment or from a patient with malaria. Quartan malaria is less severe and is preferable for Negroes. Before injection is given, care must be taken to insure that the patient is a suitable risk from a cardiorenal standpoint, hence electrocardiograph and renal function studies should be made routinely. *Contraindications* to *treatment* are: vascular hypertension, cardiac failure, cirrhosis of the liver, kidney disease, and edema. It is often necessary, however, to disregard many of these because of the seriousness of the situation. During the period of treatment, the blood count should be taken twice weekly, the urine examined daily, and the nonprotein nitrogen of the blood determined twice weekly.

After malaria is injected, fever and chills develop in five to fourteen days. The fever at the onset often remains elevated for twenty-four to forty-eight hours or longer, but usually develops into the typical tertian rhythm thereafter. In some instances, this may never develop, the fever remaining irregularly elevated throughout the course of the treatment. At least ten chills should be permitted, or preferably a total of 150 hours of fever over 100° F. If the patient is in good condition, the fever may be permitted to continue, since it seems clear that the results are better with longer periods of fever. The fever is terminated by giving quinine by mouth, 10 grains three times a day for three days and 5 grains three times a day for seven to ten days thereafter. Quinine hydrochloride may be given intravenously if the fever must be terminated quickly. The fever of malaria may be terminated with chloroquine diphosphate given as follows: 1 Gm. immediately, followed by 0.5 Gm. in six hours, and 0.5 Gm. each morning for two days. Mapharsen or Atabrine may be administered intravenously under the same circumstances. The malaria must be terminated if the nonprotein nitrogen of the blood exceeds 65 mg., if the blood count falls to two million, or if dehydration or delirium develops. Transfusions may be necessary during the treatment.

The mortality of patients with general paresis treated with malaria has been reported as from five to thirty-five per cent. There has been no mortality in a large series of patients treated (Alpers). The treatment involves a risk, but against this must be weighed the fact that death follows without proper treatment.

Because of the risk involved in malarial treatment some prefer one of the heat cabinets for elevation of temperature. The mortality with this form of induced heat is practically nil, according to its supporters, and the clinical results fully as good.

Typhoid-paratyphoid vaccine may be used in patients who cannot tolerate malaria or the hypertherm machine, but the clinical results are disappointing with this form of fever treatment.

Electrical shock treatment has been used in some cases to combat agitation and depression with reportedly good results.

V. ASYMPTOMATIC NEUROSYPHILIS

In some cases the serological evidences of neurosyphilis develop without any of the clinical symptoms of the disease. These cases are referred to as asymptomatic neurosyphilis and are discovered as a rule by accident during routine examination of the blood or spinal fluid. In the late stages of syphilis, five or more years after infection, asymptomatic neurosyphilis was found in 9.5 per cent of 2263 patients with syphilis; in 670 patients with neurosyphilis, the asymptomatic forms constituted thirty-two per cent (Merritt). They emphasize the importance of routine lumbar puncture in all patients with syphilis, since they indicate the important fact that in some cases neurosyphilis may be present without symptoms. The incidence of asymptomatic neurosyphilis is difficult to compute because relatively few studies have been made of large groups of patients without previous treatment. The discrepancies can be appreciated by a survey of Table 39.

The spinal fluid formula varies. A paretic type of spinal fluid is not un-

Table 39—Incidence of Asymptomatic Neurosyphilis

Author	Number of Patients	Incidence (Per Cent)
MOORE......	352	26.4
FINGER AND KYRLE.....	1699	28.5
MUCHA AND SATKE.....	1166	3.8 (primary stage)
		33.0 (six to twelve months)
		22.8 (two to three years)
		17.2 (three or more years)
LOMHOLT.....	204 Primary	12.0
	693 (secondary)	30.0
	156 (secondary, treated)	42.0
	454 (clinically latent)	30.0

common, and such cases were referred to among the older writers as *paresis sine paresi*. Other types of spinal fluid findings may also be encountered. Moore divides cases of asymptomatic neurosyphilis into three groups, depending on the severity of the spinal fluid findings. Group I includes patients with minimum serological abnormalities (increased cell count and/or globulin content, with other tests negative); Group II, those with fluids of an intermediate type; Group III, those with

maximal change (paretic formula). There is general agreement that spinal fluid changes increase in frequency from the first stage of incubation to the secondary stage, reaching a high point from eight to ten months after infection and then gradually falling off (Mucha and Platzer).

It is to be emphasized that patients with asymptomatic neurosyphilis are entirely symptom-free and are completely unaware of their problem. Despite this, treatment is essential, since if such cases are left to run their own course, active evidences of neurosyphilis will develop in a large percentage of instances. Moore has estimated that in Group II, symptomatic neurosyphilis develops in thirty-five per cent of the patients and in Group III, in seventy-three per cent. In the last group the probabilities favor the development of general paresis or tabes. The younger the patient and the more recent the infection, the more favorable is the prognosis during the first ten years of observation (Holm and Clark). The more strongly positive the initial spinal fluid examination, the less favorable is the prognosis. Spinal fluid improvement is a relative but not an absolute guarantee against clinical progression, and spinal fluid progression is a grave prognostic sign with respect to the development of clinical neurosyphilis.

Treatment: Asymptomatic neurosyphilis has been found to respond well to *penicillin*. For this reason, it is safe to give one or two courses of penicillin; and if the response is unsatisfactory, proceed to other forms of treatment. Penicillin exerts a favorable effect on the spinal fluid of this form of neurosyphilis, both early and late. The cell count is dramatically reduced in ten to twenty-four weeks, the protein in about six months, and the Wassermann reaction and colloidal gold more slowly. The response is better in early than in late asymptomatic neurosyphilis and in the patients with less severe types of reaction. The response is less favorable in those with strongly positive Wassermann reactions of blood and spinal fluid, and with first (paretic) zone colloidal gold curves. For this reason, it is best for the latter type of patient to combine *penicillin* and *malarial* treatment. For the less severe cases, penicillin alone suffices. For the early cases, a dose of 10,000,000 units is usually sufficient given over a period of ten days. The less favorable cases require 20 to 30,000,000 units and one hundred to one hundred fifty hours of malarial fever.

VI. SYPHILITIC OPTIC ATROPHY

Optic atrophy occurs most commonly in neurosyphilis in patients with tabes. It is found also in a small percentage of patients with general paresis and in syphilitic meningitis. Apart from these disorders, it occurs in so-called cerebral syphilis. The atrophy is of the primary type, is associated with severe loss of visual acuity and with scotomas and irregular visual field deformities, such as constriction of the visual fields, but not with hemianopsia.

The atrophy may be the result of an interstitial neuritis (syphilitic) involving the optic nerve or of an arachnoiditis. The evidence favors a neuritis involving the intracranial portion of the optic nerve. *Failure of vision* is quite apparent to the patient, who may complain of gradual visual loss over a long period of time or may develop sudden loss of vision at the onset of illness or after a long period of gradual visual loss. Beyond this, there are, as a rule, no complaints, the loss of vision either overshadowing all other symptoms, or, as is usually the case, being unassociated with other complaints. In patients with paresis, the optic atrophy is associated with other

symptoms of this disorder. The clinical features vary with the condition in which the atrophy develops. In patients with tabes and general paresis, there are well-marked evidences of these disorders. In some patients with tabes, the optic atrophy is associated only with Argyll Robertson pupils, and absent reflexes with no evidence of posterior column disease.

The findings in the blood and spinal fluid are variable and it is important to recognize that syphilitic optic atrophy is one form of neurosyphilis associated with negative serological reactions.

Untreated syphilitic optic atrophy invariably leads to complete blindness. *Blindness* develops in three years in ninety per cent of the subjects (Moore).

The results of treatment of syphilitic optic atrophy are very disappointing. Like tabes, this is an unsatisfactory form of neurosyphilis to treat. Vision can never be returned to normal and is not often improved after treatment. The object of treatment, therefore, is to prevent further advance of the optic atrophy and therefore of blindness and to improve eyesight as much as possible. Patients with unilateral atrophy or with normal or nearly normal visual acuity react best. For these purposes fever treatment is most satisfactory, either in the form of malaria or typhoid-paratyphoid injections. The usual routine treatments by means of arsenicals, mercury, bismuth, and iodides are of no value save as adjuncts to fever therapy. Penicillin has been found to be valuable in the arrest of syphilitic optic atrophy.

VII. GUMMA OF THE BRAIN

Gumma of the brain is rare. It is found in 0.5 per cent of patients with brain tumor (Alpers, Simon). Though its incidence is very low both in brain syphilis and brain tumor, it occurs with sufficient frequency to require recognition of its features.

Gumma is found usually as a solitary lesion in the brain. It is found chiefly in the cerebral hemispheres, but rare instances of gumma involving the hypophysis have been recorded. It is a well-defined, discrete lesion, has a necrotic appearing surface, is hard and fibrous, and histologically has all the features of gumma found elsewhere in the body.

The symptoms simulate those of brain tumor. Headache is the outstanding symptom and is found to be present for a relatively long period, usually several months, by the time relief is sought. This may be the only complaint, or it may be associated with a story of dimness of vision or of failing vision which is usually of relatively recent development and is much less short-lived than the headache. Convulsions, either generalized or focal, are not infrequent, loss or decrease of power over one side of the body, or other focal symptoms may either complete the picture or may be the outstanding complaint. There may be choked disc or optic neuritis, and focal signs, such as hemiplegia, hemianopsia, aphasia, or other focal signs depending upon the area damaged. The blood Wassermann reaction is often negative. The spinal fluid pressure is usually increased. The Wassermann reaction of the spinal fluid may be positive or not; uncommonly there may be a negative Wassermann reaction. The condition may exist with a negative Wassermann reaction of the blood and with a totally negative spinal fluid and with no clinical evidences of syphilis.

The diagnosis of gumma is purely conjectural and can be established only by histological verification. If, in a case of brain tumor, the Wassermann reaction of the blood is positive with the spinal fluid Wassermann reaction positive or negative, or if in such a case the spinal fluid Wassermann is positive and the blood Wassermann reaction negative, gumma of the brain may be suspected. The diagnosis can be established, however, only by surgical exploration and histological verification of the lesion. In most cases, the loss of visual acuity is so rapid, due to a syphilitic optic neuritis, that the lesion must be operated on and removed surgically in order to preserve vision. It is best in fact to operate on all subjects for the following reasons: (1) gumma of the brain cannot be diagnosed clinically with certainty; (2) it is essentially a tumor of the brain; (3) operation is necessary to preserve vision which is decreased because of the associated optic neuritis or choked disc; (4) brain tumors, usually meningiomas, may be associated at times with positive serological reactions of the blood and spinal fluid (Frazier and Alpers).

Establishment of the diagnosis histologically should be followed by intensive antisyphilitic treatment. No harm can be done by such treatment before operation as well. Large doses of iodides by mouth are most efficacious, the dosage being built up gradually. Bismuth or mercury should be given in addition.

10

Vascular Disease of the Brain

Among the vascular disorders involving the brain are numerous syndromes affecting the cerebrum and brain stem. These include meningeal hemorrhages, cerebral hemorrhage, cerebral thrombosis and embolism, and vascular spasm. Before passing to a consideration of these, it seems desirable to review briefly the pertinent factors relative to the anatomy and physiology of the cerebral vessels.

I. ANATOMY AND PHYSIOLOGY

The main arterial supply to the brain comes through the internal carotid and vertebral arteries which enter the circle of Willis and distribute blood over the cerebral hemispheres by way of the pial vessels. These in turn supply the cortex and other gray matter by means of arterioles and capillaries which arise through subdivisions of the pial arteries. Anastomoses exist between the branches of the middle, posterior, and anterior cerebral arteries. Even more important is the fact that within the cortex itself "the capillary bed is known to be a perfect network of intercommunicating vessels continuous throughout the gray matter of the cortex, so that a red cell could travel from occipital to frontal pole if it had means of locomotion" (Cobb). The veins are more commonly anastomotic than the arteries.

Variations in the circle of Willis are common. Incomplete circles with absence of one or more vessels are not very frequent, but atypical circles occur in about fifty per cent of human beings.

Quantitative studies of capillary blood supply of different parts of the brain.

chiefly of animals, reveals that the cerebral cortex is much richer in blood supply than the white matter, and that the basal ganglia have relatively rich blood supplies. The relationship between blood supply and function is not yet defined, but it has been suggested that the extent of the capillary bed is dependent on the size and number of the nerve cells and on the number of synapses and the metabolic activity of the part. Within the cerebral cortex itself there are variations in blood supply of various parts as well as of various layers. Thus, the visual cortex has a particularly rich blood supply while the layers 2 through 5 have a richer blood supply than layers 1 and 6 of the cortex.

Histologically, the cerebral arteries differ slightly from those elsewhere in the body. They possess a heavy internal elastic membrane, but no external elastica, and no elastic fibers within the adventitia. The media, moreover, is thinner and the adventitia poorly developed. The internal elastica hypertrophies and splits in old age. Around the adventitia is a perivascular space (Virchow-Robin) which is not clearly defined around small vessels, but becomes more distinct as the vessels become larger and approach the subarachnoid space. The perivascular spaces are regarded by some as analogous to the lymph spaces, but the composition of their fluid is not known and proof of this is lacking. Myelinated and non-myelinated nerve fibers are found on the arteries and on many veins of the sulci and meninges. It is doubtful as yet whether the arterioles within the cere-

450

bral tissue possess nerves, but vessels in the pia, including even the capillaries, are supplied with them. The nerves are both sensory and vasomotor. Vasoconstrictor fibers have been found on the vessels of the parietal cortex and basal ganglia in lower animals.

The blood flow in the brain is dependent upon and controlled chiefly by systemic arterial pressure, which is in turn controlled by carotid sinus mechanisms and other reflex mechanisms, particularly by regulation of blood flow through vasomotor brain stem mechanisms. By variations in carbon dioxide and oxygen content of the blood. The cerebral circulation tends to follow passively changes in arterial pressures. In addition there is an intrinsic cerebral regulation, chiefly chemical in nature, resulting in dilatation of the cerebral vessels by excess of carbon dioxide. Carbon dioxide inhalation increases intracranial blood flow. "The normal intrinsic control of the cerebral circulation is probably accomplished largely, if not entirely, by the vasodilator action of carbon dioxide, antagonizing a normally present tendency of intracranial vessels to go into a state of contraction" (Schmidt and Hendrix). In addition there is a less important vasomotor regulation of blood vessels of the brain by nervous control. Cervical sympathetic stimulation produces vasoconstriction of the pial vessels and parasympathetic stimulation causes dilatation. The vasoconstrictor nerves are about one-sixth as effective in the pia as in the skin. "The effect of alkali, heat, cold, potassium and calcium have been studied only imperfectly in animals, not at all in man. The available evidence does not indicate that any of these agents is capable of exerting more than a weak effect upon the tone of cerebral blood vessels and there is no reason to believe that any of them (including alkali and cold) can cause an appreciable vasoconstriction under physiological conditions" (Schmidt). Finally, it must be mentioned that brain tissue is particularly susceptible to oxygen lack, but the degree of resistance to oxygen deprivation varies in different portions of the nervous system, some parts being much more resistive than others. The cerebral vessels respond to vasodilators, including nitrites, choline derivatives, caffeine, theophylline and theobromine, histamine, morphine, codeine and papaverine and potassium and calcium ions. The intracranial vessels appear to be less sensitive than the extracranial to vasodilator agents. On the other hand, no drug has yet been proved capable of constricting cerebral blood vessels strongly and only a few have been proved to have any vasoconstrictor effect at all (Schmidt).

Studies on cerebral blood flow by Kety and his associates reveal interesting new findings concerning cerebral circulation. Table 40 shows the average figures in ar-

Table 40—Arterial and Venous Blood Values in Normal Subjects

(Kety)

	Normal	
	Mean	*Range*
Arterial:		
O₂ content vol. per cent..	18.	17 to 20
CO₂ content vol. per cent	50.	46 to 52
pH...................	7.42	7.38 to 7.45
pCO₂ mm. Hg..........	40.	38 to 43
Mean B.P. mm. Hg......	85.	78 to 90
Internal jugular:		
O₂ content vol. per cent..	11.	9 to 12
CO₂ content vol. per cent	55.	53 to 58
pH...................	7.37	7.33 to 7.40
pCO₂ mm. Hg..........	50.	48 to 53
Cerebral: Nutritional Index	2.8	2.3 to 3.3
Blood flow		
cc./100 Gm./min......	54.0	40 to 70
O₂ consumption		
cc./100 Gm./min......	3.3	2.6 to 4.0
Vascular resistance mm.		
Hg/cc./100 Gm./min..	1.6	1.3 to 2.0

terial and venous blood according to the studies made by this method.

The cerebral blood flow is affected by many factors:

1. It is *increased* with:
   Anoxia
   CO_2
   Papaverine
   AV angioma
   Anemia
   Epinephrine
   Pentothal anesthesia
   Sleep
   Diabetic coma
2. It is *decreased* with:
   Arteriosclerosis with hypertension
   Decreased CO_2 (hyperventilation)
   Hypotension
   Cerebral thrombosis
   Polycythemia
   Norepinephrine
   Motionless standing
   Heart failure
   Caffeine
   Aminophylline
   Histamine
3. It is *unaffected* by:
   Arteriosclerosis without hypertension
   Hypertension alone
   Stellate block

In the experimental study of cerebral anemia, various methods of ligating or occluding the vertebral and carotid arteries have been devised. However, occlusion of these vessels or even of their parent vessels as they arise from the aortic arch have failed to arrest completely the cerebral circulation in the animals. This is due to the rich anastomoses which maintain circulation by way of the spinal arteries. Because of the collateral circulation which has been called into play to various degrees, depending upon the technic of the experiments and the individual animals, discrepancies have occurred in the determination of the maximum periods of occlusion compatible with survival and of the degree of clinical and pathological changes induced by occlusion of the cerebral vessels for certain periods of time.

Weinberger, Gibbon and Gibbon devised the technic of temporary occlusion of the pulmonary artery in cats, thus producing an arrest of the circulation in the entire body and so avoiding the variable of collateral circulation. These authors found that if the circulation was arrested for less than three minutes and ten seconds no neurological disturbance ensued. If the arrest endured for three minutes and ten seconds permanent changes occurred in the cortex. When the circulatory arrest lasted three minutes and twenty-five seconds permanent alterations in behavior and psychic functions occurred and the cortex underwent softening and necrosis. Six minutes of arrest produced permanent injury to vision and sensation, and seven and one-half minutes of circulatory arrest resulted in virtually complete and permanent dementia, blindness, sensory, auditory and motor deficit with postural and reflex changes. With circulatory arrest of this duration the cerebral cortex was completely destroyed and liquefied. When the circulatory arrest persisted for eight minutes and forty-five seconds life could not be restored for more than a few hours.

Weinberger and his colleagues found that the cerebral cortex, especially the motor and visual areas of the cerebral cortex, were most vulnerable, while the olfactory, orbital, and temporal cortices were the least vulnerable. Of the cortical layers, laminae three and four were the most susceptible, while layers one and two were the least vulnerable. In the basal nuclei, the order of susceptibility, in order of decreasing vulnerability, was found to be the lateral geniculate body, the hypothalamic nuclei, the thalamic nuclei, the globus pallidus, and the caudate nucleus. The brain stem and spinal cord were uninjured by a degree of circulatory arrest compatible with survival. These findings are in agreement with those of other authors (Brown-Séquard, Gomez and Pike, and Gildea and Cobb). Kabat and Schadewald, using a different technic and employing dogs, found that periods of circulatory arrest of six minutes or less, while producing severe temporary functional changes, were followed by apparently complete clinical recovery. These authors showed that in young animals there was greater resistance to the arrest of cerebral circulation. Recently Rossen, Kabat, and Anderson studied the effects of arrest of the cerebral circulation in humans and found that loss of consciousness occurred after 6.8 seconds and that periods of arrest up to one hundred seconds did not produce objective evidence of permanent injury. The essential factor in the production of changes by arrest of cerebral circulation is the lack of oxygen. Lennox, Gibbs, and Gibbs have demonstrated that unconsciousness supervenes when the oxygen tension of the internal jugular blood is suddenly reduced to twenty-four per cent.

II. CEREBRAL HEMORRHAGE

Incidence: Hemorrhage within the brain substance is among the more common brain disorders, numbering 3.5 to five per cent of neurological diseases. It is not as common as thromboses among cerebral vascular diseases, for statistics show that thrombosis cases outnumber those of cerebral hemorrhage by a ratio of three to one or four to one. Among 407 cases of cerebral vascular lesions, cerebral thrombosis was found in 81.8 per cent, cerebral hemorrhage in fifteen per cent, and cerebral embolism in 3.2 per cent (Merritt and Aring). This is a matter of some importance, since the outlook is considerably different in the two groups of cases.

Cerebral hemorrhage is by definition hemorrhage anywhere within the brain

Table 41—Spontaneous Cerebral Hemorrhage

(*after Russell*)

	No. Cases
Hypertensive disease	232
Congenital medial defects in cerebral arteries (92 cases of aneurysm)	96
Blood diseases	36
Mycotic aneurysm	28
Vascular hamartoma	21
Arteritis (no aneurysm)	13
Neoplasms	9
Arterial degeneration (no cardio-vascular hypertrophy)	7
Various	3
Cause not found	16
Total	461

substance and includes, therefore, hemorrhage into the cerebrum, brain stem, cerebellum, or ventricles.

Etiology: Males are more frequently affected than females, the average age incidence being forty to sixty years, though cases may develop in patients much younger and older, depending on the cause. Hemorrhage is uncommon before 30 years of age, but increases in frequency in people of 50 or over.

Arteriosclerosis of the cerebral vessels is the most common cause, but it is not a *sine qua non* of hemorrhage. The cerebral vessels are normal in about one-fifth of cases. Arteriosclerosis is responsible for cerebral hemorrhage in the older age group.

Syphilis of the cerebral vessels is not as common a cause of cerebral hemorrhage as arteriosclerosis. When syphilitic vascular disease of the brain causes hemorrhage, it does so in a younger age group (thirty-five to forty-five years).

Vascular hypertension associated with cardiorenal disease, or essential or malignant hypertension is often responsible for cerebral hemorrhage. In the case of essential hypertension particularly, the hemorrhage is often multiple. Transitory increases in blood pressure in the presence of healthy or diseased blood vessels may be responsible for cerebral bleeding, as in the bouts of coughing in pertussis, fits of sneezing, or in intercourse.

Mycotic aneurysms from an embolus in a cerebral vessel in cases of endocarditis (subacute bacterial or vegetative) constitute a rare cause of cerebral hemorrhage.

Trauma may be responsible in some instances, but massive cerebral hemorrhage is not common; petechial hemorrhages are much more frequent.

Blood dyscrasias, such as purpura and leukemia, are sometimes associated with brain hemorrhage. Scurvy is also a rare cause. In these conditions the hemorrhages are multiple and variable in size.

ranging from small to large extravasations. There is no difference in the incidence of neurological complications in the different types of leukemia, such as acute myeloid leukemia, chronic myeloid leukemia, monocytic leukemia, leukosarsoma, or unclassified leukemias. The incidence of hemorrhagic and leukemic infiltration of the brain is 20 per cent higher in the chronic than in the acute forms of lymphoid and myeloid leukemia. Neurological signs and symptoms due to the leukemic disease were found in thirty-four of sixty-seven cases reported with autopsy. Among the neurological symptoms were hemiplegia and cranial nerve palsies (Leidler and Russell).

Brain tumors, particularly the glioblastomas, are often associated with hemorrhage within their substance. Hemorrhage is found in rare instances in sickle cell anemia and pernicious anemia.

Chemicals are sometimes responsible,

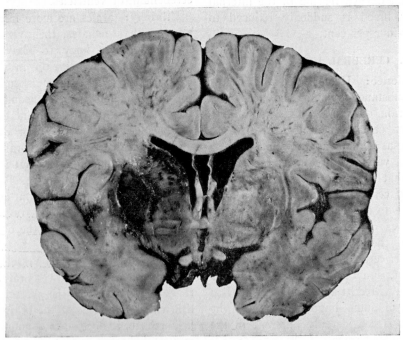

Fig. 130—*Cerebral hemorrhage,* showing the characteristic involvement of the internal capsule region and the basal ganglia adjacent to it in a patient with cerebral arteriosclerosis with hypertension.

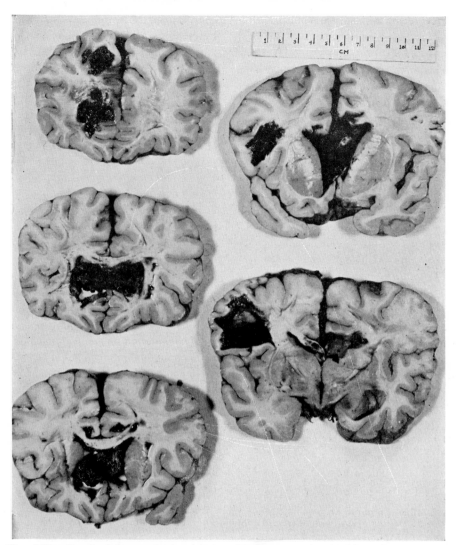

Fig. 131—*Cerebral hemorrhage,* showing bleeding in the middle cerebral artery distribution with rupture into the ventricles.

as, for example, the occurrence of hemorrhage following the injection of arsphenamine or neoarsphenamine.

Cerebral hemorrhage may develop as a result of small angiomatous malformations within the brain substance.

Congenital heart disease has been found responsible in rare instances. Cerebral hemorrhage occurs rarely in *migraine* during an attack of headache. *No cause* for the cerebral hemorrhage can be found in a small percentage of cases. Cerebral hemorrhage is sometimes found in young adults with all the features of a cerebral accident, but with no evidence of cardiac or vascular disease and no apparent cause for the hemorrhage. Cases of this sort are frequently referred to as *spontaneous cerebral hemorrhage* and in some instances have even been designated idiopathic cerebral hemorrhage. The cause of the cerebral hemorrhage in these cases is not known, but the condition has followed severe emotional stimulation, strenuous exercise, and severe vomiting following smoking of a pipe for the first time. Hypertension and cranial trauma have been responsible for the hemorrhage in some of the cases recorded.

Pathology and Pathogenesis: Hemorrhage into the brain may be massive or small, depending on the vessel which

stem, especially in the pons as well as in the cerebral hemisphere. The basal ganglia, especially those adjacent to the internal capsule, are often involved in the hemorrhage (putamen, thalamus, pallidum). In some instances, cerebral hemorrhage ruptures into the lateral ventricle and in still others into the sub-

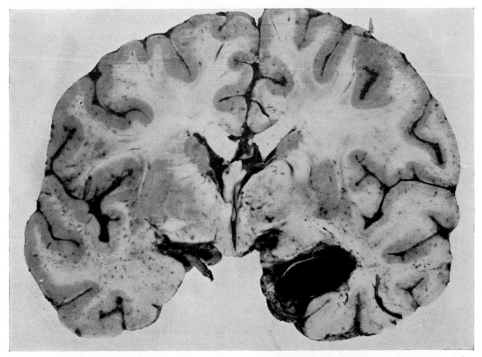

Fig. 132—*Cerebral hemorrhage,* showing a fresh hemorrhage in the hippocampal gyrus, with scattered punctate hemorrhages elsewhere.

has ruptured. It may fill most of a hemisphere or be confined to the internal capsular region. Hemorrhages are most common in the region of the internal capsule and basal ganglia, and in the cerebral hemisphere involving one or more of the branches of the middle cerebral artery. They are not so commonly encountered in the brain stem and cerebellum. Under some circumstances they are multiple, particularly in some cases of hypertension, trauma, and in blood dyscrasias. In some cases of hypertension they are apt to be found in the brain

arachnoid space, thus accounting for the bloody spinal fluid often found in hemorrhage in the brain. In rare instances, cerebral hemorrhages become encapsulated.

Histological study usually reveals fresh or clotted blood with laceration of the tissue adjacent to the hemorrhage. In the surrounding tissue are small hemorrhages, phagocytic cells, and sometimes even leukocytic infiltration.

Hemorrhage into the brain substance is almost always arterial; hence the poor outlook in almost all the cases. In rare

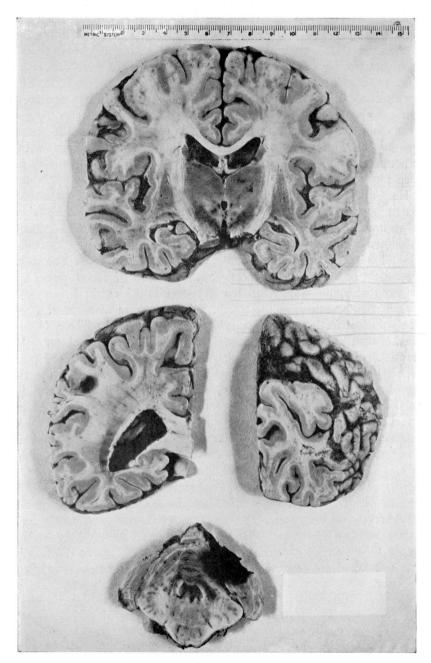

Fig. 133—*Cerebral hemorrhage*, showing multiple hemorrhages in the diencephalon, the cerebrum, and cerebellum.

instances it may be of venous origin. The *background* for the hemorrhage is found in a weakened vessel wall, either the result of a congenital aneurysm or a miliary aneurysm due to arteriosclerosis, a mycotic aneurysm from heart, lung, fat, or air emboli. In some instances, as in head injury, a direct tear of a vessel is responsible. In other cases, as in the blood dyscrasias, diapedesis is responsible.

The pathogenesis of cerebral hemorrhage is not precisely known. Many ideas have been put forth but relatively few are tenable. Among the earliest was the concept that cerebral hemorrhage was the result of rupture of a miliary aneurysm. This undoubtedly explains some cases of hemorrhage but fails to account for all. Nevertheless, the ruptured aneurysm concept is accepted quite widely at the present time. Acute necrosis of the cerebral vessels was set forth as the primary factor in hemorrhage, but the cause of the necrosis has never been clarified. Because of the fact that in not a few instances of hemorrhage and thrombosis no associated disease of the blood vessels can be found, it has been asserted that vascular accidents are preceded by spasm of the arteries within the area of hemorrhage, that this is followed by ischemia and softening of the tissue, and that hemorhage occurs within this area of necrotic tissue by necrosis of the spastic vessel itself, or by increased vascular tension and rupture of a vessel because of decreased resistance of the softened perivascular tissue.

The bleeding is regarded by some as of venous origin. "The arterioles bear the brunt of hyperpiesis; and when this system finally 'decompensates,' presumably by a process akin to vasoparalysis, abnormal tension may be transmitted from the failing arteriole to the enfeebled vein, the structure next in sequence, which

thereafter is likely to lose blood and to cause death" (Aring).

The probabilities are that no single mechanism is responsible for the bleeding, and no one mechanism can explain all instances of cerebral hemorrhage. This should be obvious from the number of causes which may produce hemorrhage into the brain. In those cases in which a weakened vessel is present, as in arteriosclerosis, or in cases with hypertension, an additional inciting factor of *sudden increase in blood pressure* by exertion is important as the immediate cause of bleeding. This may be produced by exertion of any sort — work, sexual intercourse, straining at stool, and in many other conditions. The rôle of sudden increase of blood pressure in the production of cerebral hemorrhage by causing rupture of a vessel is not definitely established. There is no doubt that in the presence of normal vessels mere elevation of the blood pressure is not sufficient to cause rupture and hemorrhage. The probabilities are, however, that in the presence of a weakened vessel as, for example, a vessel with a miliary aneurysm, or in arteriosclerosis with necrosis of the vessel wall, a sudden elevation of the blood pressure is capable of causing rupture of the weakened vessel. This mechanism is not at the basis of hemorrhage from mycotic aneurysms, trauma, and blood dyscrasias. In experimental studies on cadavers who died with cerebral arteriosclerosis, fluid was injected into both carotids and it was found that only by the application of pressure of one to $2\frac{1}{2}$ atmospheres for six minutes did rupture of vessels and destruction of brain substance by leaking fluid develop. Such pressures never occur in human cases (Lampert and Müller).

Symptoms: The onset in cerebral hemorrhage is abrupt and dramatic.

Warning symptoms, such as *dizziness*, headache, and mental confusion are found, and may be present for days or weeks before the hemorrhage develops. They are especially frequent in the cases due to hypertension. A momentary sensation of vertigo may immediately precede the development of the hemorrhage. It is not always true, however, that cerebral hemorrhage develops with dramatic suddenness. In some cases, the development of symptoms may occur over a period of hours or even days, and may simulate in this fashion the gradual occlusion of a vessel by thrombosis. This method of onset is not common, the usual case developing suddenly and explosively. Gradually developing cases are not infrequent, however, and must not be overlooked in the recognition of the condition.

Of the immediate symptoms preceding the hemorrhage, *headache* and *vomiting* are significant. Dizziness is a very common symptom at the time of onset of the attack. Severe headache occurs in a large number of patients at the onset of the attack (sixty-three per cent) and is in itself a useful sign of a vascular accident. Vomiting is said to be an important sign of cerebral hemorrhage and has been used in the differentiation of hemorrhage from thrombosis. Broadbent in 1887 asserted that vomiting occurred more frequently with cerebral hemorrhage than with other types of vascular lesions in the brain. Others assert that "vomiting, if present at the onset and if embolism is excluded, is usually indicative of cerebral hemorrhage" (Aring and Merritt).

Unconsciousness follows almost immediately after the onset. It is said to supervene in a matter of minutes in the usual case. It may be delayed, however, in some instances, and in this sense may be quite confusing in differentiating hem-

orrhage from thrombosis. Occasional instances are seen with a history of loss of power in a limb, followed by a progressive loss of power in the entire side, and a gradual lapse into unconsciousness. This may take several hours to develop. In such instances, the bleeding is probably slow and it is not until an extensive brain area has been destroyed that unconsciousness supervenes. The type of unconsciousness which ensues is profound and complete. The patient cannot be aroused, the breathing is stertorous, the pulse is rapid and full, the face flushed, and the skin clammy. The unconsciousness is so deep that the patient does not respond to pin prick or to other forms of stimulation. Sometimes it is not complete, however, and the patient may be partially aroused from his stupor. Before death ensues, the loss of consciousness becomes very profound. Some idea of the incidence of loss of consciousness in cases of cerebral hemorrhage is given in the following figures: In seventy-nine patients, 50.7 per cent were in coma at the onset of the hemorrhage and 68.1 per cent were in coma at the time of admission to the hospital (Aring and Merritt). In most patients with cerebral hemorrhage, therefore, there is complete loss of consciousness practically from the onset of the disease.

Sometimes, especially if the hemorrhage is near or in the cortex, the hemorrhage is ushered in with *convulsions* as well as unconsciousness. The convulsions may be generalized or focal but are more usually generalized. They may, however, begin as focal jacksonian convulsions but soon become generalized. Their incidence in a large series of cases has been stated as being about fifteen per cent.

The temperature may be subnormal (96° to 98° F.) or there may be a hyperthermia (101° to 102° F.). Death is not infrequently associated with a rapidly mounting temperature.

Even during the state of complete unconsciousness, neurologic signs indicating involvement of one of the hemispheres or of other parts of the brain are evident. The neck is often retracted and stiff. The head and eyes may be turned to one side in some instances, producing a postural condition referred to as conjugate deviation of the head and eyes. In a destructive lesion, such as hemorrhage, the head and eyes deviate in such a way that they look at the lesion and away from the paralysis, due to the unopposed action of the opposite cerebral hemisphere.

The usual expression of a cerebral hemorrhage is a *hemiplegia* resulting either from interruption of the pyramidal or corticospinal fibers in the cerebral hemisphere or in the internal capsule. Such a hemiplegia, as the name implies, is characterized by a loss of power of one-half of the body, the side opposite to the involved hemisphere. In a typical instance, there is loss of power of the lower facial muscles, and of the arm and leg. The facial weakness is demonstrated by a drooping of the corner of the mouth, a smoothing out of the nasiolabial fold on the affected side, and weakness in retraction of the corner of the mouth. In some instances, while the hemiplegia is still fresh, there may be a weakness of the upper group of facial muscles with inability to wrinkle the forehead on the affected side and weakness in closure of the eyelid. Such weakness, in addition to that involving the lower group of facial muscles, may simulate a peripheral facial paralysis. It is never as pronounced as the latter and disappears quickly in the course of hours or one to two days. In addition to the central facial weakness in a typical hemiplegia there may

be weakness of the palate and tongue, the palate of the affected side drooping and the tongue deviating to the hemiplegic side.

The paralysis of the limbs in cerebral hemorrhage is usually complete, with total loss of power in the arm, hand. leg, and foot. In some instances, the weakness may be partial, in which case the distal portions of the limb are usually most affected. The paralysis is, as a rule, flaccid at the onset. The flaccidity may persist until exitus or it may be followed in a few hours or days by spasticity of the affected limbs. The tendon reflexes can often not be elicited during the acute stages of shock, but in not a few cases they are overactive on the affected side from the onset. The sign of Babinski may be present or absent in the acute stages, but is usually present later. Incontinence of urine and often of feces is present from the onset. The incontinence of hemiplegia has been assumed to be the result of one of the following factors: (1) loss of consciousness or (2) mental deterioration. It may occur, however, in perfectly conscious and undeteriorated subjects, suggesting that it may be the result of other factors.

Since patients with cerebral hemorrhage are usually unconscious and frequently in deep stupor, it becomes necessary to determine the presence of a hemiplegia in a stuporous patient. This may be established by the following observations: (1) The cheek blows out on the affected side. (2) The paralyzed limbs are found to fall limp and without resistance when elevated. This sign is not always easy to interpret, since the sound limbs may fall in almost similar fashion. As a rule, the limbs of the sound side fall more gradually rather than in a heap, retaining some of their tone as they fall. (3) A useful and an almost invariable reaction is that of response to painful stimulation. If the terminal phalanx of the limb or great toe is flexed forcibly, the arm and leg will in the vast majority of cases be withdrawn even in a profoundly stuporous patient, whereas the paralyzed limbs will not be moved against the most painful stimulation. In patients with partial loss of power, stimulation such as that described will enable one to estimate the degree of loss of power in the affected limbs by determining the strength of the withdrawal in the affected and healthy limbs.

In addition to hemiplegia, other focal signs may be present, depending on the area of brain which is destroyed. *Aphasia* may be apparent if the patient is conscious. *Hemianopsia* may also be established if the patient can coöperate sufficiently. Both aphasia and hemianopsia are impossible to establish in most cases because of the loss of consciousness. *Neuroretinitis* is found in cases of malignant hypertension. *Retinal arteriosclerosis* may be found, and retinal hemorrhages are seen in some cases.

Cerebellar dyssynergia may be found in cases of cerebellar apoplexy, but this condition, due to hemorrhage in the cerebellar hemisphere, is often impossible to establish during life. The incidence of cerebellar hemorrhage without coincident cerebral hemorrhage is very low (ten cases in 17,257 necropsies or 0.0058 per cent, Michael). The appearance is that of an apoplexy, as in cerebral hemorrhage. The condition may be ushered in by sudden loss of consciousness associated with vomiting. In other cases, the development may be more gradual, with premonitory signs such as vertigo, nausea, and headache, followed by collapse and impairment of consciousness, which ensues in a few minutes or hours. If the patient remains conscious, dys-synergia of the limbs may be demonstrated. There are signs of collapse as in cerebral hemorrhage. Pyramidal signs are absent and hemiplegia not demonstrable. The spinal fluid is bloody.

Vascular *hypertension* is present in most cases, but this is not invariably the case, especially in young patients with syphilis, blood dyscrasias, or heart disease. There is frequently a leukocytosis of twelve thousand or over. The heart is often enlarged and may be fibrillating at the time of examination. It is often normal. Peripheral arteriosclerosis is found in about seventy-five per cent of cases in contrast to cerebral thrombosis, in which it is invariably present. Retinal arteriosclerosis is often present but is not constant. Albumen and casts are usually found in the urine and the blood nonprotein nitrogen may be elevated. The spinal fluid pressure is elevated and in many instances blood is present (seventy-five per cent). The absence of blood, however, does not exclude the presence of a hemorrhage. A bloody spinal fluid indicates only that the hemorrhage has penetrated either into the subarachnoid space or the ventricles. In some instances, cerebral hemorrhage has been found to be associated with a polymorphonuclear leukocytosis in the spinal fluid, simulating a meningitis. The leukocytosis usually begins within several hours after the vascular accident and disappears within the next five or six days.

Diagnosis: The problem of diagnosis in cerebral hemorrhage is of two types: It is concerned in most cases first with the problem of a patient in coma and the determination of the nature of the coma. This implies the determination of whether the coma has a cerebral basis. Having established this point, the next step is the determination of the exact nature of the cerebral disease responsible for the coma. Much depends on the exact determination of this second point, because the type of treatment will vary greatly, depending on the cause of the trouble.

As to the primary problem, the first point to be determined is whether the patient in coma has suffered from a cerebral insult. As a rule, this is not difficult to determine. The history of sudden onset, the presence of hypertension, and a previous history of cerebral symptoms will be highly suggestive in the arteriosclerotic and hypertensive cases. Coma is most frequent in hemorrhage. Convulsions occur at the onset in fifteen per cent of cases of cerebral hemorrhage, seven per cent of cases of thrombosis and nine per cent of embolism (Merritt). When such data are not available, it is necessary to exclude such common causes of coma as uremia, diabetes, and alcohol. *Uremia* will be excluded by the urinary findings and by the presence of an elevated blood urea nitrogen. It must not be forgotten, however, that many patients with cerebral hemorrhage have severe kidney disease and that an elevated blood urea is not uncommon. *Diabetes* will be excluded by the blood sugar determinations and by the absence of sugar in the urine. *Alcoholism* will reveal itself by a history of a debauch and by the smell of alcohol on the breath. The diagnosis in this condition is frequently complicated by the fact that subdural hemorrhage is not uncommonly found in alcoholics who have sustained a cranial trauma. Loss of consciousness from *cardiac disease* reveals itself by a history of cardiac trouble, definite evidence of cardiac disease, and usually decompensation. In most cases it will be necessary only to exclude these more common conditions. Cardiac disease is found in a high percentage of patients (seventy-two per cent) at the time of development of a cerebral vascular accident, either thrombosis or hemorrhage. Evidence of cardiocirculatory insufficiency is found in eighty-three per cent of patients on the basis of the past medical history, clinical examination and autopsy findings (Wilson, Rupp, Riggs, and Wilson). Hemorrhage due to *trauma* is always accompanied by a history of head injury and by external evidences of violent trauma to the skull. *Epilepsy* can be established by a previous history of convulsions. Stupor due to *barbiturates* or other sedatives can usually be determined by a history of attempted suicide or of overindulgence in drugs.

Having determined by the history of an abrupt, sudden, apoplectic onset of loss of consciousness, by the presence of a hypertension, as a rule, and by a previous history of cerebral attacks that the problem is one of cerebral origin, it is next necessary to determine the exact nature of the cerebral insult. Cerebral hemorrhage may be established as the cause of the condition in question by the sudden apoplectic onset with unconsciousness, the hypertension in many instances, the presence of hemiplegia, and the demonstration of blood in the spinal fluid. In those instances without hypertension, the other features which have been mentioned will usually suffice to establish the diagnosis. It is essential to know whether the disease is due to cerebral hemorrhage, thrombosis with softening, embolism, tumor, metastatic carcinoma, or to ventricular hemorrhage. Headache is much more common as an initial symptom of hemorrhage than of thrombosis—sixty-three per cent, hemorrhage; twenty-five per cent, embolism; and six per cent, thrombosis (Merritt).

The differentiation between *hemorrhage* and *thrombosis* is important from two standpoints: (1) prognosis, (2) treatment. This will differ for both hem-

Table 42—Differential Diagnosis of Cerebral Hemorrhage, Thrombosis, Embolism

Disease	Age	Onset	Retinal Arterio-sclerosis	Spinal Fluid	Hyper-tension	Peripheral Arterio-sclerosis	Heart Disease	Kidney Disease
CEREBRAL HEMORRHAGE	50 or more	Apoplectic, with loss of conscious-ness, vomit-ing	Often but not always present	Bloody in 75 per cent	Almost always present	Often but not always present	Frequently	Albumen or casts in urine
CEREBRAL THROMBOSIS	60 or over	Usually more gradual with premonitory symptoms and often with little or no loss of conscious-ness	Always present	Never bloody. Microscopic blood at times with red infarcts	Often but not always present	Always present	In many cases	Albumen or casts in urine
CEREBRAL EMBOLISM	Any age	Sudden, with or without loss of con-sciousness, but usually with loss	Not found	Not bloody save in cases with asso-ciated sub-arachnoid hemorrhage (15 per cent)	Not usually present	Not usually present	In most cases valvular dis-ease, mural thrombi, etc. Also pulmo-nary disease or other source of em-bolism	Not usually present

orrhage and softening. The problem is, therefore, more than of academic interest, not so much to exclude hemorrhage as to establish softening. Vascular accidents occurring in patients under fifty are more frequently due to hemorrhage, while those occurring in subjects over fifty are probably the result of thrombosis. A prolonged hyperthermia or a prolonged, persistent hypothermia is found in hemorrhage more often than in softening. A study of 245 verified cases establishes the following significant points (Aring and Merritt): Sudden, severe headache or vomiting at the onset is more frequently seen in hemorrhage. Convulsions are more frequent in hemorrhage. A dilated pupil on the paralyzed side favors hemorrhage. Unconsciousness is much more frequent in hemorrhage and signs of progression of the lesion are more characteristic of hemorrhage than thrombosis. Hyperten-

sion is more frequent in the former. The cerebrospinal fluid examination is an important aid in the differentiation. The pressure is increased much more frequently in hemorrhage, the fluid is bloody in seventy-five per cent, and rarely bloody in cases of thrombosis. The survival period is shorter in hemorrhage. In fifty per cent of the patients with cerebral hemorrhage, death ensued within four days from the time of onset.

In *embolism* the onset is sudden. The temperature response is usually high and there are severe evidences of shock. There are several points which will serve to differentiate the two conditions: In embolism, the onset is in younger people. There is usually little or no evidence of vascular disease or of hypertension. A focus of some sort, usually an endocardi-tis, is present and gives a strong clue as to the cause of the condition. While unconsciousness may be severely impaired, its disturbance is not so profound as in hemorrhage, nor does it last as long. It may be present for only a few hours or a day. The spinal fluid is bloody in fifteen per cent of cases.

Subarachnoid hemorrhage must sometimes be differentiated. These cases usually occur in younger people. The onset is with severe headache and prostration, but not usually with profound coma. As a rule there are no signs of hemiplegia, but this is not invariable. There are some cases with hemiplegia or with other focal signs. Even in these cases consciousness may not be greatly impaired. Meningeal signs are usually the only objective signs present. There is always a stiff neck and Kernig's sign, and there is always blood in the spinal fluid.

Sudden apoplectic onset of symptoms with severe loss of consciousness is not an uncommon experience in *brain tumors*. In such cases there will be a history of prodromata such as headache for a varying period of time. The presence of persistent headache in a patient with suspected vascular disease must always lead to the suspicion that tumor may be present. It is unusual for headache to persist in vascular thrombosis or embolism unless there is associated hypertension. In addition, there will be evidence of choked disc in most instances. In some cases, *metastatic carcinoma* to the brain is ushered in with loss of consciousness and an apoplectic attack. The age, the general cachexia, and the presence of a primary malignant growth establish the diagnosis. The roentgenograms in such cases will show metastases to the skull and to other bones.

Prognosis: The outlook in cases of massive cerebral hemorrhage is notably bad and it is extremely doubtful whether recovery occurs in such patients. If the hemorrhage ruptures into the ventricles, the outlook is invariably bad. Smaller hemorrhages are compatible with recovery. Clinical studies indicate that recovery occurs in cerebral hemorrhage in a small percentage of subjects, but it is a striking fact that necropsy specimens of recovered instances of cerebral hemorrhage are rare. Studies on the prognosis of cerebral hemorrhage are notoriously inaccurate. Clinical studies indicate a higher survival than post-mortem studies, but in the former it is impossible to be certain of the diagnosis and statistics differ, therefore, concerning the survival of hemorrhages. Cerebral hemorrhage is not a cause of sudden death, even when the hemorrhage extends into the ventricles. Among 109 patients, thirty-seven per cent died within twenty-four hours, seventy-five per cent died within a week, and eighty-six per cent within one month (Jones). Among 134 cases, 24.8 per cent died within twenty-four hours, 37.1 per cent within five days, thirty-eight per cent within fifteen days, 7.24 per cent within thirty days, 12.6 per cent in one to six months, 1.81 per cent within seven to twelve months (Newbill). Clinical studies of the condition are open to doubt as to accuracy of diagnosis; hence necropsy studies are more accurate and indicate that survival of cerebral hemorrhage is rare.

A feature of serious significance for outlook is deepening coma, which implies a spread of the hemorrhage. A rising temperature is of very serious import, especially if the rise is rapid. Evidence of paralysis extending to both sides is extremely grave, indicating as it does either bilateral cerebral hemorrhage or extension of the bleeding into the ventricle. Cheyne-Stokes respiration is usually serious, but it may be transitory and does not imply impending exitus. Fixed pupillary reactions are usually of serious significance. In general, poor prognostic factors in cerebral vascular disease are elevated blood pressure (over 190 systolic and 140 diastolic); prolonged duration of coma of over forty-eight hours; and Cheyne-Stokes respiration.

III. VENTRICULAR HEMORRHAGE

Types: Hemorrhage into the cerebral ventricles may be primary or secondary. The *primary* type is rare and may in-volve the lateral, third, or fourth ventri-cles without invasion of the contiguous brain substance. *Secondary* hemorrhage into the ventricular system is much more common, and results from rupture of a cerebral hemorrhage into the adjacent ventricle. By far the largest number in-volve the lateral ventricles, because of the greater incidence of cerebral hemor-rhage in the white substance of the brain. About one in six cerebral hemor-

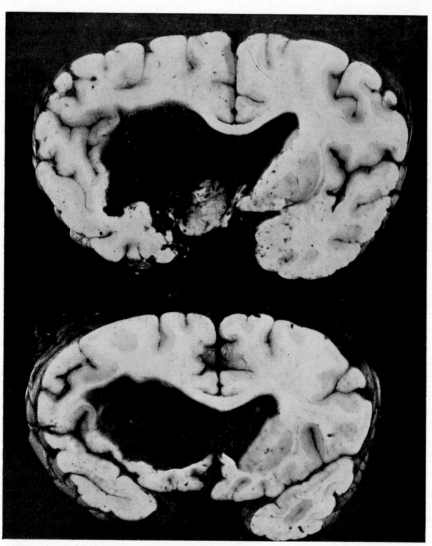

Fig. 134—*Ventricular hemorrhage.* A hemorrhage from rupture of the middle cerebral artery has spread to involve the ventricles.

rhages ruptures into the ventricle. The brain at necropsy is found to contain a large fresh hemorrhage which shows a direct connection with the lateral ventricle into which it has ruptured through the body or one of the horns. The blood is usually fresh and firm clotting has not occurred in the usual case.

Etiology: The causes of ventricular hemorrhage differ in no respect from those of cerebral hemorrhage.

Symptoms: The symptoms of ventricular hemorrhage are similar to those of cerebral hemorrhage. The condition occurs in both young and old people, usually in the older age groups. The onset is very sudden and violent with severe, intense headache and loss of consciousness practically from the beginning. It is usually so profound that the patient cannot be aroused by the most violent stimuli. Convulsions are said to be very common in the onset of ventricular hemorrhage, but studies of this specific point show that they are no more frequent than in cerebral hemorrhage. The temperature is either subnormal or elevated, just as in the case of hemorrhage into the brain. In ventricular hemorrhage there is more frequently hyperthermia due to invasion of the floor of the third ventricle by the hemorrhage. The pulse is usually feeble, stringy, and rapid. The patient is in profound *shock*. The type of motor response is variable. In some cases there is a paralysis of all four limbs (quadriplegia); in others, there may be involvement of three limbs (triplegia), or even a hemiplegia. It is not uncommon for the onset to occur with a hemiplegia, which in the course of hours develops into a triplegia or quadriplegia. Progression of this nature in an instance of bleeding into the brain is quite typical of ventricular hemorrhage. The limbs may be flaccid or there may be a com-

bination of spasticity and flaccidity. In a few cases there has been spasticity of the arms and flaccidity of the legs. There is usually stiffness of the neck and sometimes Kernig's sign. The reflexes are entirely absent in the beginning, but return slowly to an active or hyperactive state. Babinski's sign is frequently absent in the beginning, only to appear later in the course of the illness. The spinal fluid is intensely bloody in almost every case. In some cases it is almost the consistency of venous blood; in others it is a bloody spinal fluid in which the fluid is obviously mixed with blood.

Diagnosis: The diagnosis of hemorrhage into the ventricles is not difficult. The history of a sudden onset with headache, of immediate collapse with profound coma, with a paralysis of all four limbs, with blood in the spinal fluid, will be sufficient as a rule to establish the diagnosis. Progressive involvement of both sides of the body by paralysis is characteristic. The evidences of shock are even more profound than in hemorrhage confined to the brain substance. The differentiation from other diseases is similar to that of cerebral hemorrhage.

Prognosis: Practically all cases of ventricular hemorrhage are fatal. Death follows in twenty-four hours to fourteen days after the onset. It usually occurs in about two to four days in the average case. In a group of nine cases, death occurred in from twenty-four hours to sixteen days after onset (Spiller).

IV. CEREBRAL EMBOLISM

Etiology: Embolism may involve vessels of varying size and in any location in the brain. It may occur at any age, but is more frequently encountered in younger subjects than either cerebral hemorrhage or thrombosis. The chief source of emboli is in the heart, and *cardiac conditions* are therefore of the first importance in the disease. Endocarditis of various sorts serves as a source of emboli — subacute bacterial endocarditis and vegetative endocarditis. Mitral stenosis may serve as a source under two conditions: (1) when fresh vegetations are engrafted on the old endocarditis; (2) in the presence of a mural thrombus in the auricle. Coronary thrombosis, either acute or healed, is a fruitful source of embolism. Myocarditis associated with a mural thrombus may give rise to emboli in the brain. *Pulmonary diseases,* such as bronchiectasis, lung abscess, tuberculosis and bronchogenic carcinoma, serve as a source of emboli. *Fat emboli* are a rare cause, occurring secondarily to a severe injury or to trauma of the soft tissues associated with operation. *Air emboli* in divers are sometimes found to be the cause of cerebral emboli. *Thrombophlebitis* is, in rare instances, a cause of brain embolism. Cerebral embolism has been found to develop also in association with thrombosis in the carotid artery due to operative compression, in septic

Table 43—Causes of Cerebral Embolism (Autopsy Verified)

	No. Cases
RHEUMATIC HEART DISEASE WITH	
SUBACUTE BACTERIAL ENDOCARDITIS....	37
MURAL THROMBUS—LEFT VENTRICLE.....	35
INFECTIONS—ABSCESS.................	7
BRONCHIECTASIS.....................	5
SEPTICEMIA.........................	3
PATENT FORAMEN OVALE..............	2
POSTOPERATIVE......................	3
THROMBOSIS OF PULMONARY VESSELS	
AND AORTA........................	13
FRACTURES.........................	2
TOTAL........................	107

bronchopneumonia, appendicitis, pelvic abscess, puerperal sepsis, perinephritis, carbuncle, and furunculosis.

The pathway by which emboli pass from the heart or other parts of the body is not definitely known. A patent foramen ovale has usually been postulated to explain passage of the embolus from the right to the left side of the heart. This is probably true in a relatively small number of instances. More probable is the mechanism suggested by Batson, who has found that the vertebral vein system (the epidural veins, the perivertebral veins, the veins of the thoracoabdominal wall, the veins of the head and neck and the veins of the walls of the blood vessels of the extremities) is a set of valveless veins carrying blood under low pressure, providing connections with and by-passes for the portal, pulmonary, and caval system of veins, hence providing a pathway for the spread of disease between remote organs.

Symptoms: In embolism there are usually no premonitory signs, or if any are present they are of a very fleeting nature. The onset is usually extremely sudden, unattended by exertion or any other adequate cause. The patient may have turned in bed or may have been stricken when completely at rest. There is usually complete loss of consciousness, but in some instances this may be only partial, so that the patient may be aroused from his coma, or he may at times emerge spontaneously. There is, as a rule, evidence of severe collapse just as in hemorrhage with profuse perspiration, labored breathing, a rapid pulse, and incontinence. Indeed, the symptoms of embolism may so closely simulate hemorrhage that the distinction between the two is almost impossible. Convulsions frequently accompany the onset in embolism. They may be general or focal, more frequently the former. Elevation of temperature frequently accompanies the onset of embolism. Hemiplegia is usually demonstrable. Monoplegias, aphasia, hemianopsia, or other indications of brain damage may be found. General examination may reveal evidence of valvular disease of the heart, coronary disease, pulmonary disease, thrombophlebitis, or of other conditions which may serve as the source of embolus to the brain. In embolism, in short, there is in a younger person without hypertension and usually with evidence of heart disease a sudden onset of symptoms with loss of consciousness, frequently convulsions, collapse, and rise of temperature.

Diagnosis: The presence of cerebral embolism may be suspected and readily established in a patient who is known to have a source of embolus in the heart valves, the lungs, the blood vessels, or in other parts which have been indicated; who suddenly, and without apparent cause, develops evidence of a cerebral accident (unconsciousness, convulsions), and who manifests evidence of a focal cerebral lesion such as hemiplegia, aphasia, or hemianopsia. In cases of this sort, the relationship between the source of the embolus and the cerebral accident is readily apparent.

In other cases cerebral accidents develop without apparent cause in patients without hypertension, arteriosclerosis, or other reasons for cerebral vascular disease. The diagnosis of cerebral embolism in such instances is made by the demonstration of a source for the embolus after careful search for the cause of the cerebral vascular accident—an old coronary occlusion, unsuspected or overlooked heart disease, etc.

Fat embolism is a rare cause of cerebral symptoms. It results from the access of fat to the circulation, "either intrinsic fat freed through trauma or extrinsic fat or oil introduced into the organism for therapeutic or other purposes" (Warren). In the majority of instances, fat embolism results from trauma with fracture of one or more bones (91 cases out of 100, Warren), but it may occur without bone fracture, as in blast injury, burns, pressure, asphyxia, and trauma from shell fragments. In most cases, the tibia and/or femur are fractured. The incidence of fat embolism has been variously computed: 2 cases among 12,000 fractures (Darrach); 8 cases among 1000 battle casualties (Wilson and Salisbury); and 40 per cent of fat embolism in some degree in fatally burned persons (Wakeley).

The conditions necessary for entry of the embolic fat into the circulation are as follows: mobilized fat, patent and disrupted veins, and local pressure (Warren). In trauma, fat is set free from the marrow cells; in concussion, as in bomb explosions, disruption of the adipose tissues forces fat into the circulation; and in burns, the death of fat cells may liberate fat, and a pressure bandage may force it into the circulation. The total blood fat is not necessarily high in fat embolism.

Pathogenically, there is usually pulmonary edema in the acute cases; and in the cases of longer duration, there is consolidation of the lungs in addition. Petechial hemorrhages occur in the pericardium, pleura, conjunctiva, and skin. In the brain, the classical picture is that of petechial hemorrhages in the meninges and scattered throughout the brain, and minute foci of softening in the cortex and medulla.

Microscopically, there may be vascular occlusion by fat emboli without reaction, perivascular hemorrhage, or perivascular edema.

Clinically, the cases are characterized by a period of freedom from symptoms following the trauma. The diagnosis is difficult, but the condition may be suspected after the development of cerebral or pulmonary symptoms following (1) fracture or extensive injury of soft parts and (2) manipulation of a fracture.

The relationship between the vascular accident in cases of cerebral embolism and severe injuries and caisson disease is usually readily apparent.

V. CEREBRAL THROMBOSIS

Thrombosis of a cerebral vessel results in occlusion of the vessel and resultant softening of the brain tissue (encephalomalacia; infarct). In the vast majority of cases, it is arterial in origin (anemic or white infarct), but in some cases venous thrombosis occurs (hemorrhagic or red infarct). The following descriptions concern arterial thrombosis. This form of cerebral vascular disease is much more frequent than is cerebral hemorrhage, which it outnumbers in a ratio of three to one or four to one.

Etiology: Cerebral thrombosis occurs at many ages due to the variety of conditions which produce it. In most instances, it is a disease of older subjects, of fifty years or over. In some cases, as in some of the conditions listed below, it occurs in younger people.

Arteriosclerosis of the cerebral vessels is the most common cause. In a large series of patients with cerebral thrombosis, markedly sclerosed cerebral vessels were found in 74.3 per cent; moderately sclerosed vessels in 24.3 per cent. The peripheral vessels are usually sclerosed as well, but this is not invariable. *Syphilis* of the cerebral vessels is a common cause in younger subjects of 35 years or even younger. Febrile diseases, such as *typhoid fever* and *pneumonia,* are sometimes the cause of cerebral thrombosis. *Trauma* may be responsible at times. *Polycythemia vera* is commonly associated with cerebral thromboses. *Carbon monoxide* poisoning is at times responsible for the condition. Transitory and even perma-

Table 44—Causes of Cerebral Thrombosis (in Autopsy Verified Cases)

	No. Cases
CEREBRAL ARTERIOSCLEROSIS	216
DIABETES WITH ARTERIOSCLEROSIS	4
HYPERTENSION	3
PROLIFERATIVE ENDARTERITIS	6
THROMBOSIS OF THE INTERNAL CAROTID ARTERY	2
SYPHILIS	2
MENINGITIS	2
PNEUMONITIS	2
ASPHYXIA	1
COLLAGEN DISEASE	1
TOTAL	239

nent cerebral disturbances (hemiplegia, aphasia, etc.) may follow the use of *antihypertensive drugs.* The disturbances in question seem to appear more regularly when the blood pressure is lowered too quickly and too radically. Thrombosis of cerebral veins may occur rarely during the *puerperium.* They usually appear between the fourth and twenty-first day after a normal pregnancy and labor, though the onset may at times be much later. The early signs include headache, focal or generalized convulsions, monoplegia or hemiplegia. Papilledema may be present if there is obstruction of the sagittal sinus. The cerebrospinal fluid shows no abnormalities except for blood cells at times if the sagittal sinus is obstructed. Cases are usually regarded as due to cerebral embolism or as encephalitis. The condition is probably due to primary thrombosis, but it is regarded by some as embolism secondary to thrombosis of the pelvic veins. Recovery is the rule if the patient survives the initial episode, but residual signs and symptoms may persist. The mortality in the original episode is high.

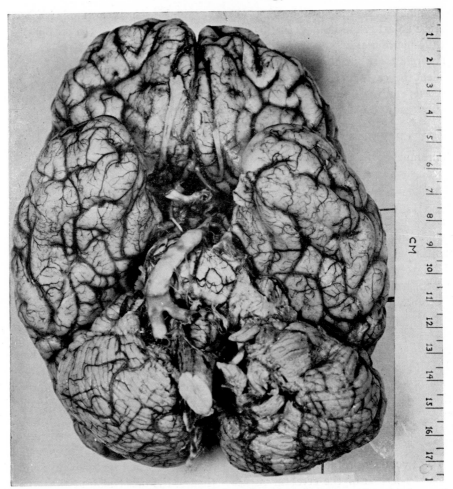

Fig. 135—_Cerebral arteriosclerosis,_ **showing the severe sclerosis of the basilar and vertebral vessels.**

Thromboangiitis obliterans (Buerger's disease) may at times involve the cerebral vessels (two per cent) and produce evidence of vascular disease, such as hemiplegia, aphasia, tics, seizures, memory disturbances, apraxia, and agnosia. Confusional episodes, excitement, and psychoses may occur. The cerebral symptoms may precede, but more commonly follow, other manifestations of the disease. The clinical course in cases of Buerger's disease of the cerebral vessels is often characterized by a history of transient cerebral phenomena, such as transitory hemiparesis. etc. The changes in the cerebral vessels are similar to those found elsewhere in the body. In rare instances, the cause of cerebral thrombosis is unassignable to a specific cause, especially in young subjects. In such instances, no cardiovascular disease is evident and in some reported cases telangiectases of the cerebral vessels have been found to be at fault.

Dissecting aneurysm of the aorta must be considered in the causation of obscure cerebral vascular disorders. Its features have been considered under spinal disorders.

Pathology: Softenings which occur as the result of arteriosclerosis are among the most commonly encountered lesions in the brain. In such cases the brain almost always shows some degree of arteriosclerosis of the large vessels of the circle of Willis. The degree of sclerosis varies in the individual case; usually it is marked. The internal carotid vessels are usually sclerosed in such cases, sometimes standing out like pipestems. In such cases the entire vessel wall is a rigid tube. The vertebral and basilar arteries are usually involved and, to a lesser degree, the posterior cerebral vessels. The middle cerebral vessels which branch off the internal carotids are among those most severely sclerosed. Sometimes the sclerosis is so severe that there is tortuosity of the vessels of the circle of Willis.

As a rule, the vessels in the pia over the cerebral hemispheres are much less affected than the vessels at the base of the brain. Occasionally, one sees a scle-rotic vessel in the pia over the cortex. It is possible in the case of the main vessels which supply the cerebral hemisphere to follow the main branch of the sclerotic anterior, middle, or posterior cerebral artery for some distance after leaving the circle of Willis, but the branches which spread over the hemisphere, i. e., the preterminal branches in the pia, are not so much affected. In the brain itself in such cases there may or may not be sclerosis of the cortical arterioles. Frequently there is little or no involvement of the vessels within the cortex itself in the presence of the most intense arteriosclerosis of the large cerebral vessels in the circle of Willis. On the other hand, there may be marked sclerosis of the cortical arterioles when there is little sclerosis of the large vessels.

In some cases there is both sclerosis of the large vessels and of the cortical arterioles. The brain in patients with

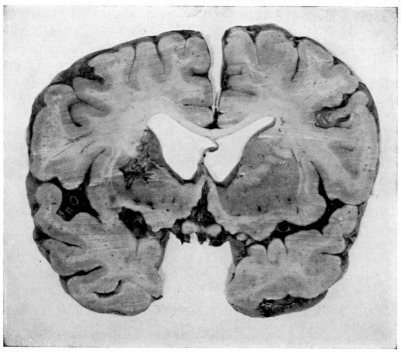

Fig. 136—*Cerebral thrombosis*, showing an old softening involving the internal capsule due to occlusion of the lenticulo-striate branch of the middle cerebral artery.

thrombotic softening shows a moderate or marked thickening of the pia-arachnoid, usually more marked in the frontal areas. The dura is thickened and often adherent to the skull. The membranes along the longitudinal sinus are especially thickened. There is usually a moderate or advanced atrophy of the brain tissue, especially in the frontal region. The atrophy becomes less marked in the more posterior parts of the brain.

One or more areas of softening of various size are invariably found in brains with intense arteriosclerosis. The localization of such areas has been worked out with considerable certainty. Thrombotic softenings in the cerebral hemispheres are most frequently found in the putamen, the caudate nucleus, the pallidum and claustrum, and finally the thalamus. Involvement of the internal capsule is present in the involvement of the basal ganglia mentioned, usually the anterior limb and knee from occlusion of the lenticulostriate and the posterior limb from involvement of the lenticulo-optic branch of the middle cerebral artery. The softenings in the putamen and other basal ganglia are usually multiple. They consist of small areas of softening, varying in size from 0.5 to 1 cm. in diameter. Sometimes most of the putamen is destroyed by the softening. Large portions of the cerebral hemisphere are softened by involvement of the anterior, middle, or posterior cerebral vessels. Less frequently softenings are found in the base of the brain. In the midbrain they are found in the floor of the aqueduct of Sylvius, causing oculomotor palsies, especially in diabetes, syphilis, and to a lesser degree in arteriosclerosis. Softenings are found in this region also involving the cerebral peduncle of one side and the opposite oculomotor nerve at its exit from the midbrain (Weber's syndrome). A similar softening involving the red nucleus and the oculomotor nerve is sometimes encountered (Benedikt's syndrome).

In the pons, softenings are found in the tegmentum under the floor of the fourth ventricle, involving the abducens and facial nerves and the pyramidal tract (Foville and Raymond-Cestan syndromes). Rarely a thrombosis of the basilar artery is encountered, producing softening of the base of the pons and much of the reticular substance under the fourth ventricle. In the medulla thromboses are found involving by softening (1) the lateral portion of the medulla (posterior-inferior cerebellar artery thrombosis) and (2) the anterior portion from thrombosis of the anterior spinal artery. These various syndromes will be discussed in a consideration of the symptoms and syndromes of cerebral softening.

The gross appearance of softenings is much the same no matter what part of the brain is affected. After occlusion of the vessel the brain tissue becomes softened. This softening may not be complete in the very first days after the occlusion, but it results later in a complete disintegration of the tissues and the formation of a cyst. In a large softening involving the cerebral hemispheres the tissue is swollen, soft to the palpating finger and has a very edematous appearance when fresh. Chemical studies indicate that the brain in vascular occlusion is actually edematous. An old area of softening will be seen as a large destructive area in the cerebral hemispheres. The tissue in this region is destroyed and the hemisphere has lost much of its bulk. It has a yellow appearance due to the collection of hemosiderin in the affected cortex. Beneath it the white matter is destroyed. There may be septa of tissue running through the destroyed area. The latter is usually collapsed, so that a large area of softening is frequently seen externally as a collapsed and destroyed region. The extent of the softened area varies, depending on the vessel which has been occluded. Anterior cerebral occlusion will cause softening in the frontal region, the middle cerebral in the lateral portion, main. Complete dissolution takes place. At the edge of the softening is a transition zone between this and the normal tissue. It is composed of numerous vessels, abnormal glial forms, and connective tissue. The vessels are not abnormal except that they are more numerous than normal. The microglia adjacent to the

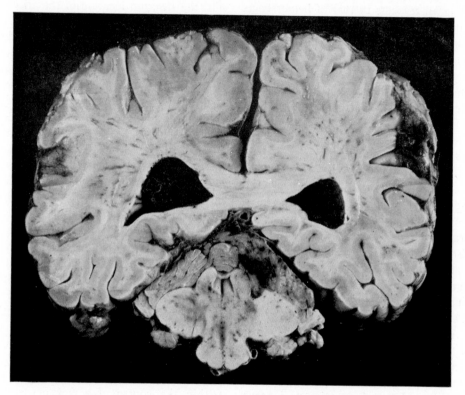

Fig. 137—*Cerebral thrombosis* involving the cerebellar hemisphere.

and the posterior cerebral in the posterior part of the cerebral hemisphere. The main branch of the middle cerebral artery may be occluded, thus causing softening of almost the entire hemisphere, but it is more usual to have occlusion of only a branch of the vessel.

The microscopic features of the softenings are quite uniform. In areas of complete softenings, the brain tissue is replaced by gitter cells which fill the destroyed area. No ganglion cells re- softened area show all sorts of abnormal forms, most of which are transition forms to gitter cells. Many of these cells contain hemosiderin pigment. The oligodendroglia are swollen. The astrocytes are at first swollen and may even assume ameboid forms. Later, astrocytes are more numerous, a definite gliosis occurs, and a glial wall is formed around the softening. The connective tissue is seen chiefly around the vessels; it does not penetrate far into the tissue. The ganglion cells are diseased around the softened area. As the softening becomes chronic, a glial-fibrous wall is formed around it.

Symptoms: The *onset* in cerebral thrombosis is usually gradual in contrast to the apoplectic development of symptoms in cerebral hemorrhage. A sudden onset is not uncommon and may be similar in all respects to that of hemorrhage, but the onset with immediate loss of consciousness is about twice as frequent in hemorrhage as in thrombosis. Premonitory symptoms are present for some time before the occlusion of the vessel occurs, but little attention is usually paid to them. They can be uncovered, however, by careful questioning. They may be found intermittently for days, weeks, or months before the cerebral accident. They consist of transient attacks of vertigo, headache, or even of mental confusion of brief duration. Cerebral thrombosis is said to develop during sleep more frequently than in the waking state, due to slowing of the circulation, but the point is of little significance, since the onset may be at any time of the day or night.

After premonitory symptoms have persisted for varying periods of time, the symptoms of actual occlusion of the vessel develop. These vary in form and quantity. *Loss of consciousness* occurs in about one-half of the cases. In many no loss of consciousness is found; in others, it may be evanescent and described as a momentary attack of dizziness or a blackout. *Convulsions* are sometimes associated with the vessel occlusion. In some instances of occlusion of a large vessel, profound stupor simulating closely that found in cerebral hemorrhage may be found.

With the disturbance of consciousness, evidences of brain damage occur, appearing usually as a *hemiplegia* with or without aphasia, but at times manifested by hemianopsia or other evidences of focal brain damage. The hemiplegia usually develops rapidly or it may unfold gradually over a number of minutes, hours, or even a few days. The onset and development is not constant and depends probably on a number of factors, among which are the rate of closure of the vessels, the size and location of the affected vessel, and the amount of brain tissue deprived of its blood supply. Sudden occlusion of a large vessel results in profound loss of consciousness and a sudden development of hemiplegia or other focal symptoms. In other instances of cerebral thrombosis, the history is forthcoming that the patient has arisen in the morning with a hemiplegia; or he has noticed development of weakness of the arm while shaving with subsequent involvement of the leg in the course of several minutes or a few hours; or he has been afflicted with weakness of the hand while at work and has found himself with a hemiplegia in the course of a few hours.

In the acute stages, the hemiplegia has the features described in cerebral hemorrhage, is often flaccid, and is frequently accompanied by aphasia. It is much more often incomplete than in hemorrhage, a hemiparesis resulting rather than a complete hemiplegia. Recovery may begin within the course of a few or several hours and may be complete in a few weeks. In the average instance, recovery begins after a few weeks and proceeds slowly over the course of months. In still other cases, it may develop over the course of a year.

As recovery occurs, the leg progresses faster than the arm. Flaccidity is replaced by spasticity. The leg is held in extension, the arm in partial flexion with the fingers adducted and flexed, the forearm flexed and pronated and the limb adducted. The gait is characteristic with the leg circumducted and dragged and with the arm and hand held in flexion. In instances in which recovery from the hemiplegia is complete, the hand and fingers recover last and may never regain their normal dexterity.

The hemiplegia may be spastic from the very onset and may not be preceded by a stage of flaccidity.

In some cases, *monoplegia* develops instead of hemiplegia. This may be manifested as weakness or paralysis of a hand or arm, or merely facial and lingual paralysis of a central type. A variety of combinations is possible, depending on the area of motor cortex which is damaged. *Aphasia* is often present in cases of cerebral thrombosis with or without hemiplegia. *Hemianopsia* sometimes develops in occipital and temporal lobe lesions.

Diagnosis: The diagnosis of cerebral thrombosis is not as a rule difficult. General examination often reveals cardiac abnormalities in cerebral thrombosis (eighty per cent), manifested usually by cardiac enlargement and in some instances fibrillation. Peripheral arteriosclerosis is almost always found. Vascular hypertension is often present but is not invariably found. Retinal arteriosclerosis is always present, its degree paralleling closely the degree of arteriosclerosis found in the cerebral vessels. A careful study of the retinal arteries is therefore important and constitutes an accurate index of the state of the large cerebral vessels. The urine in over half the cases reveals albumin or casts and there may be an increase of the nonprotein nitrogen of the blood. There may be a leukocytosis, but it is neither constant nor diagnostic. The cerebrospinal fluid may show an increase of pressure, especially during the acute cerebral episode, but it is rarely over 300 mm. of water, in contrast to cerebral hemorrhage. The fluid is clear, but may at times be xanthochromic. It is never grossly bloody, but a few red cells may be seen microscopically in some cases.

The history of premonitory symptoms, such as headache, confusion, and vertigo, followed by the development of hemiplegia, either gradual or sudden in onset, in a patient over fifty years of age with evidence of cerebral arteriosclerosis, is sufficient to establish the diagnosis of cerebral thrombosis due to sclerosis of the cerebral vessels, especially if the onset has been with incomplete loss of consciousness, a transitory loss, or no loss at all, and particularly if evidences of shock are not profound and recovery from the immediate cerebral insult appears evident. Hypertension need not be present and indeed is often absent; renal disease may or may not be found; peripheral arteriosclerosis is usually present.

Since cerebral thrombosis is most commonly due to cerebral arteriosclerosis, the condition as outlined will cover the diagnosis in the majority of instances. Those cases associated with fevers, polycythemia, head injury, etc., will be apparent from the associated condition in which they develop. Its differentiation from cerebral hemorrhage has already been considered and the main features of its development outlined. In some instances, it is extremely difficult to distinguish between slow occlusion of a vessel in older people with resultant softening and a *brain tumor*. In both instances, the history of a progressively developing lesion is striking. There is no evidence of increased pressure in the fundi or by spinal fluid manometer, but the problem is complicated by the fact that the type of tumor likely to be confused with a slowly developing thrombosis is often unassociated with signs of increased pressure. The rate of development is less rapid in tumor than in thrombosis. There is often no evidence of vascular hypertension. The distinction between the two conditions may be impossible except by air studies, but may be aided by the detection of retinal or peripheral arteriosclerosis. In rare instances, *primary thrombosis of cerebral veins occurs,* usually in the puerperium or in general and local infection. The condition is characterized by convulsions and paralysis with premonitory symptoms, such as headache, weakness, and cramps. The convulsions probably coincide with the sudden obstruction of a meningeal vein. Hemiplegia or monoplegia may be present if the obstructed vein is in the frontal area. Small amounts of blood may be found in the spinal fluid. The diagnosis is extremely difficult and has been made in most cases at postmortem examination.

Cerebral complications occur during pregnancy, producing hemiplegia and other focal signs. *"Fibrin embolism"* has been described in pregnancy, occurring in the last trimester of pregnancy, seen especially in patients having premature separation of the placenta, and attributed to excessive amounts of thromboplastin forced into the peripheral circulation.

The problem of *cerebral vascular disorders in the young* is somewhat different from that of older subjects in whom arteriosclerosis and hypertension play predominant roles. Other conditions require consideration in the young. These include heart disease (subacute bacterial endocarditis and mitral stenosis); ruptured cerebral aneurysm; hemorrhage into an angioma; delayed traumatic cerebral hemorrhage; blood dyscrasias (leukemia and purpura); injury to the carotid artery in the neck; cerebral embolism from pressure on the subclavian artery by a cervical rib; fat embolism; air embolism;

thromboangiitis obliterans; and venous thrombosis.

Neurological complications are not infrequently found in *sickle cell* anemia. The lesions are multiple and their locations variable. They consist of thromboses of the smaller vessels with congestion with sickle cells, infiltrative and degenerative changes of the vessel walls, perivascular edema, hemorrhage, and necrosis. Similar changes occur in the spinal cord. Convulsions, headache, drowsiness, vertigo, meningeal signs, aphasia, hemiplegia, confusional psychoses, and delirium may develop. The onset is usually rapid and the outlook poor. Recurrent episodes occur. The spinal fluid is usually normal, but may in some cases show increased pressure, sickle cells, xanthochromia, and increased protein.

The capillary vessels have been reported to be altered throughout the brain in *acute rheumatic fever* (Costero). Further studies indicate that lesions of intracranial vessels occur with unexpected frequency in the late stages of rheumatic heart disease, the larger and smaller arteries and veins, mainly in the leptomeninges, showing various forms of thrombosis, endarteritic proliferation, alteration of the elastic membranes and fibrosis of media and adventitia (Denst and Neuberger).

Cerebral infarcts have been found to occur frequently in patients with congenital cyanotic heart disease and in the majority of these patients are the result of vascular occlusions (Berthrong and Sabiston).

Nervous system complications may develop during the course of disease of the blood forming tissues. In *Hodgkin's disease,* spinal cord complications may occur in 10 to 14 per cent of cases. They may include evidences of spinal cord compression, posterolateral sclerosis, and root pains. Cerebral complications may appear in the form of aphasia, hemiplegia, cranial nerve paralyses, peripheral facial paralysis, vertigo, and choked disc.

In *leukemia,* central nervous system complications are found in 20.5 per cent of cases (Schwab and Weiss). They consist of cranial nerve paralyses, meningeal irritation, hemiplegia, and vertigo. In *thrombocytopenic purpura,* there may be many sorts of complications due to brain hemorrhages. These include hemiplegias, subarachnoid hemorrhage, subdural hemorrhage, and choked disc.

Polycythemia vera is frequently associated with neurological symptoms due to the associated thromboses which are found in the venous system. Focal symptoms of a varied character are frequently found, such as hemiplegia, aphasia, or hemianopsia. Choked disc is seen not infrequently and may lead to extreme difficulty in the differentiation from brain tumor, especially in the presence of focal signs. Neurological symptoms may be the first sign of the disease. *Neurogenic polycythemia,* or polycythemia occurring secondarily to neurological disorders of various sorts, is sometimes seen. It is found chiefly with diseases in the region of the hypophyseal-infundibular-diencephalic region, but it has been found also in association with cerebellar hemangioblastomas (Carpenter, Schwartz, and Walker). Encephalitis, concussion, Huntington's chorea, paralysis agitans, carbon monoxide poisoning, and pituitary tumors have been found to be associated with polycythemia. In neurogenic polycythemia, there is no enlargement of the spleen.

Hemophilia is associated with nervous system complications of many sorts (Aggeler and Lucia). Cerebral hemorrhage is occasionally encountered, and pontile hemorrhage has been recorded. Hematomyelia may develop, as well as subdural and subarachnoid hemorrhage of the spinal meninges. More frequent is subdural and subarachnoid hemorrhage in the cerebral meninges. Involvement of the facial, sciatic, femoral, peroneal, median, and ulnar nerves has been recorded in hemophilia (Aggeler and Lucia).

A variety of syndromes are encountered in cerebral thrombosis, depending on the vessel which is occluded. Occlusion of the *anterior cerebral artery* is not as common as that of the middle cerebral vessel. Various syndromes result from occlusions of the numerous branches. A thrombus in the main branch of the vessel just as it leaves the circle of Willis results in a hemiplegia of severe degree, some sensory loss over the paralyzed leg, left-sided apraxia (if the hemiplegia is right-sided), mental changes and some degree of aphasia in a left-sided lesion. Incontinence is usually present. Other occlusions of the main trunk of the anterior cerebral artery occur at various points along its course, but the signs which are produced are not very much different from those of occlusion of the main branch, and in any event have not been clearly enough defined to emphasize their distinctive features. Thus, in occlusion of the artery somewhat beyond its point of emergence from the circle of Willis, there results in addition to the signs just mentioned a grasp reflex which is due to involvement of the cerebral cortex in the region of the superior frontal convolution in its posterior part.

Any of the individual branches of the anterior cerebral artery may be occluded. From the practical standpoint by far the most important is the branch to the *paracentral lobule.* This is characterized by weakness of the opposite leg. Patients with occlusion of this branch complain chiefly of leg weakness, with slight weakness of the arm and possibly of the face.

Essentially, therefore, the lesion is a
crural monoplegia due to the fact that
the paracentral lobule gives origin to the
fibers which innervate the lower limb.
The lower limb weakness has certain
well-defined features. Thus the weakness
is greatest in the distal portions of the
limb; the foot in such cases is weakest
of all and as one ascends the leg to the
thigh the power in the affected limb
becomes increasingly greater. The reflexes are increased in the limb and there
is a Babinski sign. The weakness of the
arm may be entirely absent. Usually, it
is slight and transitory.

Lesions of the cerebral arteries, other
than the anterior cerebral, are unlikely
to cause a marked paralysis of one leg
without affecting equally severely the
arm, face, or tongue on that side. Most
of the vascular thromboses of the brain
involve the *middle cerebral artery*. Occlusion of the main trunk causes hemiplegia, hemianesthesia, expressive and
auditory-receptive aphasia, all of these
due to softening of the lateral surface of
the cerebral hemisphere. More common
is the occlusion of the lenticulostriate
branch of the middle cerebral artery,
resulting in a typical spastic hemiplegia
from the destruction of the internal capsule. Aphasia alone may develop from
thrombosis of the branch to the area
of Broca in the third frontal gyrus
or of the branch to the first temporal
gyrus.

Occlusion of the *internal carotid artery*
as a cause of hemiplegia is probably uncommon, but there are indications that
it may be more frequent than suspected.
It occurs most frequently in men, between the ages of fifty and eighty, but
cases have been reported in young subjects. It develops usually as a result of
thrombosis in an arteriosclerotic vessel,
but it may be embolic. It may follow
penetrating wounds of the neck. Trans-

ient episodes of hemiparesis, paresthesias
of the limbs of one side, aphasia or unilateral blindness may have been present
for a varying period of time prior to the
onset of the hemiplegia which characterizes the disorder. Such transient episodes
are not uncommon. The hemiplegia may
develop gradually over a period of weeks
or months, one part after another becoming weak or paralyzed, and the pic-

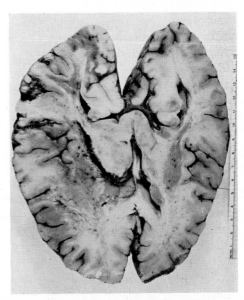

Fig. 138 — *Right internal carotid artery
thrombosis* showing the usual area of softening in the middle cerebral distribution,
with sparing of the anterior cerebral
distribution.

ture may be that of a progressive weakness involving one side of the body.
Usually the hemiplegia begins acutely
Consciousness may be impaired or lost.
Headache is common, intermittent, is
usually unilateral, and is situated often
over the eye on the side of the affected
artery. Blindness involving one eye develops in some instances on the side
opposite to the hemiplegia, and is due to
involvement of the ophthalmic artery
within the skull. In such instances
transitory episodes of blindness may occur, prior to the development of perma-

nent blindness. Hemianesthesia and homonymous hemianopsia may be found in severe cases. The diagnosis can be made with certainty only by carotid arteriography, but a presumptive diagnosis may be made in occlusion of the artery in the neck, by the absence of carotid pulsation on the affected side. In those instances in which unilateral blindness occurs the syndrome of unilateral blindness and optic atrophy of one side with hemiplegia of the opposite side is characteristic of occlusion of the internal carotid artery in the skull, with involvement of the ophthalmic artery. In most instances, the artery is occluded in the carotid sinus. The spinal fluid is clear. Roentgenograms of the skull show nothing abnormal. Occlusion of the *posterior cerebral artery* may cause hemianopsia from closure of the branch supplying the occipital lobe. The syndrome of the *anterior choroidal artery* results in hemiplegia, hemianesthesia, and hemianopsia due to destruction of the posterior limb of the internal capsule and the sensory fibers coursing through it and the visual fibers lying behind it.

Since the posterior cerebral artery supplies in part the thalamus, occlusion of the thalamic branches causes softenings in this nucleus and the production of the *thalamic syndrome*. This syndrome is characterized by (1) hemianesthesia, (2) hemichorea, (3) central pains, and (4) hemiparesis. The hemianesthesia is complete. It involves all forms of sensation: pain, heat, cold, touch, vibration, position, and muscle senses. The deeper sensations, such as position and vibration senses, are more affected than the others, but all are severely affected. In the usual case there is loss of all the sensory components. In other cases, there may be a slight appreciation of pain or temperature, though this never reaches a normal degree. In the original

cases described by Dejerine and Marie, hemichoreiform movements were regarded as an integral part of the syndrome. These are sometimes present but are not essential for the diagnosis. Usually they are absent.

Central pains are also said to be a characteristic feature of the thalamic syndrome. These pains are deep, lancinating and boring in character. They are felt deep in the soft tissues or bones. While they are sometimes present in cases of thalamic syndrome, they are by no means constant. When present, they are quite characteristic, but they are not essential for diagnosis. Much more characteristic of the sensory changes in thalamic lesions is the tendency on the part of the patient to overrespond to stimuli and to feel the effects of the stimuli long after the stimulus has ceased. Thus, pricking the anesthetic side with a pin causes a most unpleasant sensation which holds on for some time after the stimulus. Hemiparesis is not usually encountered in the average thalamic syndrome. It is sometimes found, however, and a diagnosis of thalamic syndrome must not, therefore, be excluded because of its presence. It is due probably to involvement of the adjacent internal capsule.

The syndrome of *pseudobulbar palsy* is almost always of vascular origin so that it may best be considered here. The syndrome is spoken of as pseudobulbar palsy because the bulbar symptoms, such as difficulty in swallowing, talking, etc., are due to involvement of the corticobulbar fibers in contradistinction to the bulbar paralysis in which similar symptoms result from disease of the cells in the medulla. In pseudobulbar palsy, the swallowing and speech difficulties are unassociated with atrophy of the affected muscles. In true bulbar palsy, the tongue, face, and other muscles are atrophied, show muscle fasciculations and other evidences of anterior horn cell disease due to involvement of the affected nuclei in the pons and medulla.

The cause is arteriosclerosis in the vast majority of cases. Other causes include syphilitic vascular disease, multiple sclerosis, encephalitis, porencephaly, and tuberculous meningitis. The pathological background in most cases consists of bilateral areas of softening, involving the pallidum, striatum, thalamus, and the internal capsules. The cerebral cortex is affected in over half the cases. It reveals multiple areas of cell loss, infarctions, and even minute softenings. Pseudobulbar palsy syndromes may be produced by bilateral involvement of the frontal lobes and lower portions of the motor cortex without basal ganglia disease.

The onset of the disease is usually sudden, but some cases develop gradually. The usual course consists of development of a hemiplegia in the majority of cases, but it is not unusual for cases to develop with bulbar symptoms alone, without evidence of hemiplegia, difficulty in swallowing, and talking (dysarthria particularly). After a varying period of time ranging from a few days to ten or twelve years, a subsequent attack of hemiplegia develops, or there is another episode of bulbar symptoms. The subsequent hemiplegia usually involves the opposite side, but in a small group of patients (eight to ten per cent), it involves the same side. There may be two to four attacks as a rule or as many as eight to twelve in a single subject. Often there may be complete recovery after the first attack. The bulbar symptoms consist of dysarthria, paralysis of the face, palate, and pharynx, difficulties in mastication, and paralysis of the tongue. Attacks of uncontrollable laughing or crying without suitable provocation are characteristic but do not occur in every instance.

They may be the most prominent features of the disease. The speech is nasal in type in the average patient; in others, a complete anarthria may be present. Paralysis of the vocal cord may rarely be present. Aphonia may be found. Swallowing is difficult and food is often regurgitated through the nose. Liquids are swallowed with greater difficulty than solids, though both may be greatly affected.

Despite the bulbar symptoms, no evidence of atrophy is seen involving the face, palate, or tongue, and no fibrillations are seen. The average subject reveals evidence of bilateral pyramidal tract signs. These vary, however, some patients showing only a hemiplegia with pseudobulbar symptoms, others a bilateral hemiplegia, and still others no pyramidal tract signs whatever but prominent bulbar symptoms. Other evidences of cerebral damage may be present, such as aphasia, intellectual deterioration, etc. Most patients show impairment of intellectual faculties due to cortical damage, demonstrated by loss of memory, impairment of judgment, etc.

Pseudobulbar palsy is a syndrome which is always the result of bilateral brain lesions. This is its significance of first importance. Recognition of this fundamental feature constitutes the first step in correct diagnosis of the underlying cause. It is obvious, of course, that realization of the fact that multiple foci of damage are at the basis of the symptoms will lead to certain orientations in diagnosis and prognosis different from those attributable to a single lesion. Of equal significance is the fact that the syndrome is the result usually of deep-seated lesions of the basal ganglia and capsular region. The cause, as has already been indicated, are several, but the most common is cerebral arteriosclerosis with multiple areas of softening in the brain. Other causes have been mentioned above.

Occlusions of the *basilar artery* by thrombosis or embolism have been clearly defined (Kubik and Adams). The symptoms appear suddenly and are not preceded by tangible causal factors. The first symptom is usually headache, dizziness, confusion, or coma. Difficulty in speaking and unilateral paresthesias occur in a large proportion of cases. Common findings are pupillary abnormalities, disorder of ocular movements, facial palsy, hemiplegia and/or quadriplegia, and bilateral Babinski signs. Cranial nerve palsies and contralateral hemiplegia may be combined. Not all these signs are present in every case. It is common for temporary improvement, lasting for days or hours, to occur. Death follows in the majority of cases in from two days to five weeks. A few patients survive. The spinal fluid is normal.

Disturbance of consciousness varying from slight confusion to deep coma is one of the earliest and most constant symptoms and occurs sooner or later in every case. Dizziness and headache are common. Dysarthria or other pseudobulbar symptoms is one of the most frequent and impressive manifestations. In some, there may be inability to swallow and paralysis of the tongue. Bilateral weakness of the facial muscles, emotional lability, and even pathological laughing and crying are observed. Paresthesias are sometimes present and are usually unilateral. Hemiplegia or quadriplegia is observed in every case but not always at the onset. Pupillary abnormalities are noted in almost every case, small fixed pupils being most common. Alternating facial paralysis is sometimes seen, and impairment of vision may occur. Respirations become stertorous, rapid, or Cheyne-Stokes in the terminal stages, and hyperthermia is common.

Transitory symptoms similar to those of basilar artery occlusion are reported to occur as a result of basilar artery insufficiency.

The diagnosis (Kubik and Adams) is based in most cases on the presence of bilateral involvement. Outstanding are various combinations of (1) pupillary disturbances, (2) ocular palsies and other cranial nerve palsies, (3) dysarthria, (4) bilateral extensor plantar reflexes, (5) hemiplegia or quadriplegia, and (6) commonly a marked remission of symptoms.

The clinical picture may be confused with (1) pontine hemorrhage, which is more abrupt in onset and is associated with hypertension, a bloody spinal fluid, and rapid course; (2) massive cerebral hemorrhage; (3) massive cerebral infarction; and (4) acute multiple sclerosis.

Cerebellar vascular softenings or hemorrhages are rare. In three hundred cases of cerebral vascular insults with necropsy, only twenty involved the cerebellum. Of the three cerebellar arteries—the superior cerebellar, the posterior-inferior cerebellar, and the anterior-inferior cerebellar— the first two have had their syndromes most clearly defined.

Complete occlusion of the *superior cerebellar artery* gives rise to (1) cerebellar signs on the side of the arterial occlusion, (2) involuntary movements on the homolateral side, and (3) sensory disturbances of the opposite side of the body. Not all these signs are present in every instance. The cerebellar disturbances are the most constant. The sensory disturbances and involuntary movements are less constant. In a case of superior cerebellar artery occlusion there is dyssynergia of the arm and leg, and sometimes of one of the opposite limbs. The cerebellar symptoms are as a rule quite pronounced. The involuntary movements are manifested by a coarse tremor of the arm and occasionally of the head. This tremor is quite distinctive. It is elicited on voluntary movements, is rhythmic, constant on motion and increased by emotional stimuli. It has been observed frequently in cases of this syndrome by some, but in other series it has not been so frequently encountered. As for the contralateral sensory disturbances, these are usually manifested by a loss or decreased perception of pain and temperature on the side opposite the tremor and cerebellar disturbances, due to the involvement of the spinothalamic tract which is supplied by the superior cerebellar artery. The pain and temperature disturbance involves the face, limbs, and trunk.

These are the signs one encounters in a fully developed case of superior cerebellar artery occlusion. Frequently, the syndrome is not encountered in all its manifestations. In such cases the cerebellar signs are present, with or without the tremor or the sensory disturbances. The diagnosis is not difficult in the fully developed syndrome, since no other lesion can produce a similar picture. In the less clearly defined cases, the diagnosis may be extremely difficult. Superior cerebellar artery syndromes may be encountered also in cases of infiltrating tumors of the midbrain.

Of greater practical importance is the syndrome of the *posterior inferior cerebellar artery* which is more frequently affected by occlusion than the superior cerebellar artery.

The symptomatology is quite characteristic. Most of the cases occur in males between fifty and sixty years of age. Many of the patients exhibit signs of generalized arteriosclerosis and chronic cardiovascular-renal disease. Syphilis is sometimes present and may be the cause of the vascular occlusion. Usually the cause is cerebral arteriosclerosis. Rarely it may be embolic from heart disease.

The author has seen a typical instance in Hodgkin's disease. The symptoms are striking but not dramatic. They come on suddenly without previous warning in a person who may or may not have had premonition of difficulty previously. There is usually no loss of consciousness, despite the involvement of a very vital part of the brain. There is usually marked subjective and objective vertigo, and severe nausea and vomiting at the onset of the attack.

The onset may be characterized by successive attacks of vertigo repeated at irregular intervals over a period of days. Similarly, dysesthesias, such as tingling or prickling sensations, may be felt in the ipsilateral side of the face before evidences of actual occlusion of the vessel. This is followed soon by a sensation of weakness in the arm and leg of one side, difficulty in walking due to incoordination, difficulty in swallowing, and a change in the timbre of the voice from a weak and husky voice to complete aphonia. The patient soon becomes aware also of loss of sensation on one side of the face, and possibly diplopia and ptosis of one eyelid.

The subjective symptoms are enough to force the patient to bed, but they are not as a rule attended with severe symptoms of collapse. These sometimes occur, however, and are accompanied by profuse general perspiration, tachycardia, and other signs of generalized involvement. Sometimes the patient may weather an incomplete occlusion of the artery and remain ambulatory. Usually, however, patients are forced to bed by the severe vertigo which is present at the onset and by the incoördination resulting from the cerebellar involvement. Sometimes the onset of symptoms may be with pain in the eye or on one side of the face, together with dizziness and dysphagia.

Ipsilateral Symptoms	Contralateral Symptoms
1. Loss of pain and temperature over the face	1. Loss of pain and temperature over the limbs and trunk, but not the face
2. Horner's syndrome	
3. Palatal paralysis	
4. Vocal cord paralysis	
5. Cerebellar dyssynergia of the limbs	

Examination reveals signs both ipsilateral and contralateral to the lesion. Disturbance of equilibrium is present, often with sensations of lateropulsion. Cerebellar incoördination of the arm and leg on the side of the affected vessel are constant. In addition, pain and temperature disturbances involving the face are present in practically all cases. The corneal reflex is lost. Often the disturbance of pain and temperature over the face has a lamellar arrangement, giving the so-called onion peel type of sensory loss. A Horner's syndrome is sometimes present on the side of the lesion and an ipsilateral paralysis of the palate and larynx resulting in hoarseness and difficulty in swallowing. On the opposite side of the body, involving only the limbs and trunk, is a loss of pain and temperature. In occasional cases the cervical or thoracic regions may show sparing of the sensory loss; in most cases, however, the entire opposite side of the body is affected. In addition to these characteristic signs, there may be at times loss of taste over the anterior two-thirds of the tongue, paresis of the external rectus muscle of the eye, occasional loss of sweating over the face, obstinate hiccough, involuntary micturition, and headache.

The picture of occlusion of the posterior inferior cerebellar artery is not always typical. Variations may occur (1) in the distribution of the sensory disturbances and (2) in the involvement of the cranial nerves.

The loss of pain, heat, and cold sensations may involve the opposite face, limbs, and trunk instead of the ipsilateral face and the opposite limbs and trunk. The absence of sensory loss on the same side of the face as the lesion is due to the fact that the spinal root of the trigeminal nerve fails to be supplied by the posterior inferior cerebellar artery in some instances (Stopford). "The disturbances of sensation in the half of the face opposite to the lesion must be the result of implication of the fibers arising from the opposite spinal nucleus as they lie in the deeper part of the substantia reticularis grisea" (Stopford).

In some instances, not only are the ipsilateral face and the opposite limbs and trunk involved in the sensory loss, but also the opposite side of the face.

Similarly, the involvement of cranial nerves varies. Palatal weakness may be combined with vocal cord paresis or paralysis of the same side as the lesion, or the one may exist without the other. Horner's syndrome may be absent. The variations are due to variability in the supply of the vessel (Stopford).

The prognosis is frequently good. Death follows in some cases, but many make a good recovery, either rapid or delayed. Vertigo and incoördination may persist when other symptoms have disappeared. Recurrent attacks with complete recovery from each episode are well known.

Occlusion of the *anterior spinal artery* in the medulla is very rare. It is characterized by (1) paralysis of all four limbs without involvement of the face, (2) loss of deep sensation in all the limbs, (3) peripheral paralysis of the tongue.

Thrombosis of the *vertebral artery,* producing a retro-olivary syndrome, may be confused with the posterior inferior cerebellar artery syndrome (Sheehan and Smyth). The two conditions are so similar clinically that a differentiation is often extremely difficult. The vertebral artery may be completely thrombosed, yet may give rise to fewer symptoms than such a process would warrant. The onset of the condition is similar to that which has been described for posterior-inferior cerebellar artery thrombosis, and the development is also similar. An ipsi-lateral Horner's syndrome is always pres-ent. Pain and temperature loss is found over the face, involving usually the face on the side of the lesion, but in unusual instances either the opposite or both sides of the face. The sensory impair-ment in the face is not always uniform, some parts showing loss of sensation, and others not; the first and second facial divisions may show pain and temperature loss while the third escapes, or other com-binations occur. Pain and temperature sensations are lost on the opposite side of the body, sometimes with sparing of the cervical and thoracic regions. Cere-bellar signs may be present, as well as cranial nerve signs similar to those of posterior-inferior cerebellar artery throm-bosis (aphonia, dysphagia, etc.). Weak-ness of one side of the body in addition to the other signs cited indicating pyra-midal tract involvement should lead to the presumptive diagnosis of vertebral artery thrombosis in a syndrome which resembles posterior-inferior artery occlu-sion. The differential diagnosis is almost impossible in most cases.

VI. SYNDROMES OF VASCULAR OCCLUSION

Among the many syndromes of vascu-lar occlusion are many involving the brain stem. These are the result either of hemorrhage or softening due to throm-bosis, but since they are more frequent with the latter condition and more often associated with survival when so caused, they will be considered here.

1. Midbrain Syndromes

Syndrome of the Central Gray: This syndrome affects the gray matter under the aqueduct of Sylvius in the midbrain. It involves, therefore, the nuclei of the oculomotor nerve and it is manifested clinically by (1) incomplete paralysis of the extrinsic muscles of the eyeballs. The muscles innervated by the oculomotor nucleus are all partially or totally affected. There is bilateral external strabismus due to paralysis of the internal recti inner-vated by the oculomotor nerve. Move-ments of the eyeballs upward and down-ward are limited or completely paralyzed. (2) Complete bilateral ptosis. (3) Bilat-eral loss of the pupillary light reflex due to paralysis of the sphincter iridis from involvement of the oculomotor nerve. (4) Bilateral paralysis of convergence.

Complete paralysis is more rare than cases of partial paralysis. Either type may be found in a given case. The most frequent cause is encephalitis, but com-plete isolated oculomotor paralysis has been recorded in syphilis and arterio-sclerosis. Myasthenia gravis may pro-duce a total ophthalmoplegia, but the lesion is not in the midbrain nuclei. Par-tial transient paralyses of the oculomotor nerve, due to lesions in the nuclei, are not infrequently encountered in diabetes. Similar lesions have been produced by small tumors confined to the central gray matter of the midbrain, epidemic enceph-alitis, and multiple sclerosis.

Syndrome of the Cerebral Peduncle (*Weber's Syndrome*): The syndrome of the cerebral peduncle is commonly referred to as Weber's syndrome. It is characterized by (1) complete paralysis of the oculomotor nerve on the side of the lesion. This paralysis is characterized by complete ptosis, loss of all ocular move-ments due to oculomotor innervation, external strabismus from unopposed ac-tion of the external rectus muscle, loss of the light reflex, and loss of accommodation. The oculomotor paralysis may be incomplete, but even in such cases there is not very much function of the oculomotor nerve. (2) Hemiplegia in the limbs opposite the side of the lesion. This hemiplegia is usually spastic and involves the muscles of the face and tongue as well as the limbs. There is, therefore, in a Weber syndrome paralysis of the oculomotor nerve of one side and of the limbs of the opposite side. This is a combination of signs which cannot be reproduced anywhere except in the midbrain at the cerebral peduncle. The problem in each case, therefore, is not one of diagnosis but of etiology.

By far the most common cause of Weber's syndrome is syphilis. Arteriosclerotic softening is probably rare as a cause of the syndrome. Occasionally a tumor in the interpeduncular space may produce the same group of symptoms.

Syndrome of the Tegmentum (Benedikt's Syndrome): This syndrome is characterized by the following features: (1) Complete oculomotor paralysis on the side of the lesion, causing a complete ptosis, loss of all ocular movements due to oculomotor innervation (upward, downward, and inward), external strabismus, and loss of the light and accommodation reflexes. The oculomotor paralysis is usually complete and is practically constant in the syndrome. (2) Hemichorea and hemitremor of the opposite side of the body. These involuntary movements involve both the arm and leg, but they tend to be more pronounced in the arm. They may even be present in the arm alone. The choreiform movements may be prominent or poorly developed. Cases exist without them. The tremor is by far more definite than the chorea and is of a special type. It is a coarse, irregular tremor which is present with the limb at rest but which is in-

creased under the stress of emotional or other stimuli. It is increased on voluntary motion, so that when the limb is moved the tremor assumes a very coarse type with large amplitude of the movements and with such extreme irregularity of the movements that the limb can hardly be controlled. Thus when a patient with this tremor is requested to place the finger on the nose, the tremor, which has been coarsely active at rest, becomes irregular and extremely active, so that it is impossible for the patient to hold the affected limb on the goal.

The cause of Benedikt's syndrome is either arteriosclerosis or syphilis, with softening in the tegmentum resulting from occlusion of a vessel from either cause.

2. Pontile Syndromes

Syndrome of Paralysis of Lateral Gaze (Syndrome of Foville): This syndrome is characterized by a paralysis of lateral movement of the eyeballs. Under such conditions, the eyeballs are deviated to one side and the patient is unable to move the eyes to the opposite side. There is, therefore, a complete absence of the lateral movement of the eyeballs which is due to simultaneous action of the external rectus of one side and the internal rectus of the opposite side. The paralysis may be complete, so that there is a total inability to move the eyeballs to one side; or it may be incomplete, with deviation of the eyes possible for a varying distance, sometimes great and sometimes slight. Paralysis of lateral gaze is due to a lesion in the pons involving the tegmentum of the pons near the sixth nerve nucleus. That a center for lateral gaze exists apart from the nucleus of the sixth nerve has been shown by many investigators. The evidence on which such a separate center is based is given by the following facts: (1) Lesions of the abducens nuclei exist without loss of conjugate deviation; (2) the abducens nucleus may be completely destroyed on one side, yet lateral gaze remain intact, indicating that the center for lateral gaze is independent of the abducens nucleus. Some regard the paralysis as due to a lesion of the posterior longitudinal bundle.

The cause of lateral-gaze paralysis may be softening due either to arteriosclerosis or syphilis, tumor, or encephalitis. While softening sometimes causes the difficulty, tumor is a more frequent cause of the condition.

Syndrome of Millard-Grubler: This pontile syndrome is characterized by (1) hemiplegia contralateral to the lesion, due to destruction of the pyramidal tract in the base of the pons; (2) internal strabismus due to destruction of the abducens nerve with diplopia and loss of power to rotate the eyeball outward on the side of the lesion. The resultant defect is characterized by an external rectus paralysis of one side and a hemiplegia involving the opposite side of the body. Thus a lesion in the left side of the pons producing this syndrome would cause a left abducens paralysis and a right hemiplegia. The condition is produced by vascular lesions, encephalitis, and tumors.

Syndrome of Alternating Hemiplegia: This is caused by a lesion destroying the emergent fibers or nucleus of the facial nerve and the pyramidal pathways. It is characterized by a peripheral facial paralysis of one side and a hemiplegia of the opposite side of the body. It is rarely caused by softening. It is more frequently seen in infiltrating tumors of the pons and in encephalitis from various causes.

3. Syndromes of the Medulla

Syndrome of the Pyramidal Decussation: This is a rare syndrome and is more often due to causes other than softening, such as trauma, but it is due to softening on rare occasions. It is characterized by paralysis of the arm and of the opposite leg. This paralysis is spastic and accompanied by pathological reflexes. It does not involve the face. The diagnosis is not difficult. There is only one place in which a single lesion can cause hemiplegia cruciata—the involvement of one arm and the opposite leg. This is in the lower part of the medulla at a point where the arm fibers have already crossed but the leg fibers have not yet decussated.

Syndrome of Alternating Hypoglossal Hemiplegia: This syndrome is characterized by: (1) Hemiplegia involving the arm and leg but not the face on the side opposite the lesion. It is due to involvement of the pyramid in the medulla. (2) Paralysis of the tongue on the side of the lesion. The paralysis of the tongue is peripheral in type. It is characterized by atrophy and fibrillary twitchings of half the tongue.

The syndrome is due to involvement of the pyramid and the emergent fibers of the hypoglossal nerve in the medulla. It is rarely due to basilar meningitis, and more commonly to a softening in the region mentioned. The lesion is rare.

Syndromes of the Nucleus Ambiguus: There are several syndromes which involve the nucleus ambiguus. These may be listed briefly as follows:

Syndrome of Schmidt: This is characterized by (1) ipsilateral paralysis of the larynx, causing hoarseness and (2) ipsilateral paralysis of the sternomastoid and trapezius muscles due to involvement of the spinal accessory nucleus. This results in a torticollis with an inability to turn the head, the chin pointing to the side opposite the lesion.

Syndrome of Jackson: This is characterized by (1) ipsilateral paralysis of the palate, causing difficulty in swallowing and dysarthria, (2) ipsilateral paralysis of the larynx causing hoarseness, (3) ipsilateral paralysis of the tongue accompanied by atrophy and fibrillary twitchings, and (4) ipsilateral paralysis of the sternomastoid and trapezius. This syndrome is caused by a lesion, usually softening, which involves the hypoglossal nucleus, nucleus ambiguus, and the nucleus accessorius.

Syndrome of Avellis: This syndrome is characterized by (1) ipsilateral paralysis of the vocal cord and soft palate, resulting in dysphonia (hoarseness), dysphagia and dysarthria, and (2) contralateral loss of pain and temperature in the limbs and trunk of the opposite side. The syndrome is due to a simultaneous involvement of the nucleus ambiguus and the spinothalamic tract.

VII. CEREBRAL ANEURYSMS

Cerebral aneurysms are not common. Their incidence has been variously computed at 0.5 to 1.5 per cent of necropsy

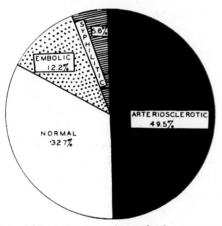

Fig. 139 — *Causes of cerebral aneurysm.* **(McDonald & Korb: Arch. Neurol. & Psychiat. 42:298, 1939.)**

material. Though they are not infrequently recognized first at necropsy, their clinical recognition is quite possible and sensitization to the possibility of aneurysm will serve to explain many an obscure case of head or face pain, ocular palsy, dimness of vision, or headache.

The aneurysms to be discussed here are the large solitary aneurysms of the brain. The miliary aneurysms associated with subarachnoid hemorrhage have been considered under that section.

Etiology: Aneurysms of the brain develop frequently from a *congenital defect* of the vessel wall, occurring usually at the point of bifurcation of cerebral vessels, resulting from a defect in the media, which is thought to be inadequately developed at the site of branching of the vessels. The media has been found to be completely absent in some instances of congenital aneurysm at arterial bifurcations, and in other instances has been found to be thinned out. In the earlier stages of development, when the larger arteries have attained a muscular coat, this is lacking in the deficient vessels, which are represented by a tube of epithelium. This concept has been widely accepted as the chief cause of cerebral aneurysms, but it fails to explain the delay in their development, as well as the mature histological structure of the aneurysmal wall. Congenital aneurysms occur in association with other congenital disorders such as polycystic disease of the kidneys, coarctation of the aorta, and anomalies of the circle of Willis. Aneurysms may develop also in association with *arteriosclerosis.* Though arteriosclerotic changes are not infrequently found in the cerebral vessels in cases of aneurysms, it does not follow that aneurysms always develop from arteriosclerosis. *Mycotic aneurysms* develop from emboli in cases of endocarditis, but they are not common. *Syphilis* is an uncommon cause of aneurysm of the brain, but it undoubtedly accounts for some cases. *Trauma* may be associated with arteriovenous aneurysms.

Cerebral aneurysm has been reported to develop at times as a result of a proliferative arteritis (Handler and Blumenthal). Rare instances of coarctation of the aorta and an associated cerebral artery aneurysm have been recorded.

Aneurysms occur at all ages. The majority of subjects are over forty years of age (fifty-four per cent) and thirty-five per cent are from twenty-one to forty years (McDonald and Korb). Males and females are about equally affected.

Pathology: Aneurysms of the brain are usually single, but they may be multiple. They vary in size from small saccular outpouchings of 0.5 mm. in diameter to large aneurysms of several centimeters (8 to 10 cm.) in cross section. The congenital aneurysms are found in the crotch between vessels, but they may arise occasionally from the main stem. The cerebral aneurysms may be divided into (1) arteriovenous aneurysms, (2) saccular aneurysms, (3) fusiform aneurysms.

The occurrence of cerebral aneurysm with aneurysm elsewhere in the body is rare. "No coexistence of intracranial aneurysms, whether single or multiple, with multiple aneurysms of other arteries such as the coronary, splenic or renal arteries has been observed" (Bigelow).

Aneurysms are found in greatest frequency in association with the anterior portion of the circle of Willis, but all parts of this vascular tree may be associated with aneurysm. Of 1023 cases of aneurysm culled from the literature, 489 or forty-eight per cent were located on the internal carotid or middle cerebral artery; 156 or fifteen per cent on the anterior communicating artery; and only 286 or twenty-eight per cent posterior to the internal carotid arteries (McDonald and Korb). They are most frequent, therefore, in association with the internal carotid and the middle cerebral arteries, but they are frequently found in association with the anterior communicating artery. They arise frequently at the junction of the internal carotid and posterior communicating arteries, at the junction of anterior communicating and anterior cerebral, or at the junction of internal carotid and middle cerebral vessels. They are not found to rise from vessels within the brain substance and they rarely if ever arise from vessels over the cerebral hemispheres. They are found practically exclusively at the base of the brain, arising from the various branches of the circle of Willis. The aneurysmal wall varies in thickness. Often the lumen is completely or almost completely occluded by the clot. In other instances, no clot is found and pulsation of the aneurysm is present.

Aneurysms of the brain may be situated above the sella turcica and thus simulate suprasellar tumors, or they may lie adjacent to the sella in the parasellar region and be confused with tumors of the sphenoid ridge.

They produce symptoms (1) by compression, and (2) by rupture. The compression symptoms result from pressure on the cranial nerves or adjacent structures, by compression of the brain tissue of the brain stem or cerebrum, or by compression of vessels and interference with circulation. They may burrow into the brain substance and form a bed therein, or they may insinuate themselves into the Sylvian fissure, between the frontal lobes, or even through the foramen magnum in the cases of aneurysms of the vertebral artery. Of the various cranial nerves which may be affected by aneurysm, the oculomotor and optic nerves are most commonly compressed, but any of the cranial nerves may be involved. The rôle of sudden increase of blood

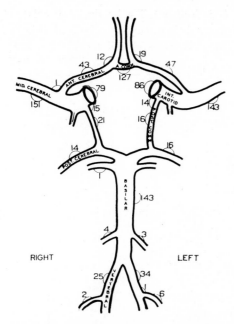

Fig. 140—*Cerebral aneurysm,* showing in diagram form the location of 1023 aneurysms in relation to the Circle of Willis. (McDonald & Korb: Arch. Neurol. & Psychiat. 42:298, 1939.)

ing fluid develop. Such pressures never occur in human cases (Lampert and Müller).

Subarachnoid hemorrhage is usually found at necropsy, since death occurs from rupture of the aneurysm. The hemorrhage is found in varying quantity over the base of the brain and may cover part or all of the cerebral hemispheres if extensive. Hemorrhage may occur directly into the lateral ventricle by rupture of a cerebral aneurysm and erosion through the temporal lobe into the inferior horn of the ventricle. Massive cerebral hemorrhage may ensue from rupture of the aneurysm into the brain tissue, usually in association with middle cerebral artery aneurysm.

On the other hand, cerebral aneurysm is not infrequently encountered at autopsy with presumably no evidence of its presence during life. Of 172 congenital cerebral aneurysms, 78 were found unruptured as an incidental find-

pressure in the production of cerebral hemorrhage by causing rupture of a vessel is not definitely established. There is no doubt that in the presence of normal vessels mere elevation of the blood pressure is not sufficient to cause rupture and hemorrhage. The probabilities are, however, that in the presence of a weakened vessel, as, for example, a vessel with a miliary aneurysm, or in arteriosclerosis with necrosis of the vessel wall, a sudden elevation of the blood pressure is capable of causing rupture of the weakened vessel. This mechanism is not at the basis of hemorrhage from mycotic aneurysms, trauma, and blood dyscrasias. In experimental studies on cadavers who died with cerebral arteriosclerosis, fluid was injected into both carotids, and it was found that only by the application of pressures of one to $2\frac{1}{2}$ atmospheres for six minutes did rupture of vessels and destruction of brain substance by leak-

Table 45—**Compilations of the aneurysms reported by eight writers to show the percentages of lesions on the anterior and posterior segments of the circle of Willis.**

Author	Total	Carotid Segment	Vertebral Segment
McDonald & Korb...	888	735 (83%)	153 (17%)
Martland...	38	27 (71%)	11 (29%)
Krayenbühl.	32	28 (87.5%)	4 (12.5%)
Richardson & Hyland.	53	42 (79%)	11 (21%)
Mitchell & Angrist...	42	34 (81%)	8 (19%)
Riggs & Rupp....	172	155 (90%)	17 (10%)
Magee.....	36	27 (75%)	9 (25%)
Courville...	91	78 (86%)	13 (14%)
	1352	1126 (83%)	226 (17%)

(From "Intracranial Aneurysms"; Hamby, Wallace B., C. C. Thomas, Springfield, Ill., 1952)

ing at autopsy (Williams, Bahn, and Sayre).

Symptoms: The symptoms of aneurysm may be divided into those due to *compression* and those resulting from

ache is frequent. The headache associated with cerebral aneurysm, where anteriorly located, is usually unilateral, recurrent, and severe, felt over the forehead and often within the eyeball. It is due prob-

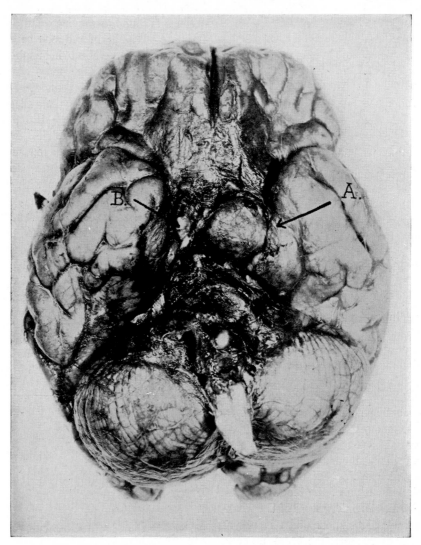

Fig. 141—*Cerebral aneurysm.* A large saccular aneurysm of the left internal carotid artery (A) and a smaller one of the right (B). Subarachnoid hemorrhage from rupture of the aneurysm.

rupture. The history has many characteristic features which suggest the presence of cerebral aneurysm. Symptoms usually extend over a moderately long period of months or years, but in cases of rupture they are exceedingly acute. *Head-*

ably to distention of the vessel or aneurysm wall and may be associated with mild leakage of blood. Aneurysm may develop without headache or pain and may be ushered in by oculomotor paralysis, indicated by diplopia, ptosis, or strabismus. A story of recurrent headache is not uncommon, the bouts of headache being separated often by long intervals of freedom from headache. Frequently analysis will indicate that the headache is in panied by a complaint of vertigo or vomiting. A history of migraine is obtained in some cases.

Associated with a bout of headache may be noted the onset of visual loss, diplopia,

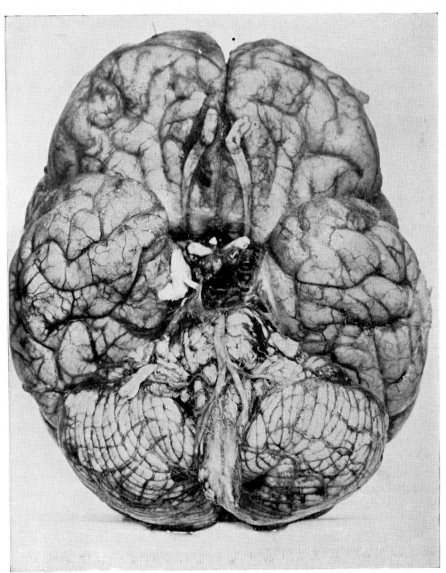

Fig. 142—*Cerebral aneurysm of the right internal carotid artery.*

reality a head pain and is often excruciating. It is at times within the eyeball, at others over the eye, or over all or part of the head. *Pain in or about the eyeballs is a frequent symptom of aneurysm.* The headache or head pain may be accom-

ptosis, tinnitus, or other symptoms, but in many instances these evidences of compression develop insidiously without reference to headache. *Paralysis of the oculomotor nerve* may follow within hours, days, or weeks after the commencement of the pain, or it may accompany the headache, and it is characterized by ptosis and loss of movement of the eyeball. Paralysis of the abducens nerve with loss of external rotation of the eyeball may develop if the aneurysm is situated posterior to the middle cerebral artery. Symptoms of rupture may ensue after a single attack of headache or they may develop after recurrent bouts over a long period of time. They are characterized by sudden, excruciating, apoplectic headache, usually accompanied by unconsciousness which may last for a varying period and be fleeting or prolonged. There may be a history of recovery from an episode of this nature.

The *focal evidences* of compression by a cerebral aneurysm vary with the position of the aneurysm.

Generally speaking, the focal signs of aneurysm concern largely evidences of ophthalmoplegia, optic nerve changes, and visual field defects, since the majority of aneurysms are found in association with the anterior portion of the circle of Willis. Other signs are found also and include loss of sensation over the first division of the trigeminal nerve, loss of the corneal reflex, deafness, and difficulty in swallowing. The ophthalmoplegias associated with aneurysm are unilateral, may be partial or complete, and may involve the oculomotor nerve alone, the oculomotor, trochlear and abducens nerves, or the abducens nerve alone. Among the most common visual field changes are (1) a scotoma on the side of the aneurysm; (2) bitemporal field defects; (3) nasal hemianopsia in the eye on the side of the aneurysm (Jefferson). It appears to be characteristic of the visual field changes associated with cerebral aneurysm that they vary from time to time and that changes which are present on one examination may assume a different or more intense pattern on another.

Visual field changes are most commonly associated with aneurysms of the internal carotid artery and less often with those of the anterior cerebral and anterior communicating arteries. Loss of vision in one eye associated with a scotoma is most commonly due to aneurysms of the internal carotid; bitemporal hemianopsia is most commonly associated with aneurysm of the internal carotid or anterior cerebral arteries, and less commonly with middle cerebral artery aneurysms; homonymous hemianopsia is most commonly caused by aneurysm of the middle cerebral or posterior cerebral arteries. Hemiparesis is not a common accompaniment of cerebral aneurysm. Papilledema occurs in ten per cent of patients with aneurysm (Dandy).

Neck stiffness and Kernig's sign are present in patients with ruptured aneurysm, due to the presence of blood in the spinal fluid. Hemiparesis or hemiplegia may be found, although they are not common, and convulsions are at times encountered. Peripheral and retinal arteriosclerosis are present in the arteriosclerotic aneurysms and evidences of syphilis in those due to syphilis. Endocarditis is sometimes found in patients with mycotic aneurysm.

In those patients in whom rupture of the aneurysm occurs, the signs are those already described in subarachnoid hemorrhage—severe, intense headache, often unconsciousness, neck stiffness, and bloody spinal fluid.

In the *suprasellar group* arising from the anterior communicating and anterior cerebral junction, gradual loss of vision is a common symptom in addition to headache, and is found with optic atrophy and bitemporal hemianopsia as in the case with suprasellar tumors. Anosmia may be found in some cases. In the *parasellar group* arising from the *internal carotid artery,* oculomotor paralysis is found, with ptosis, paralysis of movement of the eyeball, and loss of the pupillary reflexes. Pain over the eye or in the face may be present from involvement of the Gasserian ganglion and may be associated with loss of the corneal reflex. There may be and often is homonymous hemianopsia from compression of the optic tract. In other instances, aneurysms arising from the internal carotid artery may cause blindness of one eye, unilateral optic atrophy, and scotoma in the affected eye. Aneurysm of the *posterior communicating artery* simulates closely that of internal carotid artery aneurysm, with evidences of oculomotor paralysis against a background of unilateral headache. In aneurysms involving the cavernous sinus, there is complete ophthalmoplegia of the eyeball with loss of pain sensation over the forehead from involvement of the first division (ophthalmic) of the trigeminal nerve, but there is usually no loss of vision and no field defect.

Aneurysms of the *middle cerebral artery* are characterized by hemiplegia due to rupture of the aneurysm into the brain substance, producing cerebral hemorrhage (Fig. 17). They are difficult to diagnose prior to rupture and are usually announced by hemiplegia due to cerebral hemorrhage.

Aneurysms of the cavernous sinus have been divided into those producing posterior, middle, and anterior cavernous syndromes (Jefferson). The posterior cavernous syndrome is characterized by involvement of the whole trigeminal nerve, resulting in pain in the face, usually associated with oculomotor palsies, but sometimes only with abducens paralysis. The middle cavernous syndrome is characterized by pain in the first and second divisions of the trigeminal nerve, usually associated with paralysis of all the muscles to the eyeball. In the anterior cavernous syndrome, there is involvement of the first division of the trigeminal nerve with paralysis of all the muscles moving the eyeballs. This is the usual combination in a cavernous syndrome of any sort whether due to tumor, aneurysm, or infection.

Aneurysms of the *vertebral artery* may cause tinnitus and deafness, simulating a cerebellopontine angle tumor, and may be associated with difficulties in swallowing and articulation due to involvement of the vagus and hypoglossal nerves if they attain large size. They are difficult to distinguish from posterior fossa tumors.

Arteriovenous aneurysm (carotid-cavernous fistula) develops in a small number of instances, due usually to communication of the internal carotid artery and cavernous sinus, and associated with a clinical picture of pulsating exophthalmos. In some instances, aneurysm of the internal or ophthalmic artery may be at fault, or tumor of the orbit. At least seventy-five per cent of the cases are traumatic in origin, and about twenty-five per cent are spontaneous. Traumatic cases develop earlier as a rule than those of spontaneous origin, most cases of the former developing at the end of the third decade as compared with the end of the fifth decade for the latter. The outstanding symptom of the disorder is pulsating exophthalmos associated with a clearly audible bruit over the eye and head. In addition to pulsating exophthalmos, arteriovenous aneurysms may be associated with optic atrophy, choked disc, partial or complete ophthalmoplegias, cavernous sinus syndromes which may be unilateral or bilateral, and pupillary changes. The exophthalmos is not always pulsating. The diagnosis is not difficult, but decision as to the underlying condition—whether arteriovenous communication, aneurysm of the internal carotid or ophthalmic arteries, or tumor of the orbit—is often difficult. Aneurysmal types are more common in older patients, while the traumatic due to tumor and arteriovenous aneurysms. The pulsating exophthalmos develops more slowly with tumor. Treatment consists of digital compres-

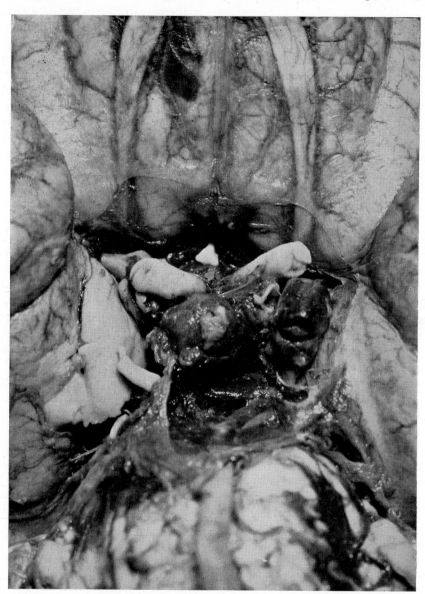

Fig. 143—*Cerebral aneurysm.* Bilateral aneurysms arising from the internal carotids and compressing the optic nerves and chiasm.

varieties are almost always arteriovenous communications. A simple aneurysm may, however, become an arteriovenous type by rupture into the cavernous sinus. Exophthalmos is greatest in the types sion of the carotid artery, about one-third of the recorded cases having been cured by this method. Ligation of the common carotid artery is beneficial. If carotid compression causes cessation of the bruit and produces no signs of cerebral anemia, beneficial results from this method may be expected. If no cessation of the bruit follows digital compression, operation is necessary.

hypothalamus and midbrain. Hydrocephalus is always present. Vascular naevi are usually present in the ipsilateral trigeminal area. Males are more commonly afflicted than females, usually before the

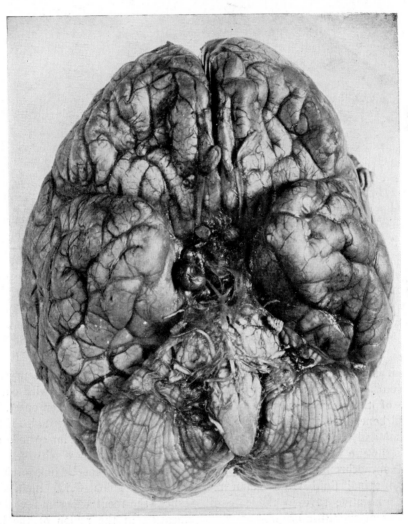

Fig. 144—*Cerebral aneurysm*. A small aneurysm arising from the posterior communicating artery and compressing the right oculomotor nerve. Death was by rupture through the adjacent temporal lobe into the inferior horn of the right lateral ventricle.

A rare form of arteriovenous aneurysm associated with a retinal arteriovenous aneurysm has been described (Wyburn-Mason). The abnormal vessels extend from the retina to the optic nerves and chiasm, and to the structures of the midbrain, extending sometimes into the

age of thirty. Visual failure, gradual or sudden, is common; and symptoms of midbrain involvement, often with a Weber syndrome, are always present.

The *roentgenogram* may reveal crescentic calcification at the base of the skull or areas of bone erosion. In many in-

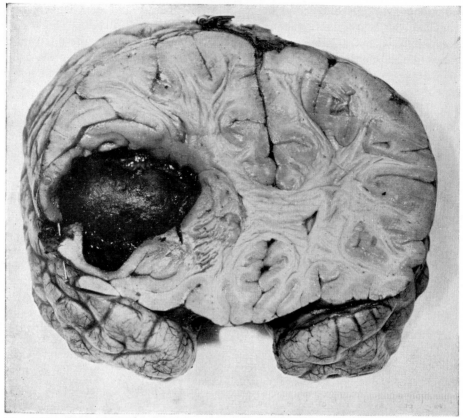

Fig. 145—*Cerebral aneurysm.* **A large middle cerebral aneurysm imbedded in the right temporal lobe and surrounded by hemorrhage.**

stances it is normal. There may be unilateral erosion of the sella turcica, or erosion of the petrous portion of the temporal bone. The *spinal fluid* pressure is normal and the fluid clear except in cases of rupture when the fluid contains blood. Xanthochromia is sometimes present. The spinal fluid Wassermann reaction is negative save in the case of aneurysms of syphilitic origin.

Diagnosis: The diagnosis of cerebral aneurysm is not an easy one, but it is a possible clinical diagnosis and often accurate. The condition may be suspected in cases with a history of recurrent headache, accompanied or followed by cranial nerve palsies. The headache is characteristic and important in diagnosis. The cranial nerve palsies may terminate in recovery with each attack or they may

be persistent. Cerebral aneurysm may be suspected in patients with ocular paralysis of painless, sudden onset. It may be presumed to be present also if there is a previous history of an episode of subarachnoid hemorrhage with severe sudden onset of headache, unconsciousness, and bloody spinal fluid. If, in such instances the roentgenogram reveals a calcification in the region of the internal carotid artery or elsewhere at the base of the skull, the suspicion is amply confirmed. Arteriography will establish the diagnosis definitely, and it is desirable to perform arteriography in most cases in order to establish the diagnosis. Instances have been recorded of verified aneurysm with negative arteriogram (Alpers and Ryan). Four cardinal points are regarded as important in the diagnosis of cerebral aneurysm (Symonds): (1) neighborhood signs, such as paralysis of the oculomotor nerve or pressure on the optic nerves, chiasm, or tracts; (2) the presence of subarachnoid hemorrhage; (3) signs of disease which might produce an aneurysm such as endocarditis and arteriosclerosis; these are absent in the case of congenital aneurysm; (4) a history indicating previous subarachnoid hemorrhage together with signs of tumor, such as compression of structures at the base of the brain.

The symptoms of cerebral aneurysm may be simulated completely by *thrombosis of the internal carotid artery*, with

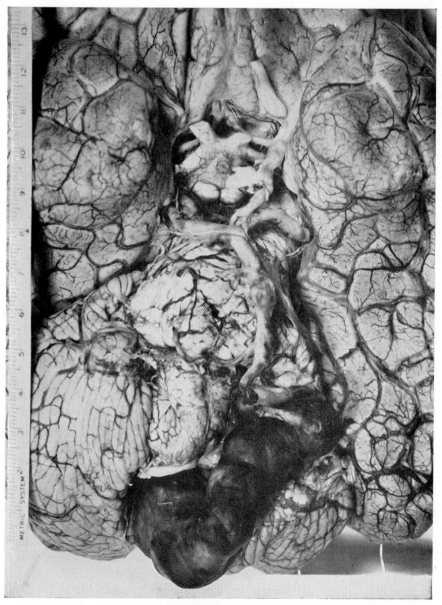

Fig. 146—*Aneurysm* **of the left vertebral artery causing symptoms of posterior fossa tumor and foramen magnum syndrome.**

a history of unilateral headache and oculomotor paralysis of varying degree. Instances of this type have been demonstrated by arteriography and confirmed at operation. Palpation of the internal carotid artery must therefore be an essential part of the examination of every patient suspected of having a cerebral aneurysm.

The separation of aneurysm from other intracranial conditions is often not easy. In those lying above the sella turcica, the condition must be differentiated from suprasellar tumors. In the latter, the history is often of longer duration, bitemporal hemianopsia more constant, and endocrine disturbances are more common than in aneurysm. Since the two conditions give rise to evidences of compression, the distinction between them may not be established until operation or necropsy, but aneurysm may be suspected if some systemic basis for it is found. Tumors in the parasellar region, the sphenoid ridge meningiomas, may be difficult to differentiate from aneurysm. Here, too, the signs may be quite similar, but the history of recurrent headache, eye and face pain is more characteristic of aneurysm than of tumor. Visual field defects such as homonymous hemianopsia are more constant in tumor. Aneurysm may simulate a cerebellopontine angle tumor if it is situated in the cerebellopontine angle. Arteriovenous anomalies may simulate aneurysm as a cause of subarachnoid hemorrhage. They are usually found over the cerebral hemispheres, and cranial nerve signs are therefore lacking. Their onset is often with seizures.

In the last analysis, aneurysm must be differentiated from tumor and from little else. The distinction may be extremely difficult, since both give rise to symptoms and signs of compression. Aneurysm may be suspected, however, if there has been a history of recurrent headaches, pains, or transient cranial nerve palsies; if there has been a previous episode of subarachnoid hemorrhage, or if there appears to be some structural basis for its development.

Prognosis: In most instances, aneurysms rupture sooner or later and give rise to evidences of subarachnoid hemorrhage. In other cases rupture fails to occur, especially in those cases in which the aneurysm is filled with clot. Often there is a history of repeated minor ruptures before a major subarachnoid hemorrhage develops. Survival may ensue from any individual episode of bleeding or there may be a fatal termination. In those cases with subarachnoid hemorrhage, survival occurs in about fifty per cent of cases. The occurrence of one attack may augur the development of others.

In a group of 47 aneurysms, 44 of which were fatal, it was found that prognosis was unfavorably influenced by previous attacks, multiple hemorrhage, mental disturbances, unconsciousness, and convulsions (Hamby).

Treatment: There is no certain cure of aneurysm. Treatment is directed toward (1) alleviation of headache, (2) improvement of cranial nerve palsies, (3) prevention of rupture. Operative procedures for aneurysm of the brain must be restricted to the large aneurysms which produce pressure symptoms. Operative procedures have been found to be of limited value in miliary aneurysm because of difficulty in disclosing the source of bleeding. Ligation of the carotid artery may give relief, but the results are variable and in some instances hemiplegia has resulted from such ligation. Ligation of the internal carotid artery has been advocated in the treatment of intracranial aneurysms. Its value is not a matter of general agreement. The process entails risk since it has been shown that ligation of the internal carotid artery is followed by a fall in intra-carotid pressure of about fifty per cent. Hemiplegia follows in some instances after ligation. The hazards of the ligation cannot be anticipated preoperatively since the test for carotid sufficiency by pressure on the internal carotid artery in the neck has been found to be unreliable, due to the difficulty in completely occluding the artery by digital compression. It is generally accepted that ligation of the artery is distinctly more hazardous in older people, but it is believed that beneficial results follow ligation of the artery in the neck for unruptured infraclinoid aneurysm in subjects under fifty years of age. Ligation of the neck of an aneurysm has been performed but is not a feasible operation in many cases. Trapping of the aneurysm intracranially by ligature is possible.

The treatment of ruptured aneurysm is the treatment of subarachnoid hemorrhage which has already been considered.

VIII. CEREBRAL VASCULAR SPASM

The problem of cerebral vascular spasm is one of great importance to the clinician and has recently attracted the attention of physiologists. There is as yet much discrepancy between the physiologists and clinicians concerning the entire problem of vascular spasm in the brain. Transient cortical symptoms, presumably of vascular origin, occur but there is some doubt as to whether these are explainable on the basis of vascular spasm alone.

Physiology: The mechanism of vascular spasm in the brain depends in part on (1) nervous mechanisms and (2) chemical mechanisms. The nervous structure for the dilatation and collapse of the cerebral vessels has been carefully worked out. The cerebral arterioles are peculiar in the relative thinness of their walls, as well as by the fact that their media is composed chiefly of collagen. Nerves have been demonstrated on the walls of the pial vessels of the cortex and to some degree along their walls in the cerebral cortex. There seems to be the fundamental structure, therefore, for the presence of a vasomotor mechanism. Stimulation of the cervical sympathetic and vagus nerves causes change in the caliber of the pial vessels. Thus, stimulation of the former causes constriction of the pial vessels, while stimulation of the vagus nerves causes vasodilatation. The effect of the cervical sympathetic is entirely unilateral, affecting the vessels of the ipsilateral hemisphere; the vagus effect is bilateral. Similar changes have been observed after the injection or local application of drugs. Thus, epinephrine, when applied locally, causes a vasoconstriction and when injected into the carotid artery produces a vasodilatation followed by vasoconstriction. Caffeine in large doses causes a constriction of the cerebral vessels. Histamine, acetylcholine, and amyl nitrite cause vasodilatation.

The effects just cited are presumed to take place by the intervention of the vasomotor mechanism in the brain. There is much doubt, however, whether this mechanism is sufficiently developed in man to produce much effect, or whether it is not in fact a very rudimentary mechanism. It has been calculated, for example, that after stimulation of the cervical sympathetic, the change in caliber of a pial vessel is only eight to ten per cent of its volume, while the change in vasodilatation is about twenty per cent. A difference in caliber of eight to ten per cent is presumably not sufficient to cause changes in the brain by anoxemia.

Because of the doubts concerning the efficacy and importance of the vasomotor mechanism in the brain, investigations have been directed to the rôle of chemical factors in causing constriction or dilatation of the vessels, acting on these directly. Schmidt has found in the medulla, hypothalamus, and parietal cortex that there is no great effect on stimulation of the cervical sympathetic, the vasodepressors, the carotid sinus, or perivertebral nerves. In the pial vessels of the parietal area there was some vasoconstriction on stimulation of the cervical sympathetic. On the other hand, in all of these areas changes in the $CO_2 = O_2$ ratio was very effective in causing changes in the caliber of the vessels. Thus, in the medulla it was found that CO_2 excess and O_2 lack caused an increase in blood flow, and that CO_2 seemed to have a specific influence in this regard. In both the hypothalamus and parietal cortex CO_2 excess and O_2 decrease caused a vasodilatation; CO_2 decrease caused a vasodilatation, and O_2 increase caused a vasoconstriction. It is, therefore, apparent from these data that vasoconstriction and vasodilatation occur under the influence of chemical stimuli, especially O_2 decrease and CO_2 increase. Further studies by Schmidt indicate that the most important intrinsic control of the cerebral circulation is a vasodilator one affected by CO_2. Schmidt asserts that "the vasodilator effect of CO_2 is the mechanism by which all of the various parts of the brain receive a blood supply proportionate to their needs." He found no evidence of the existence of an intrinsic vasomotor system.

That there is a vasomotor apparatus in the brain is unquestioned. That it causes changes in the caliber of the vessels on electrical stimulation of the cervical sympathetic and vagus nerves is equally true. The resulting change in the caliber of the vessels is not enough to produce cerebral changes as the result of anoxemia. Greater effects appear to be produced by chemical factors such as CO_2 increase and O_2 decrease. The exact decrease in blood flow as the result of these mechanisms has not been determined, but it is presumably great enough to cause changes.

Symptoms: There is a group of cases, which probably reaches large proportions, which is perhaps due to spasm of a cerebral vessel or vessels. While the evidence in favor of a sufficiently severe change in vessel caliber as a result of vasomotor changes in the cerebral vessels to produce interference with cerebral function is not convincing from the laboratory standpoint, from the clinical point of view there is, nevertheless, a large group of cases in which the clinical phenomena are explainable only on the basis of vascular spasm. Among such cases one may include transitory aphasias, hemianopsias, hemiplegias, sensory disturbances, and other signs of focal disease in the brain. These symptoms are transient and sometimes even fleeting.

The *onset* in these cases of vascular spasm is often acute, just as in cases of thrombosis or embolism; sometimes it is gradual in onset and development. Consciousness may be impaired or lost. Not infrequently there is no interference with consciousness except for a fleeting sensation of giddiness at the time of onset of the attack. There ensues quickly a complete hemiplegia, an aphasia, hemianopia, astereognosis, or other evidence of disturbance of cortical function. The characteristics of these symptoms differ in no way from those encountered in more serious cases of structural damage to the brain. Recovery may begin almost as soon as the disease begins or it may be delayed for twelve to twenty-four hours. It may proceed very rapidly, so that the signs of a complete hemiplegia may have disappeared spontaneously twenty-four to thirty-six hours after they have developed.

The *diagnosis* of cerebral vascular spasm is made largely on the basis of the transitory nature of the neurologic signs. Cerebral vascular spasm may occur in a variety of conditions, such as hypertensive states, heart disease, and arteriosclerosis. They are especially common in some types of hypertension, especially those with wide fluctuations in blood pressure. Spasm of the retinal vessels may often be observed during an attack. Distinction must be made from conditions which are capable of producing transitory cerebral episodes. *Multiple sclerosis* occurs in younger subjects and is associated with a history of evanescent symptoms involving scattered areas. Signs indicating permanent damage are usually but not always present—nystagmus, spastic paraplegia, temporal pallor of the discs, etc.

General paresis is at times associated with transitory hemiplegia, but here the clinical manifestations, such as tremors, slurred speech, mental disturbances, and the laboratory findings, are helpful. Transitory cerebral manifestations occur in occasional cases of *allergy* associated with focal brain edema. A history of allergy, urticaria, hay fever, etc., will usually lead to suspicion of this condition. *Uremia* may be associated with transient pareses, but its recognition is not difficult. Incomplete or partial *thrombosis* of a cerebral vessel may give a syndrome similar to vascular spasm, the result of the partial occlusion being a transient paresis or transient focal brain damage of other sorts. Many believe that many or most of the cerebral vascular spasms are in reality incomplete thromboses. Recovery from a thrombosis of this type is longer than can be accounted for by spasm,

while recovery from spasm is too short to be explained by incomplete thrombosis. In the long run, the degree of damage of the affected tissues is the important factor in recovery whether it be due to spasm or partial thrombosis. Spasms may occur in both healthy and diseased vessels. The objection that an arteriosclerotic vessel cannot develop spasm is true of the rigid tubes but not of vessels with scattered plaques. Its manifestations are similar to those of hemorrhage, thrombosis, or any other focal disease, except that the signs and symptoms are transient.

The problem of cerebral vascular spasm remains controversial. Recurrent transient disturbances such as hemiplegia or hemiparesis and aphasia are attributed to vascular occlusion rather than spasm (Denny-Brown) and are said to be due to occlusion of the internal carotid artery. The evidence against the occurrence of cerebral vascular spasm is stated as follows: The case against vascular spasm maintains that there is little or no physiological basis to demonstrate that vascular spasm may occur in cerebral vessels; that there is no clinical evidence for a local stimulus, without which arteries do not contract; that transitory symptoms occur in cases of mitral stenosis and auricular fibrillation, due probably to an embolus; and that the recovery of function is related to the free anastomoses between the cerebral vessels at all levels. This viewpoint is summarized as follows: "That a sudden and transient focal loss of cerebral function may be due to organic occlusion of a cerebral artery is therefore in conformity with the known facts of vascular behavior, whereas the concept of cerebral vascular spasm is not." (Pickering)

The *pathogenesis* of the symptoms is of great interest. It has been stated that the decrease in caliber of the vessels in

Table 46—Differential Diagnosis of Transient Focal Brain Disease (Hemiplegia, Aphasia, etc.)

Disease	Age	Onset	Course	Systemic Findings	Laboratory Findings
CEREBRAL VASCULAR SPASM	Any time but older age group usually	Sudden, with complete loss of power of one side or gradual extension from one part to another	Regression of symptoms in a matter of hours, usually completely	Cardiac disease, labile vasomotor system; labile blood pressure; allergy may be found	E. K. G. may be abnormal Cardiorenal disease
MULTIPLE SCLEROSIS	Younger group (19 to 40)	Sudden or gradual. Often history of previous episodes or of other transient symptoms. Other evidences of disease found on examination—pallor of discs, speech disturbances, etc.	Regression of hemiplegia and other focal signs slowly, either complete or incomplete. Takes place over period of weeks or longer, sometimes days	None of significance. Neurological examination shows evidence of multiple sclerosis	Abnormal colloidal gold curve in spinal fluid in about 50 per cent
GENERAL PARESIS	30 to 50 chiefly	Sudden as a rule. Usually hemiparesis	Regression within a few or several days	Other evidences of general paresis—irregular and sluggish or Argyll Robertson pupils; tremor of face and hands; slurred speech; overactive reflexes	Blood Wassermann positive in 90 per cent. Spinal fluid shows evidence of syphilis with paretic gold curve
ALLERGY	Any age	Sudden onset of hemiparesis or other focal signs	Rapid regression	Evidence of allergic history	Allergic reactions positive
INCOMPLETE CEREBRAL THROMBOSIS	Older subjects, over 50 as a rule	Gradual onset of hemiparesis, hemiplegia or aphasia	Slow regression over a period of days or weeks	Arteriosclerosis of peripheral and retinal vessels; often hypertension	No significant findings
BRAIN TUMOR	Adults usually, but any age	Gradual as a rule	Progressive, but rarely remissive, especially in cystic tumors and hemangiomas	Usually signs of increased intracranial pressure	High spinal fluid pressure

instances of electrical stimulation of the cervical sympathetic is only eight to ten per cent and is probably not great enough to cause any serious impairment of cerebral function. This is undoubtedly true of normal vessels, but in a diseased vessel with a thickened wall and plaque formation, a decrease in caliber of eight to ten per cent may be just enough to cause a complete occlusion of the lumen. There is the additional factor that the decrease in caliber of the vessels due to chemical stimulation is greater than that produced by elecrical stimulation and affects the intrinsic brain vessels to a much greater degree than the pial vessels. But in addition to vessel occlusion there is another very important factor to consider, and this is the time of occlusion of the vessel. A vessel which is completely occluded for only a few seconds will obviously produce few objective signs of cerebral disease but will cause fleeting subjective signs. The same vessel occluded for three or four minutes, however, will not only produce severe subjective signs but also evidences of objective disturbances due to damage of the brain cells. Animal experiments indicate that complete shutting off of the blood supply for 3½ minutes produces recoverable damage while shutting off the circulation for seven minutes produces irreversible damage. Time is, therefore, an important factor in the ultimate determination of the actual damage to the brain.

The concept of cerebral vascular spasm is unacceptable to some neurologists. *Cerebral vascular insufficiency* has been suggested as a possible mechanism to explain transitory cerebral symptoms. This is based on the belief that failure of maintenance of the systemic blood pressure is responsible for such transient signs, and restoration of the blood pressure is capable of abolishing them. Insufficiency of the cerebral circulation may develop with systemic hypotension or low cardiac output, resulting from coronary shock, antihypertensive drug, postural factors, carotid sinus syndrome, surgery and anesthetics, cardiac arrythmias, congestive heart failure, pulmonary hypertension, and gravitational states in aviation.

IX. HYPERTENSIVE ENCEPHALOPATHY

The term hypertensive encephalopathy is obviously without meaning. It has come to be applied to cases of brain damage in malignant hypertension, but it is equally applicable to any hypertensive case with brain lesions, as, for example, cerebral hemorrhage or thrombosis associated with hypertension. Since the term has found its way into the literature and has come to assume a more or less specific meaning it seems best to continue its usage despite its lack of meaning. It should be confined to cases of malignant hypertension with neuroretinitis and cerebral damage.

The symptoms of hypertensive encephalopathy have been explained by acute edema of the brain, due probably to cerebral ischemia (Volhard). The assumption is that the cerebral arterioles are more constricted than elsewhere in the body, giving rise to damage of the capillaries by anoxia, thus permitting abnormal amounts of fluid and protein to escape into the cerebral tissue. A rise in arterial pressure precedes the attacks of hypertensive encephalopathy.

The *symptomatology* concerns often a young adult with a history of headache, vomiting, convulsions, and often impairment of vision. The average age of onset is about forty years, but children and older adults (sixty years and over) may be affected. Headache, general weakness, and nervousness are the most common symptoms. The onset of symptoms is usually sudden, but is preceded in many instances by a history of headache for many months and often by attacks of vertigo. Since the brain changes in malignant hypertension vary, the symptoms are also variable. Severe headache, vomiting, and drowsiness may characterize the development of some cases, and may be associated with few or no neurological findings.

A history of headache, stupor, and of transient hemiplegia is at times encountered, and in other instances the evolution of the condition is similar to that of cerebral hemorrhage. Hemiplegia, aphasia, or other focal neurological symptoms are often found, but many cases show little on neurological examination in the absence of a history of hemiplegia or a vascular accident. A previous history of hypertension is known in most cases and may exist for months or years before the onset of symptoms. Peripheral arteriosclerosis, mild to severe in degree, is usually present. The heart is often enlarged and cardiac decompensation is not uncommon. Cardiac murmurs are frequent. The blood pressure is high; the systolic pressure is usually over 200 mm. and the diastolic 120 mm. or more.

Neuroretinitis is present in all cases, but exceptional cases have been recorded without it. The retinal arteries are sclerosed, usually severely. There appears to be no relationship between the severity of the peripheral arteriosclerosis and the hypertension, but the degree of retinal arteriosclerosis parallels closely that found in the peripheral and cerebral vessels. Papilledema occurs with the retinitis. Scotomas are frequent. Renal function is not as a rule impaired until late in the disease. The spinal fluid pressure is high in most cases, varying between 250 and 400 mm. of water. The outlook is poor, most patients dying within a period of two years.

The malignant form of hypertension can be distinguished from the benign form by the persistently high blood pressure and the rapid course. It may begin of itself or as a later stage of the benign type.

The cerebral symptoms have been defined by Rosenberg in the following categories: Those due to *cerebral edema* are characterized by severe headache, nausea, vomiting, drowsiness, and mental dullness. Those due to *multiple miliary destructive lesions* are characterized by vertigo, transient hemiplegias or aphasias, personality changes, or other transient symptoms, depending on the area of tissue destroyed. The large *cerebrovascular* accidents are characterized by the symptoms of cerebral hemorrhage already discussed. *Mixed forms* are also frequent in which cases with multiple lesions develop a large cerebrovascular accident or evidences of cerebral edema.

The *brain* in cases of malignant hypertension reveals noteworthy findings. Edema of some degree is present in all cases, in some instances severe, in others moderate. The gyri of the brain are swollen and contain an excess of fluid, accounting for the increased intracranial pressure which is found in these cases. The brain is soft and waterlogged. Often there is an excess of fluid in the ventricles. Subarachnoid hemorrhages of varying degree are found over the cerebral hemispheres or at the base of the brain. These may consist of small pools of no significance or large extravasations of blood. The cerebral cortex itself shows damage of varying degree. The cortical arterioles are thickened and sometimes hyalinized. The degree of sclerosis of these vessels parallels closely the sclerotic changes in the retinal arteries. There appears to be no relationship, however, between the condition of sclerosis of the peripheral, retinal, or cerebral arteries and the vascular hypertension. The ganglion cells of the cortex are, on the whole, well preserved; but scattered areas of cell loss are common, associated with a mild degree of gliosis. Infarct formations, large and small, are common, and are characterized by incomplete dissolution of the tissue, loss of ganglion cells, ischemic or sclerotic changes in the remaining ganglion cells, and gliosis. There may be few or many infarcts, depending on the severity of the clinical picture. Hemorrhages are likewise common. These are of two varieties: (1) massive hemorrhages similar to those found in ordinary cerebral hemorrhage; (2) punctate hemorrhages, which may be few or numerous. The hemorrhages are chiefly cerebral in location, but are frequently found in the brain stem, especially the pons and occasionally in the cerebellum.

Diagnosis: The diagnostic problem in cases of malignant hypertension concerns usually a young person with a history of headache, vomiting, and convulsions, with evidence of neuroretinitis with choked disc, often a hemiplegia or some other evidence of focal brain damage (aphasia, hemianopsia, etc.), often also signs of meningeal irritation due to subarachnoid hemorrhage, vascular hypertension, and no evidence of renal failure.

The entire picture simulates most closely a *brain tumor*, the resemblance being often so great as to make differentiation extremely difficult. The problem is increased by the fact that some forms of malignant glioma (glioblastoma multiforme) may develop with a fulminating history simulating hypertensive encephalopathy, and are often associated with hemorrhage. The onset in such cases is likely to be a little later than in vascular hypertension, in subjects of thirty-five or older. The ocular fundi, moreover, while appearing similar in the two con-

ditions, show much more evidence of retinal vascular disease in malignant hypertension. The vascular hypertension points much more preponderantly to malignant hypertension than to brain tumor. While transient vascular hypertension may occur with increased intracranial pressure, there is no evidence as yet available that a cerebral brain stem lesion, such as a tumor, can produce a steady and prolonged hypertension. Increase in blood pressure is a very rare result of brain tumor; hence the presence of a true vascular hypertension in a case of suspected hypertensive encephalopathy indicates hypertension rather than a brain tumor, no matter how closely the symptoms and findings simulate the latter. The spinal fluid pressure level is high in both instances and cannot be used as a means of differentiation. Blood in the spinal fluid is likely to favor malignant hypertension, but since hemorrhage into the tumor is common in glioblastoma multiforme it may occur in tumor as well.

Subdural hematoma is a remote possibility in some cases, but the story and findings are as a rule too fulminating to confuse with chronic subdural hematoma, while in the acute cases a history of recent trauma is always present.

Brain abscess may develop acutely and may simulate the symptoms of malignant hypertension. It will usually reveal itself by a history of sinus or mastoid infection, often with a draining ear, or by a history of a recent sinus or mastoid operation, or of recent cavernous sinus thrombosis. There may be signs of meningeal irritation and evidence of focal brain damage just as in malignant hypertension, but there is no vascular hypertension and meningeal signs, if present, are associated with polynuclear or lymphocytic cell increase in the spinal fluid rather than with blood.

X. CEREBRAL ISCHEMIA OR ANEMIA

The recognition of the manifestations of cerebral ischemia is important, since symptoms often of an obscure type are produced by the syndrome. In order to comprehend the clinical picture, some knowledge of the mechanism of the cere-

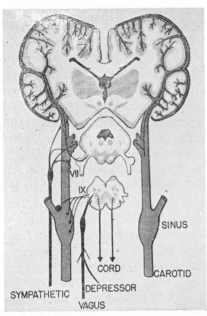

Fig. 147 — *Vasomotor control of cerebral vessels.* **Diagram showing direct vasomotor control of cerebral vessels by trunk (VII). In the medulla are indicated the extracerebral reflex mechanisms which control blood pressure and therefore cerebral blood flow. (Cobb: Williams & Wilkins Co., 1938.)**

bral circulation is essential. The older long-established conception of the cerebral circulation asserted that it was dependent on the systemic circulation, cerebral blood flow varying passively with changes in systemic blood flow. This has now been found to be erroneous. The cerebral circulation is maintained by a combination of cerebral and extracerebral factors. The *cerebral* factors have been discussed in the section on cerebral vascular spasm and consist of change in the caliber of the vessels due to chemical changes in the blood, especially

CO_2, sympathetic nerve impulses causing vasoconstriction and parasympathetic impulses causing vasodilatation. The *extracerebral* factors responsible for maintaining adequate cerebral circulation are the following: (1) carotid sinus reflexes by way of the vagus nerve to the heart and by the spinal cord and sympathetic nerves to the arteries, muscles of respiration, suprarenals and spleen; (2) aortic reflexes by the aortic depressor and vagus nerves, causing cardioinhibitory and vasodilator effects by channels through the medulla; (3) cardioinhibitory reflexes by the vagus nerve to the heart; (4) vasodilator and vasoconstrictor reflexes mediated by changes in the CO_2 and O_2 content of the blood, causing changes in the various vasomotor centers in the medulla, midbrain, hypothalamus, and cerebral cortex.

The object of the various physiological mechanisms concerned in the cerebral circulation is the maintenance of a relatively constant blood flow to the brain and one adequate for the proper functioning of cerebral mechanisms. This is accomplished by the interaction of the many reflexes already enumerated, as well as by interaction of the various organs of the body. Thus, if the blood flow to the brain is inadequate and the pressure falls in the carotid sinus, vasoconstriction takes place in other organs, the blood supply being automatically reduced in these organs and increased in the brain. Similar mechanisms are constantly at work in order to maintain adequate cerebral blood flow. Chief among the mechanisms in importance is the carotid sinus mechanism, which produces changes in cerebral blood flow dependent primarily on changes in systemic arterial pressure. Important, too, are the vasomotor mechanisms, which mediate through the various vasomotor centers in the brain stem.

Etiology: The majority of cases of cerebral ischemia are due to *cardiac* causes such as cardiac failure. Cardiac inhibition as seen in heart block is sometimes responsible. Premature ventricular contractions have been held responsible. *Hemorrhage* from various causes is capable of producing cerebral ischemia — bleeding gastric ulcer, hemorrhoids, epistaxis, intestinal tumors or ulcers, etc. The blood loss may be sudden or, as more often happens, it may be recurrent and chronic. In the former instance, the symptoms result from vasomotor collapse or shock resulting from loss of blood volume. *Secondary anemia* from various causes is often associated with symptoms of ischemia. Pernicious anemia is a common cause, but extremely low hemoglobin values (eight to ten per cent) may be found without symptoms of ischemia provided the blood volume is maintained. Leukemias and other blood dyscrasias may be responsible for ischemic symptoms.

Senile changes in the brain, *cerebral arteriolosclerosis, arterial hypertension,* and *postural hypotension* are further causes. Among other causes are *carbon monoxide* poisoning, *morphine* poisoning, *hyperinsulinism* or excessive *insulin* dosage, *anesthetics* (nitrous oxide particularly), *avitaminosis, asphyxia* from strangulation or drowning, and *cachexia.*

Symptoms: The symptoms of cerebral ischemia are usually not dramatic and the condition is often unrecognized. Chronic loss of blood from whatever cause is associated with excessive fatigue, tinnitus, dizziness, and syncopal attacks. The dizziness is usually not severe and is commonly described as a sensation of giddiness often induced by change in posture from the prone to the upright position. In cases of acute blood loss, the symptoms are more dramatic and are characterized by vertigo, unconsciousness, and often generalized convulsions.

In cerebral arteriolosclerosis, dizziness, headaches, weakness and faintness, are common symptoms of the ischemic syndrome. They are usually present on arising, disappear or subside during the day, are increased by the upright posture and improved on lying down.

The syndrome of *postural hypotension* is associated with cerebral symptoms due to ischemia. These are characterized by syncope and vertigo which appear on assuming the upright posture. Often they are precipitated by exercise. The syncope in such cases is unassociated with the extreme pallor, nausea, sweating, and slow pulse rate seen in other types of syncope. The history is characteristic. Under normal circumstances the decrease of blood flow in the brain associated with assuming the upright posture is compensated for by vasoconstriction and increased heart rate in order to maintain cerebral blood flow. This is not present in cases with postural hypotension. Systolic and diastolic pressures fall rapidly but the heart rate is unchanged. Syncope does not occur so long as the systolic pressure is as high as 50 mm. of mercury. There is an associated marked drop in diastolic blood pressure with the patient upright. The condition is due to a disorder of the sympathetic system. Since postural hypotension can be produced by destruction of the peripheral sympathetic nerves and ganglions and by extensive disease of the spinal cord, it is assumed that the difficulty is due to a lesion or lesions in the sympathetic centers or their efferent tracts in the nervous system. It cannot be ascribed to overactivity of the carotid sinus reflexes, since response to these reflexes are normal, both in horizontal and upright positions. Postural hypotension of a mild form is found in some cases of tabes.

Brief mention should be made of the *carotid sinus syndromes,* since stimulation of the carotid sinus may produce a variety of symptoms such as dizziness, unconsciousness, and convulsions. Stimulation of the sinus is produced by many conditions such as carotid-body tumors, trauma to the neck, surgery of the neck, especially thyroid surgery, ligation of the common or internal carotid artery, and tight collars.

The symptoms of carotid sinus stimulation may develop at any age. Fainting spells are the most common manifestation of the disorder, lasting as a rule from one-half to three minutes and leave no aftereffects. At times, they may last for as long as fifteen minutes and be associated with symptoms such as confusion, amnesia, and hallucinosis. Warning symptoms, such as dizziness, weakness, epigastric distress, or spots before the eyes, are common. Fainting occurs always with patients in the upright position, either sitting or standing. In some instances, there may be a history of the induction of attacks by turning the head to one side, as in the case of a motorman who developed attacks always on looking to the left; or patients may be aware that pressure on one side of the neck may cause attacks. Convulsions may accompany the fainting attacks but are not an invariable part of the picture. Many patients give evidence of unstable vasomotor systems, such as palpitation, moist palms, emotional instability, skin sensitivity, and nervousness. The heart rate is often unstable, the blood pressure fluctuates over a considerable range, the basal metabolic rate is often low (minus fifteen to minus twenty-five); hypertension and arteriosclerosis may be demonstrated at times.

Pressure over the right or left carotid sinus produces attacks identical with the spontaneous episodes in typical cases.

Depending on the degree and duration of pressure, the symptoms consist of faintness and pallor of the face, followed by unconsciousness and in most cases convulsive twitchings which develop simultaneously with unconsciousness or in some cases may precede it. Numbness and tingling are common sensations, beginning in the contralateral extremities and spreading to the whole body before fainting occurs. Loss of vision, nausea, and epigastric distress may develop. Rarely, stimulation of a hyperactive carotid sinus may be followed by serious results. Hemiplegia has been reported with prolonged stimulation of the carotid sinus by direct injury to the sinus and by pressure over the sinus in testing carotid sinus reflexes. Bilateral anterior artery thrombosis has followed immediately on carotid sinus stimulation (Marmor and Sapirstein). The following types have been described (Weiss):

1. THE VAGAL TYPE: Characterized by dizziness, faintness, and weakness resulting from cardiac systole which produces cerebral anoxemia through cardiac standstill or sinauricular or auriculoventricular block. There is an associated fall in arterial pressure and unconsciousness, which usually develops ten to twenty seconds after stimulation. Atropine and epinephrin are effective in preventing the attacks.

2. THE DEPRESSOR TYPE: Characterized by dizziness, fainting, unconsciousness, and convulsions. The symptoms are produced by cerebral anoxemia resulting from a diminution in flow of blood to to the brain. The arterial pressure falls due to vasodilatation and for this reason epinephrin is effective in aborting the attacks.

3. THE CEREBRAL TYPE: Characterized by unconsciousness and convulsions. There is no change in blood pressure or heart rate or in the total flow of blood through the brain. Denervation of the sinus or treatment of the sinus with procain prevents attacks.

Distinction must be made between the carotid sinus syndrome as described by Weiss and a hyperactive carotid sinus reflex. Most patients with an active cardioinhibitory reflex of the carotid sinus do not exhibit the manifestations of the carotid sinus syndrome (Nathansen). The former is probably the result of hypersensitivity of the vagus nerve.

XI. CHRONIC SUBCORTICAL ENCEPHALOPATHY

This is a disease originally described by Binswanger in 1894 under the title chronic progressive subcortical encephalitis. It is a rare form of cerebral arteriosclerosis, which affects the white matter but which leaves the gray matter intact. It is agreed now that the disease is not an encephalitis but is due to cerebral arteriosclerosis.

Symptoms: The *symptoms* of the disorder are not well defined, for they do not differ greatly from those of other forms of cerebral arteriosclerosis (Farnell and Globus). The disease may appear at forty but is more common at fifty or later. It is slow and insidious in onset, with progressive impairment of memory, leading to severe mental deterioration. Thus far, nothing has been observed in this mental deterioration to distinguish it from an ordinary type of cerebral arteriosclerosis. The speech soon becomes dysarthric and monotonous. Attacks of vertigo, epileptiform attacks, and repeated cerebral insults follow. Confusional and psychotic states appear. Focal signs of cerebral damage become apparent. Among these are monoplegias, aphasias, hemiplegias, and hemianopia. Emotional lability is common. Intellectual deterioration becomes more and more profound. The disease is slow and progressive in its development, but there are periods of remission in which symptoms may disappear only to become intensified at some later stage of the disease. It is not rapidly fatal. It runs a course of several years but may be fatal in the course of several months.

Pathology: The *pathology* is well defined. As already indicated, it is an atrophy and degeneration of the white matter with intact cortex. Despite severe destruction of the white matter, the cortex remains quite intact. The deeper subcortical layers are most affected, the arcuate fibers being intact. Often the destruction occurs in patches which vary both in size and distribution. Often they are sharply demarcated, but they may be less clearly defined. The diseased areas contain numerous gitter cells filled with fat. There is astrocytic hyperplasia, giving the areas a true sclerotic aspect. The changes are thought to be due to arteriosclerosis of the deeper vessels in the white matter and hence the result of nutritional disturbances.

XII. CEREBRAL ARTERIOLOSCLEROSIS

Wholly apart from the cases of cerebral arteriosclerosis associated with softenings and hemorrhage is a large group of cases involving chiefly the small arterioles of the cortex, associated with symptoms of mental deterioration and psychosis. The development and the clinical features of such cases differ materially from those of cerebral hemorrhage and thrombosis.

Pathology: The gross cerebral findings are quite constant. In most cases the dura is thickened and in some may be so firmly adherent to the calvarium that it can be separated only with great difficulty and then not without tearing the dura. The pia-arachnoid is thickened, especially along the longitudinal fissure and over the frontal regions. It becomes less pronounced over the parietal and temporal areas. In advanced cases, the pia-arachnoid membranes are seen as dense, white, fibrous membranes which are adherent to one another and to the cortex. They have a translucent appearance. In some cases the thickening is so pronounced that the gyri cannot be made out through the membranes. In early cases this membranous thickening is seen only around the larger vessels which spread out over the lateral surfaces of the brain. There is almost always atrophy of some degree. Usually a moderate degree of atrophy is present; sometimes it is pronounced or mild. In some cases there may be no atrophy whatever. The average decrease in brain weight is 100 to 150 Gm. The atrophy is almost always most marked in the frontal area but is usually found, though to a much lesser degree, in the parietal lobe. Little or no atrophy is present in the occipital lobe. The atrophy may be quite diffuse and may involve several lobes or it may be confined largely to the frontal areas. The large vessels of the circle of Willis may or may not be sclerosed. Usually there is some degree of sclerosis, but this varies widely in the individual case. The large vessels may show a mild degree of fibrosis of their walls or there may be quite pronounced evidences of sclerosis which involve all or most of the vessels of the circle of Willis, with typical plaque formation.

The microscopic picture varies widely. The pia-arachnoid shows quite definite fibrosis in all the cases. The process is one of pure fibrosis, with increased collagen and fibroblasts. There are varying numbers of large mononuclear cells in the pia-arachnoid, depending on whether there is a frank destructive process in the underlying cortex. The cellular structure of the cortex varies widely. There may be a wide variety of conditions affecting the cortical ganglion cells. In the majority of cases the following picture prevails: The cortical architecture is not disturbed. There is, however, a loss of cells which may be slight, moderate, or severe. This cellular loss is most marked in the third layer of the

cortex. It is seen as a diffuse cell loss or outfall here and there in the affected layer. There may be quite wide gaps in the cellular structure, with cells completely absent from numerous areas of the layer in question. The cell loss in the more superficial and deeper cortical layers is much less marked than in the third cortical layer. The ganglion cells themselves show a varied picture. Usually there is evidence of sclerosis of the ganglion cells. In other instances, the cells are swollen and edematous, or they may exhibit ischemic changes due to temporary occlusion of arterial blood supply. The cortical arterioles are thickened and their walls often hyalinized. There may be edematous swelling of the perivascular spaces. The astrocytes in the cortex are definitely increased in number, but there are no changes in the other glial elements.

There may be small diffuse areas of softening in the cortex and basal ganglia. Ischemic areas may also be present. These are areas of infarct formation which are of varying size and are characterized by a loss of ganglion cells, a partial gliosis, and an increased vascularity in the affected regions. In still other cases, linear softenings involving a complete cortical layer over a distance of several gyri have been described. There appears to be no relationship between the distribution or severity of the arteriosclerotic changes and the clinical symptoms.

Symptoms: The disease affects subjects usually over sixty years of age, but patients between fifty and sixty are not uncommon. The onset of symptoms is gradual. The symptoms are chiefly referable to the mental sphere. In the early stages of the disease there is noted a slight change in personality, an increased irritability, a tendency to absent-mindedness and forgetfulness. There is, as a rule, a falling off in memory and difficulty in concentration. A history of falling off of efficiency in work is common. Associated with these symptoms, which may be overlooked for some time, are vague somatic complaints, chief among which are attacks of dizziness, headache, and loss of energy. The dizzy attacks are fleeting and usually present on change of posture. Fleeting loss or impairment of consciousness is sometimes found. Generalized or focal convulsions may develop but are not common. Symptoms of the nature described may persist for months and be disregarded. If examination is made at this time there is usually found a person with evidence of sclerosis of the peripheral vessels, an appearance older than the chronological age, no vascular hypertension and as a rule no cardiorenal disease. Retinal arteriosclerosis is always present in some degree, but evidences of focal brain damage are usually absent. Tremors of the face and tongue may be present.

In more advanced stages, mental symptoms of a severe nature predominate. Confusional psychoses and signs of outspoken mental deterioration are present. Paranoid trends are common and agitated periods may also be found. Personality deviations of many sorts are frequently present. The process in general is that of a slowly progressive mental deterioration.

Diagnosis: The diagnosis of cerebral arteriosclerosis is usually easy, occurring as it does in a person of advanced age, with evidence of peripheral and retinal arteriosclerosis, and signs of mental deterioration. It simulates closely the development and findings in *general paresis*, but the distinction can be made easily by the age of onset, speech difficulties, and the serological findings. *Brain tumor* involving the frontal lobes may develop in similar fashion but is associated as a

rule with signs of increased pressure and shows no evidence of arteriosclerosis. *Senile dementia* may be difficult and almost impossible to distinguish from cerebral arteriolosclerosis, since the mental picture is quite similar in the two conditions. Senile dementia, however, tends to occur at a more advanced age. Cerebral arteriosclerosis is more likely to develop with headache, attacks of vertigo, and evidences of focal brain damage. *Confusional syndromes* from toxic causes of many sorts, such as drugs, infections, trauma, etc., are not usually confused with cerebral arteriolosclerosis.

XIII. THROMBOSIS OF THE VENOUS SINUSES

Thrombosis may involve any of the sinuses in the meninges, but some are more susceptible than others. The sinuses most frequently involved are the longitudinal, lateral, and cavernous sinuses.

Longitudinal Sinus Thrombosis: This sinus is rarely affected by thrombosis in adults. It is more often affected in infants and children as a result of infection. It is most frequently diseased in trauma, but it is involved also in infections, and in blood dyscrasias such as polycythemia vera. Sometimes it is affected secondary to disease of the paranasal sinuses and meningitis. In some instances it occurs as a terminal state of a marantic condition.

The superior longitudinal sinus receives the veins which drain the mesial aspect of the brain, as well as those which drain the superior half of the lateral surface of each hemisphere. These superior lateral veins unite in four main trunks: a frontal, a precentral, a postcentral, and an occipital. The postcentral is usually the largest. It drains the motor and sensory central gyri of the hemispheres, in addition to other important areas.

Various groups of *symptoms* result from occlusion of the sinus in its different portions, thus interfering with drainage from the various main trunks. The symptoms resulting from occlusion of the sinus at the point of entrance of the postcentral branch consist of (1) paralysis of the limbs of a special type to be noted presently, (2) disturbances of sensation, and (3) minor, probably unrelated, symptoms. The onset is sudden, with severe headache, vomiting, unconsciousness which rapidly develops into stupor, and convulsions.

The motor symptoms, paralysis of the limbs, are variable and depend both on the site and severity of the lesions. There may be involvement of both legs, all the limbs, or three or two limbs. In a group of traumatic cases, the following distribution was noted: all limbs, twenty cases; both legs and one arm, thirty-one cases; lower limbs, sixteen cases; hemiplegia, six cases; one leg, five cases (Holmes and Sargent). Involvement of one or both lower limbs is present in almost all the cases. This is easily understood when one realizes that the area first affected by the softening resulting from occlusion of the longitudinal sinus is the paracentral lobule which gives origin to the leg and foot fibers of the pyramidal system. The paralysis in these cases is more marked in the distal segments of the legs, the proximal portions being much less affected. Thus the foot and leg muscles are much more involved than those of the hip and thigh. In the upper limbs the weakness is more pronounced in the proximal segments. The reason for the latter is due to the fact that the superior cerebral vein drains the precentral gyrus to the level of the wrist innervation. Consequently, softening due to obstruction of this system will cause an escape of the hand muscles, which remain powerful despite the weakness of the rest of the limb. The paralyzed limbs are rigid. This rigidity is always more marked in the lower limbs. It comes on early, is very marked and parallels the degree of paralysis of the limbs. The reflexes are hyperactive on the paralyzed, spastic side and there is always a well-marked Babinski sign. The spasticity in many cases is so marked that it cannot be broken even with great force. Facial or lingual weakness in these patients is uncommon and usually transient.

The sensory disturbances are those of a pure cortical lesion. Pain, temperature, and touch are not affected, but some touch stimuli are not readily appreciated. On the other hand, position and passive motion are lost. Stereognostic perception is also absent (astereognosis). Two-point discrimination is lost.

In the majority of patients there is first some difficulty in passing urine or even retention, but these symptoms pass quickly. Incontinence is less frequent. Temporary paralysis of associated ocular movements (conjugate deviation) is present in some patients. Convulsions are sometimes present. The symptoms in infants and children are much less precise than in adults.

Diagnosis: This is not difficult in clear-cut cases. The presence of bilateral paralysis of the legs, more marked in the distal segments with extreme rigidity, and with the type of sensory disturbance noted previously, is sufficient to make the diagnosis in the presence of a history of trauma or infection. Sometimes a similar syndrome is caused by encapsulated brain tumors which straddle the longitudinal sinus, compressing it and the paracentral lobules. Parasagittal tumors of this type, arising from the falx cerebri, usually give signs of increased pressure, evidence of progressive disability, and monoplegic disturbances with leg weakness particularly. The syndrome can be differentiated from a paraplegia of spinal origin by the nature of the spasticity and the distribution of the loss of power in the affected limbs.

Lateral Sinus Thrombosis: Thrombosis of the lateral sinus is most commonly associated with mastoid infection, where it occurs in an incidence of about 1.5 per cent. It is found also in otitis media. It is usually associated with acute otitic and mastoid infections but may accompany chronic disease.

Symptoms: They are striking and often dramatic in onset. The history is usually that of middle ear or mastoid infection in which chills and fever suddenly develop. The temperature is of the septic variety. Tenderness of the jugular vein is frequently encountered and there may be defensive rigidity of the neck. Leukocytosis is present and anemia may develop during the course of the illness. The blood culture is positive in about fifty per cent of cases. The superficial veins may be prominent and the mastoid process swollen and tender.

The symptoms of sinus thrombosis are often obscured by the occurrence of intracranial complications of other sorts; meningitis is not an infrequent accompaniment. Brain abscess and extradural abscess are not infrequently encountered with it. The spinal fluid pressure is elevated in such instances and choked disc may be present.

Diagnosis: The *diagnosis* of lateral sinus thrombosis is not usually easy, since the condition, itself an infectious process, is etched against a background of infection, usually mastoiditis. It must be suspected in a patient with mastoid or middle ear infection in whom there is a sudden development of chills and a septic temperature. It must be suspected also in patients with mastoiditis who have been operated on, who run a persistent septic temperature despite the elimination of the mastoid infection. The diagnosis is aided by the palpation of a tender and thrombosed internal jugular vein on the suspected side. Aid is given by the *Tobey-Queckenstedt test.* Compression of the jugular vein on the healthy side produces a rapid rise in spinal fluid pressure as measured in a spinal fluid manometer. On the other hand, compression of the jugular vein on the affected side causes no rise or a very inadequate rise in spinal fluid pressure.

The problem of diagnosis of lateral sinus thrombosis is obscured and made more difficult by the occurrence often of extradural or brain abscess. The latter particularly may be associated with signs of focal brain damage, such as jacksonian convulsions, hemiparesis, etc.

Cavernous Sinus Thrombosis: This condition develops from a variety of *causes.* It may follow disease of the sinuses, especially sphenoid sinus infection. Infections around the face are particularly prone to cause the disorder; notable among these are erysipelas, cellulitis, furuncles of the face, infected furuncles in the nose, dental infections, and infections of the throat. Mastoid infection may produce cavernous sinus thrombosis. Infections of the orbit are a common source. Scalp infections and septicemia of unknown origin have been found to be associated with sinus thrombosis at times. It may accompany meningitis in some cases, but in such instances the meningitis is usually secondary to the sinus thrombosis.

Symptoms: The *symptoms* are characteristic and the condition is often bilateral. A septic temperature and leukocytosis are uniformly present. The eye is edematous, the edema extending into the facial tissues. The veins around the orbit are swollen and the affected eye is prominent and often protrudes from the orbit. A complete external ophthalmoplegia is found in characteristic cases, since the third, fourth, and sixth cranial nerves pass through the cavernous sinus. The eyeball is completely immobile and the eyelid ptosed. The corneal reflex is absent and there is loss of sensation over the supraorbital division of the trigeminal nerve, since this also traverses the cavernous sinus. Pains in the eye and over the forehead are common. Optic neuritis and papilledema are occasionally encountered. The pupillary reactions may be normal or absent and vision may likewise be normal or lost.

A chronic variety of cavernous sinus thrombosis is known, characterized by a slow development of the symptoms and signs described.

Diagnosis: The diagnosis is never difficult. The presence of an infection around the face, lips, and nares, or in the sinuses, the characteristic development of ophthalmoplegia and the septic temperature offer no obstacles to diagnosis. Meningitis may develop by extension of the infection into the meninges and may complicate the picture by the presence of signs of meningeal irritation. Abscess of the brain may develop in some cases. An encephalitis in the adjacent brain tissue is not an infrequent accompaniment of the disease. All these may produce additional symptoms and signs, but the recognition of extension of the infection to the brain is readily made.

The *prognosis* is bad even in these days of chemotherapy. Recovery is rare.

XIV. TREATMENT OF VASCULAR DISORDERS OF THE BRAIN

Cerebral Hemorrhage: Once a cerebral hemorrhage has developed the problem becomes largely one of *nursing care.* Absolute rest is, of course, imposed by the disability itself. The head and shoul-ders should be well raised. Postural drainage of the tracheobronchial tree is important. The patient should be placed on his side frequently. Mucus must be aspirated frequently. Aminophylline and atropine may be used if secretion is excessive. Excessive restlessness should be combated by mild sedatives, such as paraldehyde or bromides. The skin should be kept dry. The urinal may be kept in place in male patients to avoid contamination of the skin by urine.

Feeding becomes a serious problem because of unconsciousness; a nasal tube is, therefore, a useful procedure and permits the free administration of liquids of all sorts as well as essential vitamins. The bowels are often incontinent, but when not should be kept open by small doses of magnesium sulfate (one ounce daily) or other laxatives. Venesection may be performed in cases with hypertension, but the procedure is opposed by many. Hypertonic solutions, such as fifty per cent glucose or sucrose, may be given intravenously (50 cc. once or twice daily), but are contraindicated in patients with cardiac embarrassment. Albumin solution (25 per cent) given intravenously furnishes good nourishment and also serves to dehydrate an edematous brain. In some instances, patients with cerebral hemorrhage of relatively slow development may be operated on and the clot removed surgically with full recovery of function. *Autohemotherapy* has been advocated by some; 20 to 30 cc. of the patient's blood is withdrawn from an arm vein and injected immediately into the gluteal muscles. Clotting may be prevented by using 2 cc. of twenty-five per cent sodium citrate solution.

Cerebral Thrombosis: The general care of the skin, elevation of the head and shoulders, and the problem of feeding are precisely the same as in cerebral hemorrhage. *Caffeine* is useful in many cases in the acute stages in patients with cardiac failure, administered as caffeine sodium benzoate in doses of 0.3 to 1 gram hypodermically, depending on the requirements. *Strychnine* may be used. Patients with syphilitic vascular disease should receive *antisyphilitic treatment* as indicated in the discussion of neurosyphilis. *Prostigmine methyl sulfate* (1:2000) given intramuscularly with *atropine sulfate* (gr. ⅟₅₀) once or twice daily has been reported to give encouraging results in the treatment of spastic hemiplegias. *Injection of the stellate ganglion* by procaine has been advocated in order to combat vasoparalysis and edema (de Takats). The results of such injection are not encouraging. *Anticoagulants* are of little help in vascular thrombosis involving brain vessels. It has been suggested that these are helpful in the early days of thrombosis, but by and large they influence the course of the disorder very slightly. Vasodilators such as nicotinic acid and papaverine are helpful. It is important to maintain systemic blood pressure.

Care must be taken even during the acute stages of hemiplegia to avoid contractures. For this purpose gentle massage of the limbs is useful, with stretching of the fingers to avoid deformities. As recovery occurs, daily massage of the recovering limbs is definitely indicated to help the circulation in the paralyzed limbs. Passive movements of the limbs is valuable. The patient may be given a soft rubber ball to squeeze in order to exercise recovering power of the fingers.

One of the most important features of treatment of the hemiplegic consists of the rehabilitation program designed to educate him in the use of the paralyzed limbs. During the acute phase of the illness, before rehabilitation has begun he should have (1) a pillow in the axilla to prevent adduction contracture, (2)

foot board or posterior splint on the affected leg to prevent foot drop, (3) sand bags on the lateral aspects of the leg to prevent outward rotation, (4) passive movements of the joints twice daily. *Rehabilitation exercises* should include (1) learning to sit upright in bed by means of a rope tied to the end of the bed, (2) standing by the side of the bed using the backs of two straight-backed chairs as parallel bars, (3) passive and active movements at the joints.

Cerebral Ischemia: The treatment of ischemia of the brain depends on the underlying cause. Ischemia due to acute blood loss should be treated by lowering the head and supplying fluid to maintain blood volume. Postural hypotension patients are often helped by bandaging the lower extremities and by *ephedrine sulfate* (gr. ⅜ two or three times daily). Patients with carotid sinus hyperactivity are treated with *atropine* and *epinephrine* for the vagal type, with epinephrine for the depressor type, and with desensitization of the carotid sinus for the cerebral type. Ischemia in patients with arteriosclerosis is best treated by improving cardiac action. In patients with primary anemia, *liver, hydrochloric acid,* and *transfusions* are indicated, while those with secondary anemia require *iron* (ferrous sulfate, 2 to 3 grams daily).

In *vascular spasm, caffeine* is a useful drug given as caffeine sodium benzoate (0.3 to 1 gram) by hypodermic. *Whiskey* is also useful in small doses (one ounce) repeated as needed. *Digitalis* may be required in patients with cardiac conditions. Nitroglycerin is sometimes of value. *Nicotinic acid* in doses of 100 mg. three to six times daily is useful.

Sinus Thrombosis: Since lateral sinus thrombosis is associated with mastoid infection, *operation* of the mastoid is essential with cleaning out of the mastoid infection. *Chemotherapy* by means of one of the sulfonamide compounds is important as an adjunct to operation, but it is advocated by some instead of operation. The specific sulfonamide depends upon the causative organism. Since the condition is acute, an adequate sulfonamide level must be built up rapidly by means of intravenous dosage and maintained by oral administration. Repeated small *blood transfusions* are an important adjunct to treatment. *Ligation of the internal jugular vein* should be carried out in septic cases.

Cavernous sinus thrombosis should be treated by intensive *chemotherapy* and repeated small blood *transfusions*.

11

Tumors of the Brain

The brain is one of the commonest sites of tumor in the body. The incidence of tumor of the brain among neurological conditions of various sorts is relatively high. It is important that tumors of the brain be recognized especially since they may simulate other conditions of various types. While the actual localization of a brain tumor requires special knowledge for which the neurologist and neurosurgeon are specially trained, it is the general practitioner who has first contact with such cases. For this reason it is essential that early recognition of such tumors be made since, as is the case with tumors in other parts of the body, the best therapeutic results are obtained in cases which have been recognized early. Too frequently brain tumors come into the hands of the neurosurgeon past the time when good results may be expected from operation. Every effort must be expended therefore toward early recognition of such growths. In these days of special technics for localization of cerebral processes therefore (pneumography, arteriography, electroencephalography), the suspicion of brain tumor constitutes the first step in effective treatment.

I. TYPES OF TUMOR AND FREQUENCY

The brain is the seat of many types of tumor. Not all these types are equally benign, and each has characteristics and features of its own. Each is associated further with its own particular diagnostic and therapeutic problems, some being much more malignant than others. In Table 47 there is available a bird's-eye view of the several tumor types.

With the possible exception of the uterus, the brain is said to be the most commonly affected organ of the body (Cushing and Bailey). A survey of Table 47 reveals how numerous are the tumor types which involve the brain. Most of the tumors are primary within the brain (gliomas, adenomas, meningiomas, etc.); others involve the brain secondarily (carcinoma, sarcoma).

All parts of the brain may be involved by tumor; no area is exempt. The cerebrum and cerebellum are most frequently affected either by invasion or compression, but the brain stem is by no means uncommonly involved.

It must be apparent that the distinction between *benign* and *malignant* brain tumors, though well-founded histologically, must be regarded as relative in a clinical sense, since the most benign tumor may be regarded as clinically malignant if it is found in an inaccessible portion of the brain so that its removal is impossible.

The *location* of brain tumors varies roughly with the age of the patient. In children they are most common in the posterior fossa, especially in the cerebellum. In adults, on the other hand, they are most often found in the cerebral hemispheres, though posterior fossa involvement is not uncommon.

No *age* is exempt from tumors of the

517

Table 47—Incidence of Brain Tumors

(Afte· Cushing)

Type		Number	Percentage
Gliomas	....	862	42.6
Pituitary adenomas	....	360	17.8
Chromophobe	264		
Chromophile	73		
Mixed	23		
Meningiomas	..	271	13.2
Acoustic tumors	..	176	8.7
Congenital tumors	..	113	5.6
Craniopharyngiomas	92		
Cholesteatomas and dermoids	15		
Chordomas and teratomas	6		
Metastatic and invasive tumors	..	85	4.2
Carcinoma	56		
Sarcoma	20		
Hypernephroma	5		
Myeloma	4		
Granulomatous tumors	..	45	2.2
Tuberculomas	33		
Syphilomas	12		
Blood vessel tumors	..	41	2.0
Sarcomas (primary)	..	14	0.7
Papilloma (choroid plexus)	..	12	0.6
Miscellaneous	..	44	2.2
		2023	100.0

Table 48—Frequency of Tumors in Various Locations

(Adson)

Supratentorial 70%

Frontal lobe	16.8
Temporal lobe	13.6
Parietal lobe	11.8
Occipital lobe	2.7
Anterior fossa	5.5
Pituitary gland	2.7
Corpus callosum	11.8
Midbrain	0.9
Third ventricle	1.3
Multiple	2.3

Infratentorial 30%

Cerebellum	12.7
Fourth ventricle	6.8
Cerebellopontine angle	10.4

brain. The highest incidence is found in middle age or early adult life (twenty-five to fifty). Tumors of childhood (five to ten) are not uncommon, but their occurrence in infancy is rare. They have been found rarely in infants under one year of age. Primary brain tumors may be found also in old age.

II. GENERAL FEATURES OF THE VARIOUS TYPES OF BRAIN TUMOR

1. The Gliomas

The gliomas are infiltrating tumors which may invade any portion of the brain substance. Their accepted *classification* at present is embryological, and is based on the assumption that specific cell types of the neuroglial series predominate in various gliomas. This does not imply that the tumors are derived from embryonic cell rests of the type found in the tumor. It cannot be assumed that tumors composed predominantly of specific cell types are derived from these cells, though the assumption may be tenable. Thus, astrocytomas, though composed of astrocytes, cannot be assumed to be derived from mature astrocytic rests by this finding alone. There are tumor types such as the astrocytomas, oligodendroglioma, and medulloblastoma which are composed of pure or almost pure cell types. On the other hand, the occurrence of transitional forms, the development of benign into malignant types, and the occurrence of such tumors as the glioblastoma multiforme, which is composed of more than a single cell type, strain somewhat the validity of the concept. Because of these features attempts have been made to grade gliomas according to their malignancy, much as in the case of carcinomas. While the present day classification of gliomas proposed by Cushing and Bailey and now widely accepted leaves unsolved many problems relating to the gliomas histologically, there can be no doubt that it is useful and valuable clinically, providing as it does a sound correlation between the pathological and clinical characteristics of these tumors. The propounding of the Bailey-Cushing classification has been of untold importance in the understanding of the life history, both clinical and histological, of gliomas. A correlation of the tumor types and the embryonic level at which they are presumed to develop is of help in the understanding of brain tumors.

An effort has been made to simplify the classification of gliomas and to grade them according to their malignancy (Kernohan and Sayre). The following groups have been suggested: (1) astrocytomas (astrocytoma, astroblastoma, glioblastoma multiforme), (2) ependymomas, (3) oligodendroglioma, (4) medulloblastoma, (5) neurocytoma.

Generally speaking, the more malignant tumors are derived from the more embryonic cell types, while the more benign tumors originate from more adult or mature cell forms. Thus the medulloblastoma, which is composed of immature cells, is a malignant tumor, whereas the astrocytoma, derived from the more mature astrocyte, is a benign glioma.

Various *types* of glioma have been identified histologically and their relative incidence computed. These are of greater importance to the neurologist and neurosurgeon than to the general practitioner, but some idea of tumor types is useful even to the latter in order to emphasize the difference in their life histories. All gliomas are infiltrating and in this sense they must all be regarded as malignant tumors, regardless of the site of infiltration. Some grow rapidly and wildly and defy cure either by extirpation or irradiation or both. Noteworthy examples of this class are the medulloblastoma and the glioblastoma multiforme, long survivals of which are exceptional. The astrocytomas, on the other hand, grow slowly and are usually associated with long preoperative histories and postoperative survivals. They are much more readily amenable to bold extirpation than either of the groups already mentioned, and in the case of the cystic astrocytomas cures are not unusual. Even in solid astrocytomas complete removal is possible.

Between the slowly growing astrocytomas and the rapidly advancing glioblastoma multiforme and medulloblastoma are many other groups, some of them more benign than others. It is possible within quite accurate limits to predict the type of glioma from the nature of the clinical course, but this is not always true. Thus, it is frequently difficult to be certain whether a cerebellar tumor in a child is a medulloblastoma or an astrocytoma, though the outlook varies greatly in the two instances. The point of outstanding significance lies in the fact that though all gliomas are infiltrating tumors, they vary greatly in their clinical and histological characteristics,

Medulloblastoma (11.2 per cent): This type of glioma is found almost exclusively in the cerebellum of children, but it occurs rarely in adults in the cerebral and cerebellar hemispheres. The adult cases are more slowly growing than the cerebellar medulloblastomas of children. It is found in children of from two to ten years and very frequently between

Table 49—Types and Incidence of Gliomas

Tumor Type	Cushing	Gagel	Elvidge, Penfield & Cone	Baker	Roussy & Oberling	Total	Percentage
ASTROCYTOMA..............	255	58	55	127	119	614	37.97
GLIOBOLSTOMA MULTIFORME...	208	84	52	71	45	460	28.45
MEDULLOBLASTOMA..........	86	23	28	21	20	178	11.02
EPENDYMOMA...............	25	23	19	20	..	87	5.32
SPONGIOBLASTOMA POLARE.....	32	16	11	8	..	67	4.16
ASTROBLASTOMA.............	35	4	13	14	..	66	4.07
OLIGODENDROGLIOMA........	27	3	8	6	16	60	3.72
PINEALOMA.................	14	11	2	6	..	33	2 06
PAPILLOMA OF CHOROID PLEXUS	12	6	..	1	7	26	1.61
GANGLIONEUROMA...........	3	9	..	..	1	13	.81
NEUROEPITHELIOMA.........	2	2	3	4	2	13	.81
	699	239	191	278	210	1617	

some growing slowly and others rapidly, and they differ in their response to surgical treatment, some being hopeless and others not only hopeful but amenable to cure. For this reason some knowledge of their biological characteristics is essential for an understanding of their clinical features. In the descriptions to follow little emphasis will be placed upon their histological features, since these are accessible in greater detail in neuropathological texts.

The most common types of glioma are, therefore, the astrocytoma, the glioblastoma multiforme, and the medulloblastoma, which together constitute about seventy-five per cent or more of all gliomas. Some understanding of these main types is therefore desirable.

five and six years of age. It occurs not infrequently in pubescents or adolescents (ten to sixteen or over). The average age of appearance is about six to ten years. The cerebellar medulloblastomas give rise to a characteristic clinical course which may be detected on careful scrutiny of the facts. The story and findings will be described in detail in a consideration of the features of tumors involving the cerebellum. Here it may be stated that the clinical features correlate well with the pathological findings. Symptoms due to internal hydrocephalus from occlusion of the fourth ventricle appear early in the disease. These consist of headache. vomiting, and often of eye disturbances. Accompanying them or following them after a varying period of time appear symptoms due to destruction of the cerebellar tissue, such as incoördination of the arms or legs, and difficulty in walking.

It is usually found in the midline of cephalus of varying degree early in its development. It may, and not infrequently does, extend into the aqueduct of Sylvius and the third ventricle, and

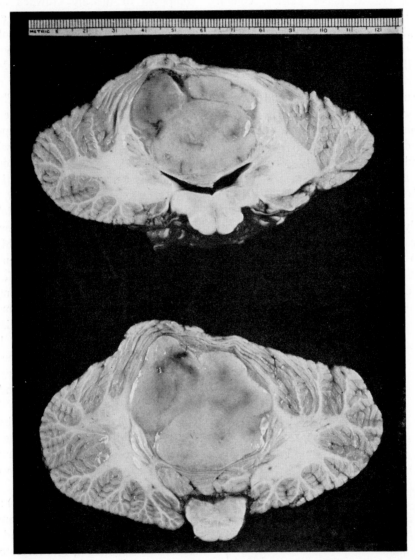

Fig. 148—*Medulloblastoma.* A large medulloblastoma occupying the vermis of the cerebellum and occluding the fourth ventricle. The clinical course was typical.

the cerebellum, involving the cerebellar vermis, but it may extend into one or both cerebellar hemispheres. It fills the fourth ventricle, occluding it completely as a rule and producing internal hydro-

may become disseminated through the subarachnoid space of the spinal canal, where it is seen as a thick pad of tumor usually covering the dorsal surface of the entire cord and extending into the subarachnoid space along its roots. Dissemination may occur also over the cerebral hemispheres along the cerebral subarachnoid space, and into the cranial nerves, causing cranial nerve palsies, convulsions, and other cerebral symptoms. Such dissemination occurs with or without manipulation of the tumor at operation. Medulloblastomas may at times invade the brain stem, but they are confined as a rule to the cerebellum and the ventricular cavities.

Grossly, the tumor appears reddish gray during life, is soft, easily compressed, and moderately vascular. It may appear at the surface of the vermis or be hidden in its depths and it gives a false impression of being sharply defined at times. In such instances it can be found to be infiltrating. It can almost always be found to be adherent to the floor of the fourth ventricle by fine strands of connective tissue, tugging on which at operation may lead to

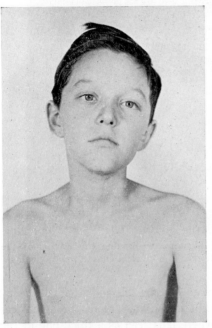

Fig. 149 — *Medulloblastoma.* Head posture in a large medulloblastoma involving the vermis and the right cerebellum.

punctate hemorrhages in the medulla. The tumor is grossly soft and can be sucked out by the neurosurgeon's suction apparatus. Histologically, the tumor is composed of densely crowded cells in streams or at times rosettes, among which is a fine reticulum and a number of small vessels sufficient to maintain blood supply without areas of necrosis. Mitoses are always present but they vary greatly in number from case to case. They are numerous in some and few in others. The cells have vesiculated carrot-shaped nuclei: the cytoplasm fails to stain with the usual cell stains. The cells of the medulloblastoma are sensitive to irradiation but their growth is never completely inactivated by irradiation. Tumors which have been subjected to irradiation show both living and dead tumor cells in histological preparations, often collagen overgrowth, and at times vessel proliferation.

The average *survival period* of medulloblastomas from the onset of symptoms, without operation or irradiation, is about eighteen to twenty-four months. Longer survival periods of two to three years have been recorded and in rare instances five-year survivals have been found. The average duration of symptoms before operation is five to twelve months. The course is rapid and malignant. The tumor is best treated by removal of as much of the tumor as is possible, followed by intensive irradiation.

Astrocytoma (35.1 per cent): This is the most common type of glioma and the most benign. It may be found in the cerebrum, cerebellum, or brain stem. It is most common in the cerebrum in adults and in the cerebellum in children. In adults it is found in subjects over thirty, while in children astrocytomas are found chiefly in the first decade of life, most of them appearing at about nine or ten years of life. It grows very slowly and not infrequently is associated with a history of symptoms extending for five or six years before relief is sought. The *history* in cases of astrocytoma is, therefore, apt to be slow and of long and growth, astrocytomas often fail to produce evidences of increased intracranial pressure until their growth has become relatively well advanced. For

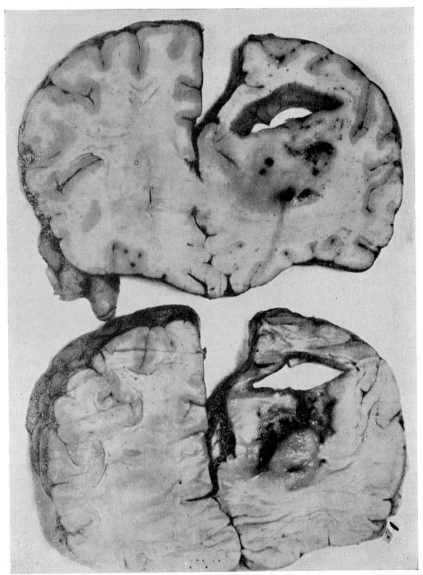

Fig. 150—*Astrocytoma* of the cystic type, showing the cystic and solid portions of tumor. In this specimen the latter predominates.

duration. Often the growth is of such an indeterminate type early in the course of the disease that little attention is paid to it. Because of the slow development this reason they often produce evidences of focal brain involvement without signs of increased pressure, such as headache and choked disc, until they have grown for some time. In a group of fifty-five verified astrocytomas, the average pre-admission history was thirty-one months (Elvidge, Penfield, Cone). Astrocytomas occur in both solid and cystic forms, the former being more common in adults and the latter in children, but both solid and cystic forms may be found in both adults and children. The astrocytomas of adults are most often solid and most common in the cerebral hemispheres, while they

type of tumor, being slowly growing, often permits the brain to adjust itself to its advance; hence signs of increased intracranial pressure are often delayed. There is frequently lack of definition between tumor and brain tissue, the former merging imperceptibly into the brain substance. The affected portion of the hemisphere is enlarged as compared with the normal side and is often firmer, sometimes even hard. The ventricular system

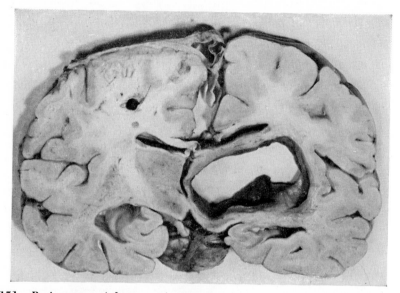

Fig. 151—*Brain tumor.* A large cystic astrocytoma occupying the basal ganglia area, showing the solid nubbin of tumor projecting from the floor of the cyst. Note the well-defined capsule and the pushed-over third ventricle.

occur much more frequently in the midline of the cerebellum in children. Despite their predominance in this region in children, the astrocytomas of childhood are less frequent than the medulloblastomas. Astrocytomas are found also in the brain stem, invading directly the structure of the base of the brain as well as the basal ganglia, third ventricle, and aqueduct of Sylvius.

The *solid* astrocytomas may be confined to a single lobe or may extend diffusely through more than one lobe or even through an entire hemisphere. This

is encroached upon and the midline structures displaced. The histological structure is characterized by a varying number of astrocytic nuclei which are round or oval and contain coarse chromatin granules loosely arranged. Large plump astrocytes constitute most of the cellular structure of some tumors. In others, giant cell forms are found. The cytoplasm can be shown by special stains to be typically astrocytic. The background of the tumor is composed of a varying number of neuroglial fibrils arranged in a loose network in some cases, in others in dense bundles, and in still others in a perivascular arrangement. The vascular architecture usually shows no abnormal forms.

The *cystic* astrocytomas are formed of varying proportions of cyst and solid tumor. Tumors of this type are well-defined and cleanly separated from the surrounding tissue. Around them is a cyst wall in which is a nubbin of solid tumor varying in size from a small pea to a large solid mass comprising most of the tumor. The cyst is filled with a fluid of high specific gravity, often yellow in color, containing large amounts of protein. The solid tumor nubbin has a typical astrocytomatous structure and the cyst wall is composed largely of neuroglial fibrils with vessels and a varying amount of collagen.

Astrocytomas run a slow benign course and not infrequently have long preoperative courses and postoperative survivals of several years. Cystic tumors are cured by complete removal of the solid portion of the tumor. The solid astrocytomas may be cured by removal of a hemisphere or all of the brain tissue invaded by the tumor. Tumors of this type have been found to extend well beyond the visible gross limits of the tumor. Postoperative survival in astrocytomas may vary from three to seven years. The cerebellar astrocytomas appear to have a longer postoperative survival than the cerebral types, probably due to the fact that more of the cerebellar cases are cystic in type. Solid astrocytomas are best treated by radical extirpation and in the case of cystic astrocytomas by removal of the mural nodule. Irradiation is of little benefit.

Glioblastoma Multiforme (29.4 per cent): This form of tumor is all too common and next to the astrocytomas is the most frequently encountered glioma of the brain. It is a highly malignant, rapidly growing tumor. It is found almost exclusively in adults of thirty-five years or over (average about forty years), though it may occur in younger adults as well. Males are more often affected than females. It is rarely encountered in children and then usually in the brain stem. The duration of symptoms before relief is sought in tumors of this type is short and the history is both rapid and in many cases apoplectic. Sudden apoplectic onset of symptoms is common in this type of tumor due to the occurrence of hemorrhage within the neoplasm. The apoplectic development of symptoms resembles closely that of vascular insults of the brain. Evidences of increased pressure are encountered early and are often of a severe degree, in contrast to astrocytomas in which increased intracranial pressure may be delayed in its appearance. In glioblastomas the growth of the tumor is so rapid that there is little capacity on the part of the brain to adjust to its advance. Symptoms are present for about six months before operation in glioblastoma multiforme, but shorter and longer durations may be encountered.

Glioblastomas are found almost entirely in the cerebral hemispheres; they may, however, invade the brain stem but are not found in the cerebellum of adults. The glioblastoma multiforme is a rapidly growing tumor, often characterized by apoplectic or sudden onset of symptoms. It frequently invades large parts of a hemisphere and not uncommonly most of a cerebral hemisphere, with consequent enlargement of the invaded brain tissue. It tends to invade the deep-seated brain structures such as the basal ganglia and not infrequently extends across the midline by way of the corpus callosum to the opposite cerebral hemisphere. In some instances, it is multiple. It is associated usually with greatly increased intracranial pressure and marked deformity of the ventricular system. Large portions of the tumor are necrotic; in some instances, the entire tumor may be necrotic. Fresh and old hemorrhages are

of many types of cells, of which the spongioblast seems to be the most common. Areas of necrosis are always found, as well as recent or old hemorrhages. Cell

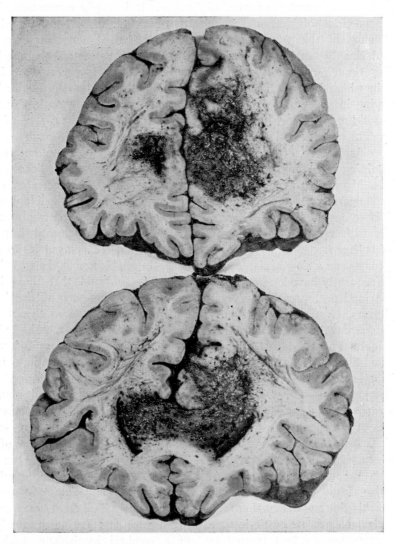

Fig. 152—*Glioblastoma multiforme,* showing the infiltration of the frontal lobes and the corpus callosum in an extensive malignant tumor of this type. The necrotic features of the tumor are well shown.

usually found within the tumor, often of large size, and it is probably these hemorrhages which account for the apoplectic onset of symptoms.

The tumors of the glioblastoma multiforme type are composed histologically

palisading and giant cells are frequent. The vessels show proliferative changes, chiefly of the adventitia, with involvement also of the intima. Glomerularlike vessel clusters are commonly seen. Mitoses are common. There is usually a collagen structure of varying degree and a deposit of neuroglial fibrils.

The average duration of symptoms before operation in tumors of this type vivals of from two to four years. There is no doubt, therefore, that the glioblastoma multiforme is a highly malignant tumor and that in our present state of

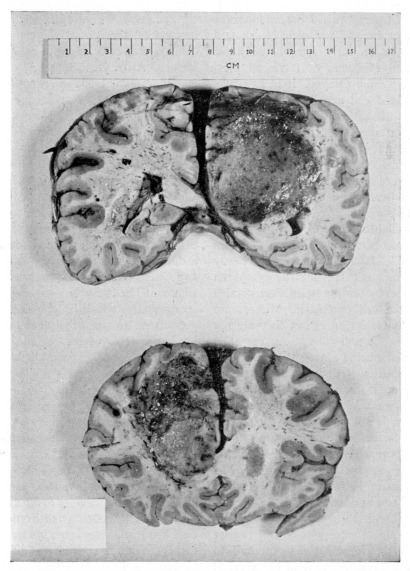

Fig. 153—*Glioblastoma multiforme* showing the large necrotic tumor in both cerebral hemispheres. The clinical history was of 6 months' duration.

is short and varies from six to ten months. Exceptional cases have had preoperative symptoms of two to three years. The average survival after operation is six to nine months, with exceptional sur-

knowledge long survivals are exceptional. It does not react to irradiation, or may do so very inadequately.

Oligodendroglioma (3.1 per cent): This form of glioma is slowly growing and is usually found in the cerebral hemisphere of adults of thirty-five or over, but has been encountered also in the brain stem. It occurs at times in children. The history is usually of long duration, often ten years or more, and in some cases even longer. Epileptic attacks appear to be an early symptom in most cases and evidences of increased pressure are usually delayed. It is, as a rule, well defined and may be found projecting into the lateral ventricles. It frequently attains large size and may give a false impression of encapsulation. The histological structure resembles oligodendroglia seen in normal tissue but is much more cellular. The tumor cells are arranged in rows or columns which are quite well defined in most cases. Blood vessels are numerous. The cells contain round nuclei with a moderately heavy chromatin structure, but the cytoplasm is not seen by routine stains. Silver stains reveal the cell cytoplasm. Mitoses are seen in some instances but they are not numerous. A fine collagenous carpet is found penetrating among the cells. Calcium is often found in this type of glioma, and is frequently visible on roentgenologic examination. The survival after operation is not long and is out of proportion to the long preoperative course; two years represents an average survival.

Ependymoma (6.17 per cent): The ependymoma is found in the cerebral hemispheres and cerebellum. In the latter situation it has a tendency to be midline involving the vermis, to project through the foramen magnum and to compress the upper part of the cervical cord. Hence it is often associated with neck pain. The tumor in the cerebellum is firm and often enucleable. In the cerebral hemispheres it may attain a large size and its connection with the ependyma of the ventricle may not be evident grossly. The histological features consist of large cells with large nuclei, arranged here and there in rosette formation around a cavity, the cells containing a ciliated surface toward the cyst lumen. Small blepharoplasten granules are seen below the cell surface. The cysts are often few in number, the rest of the tumor being composed of cells arranged in no special fashion. Astrocytes are seen. Vessels are moderately numerous and areas of necrosis are found. Symptoms are present as a rule for about one year before operation, but preoperative symptoms of three to four years are not uncommon.

Spongioblastoma Polare (4.1 per cent): This type of tumor is found chiefly in the posterior fossa involving the cerebellum and brain stem and shows a greater propensity to occur in young people. It is a slowly growing tumor with a duration of symptoms of about one to two years. Long survivals are not uncommon. The tumor is composed of polar spongioblasts which are bipolar or unipolar, tend to run in parallel rows, and lay in a fibrillar carpet.

Other Glioma Types: The *astroblastoma* (five per cent) is a glioma type which is more commonly cerebral than cerebellar and may be found in children and adults in age ranges of two to sixty years. It varies widely both in its clinical and histological characteristics, in some instances its course and development being slow and in others rapid. This type of glioma lies in malignancy between the glioblastoma multiforme on the one hand and the astrocytoma on the other, combining both malignant and benign features. It occurs most commonly in the cerebral hemispheres of adults. Grossly the astroblastomas are infiltrating, often contain hemorrhagic and necrotic areas, and may contain cysts. In cerebral cases the course is slower than in the cerebellar types, the average duration of symptoms before operation being about fourteen to twenty-two months as compared with two to six months in cerebellar cases. The type cell is an astroblast which can be seen

astroblastomas varies greatly, but survivals up to several years are recorded.

Pineal tumors (two per cent) are of two types, pinealomas and pineoblastomas.

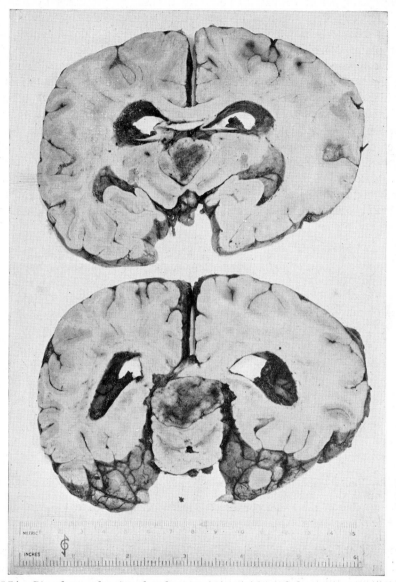

Fig. 154—*Pinealoma,* showing the characteristic position of the tumor occupying the pineal recess region and compressing the roof of the midbrain, thus producing the characteristic symptoms of increased pressure and paralysis of upward gaze.

radiating from the vessels by special stains. Mitoses are not uncommon. Vessels are numerous. Multinucleated cells are common. Survival after removal of

They are found at any age but are prone to develop in young males with signs of precocious puberty. Pinealomas are found in the region of the pineal gland, appear often to be well defined, have a granular appearance on their cut surface, have a tendency to penetrate into the third ventricle, and in rare instances may extend under the ependyma of the lateral ventricles. They compress the roof of the midbrain, particularly the region of the collicular plate. Microscopically, pinealomas are composed of large epithelioid cells and groups of lymphocytic cells, all of which lie in a connective tissue mesh. *Ganglioneuromas* are rare and are found in the cerebrum and brain stem. They are relatively slowly growing and are composed of a combination of nerve cells and neuroglial elements, the former being both mature and immature forms. *Medulloepitheliomas* are also rare and

tirely outside the brain tissue. They are attached to the overlying dura, producing symptoms of increased pressure by occupying space within the skull, giving rise to localizing symptoms by pressure on the brain tissue and by interference with circulation. At times meningiomas may undermine the brain substance, forming a deep nest and becoming almost completely covered by brain tissue, retaining, however, their dural attachment. Rarely they are malignant or multiple. Very rare instances of metastasis to the lung have been recorded. Their size varies greatly from a few centimeters in diameter to tumors six to eight inches in diameter, attaining a weight in exceptional instances of more than 800 grams.

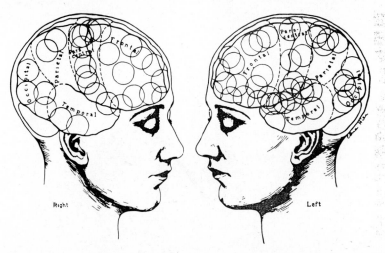

Fig. 155—*Meningioma*, showing the location of a large group of tumors of this type in relation to the cerebral hemispheres. Most of the tumors are in relation to the anterior portion of the brain. (Frazier & Alpers: Arch. Neurol. & Psychiat. 29:935, May, 1933.)

are composed of neuroepithelial cells arranged in formations resembling the primitive neural tube. They are malignant tumors.

2. Meningiomas

The meningiomas are the most benign of all brain tumors. They are encapsulated, well-defined tumors growing en-

Most meningiomas are round or global in form, but some are flat, the so-called *meningiomes en plaques*.

Meningiomas are found in various locations in the cranial cavity. Most of them are located over the cerebral hemispheres, particularly in relation to the anterior half of the cerebrum in relation to the superior longitudinal sinus or the

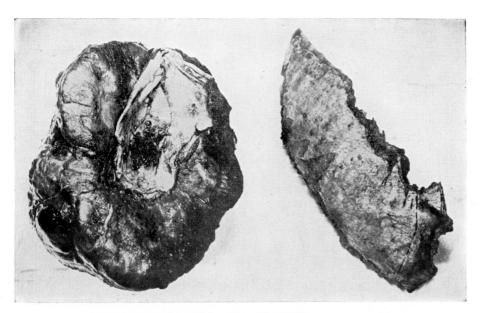

Fig. 156—*(See: Fig. 157.)*

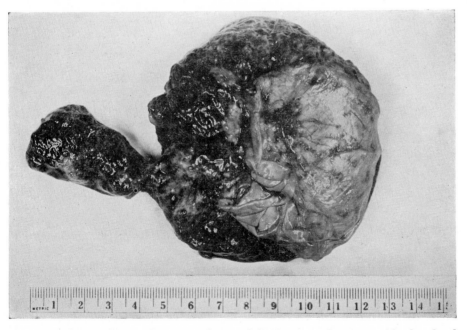

Fig. 157—*Meningioma,* showing a large globoid mass of tumor with the dural attachment invariably found in tumors of this type.

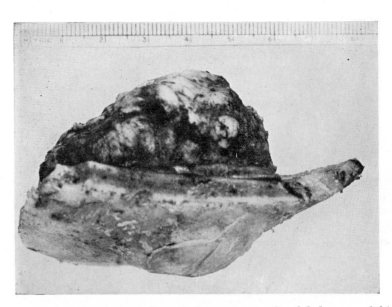

Fig. 158—*Meningioma,* showing the typical appearance of a global tumor of this type, with the overlying bone which has been eroded.

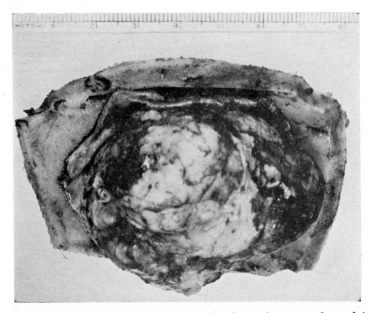

Fig. 159—*Meningioma.* A meningioma with dural attachment and overlying bone which in this case was eroded by the compressing tumor. The symptoms consisted of progressive hemiparesis with jacksonian convulsions and no evidence of increased pressure.

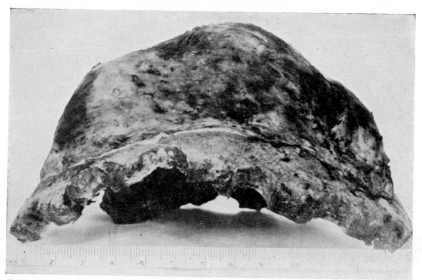

Fig. 160—*Meningioma* of the flat type, showing the overlying hyperostosis and a flat meningioma visible under the inner table of the skull.

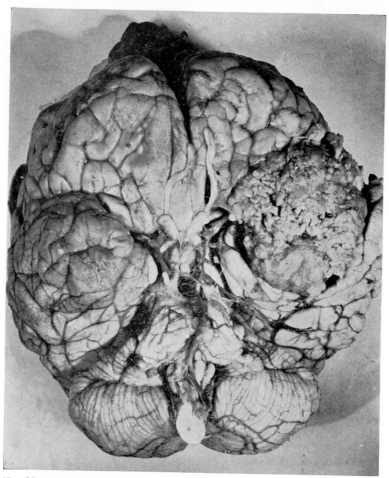

Fig. 161—*Meningioma* compressing the inferior surface of the left temporal lobe causing destruction of this region.

middle cerebral vessels. They are found not infrequently between the hemispheres attached to the falx cerebri. Still others are found at the base of the skull, in the olfactory groove area, in relation to the olfactory nerves and bulbs. Not a few are found above the sella turcica attached to the tuberculum sellae. Other locations skull, especially in the olfactory groove area and the sphenoid ridge. The bony changes consist of hyperostosis in typical instances, characterized by an overgrowth of bone associated with the tumor. Erosion of bone and dilatation of the vascular channels in the bone are also found. Proliferation of bone in ivorylike areas

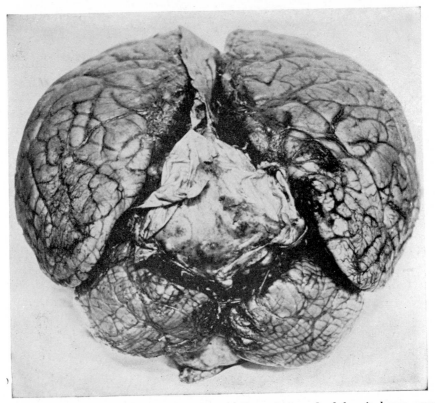

Fig. 162—*Meningioma* of the falx lying between the cerebral hemispheres, compressing these and the underlying cerebellum.

include the parasellar meningiomas attached to the lesser and greater wings of the sphenoid bones; the Gasserian ganglion; the lateral ventricles, and in some instances the posterior fossa.

In about twenty-five per cent of cases, changes are found in the bones of the skull in contact with the meningioma. Bony changes are found most commonly in the bones of the skull vault, but hyperostosis is found also in the base of the of thickening may be encountered. The cause of the local bone changes found in association with some meningiomas is not unanimously agreed upon. It is probable that the hyperostosis develops as the result of invasion of the skull of tumor cells, with consequent proliferative bone changes, though some maintain that in some instances at least the bone changes develop first and the tumor afterward.

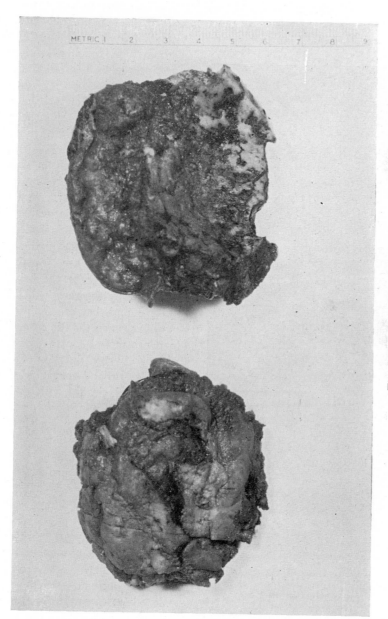

Fig. 163—(See: Fig. 164.)

Some meningiomas are firm and hard, others quite soft, and in some cases cystic formation is found. While meningiomas are usually well defined and sharply separated from the brain tissue, instances are not altogether uncommon of penetra-

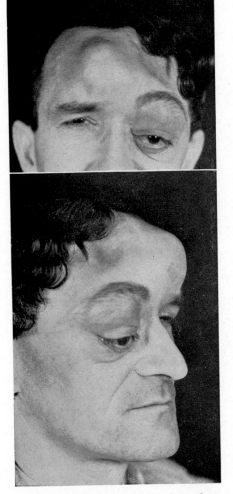

Fig. 164—*Meningioma of the frontal area illustrating the hyperostosis of the frontal bone and the underlying tumor.*

tion of meningiomas through the pia, especially in the case of the flat meningiomas. In rare instances also, they are found imbedded in the brain tissue without apparent connection with the dura. Multiple meningiomas are known to occur

and the association of meningiomas with others forms of brain tumor, such as neurofibroma, is likewise known.

Several histological types have been described — meningothelial, angioblastic, osteoblastic, chondroblastic, lipoblastic, sarcomatous, reticulin, and nonreticulin forming types. The origin of the meningiomas is still a matter of dispute. Some maintain that they originate from the fibroblasts lining the arachnoid membrane, others that they are derived from vascular structures. They are assumed by some to arise from the arachnoid villi and are found to be most numerous where these are most common. They resemble closely the arachnoid villi in their structure. Histologically, some meningiomas may assume malignant features.

Meningiomas are found chiefly in adults, the average age being forty-five years. They are rare in children and in old age, and they are slightly more common in women than in men. They run a long protracted course, giving a *history* of several years' duration of symptoms in many cases, and they tend not to recur if removed cleanly with their dural attachment. The *clinical course* of meningiomas over the cerebral hemispheres is characterized only by their slow and chronic features, but astrocytomas may also give rise to prolonged symptoms. Hence this feature is in itself not distinctive. A tumor, however, with a long protracted course may be suspected of being a meningioma, a suspicion which may in some instances be verified by the demonstration of bony changes in the skull. Recurrences develop, however, in patients in whom dural cell nests are left behind on removal.

3. Pituitary Adenomas

The pituitary adenomas are found predominantly within the sella turcica, but some are found lying above it (suprasellar adenomas). Those lying within the sella are derived from the cells of the anterior lobe of the hypophysis; no tumors are derived from the posterior lobe. Three main types are distinguishable, and these are derived from their cell counterparts in the pituitary gland. They are chromophobe, eosinophilic, and basophilic adenomas. The chromophobe adenomas are derived from the chief cells of the pituitary gland and fail to show

mon, containing both chromophobe and chromophile (eosinophilic or basophilic) elements.

The pituitary adenomas grow within the sella turcica, producing local pressure symptoms, except in the case of the basophilic adenomas, which are always microscopic and never attain large enough size to cause symptoms of pressure. The other types (chromophobe and eosinophilic), however, grow within the sella

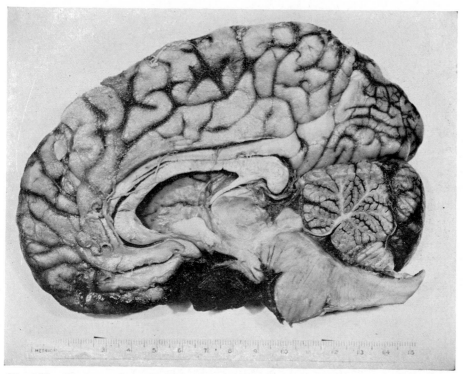

Fig. 165—*Pituitary adenoma* shown in a sagittal view of the brain. The overlying optic nerves and chiasm are compressed.

specific granules in their cytoplasm. Like their cells of origin, they are the most numerous of the adenomas, forming seventy-five per cent of all the pituitary adenomas. The eosinophilic adenomas are derived from the eosinophile cells and the basophilic adenomas from the basophile cells in the anterior lobe of the hypophysis. In addition, mixed or transitional forms of adenoma are not uncom-

confines, developing slowly, causing pressure on the optic nerves and chiasm and destroying the sella turcica and pituitary gland. The pituitary adenomas grow slowly, expanding within the sella turcica and spreading both upward and downward within its confines. They expand downward, depressing the floor of the sella turcica and impinging on the sphenoid sinus, which they may at times

completely obliterate. As they grow upward, they cause distention of the diaphragm of the sella turcica, causing it
to bulge. By this means they cause pressure on the optic nerves and chiasm. It
has been calculated that a pituitary

on the fixation of chiasm in relation to
the sella turcica. In most instances, the
optic nerves and chiasm are directly compressed as they lie above the sella turcica; in other cases, the nerves are directly compressed and the chiasm not

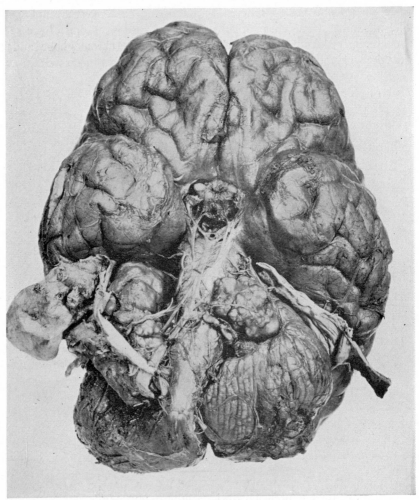

Fig. 166—*Cerebellopontine angle tumor.* Bilateral angle tumors, a large one in the
right cerebellopontine angle and a smaller one on the left.

tumor must grow and expand upward
about 10 mm. to 2 cm. before pressure is
made on the chiasm. The anterior clinoid
processes become thinned and pointed,
and the dorsum sellae may become eventually destroyed. Compression of the
optic nerve and chiasm varies, depending

quite so directly in post-fixed chiasms.
In pre-fixed chiasms, the pressure is
chiefly on the posterior part of the chiasm and the optic tract. Pressure may
not be on the chiasm in some cases,
but on the optic tract, even in adenomas
which have not burst through the dia-

phragm. Compression of the hypothalamus is not uncommon and destruction
of the hypophysis is, of course, inevitable in the course of the tumor growth.
Adenomas are soft and fleshy. In some
instances, they are cystic. They are quite

asymmetrical expansion cause pressure
on the adjacent oculomotor nerve or
other cranial nerves, or on the adjacent
uncus. They are sensitive to irradiation,
particularly in the case of the chromophobe adenomas.

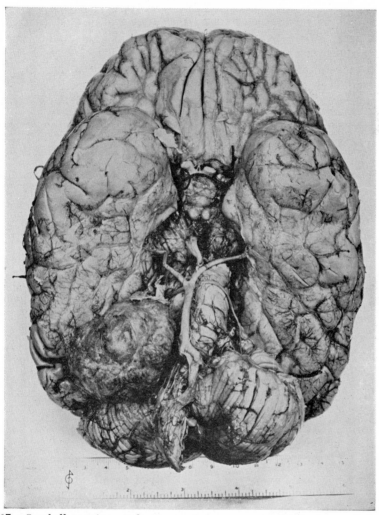

Fig. 167—*Cerebellopontine angle tumor.* A large encapsulated tumor of the right
cerebellopontine angle showing the characteristic compression of the cerebellar
hemisphere, and the compression and distortion of the brain stem.

vascular and contain many thin-walled
vascular channels. Though they grow
within the sella turcica for the most part,
they may in some instances escape into
the base of the skull by rupture through
the diaphragm sellae. They may by

Pituitary adenomas grow slowly, the
duration of symptoms averaging two to
three years before operation. They may,
however, give symptoms over a much
longer period. Their survival after treatment will be considered subsequently in

the discussion of the clinical features of the pituitary adenomas.

4. Acoustic Tumors (Neurinomas)

The acoustic tumors are among the most interesting of all the brain tumors. They are attached to the auditory nerve of one side and, in rare instances, are found bilaterally. They may develop within the auditory canal or they may form on the nerve after emergence from the brain stem. Their growth is slow and symptoms are confined, therefore, to the auditory nerve for some time. As growth proceeds, the tumor compresses the cerebellum and brain stem and produces blockage of the ventricular system by occlusion of the fourth ventricle, resulting in internal hydrocephalus. Compression of adjacent nerves is inevitable in the tumor growth, particularly the facial and trigeminal nerves, but the abducens, vagus, spinal accessory, or hypoglossal nerves may be involved. Erosion of the adjacent skull bones, especially of the petrous portion of the temporal bone,

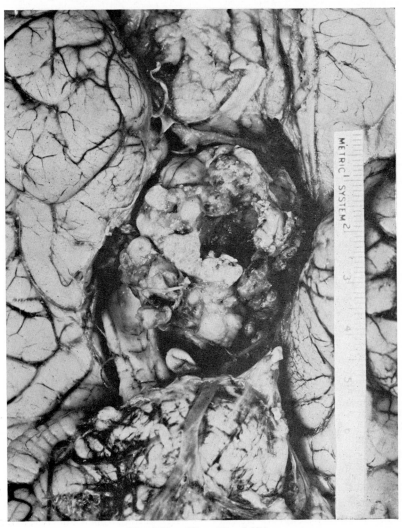

Fig. 168—(See: Fig. 169.)

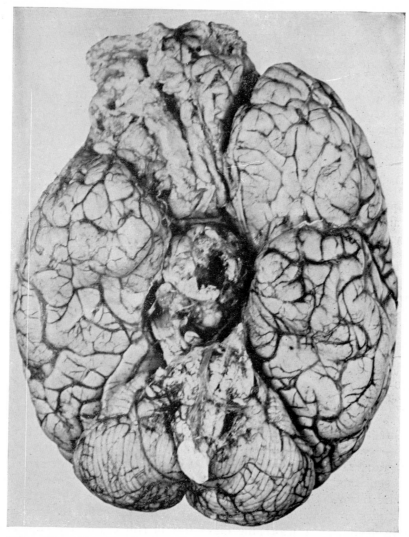

Fig. 169 — *Hypophyseal stalk tumor.* A large hypophyseal stalk tumor (cranio-pharyngioma) lying above the sella turcica and compressing the optic nerves and chiasm. The cystic character is shown through the broken capsule.

is often produced by the tumor. Tumors of the acoustic nerve are slowly growing and symptoms are usually present for several years before relief is sought.

Acoustic tumors are encapsulated and vary in size from 0.5 cm. to 3 or 4 cm. or more in length. They are attached to the auditory nerve and in the course of their development the facial nerve be-comes attached to the tumor, often being stretched over the surface. Tumors of this type are usually adherent to the structures in the cerebellopontine angle. The cut surface of the tumor is, as a rule, white and avascular, with good preservation of the tumor structure. Microscopically the tumor is composed of elongated, spindle-shaped cells with oval nuclei, forming rows and palisades and lying in a dense fibrous structure. Degeneration is found in many parts of the tumor quite often.

The acoustic tumors occupy the angle between the pons and cerebellum, but not all the lesions in the cerebellopontine angle are acoustic neuromas. Other lesions in this area include fibroblastomas, arachnoid cysts, arachnoiditis, and, on rare occasions, aneurysms.

5. Congenital Tumors

Hypophyseal Stalk Tumors: These tumors are known by many terms—craniopharyngioma, Rathke pouch tumors,

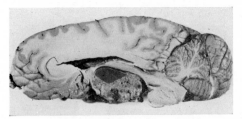

Fig. 170—*Hypophyseal stalk tumor* lying in the suprasellar area. The cystic portion is clearly shown.

bucconeural tumors, and adamantinomas. They are congenital tumors arising from the cell rests derived from the hypophyseal stalk and are, therefore, predominantly tumors of childhood. These cell structures are found on the surface of the hypophysis just under the diaphragm, immediately above it, or at the junction of the infundibulum and the hypothalamus. Most of the hypophyseal stalk tumors develop from cell rests above the sella turcica, but rarely they develop from cells within the sella, so that they may remain confined to the sella turcica throughout their course.

The majority of hypophyseal stalk tumors come to occupy a suprasellar position, compressing the optic nerves and chiasm and adjacent structures. They often attain a large size, growing downward and compressing the hypophysis, spreading upward into the anterior fossa of the skull and compressing the basilar surfaces of the frontal lobes, and expanding laterally to compress the temporal lobes. They may grow so large in rare instances as to compress the vessels of the circle of Willis in their immediate vicinity. They may, on the other hand, remain small (1 to 2 cm.). In rare instances craniopharyngiomas may be found entirely within the sella turcica and may simulate an intrasellar tumor in their clinical features. They are usually adherent to the structures at the base of the brain, sometimes loosely, but often quite firmly. They tend not infrequently to grow upward and to penetrate into the overlying third ventricle. In such instances, internal hydrocephalus develops and with it signs of increased intracranial pressure. Hypophyseal stalk tumors are usually well defined, possessing a capsule which may be thin but is more often thick and noncollapsible. Cysts are almost always present, filled with a greenish yellow fluid resembling motor oil, and containing cholesterol. The proportion of solid tumor and cyst varies. In most instances, solid tumor prevails but large portions are cystic; in others, the entire tumor may be cystic; in still others, the entire tumor is solid, but this type is uncommon. Calcification is found in seventy-five to eighty-five per cent of such tumors in sufficient quantity to cast a shadow in the roentgenogram. The sella turcica is destroyed in varying degree by the expanding tumor mass. The histological structure is composed of a branching epithelial tree with enamel buds in some cases, cysts, calcium, and an enveloping fibrous capsule.

The tumors are slowly growing with a long history of symptoms. They develop in childhood or adolescence in the majority of cases, but not uncommonly produce their first symptoms in adulthood.

Cholesteatomas: These are rare tumors found anywhere within the skull. They may be encountered in the skull are well-defined tumors, discretely separate from the brain substance, possessing a good capsule, and in some instances attached to the overlying meninges. They are composed of concentric layers of glistening, mother-of-pearl tis-

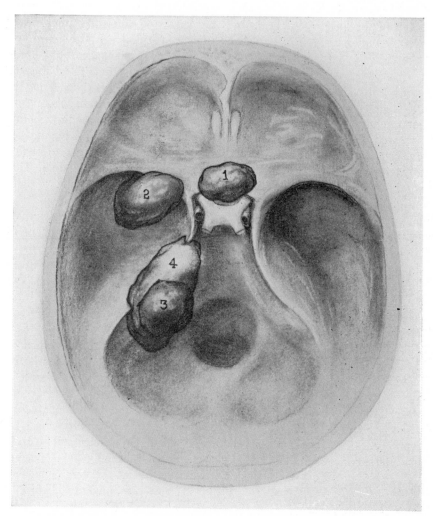

Fig. 171—*Cholesteatoma.* A view of the base of the skull showing the position of cerebral cholesteatomas. (Alpers: Amer. J. Surg. 43:55, Jan. 1939.)

with or without extension into the cranial cavity; in the cerebral hemispheres; in the cerebellopontine angle; in the pineal region, the fourth ventricle, the suprasellar region, and in the parasellar region in relation to the sphenoid bone. They sue arranged in onion peel fashion, and their histological structure reveals a fine capsule and several cell layers of a characteristic variety. Tumors of the cholesteatomatous type give rise to no characteristic clinical features; hence their recognition at present depends entirely on their pathological features.

Chordomas: These are very rare tumors, arising chiefly within the sphenoid and occipital bones, the remnants of the primitive notochord. It usually extends into the ethmoid bone and causes compression of the base of the brain by its growth. It may extend into the nasopharynx and even into the maxillary antrum.

Dermoids and Teratomas: These are rare. Their structure resembles that of similar tumors elsewhere in the body. They are well defined and possess a capsule. They are cystic, and filled with caseous material and hair. The teratomas may contain nerve fibers, brain tissue, sebaceous glands, choroid plexus, muscle, cartilage, bone, and fat. Dermoids and teratomas are found most frequently in the midline in the region of the hypophysis and pineal gland.

6. Metastatic Carcinoma

Carcinoma involving the nervous system occurs with sufficient frequency to require its consideration in many cases of brain tumor. The most fruitful sources of carcinoma to the brain are the bronchi and breast, but other sources include the prostate, kidney, thyroid, sinuses, and nasopharynx, gastrointestinal tract, and generative organs. Among 6761 cases of carcinoma, metastases were found in the

Table 50—Source of Metastatic Carcinoma to Brain
(Unpublished statistics from Mayo Clinic)
(Baker and Kiefer)

Lungs	34%
G-I tract	22%
Breast	11%
Kidneys	10%
Melanoma	8%
Thyroid gland	3%
Prostate gland	2%
Pancreas	1%
Adrenal glands	1%

nervous system in 143 cases, or 2.15 per cent (Neustaedter). Of this material, the chief sources of metastasis to the brain in order of frequency were breast, lung, pharynx and larynx, tongue, uterus, rectum and skin, bladder, hard palate, and antrum. Metastases to the brain may be single or multiple, the metastatic tumors varying in size from 0.5 to 1.0 cm. in diameter to tumors of several centimeters. They are usually well defined and grossly at least sharply separated from the brain substance. They may be found anywhere in the brain tissue, but they tend to involve the cerebral hemispheres and cerebellum much more frequently than the brain stem. They are often present in the brain without involvement of the skull bones. In rare instances, metastatic carcinoma may produce a diffuse brain involvement visible only microscopically, without gross tumor formation (carcinomatous encephalitis), and in rare cases also carcinoma may be found only in the meninges, involving the dura alone or the pia-arachnoid.

The approximate distribution of metastatic brain carcinoma as recorded in a large series of cases (Globus and Meltzer) is as follows: (1) single, massive carcinomatous metastasis, 37.2 per cent; (2) multiple carcinoma, 54.9 per cent; (3) diffuse, microscopic infiltrations, 7.9 per cent. Carcinoma metastasis to the nervous system is usually part of a general dissemination of the carcinoma, but the brain may be involved before other organs become infiltrated. Dissemination to the brain probably occurs chiefly through the blood stream, but spread by the lymph channels, may also occur especially in involvement of the meninges. In carcinoma of the nasopharynx, involvement of the brain develops by direct extension through the base of the skull or through the foramina of exit of the cranial nerves. There is usually a discrete separation between carcinoma and brain substance, the latter showing reactive changes such as gliosis and lymphocytic infiltration in the brain tissue adjacent to the carcinoma. Neurological symptoms are primary in about 25 per cent of patients with nasopharyngeal car-

cinoma. In all instances of unexplained sixth nerve palsy and in unexplained cranial nerve paralysis in general, nasopharyngeal carcinoma must always be suspected.

Metastasis of sarcoma to the nervous system is rare despite its frequency in

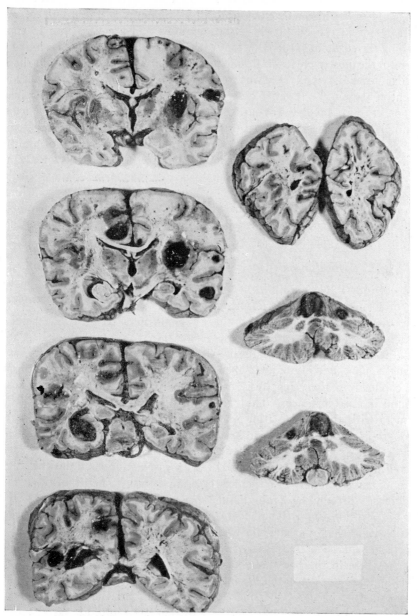

Fig. 172—*Metastatic carcinoma,* showing an example of carcinoma secondary to bronchogenic carcinoma with multiple brain metastases.

the body. Melanosarcoma from the eye or from naevi which have been tampered with spread to the brain, where they are usually disseminated in tumor masses of varying size and number. Primary sarcomas of the brain are extremely rare and are of several microscopic varieties. Primary lymphosarcoma of the brain arises extracranially either in the deep cervical lymph nodes or in the lymphatic tissue surrounding the eustachian tubes. It may extend into the posterior fossa through the basilar foramina with resulting involvement of the ninth to twelfth cranial nerves, or it may involve the middle fossa and produce pareses of the third to seventh nerves. Hypernephroma also is not infrequently associated with brain metastasis. Metastatic seminoma from the testicle to the brain has been reported. Metastasis to the brain has been observed in rare instances in mixed tumor of the parotid gland.

7. Granulomas

Tuberculomas: The brain may be the seat of a solitary tubercle or of many tubercles of varying size. Solitary brain tubercles are found in the cerebral hemispheres, the cerebellum, corpus callosum, basal ganglia, pons, and midbrain. Tuberculoma confined to the hypophysis has been found in rare instances. They are firm tumors with typical caseation seen even on gross section, grossly at least sharply defined from the brain tissue. Microscopically, they have the typical structure of tuberculomas elsewhere in the body, the surrounding brain tissue showing infiltration with lymphocytes and plasma cells chiefly around the vessels. Evidence of tuberculosis is often present elsewhere in the body, but is as often lacking or is not detectable. Tuberculous meningitis is usually found in association with the tubercle at necropsy,

but solitary tubercles may exist for some time without meningitis.

Gummas of the Brain: These tumors are extremely rare. They are found chiefly in the cerebral hemispheres, but gumma of the hypophysis has been the sixth cranial nerves. Gummas of the brain are usually solitary but may be multiple. They are the result of acquired syphilis and are very rare in congenital syphilis. Their structure is similar to that of gummas elsewhere in the body, and they are associated as a rule with positive serological reactions of the spinal fluid.

Rarely, *Schistosoma japonicum* may produce a granuloma involving the brain, giving rise to signs of brain tumor. Patients with this condition have usually been operated on for glioma. The disease is limited to Japan, Formosa, China, and the Celebes, but foreign travelers or soldiers have been afflicted and have developed brain granulomas. Fungi and parasites of many sorts may produce brain granulomas.

8. Blood Vessel Tumors

These may be of two general types (1) *vascular malformations,* and (2) true blood vessel tumors or *hemangioblastomas.* The vascular malformations include: (1) *Venous angiomas,* consisting of a collection of veins varying from a simple varix to numbers of large veins lying like a group of snakes on the surfaces of the cortex and usually associated with vascular anomalies within the cortex itself. Most, if not all, of these angiomas are wedge shaped and extend deeply into the brain. (2) *Arterial angiomas* composed of collections of arteries usually associated with the middle cerebral arteries as well. The malformation often extends deeply into the brain and may penetrate into the ventricle. Angiomas of this type are of the arteriovenous

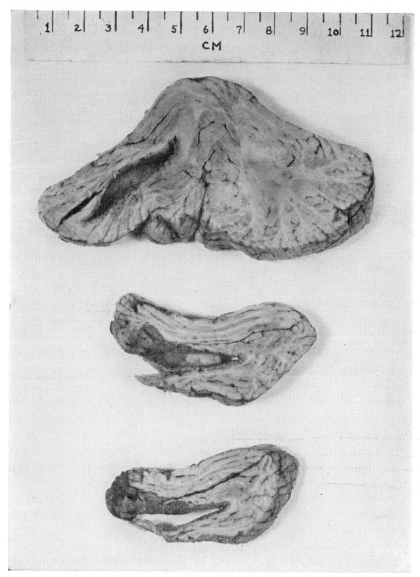

Fig. 173—*Hemangioma* of the cerebellum, showing the cystic portion of the tumor and the solid hemangioma, the darker portion.

variety and give rise to an audible bruit. They assume many forms and have been grouped into several varieties based on gross appearance. Both the venous and arterial angiomas are largely surface lesions and are frequently associated with a history of jacksonian attacks. The venous angiomas are often likely to be associated with a facial naevus in the distribution of the trigeminal nerve.

Hemangioblastomas are well defined and encapsulated tumors found chiefly within the cerebellum. They are usually cystic but they may be predominantly cystic, intermediary or largely solid. The cerebellar hemangioblastomas are sometimes but not always associated with angioma of the retina (von Hippel's disease), and in this combination are known as Lindau's disease. In this form they are usually associated with cysts of other organs—pancreas and kidney and angiomatosis of the liver. A familial incidence of the tumor and of angioma of the retina (von Hippel's disease) is usually found.

9. Miscellaneous Tumors

The brain may be involved by *choroid plexus papillomas,* arising chiefly in the lateral ventricle but from the fourth ventricle at times. These tumors are sometimes cystic but characteristically a cauliflower-like papilloma. They remain confined to the ventricle as a rule but have been known to seed to distant portions. *Cysticercus* and *echnicococcus cysts* are found on rare occasions. *Lipoma* is found rarely. Most cerebral lipomas are found at the base of the brain around the optic chiasm and diencephalon. The next most frequent site is on the corpus callosum. Rare sites include the cerebellopontine angle. They are often associated with developmental defects of the brain or cord such as spina bifida and absence of the corpus callosum. *Colloid cysts* are found in the third ventricle, derived from the paraphysis. *Simple cysts* without tumor tissue in their walls are found at times, particularly in the cerebellum but at times in the cerebrum. Their nature is not clear.

III. GENERAL SYMPTOMS AND DIAGNOSIS OF BRAIN TUMOR

The recognition of a brain tumor may be divided into three phases: the suspicion that a tumor may be present, the establishment of the diagnosis of tumor, and the precise localization of the tumor within the nervous system. The first two phases lie within the province of the general practitioner upon whom rests the responsibility of early recognition of tumor. Indeed, the general practitioner may in many instances be responsible only for the first phase of the problem, the suspicion that a tumor may be present, leaving to the neurologist the problem of determining often whether a tumor is actually present. The last phase of the problem, the localization of the tumor within the brain, is for the neurologist or neurosurgeon to determine. Much will have been accomplished if the practitioner can determine the probability of brain tumor in suspected cases.

History: The history of development of a brain tumor is essential to diagnosis and, if carefully taken, can aid greatly in diagnosis. It is characterized by a *progressive* course, signalized by the spread of symptoms from one part to another over a period of time, or by the intensification of existing symptoms. Thus, a given case may be characterized by headache, followed by visual disturbances and weakness of one side of the body, all indicative of an expanding or progressive process. In other cases, aphasia or hemiparesis may become progressively worse over a period of time.

While a progressive history is in most cases characteristic of an expanding process such as a tumor, it is by no means confined to tumor. Vascular lesions may in some instances develop by progressive stages, with gradual progression of a hemiplegia over a period of days or weeks in the case of gradual occlusion of a vessel. Degenerative processes such as Pick's lobar atrophy may give a progressive history over a long period of time, and arteriosclerotic brain disease may give a history of progressive dementia. Encephalitis may also be characterized by a story of progressive development of symptoms. All these examples serve but as exceptions, however, and tend to emphasize the fact that in the majority of cases a story of progressive brain disease is characteristic of an expanding lesion such as a brain tumor.

The history in brain tumor is in some cases intermittent, a feature which often leads to a false sense of security in diagnosis. Cystic tumors, angiomatous malformations, and sometimes meningiomas are associated with a history of advance and recession of symptoms which may be misleading and may lead to the assumption that a tumor is not present.

The onset of symptoms varies greatly and is dependent to a large extent on the nature of the tumor. Slowly growing tumors, such as the meningiomas and astrocytomas, usually give rise to a long history of symptoms extending over years, whereas tumors such as the medulloblastoma, glioblastoma multiforme, and metastatic carcinoma often develop rapidly and in the case of the glioblastoma multiforme apoplectically. The variability of onset, however, is not entirely dependent on the nature of the tumor, for location may play a significant rôle. A slowly growing tumor located in the proper area (motor cortex, brain stem) may give rise to symptoms early in the course of its development because of interference with vital structures.

Headache is a common symptom of brain tumor, but it is by no means invariably present, a fact which if kept in mind will lead to fewer errors in diagnosis. Cerebellar tumors are usually associated with headache, while in pituitary tumors headache is often lacking. Similarly, a history of headache is wanting in hemispherical tumors of many locations. These will be dealt with in greater detail subsequently.

The headache of brain tumor is likely to be constant and, save in relatively few instances, has no specific characteristics. It is general, constant, and as a rule very little affected by analgesics. It may be paroxysmal and in some instances confined to one side of the head. It is increased as a rule by any factor which increases intracranial pressure, such as coughing, sneezing, or straining. It apparently has little relation to increase of pressure within the skull, since tumors with high pressure may have no headache, while those with normal pressure may have severe headache. It is probably due to stretch on the dura and dural sinuses by the expanding brain.

Vomiting is not an invariable accompaniment of brain tumor and, save in exceptional instances, has little value in itself. It is frequently lacking even in cases with high pressure. It is often, but not always, projectile in nature and usually unassociated with nausea. When it occurs with headache it is merely confirmatory evidence of increased intracranial pressure and has little diagnostic value. At times it may herald the appearance of tumor, as in the case of the morning vomiting sometimes found in midline cerebellar tumors of childhood (medulloblastomas). Generally speaking, it has little specific value in the diagnosis of brain tumor.

Choked disc (papilledema) is an extremely important sign of tumor of the brain. It is, in the great majority of instances, due to brain tumor, but it may be caused by other conditions producing increased pressure within the skull, such as subdural hematoma and brain abscess. It is caused rarely by central nervous system syphilis, tuberculous meningitis, multiple sclerosis, high cervical cord tumors, arachnoiditis, syringomyelia, and fracture of the odontoid process. All these serve but to emphasize the fact that choked disc is caused chiefly by tumor of the brain. It is not always present; indeed, its incidence varies with the location of the tumor. Posterior fossa tumors (cerebellum, fourth ventricle, cerebellopontine angle) are usually associated with choked disc, whereas in pituitary tumors within the sella turcica it is rare. Its occurrence in tumors of other locations varies and will be considered subsequently. Choked disc is usually bilateral, but may be unilateral, varying in degree from one to several diopters of swelling. It is at times more pronounced on one side than on the other, but such inequality in elevation of the disc has no significance in indicating the side on which the tumor is located. Choked disc of one side is at times associated with optic atrophy of the opposite disc (Foster Kennedy syndrome), an association found in tumors of the base of the frontal lobe (olfactory meningiomas, suprasellar or parasellar tumors).

Visual acuity is usually not impaired in choked disc even when it is pronounced unless organization of the edema with subsequent atrophy of the nerve has taken place. Thus choked disc may be present for a long period of time with little or no loss of visual acuity. This retention of visual acuity is a valuable means of distinguishing between choked disc and optic neuritis, a differentiation which is sometimes very difficult.

The mechanism of production of choked disc is not clear. Many theories have been offered. One of the current conceptions is that the swelling is the result of pressure on the central vein of the retina with resulting venous engorgement, impairment of venous drainage, and lymph stasis. Opposed to this is the concept that choked disc results from an interrelationship between diastolic venous and diastolic arterial pressure in the retina. Thus, if retinal arterial tension is low, even a slight increase of venous pressure caused by increased intracranial pressure produces choked disc. If a high retinal arterial pressure prevails, the venous pressure must be proportionately higher to produce choked disc. In addition to these concepts, there are many others which cannot be detailed at this point.

Among other general signs of brain tumor are *bradycardia*, which, however, is not common and often occurs late in the course of the tumor growth. Its incidence has been estimated at three per cent (Rasdolsky). *Mental dullness* is sometimes noted as an accompaniment of increased pressure. *Convulsions* may be the first or an early manifestation of brain tumor. They have been found to be the first manifestation of brain tumor in eighteen per cent of cases. They may be generalized or focal in type and when generalized differ in no way from the generalized convulsions of idiopathic epilepsy. Focal convulsions may be motor or sensory in type or they may be a combination of both. Generalized convulsions have no localizing value save to indicate that the tumor must be cerebral; they never occur with cerebellar tumors. A study of 160 brain tumors with focal epilepsy indicates that this symptom occurs when tumors are close to the motor-sensory area of the cortex (White, Price, and Mixter). Moreover, brain tumor is the most likely diagnosis in the case of a middle-aged patient with focal epilepsy of recent onset, without previous history of trauma or infection. Signs of increased pressure may or may not be found with the convulsive seizures.

By far the most significant general signs of brain tumor are headache, vomiting, and choked disc, and of these headache and choked disc are most important. It is essential to bear in mind, however, that tumors may run their course without either headache or choked disc, and that headache may be encountered without choked disc, or *vice versa*.

Diagnosis: If the history has led one to suspect the presence of a brain tumor, its actual occurrence can be established by significant laboratory studies. These include:

1. *Lumbar Puncture:* If choked disc is found, lumbar puncture is unnecessary, since it is already known that increased intracranial pressure is present. Lumbar puncture is justifiable in the presence of choked disc only if the latter cannot be distinguished from optic neuritis, hypertensive neuroretinitis, or choked disc due to syphilis, in which case the serological reactions are essential.

Routine study (cells, protein, Wassermann reaction, colloidal gold) of the spinal fluid yields little information of importance in brain tumor. The cell count is almost always normal, but an increase of cells is sometimes found in gliomas near the brain surface. Protein increase is common but has no diagnostic significance save in cerebellopontine angle tumors, where it is always elevated. The fluid is at times xanthochromic. Of all the studies of the spinal fluid, the pressure yields the greatest information. It is usually increased, but normal spinal fluid pressures are not uncommon, especially in pituitary adenomas, suprasellar tumors, and gliomas of the brain stem. The spinal fluid pressure may be greatly increased, though no choked disc is present. In the absence of choked disc, lumbar puncture is important for the study of the spinal fluid pressure and routine studies. An increased spinal fluid pressure may be found in the presence of normal appearing discs. Compression of the jugular veins (Queckenstedt test) should never be practiced in a suspected or known instance of brain tumor for fear of causing herniation of the medulla through the foramen magnum.

2. *Roentgenographic Studies of the Skull:* They give valuable information in many instances. The changes to be noted are too numerous for citation. They include signs of increased intracranial pressure (impressiones digitatae, erosion of the dorsum sellae); hyperostosis or erosions; enlargement of the sella turcica, and a variety of other findings. A sign of great importance when it occurs is that of lateral displacement of the pineal gland. This gland becomes calcified quite early in many cases. It occupies a place in the midline and can be seen easily in the roentgenograms. In cerebral hemispherical tumors, especially in those of the temporal area, a calcified gland can be seen displaced beyond the midline by a tumor pressing from the opposite side. Unfortunately, the sign is not present with every tumor, so that the latter often exists without displacement of the pineal gland.

3. *Bárány Examinations:* This examination is valuable under some conditions. It is specific for cerebellopontine angle tumors, the formula of an inactive or dead labyrinth and cochlea on the side of the lesion, with an inactive vertical canal of the opposite side giving invaluable aid in the diagnosis of cerebellopontine angle tumors. Apart from this, it is of help in establishing the presence of posterior fossa tumors by the determination of the absence of shock reactions in a suspected tumor in this area (vomiting, nausea, pallor, sweating). Its usefulness apart from these instances is restricted.

4. *Electroencephalogram Tracings:* These are of great help in the detection and localization of brain tumors. Abnormal brain waves can be detected in the region occupied by the tumor, but only if the tumor is superficially placed and the cortex itself diseased. In such instances, the electroencephalogram is ninety per cent accurate as to the location of a brain tumor. Deep-seated cerebral tumors or cerebellar lesions cannot be detected at present (*v.* Electroencephalogram).

Table 51—Differential Diagnosis of Brain Tumor

Disease	Age	Onset	Signs	Laboratory Studies	Miscellaneous
CEREBRAL ARTERIOSCLEROSIS	55 or over	1. Gradual progression in some cases of cerebral thrombosis, causing progressive hemiplegia, aphasia, etc. 2. Sudden apoplectic in hemorrhage	Hemiplegia, aphasia, hemianopsia, or other signs. No increased pressure as a rule. Choked disc in cases of malignant hypertension. Retinal arteriosclerosis, cardiorenal disease, peripheral arteriosclerosis helpful	None significant	Peripheral and retinal arteriosclerosis tip the balance toward cerebral vascular disease, especially in presence of hypertensional and cardiorenal disease
SUBDURAL HEMATOMA	Adults usually but may occur in infants and children	Gradual, after head injury followed by latency, then by persistent headache. Hemiparesis, aphasia, or convulsions may develop	Choked disc often but not always. Focal signs often absent, but hemiparesis or aphasia may be found. Rarely hemianopsia	Spinal fluid pressure elevated. EEG shows abnormal electrical activity over hematoma. Pneumogram reveals shift of ventricles and distortion of ventricular system	History of head injury important but may at times be lost in the past.
BRAIN ABSCESS	Any age	History of infection in mastoids, sinuses especially. Headache, mental dullness, hemiparesis, convulsions and other symptoms may develop	Choked disc often. Homonymous hemianopsia, aphasia, hemiparesis, mental dullness, bradycardia	Spinal fluid pressure elevated and cellular increase of fluid without organisms. X-ray reveals infection of mastoids or sinuses usually	History of infection and demonstration of focus of infection all important since signs otherwise are those of tumor
ARACHNOIDITIS	Adults	Gradual, with headache	Cerebellar signs usually		No specific features. The diagnosis is established only by operation
METASTATIC CARCINOMA	50 or over usually	Sudden or gradual development of cerebral symptoms — headache, hemiplegia, etc. Usually a history of removal of malignant tumor	Choked disc may be present. Hemiplegia or other focal signs present	X-ray studies reveal carcinoma or metastasis to skull and other parts of skeleton	Diagnosis easy in presence of history of previously removed carcinoma followed by cerebral symptoms but difficult where presence of ca. is not established. It must always be suspected in older subjects with signs of brain tumor; bronchogenic carcinoma particularly

Disease	Age	Onset	Signs	Laboratory Studies	Miscellaneous
TUBERCULOMA	Children or young adults	Gradual, with headache and possibly focal symptoms such as hemiplegia, etc.	Choked disc often. Focal signs as in brain tumor. Meningeal signs at times and in these cases fever. Usually tuberculosis of lungs, mediastinal glands, genitals, kidneys, etc. demonstrable	Tuberculosis often demonstrable by X-ray in lungs, calcified glands, etc. Spinal fluid contains excess of lymphocytes and tubercle bacilli in cases with meningitis	Condition occurs in children and young people, giving rise to signs of brain tumor, with additional findings of tuberculosis in some part of body.
SYPHILITIC MENINGITIS	Adults	Acute usually, with headache, diplopia, deafness and tinnitus, dysphagia or other signs of cranial nerve involvement	Neck stiffness and Kernig's sign. Choked disc may be found. Ocular palsies, facial paralysis, deafness, palatal weakness or other cranial nerve signs	Spinal fluid shows lymphocytosis, positive Wassermann, abnormal colloidal gold curve	Headache is severe. Choked disc may be present. Multiple cranial nerve palsies, signs of meningeal irritation, and positive blood and spinal fluid reactions are important
ENCEPHALITIS	Any age	Acute, with fever, signs of systemic infection, diplopia, somnolence, convulsions in some forms	Fever, ocular palsies, other signs of brain stem involvement		
SUBARACHNOID HEMORRHAGE	Young adults or subjects 55 or over	Acute with headache, loss of consciousness	Neck stiffness and Kernig's sign. Often nothing else. Choked disc rarely	Blood in spinal fluid	Acute onset. Meningeal signs, blood in spinal fluid establish the diagnosis
LEAD POISONING	All ages	Headache, convulsions, incoördination	Hemiparesis, cerebellar incoördination, other focal signs. Choked disc not uncommon	Evidence of lead poisoning in blood smear, urine, feces, blood. Lead line seen by X-ray in children	History of exposure to lead is all important and leads to correct diagnosis. Easily missed where no such history is volunteered
HYPERTENSIVE ENCEPHALOPATHY	Young adults or older subjects	Acute, with headache, vertigo, confusional episodes	Choked disc with neuroretinitis, vascular hypertension		Presence of vascular hypertension in a young adult with neuroretinitis, without cardiorenal disease establishes the diagnosis

5. *Pneumography:* This is necessary in some cases both for diagnosis and localization. The method consists of the injection of air into the subarachnoid space by means of lumbar puncture (encephalogram) or directly into the ventricles by a trephine opening in the skull (ventriculogram), the object being to outline the ventricular system, the subarachnoid channels, and basal cisterns. Encephalography should be performed in patients without increased pressure, while ventriculography is reserved for those with choked disc and increased pressure. The deformities noted consist of a displacement of the midline structures and deformity of the ventricular system in cerebral tumors, and internal hydrocephalus in posterior fossa tumors. Other deformities occur, depending on the location of the tumor (*v.* Encephalography). Normal pneumograms may be found in patients with suspected brain tumor, which is verified later by operation or autopsy.

6. *Angiography:* This test is useful in outlining tumors and demonstrating aneurysms. It is carried out by the injection of a contrast material such as thorium dioxide into the arterial blood stream. The method is useful and has displaced air injection as a means of diagnosis in many clinics.

7. *Radioactive substances:* Radioactive substances (di-iodofluorescein) have been used in the localization of brain tumors, with a reported high incidence of accuracy. The affinity of radioactive dye for tumor tissue appears to be related to the cellularity and vascular pattern of the tumor, and concentration of the dye appears to be greater in the more malignant gliomas. Advocates of the radioactive dye method assert that it is more precise than electroencephalography and pneumography. The method has not been found to be as helpful as first reports seemed to indicate.

Ultrasound transmission has been used in the localization of brain tumors and has been said to "yield ventriculograms without air injection by utilizing a level of intensity below any known threshold of pain or damage" Ballantine *et al.*)

Differential Diagnosis: The diagnosis of brain tumor becomes possible in the presence of a history of a progressive lesion, and tenable when signs of increased pressure are present, such as choked disc, increased spinal fluid pressure, changes in the skull roentgenogram and electroencephalogram. After the presence of tumor has been established, the question of localization must be determined, a problem which will be considered later.

In some instances, brain tumor may be simulated when there is evidence of *increased intracranial pressure,* such as choked disc and increased pressure noted on spinal fluid examination, without the presence of tumor. Such symptoms have been attributed to "serous meningitis." No tumor is found at autopsy. There is often, but not invariably, a history of ear disease in such subjects. Frequently the cause of the increased pressure is not found.

In some instances, *cerebral arteriosclerosis* simulates brain tumor, giving as it does a history of a progressive hemiplegia, intellectual deterioration, or aphasia. The age incidence (fifty or over) falls within the arteriosclerotic age, retinal arteriosclerosis is present, choked disc is absent, and the spinal fluid pressure is normal. Since all these conditions may prevail in some instances of brain tumor, the diagnosis can be established in questionable cases only by pneumogram. In those instances in which retinal and peripheral arteriosclerosis are prominent and evidences of vascular hypertension and cardiorenal disease are found, the probabilities favor cerebral arteriosclerosis with cerebral thrombosis and softening. The occurrence, however, of a gradually progressive cerebral disorder may simulate brain tumor very closely. In other instances, cerebral vascular disease may be confused with tumor because of the sudden apoplectic onset of symptoms which may develop in the course of malignant gliomas, such as the glioblastoma multiforme. The presence of choked disc favors the presence of tumor, while the demonstration of vascular hypertension, cardiorenal disease, and retinal arteriosclerosis is indicative of cerebral vascular disease.

Subdural hematoma resembles brain tumor in many respects. It can be distinguished by a history of head injury either recent or remote, by mental dullness which develops and recedes, and by signs of increased pressure in most instances. The history of a head injury followed by a latent period of relative freedom from symptoms and succeeded in turn by the occurrence of headache is extremely suggestive of subdural hematoma. Mental dullness is common and hemiparesis and convulsions may develop. Signs of increased pressure are usually present. All important is a history of head injury which is usually severe but may be trivial.

Brain abscess gives all the signs of brain tumor, but in addition a very important history of infection usually in the paranasal sinuses or mastoids and a mental torpidity not usually seen in brain tumor. So important is the history and demonstration of infection that the diagnosis without it is that of brain tumor. Differentiation is important because treatment of the two conditions is radically different. Brain abscess develops most frequently in association with mastoid infection and less often after paranasal sinus disease. It is more common with chronic than with acute infections but is by no means unusual under the latter

circumstances. The history is to the effect that a patient with otitis media, mastoid or sinus infection develops after a varying period of time headache followed by or associated with evidences of focal brain damage such as hemianopsia, hemiparesis, aphasia, or other evidences of focal brain disease. Choked disc is often present but not invariably, just as in the case of brain tumor. The pulse may be slow. Mental dullness and fogginess is common and striking. The spinal fluid is under increased pressure and may show an increase of cells without the presence of organisms by smear or culture.

Metastatic carcinoma must be suspected in all patients of fifty or over with signs of increased intracranial pressure. and in those with evidence of multiple brain involvement. The diagnosis is clear in patients with a known history of carcinoma elsewhere in the body; the difficulty arises in those patients with brain tumor in whom carcinoma is not suspected. The incidence of metastasis of carcinoma to the brain is estimated at from eighteen to thirty-one per cent. Since bronchogenic carcinoma is the most common source of metastatic tumor, a roentgenographic study of the chest should be made in suspected cases. Where this is not present, more careful search for carcinoma must be made in other organs, especially the breast and kidney. Carcinoma may metastasize to the brain from any organ in the body, however. The nasopharynx as a source of carcinoma must never be overlooked in suspected cases and must not be excluded if bone destruction in the skull cannot be demonstrated. Of 454 patients with nasopharyngeal carcinoma, ocular symptoms were the first sign in 16 per cent and were present in 38 per cent of all these patients. Trigeminal symptoms with typical trigeminal face pain were found as the first symptom in 71 per cent. Metastasis to the skull is often absent and was found in fifteen of one hundred cases by Hare and Schwartz. The onset of symptoms in carcinoma is usually sudden but may be gradual and may not be associated with emaciation. Metastatic tumor to the brain has been reported fifteen years after resection of a primary breast tumor.

Tuberculoma may simulate brain tumor in every detail. It must always be suspected in persons with evidence of tuberculosis elsewhere in the body (lungs, kidneys, genital organs), but it may be present with minimal indications of tuberculosis, as in tuberculosis of the mediastinal or abdominal glands which cannot be detected clinically. It occurs most frequently in children or young adults.

Gumma is very rare. It is essentially a tumor of syphilitic origin, giving rise to signs of increased pressure like any brain tumor. It is always associated with serological evidence of syphilis in both blood and spinal fluid.

Syphilitic meningitis involving the base of the brain may resemble brain tumor closely, associated as it is with headache, internal hydrocephalus, and sometimes choked disc. The headache may be extremely severe and as intense as that of brain tumor. Neck stiffness and Kernig's sign are usually found. The onset may be acute or gradual. It can be distinguished from tumor by the multiple cranial nerve palsies and by the occurrence of positive serological reactions of the blood and spinal fluid in most but not all cases, together with cell increase in the spinal fluid and other abnormal spinal fluid tests.

Multiple sclerosis, when it is associated rarely with choked disc, simulates brain tumor, but the history of recurrence and remission of symptoms is valuable and in most instances is obtainable by a careful history. When a history of remissions is not obtainable, the diagnosis may be difficult, but it is advisable to recall that the edema of the disc in multiple sclerosis is in essence an optic neuritis and is associated with greatly decreased visual acuity and central or paracentral scotoma, findings not usually present in cases of brain tumor.

Encephalitis may at times resemble brain tumor, but the differentiation is not difficult in most instances in the presence of a history of infection and the acute development of symptoms. This does not imply that the diagnosis of encephalitis is as a rule easy. On the contrary, it may be quite difficult, but in those instances in which the onset is with fever, somnolence, and cranial nerve palsies it is possible to distinguish the presence of encephalitis. In other types which involve the cerebrum more especially there may be convulsions and hemiparesis. Choked disc is rare. The confusion with brain tumor arises not from the occurrence of choked disc in cases of encephalitis but from the occurrence of tumors which invade the brain stem and may therefore resemble cases of encephalitis. Such tumors, usually pontine gliomas or mesencephalic gliomas, develop most commonly in children, without fever, often without headache and with signs of progressive involvement of cranial nerves resulting in ocular palsies, facial paralysis, etc., together with cerebellar incoördination and paralyses of various types, such as paraplegia or hemiplegia. Choked disc is often not found throughout the course of the disease or not until late in the disorder. This type of glioma is often confused with encephalitis, from which it may be distinguished by the absence of fever, the progressive course, and the occurrence of widespread involvement of cranial nerves, pyramidal and cerebellar signs.

In some instances, *arachnoiditis* involving the cisterna magna and the pia arachnoid over the cerebellum resembles brain tumor so closely as to make the diagnosis impossible save at operation. The condition gives rise to evidences of cerebellar tumor. Arachnoiditis is found also involving the optic nerves and chiasm, but since conditions involving this area give rise to very special problems it will be considered under the discussion of pituitary tumors.

Lead poisoning, especially in children, may give rise to symptoms which resemble brain tumor very closely. The confusion is less common in adults. Choked disc, convulsions, and focal signs referable to the cerebrum or cerebellum (ataxia, reeling gait) are often present. The condition appears to be brain tumor unless some factor in the history or examination leads to the suspicion of plumbism (polychromasia, a history of eating paint, or exposure to lead fumes or liquids containing lead, etc.). In children, a lead line can be found in the long bones and the blood and urine show evidence of lead. In adults, lead encephalopathy is capable of causing a progressively developing illness which simulates brain tumor.

Subarachnoid hemorrhage is at times associated with choked disc and therefore simulates tumor in these instances. The history of abrupt onset with severe headache, the signs of meningeal irritation (neck stiffness, Kernig's sign), and the blood in the spinal fluid suffice to establish the diagnosis.

Hypertensive encephalopathy due to essential hypertension, associated with neuroretinitis and evidences of focal brain damage, such as hemiplegia, aphasia, etc., resembles tumor, especially in the presence of a history of headache. The vascular hypertension and the evidence of a neuroretinitis rather than choked disc help in the establishment of the correct diagnosis, together with indications of a vascular accident and of multiple cerebral lesions.

Chronic pulmonary insufficiency, a syndrome consisting of headache, choked disc, impairment of consciousness, confusion, and tremor and twitching of the limbs may be confused with brain tumor. It is associated with pulmonary and cardiac decompensation, the hypoxia and hypercapnia being considered primarily responsible for the neurological symptoms. Polcythemia is sometimes seen. The symptoms improve on restoration of cardiac and pulmonary compensation.

Localization of Brain Tumors: Having established the presence of a tumor of the brain, the problem next becomes one of localization. This is a discipline for the initiated and often taxes the skill of the neurologist and neurosurgeon. Despite wide knowledge, it remains impossible to localize accurately some tumors, so that pneumography is essential in order to establish the diagnosis. In the majority of subjects, however, it is possible to determine the localization of brain tumors on the basis of their clinical features alone. Only a small percentage require either encephalography or ventriculography.

For diagnostic purposes it is useful to describe the symptoms referable to involvement of various parts of the brain, but in the case of infiltrating tumors of the cerebral hemispheres it is essential to recognize that such tumors are usually not confined to a single lobe and that extension into adjacent lobes is common. Remote symptoms are not uncommon even in encapsulated tumors, such as meningiomas, due to impairment of blood supply by pressure on the vessels. The problem in instances of multiple lobe involvement is to determine the site of greatest infiltration, often a difficult problem by pure clinical means and one requiring pneumography for an answer.

Frontal Lobe Tumors: These are difficult to diagnose if by the frontal lobe is understood that part which is anterior to the motor cortex, the so-called prefrontal area. Tumors in this area are characterized mainly by disturbances referable to intellectual and personality functions. This is not to say that the frontal lobes are concerned with or are "the center" of these functions.

Tumors may involve the frontal lobes on their convex surfaces, at the base, or by pressure between the hemispheres. Those of the convex surface are most frequent. Headache is present in seventy-five per cent of cases and choked disc in about eighty per cent. The *onset* of symptoms is usually indefinite and obscure in many instances, and is often so ill-defined as to escape the attention of family and associates. A history of headache is usually obtainable and may have been present for a long period of time before relief is sought. Failing vision or blurring of vision may accompany the headache. Chief among the symptoms of frontal lobe tumor are those referable to intellectual, emotional, and personality factors. These are at times present in severe degree, in others in moderate or mild form, and in still others absent altogether. It is clear, furthermore, that while disturbances in these spheres are found chiefly with frontal lobe tumors, they may be found also with tumors in other locations, such as temporal lobe, third ventricle, hypothalamic, and hemispherical tumors elsewhere. Hence they cannot be regarded as pathognomonic of frontal lobe tumors. The symptoms are those of an organic syndrome, and in this respect differ little from other conditions associated with organic disease of the frontal lobes, such as general paresis, cerebral arteriosclerosis, and presenile and senile dementia.

In a well-pronounced instance, *memory loss* is a striking and often the earliest complaint. It concerns chiefly a loss or impairment of memory for recent events. Difficulty in concentration and in fixation of attention are also striking and accompany the memory loss. Disturbances in mathematical ability and impairment of judgment are found in well-marked cases; hence a history of poor business judgment and of unwarranted mistakes in commercial, social, and financial matters is common. These may assume many forms. Disturbances in abstract thinking and in synthesis of propositions is found in frontal lobe tumors. *Personality changes* are often noted, their striking feature consisting of a definite deviation of personality traits from those associated with the normal make-up of the patient. Irritability, irascibility, labile emotional states, indifference, euphoria, and facetiousness may become manifest. A devoted parent may become harsh and irritable with his family; a conscientious worker may care little what becomes of his business or family; a circumspect citizen may be guilty of philandering or pilfering; and a previously stable personality may develop swings of mood or facetiousness under the most trivial of provocations and in the strangest of circumstances. The number of examples may be multiplied indefinitely. The patient himself, having lost much of his sense of propriety and having developed blunting of his judgment, is little aware of his antisocial tendencies. Suspiciousness is common. Psychotic symptoms such as disorientation, delusions, and even hallucinations may be found.

Loss of power of one side of the body, progressive in nature, is an outstanding finding in tumors extending into the motor area. In some cases, difficulty in finding words is the outstanding complaint. Incontinence occasionally develops and rarely a history of excessive appetite is obtained. Often only signs of increased pressure (headache and choked disc) are present and symptoms of personality and intellectual deterioration are elicited only on direct questioning. Lapses of memory, difficulty in concentration, disturbances in mood, irritability, and personality deviations are found on examination and confirm the impressions gained from the history. These are likely to be more pronounced in bilateral involvement of the frontal lobes and with implication of the corpus callosum. Psychoses are sometimes encountered in frontal lobe tumors, characterized by confusional episodes and often delusional formations. The type of personality deviation varies greatly from case to case and resembles closely those found in general paresis — impairment of judgment, impairment of social finesse, financial peculations, and a wide variety of changes.

If the tumor involves the posterior part of the frontal lobe, particularly the posterior portion of the third frontal convolution, *aphasia* results from involvement of the left frontal lobe in right-handed persons and of the right frontal lobe in left-handed patients. The aphasia is expressive or motor in type and is characterized by complete inability to use words in advanced cases and in less severe cases by a loss or misuse of words, a tendency to substitution of letters or words, and of hesitation in the finding of words.

Involvement of the *motor cortex* by tumor results in the production of convulsions, usually motor jacksonian attacks, but at times generalized attacks. Hemiparesis, facial weakness of a central type, or monoplegia or monoparesis involving a single limb may be found. The jacksonian convulsions occurring with involvement of the motor cortex begin as a rule at a focal point, usually the face, hand (thumb), or foot, and spread from these focal parts to involve other parts of the body on the same side. They may at times be confined, however, to a single portion, such as the thumb or hand, without spread of the convulsive attack. They may or may not be associated with unconsciousness. The weakness found in motor cortex tumors may affect the entire side of the body or it may be confined to a single limb or to the face. The weakness is usually associated with spasticity of varying degree but may in some instances be flaccid.

Among other manifestations of frontal lobe involvement are symptoms which occur infrequently either alone or in conjunction with other frontal lobe signs. *Incontinence,* due to a hypertonic bladder, is encountered in a small number of instances and may be a striking and most distressing symptom. *Forced grasping occurs* in patients with involvement of the premotor area. *Tremor* often resembling that encountered in paralysis agitans is occasionally seen. Similar tremors are encountered in tumors of the temporal lobe. They are found not infrequently on the same side as the tumor. The tremor has no pathognomonic characteristics; it is often fine but may be coarse and may be static or volitional. *Ataxia* resembling closely that of cerebellar disease may develop and is more common and more pronounced in cases of bilateral frontal lobe disease. Abnormal appetite is encountered rarely.

In cases involving the basal portions of the frontal lobe, *anosmia* is found and with it optic atrophy, choked disc, or the syndrome of optic atrophy of one eye and choked disc of the other. Tumors such as meningiomas growing between the frontal lobes may give rise only to signs of pressure, or if they abut on the motor cortex, to evidences of leg or foot weakness with or without focal convulsions involving the leg or foot.

The *diagnosis of frontal lobe tumor* is difficult indeed in those instances which involve the frontal lobes in front of the motor cortex. In those patients in whom marked signs of intellectual and personality changes are found in association with signs of increased intracranial pressure, a presumptive diagnosis of frontal lobe tumor is possible, but is not conclusive. If in such instances a history of jacksonian fits is obtained, or if hemiparesis, monoplegia, or aphasia is demonstrable, frontal lobe tumor may be diagnosed with certainty. Under other circumstances, only signs of increased pressure are usually present, the indications of intellectual and personality deviations being slight. Recourse must frequently be had therefore to pneumography in order to localize the tumor. The detection of anosmia and optic atrophy will suffice as a rule to indicate involvement of the olfactory groove region.

Corpus Callosum Tumors: These are difficult to diagnose and the probabilities are that they have no distinctive clinical features. The greatest of difficulty is encountered in the separation of callosal and frontal lobe symptoms, since pure callosal tumors are rare. They are found usually in conjunction with frontal lobe tumors. *Mental disturbances* similar to those of frontal lobe tumor are common and consist of memory disturbances, difficulty in concentration, and other disturbances of intellectual function. Personality changes occur but they are probably due to frontal lobe involvement. Psychoses are common. A type of mental reaction is encountered in callosal tumors, but it is seen also in bilateral frontal lobe tumors. It consists of negativism, with a tendency to disregard requests or commands and an incapacity to respond by virtue of an inability to synthesize thoughts. Apraxia of the left hand is found in tumors involving the anterior portion of the corpus callosum. Xanthochromia, pleocytosis of the spinal fluid, and hyperthermia have been described as characteristic of a callosal syndrome. In our present state of knowledge, it seems safe to assert that no characteristic callosal syndrome is known, and that the mental symptoms encountered differ from those of the frontal lobe only in degree. Where unusually severe frontal lobe symptoms are encountered, callosal involvement may therefore be postulated.

Temporal Lobe Tumors: These evoke characteristic pictures, as a rule, if they are in the dominant left lobe; those of the right temporal area are often silent. The *onset* is characterized by a history of headache and blurred vision due to choked disc in most instances, but either or both symptoms may be lacking in twenty to twenty-five per cent of cases (Frazier). Generalized and sometimes focal convulsions are an early symptom at times, and aphasia or hemiparesis may be noted as progressive symptoms in a small number of instances. For reasons which are not clear, some cases of temporal lobe tumor may develop with a history of petit mal attacks, simulating in every respect the petit mal episodes of epilepsy. They may persist for some time before evidences of increased pressure develop. Dreamy states develop in rare instances, associated often with smacking movements of the lips. The majority of cases develop with a history of headache, blurred vision, and convulsions, with a history of one-sided weakness and aphasia developing in some instances.

Choked disc is common and occurs in about eighty per cent of the subjects.

Homonymous hemianopsia is an important finding due to interruption of the visual fibers deep in the temporal lobe. It may in early cases be a quadrantanopsia. Due to the crowding of the visual fibers in the temporal lobe, the hemianopic field cut is often through the fixation point.

Auditory-receptive, or *sensory aphasia* is an important finding in left temporal lobe tumors in right-handed persons and in the right temporal lobe in left-handed persons. Aphasia of this type is characterized by a loss or impairment of understanding of spoken words, the misuse of words without awareness of such misuse, the transposition of words, phrases, or clauses, in some instances the production of a jargon, and usually some impairment of expressive or motor speech.

Hemiparesis or *monoparesis* develops not uncommonly from invasion of the adjacent corticospinal tract.

Visual hallucinations are found in rare instances, usually in the hemianopic field. They may be formed or unformed, consisting of flashes of light, ill-defined and unidentifiable forms.

Uncinate fits characterized by unpleasant tastes and/or smells are encountered in tumors which invade the uncus region on the medial aspect of the temporal lobe. Due to herniation of the temporal lobe through the incisura of the tentorium, pressure is sometimes made on the cranial nerve and brain stem structures in some cases of temporal lobe tumor, usually those associated with a high degree of increased pressure. There results, therefore, in some patients, absence of the corneal reflex, oculomotor paralysis with ptosis of the eyelid and impairment of ocular movement, or pupillary disturbances, characterized as a rule by a dilated pupil reacting poorly or not at all to light, accommodation, and consensual responses. Tumors, usually meningiomas, lying on the greater wing of the sphenoid bone and compressing the undersurface of the temporal lobe give rise to no distinctive symptoms, hence they grow often to large size, producing only signs of increased intracranial pressure, sometimes generalized convulsions, and in some instances a unilateral nonpulsating exophthalmos.

The *diagnosis of temporal lobe tumor* is not difficult in cases characterized by auditory-receptive aphasia and homonymous hemianopsia. The localization in such instances is clear. Cases are not uncommon involving either the left or right temporal lobes with signs only of increased pressure and homonymous hemianopsia. Their distinction from occipital lobe tumors is impossible by ordinary clinical means and requires pneumography for precise localization. This is a particularly frequent occurrence in right temporal lobe tumors. Uncinate fits indicate involvement of the mesial aspect of the temporal lobe, but such fits have been described in large pituitary adenomas which have extended into the base of the skull and caused compression of the uncus and in parasellar tumors as well. The assertion that homonymous hemianopsia in temporal lobe tumors is more likely to extend through the fixation point is true only with many exceptions, since large occipital lobe tumors may produce the same defect. Similarly, the assertion that visual hallucinations are likely to be unformed in temporal lobe and formed in occipital lobe tumors has not be substantiated by extensive clinical studies.

Parietal Lobe Tumors: These give distinctive pictures as a rule, but large parts of the parietal lobe may be affected without giving indication of their involvement by tumor. The *onset* is characterized by a history of headache in many instances. Particularly characteristic are the sensory jacksonian convulsions which develop in some cases, characterized by a progressive march of sensory phenomena (numbness, prickling, etc.) from one part to another, confined as a rule to one-half or part of one-half of the body. Weakness of one side of the body may be noted and in intelligent patients a history of loss of recognition of objects in one hand. Not infrequently one finds a history of loss of recognition of the position of one leg in walking. A history of motor jacksonian convulsions is not uncommon. Pains involving the arm or leg or both is a rare complaint but is encountered at times in the life history of meningiomas.

Cortical *sensory disturbances* are encountered if the sensory cortex is affected as it is in the majority of subjects. They are characterized by loss of position sense and intact or lost vibration sense in the opposite limbs with little or no impairment of pain, heat, and cold sensations. Two-point discrimination, the recognition of differences in textures and weights, spot localization, and the recognition of numbers written on the skin are impaired or lost. Ataxia often develops as a result of the deep sensory disturbances encountered in parietal lobe tumors. *Astereognosis* is a sign of great value, but it is not present in every case. It is characterized by the loss or impairment of recognition of the shape and texture of objects in the hand opposite the side of the lesion. *Hemiparesis* or even hemiplegia may be found if the tumor impinges on the motor cortex, as it usually does. *Apraxia* is sometimes seen and at times *visual-receptive aphasia* characterized by an inability to understand written words or sentences and manifested by disturbances in reading ability.

The *diagnosis of parietal lobe tumors* is easy in patients with a fully developed syndrome of sensory jacksonian convulsions, cortical sensory disturbances, and astereognosis. In the absence of sensory fits, the diagnosis is tenable in patients with evidences of increased pressure and cortical sensory difficulties. In some subjects, large tumors may cause no objective findings of any significance and the diagnosis must be established by pneumography.

Occipital Lobe Tumors: These are not as common as those in the anterior portions of the brain. They have no distinctive *history,* as a rule, because of the fact that apart from vision, no vital functions are localized in the occipital lobe. Unless loss of vision is rapid or abrupt, there is no history of visual impairment. Rarely, motor jacksonian convulsions may develop (Frazier and Alpers). Signs of increased pressure in the form of *choked disc* are usually present and with these a *homonymous hemianopsia.* Since the latter has no distinctive features to differentiate it from a hemianopsia in the temporal lobe, the diagnosis of occipital lobe tumor must be made by pneumography unless visual-receptive aphasia is found, thus indicating a lesion at the junction of the parietal and occipital lobes.

Tumors of the Cerebellum: These are more common in children than in adults but they occur at all ages. Cerebellar tumors are practically all infiltrating; encapsulated tumors are rare.

The cerebellar tumors of childhood are chiefly medulloblastomas, with astrocytomas and ependymomas occurring with much less frequency. The *history* of onset is similar for all the tumor types, the rate of development of symptoms varying with the tumor type. The medulloblastomas develop and run their course rapidly, the astrocytomas and the ependymomas slowly. Since all these tumor types occlude the fourth ventricle because of their midline position, they first cause internal hydrocephalus and symptoms referable to increased pressure early in their course. The history concerns children between five and ten years of age as a rule. Vomiting is an early symptom, especially morning vomiting, and is particularly frequent in the medulloblastomas. It is persistent and unresponsive to ordinary dietary measures. It is often treated for some time as an ordinary gastric upset or may even be attributed to emotional factors. Headache is common, but because of the tender age of the patient is not as frequently complained of as it might otherwise be. The same is true of blurred vision, which is also common. Vomiting and headache may be the only symptoms for some time and their true significance may escape detection. As the tumor develops further, the symptoms of increased pressure are augmented by those referable to cerebellar dysfunction. Hence parents observe or there is complaint of staggering gait, difficulty in maintaining balance, and often of clumsiness of the arms or hand, noted in bringing objects to the mouth or face. By the time such symptoms develop, the tumor is well advanced. There may be a history of remission of symptoms in the case of the astrocytomas and a history of neck pain in ependymomas.

The description by Cushing of a composite history of medulloblastoma gives both a clear and concise concept of the development of symptoms. He states. "A preadolescent child previously in good health begins to complain of headache or of suboccipital discomfort and to have occasional attacks of vomiting without preliminary nausea, usually on first arising in the morning. Attendance at school meanwhile may continue but the teacher soon notices that the child is listless or inattentive and the character of its work noticeably falls off. Ere long it is apparent that there is some unwonted clumsiness of movement and awkwardness in gait. The mother may find that the child quickly outgrows its caps and she thinks the head enlarges unduly fast. In course of time, it is noticed, at home or at school, that the child's sight is impaired; or a beginning squint of one eye may be detected, even in the absence of any complaint of double vision. The family doctor, who has previously suspected some gastrointestinal disorder, may then have the eye-grounds examined and to the surprise of everyone a choked disc is found. Three or four months on the average have elapsed, and at about this stage of the malady many cases first come under hospital care."

The *head posture* is important in some cases of cerebellar tumor, though variations of head posture are by no means constant. Anterior flexion of the head is most common, the head being bent forward slightly, splinted by the contracted neck muscles, and moved in one piece with the trunk. Free movement of the head is lost. Lateral flexion is sometimes seen, resembling torticollis. In some instances, *Bruns' sign* is present. This consists of severe vertigo, nausea, and vomiting on active movement of the head, usually extension, but produced by any head movement.

Choked disc is practically always present in patients with medulloblastoma, but is not uncommon in patients with other types of cerebellar tumor with no papilledema and at times with a normal spinal fluid pressure. In a series of 159 cerebellar tumors in persons of all ages, choked disc was found in 126 (Grant and Weinberger). Signs of cerebellar dysfunction are predominant and are much more pronounced in the trunk than in the limbs, though involvement of the latter is not uncommon. The *gait* is staggering and typically cerebellar, with a wide base, the pelvis tilted forward and held stiffly, and the legs thrust forward in one piece, moving seemingly independent of the pelvis. The station is unsteady with Romberg's sign present. Standing on either foot or walking heel to toe is impossible. In advanced cases, standing and walking is altogether impossible. If the tumor is extensive *dysmetria* of the arms and legs is noted on bringing the finger to the nose or the heel to the knee. The tendon reflexes are decreased or absent, but abnormal reflexes, such as the Babinski sign, are not present. Internal strabismus is common.

The cerebellar tumors of adults may involve the midline structure or one or both of the cerebellar hemispheres. They are more commonly astrocytomas; hence they usually have a prolonged *history*. Headache and blurred vision are common complaints. Staggering and clumsiness in the use of the limbs are further complaints. Vertigo may be encountered and is likely to be more or less constant. Diplopia is found in some cases.

Choked disc is usually present. The signs of a midline tumor are similar to those described above. Tumors involving the cerebellar hemisphere are characterized by unilateral cerebellar signs. These are featured by dysmetria on finger-nose, finger-finger, and heel-knee test in the limbs on the side of the tumor. *Dyssynergia* is present on pronation-supination and patting tests. *Tremor* is often prominent, characterized by a coarse involuntary tremor which usually is absent on rest and becomes pronounced on movement (intentional tremor). Horizontal *nystagmus* is found but is by no means constant. Vertical nystagmus is occasionally found. Nystagmus is not a necessary accompaniment of a cerebellar tumor. The probabilities are that in pure cerebellar tumors, nystagmus is not present; it appears in cases with pressure on the brain stem. *Tonic fits* are rare and *skew deviation* of the eyes equally rare. *Cranial nerve* signs are not found in pure cerebellar tumors, but bilateral external rectus paralysis is sometimes found as an evidence of increased pressure late in the course of the tumor. Oculomotor paralysis may develop. Peripheral facial paralysis and absence of the corneal reflex are sometimes encountered. Rarely a cerebellar tumor may protrude into the cerebellopontine angle, causing tinnitus and loss of hearing. Visual field defects are encountered in rare cases due to the pressure of the distended third ventricle on the optic nerves and chiasm.

The diagnosis of cerebellar tumor is usually quite evident but in some cases offers real difficulties. The history is that of headache and clumsiness of limb or gait, with vertigo an occasional symptom. Signs of increased pressure are usually but not always present. In midline tumors, the cerebellar dysfunction is chiefly truncal, whereas in hemisphere tumors unilateral limb dysfunction is outstanding. In some instances, despite extensive involvement of the cerebellum, no signs referable to this organ are elicited. In such cases only pneumography can establish the proper localization. Ventriculography will disclose internal hydrocephalus with failure of visualization of the fourth ventricle.

Fourth ventricle tumors are difficult to establish in and of themselves. Their story is that of headache and vertigo, often with Bruns' symptom. Signs of increased pressure are present; beyond this there may be nothing else, and the diagnosis may be established only by pneumography.

Acoustic (Cerebellopontine Angle) Tumors: Of all brain tumors, these give a characteristic story. The typical acoustic nerve syndrome is produced by acous- and very rarely by meningeal hemorrhage involving the angle. Tumors involving the eighth nerve give a *history* extending over several years. Tinnitus is the earliest

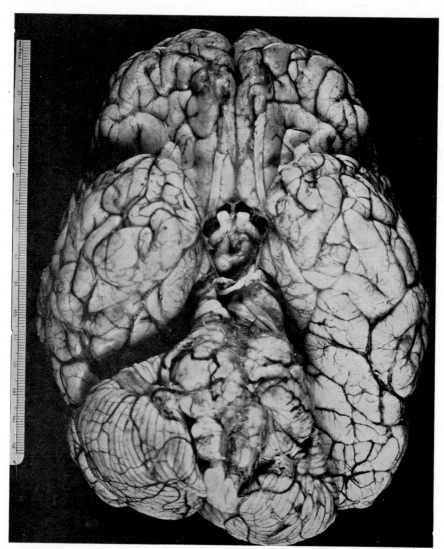

Fig. 174—*Pontile glioma.* A large infiltrating tumor of the pons and medulla, causing marked enlargement and distortion of the invaded structures. The clinical picture was that of a progressive brain stem disorder without evidences of increased pressure.

tic neuromas arising from the sheath of the acoustic nerve. The syndrome may also be caused by fibroblastomas in the cerebellopontine angle, by arachnoiditis, arachnoidal cysts, rarely by aneurysm, symptom and persists for years. Deafness follows within a varying period of time, sometimes concomitant with the onset of tinnitus; in other instances, years later. There may be no awareness of deafness in some cases, and in rare cases no deafness is present. Headache is as a rule a later symptom, but may appear early. Pain or paresthesias of the face may develop in some instances. After a varying period of time there develops a complaint of staggering gait due to compression of the cerebellum. Peripheral facial paralysis or external rectus paralysis may be noted during the course of the tumor history. Vertigo is not common in acoustic tumors, but constant or episodic vertigo may be encountered. In rare instances, face pain resembling trigeminal neuralgia occurs and in still rarer cases glossopharyngeal pain is encountered.

As in cerebellar tumors, *head posturing* is sometimes present, usually a lateral deviation but in some cases anterior flexion. *Choked disc* is usually present but cases may run their course without evidence of papilledema. An absence of the *corneal reflex* is found early in many cases. Nerve *deafness* can be demonstrated by routine and special examination. In rare instances, no evidence of nerve deafness can be demonstrated despite the intimate association of the tumor with the acoustic nerve. *Cerebellar signs* are usually prominent and are found in the ipsilateral limbs. They are featured by dyssynergia of the arm and leg, dysmetria, tremor, and the other features characteristic of cerebellar disease. *Facial* paralysis of a peripheral type is sometimes found, but is not as common as might be expected in view of the intimate relation of the tumor to the structures in the cerebellopontine angle. External rectus paralysis is an uncommon sign. Of the various laboratory tests available for diagnosis, the *Bárány test* is invaluable. This demonstrates a complete absence of responses from the cochlear and vestibular divisions of the affected auditory nerve, with absence of responses from the vertical

canal of the opposite side. An increase of the total protein in the spinal fluid is almost constant and is a valuable aid in diagnosis.

The *diagnosis* is easy in a typical instance. The history of long-standing tinnitus, deafness, headache, and finally cerebellar symptoms forms the background of a typical case, to which may be added other less usual symptoms. Supporting such a story are choked disc, an absent corneal reflex, ipsilateral cerebellar signs, typical Bárány findings, and an increase of spinal fluid proteins. Early diagnosis is important before the tumor becomes too large to remove safely. For this reason any patient with what appears to be a typical history, with an absent corneal reflex and nerve deafness, should undergo a Bárány test. It must be recalled also that rare cases may appear for years as Ménière's syndrome or may reveal no signs of nerve deafness. Atypical pictures are sometimes encountered in angle tumors. The variants include (1) normal cochlear function, or only slightly impaired function with a dead labyrinth; and (2) only decreased labyrinthine responses with loss of cochlear function.

Tumors of the globus jugulare give rise to symptoms of deafness and tinnitus and often involve other cranial nerves. They must be considered in suspected angle tumor with atypical clinical features. Aural discharge and a tumor mass in the ear are distinguishing features.

Brain Stem Tumors: They may involve any part of the base of the brain. They are infiltrating in the vast majority of cases, but in rare instances metastatic carcinoma may compress the brain stem from without. Most brain stem tumors are pontine in location, extending anteriorly into the mesencephalon or diencephalon and posteriorly into the medulla. They are usually gliomas, chiefly astrocytomas, but at times oligodendrogliomas or glioblastoma multiforme.

1. PONTINE TUMORS: These occur chiefly in children. Despite their close proximity to the ventricular system, symptoms of increased pressure are often absent. The *history* is concerned more often with an early appearance of diplopia, at times with facial numbness, and not infrequently with weakness, clumsiness in movement, or staggering gait. Headache when present is usually overshadowed by other symptoms. The durations of symptoms varies and may range from four or five weeks to several months. Generally speaking, they are of short duration before relief is sought. In many instances, *diplopia* is the initial symptom, usually associated with headache. Disturbance in gait or clumsiness in the use of the hands is noted early, but as a rule tend to follow diplopia. Weakness of the limbs is almost always found in the course of the disorder, but tends to appear late as a rule. Rarely, the first symptom may be found to be paralysis of the face or numbness involving one side of the face. Once symptoms appear, they progress steadily without letup.

The signs elicited in a typical case consist of a combination of cranial nerve, corticospinal, and cerebellar disturbances. These are found in varying combinations, but some degree of involvement of all the systems mentioned is found in every case. In some instances, cerebellar signs predominate over pyramidal; in others, the reverse is present, and in all, cranial nerve palsies are found invariably. Strangely enough, the cranial nerve paralyses are usually unilateral. *Abducens paralysis* is common. It is usually unilateral but may at times be bilateral. Absence of *corneal reflex*, impairment or loss of motor function of

the *trigeminal nerve*, and *facial paralysis* are found. The trigeminal nerve involvement is usually of a sensory type, with decrease or loss of sensation over one side of the face. Involvement of the motor division of the trigeminal nucleus is not as common, but when present re-

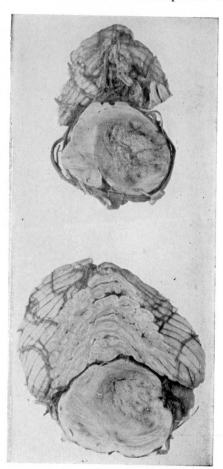

Fig. 175 — *Brain tumor.* An infiltrating tumor of the pons and midbrain implicating one-half of the brain stem structures. The subject was a child of 8 years with a history resembling encephalitis.

sults in deviation of the jaw to the paralyzed side. The facial paralysis is of a peripheral type, but some segments of the face may be more severely involved than others. At times *hypoglossal* paralysis is found if the tumor extends into the medulla. *Oculomotor* paralysis may develop if the tumor extends into the mesencephalon.

Tinnitus and *deafness* may develop in some cases and may give rise to

both sides are always present. *Sensory disturbances* are frequently lacking, but decrease or loss of pain and temperature over the opposite side of the body from spinothalamic tract invasion is sometimes

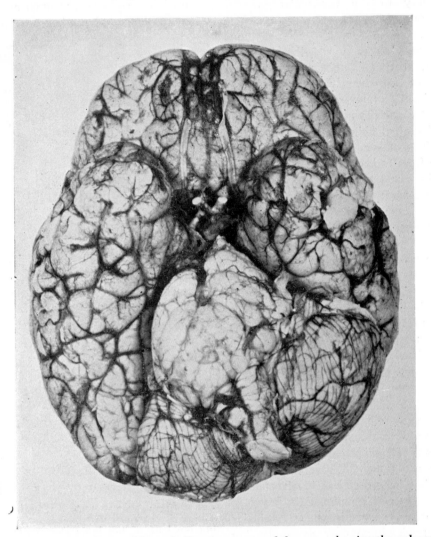

Fig. 176—Pontile glioma. A large infiltrating tumor of the pons, showing the enlargement of this structure and the verrucose appearance of the surface.

a history resembling cerebellopontine angle tumors very closely. *Pyramidal tract* disturbances are always found, and may be manifested as hemiplegia, hemiparesis, paraplegia, or quadriplegia. *Cerebellar disturbances* involving one or

found. Signs of increased pressure are frequently lacking and choked disc is as often absent as present. Increased spinal fluid pressure may be found without choked disc, or there may be no elevation of the discs. In some cases, signs of increased pressure develop only late in the disease.

The *diagnosis* is not difficult in typical cases and particularly in patients with choked disc. The progressive history and the evidence of a multiplicity of symptoms and signs (cranial nerve, pyramidal, cerebellar), all of them satisfactorily explained by a lesion confined to the pons or its environs, suffice to establish the diagnosis. Confusion arises in those patients in whom no choked disc is present, and the spinal fluid pressure normal. Such instances are likely to be confused with encephalitis, multiple sclerosis, or disseminated encephalomyelitis. From these it can be separated by the absence of fever and by the steadily progressive course. The usual patient with encephalitis will fail to show more than cranial nerve signs, the pyramidal and cerebellar disturbances being absent or minimal. Multiple sclerosis occurs in older subjects and will give a history of previous disturbances with remissions. In some instances, the course of a pontile glioma may resemble a cerebellopontine angle tumor so closely as to make clinical differentiation impossible. The Barany test in the case of a pontile glioma is not of the typical cerebellopontine variety.

2. MESENCEPHALIC TUMORS: They are rare and usually form a part of a pontine tumor. They are characterized by the progressive development of oculomotor paralysis, weakness, and cerebellar disturbances, as in the case of pontine tumors. Signs of increased pressure may be lacking. Argyll Robertson pupils may be found. Weber's or Benedict's syndrome or the syndrome of the superior cerebellar artery may be found in the mesencephalic tumors.

Third Ventricle Tumors: These fail in most instances to give characteristic symptoms. Clear distinction must be made between tumors confined to the third ventricle and those which invade the walls of the third ventricle and jut out into its cavity. The latter must be regarded as diencephalic tumors which occlude the third ventricle. The primary tumors consist of colloid cysts or solid tumors, attached to the roof of the third ventricle, the former derived from the paraphysis.

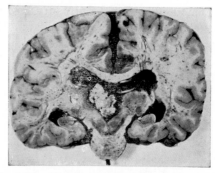

Fig. 177—*Third ventricle tumor* in which the only symptoms were headache and choked disc, with no localizing features.

The *history* is characteristic if present in typical form. It is featured by attacks of *intermittent headache* and visual disturbances, appearing with change of posture of the head, due to the occlusion of the third ventricle and the adjacent foramens of Monro by the ball-valve action of the tumor. Beyond this, there is little of value in the history. Most cases reveal only *choked disc* with no evidences of a focal lesion. Hypersomnolence, personality changes, disturbances in temperature, diabetes insipidus, periods of manic excitement and depression have been described as further symptoms, but these are found only in tumors invading the neighborhood of the third ventricle, particularly the hypothalamus. The diagnosis of primary third ventricle tumor is not tenable at present on purely clinical grounds and can be established only by pneumography. It should be suspected in all cases of brain tumor without evidences of localization.

Lateral ventricle tumors are rare. They may be primary fibroblastomas, cholesteatoma, or extensions of infiltrating gliomas. They give rise to no characteristic symptoms or signs, are associated usually with high pressure and are diagnosable only by air studies as a rule.

IV. TUMORS OF THE PITUITARY AND PITUITARY REGION

Tumors involving the pituitary region are of three types: (1) intrasellar; (2) suprasellar, and (3) parasellar.

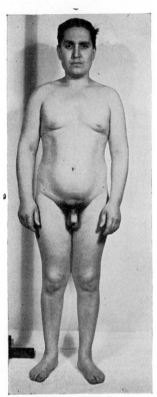

Fig. 178—*Pituitary adenoma,* showing the typical features of a hypopituitary syndrome—smooth skin, absence of facial hair, female habitus.

Intrasellar (*Primary Pituitary*) Tumors: These are of three types: (1) adenomas; (2) hypophyseal stalk tumors; (3) Rathke cleft cysts. Of these, the adenomas are by far the most numerous (ninety-nine per cent), the intrasellar

stalk tumors, and Rathke cleft cysts being very rare. The adenomas are of three types: (1) chromophobe; (2) eosinophilic; (3) basophilic; the tumor types arising from corresponding cell groups within the anterior lobe of the hypophysis. The chromophobe adenoma is associated with a hypopituitary habitus; the eosinophilic adenoma with acromegaly; the basophilic adenoma with basophilism or Cushing's syndrome. The cyst of Rathke's cleft, a rare tumor, arises from the remnants of Rathke's pouch. Hypophyseal stalk tumors are predominantly suprasellar in location but may arise within and be confined to the sella turcica. Since the adenomas are by far the most numerous of the pituitary tumors, their symptomatology will be considered as characteristic of the primary pituitary group. Of 1001 verified tumors of the brain, 101 (10 per cent) were found to be of pituitary origin (Grant).

Pituitary tumors produce their symptoms by pressure on the optic nerves and chiasm and by destruction of the pituitary gland and sella turcica. Pituitary adenomas occur chiefly between thirty and sixty years of age, but may develop anywhere from fifteen to sixty years. The *history* concerns headache and failing vision in adults, loss of vision being a more frequent first complaint than headache. Both symptoms may at times develop simultaneously. Blurring, foggy, or misty *vision* is the usual complaint, extending as a rule over several months to several years. Often a history of relief by refraction is obtained. Inability to see out of the corners of the eyes or collision with objects on either side may be noticed. In some cases, a blind spot in the visual field is noted and in others no complaints referable to vision are observed. *Headache* is a first symptom in about one-third and is present in three-fourths of the cases of pituitary adenoma.

It is usually frontal, often intense behind the eyes or in the temples, sometimes generalized, occasionally confined to one side of the head, and at times paroxysmal. Like visual loss, it has been present for some time before relief is sought. Menstrual irregularity or cessation, loss of libido and potentia, infrequent menses, gain in weight, excessive desire for sweets, polydipsia and polyuria, fatigue and loss of power may be found in varying combinations.

Optic atrophy of a primary type due to pressure of the tumor on the optic nerves is present in at least three-fourths of the patients at the time of examination. It has been estimated that a tumor within the sella turcica must rise 10 mm. to 2 cm. above the sella in the average case in order to compress the optic nerves and chiasm. The atrophy is ordinarily bilateral but it may be unilateral. The visual acuity is decreased proportionately to the atrophy in most cases, but in some (6.5 per cent) the optic discs are normal while the visual acuity is decreased. Choked disc is usually not present and is indeed rare in pituitary adenomas, but a low degree of choking (1-1.5 D) may be found in some cases. Rare cases have been recorded with high choked disc (5-6 D).

Bitemporal hemianopsia is found in the typical pituitary adenoma. It is found

Table 52—Features of Pituitary Adenomas

Type	Optic Atrophy	Bilateral Hemianopsia	Deformity of Sella Turcica	Endocrine Disturbances	Urinary Hormone Excretion
CHROMOPHOBE (Hypopituitary syndrome)	+	+	+	Amenorrhea Loss of libido Increased weight Change in skin and hair Increased sugar tolerance Decreased basal metabolism	Female sex hormone absent. 17-ketosteroids low or absent. "Corticoids" very low. Estrogens absent.
ACIDOPHILIC (Acromegaly)	+	+	+	Increased size of hands and feet Prognathism Thickening of skin Increased size of lips and tongue Enlargement of jaws and sinuses Diabetes	Female sex hormone often decreased. 17-ketosteroids normal. Estrogens decreased. Corticoids normal or increased.
BASOPHILIC (Cushing's syndrome)	0	0	0	Vascular hypertension Hirsutism Fat distributed about face, neck, shoulders, abdomen Lineae purpurae Osteoporosis Diabetes	17-ketosteroids high normal or increased. Female sex hormone usually decreased. Estrogens decreased or absent.

Table 53—Differential Diagnosis of Pituitary Tumors

Tumor	Age	Onset	Fundi	Visual Fields	Endocrine	Roentgenogram
ADENOMA (Primary)	Young adult or middle-aged	Gradual, usually with failing vision and headache. Amenorrhea, sexual impotence also	Primary optic atrophy	Bitemporal hemianopsia almost always. Occasionally homonymous hemianopsia	1. Hypopotuitary syndrome 2. Acromegaly	Ballooned out sella turcica
MENINGIOMA	Middle-aged adults	Gradually failing vision and headache Occasionally disturbance of menses or sexual power	Primary optic atrophy	Bitemporal hemianopsia	None or decreased libido or potentia	Normal sella turcica or erosion of posterior clinoids and dorsum sellae Hyperostosis of tuberculum sellae at times
ADENOMA (Suprasellar)	Middle-aged adults	Gradually failing vision and headache Occasionally disturbance of menses or sexual power	Primary optic atrophy	Bitemporal hemianopsia	None or decrease or loss of menses	Normal sella turcica or erosion of posterior clinoids and dorsum sellae
HYPOPHYSEAL STALK TUMOR	Children usually. Also in young adults	Gradually failing vision and headache. Failure of growth in children	Primary optic atrophy usually. Choked disc in some cases	Bitemporal hemianopsia	1. Infantile habitus 2. Hypopituitary habitus	Suprasellar calcification in 75 to 85 per cent. Erosion of dorsum sellae and posterior clinoids. Marked destruction in some cases

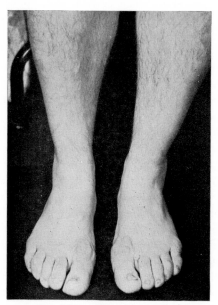

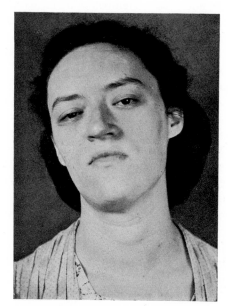

Fig. 179—*(See: Fig. 181.)*   Fig. 180—*(See: Fig. 181.)*

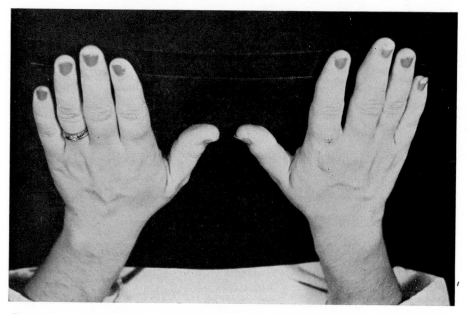

Fig. 181—*Acromegaly* in a patient with a large eosinophilic adenoma of the pituitary, showing the typical spade-like hands and feet and the coarse enlarged facial features.

in seventy-five to eighty per cent of cases of adenoma. Hemianopsia is usually found in conjunction with optic atrophy, but patients are encountered in whom the optic discs are normal while bitemporal hemianopsia for color or form is present. *Homonymous hemianopsia* is found in six to sixteen per cent of patients due to irregular pressure on the optic tracts by the expanding tumor. Normal visual fields are found in rare instances, particularly early in the disease. *Scotomas* occur in about 15 per cent of patients, usually central, resulting from retrochiasmal extension of the adenoma.

Enlargement of the sella turcica is found invariably in patients with primary pituitary tumor, the degree varying with the size of the tumor. The typical deformity consists of enlargement of the anteroposterior diameter and the depth of the sella turcica, with pointing and thinning of the anterior clinoid processes and destruction of the posterior clinoids and dorsum sellae. The floor of the sella is compressed and ballooned out. The degree of sellar enlargement varies from slight enlargement to pronounced ballooning.

Endocrine disturbances are found also in pituitary tumors. The impairment of anterior pituitary function, as measured by various tests, varies from none at all to severe panhypituitarism, depending on the degree of damage to the gland. The pituitary hormones are not equally affected, thus producing various combinations of hypothyroid, hypoadrenocortical, and hypogonadal manifestations. Hypopituitary syndromes of the Froeh-

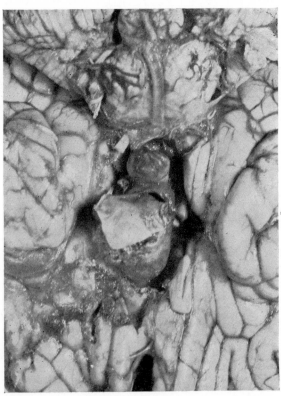

Fig. 182—*Pituitary adenoma.* A large adenoma of the pituitary, compressing the optic nerve and chiasm.

lich type are found in chromophobe adenomas. This is featured by a depression of sexual function, adiposity,

Acromegalic syndromes are found with eosinophilic adenomas and are featured by enlargement of the jaw, protrusion of

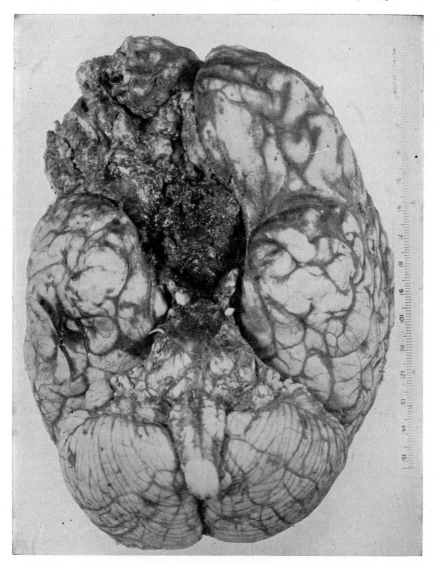

Fig. 183—*Suprasellar meningioma.* A large suprasellar meningioma in a young girl of 18. The tumor is covered with hemorrhage because of previous operation. The optic nerves and chiasm are not seen and are covered by tumor.

atrophic changes in the skin and hair, decreased metabolic rate, and high carbohydrate tolerance. The skin is smooth and delicate, the hair soft, the facial hair scanty, the pubic hair sparse and of female type, and the basal metabolism low.

the lower jaw, prominence of the eyebrows, enlargement of the hands and feet, thickening and wrinkling of the skin of the forehead and face, enlargement of the nose and lips and of the frontal sinuses.

Basophilism is associated with a basophilic tumor which is always microscopic and never gives rise to evidences of pressure on the optic nerves and chiasm (optic atrophy and bitemporal hemianopsia). It is featured by hypertension anemia, hirsutism, fat deposits about the neck, shoulder girdles, and abdomen with purple lineae striae, osteoporosis, and decreased sexual activity. Basophilism may be produced by adrenal cortical tumors and tumors of the ovary. The demonstration of a substance resembling the hormone of the adrenal cortex in the blood and urine of patients with basophilism has been regarded as evidence of its adrenocortical rather than its pituitary nature (Anderson and Haymaker). Recent studies indicate that basophilism may be primarily adrenal in origin.

If pituitary tumors extend beyond the confines of the sella turcica they may cause symptoms referable to the brain stem, such as oculomotor palsies, trigeminal pain, and uncinate fits. A cavernous sinus syndrome (ptosis, complete external ophthalmoplegia, loss of sensation in the first trigeminal division) is encountered in rare cases.

The *diagnosis of pituitary tumor* is not difficult in typical cases. The history of failing vision and headache over an extensive period, and the findings of optic atrophy, bitemporal hemianopsia, endocrine disturbances, and enlargement of the sella turcica in typical cases make the diagnosis simple. Early cases are difficult to diagnose, but a patient with a history of failing vision and headache should have the benefit of roentgenographic studies of the skull and visual field studies. The main problem lies in the detection of cases early, before optic atrophy and visual acuity are lost beyond repair. Since pituitary adenomas are highly vascular tumors, hemorrhage may occur in them, often with dramatic suddenness, in a patient not previously suspected of having a pituitary tumor. The resulting symptoms simulate those of cerebral hemorrhage, with severe headache, nausea, vomiting, neck stiffness, drowsiness and confusion, and elevation of temperature. Rapid loss of vision or total loss of vision is characteristic. The spinal fluid is bloody. The condition is differentiated from cerebral and subarachnoid hemorrhage by the disclosure of a large sella turcica on roentgen examination of the skull.

Suprasellar Tumors: These are of various *types*. The most common include adenomas, meningiomas, and hypophyseal stalk tumors. In addition, suprasellar lesions include aneurysm from the anterior cerebral, internal carotid, or anterior communicating arteries, arachnoiditis, and glioma of the optic chiasm.

The *history* of onset concerns loss of vision and headache extending over a relatively long period of time. Menstrual disturbances and loss of libido may be included in the history. The cardinal signs caused by tumors or other lesions in the suprasellar area are *optic atrophy* of a primary type and *bitemporal hemianopsia*. The *Foster Kennedy syndrome*, consisting of optic atrophy with scotoma of one eye and choked disc of the other eye, is found in suprasellar tumors, chiefly in tumors of the base of the frontal lobe (olfactory meningiomas), but it has been recorded also in parasellar tumors (sphenoid ridge meningiomas), in arachnoiditis of the chiasmal and prechiasmal region, and in aneurysm. The nature of the optic nerve changes demands that the offending process must involve the optic nerve prechiasmally. The visual field defects are not always those of a bitemporal hemianopsia. Homonymous hemianopsia is found at times and even quadrantanopsias are encountered.

Roentgenographic changes in the sella turcica are not of the same variety as in primary pituitary tumor and are not essential to diagnosis. They consist of erosion of the dorsum sellae and posterior clinoid processes in most cases. Erosion of one side of the sella turcica may be found, and a completely normal sella is not unusual. In doubtful cases, suprasellar tumors may be diagnosed accurately by pneumogram, the defect consisting of obliteration of the cisterna chiasmatis. Marked destruction of the sella may be found in some instances of hypophyseal stalk tumor. In seventy-five to eighty-five per cent of stalk tumors, a calcified shadow is seen above the sella turcica. *Endocrine changes* are not constant. The suprasellar meningiomas and adenomas may be associated with menstrual disturbances or loss of libido. The hypophyseal stalk tumors, developing as they usually do in childhood, are associated with delayed growth and a picture of infantilism.

The *hypophyseal stalk tumors* (craniopharyngiomas) occur chiefly in children and young adolescents but they may be found also in adults. The history varies in length from several months to one or more years and is concerned with headache, failing or loss of vision, failure of growth or peculiarity of development. Headache is the most frequent complaint, either alone or associated with dimness of vision, while failure of vision and arrest of growth are common features of the history. The headache is usually frontal but may be occipital or in the vertex. In a series of fourteen cases, it was present in every instance, usually as the first symptom, but in some appearing late in the disorder (Frazier and Alpers). Mental symptoms may be the first manifestation of a craniopharyngioma, but the type of mental symptoms is varied and has no specific significance (Riser).

Examination reveals primary optic atrophy in some patients and choked disc in others, the incidence of the two conditions being about equal. Optic atrophy is said to be more common in older subjects and choked disc in younger patients. This is not always true. Visual field changes are almost invariably present and consist usually of bitemporal hemianopsia, with homonymous hemianopsia, bitemporal quadrantanopsia, and binasal hemianopsia in other instances. In rare cases the visual fields may be normal. Endocrine disturbances are more common in children and adolescents than in those over twenty years of age. Hypopituitary manifestations predominate, with evidence of the *Froelich syndrome* appearing most frequently. Manifestations of failure of growth occur frequently, giving rise to symptoms of dwarfism. Somnolence is common. Scanty hair, feminine distribution of pubic hair, loss of sexual vigor, and amenorrhea are common among adult patients. In young patients, a normal pubescent period is rare and a history of normal development of menstruation in female patients is rare. Roentgenograms reveal various disorders. Calcification above the sella turcica is found in seventy-five to eighty-five per cent of cases. Erosion of the dorsum sellae and the posterior clinoid processes is common. Enlargement of the sella turcica by erosion from above is not uncommon.

The *diagnosis of a suprasellar tumor* is dependent on the findings of the chiasmal syndrome, consisting of optic atrophy and bitemporal hemianopsia against a historical background of headache and failing vision. The occurrence of roentgenographic changes and endocrine disturbances is not essential to the diagnosis, though these are helpful if present. The problem in such cases is concerned largely with the question of vision. The presenting symptom in most instances has to do with headache and failing vision, a combination of symptoms which in many patients is regarded as due to almost anything but tumor in the supra-sellar or sellar region. In a large number of cases, the assumption is still made that failing vision is due to refractive errors, sinus disease, or some systemic affliction. bination of symptoms may develop in sinus disease, but sinus infection is a much less common cause than tumor and is not associated with a bitemporal hem-ianopsia. (2) *Progressively failing vision*

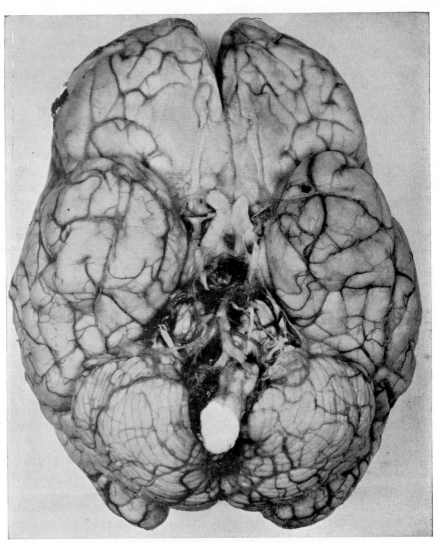

Fig. 184—*Suprasellar meningioma,* showing the remains of a tumor in this region, compressing the posterior portion of the chiasmal region.

Mistakes in diagnosis will be avoided if the following facts are kept in mind: (1) *Headache* associated with blurred vision or failing vision must always be assumed to result from tumor until this assumption is disproved. A similar com- must always be assumed to result from a tumor or a compressing lesion of other sort in the region of the sella turcica until proved otherwise. Only in this way can operative lesions be detected and mistakes in diagnosis avoided.

Headache and failing vision must therefore be assumed to be due to tumor in the region of the sella turcica and must lead to examination of the visual fields and roentgenograms of the sella turcica. If it is found that optic atrophy and bitemporal hemianopsia are present, the diagnosis of a suprasellar lesion must be made, regardless of the state of the sella turcica or the presence or absence of endocrine symptoms. The sella turcica may be completely normal or show only minor changes, such as erosion of the dorsum sellae and posterior clinoids; or it may be enlarged and above it may be seen distinct calcification. Endocrine disturbances may be completely lacking or there may be only a history of scanty menses or of failing sexual powers. Scotomatous defects may occur in the visual fields in instances of suprasellar tumor. In such cases, if the onset is acute, the occurrence of scotomas and rapid failure of vision may simulate closely acute multiple sclerosis. The occurrence of headache will usually force the assumption of a suprasellar tumor. This may be confirmed by x-ray of the skull, which may show deformity of the sella turcica, or it may be established only by pneumogram. In any event, it must be clear that a diagnosis of a suprasellar tumor requires only optic atrophy and bitemporal hemianopsia for confirmation.

Other conditions, such as syphilitic optic atrophy, multiple sclerosis, etc., may cause atrophy of the optic nerve, but not hemianopic field cuts, whether these be bitemporal or homonymous in nature. It must not be forgotten that suprasellar tumors may at times grow asymmetrically and compress only one optic nerve, giving rise to unilateral blindness and optic atrophy before the opposite eye becomes involved. Chiasmal symptoms may rarely be the result of tumors originating in the pineal region, with diabetes insipidus as the outstanding complaint (Horrax and Wyatt). The meningiomas and adenomas occur in adults of 30 or over. The hypophyseal stalk tumors are most common in children and young adults, and in addition to the chiasmal syndrome findings are associated with deformity of the sella turcica, a calcified shadow above the sella, and endocrine disturbances. In some instances, the sella turcica may be normal and the endocrine changes minimal. Aneurysm is characterized by a sudden onset of head pain or of pain behind the eyes, usually recurrent and often associated with extraocular palsies and subarachnoid hemorrhage. Arachnoiditis is difficult if not impossible to diagnose clinically and is discovered at operation in instances regarded as suprasellar tumor.

Caution must be exercised in cases with the symptomatology described for suprasellar tumors, in not attributing the findings to *sinus disease*. Infections of the sphenoid and ethmoid sinuses or of the maxillaries and frontals are an uncommon cause of optic atrophy and in any event are not capable of causing atrophy and bitemporal hemianopsia except in rare instances when they may be responsible for arachnoiditis involving the optic nerves and chiasm. In any case of suspected suprasellar tumor, the diagnosis of sinus disease must be reached only with extreme caution. *Retrobulbar neuritis* may at times be confused, but the acute onset with eye or head pain, the rapid loss of vision, the presence of scotoma, and the tendency to be unilateral in many cases should lead to the proper orientation and should result in a search for the cause of the neuritis among infections, degenerative and systemic disorders of many sorts.

Among the conditions requiring differentiation from suprasellar tumors are those associated with primary optic atrophy. Chief among these is *syphilitic optic atrophy,* which is confused because of the sluggishly reacting pupils which accompany optic atrophy, but largely because headache is disregarded in the evaluation of the symptoms. Confusion is created further by the fact that syphilitic optic atrophy may at times be associated with a negative spinal fluid Wassermann or completely negative spinal fluid reactions, a situation which leads to a false sense of security in the treatment of optic atrophy. In those cases with positive serological reactions, the diagnosis of syphilitic optic atrophy is clear. In those instances due to tabes dorsalis, the diagnosis is not difficult. In other instances, the diagnosis must be seriously questioned if headache and progressive loss of vision predominate. The latter distinction should not be too strongly emphasized, since the visual loss in syphilitic optic atrophy is progressive, complete blindness ensuing in ninety per cent of untreated cases in three years. *Multiple sclerosis* may be associated with optic atrophy, but in most instances it offers no real difficulties in diagnosis, since the history of appearance and disappearance of symptoms and the evidences of disseminated lesions suffice to establish the correct diagnosis.

Loss of vision and optic atrophy following *hemorrhage* is not common, but it occurs with sufficient frequency so that it is of practical importance. Two main groups of cases are distinguishable (Tidy): (1) those in which the visual disturbance follows closely or immediately the hemorrhage, and (2) those in which loss of vision follows hemorrhage after a varying interval. It is probable that hemorrhage in itself is not sufficient to cause visual loss, since blindness does not develop in hemorrhage in a normal subject. The sites of

the hemorrhage responsible for visual disturbances are given as follows: gastric ulcer, thirty-six per cent; uterus, twenty-five per cent; epistaxis, seven per cent; bloodletting, twenty-five per cent; wounds, five per cent (Fries). A single profuse hemorrhage never causes blindness; repeated hemorrhages are required, but the bleeding preceding the visual loss is usually profuse. The blindness may be noticed immediately following a hemorrhage or an interval of three to eight days may pass before visual disturbances are noted. Instances are recorded of intervals of eighteen and twenty days. In thirty-three per cent the blindness is complete and permanent in both eyes; in fifty per cent there is no improvement from the maximum loss; about ten per cent recover good or complete vision (Tidy). The visual fields show paracentral scotomata or sectorlike defects. Ophthalmoscopic examination reveals swelling of the optic disc shortly after the onset of the symptoms; the swelling may vary from one to several diopters. Optic atrophy later follows.

Parasellar Tumors: These are of three main varieties: meningiomas, aneurysms, and metastatic carcinoma, of which the meningiomas are the most frequent. Parasellar tumors may be located immediately adjacent to the sella turcica on the lesser wing of the sphenoid bone or at a distance on the greater wing. Of these the clinical features of the lesser wing tumors are better known. Their *history* differs in important respects from those of the intrasellar and suprasellar groups. Headache is prominent, is usually frontal, and is at times unilateral and described as a pain experienced chiefly over the eye. Failing vision is a prominent symptom and usually accompanies the headache, but may be the only symptom for some time.

Ptosis of the eyelid, diplopia, and unilateral nonpulsating exophthalmos are further symptoms. Patients may become aware, therefore, of drooping of the eyelid, protrusion of the eyeball, and in some instances loss of movement of one eyeball. Pain in the face may develop in patients in whom the adjacent trigeminal ganglion is compressed.

Primary optic atrophy is found frequently, and in the case of small tumors may be unilateral. The syndrome of choked disc of one side and optic atrophy of the opposite side is not infrequent. Normal optic nerves are also encountered. *Homonymous hemianopsia* from pressure on the optic tract is found in practically all instances. In those instances in which the tumor has grown to sufficient size to compress the chiasm, bitemporal hemianopsia may be encountered. *Oculomotor* paralysis from pressure on the adjacent oculomotor nerve is not uncommon (ptosis, external strabismus). Nonpulsating *unilateral* exophthalmos is found in some cases. A cavernous sinus syndrome may be encountered. *Roentgenographic changes*, when present, may consist of unilateral erosion of the sella turcica; erosion of the optic foramen; erosion of the dorsum sellae and posterior clinoids, erosion or hyperostosis of the sphenoid ridge and distortion of the orbital or sphenoid fissure; or there may be a calcified shadow to one side of the sella turcica.

The *diagnosis* depends on the presence of optic atrophy with homonymous hemianopsia, though this may be produced at times by an intrasellar tumor. The latter will be associated with a typical enlargement of the sella turcica. Clinching findings are the evidences of involvement of parasellar structures, such as the oculomotor nerve, nonpulsating exophthalmos, and changes in the sella turcica, sphenoidal fissure, or sphenoid ridge. Meningioma is associated with a slowly progressive history; aneurysm and carcinoma with abrupt onset.

Most parasellar tumors involving the lesser wing of the sphenoid bone are meningiomas. The clinical picture is in most cases typical, but variations are not unusual. In the average case there will be found a primary optic atrophy and a homonymous hemianopsia, often without changes in the sella turcica. In other instances, there may be in addition evidence of paralysis of the oculomotor nerve of one side, with resulting external strabismus and paralysis in upward, downward, and inward movement of the eyeball, associated with ptosis.

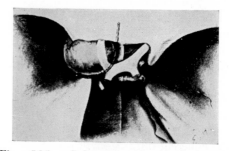

Fig. 185 — *Sphenoid ridge meningioma* showing a tumor on the lesser wing of the sphenoid bone, compressing the optic nerve and tract, giving rise to the characteristic clinical features of a tumor in this area. (Alpers & Groff: Arch. Neurol. & Psychiat. 31:713, April 1934.)

In still other instances, if the tumor encroaches on the cavernous sinus, there may result complete or almost complete paralysis of one eyeball. One group of tumors occupying the sphenoid ridge is accompanied by unilateral nonpulsating exophthalmos, but it must not be assumed that all sphenoid ridge tumors must be associated with this finding.

Gasserian ganglion tumors are in reality parasellar tumors. They are characterized by pain in the face similar to that of trigeminal neuralgia but apt to be less paroxysmal and more constant and to be associated with paresthesias and sensation of numbness in the face. Examination reveals absence of the corneal reflex, loss or decrease of pain sensation over part or all of the face. Evidences of increased pressure may be present or absent.

V. TREATMENT OF BRAIN TUMORS

The treatment of brain tumors is a surgical problem, aided in the cases of some tumors by irradiation. Since brain tumors vary greatly in malignancy, treatment of the various tumor types must be an individual problem. Good treatment in brain tumors, as in tumors elsewhere in the body, is dependent on early diagnosis before the tumor becomes an unmanageable surgical problem.

The only effective treatment of *meningiomas* is removal not only of the tumor but of its dural attachment as well. Where removal is complete, no recurrence occurs. In cases with recurrence, nests of tumor cells have been left in the adherent dura. Convulsions may persist after removal of a meningioma due to the cortical injury before operation and incident to removal. Irradiation is ineffective in the treatment of meningiomas.

Operative treatment of the *gliomas* is dependent on several factors: (1) the size of the tumor; (2) the position of the tumor, and (3) the nature of the glioma. Of the various types of glioma, the cystic astrocytomas are most amenable to treatment. If the solid tumor nubbin can be removed *in toto*, no recurrence develops and a complete cure can be expected. Solid astrocytomas, if removed completely, may develop no recurrence, but excision must be made well beyond the grossly apparent confines of the tumor. The operative results in the

case of the glioblastoma multiforme are almost uniformly bad save in rare instances of survival. Similarly, removal of the medulloblastomas is purely palliative, complete extirpation being usually impossible because of their close proximity to the fourth ventricle. Life may be prolonged, however, by irradiation of the tumor.

Irradiation of the gliomas is in general ineffective as a means of treatment in itself. It is valuable in the case of some tumors only as a supportive treatment after partial operative removal or in the case of inaccessible tumors. The medulloblastomas are radiosensitive, but irradiation results only in the extinction of some of the tumor cells. Complete destruction of the tumor never results. Some recession of symptoms may follow irradiation of astrocytomas, but the effect is never striking. Irradiation has no effect on the glioblastomas.

The treatment of *pituitary adenomas* is concerned with the preservation of vision and the prevention of failure of vision in cases with adequate or normal sight. Two types of treatment are available—operation and irradiation. The proponents of irradiation point to the absence of fatality by this method, while the advocates of surgery point out that the mortality is less than five per cent. The use of irradiation may result in valuable time lost in the preservation of vision, according to its opponents, while its advocates indicate that remission of symptoms and signs can be obtained in fifty per cent of chromophobe adenomas. The chromophile adenomas are less susceptible to roentgen therapy than the chromophobe type.

It is difficult to establish set rules concerning the use of surgery or irradiation in the treatment of pituitary adenomas. In patients with definite optic atrophy and clear evidences of pressure on the optic nerves and chiasm, operation is preferable in order to relieve the compression already existent and to prevent further compression and hence greater visual loss.

Roentgen therapy is best reserved for the following types of cases:

1. Early cases:
   (a) Cases with no optic atrophy, but with hemianopsia, with little or no loss of visual acuity.
   (b) Cases with early optic atrophy with hemianopsia, but with normal or near normal visual acuity.
2. Postoperative treatment.
3. Cases in which operation is refused.

"If the visual acuity is better than % in each eye, and if the atrophy of the optic nerve is not advanced, irradiation therapy is indicated, regardless of changes in the visual field or the sella. However, if visual acuity is less than % in either eye, especially if the impairment in vision has advanced with any speed, say, in less than six months, to a complete unilateral or bilateral cut of the temporal field, and if atrophy of the optic nerve is pronounced in either eye, then surgical intervention must be seriously considered" (Grant).

When irradiation is used, it should be followed carefully for its effect on the optic nerve, visual fields, and visual acuity. Any indication of advance in any of these factors should mean substitution of operation for roentgen therapy in order to preserve vision. Frequent ophthalmoscopic and visual field studies are necessary in order to prevent visual loss.

It may be objected that the early cases suggested for irradiation are precisely the ones best suited for operation since pressure effects at least. Since roentgen treatment is efficacious in many cases, a trial of such treatment in early cases appears advisable, especially if they can be studied adequately to prevent irrep-

arable visual loss. That these studies are essential is clear from the fact that it is not possible to predict from the clinical studies whether vision is still recoverable and when it will become permanent.

Most patients with pituitary adenoma require operation, since the indications of pressure and visual loss are usually well advanced by the time they appear for treatment. Operation followed by irradiation may be followed by remission of symptoms of ten to twenty years. In acidophilic adenomas associated with acromegaly, operation brings good relief of the visual disturbances but none for the endocrine disorders. Cystic adenomas of the pituitary are not susceptible to irradiation.

Hypophyseal stalk tumors may be removed completely if small. In the case of larger tumors, complete removal is impossible because of their adherence to the brain stem structures. Emptying of the cystic contents of the tumor often gives no relief because the cyst wall is so thick as not to collapse when emptied. Irradiation is said to help in some tumors of this type.

Metastatic carcinoma to the brain, if found to be solitary, is an operable lesion, provided there are no evidences of metastasis elsewhere in the body and the condition of the patient is such as to assume that operation may result in survival of sufficient length to justify a craniotomy. The condition is inoperable if there is widespread metastasis, or evidence of multiple metastases to the brain. *Tuberculoma* is an inoperable lesion. *Gumma* of the brain, though rare, is frequently so large that it causes signs of brain tumor and must be treated by surgical removal before antisyphilitic treatment is effective. Cystic *hemangioblastomas* are favorable tumors for removal, similar to the cystic astrocytomas. The venous and arterial angiomas are not favorable lesions for operation and little can be done with them at present. The telangiectases and venous angiomas respond favorably at times to irradiation. *Brain stem* gliomas are inoperable, but partial relief of symptoms may be obtained at times by irradiation.

Prognosis: The outlook in the case of brain tumors varies with the type and location of the tumor. *Meningiomas* if removed cleanly do not recur. Recurrence occurs, however, at times many years after removal if removal is not complete. Much depends on the position of the tumor and on the question of whether removal has been complete. *Gliomas* vary in their outlook. Long survivals are not infrequent in the astrocytomas, especially in the cystic astrocytomas of the cerebellum and cerebrum. Survivals of over twenty years have been recorded in the Cushing series. If complete removal of the solid portion of the tumor is made, survival for an indefinite period follows. The solid astrocytomas vary in their growth rate; an average survival of thirty-seven months was reported for such a group by Cairns. The glioblastoma multiforme is associated with a short survival averaging six to seven months, but survivals of over a year have been recorded and one of over four years (Eisenhardt). Patients with medulloblastomas similarly have a poor outlook, surviving operation for an average of about thirteen months. In other gliomas, the outlook varies, depending on the degree of malignancy.

The *pituitary adenomas* vary in outlook. Studies by Henderson of the Cushing series of 338 adenomas indicate that patients with chromophobe adenomas may survive for a long time (twenty years), but that rapid recurrence may frequently occur. Many patients are improved from ten to twenty years, but ninety-five per cent of those with a recurrence showed indications of it within five years after operation. Eosinophilic adenomas associated with acromegaly respond well to treatment in so far as local pressure effects on vision is concerned but do not respond in so far as the endocrine disturbances are concerned. Good results may be expected in the *acoustic neuromas* if they are removed early enough. While survival after removal of *metastatic carcinoma* is short, averaging two to six months, survivals of two years or slightly longer have been recorded.

It should be emphasized that while tumors may be removed completely, the end results of operation may be totally unsatisfactory. A complete extirpation may be without avail if it leaves its victim blind, paralyzed, or ataxic. It is essential, therefore, that diagnosis be made early and that patients be brought to the surgeon in good time, so that beneficial effects from operation may be possible.

12

Abscess of the Brain

I. CAUSES OF BRAIN ABSCESS

Abscess of the brain, though low in incidence among general medical conditions, is high in occurrence in some forms of infection in the body. Its *incidence* has been estimated at 1.3 per cent (Evans) of a large number of hospital admissions, but it is unfortunately not uncommon in diseases of the sinuses and mastoids. Fortunately, the occurrence of brain abscess has been materially reduced since the use of chemotherapy and antibiotics, largely as a result of the decreased incidence of sinuses, ear, and mastoid infections. Brain abscess has now come to be rare. It may be an acute or chronic condition, and when acute it gives rise to extremely difficult problems of diagnosis and treatment. No *age* is exempt from brain abscess. Its greatest incidence is between the ages of ten and thirty-five, but it may occur in young children and in adults over thirty-five. It is uncommon in aged subjects.

Table 54—Causes of Brain Abscess

1. OTOGENOUS (40 to 50 per cent):
   Mastoiditis
   Otitis media

2. SINUS (7 to 10 per cent)
   Frontal sinus
   Maxillary sinus
   Sphenoid and ethmoid sinuses

3. TRAUMA (4 to 5 per cent):
   Bullet wounds
   Depressed fractures
   Stab wounds

4. METASTATIC (2 to 24 per cent):
   Pulmonary infection:
     Bronchiectasis
     Lung abscess
     Empyema
   Endocarditis
   Tuberculosis
   Actinomycosis
   Amebic dysentery
   Tonsillitis (tonsillectomy)
   Appendicitis
   Pyelonephritis
   Septic abortion
   Osteomyelitis
   Tooth extraction

5. MISCELLANEOUS:
   Infections of orbit
   Cavernous sinus thrombosis
   Furunculosis
   Osteomyelitis of skull
   Infections of face:
     Abscess of eyelids
     Abscess of lips
     Parotitis
     Tonsillitis

Etiology: Brain abscess is almost always secondary to infection elsewhere in the body, a fact which looms large in the suspicion and diagnosis of the condition. In a small percentage of cases, no focus of infection can be found. These cases, referred to as *cryptogenic* abscesses, may have resulted from infections either undiscovered or completely healed. In the vast majority of cases, brain abscess is the result of infection in the paranasal *sinuses* and *mastoids*. The mastoids are more frequently the source of brain abscess than the sinuses, though the latter are by no means an infrequent source.

585

About forty to fifty per cent of all brain abscesses are otogenic in origin, but statistics of their incidence in many series of cases varies between thirty and eighty per cent. About seven to ten per cent are the result of sinus disease. Regarded in another light, the incidence of brain abscess in ear disease is 6.3 per cent (Wilson). Of the various types of ear disease associated with brain abscesses, acute and chronic mastoiditis are the most prolific sources. Otitis media may sometimes be responsible. Of the paranasal sinuses, frontal sinus infection is the most common focus, but infection of the maxillary sinus, sphenoids, or ethmoids may be associated with brain abscess. Multiple sinus disease is not uncommon.

Metastatic brain abscess may be defined as an abscess arising from a source of infection remote from the brain. Abscesses of this nature may be divided into four groups; (1) pleuropulmonary, the abscess arising from disease of the pleura and lungs, particularly bronchiectasis, (2) those arising from pelvic, abdominal and skin infections, (3) those of cardiac origin, resulting from acute, subacute, or chronic bacterial endocarditis, (4) those in which no primary source of origin can be demonstrated (Gates, Kernohan, and Craig). It appears to be true that in any large group of cases of brain abscess there will be some instances in which the primary infection resolves and is not demonstrable at the time of development of the brain abscess. The incidence of metastatic brain abscess is reported as thirty-eight per cent of all brain abscesses (Gates, Kernohan, & Craig). It is believed that the abscess results from transient bacteremia occurring in the course of the infection. Pneumonectomy in cases of bronchiectasis is at times complicated by the condition. Pulmonary tuberculosis and actinomycosis of the lungs may rarely be responsible for a metastatic brain abscess. Amebic dysentery is also a rare cause. Vegetative endocarditis is a much less common source of metastatic abscess than is pulmonary infection.

In rare instances, congenital heart disease is associated with so-called *paradoxical brain abscess*. Paradoxical brain abscess may develop with many varieties of heart disease. An analysis of thirty-three cases of congenital heart disease associated with brain abscess revealed the condition to be associated with the following types of heart disease (Hanna). The mechanism in these

Tetralogy of Fallot	17
Patent foramen ovale, or interstrial septal defect	8
Basal interventricular septal defect	5
Basal interventricular septal defect and patent foramen ovale	1
Eisenmenger complex	1
Cor triloculare biatrium	1

cases is not known; antecedent infection, the extraction of teeth, and other factors appear to have preceded occurrence of the reported abscess. In the cases of congenital heart disease associated with brain abscess, bacterial endocarditis is usually absent. This seems to be due to the fact that "in every instance, there existed the possibility of venous blood being recirculated through the systemic circulation without first passing through the lungs. In this way, the organisms of a transient bacteremia, originating at the site of an infected tooth socket, tonsils, the upper respiratory tract, or elsewhere, might avoid the infiltration by the pulmonary capillaries and pass, either in the free state or encased in fibrin, into the aorta and thence into the brain" (Gates, Rogers, and Edwards). Metastatic brain abscess has been found secondarily to abscess of the liver, appendicitis, pyelonephritis, puerperal sepsis, septic abortion, and osteomyelitis of the long bones.

Infections of the *face* resulting in cavernous sinus thrombosis may terminate in brain abscess by retrograde extension of the infection from the cavernous sinus into the brain. *Trauma* is a source in some instances. The incidence of traumatic brain abscess varies greatly. Traumatic abscesses develop in four or five per cent of brain abscesses in civil life. They are considerably more frequent in time of war. Brain abscess in such instances results from the introduction of infection by penetrating missiles or bodies, as in bullet wounds, stab wounds, and depressed fractures. In such cases there is invariably penetration of the missile or foreign body through the dura into the brain substance. *Furunculosis* has been found as a source of brain abscess in rare instances. Extraction of abscessed *teeth* with resulting osteomyelitis of the jaw and septicemia has been found responsible in rare instances. Direct transplantation of organisms into the brain with subsequent abscess formation occurs as the result of sinus operation in some cases. *Tonsillectomy* rarely is associated with complicating lung abscess and brain abscess. *Infections of the face* or *orbit* may result in brain abscess by retrograde thrombophlebitis. *Osteomyelitis of the skull* may be followed by extradural or subdural abscess and abscess of the brain.

Pathogenesis: Brain abscess may develop by three main mechanisms: (1) retrograde phlebitis; (2) direct extension; (3) *via* the blood stream. The first two mechanisms function largely in abscesses associated with sinus and ear disease; the last in metastatic abscesses from the lungs, heart, or other distant sources.

In sinus infection, the pathways responsible for the production of brain abscess are chiefly two: retrograde phlebitis and direct extension. Retrograde infection is most common in acute sinus disease, as in the cases of sinus infection and abscess, associated with swimming; in chronic sinus infection, either mechanism may be responsible. The pathway usually responsible in acute cases is by the diploic veins, which spread upward from the region of the frontal sinus.

The pathways of infection in otogenic abscess are many. Infection may reach the brain from otitis media or mastoid infection by one of the following routes (Yaskin): (1) from the antrum through the tegmen tympani; (2) by way of the superior semicircular canal; (3) by way of the zygomatic cells; (4) by retrograde extension along venous channels; (5) by the internal auditory meatus; (6) by thrombosis of the lateral sinus.

Pathology: Any part of the brain may be the seat of abscess, but the temporal lobe, the cerebellum, and the frontal lobes are most commonly involved. Parietal and occipital lobe abscesses are less common. Brain stem abscess is extremely rare. Cerebellar abscess is not as common as cerebral abscess; for every three cerebral abscesses, two are found in the cerebellum. Next to the temporal lobe however, the cerebellum is the most common seat of brain abscess. Frontal lobe abscess usually follows sinus infection but may develop following ear disease. Temporal lobe abscess is most common with ear infections but may develop as a result of sinus disease. Generally speaking, abscess develops on the side of the source of infection, a left frontal sinus or mastoid infection being associated with a left frontal or temporal lobe abscess. Abscess in the opposite cerebral hemisphere is not uncommon, however; hence left mastoid or sinus infection may be found with a right cerebral or cerebellar abscess.

Most abscesses of the brain are solitary, but some are multiple. This is especially true of the metastatic abscesses. Some are multiloculated, composed of several chambers, each separated from the adjacent chamber by a well-formed diaphragm of tissue.

Brain abscess develops histologically as an encephalitis composed of bacteria, polymorphonuclear leukocytes, glial reaction, and arteritis. From this focus there develops further infection associated with an outpouring of leukocytes and the formation of an abscess similar to that which is found elsewhere in the body. In the very early stages, the focus of leukocytes is surrounded by dilated blood vessels and perivascular infiltration. On the fringe of the abscess an active encephalitis is found in the adjacent brain tissue, characterized by free leukocytes in the brain, perivascular infiltrations with polymorphonuclear cells, punctate hemorrhages, colonies of bacteria, and evidences of arteritis.

As the infection develops, effort is made by the surrounding brain tissue to envelop the abscess by the formation of a capsule. This is usually more abortive and less complete in the case of brain abscess than in instances of abscess elsewhere in the body. The capsule develops chiefly from the collagen of the blood vessels, and, according to some writers, from the lymphocytes, aided ineffectively by the glial tissue, particularly the astrocytes. If the abscess is close to the brain surface, collagen may be contributed by the overlying meninges.

No specific knowledge is at hand concerning the time necessary for encapsulation of a brain abscess, but in the average instance three to four weeks have been found sufficient for adequate encapsulation (Alpers). This is variable, however, dependent on many factors. In some cases good encapsulation is found in twelve to fourteen days; in others, inadequate walling off of the infection is found after six to twelve months.

Despite good encapsulation, there still remains in most brain abscesses a pericapsular encephalitis which serves as an active source of infection in many instances. This factor is given too little value in the treatment of brain abscess. Encapsulation is dependent on (1) the nature and virulence of the organism; (2) the resistance of the host; (3) the association of factors such as septicemia. It has been found that aerobic organisms are better capsule formers than the anaerobic group, and that the streptococci are more prone to form capsules than staphylococci. A local meningitis is associated with most brain abscesses and generalized meningitis develops as a complication in some cases. The local meningitis is reactive and sterile.

Organisms of many types are found to produce brain abscess, and may be found in pure or mixed cultures. The most common organisms are the streptococcus and pneumococcus with the staphylococcus a weak third. The streptococcus has been found most often (Alpers), but a recent study of 48 cases of brain abscess reveals the staphylococcus as the predominating organism (McFarlan). Among other organisms which have been recorded are B. coli, B. typhosus, B. pyocyaneus, B. influenzae, B. proteus, and Clostridium welchii. Actinomyces have been found.

II. SYMPTOMS OF BRAIN ABSCESS

The symptoms of brain abscess, like those of tumor, may be divided into general and focal manifestations, the former having to do with the recognition of the presence of abscess and the latter with its precise localization.

Since brain abscesses may be acute or chronic, their onset varies accordingly. In some, the development of symptoms is abrupt and almost apoplectic, particularly in cases of metastatic abscess;

in others, it is slow and gradual, resembling the progression of symptoms encountered in brain tumor. The onset in metastatic abscess is usually apoplectiform in character with sudden headache, vomiting, or dizziness. The development of symptoms in traumatic abscess may be rapid or may unfold gradually after months or years. The onset in acute sinus or ear disease is often obscured by stances, it may be experienced as a unilateral head pain. It is not uncommonly associated with vomiting, especially in the presence of cerebellar abscess. *Vertigo* may usher in the appearance of abscess, either alone or in association with headache, and may persist for some time. *Choked disc* is found in about fifty to sixty per cent of all brain abscesses, but is more frequent when the abscess is in

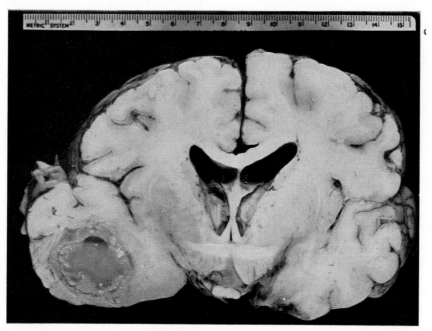

Fig. 186—*Brain abscess.* A well-defined and well-encapsulated brain abscess of the right temporal lobe from a patient having chronic mastoid infection with symptoms of ten months' duration.

the sinus or ear symptoms, making the detection and appraisal of cerebral symptoms difficult. In chronic ear and sinus conditions, the development of symptoms is gradual but may at times be acute, following an exacerbation of the ear or sinus condition. Those of chronic abscess unfold over a period of several months or years. *Headache* is usually present and is found early in abscess as in tumor. It may be constant or intermittent, is increased by straining of any sort and is uninfluenced by medication. In some instances, it may be experienced as a some locations than in others. It has been found in 63.6 per cent of a group of forty-four brain abscesses (Cowan). It is most common in association with cerebellar abscess and appears to be more frequent in abscess of the frontal lobe than in that of the temporal lobe. Despite the high incidence reported in some series (over fifty per cent), it has been found in much lower incidence by others (thirty-five per cent).

Most abscesses of the brain are associated with a peculiar *mental state* difficult to describe because it is manifested often only by a slight deviation from the normal, but the change is definite to the practiced eye. It is characterized by a torpidity which manifests itself by dullness, slowness of reaction, seeming indifference, and a tendency to somnolence. The responses to questions may be delayed slightly or severely, giving the impression of lack of interest, and general

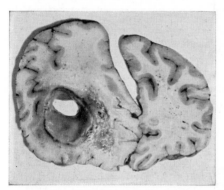

Fig. 187—*Brain abscess.* A brain abscess in the right frontal lobe showing the marked swelling of the surrounding brain, the pushing over of the midline structures and the well-defined capsule in an abscess with symptoms of only four weeks' duration.

cerebration is retarded. These changes may be slight in degree or so pronounced as to be obvious to any observer. They are described frequently as toxic.

Bradycardia is present in a large portion of cases, its incidence being estimated as high as seventy-five per cent (Rasdolsky). It is frequently not present early in the course of abscess formation, making its appearance in the well-advanced or late stages. It is by no means a constant sign. It may be present in some stages of abscess and not in others, or it may be totally lacking.

The *pulse,* moreover, may be constantly slow, varying from forty to sixty per minute, or it may be slow at times and tend to be normal at others. A *chill* may mark the onset in some cases

and *convulsions,* either focal or generalized, in others. Chills are more prone to occur in acute abscesses. *Fever* is present in acute abscesses, but its significance is often obscured by the presence of acute infection elsewhere. It is uncommon in chronic abscesses, the temperature in these instances being normal or frequently subnormal. The *spinal fluid* pressure is usually increased, even in patients without choked disc. The cell count is often normal. It may be moderately increased due to the local meningeal reaction above an abscess (fifty to five hundred lymphocytes). The fluid is sterile. In some cases the abscess may be associated with a severe meningeal reaction due to rupture of the abscess into the subarachnoid space. In such instances, bacteria are found in the spinal fluid. *Meningeal signs* are absent in chronic cases and in most acute cases except in those associated with a generalized meningeal exudate. Leukocytosis is not prominent.

Having established the presence of a brain abscess, either acute or chronic, by the occurrence of headache, choked disc, mental torpidity, bradycardia, and the other symptoms listed above, the problem then becomes one of localization of the abscess. In this respect the problem in brain abscess differs in no way from that of brain tumor.

Temporal lobe abscess is the most frequent of all brain abscesses and is usually associated with ear infection or infection of the mastoid. It may develop secondarily to sinus infection. It may result from acute or chronic infection, but is more commonly associated with chronic ear disease in which there has been an acute exacerbation of symptoms. Thus temporal lobe abscess may follow acute otitis media or acute mastoiditis, or it may result from a long-standing otitis or mastoid infection. A not uncommon history is that of a draining ear for several years followed by cessation of the drainage, followed in turn by a recurrence of running ear. The onset of cerebral symp-

unfortunately cannot always be demonstrated, usually because the patient's mental or physical condition makes it impossible. It is not always present in

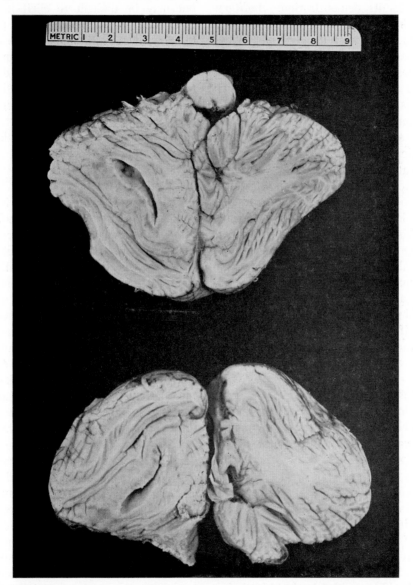

Fig. 188—*Brain abscess.* A collapsed abscess cavity in the cerebellum, with poorly defined walls and with clinical symptoms of eight weeks' duration. The source lay in an infected mastoid.

toms may be associated with the cessation or recurrence of drainage. Abscess of the temporal lobe is often associated with *homonymous hemianopsia.* This

any event even in cases in which field studies can be made. Its incidence has been found to vary in different series from thirty-three to sixty-six per cent.

Its occurrence is of such great significance, however, that it should always be sought early in suspected cases of abscess before the clouded mental state precludes its demonstration. *Auditory-receptive aphasia* is a valuable sign if present. A central *facial weakness* can be demonstrated in many instances and at times a *hemiparesis* is present. Ocular palsies are sometimes seen, especially if there is an associated petrositis.

Frontal lobe abscess usually results from sinus disease, either acute or chronic, and is most frequently the result of frontal sinusitis, though sphenoiditis, ethmoiditis, and maxillary sinusitis may be associated with frontal lobe abscess. There is often a history of onset of acute sinusitis following swimming or diving, leading eventually to evidences of acute brain abscess. In some cases acute sinusitis may be associated with an extradural abscess and osteomyelitis of the frontal bone. *Expressive aphasia* may occur if the abscess is in the left frontal lobe and posterior. *Hemiparesis* or *hemiplegia* are occasionally encountered, as well as jacksonian or generalized convulsions.

In rare instances, abscess may involve the parietal or occipital lobe, giving rise to a cortical sensory syndrome in the first instance and to a homonymous hemianopsia in the second.

Cerebellar abscess, next to abscess of the temporal lobe, is the most frequent of brain abscesses. It is usually the result of ear infection. Acute cerebellar abscess is usually associated with extradural abscess or thrombophlebitis; chronic abscess with labyrinthitis. Infection reaches the cerebellum from the mastoid by (1) the labyrinth; (2) lateral sinus thrombosis; (3) caries of the petrous bone; (4) the internal auditory canal (Eagleton). Cerebellar abscesses are usually single but may be multiple.

Headache is constant and the incidence of choked disc high. Cranial nerve palsies are common. Cerebellar signs are often demonstrable in the chronic cases but may be difficult to elicit in acute cases due to inability of the patient to carry out the demands of a neurological examination. For this reason, cerebellar abscess is frequently most difficult to diagnose. Since it often follows a labyrinthitis, a history of this condition may lead to the suspicion of a cerebellar abscess, though the signs may be lacking to confirm the diagnosis.

III. DIAGNOSIS OF BRAIN ABSCESS

The diagnosis of brain abscess is often difficult, particularly in acute conditions. More than almost any other neurological condition, it requires careful daily observation in the acute cases and a cautious synthesis of data in all instances.

Since brain abscess is in effect a brain tumor with an infection, the history of an infection looms large in the diagnosis. In the absence of a history of sinus, ear, or chest infection, the diagnosis in chronic cases is usually brain tumor. The presence of infection in acute brain abscess is always obvious. These facts serve but to emphasize the importance of the overt fact that a *history of infection* is a prerequisite for the diagnosis of brain abscess. It may be impossible at times to obtain a history of infection because the patient is too ill to give the necessary information or because the infection may have been so slight as to pass unnoticed. Infection may involve sinuses and mastoid or there may be a pansinusitis; moreover, and this is true in the chronic cases particularly, the evidence of abscess may first become apparent after ear and sinus infections clear up. On the other hand, abscess may be present with an intact tympanic membrane or in the absence of a recent ear discharge.

The detection of an acute brain abscess is a challenge to careful observation. The difficulty lies primarily in the fact that an acute abscess is engrafted on a background of another acute illness, such as acute sinusitis, otitis media, or mastoiditis. Its early manifestations tend to be obscured, therefore, by evidence of an-conditions, and may be confirmed by the demonstration of focal brain signs or by signs of increased intracranial pressure. Such a patient, were he to develop a chill, a further rise in temperature, headache, bradycardia, and a convulsion, and were he to show a homonymous hemianopsia, aphasia, hemiparesis, or other focal

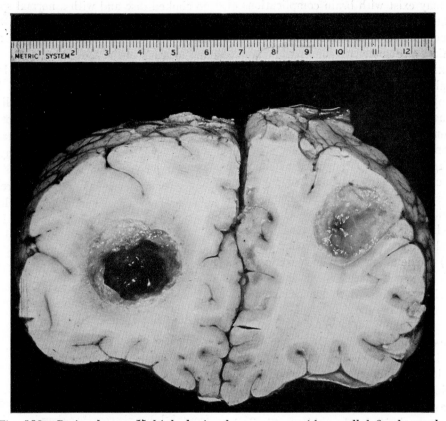

Fig. 189—*Brain abscess*. **Multiple brain abscesses, one with a well-defined capsule and the other poorly delimited, from bronchiectasis of long standing.**

other serious illness, some of the symptoms of which, such as headache and fever, are common to both conditions. The situation as it presents itself is that of a patient with acute sinus or ear disease, who appears to be sicker than he should be with either of these conditions, and who, despite adequate surgical or chemical methods of treatment, fails to respond by improvement. A brain complication may be suspected under these brain sign, could under such circumstances be regarded rightfully as having developed a brain abscess.

The problem becomes easy in those cases in which *choked disc* is found, for abscess can be assumed whether or not focal brain signs are present. In the absence of choked disc, an elevated spinal fluid pressure of 200 mm. or over of water points to a possible abscess but is not proof in itself. since a high pressure may be produced by the brain edema which accompanies other complications such as meningitis, encephalitis, etc. It may be desirable at this point to emphasize the fact that while choked disc is an important finding in support of the supposition that brain abscess is present, it is by no means pathognomonic. It may exist with brain complications of other sorts, such as meningitis, otitic hydrocephalus, or arachnoiditis. The conditions are somewhat different in metastatic abscess, for in these cases the cerebral complication is ushered in by an apoplectic onset characterized by headache, vertigo, and chill, and is followed soon by definite evidence of focal brain damage.

The problem of diagnosis of subacute or chronic brain abscess differs from that of acute abscess. It is customary to describe four stages in the development of such an abscess, (1) the onset of cerebral infection; (2) the latent period; (3) the development of suppuration; and (4) the encapsulation of the abscess. Such a categorical and artificial classification is hardly ever demonstrable in actual practice. The onset of infection, the stage of acute encephalitis, is usually so indefinite as to be easily overlooked, or it may be completely obscured by the evidences of infection elsewhere, as in the sinuses or mastoids. In other instances, however, it is clearly evident. Similarly with the period of latency. In the majority of instances, a chronic abscess develops against a background of sinus or ear infection, or, in other instances, of pulmonary infection. Overt symptoms appear chiefly when the abscess is moderately well developed and are similar to those of a brain tumor — headache, choked disc, bradycardia, progressive focal signs, and the mental obtundity seen so frequently in brain abscess. As a rule, the source of infection is known

to the patient and develops in the history without prodding. Not infrequently, however, the presence of infection in the sinuses, ear, or chest are demonstrated only on examination and call attention to the possibility of brain abscess. It is important to recognize the fact that brain abscess, like brain tumor, may exist with no choked disc and with a normal spinal fluid pressure. In such cases, only *pneumography* can determine the presence and location of the abscess.

If ear disease is present and a brain abscess is suspected, the temporal lobe on the side of the ear infection is likely to be involved. That this is not an invariable rule, however, is demonstrated by the fact that ear infection may be associated with frontal lobe abscess and rarely by abscess of the opposite cerebral hemisphere. The signs of greatest localizing significance are homonymous hemianopsia (about fifty per cent), sensory (auditory-receptive) aphasia, and a central facial weakness. None of these signs may be present, however, or the patient may be so ill as to render their demonstration impossible. In these cases, only ventriculography can determine the location. In the presence of sinus disease, frontal abscess is most common, but temporal lobe abscess is possible. The signs of greatest value in the localization of frontal lobe abscess are hemiparesis or hemiplegia, motor (expressive) aphasia, and jacksonian convulsions. Cerebellar abscess, as has been indicated, is often extremely difficult to diagnose but may be suspected in the presence of ear infection and a history of labyrinthitis.

Ventriculography may be necessary in cases of suspected or known abscess which are difficult to diagnose. While there may be risk involved in the procedure, the exigencies of the situation are such as to justify such an examination

IV. DIFFERENTIAL DIAGNOSIS OF BRAIN ABSCESS

Of the various conditions with which brain abscess may be confused, *meningitis* is among the most important. In some instances, the distinction becomes extremely difficult when abscess and meningitis coexist as sometimes happens when an abscess ruptures into the subarachnoid space. The distinction is important because of the difference in treatment required for meningitis and abscess, the former being medical, the latter surgical. Meningeal signs are well pronounced in meningitis and usually absent in abscess; choked disc is usually present in abscess and may be absent in meningitis; the fever tends to be of a septic type in meningitis and the pulse rapid; the cell count of the spinal fluid is greatly increased in meningitis (one thousand or over) and the fluid contains bacteria by smear and culture, while that of abscess is sterile and the cell count low. In cases in which abscess and meningitis coexist the distinction is not of too great importance, since the problem is that of control of the meningitis before treatment of the abscess.

Extradural abscess sometimes offers difficulties in acute ear and sinus conditions. It is an extremely difficult condition to diagnose and is revealed largely by exploration. Excessive headache over and above that of the underlying condition, meningeal signs, and prolonged fever are suspicious features. The presence of osteomyelitis of the bone and edema of the forehead extending to the hairline are important confirmatory findings. In ear diseases particularly, *lateral* sinus thrombosis requires differentiation from abscess. In most instances, the sudden onset of headache, chills, spiking fever with sweats, leukocytosis, and tenderness of the jugular vein, offer rather distinctive features. Though many of these symptoms are common to sinus thrombosis and abscess, the irregular fever, the chills, and the neck tenderness usually suffice to establish the diagnosis. In many instances, however, the distinc-

Table 55—Differential Diagnosis of Brain Abscess

	Brain Abscess	Brain Tumor	Purulent Meningitis	Lateral Sinus Thrombosis	Labyrinthitis
ONSET	Acute or chronic	Usually chronic May be acute	Acute	Acute	Usually acute
INFECTION	Present	Absent	Present	Present	Usually present; often absent
HEADACHE	Usually present	Usually present	Present	Usually present	Absent
CHOKED DISC	Usually present	Usually present	Absent	Absent	Absent
PULSE	Usually slow	Usually unaffected	Rapid	Rapid	Unchanged
MENTAL STATE	Usually befuddled	Unchanged as a rule	Unchanged, stupor or confusion	Unchanged	Unchanged
SPINAL FLUID	Increased pressure. Cells 50–500 lymphocytes	Increased pressure. No change in cells	Cells greatly increased, to 10,000 (polymorphonuclears)	Unchanged	Unchanged

tion is made clear only on operation and exposure of the thrombosed sinus.

Labyrinthitis also offers difficulties, especially in cerebellar abscess. The onset of labyrinthitis may be acute or slow and is associated with intense vertigo which is episodic and postural. Headache and focal brain signs are absent. While lurching of gait is present in labyrinthitis, it is found in association with vertigo. In cerebellar abscess, gait and other disturbances of incoördination are constant and develop independently of episodes of vertigo. The incoördination associated with cerebellar abscess, therefore, is found without a history of vertigo which accompanies the unsteady gait. Vertigo is often present in cerebellar abscess histories, but careful inquiry will reveal that the reeling and lurching which constitute a prominent feature of cerebellar abscess are independent of attacks of vertigo. In labyrinthitis, on the other hand, vertigo invariably accompanies the gait difficulties. Deafness usually accompanies labyrinthitis and free intervals in which no vertigo is present is characteristic of the condition.

Brain tumor is a problem only when no history of infection is obtained or in those cases in which no focus of infection is found on examination. The developmental history of abscess simulates so closely that of tumor, that in the absence of infection by history or examination, the diagnosis is brain tumor. The operative treatment of the two conditions is so different that the diagnostic distinction is essential. Associated at times with ear disease particularly are a number of conditions described variously as *circumscribed serous meningitis, arachnoiditis,* and *otitic hydrocephalus,* all of which are variants of a single condition, to wit: arachnoiditis or localized meningitis, which in some instances is associated with focal collections of fluid in the subarachnoid space (circumscribed serous meningitis). Otitic hydrocephalus is an external hydrocephalus associated with acute or chronic otitis media, with or without meningitis and characterized by the occurrence, chiefly in children or adolescents, of intermittent headache and choked disc, occasionally by abducens paralysis, and by a spinal fluid under pressure but without excess of cells or protein. The outcome is usually recovery with removal of focus of infection in the ear and repeated lumbar puncture. Distinction is made from abscess by absence of constant headache or focal brain signs.

V. TREATMENT OF BRAIN ABSCESS

The treatment of brain abscess is *surgical* and the methods of treatment by no means uniform. Tapping of the abscess appears to give the best result, but wide exposure of the abscess and even removal have their advocates. Careful analysis of one hundred cases of brain abscess by Grant reveals the fact that forty-seven of the patients recovered while fifty-three died. The best results appear to be obtained by more conservative methods of treatment, such as tap, or tap and drainage of the abscess through trephine openings in the skull. Craniotomy or craniectomy has not produced as good results as trephine and tap.

Excision of cerebellar abscess with the aid of *penicillin* has been found to be both a safe and remedial procedure (Pennybacker). Radical treatment of brain abscess has been made more available by the use of the *sulfonamides* and *antibiotics,* with the result that removal of abscess walls with necrotic tissue, associated with primary closure without drainage, has become possible through the use of the sulfonamides and penicillin with good results (McCarthy and Griffin).

An important aspect of treatment which cannot be neglected is the elimination of the focus of infection responsible for the abscess, whether in the mastoids, sinuses, or other areas. Unless this is done, the possibility persists that recurrence of the abscess may follow. Whether the focus is to be eliminated before or after operation on the abscess requires careful analysis of each case. In the majority of instances, the abscess will be operated on first and the mastoid or sinus infection subsequently. There are strong advocates, however, of the elimination first of the focus of infection, followed subsequently by drainage of the abscess. The time for operation is of great importance and requires good judgment. Penicillin and the sulfonamides constitute important adjuncts in treatment, and intensive treatment with these drugs is important in every case of brain abscess. Their effect may be negligible in cases of encapsulated abscess.

Operation is harmful unless the abscess has become encapsulated, and the constant observation of the patient for the correlation of symptoms and the histological processes going on in the brain is always difficult and sometimes impossible. This aspect of the treatment requires the careful observation of both the medical and surgical aspects of the problem. Intensive chemotherapy with appropriate sulfonamide drugs is invaluable in combating the infection and in making possible reactive processes on the part of the patient so that encapsulation appears complete as judged by the clinical symptoms. No specific criteria for judgment of this process are known, but encapsulation may be said to take place when acute symptoms subside, when constitutional symptoms of a severe nature recede, and when evidences of focal involvement of the brain become definite. None of these criteria are specific. Were

this so, the entire problem of when to operate in brain abscess would be greatly simplified. It may be said, however, that *recession of acute systemic symptoms* indicate probably a successful effort on the part of the patient to overcome the infection. To this extent it may be possible to correlate symptoms and pathology and to assert that encapsulation is at least in process of formation during this period.

The outlook, both immediate and remote, in cases of brain abscess varies greatly from series to series. It is dependent on the virulence of the infection, the time of operation, and the method of attack. Provided the abscess has been attacked properly and the infection not too virulent, the outlook for recovery is good. The mortality remains high, however, in an over-all view of brain abscess. Paralyses, hemianopsias, and other disabling symptoms are likely very often to be persistent in greater or lesser degree due to destructive tendencies of abscess. Recurrence of the abscess is sometimes encountered due to refilling.

VI. PETROSITIS (Suppuration of the Petrous Pyramid)

Petrositis, or suppuration of the petrous pyramid, results from acute or chronic mastoid disease but is much more common with acute infections. The underlying condition is either an osteitis or osteomyelitis of the petrous tip in the temporal bone, usually an osteitis.

Symptoms: The *symptom* background is set as a rule in an acute mastoiditis. Following mastoidectomy, the temperature generally returns to normal, the middle ear discharge ceases, and the mastoid begins to heal, when the patient begins to complain of pain in the eye on the side of the lesion. The eye pain is a quite constant feature of the illness and usually the first symptom. It is a deep pain, experienced in and behind the eye, and often worse at night. The pain as a rule is constant with severe exacerbations, but it may be intermittent. It may develop early in the disease, coincident with or early in the development of the symptoms of otitis or mastoid infection, or, as is generally the case, after mastoid operation. In the latter eventuality, it may make its appearance within a day or weeks after operation. It may be absent. Coincident with the development of eye pain, the middle ear very frequently begins to discharge profusely and the patient develops fever (99° to 102° F.).

The presence of an ear discharge is not constant, however. The discharge may be scant or there are instances in which pain following acute otitis or mastoidectomy is associated with no discharge from the middle ear and a healed mastoidectomy wound. Chronic suppurative lesions of the pyramid may occur with no discharge from the ear. Pain in the face may be experienced, diplopia and transient facial paralysis may be noted. Examination usually reveals a profuse discharge from the ear and frequently an abducens paralysis with the eye held in internal rotation. This is not constant, however. When present it is found on the side of the discharging ear. Some maintain that abducens paralysis is not a part of the petrositis symptomatology. Transient facial paralysis, generally the central type, may be present. Vertigo is an inconstant complaint due to accompanying labyrinthitis and nystagmus may be encountered but it is by no means constant. Rarely, hoarseness and difficulty in swallowing have been recorded. Moderate leukocytosis is present (ten to thirteen thousand) and usually a secondary anemia. The spinal fluid reveals no abnormalities. Roentgenograms of the petrous pyramid reveal increased density or clouding and evidence of an osteitis or osteomyelitis.

Diagnosis: The *diagnosis* of petrositis may be made on the basis of the development of ocular pain following mastoiditis or mastoidectomy, usually an abducens paralysis, low grade fever, and the demonstration of changes in the petrous apex on roentgenologic examination. The diagnosis cannot be made by the roentgenologic findings alone but requires correlation of both clinical and roentgenologic findings. The occurrence of eye and face pain is not in itself tacit evidence of petrositis. Occurring during the course of mastoiditis or after mastoidectomy, it may be the result of postoperative pain, pain due to sinus disease, lateral sinus thrombosis, or meningitis.

Eye pain within and behind the eye is regarded by many as a distinctive and diagnostic feature of infection of the petrous apex, but in many recorded instances the pain has not been typical and has been found in the frontal region and around the eye. It has been found in other instances referred to the temple, the teeth, the face, the ear, and in rare cases to the back of the skull. Similarly, the presence of an abducens paralysis under similar conditions may result from meningitis, sinus thrombosis, labyrinthitis, brain abscess, and infection of the sphenoid bone. The time of development of an abducens palsy is of some importance in diagnosis. Its development during the persistent pain after healed mastoidectomy is regarded by some as a sign of disease of the petrous tip and is of greater significance than an abducens paralysis which supervenes within a few days after the onset of an acute otitis or mastoiditis. Moreover, petrositis may develop without abducens paralysis.

The condition must be distinguished from the *Gradenigo syndrome*, which is characterized by ocular pain, and abducens paralysis occurring during mastoid infection and terminating in recovery. It is probable that most cases of this syndrome are in truth petrositis. Disease of the *sinuses* can be usually distinguished easily by its typical history and its characteristic clinical and roentgenologic findings. Eye and face pain may develop at times during the course of a *temporal lobe abscess*, but this may be differentiated by evidence of increased pressure such as choked disc, homonymous hemianopsia, and aphasia. *Labyrinthitis* may be differentiated by the intense vertigo, nystagmus, and negative roentgenologic findings. Infection in the lateral, cavernous, superior, and inferior petrosal sinuses may be associated with face pain and abducens paralysis in all save lateral sinus thrombosis. All these conditions are sufficiently distinctive to make differentiation relatively easy.

13

Cranial Trauma

I. BLOWS TO THE HEAD

Blows to the head produce many sorts of injuries, each with its specific diagnostic and therapeutic problems. Head injury is, of course, considerably more common in warfare than in civil life, but its incidence in the latter has become increasingly greater with the advent and development of the age of mechanization. Head injuries constitute almost 6 per cent of wounds sustained in warfare. Industrial hazards and automobiles have been responsible for a decided increase in the occurrence of head injury, and, all things considered, are as prolific as injuries by missiles in the production of cranial trauma. Almost three-fourths of all head injuries in civil life are caused by the automobile. Since the advent of the automobile, furthermore, the incidence of head injuries has increased to 2.5 per cent as compared with 0.86 per cent before its advent. United States census reports (1936) indicate a death rate of 27.8 per one hundred thousand of automobile accidents and of 28.5 per one hundred thousand for traumatisms of other sorts. The proper diagnosis of head injuries constitutes, therefore, one of the major medical problems of the day and demands of the general practitioner and the specialist careful observation both for diagnosis and treatment.

Head injuries are of two main types: (1) *Closed head injuries*, characterized by absence of exposure of the brain contents as a result of cranial trauma. In this group is included all cases of concussion, contusion, laceration, hemorrhage, and other conditions consequent to trauma, with or without associated skull fracture, in which the skull has not been penetrated and the brain contents exposed. (2) *Open head injuries*, characterized by exposure of the brain contents by a compound fracture due to penetration by a missile or by other objects.

Injury to the head may result in (1) fracture of the skull; (2) hemorrhage; (3) laceration and contusion; (4) concussion. These will be considered separately, but since hemorrhage has already been discussed in affections of the meninges it will not be reviewed here.

The symptoms resulting from head injury are due largely to the effects of the injury on the brain. The effects upon the bony structures are purely secondary and incidental. Much more important is what happens to the brain itself than what occurs in the skull. From this it must not be inferred that the skull changes are entirely unimportant, since only six per cent of cases of skull fracture are unassociated with evidence of brain injury (Mock) and depressed or compound fractures of the skull are matters of serious significance. With all this, it may still be said, however, that the injury to the brain is of much greater consequence than the injury to the skull. Contusion and laceration of the brain, concussion, subdural and subarachnoid hemorrhage, may all develop without skull fracture. Hence it is clear that brain injuries of both minor and major degree develop without skull injury. For this reason the assessment of a head injury must consist primarily of an analysis of the degree of damage to the brain, regardless of what has occurred to the skull. Because of the occurrence of brain damage of various degrees without skull injury, the tendency to measure the severity of the brain injury by the occurrence of skull fracture must be regarded as inadequate.

While skull fracture may be commonly associated with brain injury, its presence reveals nothing of the underlying brain damage, for it may be associated with no damage at all, with minor damage, or with severe injury which may result in death. Three exceptions to this assertion are of importance and indicate conditions in which the injury to the skull is of great clinical significance. These are: (1) Compound fractures. (2) Depressed fractures. In both of these conditions, what has developed in the brain is a direct consequence of what has occurred in the skull. Brain damage is almost always but not invariably found in both conditions and it is essential in an evaluation of treatment of these conditions to know not only whether the brain is damaged, but if damaged, what the condition of the bony structure is. (3) Extradural hemorrhage. Since this is almost invariably associated with fracture of the skull, it is important when such a diagnosis is suspected to know whether a linear skull fracture is present.

The mortality from head injuries is a matter of some significance but is variously estimated, depending on the source of the material. A general mortality rate of 6.9 per cent is reported in 754 cases of head injury (Bulynin), and of five per cent in 554 cases (Pickles). General mortality rates of 17.7 per cent (Wright) and 17.8 per cent (Fay) have been recorded. The mortality from head injury rises with increase in age, the incidence of death being definitely higher in older subjects. Of greater value would be comparable figures of the incidence of mortality in the various types of head injury, but these are difficult to obtain. Mock reports an average mortality rate of ten per cent for serious head injuries, an average death rate of thirty per cent for proved skull fractures, and estimates that three hundred people are being killed each day by brain injuries.

General Symptoms of Cranial Trauma: Head injury, regardless of type, is followed by a group of symptoms which may be regarded as common to all forms of cranial trauma. Not all the symptoms may be found in every patient, but most of them are present in the majority of instances.

Unconsciousness or *impairment of consciousness* is found in every head injury of any degree of severity. Its recognition is of importance particularly in the evaluation of posttraumatic sequelae. The determination whether posttraumatic sequelae are of psychogenic or structural origin will be influenced in part by the demonstration of loss of consciousness at the time of the acute injury and the evaluation of the degree of this loss. Many psychogenic problems following head injury have had little or no loss or impairment of consciousness, and reveal a series of complaints entirely disproportionate to the degree of injury. Unconsciousness may be extremely slight, moderate, or profound in degree. It is variously described in the milder instances as a feeling of being dazed, or as being able to hear but not to understand what occurred in the environment, while in more severe examples it varies from a loss of contact with the surroundings with awareness but not identification of happenings, to complete stupor and coma. It is generally agreed that the greater the depth and the longer the duration of unconsciousness the more severe the head injury, and that the duration of loss of consciousness is the most reliable basis for classification of the severity of the head injury. Recent studies indicate that the most accurate index of the disturbance of consciousness in head injury is the degree of disorientation, especially the disorientation in time (Moore and Ruesch), and the duration of posttraumatic amnesia (duration of coma and disorientation) is probably the best index of the general disturbance of the brain caused by the injury (Symonds). On the other hand, severe brain injuries may at times develop with only slight or even no apparent loss of consciousness, while profound loss of consciousness of long duration may be followed by no serious consequences. The cause of the unconsciousness in head injuries is not definitely known.

Headache is an accompaniment of almost all acute head injuries. Its intensity and duration vary greatly. It is generalized and in severe cases associated with nausea and vomiting. It may be fleeting or it may persist for some time after the injury. It is not in itself a reliable index of the severity of the head injury. It may be found in severe degree in concussion as well as in instances of meningeal hemorrhage. Conversely, it may be only slight or even trivial in severe injuries. Its persistence following head injury is important and must always lead to search for the reason for its presence, whether it be due to subdural hematoma, external hydrocephalus, a postconcussional state, or psychogenic causes. In the acute state it has no pathognomonic features except in cases of subarachnoid hemorrhage, in which it is accompanied by evidences of meningeal irritation. To all outward appearances, the headache of concussion, contusion, and of subdural or extradural hemorrhage is similar in all respects.

Vertigo is second only to headache as a symptom of acute head injury and is also a persistent sequel in numerous instances. It is a true vertigo, either subjective or objective in nature, aggravated as a rule by change in posture, and accompanied sometimes by tinnitus. It disappears usually within a short time after the head injury, but it may persist for long periods and become a major problem after the acute head injury has subsided. Its posttraumatic features will be considered subsequently.

Associated with head injury is frequently a varying degree of *confusion* which may become severe enough at times to express itself in delirium. Transient confusion is common in concussion. More severe degrees may develop in contusions, lacerations, and meningeal hemorrhage, and may persist for days. The confusion may persist in some instances long after the effects of the acute head injury have worn off.

Changes in body temperature are common. Hyperthermia of moderate degree (99° to 100° F.) is common. High temperatures are found in extradural hemorrhage and as a terminal sign in severe cases of trauma. Hypothermia is not uncommon, and in many cases also the temperature may be normal. The *pulse* rate is usually elevated but bradycardia is often noted. It has no diagnostic significance in itself. The *respirations* are as a rule increased but may be profoundly depressed and irregular. The respirations may be forced and labored in instances of severe injury or they may be periodic and of the Cheyne-Stokes variety in other cases. The *blood pressure* falls in severe cases with profound shock. It is elevated in the late stages of extradural hemorrhage.

Next to the degree and duration of unconsciousness, marked changes in the body temperature and in respiratory rate are the best index of the severity of brain injuries. The severity of the head injury cannot be assessed from the vital signs alone, but much help can be obtained from them in association with other criteria. No single sign is in itself conclusive, but, as has been stated, the degree and duration of loss of consciousness is the most valuable single sign. Among 373 cases of head injury, the signs of grave prognostic significance were found to be a temperature of over 103° F., irregular, labored, or periodic respirations; a compound fracture; pupillary abnormalities; and severe paralysis. Signs that the injury probably was severe were a temperature of 100° to 103° F.; a pulse rate over one hundred; a respiratory rate over twenty-eight; a systolic blood pressure under 90 mm.; a pulse pressure under 30 mm. or over 70 mm.; fracture of the skull, convulsions, and mild neurological signs (Pilcher and Angelucci). Of good significance are a normal temperature and respiratory rate and absence of skull fracture. That these cannot be assessed as isolated signs is shown by the fact that in a study of 151 cases of cranial trauma with necropsy findings, the majority with profound head injury revealed no significant changes in blood pressure and pulse rate during the period of hospitalization. This serves but to emphasize the highly important point in the management of head injuries, that an evaluation of the injury must take into consideration all features of the clinical problem, and that no single symptom or few symptoms can be relied upon to gauge the seriousness of the brain injury.

All cases of head injury are associated with some degree of shock, the more severe the injury the greater being the evidence of shock. It is generally agreed that the manifestations which accompany head injuries are analogous to those of surgical shock. In mild cases of head injury, only fragments of the total picture of shock are found, but in severe instances the expression of shock is well marked, with coldness, pallor, sweating, and failure of blood pressure on the venous side of the circulation. It is this feature of head injuries which must be recognized clearly in order to approach properly the problem of treatment, for it is shock, partial or complete, which must always be combated in every case of injury to the brain.

Pathology of Cranial Trauma: Injury to the head is associated with a number of possible brain changes. In a large percentage of cases, skull fracture is present, usually a linear fracture, but in some instances depressed, compound, or comminuted, depending on the nature of the injury. This may be the only manifestation of the head injury, and may be unassociated with evidences of brain injury.

Meningeal hemorrhage is common in cranial trauma of varying intensities. It is manifested usually by bleeding into the subarachnoid space, the extent of the subarachnoid hemorrhage, varying from a thin localized film over scattered areas of the cortex, to a thick pad of hemorrhage covering the base of the brain or the cerebral hemispheres. The bleeding in such instances is usually confined to the subarachnoid space, but may be associated with punctate hemorrhages in the underlying brain, or in scattered portions of the brain or brain stem. In the majority of instances, subarachnoid hemorrhage is unassociated with changes in the brain. Thin films of subarachnoid hemorrhage are readily absorbed and offer no problems; thicker layers of hemorrhage may become organized and may be responsible for pia-arachnoid fibrosis over the base of the brain or the vertex.

In addition to subarachnoid hemorrhage, both subdural and extradural hemorrhage may follow head injury. Subdural hemorrhage is often found without fracture of the skull, extradural hemorrhage is practically invariably found with skull fractures. Subdural bleeding develops from tear of a cortical vein with subsequent bleeding into the subdural space. The development of the subdural hematoma has already been described (v. Meningeal Hemorrhage). Extradural hemorrhage is usually of arterial origin from rupture of the middle meningeal artery, but may be of venous origin at times due to bleeding from the large venous sinuses of the dura (v. Meningeal Hemorrhage). Large cerebral hemorrhage is rare in head injury, but when found is part of a very extensive brain injury, associated with skull fracture. Punctate or conglomerate hemorrhages may be found in the brain stem or in the cerebral hemisphere in cases of severe head injury. Pontine hemorrhages are not uncommon in severe brain injuries.

The concept of vasoparalysis of the central nervous system, or "central vasoparalysis" (Scheinker), has been offered as an explanation of vascular brain changes which occur in trauma, intoxications, and as a result of chemical irritants. The morphological features of the condition include: "(1) maximal distention of the smaller veins and capillaries, associated with signs of stasis; (2) degenerative changes or complete necrosis of the vessel wall, with an increase in permeability for serous fluid and red blood cells; and (3) distention of the perivascular spaces" (Scheinker). Changes develop in the surrounding parenchyma as a result of the vasoparalysis. These consist of demyelination, swelling of the axis cylinders, and changes in the nerve cells.

"As the result of trauma, vasoparalysis occurs in some unknown manner, and the smaller veins and capillaries dilate to such an extent that actual slowing of the blood stream and partial or complete stasis results" (Scheinker). The action causing the vasoparalysis is indirect and can be transmitted to distant parts of the vascular tree, far removed from the site of the trauma. Following the vasoparalysis, slowed circulation results, leading to the accumulation of carbon dioxide and other metabolites. Further dilatation occurs as a result of the action of the accumulated carbon dioxide, causing increased permeability of the vessel wall. Degeneration and necrosis of the vessel wall may occur if the alterations are severe.

The most essential factor in the production of the changes in vasoparalysis is the increased permeability of the vessel wall with resulting escape of solid and fluid constituents of the vessels, and the accumulation in the widely distended perivascular spaces of serous fluid and red blood cells. The increased permeability is aided by the hypoxia which ensues from the retarded circulation.

The persistence of vasoparalysis over a prolonged period of time may lead to venous thrombosis in intact veins due to the slowing of the blood stream. In such instances, no damage to the vessel wall is demonstrable, and the changes in the surrounding tissue are similar to those observed in softenings from vascular occlusion.

The brain itself reacts to injury in many fashions. Edema is assumed to be present in every instance of brain injury of any severity. This, however, is not generally agreed upon. Unfortunately, the term "brain edema" is very loosely used, mere brain swelling or wetness being accepted loosely as edema. The application of chemical, physical, and histological criteria of brain edema throws doubt on its occurrence in severe degree in most cases of trauma. Studies of brain volume in dogs indicates an increase within a few hours after head injury, reaching a maximum by the sixth day and subsiding by the sixteenth (Fisanovich). The brain in the human appears swollen at necropsy, the gyri puffed, and the sulci often obliterated. This appearance has been regarded as due to edema of the brain consequent on the trauma. It is important, however, to keep clearly in mind that swelling of the brain and wetness of its surface need have nothing to do with edema. Indeed, the edematous brain may not appear wet on section. Investigations have shown in fact that injured brains contain less water but more blood than normal brains (Shapiro and Jackson). Measurement of the fluid content of brain tissue of animals subjected to trauma failed to reveal an increase sufficient to cause a significant rise in spinal fluid pressure (Pilcher). An increase in the fluid of the gray matter of dogs has been found after cranial trauma, but without evidence of marked cerebral edema (Pilcher). Histological studies of thirty-one traumatized brains failed to reveal evidence of generalized posttraumatic edema but showed edema limited to the neighborhood of the bruised area (Greenfield).

The issue of brain edema in head injury has not been settled, and it is still a matter of controversy whether edema is to be found after cranial trauma. Study of the cerebral hemispheres of kittens and cats reveals that there is edema of the brain after cerebral concussion, due to increased water content (Kollros). Other experimental studies reveal that concussion is associated with edema and congestion of the brain, fluid being extravasated through permeable, anoxic, capillary membranes (White, Brooks, Goldthwaite, and Adams).

Moderately severe or severe head injuries are associated often with contusions of the brain and with laceration of the brain tissue, characterized by punctate hemorrhage into the area of contusion, destruction of ganglion cells, myelin, and axis cylinders, and by the subsequent formation of a fibrous glial scar which may be the source of posttraumatic sequelae such as headache, vertigo, or convulsions. In patients with extensive brain injury due to penetrating wounds, scar formation or cerebral cicatrix develops. The lacerations and contusions which develop after head injury are found under the site of the injury or may be some distance removed from it. The contusions and lacerations of the frontal pole and the undersurface of the frontal and temporal lobes are, so to speak, injuries at a distance. *Contrecoup* injuries are common, resulting in the development of contusions in the cerebral hemisphere opposite the site of injury, or in the occurrence of subdural hemorrhage over the opposite hemisphere. The reason for *contrecoup* injuries is not definitely known.

Brain abscess develops in cases of head injury due to penetrating missiles with penetration of the dura by the bullet, fragment of bone, or other foreign object. Extradural and subdural abscess may develop at times.

The late effects of brain injury are not well-defined from the pathological standpoint. That late complications, such as abscess and scar, ensue is well known, but it is not clear what changes if any develop in the brain in instances of head injury without objective neurological signs, but with many subjective symptoms. Some indication of what takes place is found in electroencephalogram studies, but histological studies are lacking.

stitute a reliable index of the severity of the injury. Studies of the brain waves in head injuries indicate clearly that abnormal waves develop in the brain following trauma. Furthermore, it is evident that the degree of elec-

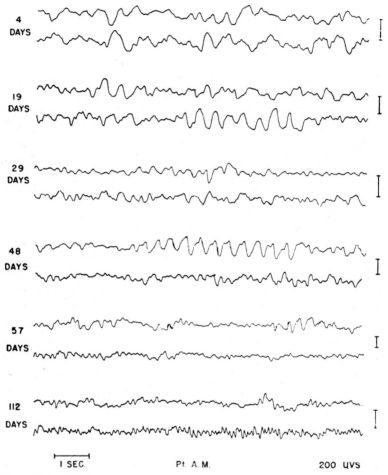

4 DAYS

19 DAYS

29 DAYS

48 DAYS

57 DAYS

112 DAYS

I SEC.   Pt. A. M.   200 UVS

Fig. 190—*Electroencephalograms* from a patient with severe head injury, cerebral concussion and contusion, and subarachnoid hemorrhage. After the injury continuous, irregular slow waves were followed by progression toward regularity of frequency and rhythm.

Electroencephalography has come to assume a greater and greater rôle in the interpretation of the effects of head injuries and the probabilities are that it will become increasingly important as more data is accumulated. The EEG abnormality in head injury is said to con-

trical abnormality parallels in general the clinical condition of the patient and the degree of injury of the brain. Concussion has been found to be associated with a diminution or cessation of the electrical activity of the entire cerebral hemisphere. Clinical improvement is followed by diminution or disappearance of the electrical abnormalities, but severe head injuries may be followed in some instances by persistence of electroencephalographic changes several years after the injury. There is, however, often a striking lack of relationship between recovery of the EEG and of the patient, and this discrepancy shows that recovery depends on other potent factors, including the basic pre-traumatic personality and

soldiers was found in sixty-seven per cent (Williams). Efforts to correlate the persistence of abnormal electroencephalographic changes and posttraumatic states suspected of being psychogenic have not as yet been conclusive.

II. FRACTURES OF THE SKULL

Types: Skull fractures may be (1) linear; (2) comminuted; (3) compound,

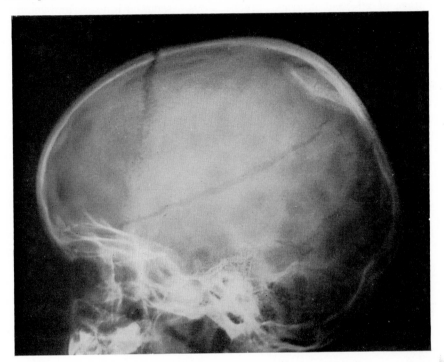

Fig. 191—*Cranial trauma.* **A large linear fracture of the frontoparietal region, without displacement of the bone.**

environmental stress as well as on the kind and severity of the injury. Focal damage of the cerebral cortex is associated with focal electrical changes. Hysteria and malingering are unassociated with abnormal electroencephalograms. Subdural hematoma is associated with a quiet or silent record over the area of hemorrhage.

Positive correlation of abnormalities in the electroencephalogram, the severity of the injury and the persistence of symptoms in a group of eighty-seven invalided

or (4) depressed. They may be primarily fractures involving the vault or the base of the skull. Under some circumstances, they may involve both the vault and the base, extending from the temporal bone into the middle fossa, from the occipital bone into the foramen magnum, or from the frontal bone into the anterior fossa.

A blow to the skull is followed by a depression at the site of the blow, whether or not fracture ensues. The uniform development of this transitory distortion has been demonstrated clearly by cathode ray oscillograph (Gurdjian).

Frequency: The frequency of skull fractures is difficult to evaluate and estimates vary widely. Among a group of 13,055 fractures, 445 or 3.3 per cent were found to involve the skull (Pancoast, Pendergrass, Schaeffer). Other estimates place the incidence at seven per cent. Fractures of the skull are found in a high percentage of all head injuries. Precise figures are difficult to obtain because many fractures involving the base of the skull are not visible by roentgenography.

Mortality: The outlook in cases of skull fracture is difficult to evaluate, since it is the condition of the underlying brain tissue which is of greater significance than the condition of the skull. This must not be taken to mean,

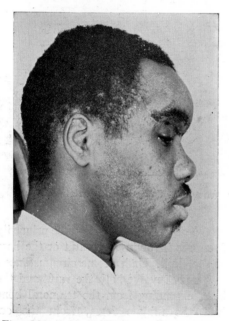

Fig. 192 — *Skull fracture* resulting from the shearing action of a steam shovel, resulting in almost complete removal of the frontal bones. The separation of the skull bones resulting from the fracture is clearly illustrated by the bulging of the forehead. The patient suffered moderate transitory headache.

however, that skull fracture is a benign and harmless injury without a respectable mortality rate. Simple linear fractures without injury to the brain probably have a low mortality. A mortality rate of ten to twelve per cent is regarded as inevitable in fractures of all types due to the occurrence of shock, the presence of massive cerebral lesions, small hemorrhages in vital centers, serious associated injuries, and complicating diseases (Mock). Among 258 persons with head injury, thirty-one per cent died (Bulynin). The mortality is distinctly higher for fractures involving the base of the skull than for those of the vault.

Linear Fractures of the Vault: The posterior (occipital) and lateral (temporal, parietal) portions of the skull are more often involved by fracture than the frontal areas, though the incidence of the latter is not low. Among 445 skull fractures, 120 were frontal, 239 occipital seventy-six posterior fossa, and ten were at the base of the skull (Pancoast, *et al.*). The incidence of the location of skull fractures varies widely from one series to another. Roughly estimated, about one-half of the vault fractures involve the lateral aspects of the skull, about one-third the posterior portions, and about one-sixth the frontal areas. If the fracture line is long, it may extend from the vault into the base of the skull.

Skull fracture is associated with a varying *period of unconsciousness* which may be fleeting in some instances or may persist for several hours or longer in others, depending on the degree of brain injury. In fractures uncomplicated by injury to the brain tissue, the period of unconsciousness is not usually long. *Headache* is always present, and constitutes the chief problem in many cases. Not uncommonly, skull fracture may be found with few or no symptoms of injury.

Nausea and vomiting are often seen. *Confusion and delirium* are often found for varying periods of time, and tend to be more prolonged in severe cases. Outward *evidences of injury* are practically always present in the form of scalp or face wounds. The pulse is rapid but may be slow in some instances, the respirations increased, and the temperature may

place in most cases without sequelae. In some, persistent headache or vertigo may follow.

Depressed Fractures: In a small percentage of cases, fractures of the vault are depressed in character. The depression in civil life may be found with intact scalp or in association with a compound fracture. In warfare, depressed fractures

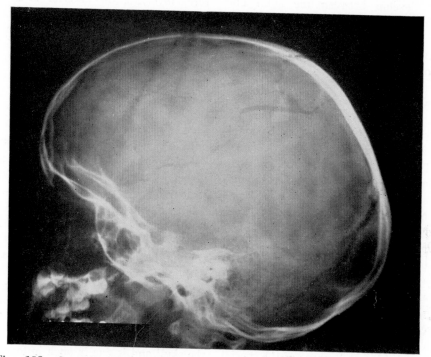

Fig. 193—*Cranial trauma.* A linear fracture of the frontoparietal area with depression and displacement of bone in the parietal region.

be slightly elevated. Neck stiffness is present in subjects with hemorrhage into the meninges and a bloody spinal fluid may be obtained on lumbar tap of such patients. The *spinal fluid* in the majority of subjects is clear and may be under increased pressure.

Recovery from the acute episode is fast in most instances, provided that the skull fracture is unassociated with injury of the brain or the meninges. Consciousness is regained and headache becomes more prominent. Recovery takes

are almost always compound. They result from blows with a blunt object, a blackjack, the head of a cane, a stone, etc. Most depressed fractures are found in the frontal regions of the skull. The degree of injury varies. There may be only slight depression without pressure on the brain substance, or severe depression with fracture and depression of the inner table of the skull with laceration of the underlying brain and meninges, and with bone spicules driven into the brain tissue.

In this type of fracture particularly, the damage to the underlying brain tissue is most important. Some subjects escape without brain injury; most of them suffer lacerations and contusion. Many of these develop meningeal adhesions or brain scars later, some of which serve as foci for the development of epileptic attacks. As a result of the laceration, firm adhesions develop between the skull and meninges, the meninges and brain, and scar tissue is found in the underlying lacerated brain substances.

Not all depressed fractures are associated with injury of the brain tissue. Many, however, are, and when this occurs, evidence of focal brain damage is invariably present. This may be manifested as a monoplegia, such as facial, hand, or arm weakness, as aphasia, or as a convulsive attack. The general symptoms of brain trauma, such as headache, loss of consciousness, vomiting, and confusion, are always present. Blood is found in varying amounts in the spinal fluid due to laceration of the meninges and the brain. Roentgenograms of the skull will reveal the depressed fracture, a diagnosis often not easily made by palpation because of confusion of the edge of a hematoma beneath the scalp with a depressed fragment of bone. Because of the special problems created by the depression of the bony fragment and the injury of the brain tissue, the treatment of a depressed fracture differs from that of a simple linear fracture. This will be considered subsequently.

Fracture of the Base: The occurrence of fractures of the base of the skull is difficult to estimate, since in many the fracture line cannot be demonstrated by the roentgenogram. It has been estimated that only fifty per cent of fractures at the base are visible by this method, and base fractures are therefore frequently overlooked. Reliance must be placed, therefore, upon their clinical features and less upon their demonstration by roentgenogram.

The majority of base fractures are found to involve the anterior and middle fossae of the skull, especially affecting the frontal and temporal bones. Some base fractures involve the posterior fossa.

1. *Anterior Fossa Fracture:* Fractures involving the anterior fossa may result from (1) extension of a linear fracture of the frontal bone into the anterior fossa, or (2) primary involvement of the anterior fossa with or without extension into the vault.

The fracture line in such cases may involve (1) the orbital plate alone or in conjunction with other parts of the anterior portion of the base of the skull; (2) the paranasal sinuses—frontal, maxillary, or ethmoid; (3) the ethmoid plate region.

The symptoms of anterior fossa fracture include, of course, those referable to all head injuries; namely, a history of trauma, headache, and a variable period of loss of consciousness.

Bleeding from the nose is only suggestive of a fracture in this region. It is found frequently in patients with head injury without fracture of the base of the skull and is due in such instances to damage to the mucous membranes of the nose or to fracture of the nasal bones. Nose bleeding may be suspected as being due to fracture of the anterior fossa when it is persistent as a steady flow for several hours.

Orbital ecchymosis is suggestive of a fracture line through the orbital plate forming the roof of the orbit. This is a fragile plate of bone, easily fractured. The orbital ecchymosis of anterior fossa fractures is confined to the upper and lower lids, is sharply demarcated, associated with swelling, and does not extend into the surrounding tissue. In cases of direct blows to the orbital region, the ecchymosis resembles the ordinary "black eye," the discoloration and swelling involving not only the eyelids but the adjacent face as well.

Leakage of spinal fluid is, of course, bona fide evidence that a fracture of the anterior fossa is present, involving the region of the cribriform plate. Spinal fluid leakage occurs as a rule after a head-on injury to the forehead or sometimes to the face, and is usually associated with a depressed frontal fracture or a linear fracture extending into the cribriform plate region. The spinal fluid leak is due to rupture of the arachnoid membrane and dura, permitting fluid to escape through the nose. It may be seen as a clear watery discharge, escaping in a steady drip or mixed with blood, in which case it is found as a pinkish discharge from the nose. The discharge appears to be increased on sitting up.

Spinal fluid leakage usually develops as a result of acute head injury, but it may develop spontaneously late in the course of the fracture. Delayed leakage of this variety results from rupture of the dura and arachnoid which has been torn and then sealed off again during the course of the acute injury. Violent sneezing or nose blowing reopens the sealed-off area. Spontaneous leakage of fluid usually heals spontaneously but is apt to continue indefinitely and can only be helped in such instances by repair of the dural laceration by suture or fascial transplant. This must be performed as promptly as possible to prevent the development of meningitis.

Injury to the optic nerve may result from anterior fossa fractures. Primary optic atrophy may develop on one or both sides and may be complete or incomplete. The light reflex is lost early in such cases. In rare instances, the optic chiasm may be torn and visual field defects ensue. In patients with extensive hemorrhage into the orbit, complete ophthalmoplegia may result with ptosis of the eyelid, dilatation of the pupil, inactivity of the pupil to light and in accommodation, and loss of movement of the eyeball.

Signs of *meningeal irritation* (Kernig's sign, neck stiffness) are almost always found, due to the presence of blood in the spinal fluid. In some cases, a purulent meningitis may develop rapidly and may be associated with high fever. Meningitis is most apt to develop if the fracture line passes through the nasal sinuses, but occurs also by ascending infection from the nose when there is fracture of the cribriform plate.

Pneumencephaly or air in the brain develops sometimes in patients with dural tears and cribriform plate fractures, and results from aspiration of air, by sneezing or blowing the nose, into the ventricles, under the dura, or into the brain itself. The air is usually subdural, but if a cerebral laceration is present, air may enter the ventricle through this tear. It is associated with severe headache and even unconsciousness. Roentgenograms of the skull will reveal the presence of air. The dural laceration must be repaired in order to relieve the condition. Failure to do so results in the aspiration of more air into the cranial cavity or brain so long as the dural defect remains open.

2. Middle Fossa Fracture: Not infrequently fractures involve the petrous portion of the temporal bone, either by extension of a long vault fracture or by primary involvement of this portion of the temporal bone. In the latter instance, the fracture line is usually not visible by roentgenogram and external evidences of the fracture must be relied on for diagnosis.

Bleeding from the ear is a frequent symptom, but it is not diagnostic of middle fossa fracture. It results usually from tearing of the tympanic membrane due to the injury or from a laceration of the external auditory canal. These are by far the most common causes of bleeding from the ear due to head injury. The presence of ecchymosis over the tip of the mastoid bone (Battle's sign) will confirm the impression of a temporal bone fracture.

Spinal fluid leakage from the ear establishes a middle fossa fracture definitely. It is caused by a tear of the dura and arachnoid adjacent to the temporal bone, the fluid escaping through a ruptured tympanic membrane into the external ear. It is seen as a leakage of pure fluid or as a pinkish fluid due to admixture with blood. The leakage stops frequently after thirty-six to forty-eight hours, but may persist in some cases.

Paralysis of the facial nerve may follow in some cases if the fracture extends into the fallopian canal. This is a typical peripheral facial paralysis which may result from a tear of the nerve or from hemorrhage into the sheath. The facial paralysis may develop immediately and in such cases is due to a laceration of the facial nerve. In some instances, the paralysis develops gradually or late (two or three weeks after fracture), due to choking of the nerve by scar tissue. The paralysis is typical, with loss of power of the forehead muscles, inability to close the eyelid, and loss of power of the muscles of facial expression. Most cases of facial paralysis gradually develop after middle fossa fracture recovery, but if the nerve is torn permanent paralysis results unless the nerve is repaired. The facial paralysis may develop within a few days or a few weeks and may recover within six to eight weeks to three to four months.

Diplopia and *external strabismus* are sometimes seen. *Tinnitus* and *deafness* may develop, with partial or complete deafness. Tinnitus is usually permanent and evades successful treatment. *Vertigo* is a common symptom, due to hemorrhage into the labyrinth. It is, as a rule, true vertigo of a subjective or objective type, often associated with nausea and vomiting. It tends to disappear in two to four weeks but may persist as a permanent disability. Signs of *meningeal irritation* are often present due to the presence of blood in the spinal fluid. In subjects with otorrhea, purulent meningitis may ensue.

Compound Fractures and Penetrating Wounds: Penetrating wounds of the skull are of greatest importance in war but are significant also in civil practice. Penetrating wounds of the skull may escape without penetration of the dura; or the dura may be penetrated and with it fragments of bone driven into the brain, together with the extrusion of brain tissue; or there may be penetration of the bullet or bone fragments into the cerebral ventricles or the nasal sinuses.

The brain injury in such cases is characterized by scar formation of the brain at the site of injury with firm adherence of the meninges to the edges of the skull opening. In the acute stages of the injury there is extensive laceration of the meninges and brain with numerous hemorrhages not only adjacent to the path of the missile but scattered in the brain tissue at considerable distance from the injury as well. In addition, there is extensive scar formation along the path of the missile. As in other brain scars, there is a distortion of the brain tissue and a displacement of the lateral ventricle due to the contraction of the cicatrix. The symptoms due to penetrating wounds are the result of (1) the penetration of the missile; (2) the tissue destruction; (3) the scar formation at the point of entry and along the course of the bullet or other penetrating object.

The severity of the symptoms depends to a large extent on the severity of the injury of the brain tissue. *Unconsciousness* in varying degree is present in almost all cases. It is not always present, however, even in severe penetrating injuries. Headache, vertigo, vomiting, bradycardia, and hyperthermia are common. Focal symptoms of various sorts develop, depending on the areas of destruction of brain tissue. Memory loss, personality changes, and aphasia may result from frontal lobe injury. *Focal brain damage* is much more frequent than in closed head injuries. Hemiplegia or monoplegia are found, the latter involving face, arm, or leg in various combinations. Blindness or oculomotor paralysis may develop if the missile penetrates the orbit. Hemianopsia from involvement of the temporal or occipital lobes is sometimes present after gunshot injury. Penetrating skull wounds show a strong tendency to spontaneous recovery.

More important even than the acute symptoms are the *late symptoms* and sequelae of gunshot wounds. Among the late symptoms may be listed vertigo, depression, amnesia, memory defect, and personality changes which often disappear in three to nine months. Among the *sequelae* of importance are (1) cranial defects, which often require repair by cranioplasty; (2) convulsions, which may develop as late as fifteen years after gunshot wounds, but are found more usually from two to five years after the accident. They are usually generalized, but may be focal or jacksonian seizures, and they are similar in their features to convulsions of idiopathic epilepsy. Their frequency varies from an occasional convulsive attack occurring once a year or even less to numerous attacks. They result usually from cerebral scars, but

they may develop also as a result of generalized brain injury in the form of punctate hemorrhages or ischemic areas with resulting small scar formations. (3) Arteriovenous aneurysm may develop after gunshot injury, usually in the cavernous sinus region. It is characterized by pulsating exophthalmos, oculomotor paralyses varying from weakness of the external rectus muscle and slight palsy of other eye movements to complete ophthalmoplegia, hypalgesia over the first division of the trigeminal nerve, and a to-and-fro bruit heard not only over the eyeball but over other parts of the skull as well.

The problem in penetrating and compound wounds of the skull is concerned largely with the *question of management*. It is generally agreed that immediate surgical intervention is not necessary in most cases, and that both in civil and war cases the immediate problem is the arrest of hemorrhage and the care of shock, the prevention and limitation of infection of the wound, the maintenance of brain damage to a minimum, and the prevention of sequelae. Complete debridement of the wound is essential within forty-eight hours of injury, the mortality rate increasing after this period. Experience in World War II has shown that operation may be delayed as long as forty-eight hours and that hasty operations are harmful. Munro believes that surgical intervention after forty-eight hours has a prohibitively high rate of infection. Sulfonamides should be given by mouth for at least forty-eight hours. One of the sulfonamide compounds may be sprinkled on the wound and brain as soon after injury as possible, but sulfathiazole should not be dusted on the brain because of the tendency to produce convulsions. Since compound fractures of the skull are open wounds, every effort must be made to convert them into closed wounds with a minimum degree of damage to the brain and without infection. Debridement of the wound, therefore, must be complete and must avoid infection and the increase of the already existent brain damage. Bone need not be removed unnecessarily, the dura should not be opened if it is undamaged, and deeply seated missiles should not be sought after for fear of introducing infection and damaging tissue. In 130 patients operated on with special attention to the care of shock, complete debridement, and the prevention of infection, the mortality rate was only 9.2 per cent and postoperative sepsis only 7.6 per cent (Munro).

III. CEREBRAL CONCUSSION

There is no general agreement as to what should be included among cases of head injury referred to as cerebral concussion. The generally accepted view among most neurologists is that cerebral concussion is a condition characterized by transitory unconsciousness, with no evidence of structural brain damage. Some include cases also of cerebral contusion among those of concussion, but it seems best to reserve the term for cases with complete clinical recovery. It would be ideal, of course, to include under cerebral concussion only those cases which have no evidence of brain injury. It is precisely this data, however, which is lacking, since not enough is known of the concussed brain to say that no visible damage is found in any instance of the disorder. Hence the criterion must be clinical recovery. This is true, of course, of other forms of brain injury, such as subarachnoid hemorrhage, contusion, etc., but in all these instances evidence of brain damage is present as shown by hemorrhage in the spinal fluid, signs of focal brain damage, etc. It is possible that in concussion the brain damage is of a totally different nature, being pri-

marily an interference with the physical-chemical cell relationship and an interference, therefore, with cell function on this basis.

Pathology: The *pathology* of cerebral concussion is not known definitely, a situation which is responsible for much of the uncertainty which exists concerning the nature of the condition. Most cerebral concussion patients recover, so that no study is possible of the nervous system in the condition. Of those which die and show brain changes, death has ensued too rapidly to permit a correlation of symptoms and damage. Most of the patients show no evidence of brain damage.

In experimentally produced concussion in guinea pigs, cats, and monkeys, chromatolysis of certain neurons was found to occur within twenty-four hours (Windle, Groat, and Magoun). Changes were most constant in the lateral vestibular nuclei and the scattered large neurons of the brain stem tegmentum. The red nuclei, the nuclei of the trigeminal tract, the medial vestibular, and cochlear nuclei became involved. The large pyramidal cells of the cerebral cortex showed alterations but no chromatolysis. In some, punctate perivascular hemorrhages have been found scattered in the cerebral cortex and white matter and in the medulla. Recent physiological investigations (Denny-Brown and Russell) indicate that concussion may be produced by a physiological mechanism in which acceleration of the head and depression of medullary mechanisms play an important rôle. Pure concussion, according to their investigations, can be produced by subjecting an animal's head to a rate of change of velocity (acceleration concussion) of approximately twenty-eight feet (865 cm.) per second.

According to these studies of experimental concussion in cats, dogs, and monkeys, the condition is regarded as a direct traumatic paralysis of nervous function without vascular lesion, persisting for a varying period, depending on the type and severity of the injury. There ensues transient reflex paralysis of the respiratory and vasomotor mechanisms and of the reflex mechanisms of the pons and medulla. Concussion due to acceleration is not associated with change in intracranial pressure. Failure of blood pressure in severe head injury is identical with surgical shock and is associated with peripheral vasoconstriction and paralysis of the venous side of the circulation. Death in such concussion is due to failure of the blood pressure through failure of the vasomotor centers or from lack of recovery from the effect on the vasoglossopharyngeal mechanisms.

Opposed to the paralytic concept of concussion is that which maintains that concussion is associated with evidence of diffuse stimulation of nerve cells and that it is due to stimulative rather than paralytic factors (Walker). The loss of consciousness and the other phenomena of concussion are attributed to paralytic effects on the nerve cells of the hypothalamus (Jefferson).

Shear strain rather than acceleration is regarded as the chief mechanism of brain injuries (Halborn). According to this concept, five properties of brain tissue must be considered in the understanding of brain injuries. These are: (1) its comparatively uniform density; (2) its extreme incompressibility; (3) its small resistance to changes in shape; (4) its feeble rigidity as compared with the skull; (5) the shape of the brain and the skull. Shear strain may be associated with or without distortion of the skull. The skull reacts to a direct blow by indentation or fracture and in either event the shear strain is superficial and confined to the area of depression or fracture. The chief sources of brain injury are rotational acceleration forces. A blow on the occiput with forward rotation causes a large amount of shear strain in the anterior part of the temporal lobe. Rotation in the horizontal plane produced by a blow near the upper jaw or temples causes most strain at the sides of the convexities. Collision of the head with stationary objects is more likely to cause rotation than impact by moving objects. Other concepts concerning the mechanism of concussion maintain that at the time of injury there is compression of the brain, a diminution in its volume, squeezing of the spinal fluid out of the perivascular and perineuronal spaces and deprivation therefore of food substances of the nerve cells. Still others believe that the damage is to the vegetative centers in the hypothalamus, the blow being transmitted through the ventricular fluid.

Study of the enzymes of the spinal fluid reveals that following concussion there is a splitting of nucleic acids, the origin of the enzymes responsible for the reaction probably being in the brain tissue (Spiegel).

Symptoms: The *symptoms* of cerebral concussion are characterized by headache, by loss of consciousness of some degree and by retrograde amnesia for the accident. This may be a fleeting feeling of being dazed or it may be a total loss of consciousness lasting for several minutes to several hours (six to forty-eight hours). The assumption is made, as a rule, that if the loss of consciousness lasts for an appreciable length of time, cerebral contusion or laceration must be present, but complete recovery in those cases without evidence of local brain damage makes such an assumption doubtful.

The description of the symptoms of

concussion is difficult to fit into a single pattern. In very *mild cases,* the result of the head injury may be merely a dazed feeling in which the patient is incapacitated for a few to several minutes, feels cold and nauseated, shows some change in the pulse, but is able to resume his activities in a short time, either with complete recovery or with a feeling of haziness which gradually wears off. In *more severe cases* there is more prolonged loss of consciousness from which the patient gradually emerges. There is usually loss of memory for the accident; and there may be a slight temperature elevation, bradycardia, and a slight fall in blood pressure. *Headache* is present in almost all cases, sometimes mild, at other times severe. It, too, disappears gradually but may persist as a stubborn sequel of the injury. It is made worse by sitting up and by increasing intracranial pressure by coughing, sneezing, or other means.

Vertigo is also a distressing though not a constant complaint after cerebral concussion. It may be a severe episodic vertigo occurring in attacks or it may be mild. It is usually aggravated by change of posture. It tends to disappear in most cases, but may persist. As the patient emerges from his unconsciousness, he exhibits some degree of confusion, either of a mild or severe degree. This may consist of disorientation and memory disturbance or it may be so severe as to produce delirium, severe confusion, and other psychotic states. This, too, clears up in the majority of cases within a few weeks. Neurological examination reveals nothing, either during the acute stages or later. The general picture is that of a person in shock, the depth of the latter depending on the severity of the injury. Coldness of the skin is usually found, the skin may be wet due to a cold perspiration, the pulse

is rapid but sometimes slowed, the respirations are increased, and the temperature is normal, slightly elevated or slightly decreased. Leukopenia is claimed by some to be part of the concussion syndrome. The spinal fluid pressure may be increased in the acute stage due to brain edema, but no other abnormalities are found in the spinal fluid. The electroencephalogram is said to be abnormal in cases of concussion, these abnormal waves persisting and permitting differentiation between organic and psychogenic posttraumatic states. The brain in experimental cerebral concussion is associated with diminution or cessation of the electrical activity of the whole cerebral hemispheres as seen in the electroencephalogram.

"Punch drunk" or traumatic encephalopathy offers a good example of the effects of concussion. This condition is seen in fighters who have been subjected to constant battering and is characterized by interference with intellectual functions, producing slowness of thought, memory loss, personality changes, and even episodes of confusion. The condition is the result of repeated cerebral concussions from blows to the head.

Diagnosis: The *diagnosis* of concussion is made in retrospect after the patient has recovered or after it is clear that he has no indication of damage to the brain. It might be assumed if concussion is unassociated with visible brain damage, that no aftereffects should follow. This, of course, is not the case, since transient damage of a physiochemical nature may follow without changes in the brain structure. It is possible that in the patients with aftereffects or permanent sequelae, damage of an ischemic or hemorrhagic nature does occur independent of the primary physiochemical change. It is impossible to assert in the acute stages of the head injury while the patient is still unconscious that cerebral concussion is present. This can be done only when emergence from unconsciousness occurs. In this sense the diagnosis of cerebral concussion becomes a diagnosis by exclusion. In patients with prolonged unconsciousness, extradural or subdural hemorrhage may be confused with concussion. In the former patients, the stupor tends to become more pronounced with time, while in concussion it tends to lessen and clear up. Blood in the spinal fluid will help in establishing a diagnosis of subdural hematoma if this is suspected, since acute subdural hemorrhage due to trauma often ruptures into the subarachnoid space. A tendency to elevation of temperature, falling pulse, and rising blood pressure favors extradural hemorrhage. Increase in the depth of the unconsciousness also favors hemorrhage as opposed to concussion.

Prognosis: The *prognosis* of concussion cannot be gauged with accuracy because various writers include in the condition not only pure concussion but also cases of contusion and laceration as well. Certain general principles may be established, however. Among these are the following: Most patients with concussion recover within a few days to several weeks (eight to ten weeks), depending upon the severity of the injury. In some patients recovery is slower and may take place anywhere up to six months. In others, permanent disability ensues, the figures varying from sixteen to twenty-five per cent in different clinics. Recovery tends to be slower and after-effects more numerous in older people beyond the ages of forty-five to fifty. Generally speaking, the longer the period of unconsciousness the more severe and the more prolonged the symptoms, and the greater the tendency to sequelae. Complete and quite rapid recovery,

however, may follow a severe injury and incomplete recovery a comparatively insignificant trauma. The presence of compensation factors retards recovery in many instances, patients using their symptoms unconsciously to justify their claims. Symond asserts that after a period of unconsciousness up to one hour, nineteen out of twenty persons will be back at full work within two months. If stupor persists longer than twenty-four hours, the chances are against the patient being fit for work within two months, but eight of ten patients will be able to return to full work within six months.

IV. CEREBRAL CONTUSION AND LACERATION

The distinction between concussion and cerebral contusion or laceration is one of degree. Many authors include the latter in the concussion group. The incidence of contusion and laceration is 43 per cent of a large group of head injuries (Munro).

The *pathology* of contusion and laceration is more definite than that of concussion. Contusions and lacerations may be present with or without skull fracture. Their location varies depending on the site of injury, but they may be found anywhere in the cerebral hemispheres. The base of the frontal lobes and the tip of the temporal lobes are sites of predilection. Contusion is characterized by hemorrhage into the brain substance. These are discrete or confluent and confined to the cortex or spread into the white matter. The brain in such areas has a bluish cyanotic appearance. Hemorrhage is found in the meninges in these areas. Tear of the affected tissue is found when laceration is present. Microscopic examination shows small hemorrhages around vessels with destruction of the adjacent brain tissue. Scar formation develops in these areas on recovery, due to the development of gliosis and adherence of the meninges to the contused and lacerated area.

The *symptoms* are similar to those of concussion. Shock in varying degrees is present, depending on the severity of the injury. Unconsciousness is the rule and is likewise variable in degree and duration. Headache and vertigo are prominent symptoms. Convulsions may occur at times as a result of contusion and laceration. Neurological examination is often negative, but may reveal evidence of focal damage, such as monoplegia or hemiplegia, providing the laceration is in the proper location. The spinal fluid is found often to contain blood, and is under increased pressure in most but not in all cases. Roentgenograms of the skull may show evidence of fracture.

The *diagnosis* as opposed to concussion is more clean cut. Contusion or laceration, or both, may be established when (1) unconsciousness is unusually prolonged and sequelae present; (2) blood is found in the spinal fluid; (3) evidences of focal damage are present.

V. BLAST INJURIES

Blast injuries have assumed importance as a result of experiences in World War II. They are of three types: (1) *atmospheric* blast injuries resulting from a wave generated by an explosion; (2) *immersion* blast injuries resulting from a shock wave under water; and (3) *solid* blast injuries due to a wave transmitted through a solid structure, such as a steel deck.

The *symptoms* resulting from blast resemble those of concussion. In rare instances, subdural hematoma may follow. Opinions are divided concerning the importance of blast as a cause of cerebral symptoms, one group of investigators maintaining that symptoms occur referable to blast, while others believe that

blast is incapable of causing specific damage to the nervous system (Denny-Brown), and that 90 per cent of the cases so diagnosed are in reality acute hysterical-anxiety syndromes (Schwab).

Atmospheric blast is associated with severe pulmonary damage in the form of hemorrhage, and little or no evidence of brain damage. Despite the latter, symptoms such as headache, backache, confusional states, personality change, and subdural hematoma have been described.

Immersion blast is characterized by the fact that the portion of the body submerged in water is more seriously injured than that exposed to air, and the surface of the body toward the source of the blast is injured more severely than that portion away from the blast. Brain damage is not significant in immersion blast.

VI. MENINGEAL AND CEREBRAL HEMORRHAGE

Meningeal Hemorrhage: Hemorrhage into the meninges is not uncommon after head injury. Such hemorrhage may be extradural, subdural, or subarachnoid. These have already been considered in detail and the reader is referred for a discussion of them to Chapter 5 (Diseases of the Meninges).

Mention should be made of the intracranial hematomas encountered in warfare as compared with those of civil life. Only 83 hematomas were found in a group of 2000 missile wounds. A study of these cases reveals that the hematomas of warfare differ from those of civil life in the following respects: (1) they are not progressive; (2) cerebral compression is less important as a cause of death than direct neural damage inflicted by the missile; (3) the lucid interval is often absent because of the severity of the original brain lesion; and (4) neurological signs in excess of what might be expected from the radiographic appearances are of value in reaching a diagnosis, but slow pulse and raised blood pressure are not.

Subarachnoid Hemorrhage: Hemorrhage in the subarachnoid space following head injury may occur under a variety of circumstances. It may be present with or without fracture of the skull. It may occur with fractures of the vault or the base of the skull, with laceration and contusion of the brain, in association with subdural hemorrhage or with hemorrhage into the brain. It may and most often does occur without associated brain injury.

The *symptoms* are quite uniform. Unconsciousness in some degree is always present. Evidences of shock are seen. The temperature is often slightly elevated (100° F.), but in some instances may be higher (102° to 103° F.). Headache is constant and often very severe. Signs of meningeal irritation (neck stiffness and/or Kernig's sign) are present but in rare instances may be absent. Focal signs of brain damage are usually absent when the hemorrhage is chiefly over the cerebral hemisphere but hemiparesis or monoplegias may be seen. Cranial nerve palsies may be found when the hemorrhage involves the base of the brain. Optic atrophy or optic neuritis develops in rare instances when the hemorrhage involves the sheath of the optic nerve. Oculomotor palsies in varying degree are sometimes seen. Peripheral facial paralysis may be found.

The spinal fluid is always bloody. It may show an admixture of blood and spinal fluid in less severe cases or simulate venous blood in more severe instances. The spinal fluid pressure is elevated as a rule.

The condition clears up without sequelae in most cases, but severe headache or vertigo may follow in some instances. In those patients in whom the subarachnoid hemorrhage is part of a generalized severe brain injury, recovery does not follow, but in instances of uncomplicated subarachnoid hemorrhage recovery is the rule.

Cerebral Hemorrhage: In rare instances, head injury may be associated with massive hemorrhage into the brain substance similar to that found in apoplexy. Such cases are usually associated with very severe head injury and with skull fracture, though in rare cases no fracture of the skull is found. In such patients, the problem always arises whether the brain hemorrhage preceded the head injury or followed it. The symptoms are similar to those of cerebral hemorrhage.

Hemorrhages into the brain stem, especially the pons, are often found in brain hemorrhage following trauma.

In very rare instances, *delayed cerebral hemorrhage* is found following head injury. These are of two varieties, early and late. In the early type, the hemorrhage occurs within a few weeks of the injury, probably as a result of traumatic weakening of an arterial wall. In the late variety, the interval between injury and apoplexy may be several months or even years. The mechanism in this type is assumed to be hemorrhage into a cyst resulting from intracerebral hemorrhage at the time of injury.

VII. THE AFTEREFFECTS OF HEAD INJURY

Head injuries may be associated with a number of aftereffects. These are of many varieties and include such conditions as the posttraumatic syndrome, hemorrhage, infection, pneumocele, and convulsive states.

Posttraumatic Syndrome: For want of a better term, a well-defined group of symptoms easily recognized by all is referred to as the posttraumatic syndrome or often as the postconcussional syndrome. The latter term is less preferable since the symptoms may develop following concussion, contusion, or more severe states following head injury. It is also stigmatized as posttraumatic neurosis. Of all the sequelae of head injury, it is the most difficult to cope with, since the symptoms are usually not associated with definite signs of nervous system damage. The problem in such instances is invariably that of psychogenic versus organic or structural, and the issue is decided often on the preconceived prejudices of the examiner.

A few facts must be emphasized as pertinent to the problem of the posttraumatic syndrome. These are: (1) The symptoms which comprise this syndrome may develop after trivial head injuries or after severe injuries. (2) The syndrome is composed entirely of subjective complaints, such as headache, vertigo, fatigue, insomnia, and anxiety. For these there is no objective proof; hence everything depends on the evaluation of the examining physician. (3) The symptoms persist for a varying period of time, but this variability cannot be used as a measuring rod to judge of the psychogenic or structural features of the problem.

The symptoms which characterize the posttraumatic syndrome are almost uniform in their expression and stereotyped in their manifestations. *Headache* is often prominent; *dizziness* is found in many instances. Headache, however, usually dominates the picture, is resistant to all forms of therapy, and is persistent. Associated with it is *easy fatigue,* often a feeling of ill-defined tension, lack of appetite, insomnia, marked anxiety, disturbance of memory, and a variable number of nonspecific symptoms.

Headache is one of the commonest of the posttraumatic sequelae. It clears up in most of the patients soon after the injury but is persistent in others. It may follow concussion, skull fracture, menin-

geal hemorrhage or indeed any type of injury. While headache is apt to follow more frequently severe head injury, it is not uncommonly found after mild or insignificant head trauma. Headache was not significantly more common in patients in the posttraumatic period in cases with increased spinal-fluid pressure or bloody spinal fluid (Friedman and Merritt). Some believe that adequate prolonged rest will prevent posttraumatic headaches to a large degree: others see no association between the two It is the most persistent of the symptoms following head injury. It has specific characteristics. Thus it is usually described as constant, generalized and is often affected by change of posture of the head or by increasing intracranial pressure. In many instances, it may be localized at the point of injury. It may be paroxysmal, lasting from one to three hours at a time. It is aggravated by mental and physical effort.

In many instances, posttraumatic headache tends to disappear gradually; in others, it continues indefinitely. In the cases with an organic basis, the headache is due to meningeal adhesions which produce the symptom by traction on the dural sinuses. In some patients, the headache is of psychogenic origin and under such conditions compensation litigation is apt to aggravate and prolong it. The treatment of posttraumatic headache is difficult. Some patients respond to insufflation of air into the brain in order to break up the adhesions; others recover slowly; a small percentage do not recover. In those in whom compensation is a factor, equitable settlement of the case should be carried out as promptly as possible. Psychotherapy may be necessary despite settlement.

Vertigo is fully as common as headache after injury and is often combined with it. It disappears within two weeks to two months in the majority of cases. In others it is persistent. Most cases of posttraumatic "dizziness" are not in reality vertigo, but are ill-defined sensations often described as dizziness. "Dizziness" of this sort is constant, unaffected by posture and vegetative symptoms, and is apt to be part of a number of other somatic complaints of psychogenic origin. Whether such cases are due to structural damage or not must be decided on the facts in each case. In many patients, they are not due to organic damage to the brain. True vertigo is found sometimes after trauma and has all the features of true dizziness. It is usually episodic, appears on change of posture of the head or body, and is associated with nausea or vomiting. Such vertigo results usually from hemorrhage into the labyrinths but may be due to brain stem involvement. The treatment of posttraumatic vertigo is that of vertigo due to other causes (q.v.).

Associated with headache and vertigo are often fatigability, sleeplessness, general anxiety, dyspepsia, difficulty in concentration, depression, and a variety of other symptoms.

The handling of the symptoms referred to as the posttraumatic syndrome requires great patience and understanding The symptoms must be regarded as due to a mixture of structural damage and the emotional reaction thereto. A judicious appraisal of the problem requires a proper appreciation of the pretraumatic personality and constitution, the severity of the general injury to the brain, the residual intellectual and physical state, and the nature and degree of persistent anxiety (Denny-Brown). Too little attention has been directed to the personality structure prior to the head injury, a factor which must be evaluated carefully in order to appraise fairly the residual anxiety. Attention to this factor will reveal often an unstable emotional structure, in which case the symptoms should be regarded as chiefly or entirely of psychogenic origin. In the absence of proof of a previously unstable personality, it is hazardous to assume that the symptoms are of purely psychogenic origin. Efforts to explain the reasons for the anxiety and the constellation of symptoms following head injury have not been fruitful. Studies indicate that the longer the period of posttraumatic amnesia, the greater the tendency to persistence of symptoms and the development of invalidism. No correlation appears to exist between the length and degree of unconsciousness and the severity of the injury and the development of the posttraumatic syndrome. Nor is it possible to assert arbitrarily that the symptoms which comprise the posttraumatic state are due to structural damage up to an arbitrary period such as six months following injury, after which they must be assumed to be psychogenic in origin.

A careful follow-up study of a large group of head injuries (200) showed the following (Denny-Brown): Factors of bad prognostic significance for return to work in two months were: disorientation, one to seven days; transient abnormality in EEG; initial restlessness or excitement; abnormality in reflexes; other disease or injury; questions of compensation or litigation; fracture of the skull; blood in spinal fluid in first two days; initial apathy; defect in intellectual performance late in hospital stay; age over forty years. Factors of bad prognostic significance for return in six months were: disorientation, one to seven days; laceration of scalp with compound fracture; initial apathy; age over forty years; injury to other parts; blood in spinal fluid in first two days; fracture of skull; abnormality in reflexes, initial emotional disturbance; other disease; abnormality of EEG; questions of compensation or litigation. Post-concussional symptoms, where chronic, occur in a large number of subjects who were neurotic prior to the accident (Guttmann). This view is held by many.

The most effective *treatment* of the condition must of necessity be prophylactic. After careful study and appraisal of the head injury, if nothing of a serious nature is found, the problem should be discussed frankly with the patient, an effort being made to relieve all anxiety concerning the trauma. Many patients can be saved by this procedure. Once the syndrome becomes established, efforts at rehabilitation become extremely difficult and are often hampered by problems of compensation, interfering lawyers, fear of insanity, and other factors. Prolonged reëducation is required in such cases. Encephalogram has been found helpful in dispelling the headache in some cases.

Convulsions: Epileptic attacks following head injury usually follow penetrating wounds of the skull with subsequent scar formation of the brain. In a small percentage of cases they follow brain injuries without evidence of fracture. There is a high incidence of seizures in patients with penetration of the dura; laceration of the brain by bone fragments or missiles; healed brain abscesses, and severe meningocerebral laceration. Seizures are usually not found in closed head injuries (except in rare subjects with a dural scar as the result of contusion); subdural meningitis (except rarely where there is a meningeal scar); simple meningitis, and chronic internal hydrocephalus (Penfield). Seizures are twice as frequent in persons whose dura has been penetrated (Ascroft). The incidence of posttraumatic convulsions is hard to establish, since most statistics are on the basis of gunshot wounds in war. The incidence is variously computed at from 2.5 to 34 per cent of craniocerebral in-

juries. In a series of 630 patients with head injury, traumatic epilepsy was found in 8.4 per cent (Denny-Brown).

Convulsions may develop within a few hours or several years after a head injury. In the latter case, it is always difficult to assess the rôle played by the

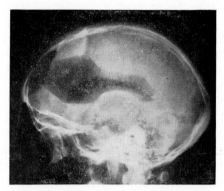

Fig. 194—*(See: Fig. 195.)*

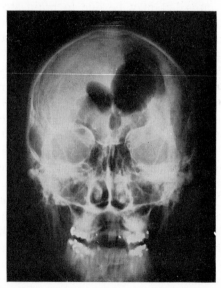

Fig. 195—*Cranial trauma.* A large porencephalic cyst in the left frontal lobe following a severe penetrating head injury and scar formation.

injury. As a rule, convulsions develop within a few weeks after injury, but when delayed they develop twelve to eighteen months after injury, but their appearance ten to twenty years after a bullet wound of the skull or after scar from a depressed fracture is not unusual. Investigations indicate clearly that the possibility of the development of convulsions is greater in head injuries in which the dura has been penetrated than in those in which the dura is intact. A review of 317 cases of gunshot wounds of the head in the war of 1914 to 1918 reveals the fact that convulsions were twice as frequent in patients whose dura had been penetrated (forty-five per cent) as in patients whose dura was intact (twenty-three per cent) (Ascroft). Convulsions are much less common in nonpenetrating wounds of the skull. The presence of infection undoubtedly increases the possibility of convulsions, but there is no evidence that the removal of a metallic foreign body reduces the liability to epilepsy. Convulsive seizures, furthermore, are more common in injuries involving the sensorimotor cortex than in wounds elsewhere in the brain.

The convulsive seizures which develop following penetrating missiles or after depressed fractures of the skull, occur as the result of meningocerebral adhesions or of scar formation within the brain substance. In the former instance, dense adhesions are found between dura, underlying arachnoid, and the cerebral cortex, with glial proliferation and ganglion cell degeneration in the superficial cortical layers. In the latter instance, there is a firm, dense meningeal scar associated with a hard glial scar in the cortex due to penetration of the missile through the dura. In both instances, the scar formation acts as a trigger to set off the convulsive seizures.

Most of the seizures resulting from penetrating skull wounds are typical *generalized convulsions;* fewer are focal jacksonian attacks; very few if any are of the petit mal type. Most of the attacks are diurnal, but nocturnal seizures may occur. Examination reveals nothing of significance in many instances. In others there may be residuals of an old hemiplegia, monoplegia, hemianopsia, or other cerebral defect. Electroencephalogram will reveal abnormal waves in the area of focal damage. Pneumogram reveals dilatation of the lateral ventricle of one side, with pulling over of the ventricle to the side of the scar. In other instances, meningocerebral adhesions may be seen, associated with cortical atrophy and dilatation of the ventricles.

The possibility of disappearance of the epileptic attacks is greater in seizures which begin in the first few weeks after injury and becomes less in instances which develop in the first two years after trauma. *Medical treatment* offers the best results (*v.* Chapter 13). In a small percentage of patients (twenty-five out of 165), removal of the cortical scar resulted in complete eradication of the attacks (Penfield). The problem of treatment is governed largely by the fact that removal of the scar or dissolution of the adhesions responsible for the attacks, is followed by stoppage of the convulsions in only a small percentage of cases. For this reason medical treatment with one of the anticonvulsants should be given a thorough trial before operation is contemplated. If the attacks are well controlled by medication, there is no need for operation, but if drug treatment is ineffective, removal of the scar responsible for the attacks should be advised.

Mental symptoms of various sorts develop after head injuries. These include delirium, personality disorders, mental deterioration, memory disturbances, and confusional syndromes (Korsakoff psychosis). The incidence of posttraumatic psychoses is difficult to estimate, but their incidence is low. They represented 0.6 per cent of all admissions to mental hospitals in 1936. Males are more often affected and adults are more apt to suffer than children.

Cranial Nerves: The cranial nerves are injured under many circumstances in head injury. The *olfactory* nerve is injured usually only in persons having severe injury, particularly in association with ethmoid plate fractures and injuries of the base of the frontal lobe. The *optic* nerve is injured under many circumstances, with resulting loss of vision, either partial or complete. Usually the head injury is severe. Hemorrhage may develop in the optic sheath; the nerve may be compressed by callus forming along a fracture line in the optic foramen; or adhesive arachnoiditis may develop late after injury and may cause optic atrophy and visual field changes. Rare instances of direct injury of the optic chiasm with softening have been reported. Blindness may develop immediately, with recovery in four weeks. The symptoms are usually unilateral. There may be complete or partial blindness with scotomas or sector defects and pallor of the nerve.

The *facial* nerve is injured especially in fractures through the petrous portion of the temporal bone. It may be completely severed; hemorrhage may develop within the sheath of the nerve; or infection may develop following basilar fracture through an infected mastoid. The paralysis of the face is typically of the peripheral type. Delayed facial paralysis almost always is followed by complete recovery. The outlook is not as favorable in cases of immediate paralysis (Turner). The *auditory* nerve is frequently injured, especially in fractures involving the petrous portion of the temporal bone. Deafness and tinnitus, particularly the latter, are common posttraumatic symptoms. Vertigo is common after trauma.

Miscellaneous: Meningitis and brain abscess may develop after head injury. Subdural and extradural abscess are also found after trauma.

Pneumocele is a rare complication after head injury. It follows ethmoid plate fracture or fracture through the paranasal sinuses, and is associated with leakage of spinal fluid. Because of rupture of the dura and arachnoid a direct communication is established with the cranial cavity and remains patent. Air is insufflated into the cranial cavity and roentgenograms reveal air within the skull and ventricles.

Dilatation of the cerebral ventricles follows head injury and is of three types (Northfield): (1) a local bulging of the ventricle resembling a diverticulum; (2) enlargement of the whole of one lateral ventricle; (3) general symmetrical enlargement of the ventricles without involvement of the third and fourth ventricles. The degree of ventricular dilatation is greatest in those who have sustained severe head injuries. The dilatation of the ventricles may result from disturbances of the cerebrospinal fluid system, or from atrophy of the brain itself (hydrocephalus *ex vacuo*).

Localized hydrocephalus has been found following penetrating wounds of the skull. Complete obliteration of the body of the lateral ventricle may develop after parietal wounds involving the ventricle, the obstructed inferior horn expanding to form an enormous cyst with symptoms resembling brain abscess in the wound track. The condition responds to the reestablishment of communication between the inferior horn and the lateral ventricle, together with coagulation of the choroid plexus of the inferior horn.

Injuries to the hypophyseal-hypothalamic region results rarely in diabetes insipidus. In rare instances, parkinsonism has followed head injury due to injury of the basal ganglia.

Intracranial hypotension has been emphasized as occurring at times and is often unrecognized. It is said to occur in the following conditions: (1) post-traumatic, with or without leakage of spinal fluid to the outside or into the subdural space, (2) postoperative, (3) secondary to surgical or medical pro-cedures, (4) following radiotherapy, (5) primary hypotension. The condition is manifested by coma, hemiplegia, convul-sions, and at times mental symptoms. The diagnosis cannot be made on clinical grounds alone or by lumbar puncture. Trephining is necessary to demonstrate the collapse of the brain.

Prognosis: A study of cases of head injury illustrates the following factors in prognosis: (1) the severity of the injury is the most important factor in prognosis: (2) equally important is the age of the patient, the prognosis being worse in sub-jects over forty; (3) bloody spinal fluid worsens the outlook because of the fre-quent association of contusion and lacer-ation; (4) associated injuries of the chest, spine, and spinal cord are bad prognostic features, as are preexisting cardiovascu-lar and renal diseases; and (5) acute medical complications worsen the prog-nosis.

VIII. TREATMENT

Closed Head Injury: Certain gen-eral measures may be used in all patients having head injury; specific types of in-jury require special forms of treatment. For many patients only general treat-ment is necessary. Important general principles can be applied nevertheless in all cases. The following should always be observed:

1. The treatment of head injury must be an individualized problem. Much harm has been done by attempts to re-duce to rigid formulae the handling of all head injury cases. In each case it is essential that a diagnosis be made as rapidly as possible in order to determine the best course of treatment. The han-dling of a patient with cerebral concus-sion will be different from one with sub-arachnoid or extradural hemorrhage, and the treatment of every patient having concussion will not be the same. Thus some may require lumbar puncture, others dehydration, and still others fluid. The approach to each problem of head injury must remain, therefore, an indi-vidual one, each case must be handled on its own merits, and individual prob-lems within each case treated accord-ingly.

2. The patient should be moved as little as possible, especially if he is in shock of moderate or severe degree.

3. Avoidance of doing too much for the patient. Under many circumstances the less done for him the better.

Elevation of the head from fifteen to forty-five degrees is desirable. The skin should be kept dry, especially when there is urinary incontinence, in order to pre-vent bedsores.

The *temperature, pulse, respirations,* and *blood pressure* should be taken as often as it appears indicated. Usually, this is not necessary more often than every three hours. In patients with pro-longed unconsciousness and those in se-vere shock, they should be taken every hour until the severe acute effects of the injury are over. In patients with sus-pected extradural hemorrhage, they may be taken even more frequently.

Rest is imperative. Most subjects will rest quietly, but marked restlessness is found in many instances. This is best combated by sedation, which is prefer-able to restraints, since the constant pulling against the latter raises intracranial pressure and does not help bleeding if it is present. *Morphine* should be avoided because of depression of respiration. *Paraldehyde* (3 or 4 drachms) may be given by mouth, nasal tube, or rectum and may be repeated as often as necessary. *Barbiturates* may be given if the restlessness is extreme. Sodium Amytal, grains 7½, intravenously, is effective and may be repeated if it does not control the restlessness. Luminal sodium (grains 1½ to 3), intravenously, may be used. Phenobarbital may be given by mouth if the patient is conscious. *Bromides* (grains 15 to 30) and *chloral hydrate* (grains 20 to 30) may be used but are not as desirable as other forms of sedation because of their depressing effect.

Heat applied externally is often necessary, especially in patients with decreased temperatures. Patients should be placed between blankets if possible.

The administration of *fluids* is important. It is the custom in many clinics to give hypertonic solutions routinely for dehydration on the assumption that the brain in every patient with head injury is edematous. This is not supported by the facts and many patients not only do not require dehydration but need fluids instead. It has already been pointed out that there is some difference of opinion concerning the occurrence of brain edema in head injury. Edema reaches its height twelve to twenty-four hours after injury, persists for one or two days and then recedes (Oldberg). Treatment for edema is, therefore, indicated between the twelfth and seventy-second hour. After this period the persistence of coma or of increased pressure cannot be regarded as due to brain edema. In patients with increased pressure as measured by spinal fluid manometer, it is advisable to give *hypertonic solution* (100 cc. of fifty per cent dextrose or sucrose intravenously). Magnesium sulfate by mouth

may be sufficient in some cases. Concentrated serum has been used with good results in some instances, and magnesium sulfate by rectum by slow drip is advocated by some. This may be repeated if necessary in the course of twenty-four hours. Care must be taken to note the appearance of the skin and mucous membranes, since more harm than good can be done by too active dehydration.

In patients who need fluid, this can be supplied by nasal tube or by subcutaneous administration of saline (500 to 1000 cc.). Dried human *plasma* has been found to be useful in proper solution given intravenously. *Caffeine sodiobenzoate* (grains 7½) may be given intravenously every four hours for active dehydration or caffeine citrate (grain 1) by mouth three or four times a day is useful.

The *diet* should consist only of liquids which may be reënforced with the proper vitamins and should consist of at least 2000 cc. daily except in patients in whom dehydration is desired, when it can be reduced to a daily intake of 1200 cc. or, in extreme cases, to 1000 cc. In unconscious patients, feeding may be carried out by nasal tubes.

Lumbar puncture is not necessary as a routine procedure. The ordinary patient having concussion can do without it. It should be performed as a diagnostic measure under the following circumstances: (1) when signs of meningeal irritation are present, for the establishment of a diagnosis of subarachnoid hemorrhage or when meningitis is suspected; (2) to determine the presence of increased pressure when subdural hemorrhage, extradural hemorrhage, or edema is suspected; (3) as a diagnostic measure in doubtful cases when there is prolonged unconsciousness.

Roentgenograms of the skull are not necessary as a routine procedure and add nothing to the understanding of the average case. They may wait until after the acute effects of the injury have worn off. In suspected extradural hemorrhage, the patient may be moved for a skull roentgenologic examination, since the presence of a fracture line across the middle meningeal groove helps greatly in the establishment of a diagnosis. Routine roentgenogram of the skull should be taken eventually in all cases of head injury for diagnostic and medicolegal purposes.

The length of stay in bed must be handled individually. Patients with mild head injury may be kept in bed for two or three days and returned to work in seven to ten days. Patients with more severe injury must remain in bed for two to three weeks and may not return to work for months. No general rule is applicable and each case must be handled individually.

Fractures of the Skull: Lacerations of the scalp should be cleaned carefully and tetanus antitoxin given. Sulfonamide powder should be applied to the wound.

Linear skull fractures require no special treatment beyond the general measures already referred to. *Depressed* skull fractures require careful cleaning of the skin and debridement if they are compound. Sulfonamide derivatives may be applied to the meninges and brain tissue. The sulfonamide drugs are well tolerated when applied to the scalp, meninges, and cortex, but sulfathiazole should not be applied to the cortex directly because of its tendency to produce convulsions.

Ethmoid plate fractures with spinal fluid leakage require the following: (1) repeated removal of clots from the nose; (2) prevention of nose blowing to avoid ascending infection into the meninges; (3) avoidance of lumbar puncture so that infection may not be sucked back into the meninges; (4) administration of sulfonamides or penicillin as a preventive against infection. Most fluid leaks will clear up spontaneously; those which persist require surgical repair.

Petrous bone fractures with spinal fluid leakage are handled as follows: (1) The ear and ear canal are covered with a bland disinfectant, such as Mercurochrome, and a sterile gauze applied. This should be changed frequently as it becomes saturated with fluid. (2) No lumbar puncture should be performed. (3) Sulfonamides should be administered. Most cases will clear up spontaneously on this régime; some patients will develop a purulent meningitis.

Hemorrhage of the Meninges: Extradural hemorrhage must be treated surgically by clipping off the bleeding meningeal artery. The treatment of *subdural hemorrhage* is also surgical. *Subarachnoid hemorrhage* should be treated by repeated lumbar punctures daily until the spinal fluid is xanthochromic or clear. This is done for two purposes: (1) to prevent organization of the hemorrhage and the development of pia-arachnoid adhesions; (2) to relieve headache, a very effective means in such cases. Where the spinal fluid pressure is high, it is a good working principle to remove only enough fluid to reduce the pressure by one-half. If the spinal fluid pressure is normal, as much fluid may be taken as will drain off.

14

Epilepsy and Convulsive States

I. DEFINITION AND CLASSIFICATION

Epilepsy is a condition characterized by recurrent seizures of various types associated with disturbance of consciousness, and accompanied by evidence of electrical discharge from the cortical cells. The epileptic attack is featured, therefore, by a discharge from the cortical ganglion cells, an assumption which is supported both by the clinical features of focal and generalized convulsions and by the brain waves which can be recorded by the electroencephalograph.

The incidence of epilepsy is difficult to estimate, but it is generally asserted that the incidence is 0.5 per cent of the total population of the United States, giving a total figure of six hundred thousand epileptics in this country. These figures taken from the military draft of 1917, are probably low, but they serve as a minimum figure of incidence of epilepsy in the United States. It is estimated now that there are about 900,000 epileptic persons in the United States (Lennox).

Two main groups of epilepsy may be distinguished: (1) *idiopathic, cryptogenic, genuine,* or *essential* epilepsy, for which no specific cause is known; (2) *symptomatic* or *secondary* epilepsy, produced by a variety of conditions. The idiopathic type has long been regarded as a special form of epilepsy of unknown origin, but the present-day tendency is to regard it as another form of symptomatic epilepsy for which no cause has yet been disclosed. Just as in the other forms of symptomatic epilepsy for which a cause has been found, so, too, in so-called idiopathic epilepsy will a specific cause be disclosed in due time. Whether this viewpoint is justified can be determined only by future studies. Practically speaking, in our present state of knowledge, it is both justifiable and necessary to divide cases of epilepsy into a large idiopathic group for which no cause can be found after careful study, and a symptomatic group for which specific causes are known.

The use of the term *epileptiform* to describe seizures of a symptomatic nature serves no useful purpose. Such attacks have features similar to those of typical epileptic seizures and should therefore be spoken of as epileptic. The inference in the use of the term epileptiform is that the convulsive state is not typically epileptic, that it is not idiopathic in type, or that it is secondary to some specific cause, in which case it is best referred to as symptomatic epilepsy.

II. GENERAL CHARACTERISTICS OF ATTACKS

Since attacks of one or another sort are the distinctive feature of epilepsy, it seems desirable to describe their characteristics. Epileptic episodes have been variously termed convulsions, seizures, fits, and attacks. None of these terms is entirely satisfactory and many of them are used interchangeably. Since the attacks vary greatly in nature, none of the features to be described are common to them all.

Aura: An aura or warning of an impending attack is found in many major seizures, but is not invariably present by any means. It is usually absent in minor seizures and in focal jacksonian attacks.

Loss of Consciousness: All major epileptic attacks are characterized by loss of consciousness. This varies in duration from several seconds to several minutes, but in such attacks loss of consciousness is always present and serves to differentiate true epileptic attacks from hysterical fits or other conditions simulating epileptic attacks. Loss of consciousness in some degree is always present in minor attacks as well. This may be only a temporary impairment of consciousness or it may be a complete loss, but some degree of impairment of consciousness is present always in minor or petit mal episodes in epilepsy. The impairment of consciousness may be difficult to establish in minor attacks and patients usually assert that consciousness is not lost. Careful inquiry, however, will reveal always some impairment of consciousness interfering momentarily with intellectual functions but often of such minor degree as to be disregarded by the patient. There may be a staring off into space for a split second, an interruption in conversation for a brief space, or some similar interruption of consciousness.

Impairment or loss of consciousness, however, is not found in all types of epilepsy. Focal jacksonian attacks, whether motor or sensory, are not infrequently associated with no disturbance of consciousness. Loss or impairment of consciousness is not found in psychomotor or temporal lobe seizures, but there is an associated amnesia for the seizure, and

an unawareness of the fact that it has occurred.

Motor Movements: Movements of the limbs in an epileptic attack are found regularly in major or grand mal seizures, and in jacksonian motor attacks. They are found at times in sensory jacksonian attacks in which the cortical discharge has spread into the adjacent motor cortex. Myoclonic jerks are sometimes seen in petit mal seizures. Automatic movements—rubbing of the hands, chewing or champing movements, and automatisms of other sorts—are seen in psychomotor and temporal lobe seizures. In petit mal seizures, motor movements are not seen. Movements of the limbs are usually clonic, but may be tonic in grand mal seizures, and are clonic in motor jacksonian seizures.

Miscellaneous Features: In many major seizures, *incontinence of urine* accompanies the attack, but this is by no means constant. It may occur in motor jacksonian fits as well. *Tongue biting* is common but not invariable in major attacks. Following the attack there may develop headache, confusion, drowsiness, or automatic states of various sorts. These are much more common after generalized convulsions than other types of seizures.

Types of Attack: Epilepsy is characterized by the occurrence of a variety of seizures, each with its distinctive features. Some of these may coexist in the same patient; often pure cultures of seizures of one type or another are found. Thus grand mal attacks are often interspersed with petit mal episodes and rarely with uncinate fits. Motor and sensory jacksonian attacks may be found in the same patient; or motor jacksonian seizures may be found in persons with generalized epileptic attacks.

The following types of seizures may be distinguished:

Motor:
  Major (grand mal)
  Jacksonian (motor)
  Status epilepticus
Sensory:
  Jacksonian (sensory)
  Uncinate
Psychical:
  Petit mal
  Dreamy state
  Automatisms or psychical attacks

Based on their clinical and physiological studies in human subjects in whom stimulation of the cerebral cortex was carried out, Penfield and Jasper give the following classification of seizures with the localization of the discharge which produces them:

CLINICAL TYPE	LOCALIZATION
Somatic Motor	
1. Generalized seizure (grand mal)	Complete motor
2. Jacksonian seizure (local motor)	Pre-Rolandic gyrus
3. Masticatory seizure	Lower Rolandic
4. Simple adversive seizure	Frontal
5. Tonic postural seizure (decerebrate opisthotonic)	Brain stem
Somatic Sensory (Auras)	
6. Somatosensory seizure	Post-Rolandic gyrus
7. Visual seizure	Occipital
8. Auditory seizure	Temporal
9. Vertiginous seizure	Temporal
10. Olfactory seizure	Infratemporal
Visceral	
11. Autonomic seizure	Diencephalic
Psychical	
12. Dreamy state seizure	Temporal
13. Petit mal	
14. Automatism (ictal and post-ictal)	
15. Psychotic states (secondary)	

It is clear from this grouping that the classification of epileptic attacks may be made very broad and that even more detailed classifications are possible. The point in common with all attacks is their tendency to recurrence and the development of unconsciousness during most, but not all, seizures. Though many types of seizures are possible, the epileptic develops, as a rule, his own predominant type, whether these be grand mal or petit mal seizures, or seizures of a special type. Grand mal or generalized attacks may appear exclusively or almost exclusively, and petit mal attacks are found not infrequently in pure culture. It is not uncommon, however, for patients to develop more than one type of epileptic attack; hence the occurrence of grand mal and petit mal seizures in a single subject is a matter of common experience, while the intermingling of other types of attack is also not infrequently found.

III. GENERALIZED SEIZURES
(Grand Mal)

These are characterized by the presence of (1) an *aura*, (2) *convulsion,* and (3) *postconvulsive state.*

Aura: Attacks are usually but not always ushered in by an *aura* which is the first indication of the impending seizure. An aura may be defined as a sensory experience preceding the epileptic convulsion. In many instances, the seizures develop without an aura, the convulsion being the first manifestation of the fit. The aura may often give an indication of the origin of the epileptic discharge. The incidence of auras has been variously computed. Among 1145 cases of epilepsy, auras were found in fifty-seven per cent (Gowers). They may be said to occur, therefore, in about one-half of the patients with epilepsy. Their type varies greatly, and many terms are used by patients to describe the sensation experienced. The most frequent type of warning is the epigastric aura (Gowers); on the other hand, among 750 patients with epilepsy one-fourth defined their auras in nondescript terms, such as a "queer feeling," "dizziness," "numbness," etc. One-sixth had abdominal warnings, such as nausea (Lennox). Auras are frequently disregarded by the physician, more attention being given to the more spectacular convulsive attack. They are significant for two reasons: (1) They may give an indication of the point of onset of the attack in the cerebral cortex. The aura is regarded by some as the attack itself and not the forerunner of the attack. It is regarded as the first phase of the epileptic discharge in the cortex (Antoni). (2) They give a warning to the patient who in many instances, but not always, is able to protect himself against a fall by lying or sitting down. The aura in epileptic fits is of various types and may differ in the same patient. They may be somatic, visceral, or special sense auras.

Somatic auras differ in type and distribution. They consist often of feelings of numbness, "pins and needles" sensations, tingling, or other forms of paresthesia involving the extremities or traveling up the trunk. Tingling and numbness are the most common of the somatic auras. Occasionally generalized somatic auras are described as sudden feelings of numbness or tingling throughout the body. True pain is probably never experienced as an epileptic aura. Somatic auras of the type described are caused by discharges in the postcentral gyrus (Areas 3, 1, and 2) (Penfield and Jasper).

Visceral auras may be referred to any of the viscera. Epigastric sensations of many sorts are common. They consist of a feeling of fullness or emptiness of the stomach, cramps in the epigastrium, and of indefinable sensations of many sorts. Nausea occasionally occurs as an epileptic aura. From the epigastrium the auras usually ascend over the trunk to the neck or head. They have no localizing value so far as the cortex is concerned, since they may be produced by stimulation of the cortex at many points. Abdominal pain as a symptom of epilepsy has been described (Moore), and it appears to be dependent upon discharges from areas of the cerebral cortex which are capable of producing disturbances of gastric motility (Areas 6, 5, and 3). Changes have been observed in the EEG in such cases, which may be of the idiopathic or symptomatic type. The abdominal pain may be an aura or may constitute the attack.

Palpitation, shortness of breath, a sensation of strangling, and other visceral sensations are sometimes felt. Headache or a sense of fullness in the head are common. Auras referable to the special senses are not uncommon. These consist of tinnitus, vertigo, unpleasant smells or tastes, and visual phenomena of various sorts. Visual auras may be experienced as a sense of darkness before the eyes, lights, stars, whirling and moving lights and colored lights (Penfield and Jasper). They may be followed by dizziness or a humming sensation in the ears. Visual hallucinations occur as auras in epileptic seizures due to disease of the temporo-occipital region. They are usually unconnected with previous experiences, but in rare instances may be equivalent to a reenactment of vivid emotional experiences (Robinson and Watt) due presumably to involvement of Area 19. Pain in the eyeball may precede or follow a seizure. Macropsia and micropsia may be found. Visual auras have their origin in the calcarine cortex. Auditory sensations such as humming or buzzing, may precede a major attack and are usually associated with dizziness. Dizziness alone may be experienced as an epileptic aura. Olfactory auras consisting of disagreeable or disgusting odors are rare.

Convulsion: After the aura, the *convulsive seizure* develops immediately as a rule, though there may be a latency of seconds or minutes between one and the other. Unconsciousness supervenes at once after the aura, but in some cases it appears even before the aura is completed. With the onset of unconsciousness there follows the convulsive state which characterizes the epileptic fit. A shrill cry may initiate the attack and the patient falls to the ground with the development of unconsciousness. The body is thrown first into a tonic state, the entire body becoming rigid with the arms and legs extended. The jaws are firmly clenched, the head retracted and often rolled from side to side, the eyeballs rolled up, respirations cease, and the face is flushed or cyanotic. The bladder or bowels may be emptied during this tonic phase of the attack. Following the tonic phase, which may be very brief or may last for half a minute, there follows the clonic phase during which the head jerks forcibly, the arms and legs contract and relax vigorously in forcible clonic movements, the jaws jerk, saliva pours from the mouth, the tongue may be bitten, the breathing is noisy and stertorous, the body is covered with a profuse sweat, and the bladder or bowel or both may be emptied. The convulsive seizure may last for one to ten minutes, the clonic movements becoming gradually less vigorous and finally ceasing entirely, the thrashing movements of the head and the rolling of the eyes disappearing, the breathing becoming less forced and more regular, and the entire fit ending eventually in a complete letdown or relaxation which may be followed by deep sleep lasting for minutes or hours, by confusion, or by no aftereffects whatever.

The convulsion in grand mal attacks is generalized, involving all the limbs. It is usually associated with clonic movements of the limbs and trunk, but tonic seizures are not uncommon. Attacks may be completely tonic, with few or no clonic movements, or they may begin as tonic seizures and break down into clonic movements, which is the invariable pattern in generalized seizures. The convulsion develops usually in all the limbs simultaneously, but may begin in one limb and spread rapidly to the others. A generalized attack may begin simultaneously in all the limbs or it may start as a focal motor attack and spread to involve the entire body. The probabilities are that a generalized attack begins simultaneously in both motor cortices, with resulting discharge in both sides of the brain. In those cases which begin as focal attacks, the discharge must originate first in the opposite motor cortex and spread to the other side.

Postconvulsive State: Following the convulsion comes the *postconvulsive state*, during which the patient may drop off into a deep sleep lasting several minutes to several hours. Following this he may awake completely clear or confused. In other instances, the convulsive seizure may be succeeded immediately by confusion lasting for minutes or for several hours. *Headache* is not an uncommon sequel after generalized convulsions and may last for minutes or hours after the attack. In most cases, the only sequel of which the patient is himself aware is a feeling of general *muscular soreness* which constitutes for him the only indication that he has suffered from an attack. Vomiting sometimes follows. Automatic phenomena of many sorts may follow a convulsion (undressing, kleptomania, etc.) and fugue states may sometimes develop. *Psychotic states* may follow seizures at times. In many cases the fit is succeeded by no sequelae of significance and it is not uncommon to obtain a history of patients proceeding with their occupations immediately after a seizure as if nothing had occurred.

Status Epilepticus: Grand mal or generalized seizures may continue in some instances for hours without cessation of the attacks. This condition is known as *status epilepticus*. The attacks in this state may follow one another in rapid succession or at lengthier intervals, but they persist for hours or even days unless checked by medication. Status epilepticus may develop in both the idiopathic and the symptomatic types of epilepsy and has no particular significance save that the cerebral cortex under such conditions is in a state of greatly increased irritability. Death may ensue in status epilepticus, and the condition must therefore be regarded as a serious omen.

Generalized Major Convulsions: Generalized major convulsions have no localizing significance. They indicate merely an increased irritability of the cortex, though they take their origin in motor discharge in or through the motor cortex. In this connection it is essential to recognize the fact that generalized convulsions may be found resulting from focal brain disease, without a history of focal jacksonian convulsions, or with such a history. In the latter case, the generalized convulsion may develop following an initial jacksonian attack, or seizures may begin as focal attacks and later in the course of the disease become generalized. Some types of lesions, as, for example, tumors of the temporal lobe, are prone to be associated with generalized convulsions, but the convulsion in itself fails to point to disease of the temporal lobe. Generalized seizures occur most often in idiopathic epilepsy, but they may be the first manifestations of symptomatic epilepsy. They may be the first symptom of general paresis, brain

tumor and other disease of the brain. While they have no localizing significance, therefore, they may indicate structural brain disease, especially where they appear for the first time in adults, with no previous history of seizures in infancy or childhood.

IV. FOCAL SEIZURES

Motor Jacksonian Seizures: These are focal clonic convulsions characterized by movements of a limb, part of a limb, both limbs of one side of the body, or of the muscles of the face. They are, therefore, associated with local movements. The pattern of involvement varies greatly, depending upon the area of the motor cortex which is discharging. The convulsive movements may be confined to a small part (thumb, hand, etc.) or spread to involve one entire side of the body, and is not always the same in an individual case. At times convulsions may begin focally and become generalized. Unconsciousness or some impairment of consciousness is not usually found in motor jacksonian attacks, but this is not constant. The majority of cases are found with no impairment of consciousness whatever, unless they are followed by generalized seizures.

Jacksonian convulsions begin as a rule from one of three foci: the thumb and index fingers, the angle of the mouth, or the great toe and foot, in this order of frequency (Walshe). Following the initial discharge from one of these foci there develops a march of movement from one member to different members of the same side of the body; e. g., from thumb to fingers to wrist to arm to face. The march of the attack is conditioned by the representation of the various parts in the motor cortex. Attacks beginning in the arm most often appear first in the thumb and index finger, spreading from this point up the forearm to the arm; if the attack spreads to the leg from this point, the proximal portion of the limb is first affected, the attack spreading out to the foot, thus, thigh, leg, foot, and toes. Or, to put the matter more simply, an attack beginning in the hand passes up the arm and down the leg. Attacks beginning in the leg start in the great toe and extend up the leg, and if they involve the arm, extend down the arm. Attacks involving the face begin usually at the angle of the mouth. Not infrequently a seizure may involve the whole arm initially.

Jacksonian attacks are clonic in nature but may be tonic at first for a period of a few seconds. Flexor movements are produced by the seizures. Consciousness is not impaired if the convulsion remains restricted, but it may be lost or impaired with spread of the convulsion. Postconvulsive paralysis may follow the attack; it may be so brief as to escape detection or it may persist for a varying length of time. A Babinski sign may be elicited after a seizure involving the foot.

A special type of focal attack is that referred to as conjugate deviation of the head and eyes (simple adversive seizure). This is characterized by turning of the head, usually followed by turning of the whole body in the same direction and by conjugate deviation of the eyes in the same direction. The deviation of the head and eyes is away from the hemisphere in which the epileptic discharge occurs. The attack occurs frequently without other evidences of epileptic convulsion except for loss of consciousness, but it may develop into a generalized convulsion under some circumstances. It is due to involvement of the frontal lobe. Thus, deviation of the head and eyes to the right is due to involvement of the left frontal lobe and *vice versa*.

Physiologically speaking, there is little reason to differentiate between focal and generalized convulsions, since all convul-

sions must develop through the motor cortex. Clinically, however, focal motor jacksonian seizures are of great importance. They indicate usually a lesion in the opposite motor cortex. They may, however, be associated with disease elsewhere in the brain (occipital or temporal lobes) causing irritability of the motor cortex and a focal convulsion.

Sensory Jacksonian Seizures: Focal sensory jacksonian attacks are not as common as their motor counterpart. They are characterized by sensory experiences distributed in parts of the body similar to the motor attacks, and by a similar march of the sensory phenomena. The attacks may persist in the sensory sphere only, or they may, and often do, spread to the adjacent motor cortex, causing movements of the corresponding limb or that part of the limb which is affected by the sensory attack. They may or may not be associated with impairment of consciousness. The sensations described vary greatly — numbness, tingling, prickling, and even vague painful sensations. They indicate involvement of the opposite sensory cortex in the parietal lobe by some focal disease process.

V. PETIT MAL

In contrast to the generalized or grand mal seizures stand the petit mal attacks. These may occur alone in pure culture, they may predominate over generalized attacks in a particular case, or they may be interspersed among the grand mal seizures. They are characterized by a fleeting impairment of consciousness without convulsive movements, following which there is usually a complete return to normal as if nothing had occurred. Petit mal attacks often occur in conjunction with grand mal spells, but they may be found in pure culture without indication of grand mal attacks at any time during the course of the disease. Not a few cases of epilepsy in fact are found with only petit mal seizures.

Petit mal episodes develop as a rule without an aura. The type of sensation varies; there is often a fleeting staring off into space, accompanied by a pallor of the face, or a blank look during conversation with perfect continuance of the conversation after the attack has passed. In other instances, loss of the thread of conversation develops. Attacks may develop during walking, swimming, riding a bicycle or other acts, and all of these activities may be continued during petit mal as if nothing had occurred. In other instances, objects may be dropped from the hands during an attack. So slight are the manifestations of a petit mal attack that they are usually unrecognized by others unless some overt act such as dropping of an object occurs during an episode. The patient himself is usually aware of the attack, but it is not unusual to find even intelligent patients who are completely unaware of their episodes.

Petit mal attacks tend to be more prominent during childhood; when present, they occur more frequently than grand mal convulsive seizures; they are associated with little, if any, mental impairment (Lennox). Their frequency may vary from a few to ten, fifty, or even a hundred or more a day. Status epilepticus of the petit mal variety is rare. It is reported to occur in 3 per cent of persons having epilepsy. They may be experienced daily or occur at infrequent intervals, and last five to thirty seconds or from one to two minutes. Generally speaking, they are apt to occur at relatively frequent intervals and in moderate frequency. They begin and end abruptly. Attacks are described often as dizziness, mental confusion, blankness, and by many other terms. The subject is usually immobile. Slight motor twitches may be seen, but these are not convulsive in nature. In still other instances, the attack is characterized by complete loss of consciousness and fall without the occurrence of motor components. Seizures are apt to occur after arising. They may be precipitated by emotion, excitement, or menstruation, and are less frequent during physical or mental activity.

Impairment of consciousness is always present in true petit mal attacks. The story is often given that patients in such attacks are aware of voices in the surroundings or of what is going on in the environment, but careful inquiry will demonstrate either that there is no awareness of what has been said under such circumstances, or that at some point in the attack consciousness has been impaired or lost for a very brief period. The issue is of great importance, since the distinction must be made at times between attacks of vertigo and petit mal seizures, impairment of consciousness indicating definitely a petit mal seizure. A similar distinction must be made often between psychogenic episodes and petit mal epileptic attacks; here, too, impairment of consciousness points definitely away from a psychogenic origin.

Petit mal attacks have no specific localizing significance. They may at times be the first indication of temporal lobe tumor or hypoglycemia. Petit mal is rarely associated with brain trauma or significant brain damage.

VI. TEMPORAL LOBE SEIZURES
(Psychomotor Seizures)

The group of psychomotor or psychic seizures has come to be referred to in general as temporal lobe seizures, due to disclosure by the EEG that many of the seizures of this type are associated with abnormal EEG records, especially in the anterior part of the temporal lobe. Included among temporal lobe seizures are automatisms, uncinate fits, illusions of various types and hallucinatory experiences.

Temporal lobe seizure constitutes a relatively loose term, since the clinical pattern of temporal lobe seizure varies greatly, depending on the situation and mode of spread of the discharge. There is a close correlation between temporal lobe seizures and the demonstration of a temporal lobe focus by the EEG, either by sleep EEG or by special activating measures.

The *incidence* of psychomotor seizures varies within wide limits. They have been found in six per cent of 1900 office patients (Lennox); in about one of every five patients with epilepsy, representing about one-half of all patients with seizures of focal cortical origin (Jasper); and in about one-third of adult epileptics either in pure form or in association with convulsive seizures (Bailey and Gibbs). Under some circumstances, attacks of a psychomotor nature develop with or without alteration of consciousness. The problems of psychomotor seizures require a good deal of clarification. The term psychic equivalent or epileptic equivalent has little meaning if the assumption is that the psychic manifestations are the equivalent of a seizure without in fact being a seizure. It seems obvious that the attacks in question must constitute an epileptic attack or not, and that the tendency to regard them as equivalents of attacks has little meaning. The assumption is made in the case of psychomotor seizures that an epileptic discharge is capable of producing psychic reactions which are in the nature of an epileptic discharge unassociated with convulsions, but with some impairment of consciousness. That these are in fact epileptic attacks is shown by the following evidence: (1) They are found in patients with other forms of epileptic

attack though they may occur as the only manifestation of seizures. (2) They are associated usually but not always with impairment of consciousness. (3) They are associated with special types of brain waves in the electroencephalogram (Gibbs and Gibbs). By sleep EEG records special waves are disclosed in the temporal lobe. These are found in such records in about ninety per cent of temporal lobe seizures. The cortical discharges in temporal lobe epilepsy as revealed by the EEG may be localized in any portion of the temporal lobe or of the neighboring regions. They may be found in the anterior portion of the temporal lobe, on the lateral surface, the inferomedian surface (apex, uncus, limen insulae), or in the posterior orbital region backward along the entire length of the hippocampal gyrus into the amygdala and hippocampus (Gastaut). (4) They respond to anticonvulsant drugs.

The attacks may consist of *temper outbursts* or more particularly of *automatisms* of various sorts.

True amnesia for all that occurred is characteristic of an attack of temporal lobe epilepsy, with no evidence of unconsciousness during the episode. In such psychomotor seizures or temporal lobe automatisms the patient may move about, be confused or may even carry out complicated activity.

Paroxysmal gastrointestinal, cardiorespiratory, or genitourinary symptoms may occur as an aura or as a manifestation of psychomotor or temporal lobe seizures.

Psychomotor seizures are frequently confused with petit mal episodes. Their duration is longer, the seizure lasting for minutes, as compared with seconds for the petit mal seizure, and they are often associated with automatisms. These appear in great variety and are characterized by the performance of simple or complex acts without the conscious knowledge of the patient, at times to his embarrassment. They may consist of turning around and clapping hands, undressing, and a number of other acts. "Alterations in behavior and inability to reason have been found to occur in patients coincidentally with the appearance of alterations in cerebral potential as detected by the electroencephalograph which suggested transient epileptic discharge" (Penfield and Erickson). Attacks characterized by behavior automatisms occurred in 78 per cent of 155 patients operated on for temporal lobe seizures (Feindel and Penfield). The area responsible for the irritation of behavior automatism "appears to centre in the periamygdaloid region" which includes uncus, amygdaloid nucleus, ventral claustrum, and the temporoinsular cortex in the anterior part of the sylvian fissure (Feindel and Penfield). *Compulsive laughter* has been reported as the only feature of an epileptic attack. It probably represents a psychic type of seizure

Three types of psychomotor seizures may be differentiated: (1) those shown by persons with the classical types of epilepsy; (2) those occurring before convulsions, and (3) those which in themselves constitute epileptic manifestations. Hypnotic-like states, excitements, and depressions may develop during psychic attacks. Crimes and misdemeanors may be committed during attacks; these include arson, theft, even manslaughter and exhibitionism. Memory for the happenings which have transpired during an attack is usually vague or lost, and many patients in whom the condition is unrecognized are regarded as hysterical or as ordinary criminals. The significant diagnostic point in such instances consists of the occurrence of automatisms with impairment of consciousness, a feature which can be determined by a careful history and a study of the personality. Distinction between epileptic automatisms and malingering is sometimes very difficult and is of great medicolegal importance. The occurrence of impairment of unconsciousness and of abnormal brain waves by electroencephalogram are helpful in making the distinction, but a careful analysis of the social and personality factors involved is essential.

Two types of lesions are found in temporal lobe epilepsy: (1) focal, due to tumors, glial scars, meningeal adhesions, aneurysms, and meningocortical scars; (2) diffuse, represented by cortical atrophy of varying degree and extent, involving many cerebral gyri and in the more severe lesions extending into the subcortical structures. The causes of the diffuse lesions are represented by compression of the head during birth, cerebral edema, and closed head injuries.

Uncinate Fits: These are found rarely and are characterized by disagreeable odors or tastes often associated with tasting movements of the lips and tongue and with impairment of consciousness. "In cases of this group, there is at the onset of the paroxysms a crude sensation of smell or one of taste, or there are movements of chewing, smacking of the lips, etc. (sometimes there is spitting). In some of the cases of this group there is a warning of what is known as the epigastric sensation, a crude development of a systemic sensation; this warning sometimes occurs along with a crude sensation of smell or with the chewing, etc.. movements" (Jackson). Attacks of this type may develop in idiopathic epilepsy or may be the only manifestation of symptomatic epilepsy. They indicate disease of the uncus region in the temporal lobe.

Dreamy States: This is an uncommon form of epileptic seizure characterized by some disturbance of consciousness with a sense of reminiscence or recollection, a sense of strangeness, and a sense of seeing things far away or near at hand (Jackson).

Penfield and Jasper include in dreamy state seizures two types of reaction: (1) illusional seizures; (2) hallucinatory seizures. *Illusional seizures* may occur alone or they may usher in a larger epileptic attack. The patient in his attacks is in touch with his environment but fails to interpret his experiences properly. Such a seizure may have to do only with (1) visual perception; the things seen for the moment may seem larger and near (macropsia) or smaller and more distant (micropsia); or (2) there may occur a similar alteration in auditory perception (auditory illusion); sounds may seem suddenly louder than they should (macracusia), although the significance of these sounds is still not understood; (3) the patient may have a sudden illusion of memory. He has a feeling that he remembers his environment, that he has been here before or experienced all this at another time, a feeling of familiarity, a sense of *'deja vu'*; (4) there may be an illusion of remoteness, a sudden feeling of strangeness or of unreality; he may feel as though he were far away and yet can perceive the scene, may seem to see himself and know what is happening to his body, as though he were a secondary observer.

The *hallucinatory seizures* resemble true dreams and are not altered perceptions. The hallucinatory phenomena seen with epileptic seizures differ from those encountered in mental disease. They are not as well formed as the latter and involve chiefly vision and hearing. Auditory hallucinations occur infrequently and are usually associated with visual experiences. The visual hallucinations often are described as a reminiscence or as a complex memory. Associated with the dreamy states are often found chewing and tasting movements and epigastric aura. Dreamy states result from disease of the temporal lobe, probably the uncus region (Jackson), but Penfield and Erickson find them associated with lesions deep within or beneath the temporal lobe.

VII. MISCELLANEOUS

Diencephalic Autonomic Seizures: These are rare seizures due to a focal epileptic discharge in the vicinity of the dorsal nucleus of the thalamus on one or both sides. They are characterized by vasodilatation, sudden rise in blood pressure, lachrymation, diaphoresis, salivation, dilatation or contraction of the pupils, protrusion of the eyes, increase of rate and pressure of the pulse, marked retardation of the respiratory rate, hiccoughing, transient shivering, sometimes incontinence of urine, and fall of the temperature well below normal.

Tonic Seizures: These are usually of brief duration and are characterized by extension of the arms and pronation of the hands, together with extension of the legs and strong plantar flexion of the feet. The attitude is that of decerebrate rigidity. Attacks of this sort are usually described as cerebellar fits, since they are encountered at times in cerebellar tumor. The tonic attacks referred to are dependent on mechanisms in the brain stem from the mesencephalon to the spinal cord and are not due to discharge within the cerebellum. Other tonic attacks in one or two limbs, characterized by tonic spasms, have been described under the term subcortical epilepsy or striate epilepsy. The cause of such attacks is not known, but they have been described in lesions of the corpus striatum.

Mental Deterioration: In epilepsy this is a matter of extreme importance, since there is a tendency to regard all cases of epilepsy as terminating eventually in deterioration. Comparable studies reveal, however, that the incidence of deterioration is much less among cases in private practice (ten per cent) than in institutionalized epileptic patients (eighty to eighty-five per cent). Deterioration appears to be much more frequent in those with grand mal attacks than in those with petit mal episodes. However, there seems to be no relationship between the number and severity of grand mal seizures and the mental deterioration. Studies have revealed that the possibility of deterioration is greater in persons with lower mental quotients to start with and in those persons in whom the seizures begin early in life. Equivalent studies demonstrate that convulsions appear earlier among deteriorated than non-deteriorated patients.

A study of 449 persons with symptomatic epilepsy and 1456 essential epileptics reveals that twenty-six per cent of the symptomatic group and ten per cent of the essential group showed definite deterioration though the former group had fewer seizures (Lennox). If in the two groups those who were deficient at birth are eliminated, the disparity is twelve per cent and six per cent. The same study revealed that serious deterioration is more manifest in all ages in the symptomatic group, but the difference is greatest if the seizures began late in life. It seems apparent, therefore, that deterioration is greater in persons with symptomatic epilepsy. A false type of deterioration is seen in many patients due to a retardation of mental reactions following anticonvulsant drugs of a sedative type. Discontinuance of the drug results in great improvement of the retardation.

About 10 per cent of epileptic persons become too dull to be employed, and about one third are not fit subjects either for training or for employment in the following types of work: (1) occupations in which the lives of others may be endangered; (2) in the operation of machinery of such a nature or work at such a height that temporary loss of consciousness might injure the patient.

VIII. PHYSIOPATHOLOGICAL MECHANISMS IN EPILEPSY

The precise factors involved in the production of convulsions have yet to be determined. Several mechanisms have been held responsible, but no single factor seems to explain all the clinical facts. It is conceivable that more than one mechanism may be at work in different cases. Among the many mechanisms which have been propounded to explain the occurrence of epileptic seizures are the following (Cobb): (1) direct irritation; (2) congenital defect; (3) tissue destruction; (4) increased intracranial pressure; (5) congestion; (6) hydration; (7) dehydration; (8) vasoconstriction; (9) increased permeability; (10) asphyxia; (11) alkalosis.

Epilepsy or the epileptic seizure or attack is characterized by the occurrence of a neuronal discharge beginning as a local discharge which spreads along neuronal pathways. The local discharge which initiates the attack occurs in the motor cortex, is excessive, and spreads quickly to produce the convulsive seizure. This much is definite. Proof of the contention is given by the evidence of discharge during the course of seizures, as shown by the brain waves recorded by the electroencephalograph. The point at issue seems to be the determination of the mechanism which sets off the discharge responsible for the convulsive attack. On this point there is no evidence which seems to indicate that any one factor is largely responsible for the firing off of seizures. More than one mechanism may be capable of producing epileptic attacks and it is even possible that more than one mechanism may be operative in a single case. Irritation or stimulation of the cortical ganglion cells may be responsible in cerebral scars, brain tumor, or encephalitis; anoxemia is at fault in carbon monoxide poisoning; and still other factors may be found to be responsible in other instances.

Of the many mechanisms detailed here four principal factors may be mentioned as being of importance in the precipitation of epileptic attacks. These are: (1) anoxemia; (2) changes in acid-base equilibrium; (3) alterations in nerve conduction; (4) changes in cerebral blood flow.

The rôle of *anoxemia* in the production of convulsions is enticing. It is difficult to prove, though there is much fruitless speculation concerning its rôle not only in the production of convulsions, but of other cortical symptoms. There is relatively little evidence that anoxemia plays a rôle in epileptics, but convulsions can be produced in animals by ligating the arteries supplying the brain and by limiting the oxygen intake. In humans, mechanical asphyxia, as in strangulation, produces convulsions, and the same is true of carbon monoxide poisoning. Seizures occur in Stokes-Adams syndrome, provided the heart block lasts long enough (seventeen seconds). Transient anoxemia in cerebral vascular spasm may produce seizures if the impairment of circulation is long enough. Convulsions may be produced in animals by ligating the carotid sinus associated with a sharp fall in blood pressure. It is clearly evident that the anoxemia associated with the examples cited accounts for relatively few examples of epilepsy and certainly cannot be held responsible on the basis of present evidence for the convulsive attacks of habitual epileptics.

Vascular mechanisms may be important in the steps leading up to an epileptic discharge but are not involved in the mechanism of the discharge (Penfield and Erickson). No changes occur in the general cerebral circulation; those which develop take place at the point of discharge responsible for the convulsion. Seizures in the human and in experimental animals are followed in a few seconds by increased blood flow through the gray matter in which the discharge is occurring, and is likely to be associated with cessation of visible arterial pulsation until toward the close of the seizure, when such pulsation reappears and becomes more violent (Penfield and Erickson). Vasoconstriction and shrinking of the brain do not occur during a seizure. Ischemia is apparently irritating to nerve cells and may set off convulsive attacks. Convulsions may be associated with vascular spasm in the brain, Raynaud's disease, anoxia, and with angioneurotic edema.

"Certain circulatory changes are associated with all epileptic seizures, whether induced or spontaneous and whether in man or in experimental animals. A few seconds after onset of discharge there is marked increase of blood flow through the gray matter in which the discharge is occurring, but not involving all ganglionic areas even when the attack is said to be generalized. This increased blood flow is due to dilatation of the cerebral vessels by a substance formed in the tissue (such as carbon dioxide or perhaps an unidentified substance) by the overactivity of the discharging ganglion cells.

"This sudden opening of the vascular bed decreases resistance to flow through the tissue and is apt to be associated with cessation of visible arterial pulsation until toward the close of the seizure, when such pulsation reappears and becomes more evident.

"Hyperemia of the brain is an infrequent but significant sequel to seizures. It appears in those areas involved by maximum discharge and resembles the reactive cerebral hyperemia that appears throughout the brain as the result of experimental asphyxia. Postictal hyperemia, therefore, seems to be due to asphyxia of ganglion cells resulting from the inadequacy of the circulatory increase to compensate for the great advance in metabolic activity of the ganglion cells during discharge.

"Vasoconstriction and shrinkage of the brain do not occur during a seizure. . . . These evidences of instability of circulation, as well as the hyperemia occasionally seen in cerebral scars, may well play an important rôle in the mechanism which leads up to the spontaneous discharges within the brain of the epileptic but are not involved in the mechanism of the discharge. Each epileptic seizure is produced by a primary neuronal discharge and the discharge causes a secondary alteration in intracerebral circulation" (Penfield and Erickson).

There appears to be no causal relationship between changes in cerebral blood flow and occurrence of epileptic seizures. Disturbance of *acid-base equilibrium* may be important. Alkalosis tends to induce fits and acidosis to inhibit them. The production of convulsions by an alkalosis induced by hyperventilation is well known and is accompanied by changes in the brain waves as seen by electroencephalograph. Local changes in pH have been found in the cerebral cortex in experimentally produced convulsions. The alkali reserve is normal in epilepsy and the pH of the blood and spinal fluid is normal between attacks. There is evidence to indicate that there may be a shift of the blood pH to the alkaline side immediately before an attack. In experimentally induced convulsions, there is a shift of electrolytes in cerebral cortical neurons, with a loss of potassium and a gain of sodium (Colfer). An accumulation of acetylcholine may precipitate seizures. An increase in tension of CO_2 of the blood induces seizures.

Indications that the epileptic seizure is associated with *disturbances in neuronal activity* are found in the recent accumulated work on the electroencephalogram in epilepsy. "In an epileptic seizure, there is paralysis of normal function of gray matter throughout the area of ganglionic spread of the epileptic discharge" (Penfield and Jasper). Gibbs, Gibbs, and Lennox define epilepsy as a *paroxysmal cerebral dysrhythmia* behind which lies probably chemical or physicochemical abnormalities of the nerve cells resulting in abnormal and excessive discharge. Their reasons for regarding epilepsy as a "disordered functioning of the rate-regulating mechanisms of the brain" are as follows: "Grand mal epilepsy is characterized by extreme acceleration of the electrical activity of the cortex; psychomotor attacks by extreme slowing of this activity, and petit mal, by alternation of fast and slow activity."

Convulsive activity of the brain is accompanied by an increase in the rate of glucose utilization, involving also an increased rate of utilization of high-energy phosphates. Studies of Metrazol convulsions indicate that the cerebral lactic acid level is increased during the convulsive discharge, that a partial breakdown of phosphocreatine occurs during seizures, and that the cerebral glycogen remains unchanged during seizures (Gurdjian).

Hydration of the brain and *increased intracranial pressure* have been mentioned as factors in determining the onset of seizures. A sudden increase of intracranial pressure is capable of producing a convulsion, but chronically elevated pressure does not cause seizures. The introduction of air too rapidly and at too high pressure can precipitate attacks.

Convulsions may be produced in animals by water intoxication. They may also be produced in epileptics within twelve to forty-eight hours after sudden water storage (McQuarrie), but nonepileptics fail to develop convulsions under the same conditions. Dehydration regimes, moreover, have been found helpful in the control of convulsions. There is no good evidence, however, that abnormalities of water metabolism are an invariable causative factor in all cases of epilepsy.

IX. PATHOLOGY OF EPILEPSY

A clear distinction must be made between idiopathic and symptomatic epilepsy. In the latter are numerous diseased conditions which accompany the epilepsy. For idiopathic epilepsy, no specific brain changes have been found. The brain grossly appears normal in most instances. Pia-arachnoid thickening, atrophy of the frontal or other gyri, and dilatation of the ventricles are sometimes found, but these have no specific significance. The brain weight is usually normal but may be decreased, especially in institutionalized deteriorated epileptics. The microscopic findings, such as the varied types of changes in the ganglion cells and the ischemic and sclerotic cell changes in Ammon's horn of the temporal lobe, are nonspecific and are found in conditions other than epilepsy. Among the histological findings in the brain described in epilepsy are sclerosis of Ammon's horn, marginal sclerosis of the cortex, and degeneration of the Purkinje cells of the cerebellum. Ischemic necrosis has been found in the occipital lobe in epileptics, in the thalamus, dentate nucleus, and inferior olive. The significance of these ischemic changes is not known, but it seems more probable that they are the result rather than the cause of the

vascular changes associated with the convulsive attack. All things considered, study of the brain has failed to reveal changes which can be regarded as characteristic for epilepsy.

Similarly, no specific or constant changes are found in the blood, urine, spinal fluid, or other laboratory examinations. The blood count in epilepsy is normal. The spinal fluid shows no abnormalities; the cell count is normal as a rule, but may be slightly increased in about four per cent of cases; the spinal fluid pressure is normal but is increased during a seizure; the total protein is slightly increased in a small percentage of cases. Blood sugar studies are not abnormal and sugar tolerance curves reveal nothing. The basal metabolic rate is normal in the usual case. Other chemical studies, such as the calcium and phosphorus content of the blood, show no deviation from normal. Similarly, no changes have been found in the acid-base equilibrium in epileptics in the intervals between attacks. Changes are found to occur on the acid side, however, during a seizure.

X. CAUSES

The cause of idiopathic epilepsy is unknown. In a large number of instances, however, epileptic seizures are symptomatic both in children and adults. In a study of 1648 patients with a diagnosis of epilepsy, 535 or 32.4 per cent gave evidence of an organic lesion of the brain prior to the first seizure (Smith, Robinson, and Lennox). The causes were found to be as follows: prenatal, 13.3 per cent; natal conditions, 30.1 per cent; postnatal trauma, 20.7 per cent; infections, 17.2 per cent; other conditions, 6.4 per cent; unassigned, 12.3 per cent. The conditions which may produce symptomatic epilepsy include the following:

Congenital:
  Cerebral aplasia
  Birth injuries
  Congenital syphilis
  Congenital idiocy
  Porencephalic cyst
  Cerebromacular degeneration
  Cerebral hemiatrophy
  Tuberous sclerosis

Degenerative:
  Lobar atrophy (Pick's disease)
  Presenile dementia (Alzheimer's disease)
  Multiple sclerosis

Inflammations:
  Encephalitis, epidemic
  Encephalitis, syphilitic (general paresis)
  Meningitis
  Brain abscess
  Parasitic disease—hydatid cyst and cysticercosis
  Arachnoiditis

Vascular ·
  Arteriosclerosis
  Cerebral thrombosis, hemorrhage, and embolism
  Cerebral vascular spasm
  Sinus thrombosis
  Raynaud's disease
  Angioneurotic edema
  Cerebral aneurysm

Traumatic:
  Cerebral contusion and laceration
  Cerebral cicatrix
  Subarachnoid hemorrhage
  Subdural hematoma
  Middle meningeal hemorrhage
  Electrical shock treatment

Tumor:
  Gliomas
  Meningioma
  Metastatic carcinoma
  Tuberculoma

General Somatic Diseases
  Acute fever (children)
  Protein sensitization
  Heat stroke
  Hyperventilation (alkalosis)
  Hypertension
  Subacute bacterial endocarditis
  Stokes-Adams' syndrome
  Carotid sinus syndrome
  Uremia
  Hypoglycemia
  Hypoparathyroidism
  Blood dyscrasias

Intoxications:
  Botulism
  Tetanus
  Toxemia of pregnancy
  Water
  Alcohol
  Cocaine
  Camphor
  Lead
  Epinephrine
  Arsphenamine
  Picrotoxin
  Magnesium sulfate
  Strychnine
  Absinth
  Thujone
  Caffeine
  Ergot
  Nicotine
  Anesthesia

It is clear from the above list of conditions which may give rise to epileptic seizures that many diseases may at one time or another be the cause of epileptic convulsions. It would be impossible to indicate *seriatim* the occurrence of fits in this long list of causes. It is possible only to say that in some of the conditions cited convulsions occur rarely; in others, they are common. It is sufficient in general to recognize the fact that a wide variety of diseases may be associated with convulsions at one time or another during life.

The development of convulsions during *infancy* is common. In many instances, they occur with fevers, teething, gastrointestinal upsets, or with other systemic disease. It has been held in the past that infantile convulsions of this nature have no significance, that they are the equivalent of a chill in an adult, and that they rarely recur. That they are not without significance is shown by a study of epileptic patients, fifty-one per cent of whom had convulsions prior to four years of age (Thom). About twelve per cent of infantile convulsions are followed by recurrence (Shanks). Of these fifty per cent are associated with an abnormal

EEG in adult life. Less than half the cases of infantile convulsions are due to primary disease of the nervous system (Shanks). About twenty per cent of patients whose seizures began at puberty or later had an isolated convulsion as an infant (Lennox). Febrile convulsions in children may therefore presage recurrent cur with high fever, and half of the children have a family history of convulsions, usually infantile or isolated (Lennox). An abnormal EEG usually increases the likelihood of recurrence of convulsions. The EEG is usually normal in febrile convulsions, (seventy-one per cent, Lennox).

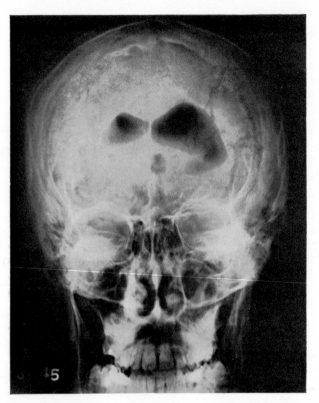

Fig. 196—Epilepsy developing immediately after a boy of 14 was struck by lightning. Note the enlargement of the ventricles, especially that of the left, due to atrophy of the brain substance.

idiopathic convulsions. This outcome is more apt to occur in the presence of a history of an atypical age of onset (before one or after three), of frequent or severe convulsions with prolonged fever, of an abnormal birth, of a family history of epilepsy or convulsions on both sides of the family, and in the presence of an abnormal EEG (Lennox). Febrile convulsions in childhood almost always oc- It is possible that in many instances of infantile convulsions attributed to fever, gastrointestinal upsets or teething, actual brain changes may be present but undetected and must therefore be searched for carefully. In any event, the convulsions of infancy cannot be said to be of no significance, even when associated with time-honored factors such as fever, etc. Careful studies indicate that among epileptics the incidence of convulsions in infancy is high, though it does not naturally follow that all epileptic attacks in infancy will be heard from later in life. It is believed by some that the term febrile convulsions should be restricted to cases with repeated convulsions during fevers and only with fevers (Gibbs). There is, in such instances, a high hereditary factor and a low EEG abnormality. A positive family history of convulsions with a febrile illness, ceasing in childhood and not recurring in adult life, confirms the diagnosis, as does a normal EEG.

The infantile convulsions referred to are presumably unmotivated, save by fever, teething, etc. In many other instances, however, convulsions occur in infancy as the direct result of birth injury, cerebral diplegia, or congenital defects. Birth injury may cause punctate hemorrhages, lacerations, or scars, all of which may cause convulsions in infancy and be followed by recurrent attacks later.

Cerebral diplegia (Little's disease) may be associated with convulsions, but in a lower incidence than might be expected. *Cerebral hemiatrophy* is frequently associated with convulsions, while in *amaurotic family idiocy* (Tay-Sachs disease) convulsions form a prominent and often an early symptom. In *tuberous sclerosis,* convulsions form an important and essential feature of the disease and, in most cases, constitute the first symptom. Convulsions develop frequently also in association with *cerebral agenesis* in its many forms. They are found consistently in *Sturge-Weber's disease,* which occurs in infants and is found associated with facial naevus, vascular changes in the eye of the same side, angiomatous malformation of the pia, intracerebral calcification and epilepsy, both generalized and focal. Epilepsy is found also in a rare disorder entitled *cerebral calcification epilepsy* (Geyelin and Penfield) characterized by convulsions and intracerebral calcification.

Convulsions occur occasionally in *multiple sclerosis*; when they do, they are usually generalized, but focal convulsion may occur. Recent studies show an incidence of convulsions in about six per cent of cases of multiple sclerosis. Seizures may usher in an attack of *cerebral hemorrhage* and occur in generalized *cerebral arteriolosclerosis* (fourteen to fifteen per cent) in persons of advanced age. The problem of arteriolosclerosis in the production of convulsions is important since it is well recognized that convulsions may be associated in older subjects with this condition. The convulsions develop in subjects with normal blood pressure or in those with hypertension. They are usually generalized but may be focal.

Convulsions occur also in *heart block* (Stokes-Adams syndrome) and in *paroxysmal tachycardia*. The Stokes-Adams syndrome, consisting of syncope and convulsive seizures, occurs in patients with slow heart rates. The convulsions in this condition result from any alteration in the cardiac mechanism causing sudden drastic reduction of cardiac output and cerebral blood flow. They occur under the following circumstances: (1) during transition from partial to complete AV block; (2) during the maintenance of complete AV block; (3) in transient ventricular flutter-fibrillation and, more rarely, cardiac arrest; (4) in patients with the cardio-inhibitory type of carotid sinus syncope, from vagal stimulation due to various factors resulting in episodes of ventricular standstill; (5) in depression of the cardiac pacemakers by quinidine, procaine amide, or potassium in subjects with AV block and other states associated with slow heart rates (Bellet). Convulsions may develop also in a hyperactive *carotid sinus* reflex, usually within twelve seconds following pressure on the carotid sinus. They may develop in embolic encephalitis associated with *subacute bacterial endocarditis* or *mitral stenosis* or in cerebral ischemia associated with *myocardial disease* or *Raynaud's disease*. They have been found also in *thromboangiitis obliterans* affecting the cerebral vessels. They occur in *subdural hematomas* but not as a rule as the initial symptom. Their incidence is placed at from ten to twenty-five per cent; convulsive seizures probably occur closer to the higher figure in subdural hematoma.

Convulsions are not uncommon in *presenile dementia* (Alzheimer's disease) and they occur both in this disease and in *lobar atrophy* (Pick's disease). They are found also in *Huntington's chorea* rarely, in *Schilder's disease* and *Friedreich's ataxia*.

Epilepsy following *head injury* is usually caused by a penetrating wound followed by scar formation. It may at times follow closed head injuries in from two to twenty years and may be generalized or focal. Its incidence varies greatly (*v.* Cranial Trauma). It has been suggested that the incidence of seizures increases as the length of the period of posttraumatic amnesia grows longer. In posttraumatic epilepsy there is reported to be a tendency for the seizures to decrease spontaneously after two to three years and to cease after four to five years in about forty-five per cent of cases. This appears to hold true of seizures developing early or late after the head injury.

Seizures occur frequently with *porencephalic cysts;* they are often focal but may be generalized even in the presence of a focal lesion such as porencephaly. It is a curious feature of porencephalic cyst that the occurrence of convulsions may be long delayed, though the cyst presumably was of congenital origin. Whether congenital, posttraumatic, or postvascular, porencephaly may be present for some time before convulsions or other evidences of its presence become manifest.

Brain tumors are commonly associated with seizures and must always be suspected when attacks develop in adults. Convulsions are often the first symptom of brain tumor. Convulsions are found particularly in tumors involving the cerebral hemispheres, especially in tumors of the temporal and frontal lobes. They occur with both infiltrating and encapsulated tumors. They are not found in posterior fossa tumors. Convulsions do not occur in pituitary tumors unless they escape from the sella turcica and compress the brain. Suprasellar tumors may cause convulsions by pressure on the frontal or temporal lobes. Seizures occur in supratentorial tumors in twenty to forty-five per cent of cases, the figures varying for different series (30.9 per cent, Sargent; 21.4 per cent, Parker; thirty-nine per cent, Dowman and Smith; 25.7 per cent, Ley and Walker). Of the various types of brain tumor, seizures occur chiefly among the meningiomas, astrocytomas, and oligodendrogliomas. Seizures occur in a relatively high incidence of cases in *brain abscess* (twelve to fifteen per cent) but not usually as an initial symptom. They are more common in cases of abscess of the frontal and temporal lobes. *Idiopathic hypoparathyroidism* is a rare cause of seizures. It is characterized by low serum calcium, elevated serum phosphorus, normal serum alkaline phosphatase, and the absence of radiological evidence of rickets or osteomalacia. Dental defects, cataracts, trophic changes in the nails, and symmetrical cerebral calcification are often present. Papilledema is sometimes found in association with the hypocalcemia. The seizures occurring in idiopathic hypoparathyroidism are generalized. Not all patients with hypocalcemia develop seizures and the reason for their occurrence in some cases and not in others is not known. The electroencephalogram has been reported to be abnormal.

Seizures may develop in some instances for the first time following *electrical shock treatment*. They may be recurrent, once initiated, but it has been asserted that their incidence after shock treatment is no greater than in the normal population (Kalinowsky).

Cerebral vascular spasm may be associated with either general or focal convulsions and *subarachnoid hemorrhage* is at times associated with generalized seizures. Convulsions may be the first sign of *general paresis,* a point which should always be recalled in an adult with sudden onset of convulsions. Seizures occur in ten to twenty-five per cent of cases of general paresis. They are found also in *acute syphilitic meningitis,* in vascular forms of neurosyphilis, and in *congenital syphilis.*

Seizures are the most frequent central nervous system manifestation in *lupus erythematosus.* They may precede recognizable symptoms of the latter by years. Seizures may occur in chronic *recurrent malaria.* Seizures often regarded as idiopathic may occur as a result of *rheumatic heart disease.* They usually develop in adults and the diagnosis is possible if rheumatic heart disease is present and if there is a history of rheumatic fever. The EEG is not specific. There is usually a latency of several years between the acute rheumatic disease and the occurrence of the seizures (Whitman and Karnosh).

Epileptic seizures are not uncommon also in cases of chronic *alcoholism,* but it is still undetermined whether they develop because of the alcoholism or whether they result from extraneous causes unassociated with the alcoholism. Chronic alcoholism is a rare cause of epilepsy. Alcohol in any form, however, may precipitate convulsions and must be avoided by epileptics. The problem of the relationship of alcohol to the production of convulsions has long been a matter of investigation. Alcohol is capable of precipitating convulsive attacks in those subject to seizures. but it is a rare cause of convulsions. Alcohol is said to precipitate generalized seizures more frequently in instances of symptomatic epilepsy and particularly in petit mal and psychomotor seizures. There are patients who have convulsions only when intoxicated: the problem of causation is a little more complicated in such instances, but even here alcohol probably is only a precipitant. Among a group of 1254 patients with epilepsy, alcohol was found to be a precipitating factor in six per cent and in twenty-one per cent of those who used alcohol (Lennox). A study of the EEG in chronic alcoholism with seizures reveals a low incidence of abnormalities.

Lead encephalopathy is associated with convulsions in both children and adults. In children, convulsions may usher in the signs of plumbism. The incidence of convulsions in the various forms of *encephalitis* is difficult to define. They are rare following lethargic encephalitis and their occurrence after the many forms of disseminated encephalomyelitis is also uncommon. Convulsions develop frequently in *encephalitis periaxialis diffusa* (Schilder). They have been reported following measles, pertussis. varicella, and mumps encephalitis. Convulsions occur in *meningitis.*

Seizures may develop during the course of *general anesthesia.* An EEG study of twenty-two patients indicates that the anesthetic convulsions differ in no way from the epileptic seizure and that they are the result of an inborn but latent epileptic liability (Williams and Sweet).

XI. GENERAL SYMPTOMATOLOGY

Epilepsy may develop at any *age*. In the idiopathic variety, the onset is often in infancy, but the appearance of seizures in childhood, puberty, or later is not uncommon. They are prone to appear especially at puberty between the ages of ten and fifteen. While seizures occurring for the first time in adult life must always be suspected of being of symptomatic origin, it is not at all unusual to find that they are idiopathic in type or at least that no cause can be found for their development. Epilepsy may develop late in life (sixty to seventy years) due to cerebral arteriosclerosis and to subsequent brain changes. This is often spoken of as senile epilepsy. In general, the symptomatic epilepsies are apt to appear at a later date than seizures of the idiopathic variety, the time of appearance depending, of course, on the cause.

The occurrence of epilepsy in middle or later life, due to no known cause, appears to be more common than is generally conceded. Among 602 cases of epilepsy followed over a period of eighteen years, the onset of convulsions was found to be as follows (Nattras): before ten years, twenty-two per cent; ages eleven to twenty, thirty-one per cent; ages twenty-one to thirty, twenty-two per cent; ages thirty-one to forty, twelve per cent; over forty, thirteen per cent (eighty-one patients). Epilepsy of undetermined origin may develop, therefore, in later life and is not uncommon at such times. The incidence as to *sex* has no significant meaning. Both sexes are subject to seizures, large series of cases

indicating no outstanding predominance of either sex. In a group of noninstitutional epileptics, fifty-eight per cent were found to be males and forty-two per cent females.

The problem of *heredity* in epilepsy has baffled neurologists for many years. Idiopathic epilepsy was at one time regarded as widely inherited. Statistical studies of inheritance of epilepsy are at such wide variance with one another that it is difficult to evaluate them. Moreover, they are open to the criticism that studies of institutionalized epileptics and those seen in private practice are probably not comparable for statistical purposes. A history of seizures was obtained for 3.2 per cent of 20,000 near relatives of 4231 epileptics (Lennox). Seizures were found in eight per cent of the immediate family of one thousand epileptics and in 13.2 per cent of all known relatives (Himler). On the other hand, a history of convulsions was found in twenty-eight per cent of two hundred cases of epilepsy and in only ten per cent of a control series (Brain). Among one thousand patients with epilepsy, a history of convulsive seizures was found in 18.1 per cent in the immediate families (Stein). When these figures were corrected to include parents, siblings, and children, the incidence was 3.7 per cent for epileptics and 1.3 per cent for controls. On the other hand, it is asserted that "statistical studies have agreed that not more than twenty per cent of patients give a history of seizures in any known relative" (Lennox).

The incidence of epilepsy has been studied in identical twins and has been found to be high in such twins with seizures. A study of 253 pairs of twins reveals that in identical (uniovular) twins, epilepsy developed in both twins in 66.6 per cent, while in fraternal (binovular) twins, both individuals were epileptic in only

3.15 per cent (Conrad). In a group of 122 twin pairs affected with seizures, without evidence of prior brain damage, both twins were epileptic in eighty-four per cent of one-egg and ten per cent of two-egg twins. A study of brain waves in the families of epileptics by means of the electroencephalogram reveals an incidence of sixty per cent of abnormal brain waves (Lennox). It is uncertain whether this indicates that the tendency to inheritance of epilepsy is found in sixty per cent of cases. "The genetic factor in epilepsy is probably no greater than it is in many other common diseases" (Lennox). No hereditary factor has been disclosed in cases of symptomatic epilepsy.

The possibility of the development of epilepsy in offspring becomes one chance in one hundred if in the affected parents (1) a history of evidence of brain injury antedated the seizures, (2) there is an absence of epilepsy or migraine in blood relatives, (3) the seizures began later than infancy or childhood, (4) the mentality of the patient was normal at birth, and (5) there is no predisposition to seizures in the spouse (Lennox).

The *occurrence* of epileptic attacks varies greatly from case to case. In some instances, seizures may be few during the course of the patient's lifetime and may occur at widely separated intervals. An analysis of a group of patients who had only one to three seizures in their lifetime reveals that three groups may be distinguished: (1) Those in whom the seizure was frequently associated with excess alcoholic intake. These had a bilaterally synchronous three per second wave and spike abnormality in the EEG. (2) Those in whom the seizures were precipitated by fatigue and emotional and physical stress. The EEG revealed a diffuse dysrhythmia. (3) Those in whom the seizures were associated with

stress. The EEG revealed bilaterally synchronous 6 per second activity (Kershman). In others, they may appear several times a week or almost daily, and in rare instances there may be only a few attacks during a lifetime. Convulsions may develop in infancy during fevers and never be heard from again. Seizures may fade out during adult life, but it is difficult to estimate the incidence of such disappearance of convulsions.

Seizures may occur during the day, night (sleep), or both day or night (sleep). In idiopathic cases there is no relationship to specific factors, such as fatigue, appetite, etc. Diurnal attacks may develop at any time but are more common in the morning shortly after arising. Nocturnal attacks are frequent, appearing especially in the early hours before waking or soon after falling asleep. The seizures occurring during sleep may develop in sleep at any time, both day and night, and are not strictly nocturnal attacks. Convulsions are often more common during the menstrual and premenstrual periods, but there is no known significance of this feature of their incidence.

Seizures may at times be precipitated by psychical trauma of many sorts, such as the barking of a dog, a sudden noise, or severe emotional strain. Included in this group should probably be those cases of musicogenic epilepsy in which epileptic attacks are precipitated by the sound of a musical instrument.

Physical examination often reveals nothing in idiopathic epilepsy, but abnormalities of one sort or another have been reported. Among these are visceroptosis, constipation, and diminished respiratory ventilation seen in a deficit of oxygen saturation of the blood. Generally speaking, the routine physical examination in cases of idiopathic epilepsy reveals nothing significant.

Routine neurological examination is invariably negative except in cases of symptomatic epilepsy, the findings in these cases depending on the location and nature of the underlying damage.

XII. DIAGNOSIS

The primary step in diagnosis is the recognition of the occurrence of seizures. whether these are grand mal, petit mal, psychomotor, or focal. For this, one is almost entirely dependent on the history of the description of the attacks, in which the patient is often of little help, since he is unaware of the nature of the attack during the period of unconsciousness. It is essential in both grand mal and petit mal attacks to be certain that unconsciousness or impairment of consciousness has been present during the seizure. It is also important in grand mal seizures to satisfy oneself concerning the presence of clonic movements, frothing at the mouth, tongue biting, incontinence, and the postconvulsive state.

Great care must be exercised in determining the nature of petit mal spells, since these may simulate other disturbances; in these, the occurrence of impairment of consciousness is important. In most instances, a reliable description can be obtained only from relatives or from others who have had occasion to observe them. It is sometimes difficult to decide whether unconsciousness is present in the seizures, since they are usually seen by untrained observers. In the case of petit mal spells, the patient is usually the best witness and can as a rule be relied on to give a good account of the attacks. It is important to establish the presence of fleeting impairment of consciousness in such episodes in order to distinguish them from attacks of vertigo and hysteria. Though a history of impairment or loss of consciousness is important in many seizures, it is essential to recognize that seizures may occur without loss of consciousness. Among these are jacksonian seizures and temporal lobe seizures. The occurrence of jacksonian seizures must usually be established by direct questioning, since untrained observers are unaware of their significance and will not, as a rule, volunteer this very significant information. A history of previous medication, such as bromides or phenobarbital, often gives a clue as to the nature of the condition.

Having established the fact that true seizures are present, the problem then becomes one of determining whether the seizures are idiopathic or symptomatic in nature. The diagnosis of idiopathic epilepsy is made on the basis of the following criteria: (1) a history of seizures beginning usually in childhood or adolescence, but in adult life in some instances; (2) the absence of findings by physical or neurological examination except in some cases where there are obvious evidences of mental deterioration; (3) the absence of significant laboratory findings; (4) an abnormal electroencephalogram. In idiopathic epilepsy, there are no abnormalities on physical, neurological, or laboratory examination and it is precisely because of these negative findings that such cases are classified as idiopathic, there being no clue as to a possible cause.

In symptomatic epilepsy, on the other hand, indications of an underlying cause are present either in the history (trauma, encephalitis, syphilis, etc.), the neurological examination, which shows as a rule abnormal findings of some degree, or in laboratory studies, such as positive serological tests, hypoglycemic sugar tolerance curves, depressed skull fractures, or abnormal encephalogram demonstrating evidence of a focal brain lesion. The occurrence of abnormal findings indicating an underlying cause always points to a symptomatic type of epilepsy. On the other hand, the neurological examination may often be negative even in cases with focal lesions and it often happens that the EEG may reveal an epileptogenic focus in the absence of abnormal neurological findings or of a history of focal seizures. The best clue to localization of an epileptogenic zone is the seizure pattern. The greatest supplementary aid is the EEG.

The *electroencephalogram* (EEG) is of great help in the diagnosis of epilepsy. By means of electrodes placed on the scalp or on the periosteum, it is possible to record electrical activity of the brain by means of brain waves which are then greatly amplified and recorded. Such brain waves are known to have a normal rhythm or pattern, but many individual differences are found. Alpha, beta, gamma, and delta waves are differentiated, all with characteristic amplitudes. The EEG is affected by sleep, vision, and abnormal brain processes, such as tumor, cyst, cicatrix, hematoma, etc. Abnormal rhythms, notably slow rhythms (delta waves), are found in a variety of conditions—brain edema, coma, stupor, acute degenerative processes; small discrete lesions are often missed, and brain stem and posterior fossa lesions are difficult to detect. Normal rhythms are lost in states of emotional tension and excitement. Brain waves are slowed by sleep, sedative, and low carbon dioxide tension, and are increased by fright, sensory stimulation, and high carbon dioxide tension.

Abnormal rhythms and frequencies of brain waves as seen in the EEG are found in epilepsy. These are generalized in the idiopathic type and focal in the symptomatic variety. They are found between attacks, are increased by hyperventilation, and are depressed by sedative medication. Abnormal EEG records have been found in epilepsy during sleep

(Gibbs and Gibbs). According to some investigators (Gibbs, Gibbs, and Lennox) characteristic brain waves are found for each type of fit. Grand mal (generalized) seizures are characterized by bursts of diffuse multiple spikes and sharp waves; jacksonian seizures are featured by localized sharp waves; petit mal attacks are associated with wave and spike patterns of a characteristic nature, most marked in the frontal areas; psychic seizures likewise have characteristic patterns of rhythmic slow waves. Other investigators question the specificity of certain types of brain waves for specific types of seizures, maintaining that no diagnosis of the type of seizures can be made from the brain wave pattern.

Justification for the use of specific terms to describe the electroencephalographic tracings, in order to correlate them with their clinical counterparts, is given by their leading proponents, Gibbs, Gibbs, and Lennox. Their reasons are as follows:

"During a typical clinical petit mal seizure, the electroencephalogram shows high voltage alternate waves and spikes which recur at the rate of approximately three per second; during a clinical grand mal seizure, the record shows fast waves of increased amplitude, and during a clinical psychomotor seizure, the record shows high voltage four to six per second waves, many of which have flat tops."

Specific seizures appear, therefore, to have specific types of brain patterns. The advisability of assigning such specific patterns to definite seizures has been questioned on the basis that it is not always possible to correlate the type of wave with the type of seizure. Despite such objections, it is clear that the classification of Gibbs, Gibbs, and Lennox is useful. They state that "the electrical pattern during a seizure is distinctive for each of the three main types of seizures,

When seizure discharges appear in the routine electroencephalogram, they tend to correspond to a type of clinical seizure already reported in that case. This correspondence is greatest for petit mal seizures, less evident for psychomotor types of seizure; though in the latter, if grand mal seizures are present, the EEG record may be predominantly that associated with grand mal attacks.

"In about forty-eight per cent of persons with a history of seizures, a routine

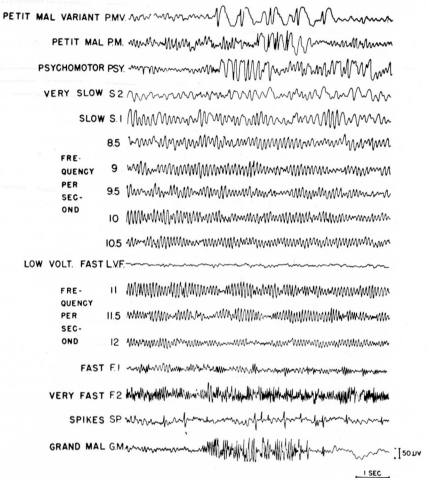

PETIT MAL VARIANT P.M.V.

PETIT MAL P.M.

PSYCHOMOTOR PSY.

VERY SLOW S.2

SLOW S.1

8.5

FRE-
QUENCY   9

PER
SEC-   9.5
OND

10

10.5

LOW VOLT. FAST L.V.F.

FRE-   11
QUENCY

PER   11.5
SEC-
OND   12

FAST F.1

VERY FAST F.2

SPIKES SP.

GRAND MAL G.M.

50 μV

1 SEC

Fig. 197—*Epilepsy*. EEG patterns in the various types of seizure. (Gibbs, *et al.*)

seizures, and least evident for grand mal seizures." Clinical experience indicates clearly that there is often no correlation between seizure type and EEG records. Major seizures may reveal in interseizure records a predominance of the petit mal type of EEG record with few or no fast waves. The highest correlation appears to be between the petit mal and psychic electroencephalogram is of great value in diagnosis, and in about forty-two per cent it is of little or no value" (Gibbs, Gibbs, and Lennox). This assertion is made on the basis of a large number of interseizure records in which it was found that in thirteen per cent of clinically diagnosed epilepsy the routine electroencephalogram was perfectly normal,

Table 56—Types of Seizures, Electroencephalographic Patterns, and Therapy

(After Lennox)

Type of Seizure	Chief Characteristic	Electroencephalogram		Therapy In Order of Choice
		In Seizure	*Interseizure*	
JACKSONIAN	"March" of sensation or motion, consciousness retained	High voltage fast discharge beginning locally and spreading	Usually normal	Surgical removal of discharge focus Phenytoin sodium Mesantoin, phenobarbital, or others
FOCAL CONVULSION	One-sided convulsion or localized symptoms initiating generalized convulsion—consciousness lost	High voltage fast waves beginning locally	Focus of seizure discharge; slow waves or spikes	Possibly neurosurgery Phenytoin sodium Mesantoin, phenobarbital, or others
GRAND MAL	Generalized tonic-clonic convulsion, consciousness lost	Generalized continuous high voltage fast waves or spikes	Seizure discharge —18% Waves, slow or fast —64% Normal —18%	Phenytoin sodium Mesantoin, phenobarbital, bromides, or others
PSYCHOMOTOR (psychic equivalent)	Period of amnesia, with or without tonic muscular spasm or contortions	Generalized high voltage slow waves, perhaps square-topped	Seizure discharge —49% Waves, slow or fast —36% Normal —15%	Phenytoin sodium, along or combined with tridione
PETIT MAL (pyknoepilepsy)	Transient lapse of consciousness, minimal rhythmic jerking at three per second	Generalized high voltage, "dart and dome," at 3 per second	"Dart and dome" 82% Other abnormalities —10% Normal —8%	Tridione, preeminently effective Ketosis Caffeine Mebaral Amphetamine sulfate may be tried
MYOCLONIC JERKS	Lightning-like jerk of extremities with consciousness probably retained	If anything, single petit mal, "dart and dome"	Possibly isolated, "dart and dome"	
AKINETIC	Sudden loss of posture with falling or nodding	Often series of high voltage 2 per second waves or slow spike and wave —frequently localized—pronounced dysrhythmia often not accompanied by clinical symptoms.		
AUTONOMIC (diencephalic)	Pallor, flushing, palpitation, sweating, giddiness, nausea, etc., consciousness retained	Usually normal, even during seizure, or random slowing		Possibly phenobarbital or amphetamine sulfate

while in twenty-nine per cent it was not sufficiently abnormal to be indicative. The possibility of obtaining an abnormal electroencephalogram record appears to be directly proportional to the severity and number of the seizures. Patients with a normal EEG pattern are likely to have rare seizures (Gibbs). Records made *during* a seizure are practically always abnormal. Anticonvulsant drugs only rarely obliterate all abnormal brain waves.

The electroencephalogram is said to be abnormal in eighty-five per cent of cases of epilepsy, the other fifteen per cent showing normal brain waves. Abnormal brain waves are found in ten per cent of normal subjects. While most investigators maintain that abnormal brain waves are found in a high percentage of patients between fits. Williams found them in only forty per cent. He found also that abnormal electroencephalograms were found in fifty-five per cent of patients with grand mal seizures, sixty per cent in those with petit mal seizures, eighty-three per cent in psychomotor attacks, and ninety per cent in patients with mixed types of seizures. The occurrence of paroxysmal outbursts of activity in the EEG, however transient, probably represents epileptic activity (Williams). Under such circumstances it is believed that a liability to epilepsy exists, even in the absence of fits, provided that the outbursts are paroxysmal.

There is no agreement concerning the following: (1) the incidence of abnormal brain waves in interseizure records in the various forms of epilepsy, except to indicate that the highest incidence of abnormality is in the petit mal type of seizure (85 per cent), the next highest in the psychic seizures (42 to 83 per cent), and the lowest in grand mal seizures; (2) the incidence of normal EEG records in inter-seizure records, estimates varying from 15 to 20 per cent.

It is clear that for clinical purposes the diagnosis of epilepsy cannot rest on the EEG alone in view of the normal inter-seizure records in 15 to 20 per cent. The diagnosis must depend on clinical observation, using the EEG as a correlative examination.

In patients with normal interseizure records, it appears true that these occur in seizures of later onset; in seizures that are more frequently nocturnal and fewer in number; and patients with such records require less treatment and have a better outlook (Abbott and Schwab).

Electrocorticography, the tracings obtained from the exposed cerebral cortex, differ from those obtained from the scalp in two characteristics; (1) the amplitude of the cortical activity is 3-4 times greater; (2) rapid oscillations in electrical activity are not distorted and hence appear as spikes. It has been said that the ECG is dependent on the cyto-architecture of the cortex and that different areas have typical frequencies and patterns. Though recognition of an area by its rhythm is possible at times, such prediction is said to be no better than chance (Marshall and Walker). Anesthesia affects the ECG. Ether causes marked slowing of the cortical frequencies with some increase in amplitude. Pentothal augments the frequency and amplitude. Electrocorticography is particularly valuable in the localization of epileptogenic foci.

The distinction between a *faint* and an epileptic seizure is often difficult clinically. The symptom common to the two conditions is loss of consciousness. Faints occur usually in the erect posture. They develop as the result of interference with vascular mechanisms, as in orthostatic hypotension, cardiac arrest, carotid sinus stimulation, and under emotional stress. The failure to develop convulsive twitchings is not a valid means of differentiation between a fit and a seizure since many seizures develop without convulsive movements. The occurrence of convulsive twitchings, as also the development of incontinence, favors an epileptic seizure. The demonstration of an aura also favors an epileptic seizure. People in faints always fall; those subject to seizures often develop impairment of consciousness without a fall. Efforts to relate faints to seizures in the majority of instances are inconclusive. Though syncope and epilepsy may occur in the same family or same individual, syncope is not a special form of epilepsy. Fast rhythms in the frontal lobes have been found in patients with syncope.

XIII. ABERRANT FORMS OF EPILEPSY

Among the many *aberrant forms* of epilepsy are myoclonus epilepsy, a tonic form, epilepsy partialis continua, pyknolepsy, and reflex epilepsy.

Myoclonus Epilepsy: *Myoclonus epilepsy* is rare and is characterized by the violent contraction of muscle groups, generalized or local on one or both sides of the body, involving limbs and/or trunk, sufficiently violent to cause the dropping of objects, catapulting of the patient to the floor, etc. They are usually intermittent but may be constant. Several types of myoclonus epilepsy have been described, the most definite of which are: (1) intermittent myoclonus (Lundborg), and (2) progressive familial myoclonus (Unverricht). The first type consists of intermittent myoclonic contractions. It is not progressive. The familial type of Unverricht is inherited as a recessive Mendelian character, appears most often in girls before puberty, usually with generalized epileptic attacks. After a period of one to five years, the second stage of myoclonus develops, char-

acterized by muscle twitchings which increase in intensity and frequency and gradually involve the entire body. Intelligence becomes impaired until severe dementia develops. The disease lasts from ten to twenty years, death ensuing often from involvement of the bulbar muscles. Ataxia, tremor, dyssynergia, and other signs of disease of the brain develop. Pathologically, there is degeneration of the cells in the dentate nucleus of the cerebellum, thalamus, nucleus ruber, substantia nigra, and other basal ganglia. Inclusion bodies are found within the ganglion cells in the affected areas.

Tonic Epilepsy: *Tonic epilepsy* without clonic features is characterized by a tonic contraction of all the limbs with arching of the back and opisthotonus. Seizures of this nature in pure form are found in cerebellar and mesencephalic disease (tumor, softening). In cerebellar disease, they are associated with "skew deviation" of the eyes, one eye looking up and out, the other down and in. A special form of tonic epilepsy has been recorded as striatal epilepsy, involving usually one or more limbs. The term is ill defined and until further confirmation is possible cannot be regarded as a special form of epilepsy.

Epilepsia Partialis Continua: *Partial continuous epilepsy* is a form of attack characterized by the occurrence of continuous muscular twitchings in some part of the body. The attacks may occur between generalized seizures in cases of epilepsy, or they may develop independently of other forms of seizures. In the latter case, their significance is frequently overlooked. The movements may affect the eyelid, a portion of the face, the thumb, a finger, part of an arm or forearm, or other muscle groups. They consist of constant twitchings of the muscle involved, the term partial continuous epilepsy designating the two main features of this form of attack: (1) the partial involvement of a limb or even of part of a muscle; (2) the continuous movement of the muscle. The latter may continue for hours or days. This form of epilepsy is not associated with loss or impairment of consciousness and is not followed usually by loss of power of the affected muscles. It results from processes which affect the motor cortex—tumor, abscess, syphilis, encephalitis, metastatic carcinoma.

Pyknolepsy: This is a term given to a variety of epilepsy found in children (five to twelve years), characterized by numerous blank episodes simulating petit mal, occurring in rapid succession many times a day. During these spells the stare is vacant for a few seconds, following which the child resumes his activities without interruption. The attacks are unassociated with motor twitchings and cease after months or years without the development of other signs of epilepsy. The attacks are similar to petit mal and differ from the usual variety only by their numbers and their complete disappearance in the course of time. It is doubtful, in fact, whether it is justifiable to regard pyknolepsy as a special variety of epilepsy. It is best regarded as a form of petit mal. It does not respond to the usual sedative treatment of epilepsy, such as bromides, phenobarbital, etc.

Diencephalic Epilepsy: This form has been described (Penfield) as due to damage of the diencephalon by brain tumor. Attacks of this nature are characterized largely by vegetative phenomena, such as lacrimation, diaphoresis, vasodilatation, rise in blood pressure, salivation, dilatation or contraction of the pupils, increased pulse rate, protrusion of the eyeballs, bradypnea, hiccuping, transient shivering, Cheyne-Stokes respirations, and rare loss of consciousness.

Reflex Epilepsy: This term has been widely used in medical parlance to indicate those cases of epilepsy which are precipitated by sensory stimulation of many sorts. The term is a poor one, since it implies a special category of epilepsy. It would be preferable to speak of reflexly precipitated epilepsy rather than reflex epilepsy, since fundamentally the affected subjects are epileptics in whom seizures are precipitated by sensory stimulation. The most frequent examples of this form of epilepsy are seen in those cases which are precipitated by music and noises of various sorts. Pleural epilepsy, convulsive seizure on puncture of the pleura, is an example of reflex epilepsy. Included also are those instances referred to as musicogenic epilepsy in which the spells are precipitated by hearing music. Emotional stimulation may precipitate epileptic attacks. Reflex epilepsy is precipitated in rare instances by a visual stimulus or by photic stimulation. In one instance, petit mal episodes were caused by a tap on the shoulder, and a small hemangioma was removed from the motor cortex (Forster). In instances of reflex epilepsy the suddenness and unexpectedness of the stimulus is constant. The type of stimulus varies and may consist of music, sudden noise, a moving object, and visual stimuli of many sorts.

XIV. TREATMENT

The purpose of treatment is control of the seizures. To attain this end it is necessary to make certain of the following: (1) proper identification of the seizure by careful history, since some of the drugs available are much more effective in some forms of epilepsy than in others; (2) careful neurological evaluation in order to separate idiopathic and symptomatic cases; and (3) the establishment of adequate drug therapy.

After choice of the drug or drugs to be used in a particular instance, it is best to begin with a minimum dose and to increase this gradually to the point of greatest effect and fewest side reactions of the drug. More than one drug may be used in the control of seizures, when seizures are difficult to control or when more than a single type of seizure is present.

Failures in treatment result from improper recognition of the type of seizure, and consequently improper selection of drugs, failure to give drugs in sufficient dosage, and too frequent shifting of drugs.

The treatment of epilepsy must be directed toward care of the general health as well as of the seizures. A nutritious diet is important. Diets as a therapeutic measure in epilepsy have less value than drugs. While many sorts of diets have been used, only the *ketogenic diet* has any value. This produces essentially an acidosis. Fat is increased in the diet and carbohydrate and protein diminished; effective ratios of fat to carbohydrate and protein are three to one or four to one. This form of dietary treatment is especially effective in children. It has the disadvantage of being extremely unpalatable as a steady diet and of losing its efficacy in the course of time. The restriction of *fluids* to 1000 to 1500 cc. daily for all forms of fluid is said to have some value in the treatment of epilepsy, and is advocated strongly by some investigators. It is not necessary to restrict fluids in the average case except in those instances in which there seems to be a clear relationship between fluid intake and the precipitation of attacks. In such instances, the total fluid intake per diem should be restricted. Routine restriction, however, is unnecessary and accomplishes little in the average case.

Alcohol in any form must be avoided, since it is common experience that alcohol, whether in the form of hard liquor, wine, or beer, tends to precipitate attacks. There should be no deviation from this dictum. *Tobacco* need not be restricted save in instances of obvious abuse. *Coffee* should be restricted to moderate intake and in cases of abuse should be eliminated entirely. *Constipation* should be avoided, since it is a common precipitating factor of epileptic attacks.

The problem of *physical activities* must be answered in every case of epilepsy, especially in the case of younger patients. It is a safe rule that no physical activities should be permitted which will tend to harm the patient. Bicycle riding, swimming, climbing, or other activities in which serious physical harm might result if a seizure were to develop during their course, should all be eschewed. These need not be eliminated in all cases of epilepsy, however. It is obvious that patients whose attacks are entirely nocturnal may engage safely in physical exercise; the same holds true of those instances in which attacks are so widely scattered as to eliminate the possibility of bodily injury. For the average patient whose seizures occur unpredictably despite treatment, physical activities which might cause injury must be avoided. Physical exercise is not only desirable but valuable in all instances, the object in such cases being to enlarge chest volume and increase aeration.

Occupations which may produce injury must be avoided; thus epileptics should not be permitted to work with machinery when there is a distinct possibility of the development of attacks while doing so. Efforts should be made, therefore, to place them in occupations which do not jeopardize their lives. Care must be directed also to the *emotional* factors in epilepsy. Freedom from anxiety and the elimination of extreme emotional reactions must be obtained. Epileptics are sensitive of their attacks, are apt to regard themselves as stigmatized, and develop, therefore, unhealthy reactions to their illness. All this should be handled by open discussion with the patient if his intelligence will permit it, with the object in mind of establishing a healthier adjustment to his affliction. Reading material which illustrates these points by accounts of famous characters in history who have been epileptic is extremely helpful.

Every effort must be made to make the epileptic feel in no way different from his companions, and he must therefore be urged to engage in all activities short of those which may bring him harm. A follow-up study of college students with epilepsy provides evidence that the presence of seizures in persons with higher intelligence need not constitute a barrier to academic training, social adjustments, or to work after leaving college. Sufferers with epilepsy are not excluded from colleges, as indicated by the results of a poll of 1700 colleges. Physical abnormalities of any sort should be eradicated.

Table 57—Drug Treatment of Epilepsy

Drug	Dosage	Field of Greatest Use	Side Reactions
PHENOBARBITAL	1½ to 6 or 7 or even 10 gr. daily	Major seizures	Dermatitis, apathy, drowsiness, sluggishness, mental dullness, irritability, asthenia
DILANTIN SODIUM	3 to 9 gr. daily	Major seizures and psychomotor attacks	Gastric distress, nausea, vertigo, ataxia, tremor, blurred vision, diplopia, drowsiness, insomnia, irritability, hyperplasia of gums, dermatitis, purpura
MESANTOIN	3 to 9 gr. daily	Alone, or as adjunct to other drugs, on in cases intolerant to other drugs	Dermatitis; drowsiness uncommon; aplastic anemia rare
BROMIDES	30 to 45 gr. daily	Major seizures	Acne, mental sluggishness, depression; bromide intoxication in some cases
MEBARAL	1½ to 9 gr. daily	Major seizures Minor attacks in some instances	Drowsiness
MILONTIN	0.5 Gm. 3 to 6 times daily	Petit mal	Nausea, vomiting, dizziness, drowsiness
TRIDIONE	0.3 Gm. 3 to 6 times daily	Petit mal	Photophobia, dizziness, gastric distress
MYSOLINE	0.25 Gm. 3 to 6 times daily	Grand mal and psychomotor seizures	Drowsiness, atoxia, nausea, vomiting, dizziness

The problem of *marriage* often arises. While some states regard marriage of an epileptic as illegal, there is no reason why a person with epilepsy should not marry except in the case of obvious mental deterioration. The question whether an epileptic should have children must be discussed frankly and the known facts made clear (*v.* Heredity). The decision regarding children must then be left to those directly involved. When both parents have epilepsy, or a history of epilepsy in the family, having children should be discouraged. In the case of adoption of children, care must be taken that there is no history of epilepsy in the children's parents. The distress of parents faced with epilepsy in an adopted child is not difficult to imagine.

The treatment of the seizures is, of course, symptomatic, since the cause of essential epilepsy is not known. For such treatment, the most efficacious drugs are phenobarbital, Dilantin Sodium, and bromides. Of these diphenylhydantoin sodium (Dilantin Sodium) and phenobarbital are the most useful for all types of seizures except petit mal. The choice of one drug as compared with another is often difficult. When seizures are infrequent, phenobarbital is the drug of choice. When they occur frequently, Dilantin Sodium is to be preferred. Often the two are combined, or other drugs may be given with either Dilantin Sodium or phenobarbital.

The drug treatment of epilepsy must be guided by a few general principles which will be found useful in the handling of the seizures. These may be summarized as follows: (1) The drugs which are most efficacious in treatment are often associated with the development of a tolerance on the part of the patient. Hence it becomes necessary from time to time to increase the dosage or to stagger the drugs in use. In the latter case, the substitution of one drug for another must always be carried out gradually lest attacks be precipitated by too rapid withdrawal. (2) It is essential that the drugs in use be given with an eye to the seizure rhythm. For this reason it is best to concentrate the dosage of the drug at those times when seizures are most prevalent. For nocturnal and sleep attacks, the drug should be given chiefly in the latter part of the day and before retiring; for women whose attacks occur chiefly around the menstrual periods, increased dosage should be given a week prior to and following the menses. (3) The dosage of the drug or drugs used in the treatment must be built up gradually. It is best to begin with small doses and to increase these gradually until the optimum dose has been reached. For this reason it is necessary to see the patient repeatedly, until it is certain that the type of drug or drugs and their dosage is suitable to the patient and his type of seizure or seizures. (4) Drugs, when given, should be administered in doses which will if possible control the seizures. To this end, large doses are preferable to small. The tolerance of the epileptic will be found to be surprisingly high for most anticonvulsants. Where large doses of drug are required, it is often better to compromise and to be satisfied with incomplete control of the seizures in order to avoid toxic drug effects. It is better to have an occasional seizure than a drowsy, confused patient. (5) Once the optimum dosage has been ascertained, it should be continued indefinitely until good reasons are found for changing it. These include tolerance to the drug, the development of side reactions, or freedom from seizures. The dosage of the drug should not be decreased until the patient has been free from seizures for a long period of time, preferably a year. Under these circumstances, the dosage may be decreased gradually by removing one dose when it is least needed, but the drug must not under any circumstances be withdrawn at once for fear of precipitating seizures or status epilepticus.

Dilantin Sodium (diphenylhydantoin sodium): This is a most useful anticonvulsant and has the advantage of not producing a sedative effect. It may be given without fear of causing the drowsiness and letdown feeling which often follows the use of phenobarbital and bromides. Best results with the drug are obtained only if it is given to the threshold of tolerance; hence it must be administered in doses just short of the toxic dosage for the individual patient. The difference between the effective and toxic dose may be very slight. What this dosage is must be worked out individually. It is given in doses of 1½ grains three or four a day as an average dose, but it may be given as often as five to six times a day. Children may be started on 1½ grains once or twice daily and the subsequent dosage adjusted according to the therapeutic response. Very young children may be given ½ grain twice daily. It should be given at times of the day when the seizures are most frequent. If it is started in a patient who has been taking phenobarbital or bromides, the latter drugs should be withdrawn gradually over the course of several days. Dilantin Sodium is particularly efficacious in major seizures and in the psychic attacks of epilepsy, but is not so effectual for the minor episodes.

Convulsions were relieved in about sixty per cent of epileptics treated with Dilantin Sodium and followed for two months to two years. It must frequently be given with phenobarbital or bromides, preferably the former, in combinations which can only be worked out for each individual case. In those cases in which Dilantin Sodium alone is incapable of controlling seizures, it is best given with phenobarbital. Experience has shown that in such instances full doses of both drugs must be used, for Dilantin 3 to 9 grains daily and for phenobarbital, 1 to 3¾ grains daily (Merritt and Brenner).

Of one hundred epileptic patients treated with Dilantin Sodium and phenobarbital, eight of fifty-six with grand mal seizures showed marked improvement of the grand mal seizures, twelve moderate improvement, sixteen were questionable, and twenty showed no improvement. Petit mal and psychomotor seizures were not affected (Merritt and Brenner). Toxic symptoms sometimes develop following the use of Dilantin Sodium; they consist of gastric distress, vertigo, ataxia, tremor, blurred vision, diplopia, nausea, irritability, hypertrophy of the gums, dermatitis, hirsutism, and purpura. In some instances, Dilantin Sodium causes drowsiness and a letdown feeling which makes it necessary to stop the drug. Nystagmus often develops. At times, cerebellar signs, with unsteady gait and intention tremor, occur. Most of the side reactions disappear after cessation of the drug. If on renewal the same symptoms reappear, the drug should be stopped, and not renewed.

Mesantoin (methyl, phenyl ethyl hydantoin): Because of the toxic effects of Dilantin Sodium in some cases, another form of hydantionate has been developed, known as "Mesantoin." It is dispensed as a tablet in doses of 1¼ grains, and given three to six times daily. It is said to be more effective than Dilantin Sodium, and to cause a reduction in the number of seizures in 90 per cent (Kozol) and in 60 per cent (Loscalzo). It is not as reliable a drug as Dilantin Sodium in the reduction of seizures, but it is a useful adjunct in treatment of the following patients: (1) those who are intolerant to

Dilantin Sodium, and (2) those who cannot be controlled by other forms of treatment. In some instances, it may be used alone. Toxic effects are less frequent than with Dilantin Sodium. Ataxia and gum hyperplasia are rare, and drowsiness appears only in high doses. Exfoliative dermatitis may develop. Aplastic anemia, agranulocytosis, and pancytopenia have been reported.

Phenobarbital: This is also a most useful drug; many still regard it as the most useful. It is given in doses varying from ½ to 1½ grains, given sufficiently often to control seizures. It is frequently not given in large enough dosage. Epileptic patients are capable of tolerating large doses of the drug, the amount varying with the individual patient from 1½ to 6 or 7 grains a day. Among the toxic reactions of the drug are dermatitis, apathy, drowsiness, sluggishness, mental dullness, irritability, and asthenia. These may be so pronounced as to preclude use of the drug. Drowsiness and asthenia are the most disturbing of the side reactions. At times prolonged use of the drug results in mental sluggishness which may simulate deterioration. It is possible that the feeling of well-being and the brightness described after the use of Dilantin Sodium is due not so much to the effects of this drug as to the release from the effects of phenobarbital. Despite all this, phenobarbital causes toxic effects in a surprisingly small percentage of instances when one considers its widespread use. The efficacy of phenobarbital in controlling seizures is difficult to evaluate, figures varying from thirty to eighty per cent.

Amphetamine sulfate, 10 mg. two or three times a day, is valuable in counteracting the drowsiness, but is not always successful. Phenobarbital must often be given with Dilantin Sodium or bromides in order to produce its best effects.

Bromides: They still constitute a useful means of controlling seizures, but they have been largely replaced by other drugs. Their lack of popularity is due to the greater and easier tendency to side effects than in most of the other drugs used in the treatment of epilepsy. Bromides may be used as the basic treatment of epilepsy and in some cases which respond inadequately to phenobarbital and Dilantin Sodium they are ideal. They are also extremely valuable as a change when tolerance has been developed to other drugs. They may be used in the form of sodium, potassium, or strontium bromide, the first named being most widely used. The dosage varies from 10 to 15 grains three times a day; larger doses may be necessary in some cases.

The drug may be given for indefinite periods, but it is apt to produce unpleasant side reactions which limit its value. These include acne, mental sluggishness, and depression. A blood bromide level of 150 to 200 mg. is necessary to keep patients free from attacks. Bromides are heaped up slowly in the body and are excreted slowly, chiefly in the urine. It has been found that the efficacy of bromide administration is greatly enhanced if the chloride intake is controlled. For this reason it is advisable to limit the intake of sodium chloride to 6 or 7 Gm. per day, or in some cases to a minimum of 4 to 5 Gm. daily. The efficacy of bromides in controlling seizures is hard to estimate. Remissions over one year were produced in 71.7 per cent of eighty-five private patients treated with sodium bromide (Pollock). A combination of bromide and phenobarbital may be used to control spells.

Mebaral (nephobarbital): Mebaral is useful in some cases of epilepsy in doses of ½ to 1 grain three times a day or, in other instances, 3 grains three times a day. It is more effective in grand mal than in petit mal seizures, but in the author's experience has often been found useful in the latter. If the drug is used as a substitute for phenobarbital it should be given in double the dosage of the latter drug.

Mysoline (primidone) : This is useful in the control of grand mal and to a lesser extent in psychomotor seizures. It is given in doses of 250 mg. tablets, and 4 to 6 tablets may be given daily. Drowsiness, ataxia, nausea, vomiting, and dizziness are the toxic manifestations of the drug. Of these, drowsiness is the most serious offender. It is therefore necessary to begin dosages with $\frac{1}{4}$ or $\frac{1}{2}$ tablets, gradually increasing the dose. Even under these circumstances, drowsiness is common. Persistence with the use of the drug for seven to ten days usually overcomes the drowsiness, but for effective control of seizures the drug must be used in doses which produce unpleasant effects. For this reason it is usually combined with Dilantin Sodium or Mesantoin.

Tridione: Tridione (trimethadione) is effective in petit mal, but is helpless against grand mal seizures. Improvement has been noted in 83 per cent of patients, 31 per cent being completely relieved of seizures. It is not effective in psychic seizures. It appears to be more valuable in children than adults. It is given in capsules of 0.3 Gm. The dose for adults is 0.9 (3 capsules) to 1.8 Gm. (6 capsules) per day. For children, the dose is 0.3 Gm. daily for infants; 0.6 Gm. daily for children of two to four years; and 0.9 Gm. daily for children five years and older.

Photophobia and gastric distress may follow use of the drug, but they disappear either with withdrawal of the drug or reduction in dose. In the former case, the drug may be renewed in lower doses.

Tridione has a tendency to affect the blood-forming organs, and to produce agranulocytosis and anemia. It is essential, therefore, that blood counts be done at weekly intervals during the first month of treatment. If there is no change in the blood picture, the drug may be continued and blood studies made at monthly intervals thereafter. If changes in the blood are found, the drug must be withdrawn and not renewed.

Paradione (paramethadione) : This may be used instead of Tridione if the latter cannot be tolerated. It is used in the same dosage as Tridione.

Milontin (Phensuximide) : This may be used in the treatment of petit mal when Tridione or Paradione are ineffective. It is given in dosages of 0.5 Gm. three times daily, increasing by 0.5 Gm. as needed. It may be given in total dosages of 2 to 3 Gm. daily. Unpleasant side-effects are nausea, vomiting, dizziness, and drowsiness.

Phenurone: *Phenacetylurea* has been found to be a useful adjunct in the treatment of seizures. It is given in doses of 0.5 gm. three to six times daily. It may be used alone or in conjunction with other drugs. Its greatest value has been found in the treatment of psychomotor seizures, but it has also been reported to be useful in the treatment of petit mal. It is often associated with unpleasant side-reactions. These include depression, sometimes severe in degree; anorexia, weight loss, liver damage; skin reactions; and hematopoietic reactions.

Status Epilepticus: *Status epilepticus* represents a special problem both in treatment and diagnosis. The first indication in a patient with repeated convulsions is to stop the convulsions as quickly as possible. After this has been accomplished, the problem of causation may be investigated, an effort being made to determine whether the condition is due to idiopathic or symptomatic epilepsy, just as in the case of the isolated attack. For status epilepticus it is necessary to give sedatives intravenously or intramuscularly. For this purpose sodium phenobarbital (gr. 1½) is the most useful drug. One dose of the drug may not be sufficient to control the convulsions; hence it may be repeated in one or two hours. Paraldehyde may be given in doses of 4 to 6 drachms by nasal tube or rectally to control the seizures. Intravenous paraldehyde (2 cc.) is often valuable in the treatment of status epilepticus. The drug may be given intramuscularly, 8-10 cc. as an initial dose and 5 cc. every half hour until the seizures cease. *Magnesium sulfate* (twenty-five per cent) intravenously in dosages of 10 cc. may be efficacious in terminating status epilepticus. Despite all efforts to control seizures by drugs in status epilepticus, the convulsions may continue; in such cases, ether or Avertin may be necessary to stop the convulsions.

The Surgical Treatment of Epilepsy: Surgery is confined to those cases in which a specific cause is found, such as brain tumor or cortical scar, and consists of removal of the tumor or scar. Convulsions may persist even after complete removal of either tumor or scar and drug treatment may therefore be necessary as a postoperative treatment. No operation for the relief of essential epilepsy offers any hope of permanent cure.

The operative treatment of epilepsy has been authoritatively summarized by Penfield and Erickson. They find that the best results from operation are obtained in patients with a removable localized lesion in an otherwise normal brain. Excision of meningocerebral scars due to trauma or infections gives better average results than excision of a simple local cerebral lesion. Excision of focal microgyria gives very encouraging results. Excision of intracerebral arteriovenous aneurysm in a block seems to give a good prognosis for cessation of attacks. Excision of scars left behind by arterial occlusion gives a good prognosis provided fairly complete removal of the damaged area is feasible. Scars situated in the frontal lobe seem to respond particularly favorably. The duration of the lesion and the age of the patient have no influence on the results. Operations for separation of adhesions give only poor results.

The results of operation for epilepsy as given by Penfield and Erickson are as follows: In patients with meningocerebral cicatrix, removal of the scar resulted in complete cures in 22.5 per cent and 22.5 per cent more were three-fourths improved or better. In patients with cerebral cicatrix, nineteen per cent had complete freedom from attacks and twenty-one per cent were three-fourths improved or better.

The removal of epileptogenic foci by operation offers help in the control of seizures. If it has been demonstrated that such a focus exists, excision offers a good chance of complete or almost complete control of the seizures (thirty-three of fifty-nine cases, Penfield and Steelman). The cause of the focal lesion is most often head injury, second, birth injuries, and third, local infection. The patients with focal seizures have in common the presence of a zone or area of ganglion cells in which the circulation has been interfered with. The actual focus in which the epileptic discharge originates is to be found in this peripheral and partially destroyed zone. Partia anoxemia produces in ganglion cells an abnormal state in which spontaneous neuronal activity is increased. This increase may be called the epileptogenic factor. For effective surgical therapy the epileptogenic focus must be removed, in addition to the scar, cyst, or tumor (Penfield).

There is, therefore, a considerable percentage of patients having operative organic cerebral lesions with epilepsy who do not improve or who improve only partially. For this reason it is advisable in the handling of a problem of this sort first to give a thorough trial of medical treatment. If this fails to control the convulsions either immediately or remotely, operation may be performed. If the convulsions are controlled by medical treatment, no surgery is indicated, since all has been attained that can be hoped for from operation. Penfield and Erickson assert that where an objective lesion of the brain can be demonstrated as the cause of a seizure, permanent disappearance of attacks never occurs with or without medication. Since permanent disappearance is attainable in only a small percentage of cases by operation, much can be hoped for by medical treatment in many cases in the partial disappearance of the attacks.

Surgical treatment of *temporal lobe* seizures is advocated in some instances and is reported as encouraging (Penfield and Flanigin), with fifty-seven per cent success. The treatment should be reserved for patients who have failed to respond to medical treatment. A study of 120 cases of temporal lobe epilepsy (Earle, Baldwin, and Penfield) revealed the following causes: (1) birth injury (twenty-five cases), (2) anoxic injury at or near the time of birth (twenty-one cases), (3) postnatal head injury (thirty-two cases), (4) infection or neoplasm (thirty cases). Gross lesions of the brain consisted of slight atrophy or toughness of a single gyrus to atrophy of the entire temporal lobe and adjacent cortex. His-

tological study revealed diffuse increase in astrocytes in the atrophic cortex and loss of neurons in some instances, with cystic degeneration.

XV. NARCOLEPSY

Allied to epilepsy is a condition referred to as narcolepsy, which includes a variety of ill-defined entities. Narcolepsy is characterized by attacks of hypersomnolence and cataplexy, either in combination or alone. It is customary to separate cases of narcolepsy into two groups: (1) idiopathic, of unknown origin; (2) symptomatic, secondary to known causes.

There is some doubt as to what to include in the narcolepsy group. By definition, only those cases with somnolence and cataplexy should be placed in this group, but in practice there have been included cases only with somnolence. It has been found that most of the cases with somnolence alone are symptomatic, while those with both somnolence and cataplexy are idiopathic.

Etiology: Narcolepsy may develop either in males or females but seems to affect males more frequently. The onset is usually from ten to twenty years of age but patients over twenty are not uncommon. Of the conditions which have been found associated with narcolepsy, encephalitis, brain tumor, and trauma deserve particular mention. Cranial trauma is regarded by some as a particularly important cause of narcolepsy. No specific cause can be found for many cases.

Symptoms: The onset in most cases of narcolepsy is early in life, but in cases secondary to tumors, etc., the onset is delayed. Periods of *hypersomnolence* are striking and may exist with or without cataplectic attacks. The afflicted person complains of inability to stay awake and of falling asleep under a variety of circumstances—at the table, in church, during conversation, over studies, etc. The sleep may be very short, a mere nod, or may continue for some time—half an hour or several hours—and may resemble a deep sleep. Consciousness is variously impaired from awareness of what goes on in the surroundings to a complete loss of consciousness. Equally as characteristic are the attacks of *cataplexy*, which may occur with or without the attacks of somnolence. These are characterized by attacks of weakness of the limbs and complete loss of muscle tone. They are precipitated by emotional stimuli of various sorts—laughter, fear, anxiety, anger, etc. —but are particularly prone to be produced by laughter. During such attacks, patients complain of a feeling of weakness in the knees and trunk on laughing or other emotional stimulation, frequently but not invariably associated with falling. Fragmentary attacks are not uncommon, characterized by sensations of weakness in the knees, arms, or trunk, but without falling. *Diplopia* may occur in narcolepsy just before the attack of sleep or just after awakening. It may be present as an isolated symptom of the disorder.

The attacks of somnolence and cataplexy are persistent and do not disappear spontaneously. Physical examination often reveals nothing. Endocrine disturbances sometimes occur, as, for example, hypopituitary and hypothyroid states. Obesity is not an uncommon accompaniment. No findings can be elicited on neurological examination in many cases, but in some instances, as in encephalitis, tumor, etc., evidences of nervous system disease may be found. Laboratory examinations reveal nothing significant in most cases.

Associated with narcolepsy is a strange phenomenon known as *sleep paralysis,* which has been described under a number of terms such as "delayed psychomotor awakening," "predormitial and postdormitial paralysis," and "cataplexy of awakening." In some instances, the condition occurs without associated narcolepsy (Rushton). The condition is characterized by a benign transient paralysis at the beginning or end of sleep, usually associated with no impairment of consciousness. Paralysis is usually complete, but movements of the eyes and ability to speak may be retained. The paralysis varies in duration from a few minutes to two hours or more. Recovery is usually spontaneous, but it may be induced by a light touch or vigorous shaking. The patient is aware of his predicament throughout the period of paralysis and often exhibits extreme anxiety and fear of death. The condition may begin in childhood and persist until old age without serious effects. Sleep paralysis may at times be replaced by sleepwalking. The cause of the condition is not known.

The *Kleine-Levin syndrome* is a rare disorder characterized by occurrence in males usually in the second decade, periodic attacks of abnormal sleep lasting for several days, excessive hunger during such periods, motor unrest, irritability, and mild mental confusion. Between attacks, patients are normal. The reported cases reveal no evidence of encephalitis or narcolepsy, and the EEG is normal. The cause of the condition is unknown.

Diagnosis: The diagnosis is easy in typical cases, the attacks of hypersomnolence and cataplexy being typical. It is sometimes difficult to separate some cases of narcolepsy from *epilepsy,* especially cases with petit mal. The distinction between narcolepsy and epilepsy is so difficult at times that there are those who believe that the two conditions are the same. Efforts to settle the issue by study of the EEG are inconclusive. In most instances, the EEG pattern is normal; but in some cases, abnormal but not paroxysmal records are found (Finley and Dines). On the other hand, the EEG tracings in other cases of narcolepsy were found to be similar to those obtained in epilepsy (Cohn and Cruvant).

Not infrequently minor attacks of epilepsy occur with the narcoleptic attacks and serve as proof of the contention of many that narcolepsy is a variety of epilepsy. Many features of the attack are like epilepsy (periodicity, impairment of consciousness), but the best evidence appears to regard narcolepsy as an entity distinct from epilepsy. The distinction from minor attacks is easy in those patients with cataplexy, but in patients with somnolence only, the differentiation is much more difficult. The association of major seizures, the dissimilarity of minor attacks to sleep, and the electroencephalogram will be helpful in doubtful cases. In other instances, narcolepsy must be distinguished from cases of hysteria with attacks of catalepsy or from other psychogenic conditions with similar attacks. The social history and the personality study will usually reveal the fact that episodes of this nature develop under circumstances of emotional stress in unstable personalities and are in reality conversion symptoms. While cataplectic attacks occur as a result of emotional stimuli, the association of a single stimulus with the episode is not as definite in psychogenic attacks.

Treatment: Many cases persist for several years (twenty to twenty-five years); some are said to disappear spontaneously. The most effective drug in the treatment of narcolepsy is *amphetamine* (Benzedrine) *sulfate.* The dosage must be individualized and varies widely from case to case. Since the attacks occur at almost any time, the dosage must be spread through the day, but the drug should not be given later than four o'clock in order to prevent wakefulness at night. In mild cases, 10 mg. given three or four times a day is sufficient. In more severe cases, 20 to 30 mg. four or five times a day may be given safely. The drug may be given for long periods in such patients without harmful effects, but there appears to be a variability in the susceptibility to the drug on the part of patients and side symptoms, such as restlessness, nervousness, excitability, or depression may develop after small dosage in some patients or not at all in others. No cases of addiction among narcoleptics have been recorded. Because of the fact that tolerance to the drug develops after prolonged administration, it seems best to stagger the drug with other medication. The effect of amphetamine is better on the cataplectic symptoms than on the attacks of drowsiness, but in some cases the latter are greatly improved by the use of the drug. In a few instances, the drug has been given to patients having vascular hypertension with narcoleptic attacks without harmful effects.

In some patients, *ephedrine sulfate* has a better effect than amphetamine. The dosage of this drug varies from ⅜ to ¾ grain two to four times a day. Alternate doses of amphetamine and ephedrine may be efficacious in some cases. *Desoxyephedrine hydrochloride* (2.5 mg.) in doses of two to eight tablets a day was found to be efficacious in the treatment of narcolepsy (Eaton). *Metrazol,* gr. 1½ once or twice daily, may be helpful as an accessory treatment. The cataplexy has been found to respond to *potassium chloride* in doses of 30 to 75 gr. daily.

15

Extrapyramidal Diseases

Among the diseases of the nervous system involving the motor apparatus are those which implicate the extrapyramidal system. These include such important disorders as chorea, paralysis agitans, progressive lenticular degeneration, and other disorders. They include both hyper- and hypokinetic disorders.

I. DEFINITION

The motor systems in the body are divisible into two main groups: (1) the pyramidal system, and (2) parapyramidal, or extrapyramidal, system. The pyramidal system is composed of the cells and fibers of the pyramidal or corticospinal pathways. These fibers originate in the cells of the opposite motor cortex (Area 4), to a lesser degree from the cells of the same side and from cells in other portions of the cortex. They pass through the internal capsule and brain stem to be distributed to the anterior horn cells at various levels of the spinal cord. This is the main motor pathway for voluntary movement. In contrast to it stands the extrapyramidal system, which is composed of the basal ganglia and the extrapyramidal motor cortex and includes the motor pathways of the brain and brain stem exclusive of the pyramidal pathways.

If the pyramids in the medulla in cats or monkeys are sectioned, all the fibers of the pyramidal pathway are interrupted. Cortical stimulation of parts of the cerebrum will elicit motor reactions of various types despite the fact that the pyramidal pathways are interrupted. It has long been recognized that stimulation of cortical areas outside of the precentral motor gyrus was capable of eliciting movements. The cortical areas from which such movements are elicited are referred to as the extrapyramidal cortical areas. Their precise cortical projections are not yet definitely known, nor are the precise portions of the cortex subserving extrapyramidal functions completely identified. Some of them, however, are known; others will probably be added as the relationship between the cerebral cortex and the extrapyramidal basal ganglia system becomes clarified.

Included among the extrapyramidal cortical areas are Areas 6, 8, 19, 3, 1, 2, and 5 (Fig. 198). Stimulation of Area 6 in its various portions causes movements of many types. Stereotyped movements are elicited, often associated with turning of the head and torsion of the body, persisting after removal of the motor area (Area 4), and disappearing only after Area 6 is undercut. Other parts of Area 6 (6aα and 6bα) yield movements of the mouth, salivation and chewing, and inhibition of respiratory movements (6bβ). Stimulation of Area 8 causes conjugate deviation of the eyes. Areas 3, 2, and 1 facilitate movements from Area 4. Important also are the suppressor areas of the cortex and the reticular substance and pathways. The suppressor areas of the cerebral cortex are in connection with the caudate nucleus and the reticular substance of the medulla (*v.* Chapter 3).

In the human, two types of extrapyramidal fields may be differentiated (Foerster): (1) those which produce turning of the head, trunk, and extremities, with or without deviation of the eyes, to the opposite side; (2) those which cause deviation of the eyes only.

movements are elicited from stimulation of frontal and parietal lobes and from the region of the ectosylvian gyrus and the suprasylvian gyrus (Tower). The cortical extrapyramidal activity elicited by stimulation of the cortex was very nearly equivalent to the total activity of the decorticate cat and Tower concludes that the stimulation of extrapyramidal path-

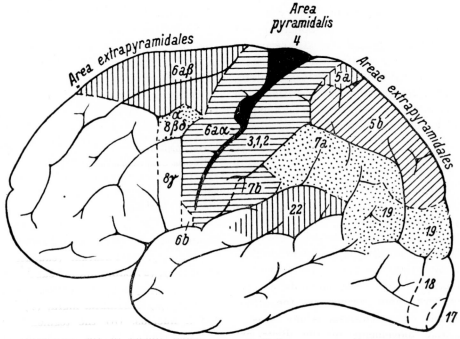

Fig. 198—*Cerebral cortex,* showing the motor pyramidal and extrapyramidal cortical areas. (After Foerster.)

The first type of movement was obtained from the anterior and posterior parts of Area 6, the postcentral gyrus, the anterior part of the superior parietal lobule, and the superior temporal gyrus. The eye movements were obtained from Area 8 of the frontal lobe, the posterior part of the superior parietal lobule and Area 39 (gyrus angularis) and Area 19 of the occipital lobe. Similar areas have been established in general in the monkey.

After section of the pyramids contraction of skeletal muscle is possible on stimulation of the cerebral cortex. In the cat,

ways in the cat elicits patterns of activity determined entirely by the integration of subcortical centers. All the patterns of movement elicited on stimulation of the cortex in the cat with bilateral pyramidal section are also observed in the decorticate cat. The problem is different in the monkey, for here "electrical stimulation of the cortical surface of the monkey after surgical division of the pyramids so far has never elicited all the patterns of movement observed in the unanesthetized chronic preparation, as it did in the cat" (Hines).

Ablation of extrapyramidal cortical areas yields instructive results. The result of ablation of Area 6 has been referred to (Chapter 3). Ablation of Area 6 in monkeys and chimpanzees causes disturbances in skilled movements and a cataleptic type of rigidity, and increase of the deep reflexes. All the changes except the disturbance of skilled movements are transient. "When Area 6 is removed after ablation of Area 4, great increase is observed in movement disability; any existing spasticity is greatly augmented; deep reflexes become uniformly exaggerated, and specific neurological signs, such as those of Rossolimo (toes), Hoffman (fingers), and the fanning sign of Babinski, all appear and, in the chimpanzee, remain permanently" (Fulton). Removal of all of Area 6 and the anterior border of Area 4 caused paralysis, a grasp reflex which gradually disappeared, clonus, brisk reflexes, and hypertonus (Hines).

Section of the pyramids (Tower) in cats causes paralysis below the level of the lesion, with decrease in tone greater in the proximal muscles and paralysis more serious in the distal muscles. The paralysis is not spastic, discrete movements of the digits are lost, and the tendon reflexes are slow and pendular, resembling those found in disease of the cerebellum. Complete removal of either the occipital or temporal lobes has no effect on the control of movement (Klüver and Bucy). Removal of the parietal lobe is followed by disturbance in the fine movements of distal segments, and by poor adjustment in the range and direction of movements (Kennard and Kessler). Removal of Area 6 results also in forced grasping and groping. In a few human cases the symptom has been recorded with disease of Area 6. Removal of Area 6 has in some instances resulted in the abolition of choreo-athe-tosis (Bucy) suggesting that athetosis depends for its expression on intact extra-pyramidal pathways.

II. ANATOMY AND FUNCTIONS

The extrapyramidal system is composed of the basal ganglia plus portions of the cerebral cortex which have connections with the basal ganglia. The basal ganglia are a group of large gray masses deeply situated in the brain tissue. There is no unanimity concerning the nuclear masses to be included among the basal ganglia. A comprehensive classification includes the following:

Caudate }
Putamen } Striatum
Pallidum (Globus Pallidus)
Thalamus
Hypothalamus
Nucleus Subthalamicum
    (Corpus Luysii)
Red Nucleus
Substantia Nigra
Reticular formation of the midbrain

Another classification (Papez) includes: (1) the striatum (caudate and putamen), (2) pallidum, (3) subthalamic nucleus, (4) prerubral nucleus, (5) red nucleus, (6) substantia nigra, (7) interstitial nucleus, (8) the tegmental and reticular nuclei of the midbrain. Still other groupings have been suggested, but the first classification given will be followed, since it covers the main nuclear masses referred to as the basal ganglia.

The nuclei comprising the basal ganglia are varied in structure as well as function. The *striatum* (caudate and putamen) is composed of large numbers of small ganglion cells among which are interspersed large ganglion cells of a motor type. The small ganglion cells are receptive, sending processes from one part of the striatum to another. The large ganglion cells give rise to axones terminating in the pallidum, and substantia nigra. The *pallidum* contains only

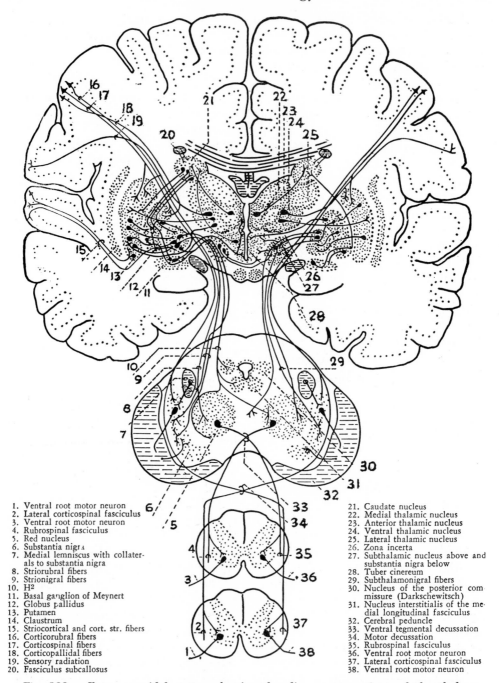

1. Ventral root motor neuron
2. Lateral corticospinal fasciculus
3. Ventral root motor neuron
4. Rubrospinal fasciculus
5. Red nucleus
6. Substantia nigra
7. Medial lemniscus with collaterals to substantia nigra
8. Striorubral fibers
9. Strionigral fibers
10. H²
11. Basal ganglion of Meynert
12. Globus pallidus
13. Putamen
14. Claustrum
15. Striocortical and cort. str. fibers
16. Corticorubral fibers
17. Corticospinal fibers
18. Corticopallidal fibers
19. Sensory radiation
20. Fasciculus subcallosus

21. Caudate nucleus
22. Medial thalamic nucleus
23. Anterior thalamic nucleus
24. Ventral thalamic nucleus
25. Lateral thalamic nucleus
26. Zona incerta
27. Subthalamic nucleus above and
    substantia nigra below
28. Tuber cinereum
29. Subthalamonigral fibers
30. Nucleus of the posterior com-
    missure (Darkschewitsch)
31. Nucleus interstitialis of the me-
    dial longitudinal fasciculus
32. Cerebral peduncle
33. Ventral tegmental decussation
34. Motor decussation
35. Rubrospinal fasciculus
36. Ventral root motor neuron
37. Lateral corticospinal fasciculus
38. Ventral root motor neuron

Fig. 199 — *Extrapyramidal system* showing the diverse connections of the thala-
mostriatal, striothalamic, and corticostriatal pathways. (Huber and Crosby: Macmillan Co., N. Y.)

scattered large motor ganglion cells, which give rise to nerve fibers entering the ansa lenticularis to be distributed to the red nucleus, substantia nigra, and the hypothalamus. Closely connected with the pallidum is the *corpus subthal-* rubro-thalamic system and large multipolar ganglion cells which give rise to the rubrospinal tract.

The basal ganglia have rich connections with one another and with other parts of the brain stem. The intricacy

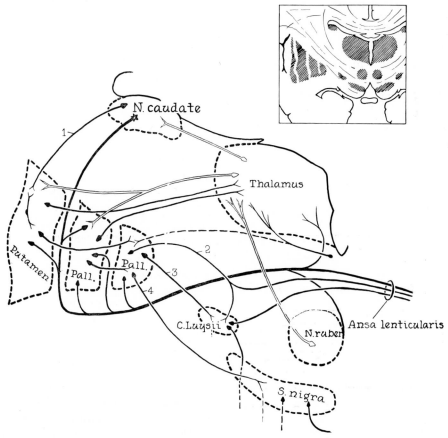

Fig. 200—*Basal ganglia,* showing their afferent and efferent connections with one another and the formation of the ansa lenticularis; efferent solid lines, afferent double lines.

amicum (corpus Luysii) which contains ganglion cells similar to those found in the pallidum. It lies in close connection with the latter. The *substantia nigra* in its zona compacta has multipolar ganglion cells which contain melanin pigment. A portion of the substantia nigra, the zona reticulata, is unpigmented. The *nucleus ruber* contains many small ganglion cells forming part of the dentato- of these connections is seen in the following fiber connections of the basal ganglia: The *corpus striatum* (caudate and putamen) is in relation to the subcallosal bundle and the external capsule. It gives origin to the striopallidal and strionigral fibers, which synapse in the pallidum and substantia nigra. The striatum has no direct connection with the cerebral cortex. It receives fibers from the thalamus and is in indirect connection with the cortex by this means. The *substantia nigra* has efferent connections with the tegmentum of the midbrain, which connects in turn with the inferior olive and cerebellar cortex. It also has connections with the pallidum and thalamus. The *pallidum* receives afferent fibers chiefly from the medial nucleus of the thalamus. It sends efferent fibers by way of the ansa lenticularis to the prerubral field, the hypothalamus, the nucleus subthalamicum, substantia nigra, and the ventral nucleus of the thalamus. It has connections with the tuber cinereum and by Forel's bundle H 2 with the nucleus ruber. Connections are described with the pes pedunculi and the tegmentum. "The globus pallidus discharges through three chief circuits. These are (1) fibers to the red nucleus, (2) fibers to the substantia nigra, and (3) fibers to the corpus subthalamicum and its vicinity, which may be regarded as homologous with the reticular formation more caudally" (Mettler). The *red nucleus* gives origin to the rubrospinal, rubro-oculomotor, and rubroreticulo-olivary tracts.

It is apparent, therefore, that the basal ganglia are in rich connection with one another. The striatum (caudate and putamen) is connected with the pallidum and substantia nigra; the pallidum with the thalamus afferently and efferently by way of the ansa lenticularis with the red nucleus, the hypothalamus, the nucleus subthalamicum (luys), and the thalamus; the substantia nigra with the tegmentum of the midbrain; the red nucleus afferently with the cerebellum by way of the superior cerebellar peduncle and efferently giving rise to the rubrospinal and other pathways.

It has long been a problem as to the nature of the connections of the basal ganglia with the cortex, and whether cortical connections are present between some or all of the basal ganglia and the cerebrum. Present investigations indicate that such connections are to be found and that the basal ganglia are actually in the closest possible functional relation with the motor mechanisms of the cerebral cortex (Kennard and Fulton). Connections of the striatum with the cerebral cortex are still uncertain, but the existence of connections between the cerebrum and the substantia nigra have been amply shown. Connections of the caudate nucleus with the cortex by way of the internal capsule have been described (Cajal), and others have suggested connections between putamen and cortex (Economo, Kodama), the latter by way of the subcallosal bundle. The striatum is presumed to be connected with the frontal cortex by means of the subcallosal bundle, but clinching evidence for this seems still to be lacking.

In the human the number of extrapyramidal cortical connections is less elaborate than those described in the monkey. They include (1) corticopontine fibers originating from the orbital and middle frontal gyri, the middle and inferior temporal gyri, the gyrus angularis and the superior parietal lobule; (2) corticonigral fibers to the substantia nigra, originating from the Rolandic region, the foot of the first frontal gyrus, and the opercular region of the frontal and parietal lobes; (3) corticothalamic fibers to the thalamus, coming from the middle and inferior frontal gyri, from the medial surface of the frontal lobe and the precuneus. In the monkey, the parietal and temporal lobes give rise to fibers destined for the nucleus ruber, substantia nigra, and the tegmentum of the medulla. Corticomesencephalic connections have also been found from the parietal and occipital lobes to the superior colliculus and from the temporal lobe to the inferior colliculus. Other connections have been found from Area 8 to the tegmentum of the medulla and to the substantia nigra; from Area 9 to the lateral thalamic nucleus, to the nucleus ruber, and to the pontine nuclei, and from the prefrontal region to the thalamus, tegmentum of the midbrain, pons, and substantia nigra.

The *functions* of masses of gray matter as large as the basal ganglia, occupying an important part of the brain substance, should be much more evident than they are. Actually, much remains to be known concerning their precise function. The functions of the extrapyramidal system have been summarized as follows (Bucy): (1) the production of integrated primary movements of the skeletal musculature, (2) the integration of associated movements, (3) the control and inhibition of postural reflexes, (4) the suppression of electrical activity in other areas of the cortex, (5) the imperfect and partial control of visceral and vegetative functions.

The striatum serves as an inhibitory mechanism (Mettler) acting apparently on the cerebral cortex by inhibiting bodily movement. The functions of the pallidum are not definitely known. It is apparently inexcitable on stimulation. It has been found that in the absence of the cerebral cortex the striatum and pallidum have no effect on locomotion or postural adjustments. So closely interrelated are the functions of the cortex and basal ganglia that no definite function can be assigned the basal ganglia independent of cortical action. The putamen and pallidum have been found to be inexcitable on electrical stimulation.

The functional interrelationship of the pyramidal and extrapyramidal systems is not definitely established and much remains to be clarified concerning the problem. The pyramidal system may be said to deal with finer adjustments of movement, shown particularly in the fine

movements performed by the thumb and digits. It is a voluntary system which is said to be entirely excitatory (Tower). The extrapyramidal system is concerned with more stereotyped movements and postural mechanisms in the brain stem, controlled and modified by the extrapyramidal cortical areas.

So close is the functional relationship between the pyramidal and extrapyramidal systems that it is hardly possible to consider one without the other. "As far as the striatum is concerned, all the evidence indicates that it is an inhibitory mechanism. Stimulation of it produces inhibition and removal of significant portions of it results in marked release phenomena. Since cortical stimulation, after the pyramids are cut, results in an inhibition which can be markedly reduced by narcotizing the caudate, since lesions of the caudate includes all the release phenomena which can be elicited on cortical removal, and since fibers pass from the frontal cortex to the neostriatum, we feel justified in concluding that the caudate is under some degree of cortical control which serves to inhibit bodily movement and that, conversely, we may say that at least some of the inhibitory power of the cortex is exerted through and by means of the caudate" (Mettler and Mettler).

Stimulation of the pallidum has been for the most part without results and the pallidum has been regarded as inexcitable. Recent studies (Mettler and Mettler) indicate that stimulation of the pallidum in cats causes "a positive motor effect of an extensor nature" in the forelimb of the same side. Stimulation of the subthalamic region causes contraction of the midline musculature of the opposite side of the body, while stimulation of the red nucleus region causes curvature toward the side stimulated. Stimulation of the substantia nigra pro duces an increase in extensor tone of the opposite side of the body chiefly but also of the same side (Mettler and Mettler).

Pathological and clinicopathological studies have thrown some light on the functions of the extrapyramidal and basal ganglia system. These have been concerned largely with study of involuntary movements, such as chorea and athetosis, and with the disturbances of muscle tone as found in paralysis agitans. *Chorea* has been found to be associated with disease, particularly of the striatum, but it has been found also in conjunction with lesions of the thalamus, nucleus ruber, corpus subthalamicum, superior cerebellar peduncle, ansa lenticularis, and postcentral gyrus. The evidence for the striatal pathogenesis of chorea is not complete, but the lesions found in Huntington's chorea, in manganese poisoning, chorea gravidarum, and in some cases of symptomatic chorea following diphtheria and other infectious diseases, indicates that there is widespread disease of the striatum in chorea and that it affects chiefly the small cells of the striatum. Opposed to this evidence is the frequent occurrence of vascular lesions of the striatum without the production of chorea.

From these observations of striatal disease in chorea has arisen the concept that chorea is generated in the basal ganglia independent of the cerebral cortex. "Chorea is to be regarded as an ataxia of pallidal functions conditioned by the striatum, especially by the omission of the small receptive and associative ganglion cell elements of the striatum" (Jakob). This view regards the origin of the choreiform movement, therefore, as being within the basal ganglia system, particularly the striatum. Opposed to this observation is the fact that the choreiform movement depends upon an intact corticospinal pathway for its expression and that a lesion of this path-

way results in the elimination of the choreiform movement. This fact, in addition to observations of chorea due to lesions elsewhere than in the striatal system (postcentral gyrus, ansa lenticularis, corpus subthalamicum, thalamus, etc.), has led to the assertion that chorea is a release phenomenon whereby cortical activity acts unopposed in the presence of lesions in the basal ganglia system.

Of particular importance is the observation of circumscribed atrophy of the opposite postcentral gyrus in a case of senile hemichorea, without involvement of the striatum (Wilson). Chorea and athetosis are regarded by Wilson as being "exteriorized *via* the corticospinal tracts and that behind their appearance is an afferent disorder of regulation, producing choreiform and athetoid movements, ataxia, or incoördination, and hypotonia. This afferent disorder . . . is attributable to lesions situated on the cerebello-mesencephalo-thalamo-cortical path." This view maintains, therefore, that chorea may be produced by lesions anywhere along the cerebello-mesencephalo-thalamo-cortical pathway and the evidence in disease conditions appears to support it. While it is impossible to maintain that chorea is caused by a lesion of the striatum, it is justifiable on the basis of the evidence to assert that the striatum is commonly diseased in chorea, more commonly than other portions of the brain or brain stem. The production of the choreiform movement, however, is brought about by the unopposed activity of other portions of the brain released by the disease of the striatum.

The problem of *athetosis* is even more complex than that of chorea. Relatively less is known concerning the brain changes in athetosis. The most frequent cause of infantile and juvenile athetosis is congenital malformation (status marmoratus) of the striatum (Alexander). In some instances, it results from birth injury which produces destructive lesions of the putamen and pallidum, or by vascular disease in early infancy and childhood. In adults, athetosis develops in disease of the putamen and pallidum in progressive lenticular degeneration, in hemorrhage, softening, tumor, or encephalitis involving usually putamen and pallidum, but in some instances the thalamus and hypothalamus. It has been asserted that "athetoid movements in the adult are found only in cases in which there are lesions in the pallidum" (Jakob). In any event the evidence points to the implication of the putamen and pallidum in adults and of the striatum in infants in the production of athetosis. That this, too, like chorea, must be regarded as a release phenomenon is shown by the cases of athetosis which are relieved by removal of the opposite motor cortex. These demonstrate also the close and intimate relationship between the pyramidal and extrapyramidal systems.

Several instances of removal of the motor cortex in patients with athetosis (Horsley, Sachs, Bucy) have demonstrated the fact that the involuntary movements can be eliminated by removal of the opposite Areas 4 and 6 and that these areas are the effector pathways for production of athetotic movements. "Extirpation of the precentral region is an effective form of treatment for the involuntary movements of choreo-athetosis or of tremor, either at rest or in association with voluntary movement. The extirpation will be most effective when it includes both Areas 4 and 6 of Brodmann and when every effort has been made to include all of the representation of the extremity concerned" (Bucy).

III. CLINICAL DISORDERS

The diseases resulting from involvement of the extrapyramidal system have to do essentially with disorders of movement. They may be grouped as follows:

1. *Hyperkinetic:*
   Huntington's chorea
   Athetosis
   Hemiballism (hemichorea)
   Myoclonias
   Dystonia musculorum deformans

2. *Hypokinetic—Hyperkinetic:*
   Progressive lenticular degeneration
   Pseudosclerosis (Westphal-Jakob)
   Paralysis agitans

While grouping into hyper- and hypokinetic types is not altogether accurate because of a merging of one type with the other in most instances, the classification offers nevertheless an outline of the types of disorders with involvement of the basal ganglia.

IV. PARALYSIS AGITANS *(Parkinson's Disease; Parkinsonism; Shaking Palsy)*

Nomenclature: Paralysis agitans was first described in older people by James Parkinson in 1817, and was called by him the shaking palsy, the term paralysis agitans being given to it later. For many years the disease seemed clearly defined clinically, but with the advent of epidemic encephalitis of the lethargic type, many sequels developed in young people which simulated closely in their clinical features the cases of paralysis agitans in older patients. The encephalitic cases came to be termed postencephalitic parkinsonism or simply parkinsonism, the inference developing in time that the term parkinsonism was synonymous with the encephalitic group, while paralysis agitans was reserved for the older group. From this also grew the concept that every case of paralysis agitans represented a chronic encephalitis whether recognized or not. a concept entirely unjustified by the facts. The term "idiopathic" came into use in order to distinguish the genuine cases of paralysis agitans from the postencephalitic type.

Actually, the term "paralysis agitans" or "parkinsonism" is used interchangeably for the two groups of cases. Of the two terms, paralysis agitans is to be preferred to parkinsonism or Parkinson's disease. Since paralysis agitans is in the majority of cases due to (1) encephalitis, (2) senile brain changes, and (3) arteriosclerosis, the diagnosis of the disorder should always be modified to indicate the causative factor, as, for example, postencephalitic paralysis agitans, senile or arteriosclerotic paralysis agitans.

Paralysis agitans may with reason be regarded as a disorder occurring in the following forms:

1. Senile, idiopathic, or genuine paralysis agitans.
2. Symptomatic paralysis agitans:
    (a) Postencephalitic.
    (b) Vascular: Arteriosclerotic.
    (c) Toxic: Manganese, carbon monoxide, carbon disulfide.
    (d) Tumors.

The senile group which corresponds to the group described by Parkinson in older people has nothing whatever to do with senile disease of the brain in its commonly accepted form (senile dementia, senility). The term is used here in order (1) to indicate the occurrence of this degenerative form of the disease in the senile or presenile period, and (2) to distinguish it from the encephalitic and other forms.

Etiology: The senile form occurs usually at fifty to sixty years of age, but may develop after forty years of age or beyond sixty. A juvenile form has been described, occurring in the second decade of life. The encephalitic forms are found at all ages, but usually in young people of fifteen years or more, well below the age onset of the senile form. The arteriosclerotic variety appears at about the same age level as the senile form. Men are much more commonly afflicted than women in the senile and arteriosclerotic varieties, but in the encephalitic type the incidence is more evenly divided. Negroes are rarely affected.

The precise cause is not known for the senile form. The process is degenerative, involving the cells of the basal ganglia, the cause of the degenerative process being unknown. The influence of heredity has been carefully investigated. It is not an important influence in most cases of the senile form, but a tendency for the disease to occur in families has been noted by many investigators. It was found in more than one member of a family in fifteen per cent (Gowers) and in forty-five of seventy-two cases (Allan). In the encephalitic variety, the cause seems to be the infection which produces encephalitis lethargica. Other forms of encephalitis are on very rare occasions associated with a paralysis agitans syndrome, among them being syphilis, measles, chickenpox, scarlet fever, typhus, pertussis, and mumps.

A paralysis agitans syndrome is sometimes seen following manganese poisoning, and in lead, carbon monoxide, and carbon disulfide intoxication. Trauma has been cited as a cause in some cases, but actual proof is lacking that head injury may cause the disease in some cases. Instances have been reported of cases of paralysis agitans in which head injury appears to have precipitated the symptoms of the disease. The disease is reported to have followed electrical shock in some instances. While many instances of paralysis agitans following trauma have been reported, it is not satisfactorily shown that there is a direct relationship between head injury and the paralysis agitans syndrome. Brain tumor not infrequently invades the basal ganglia area but very rarely causes a paralysis agitans syndrome. Paralysis agitans has been attributed frequently to emotional factors, but there is no good evidence that emotional strain is capable of producing a genuine paralysis agitans syndrome. Those cases which have been reported following emotional strain have been characterized chiefly by tremor which may in itself be of psychogenic origin; none have shown rigidity.

Pathology: Paralysis agitans is associated with disease of the basal ganglia. This is definite and uncontested. There is wide diversity of opinion, however, concerning the precise location within the basal ganglia of the pathological process. The disease process affects chiefly the striatum (caudate and putamen), the pallidum, and substantia nigra. Lesions have also been found in the corpus subthalamicum, medulla, hypothalamus, central gray matter around the aqueduct and third ventricle, and cerebral cortex. The entire basal ganglionic system is affected, therefore, but in varying degrees. The striatum, pallidum, and substantia nigra suffer most, but it must be emphasized that all parts of the basal ganglia are affected. The disease has been said to involve more particularly the striatum and pallidum in the senile type, and the substantia nigra in the postencephalitic variety. This concept, however, has been found not to be tenable and recent studies have shown that the substantia nigra is almost invariably damaged in both forms of the disease, that the lesions are widespread and not limited to the substantia nigra, and that the pyramidal system is spared.

It seems evident, therefore, that all the basal ganglia are diseased in varying degree in paralysis agitans (striatum, pallidum, subthalamicum, substantia nigra) but that the substantia nigra is most often and most profoundly affected. The cerebral cortex (frontal lobes) has been found to be diseased in both the senile and encephalitic varieties when careful studies have been made of it.

The histological process in senile paralysis agitans is purely degenerative and consists of loss or disease of the ganglion cells in the basal ganglia, with glial replacement, and demyelination. In the postencephalitic variety cell loss is found, usually associated with lymphocytic infiltration into the tissues and perivascular infiltration with lymphocytes. These are particularly impressive in the acute stages of the encephalitis. After recovery from this phase, the inflammatory process recedes for the most part, so that evidence of its presence is often not great in the brains of many patients with postencephalitic paralysis agitans. In some instances, it has disappeared completely, only the degenerative changes being present.

Vessel changes are common in the arteriosclerotic variety of paralysis agitans. These consist of sclerosis and calcification of the vessel walls. The brain tissue in the arteriosclerotic cases shows cell loss, lacunae and distintegration of the gray and white matter. The pallidum and substantia nigra are predominantly affected, but all parts of the basal ganglionic system participate.

Symptoms: The development of paralysis agitans is gradual and insidious in the vast majority of cases, the appearance of the disease being so slow as to escape detection in its earliest manifestations. The symptoms may develop over a period of months or years. _Tremor_ is commonly the first symptom to attract attention. It may involve one or both hands and may be particularly noticeable in writing, a common complaint being inability to write without shaking. _Slowness of movement_ is also an early symptom but is not as frequently a source of complaint as tremor. It is manifested by inability to move around as easily as normally, by increased slowness in performing all sorts of acts, such as dressing, etc. _Fatigue_ is a common complaint and it is not unusual for patients to make this their main source of difficulty. At times more unusual complaints bring the patient to the physician for relief. Among these are awareness of difficulty with speech or of change in the appearance of the features. *Pain* in one or both arms is not uncommonly found in paralysis agitans and may be an early manifestation.

The manifestations of paralysis agitans are usually bilateral, but it is not at all uncommon for them to be unilateral, either in the beginning of the illness or throughout its course. Symptoms may be confined to a single limb, in some instances for a long period before extension to other parts. It is not uncommon to obtain a history of progression from one limb to another during the course of the disease until all are eventually implicated. The signs are usually a combination of tremor and rigidity, but it is common to find patients with much tremor and little rigidity and others with much rigidity and little tremor.

An over-all picture of the disease indicates that it progresses slowly and the findings vary with the stage of development of the disorder. The face is immobile, the arm or arms fail to swing in walking, and the fingers move in the typical tremor in early cases. In advanced cases, the facies are immobile, the body is bent forward, the arms are slightly flexed, tremor is usually present in the fingers, the gait is shuffling and often festinating; there is moderate to severe rigidity of the musculature and relative weakness of the muscles, the voice is low and eventually almost inaudible, and saliva drains profusely from the corners of the mouth. As the disease advances, the rigidity becomes greater, the tremor more severe, until the patient is confined to a chair or bed. Even feeding becomes impossible. Death is due to an intercurrent infection, such as pneumonia.

The *tremor* may be unilateral or bilateral and involves the fingers and hands much more often than the arms and forearms. It is characteristically seen in the distal portions of the limbs, but it may in severe cases involve the forearms and arms. It is rhythmical, usually coarse, occurs at a rate of four to seven per second, and in the hands is characterized by a posture of adduction of the thumb and fingers with a rhythmical rubbing of fingers and thumb, producing the so-called *pill rolling tremor*. Flexion and extension movements are not uncommon. The tremor is said to be present at rest (static tremor) and to disappear temporarily on movement. Movement abolishes the tremor temporarily; soon after the limb is moved and has come to rest, the tremor reappears. This is true in many instances, but it is by no means characteristic, for many cases are found in which the tremor not only persists during movement but may at times be increased by it. The tremor may, in advanced cases, involve the lips and face. Coarse, rhythmical tremor involving the head is quite common and often very distressing. Tremor of the legs is much less common than in the hands. It usually involves the calves but may spread to the thighs. All tremors are increased by emotional stress, fatigue, and anxiety, and disappear during sleep.

Rigidity in some degree is present in all cases of paralysis agitans. It is a state of increased tension of the muscles, causing resistance to passive motion. It may be present for a long time in only one arm or in one arm and leg. It usually involves all the limbs. It is detected by the resistance to passive movement and by the *cogwheel sign*, a sensation as if moving the muscle over a ratchet. This sign is present early and is important to recognize; it is elicited by slow passive pronation and supination or flexion and extension of the forearm on the arm. An early sign also is the loss of normal swinging of the arm in walking. Still another is the loss of capacity to perform rapid movements as in repeated striking of the forefinger against the thumb. A manifestation of the rigidity is seen in the typical *gait*, which in the early stages is slowed and associated with failure to swing the arm naturally. Later the gait becomes shuffling, the body bent forward, the arms and legs slightly flexed. Often there is difficulty in starting the act of walking and once initiated there may be a propulsion with inability to hold back. The patient under these cir-

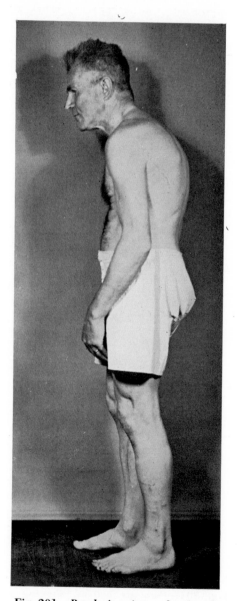
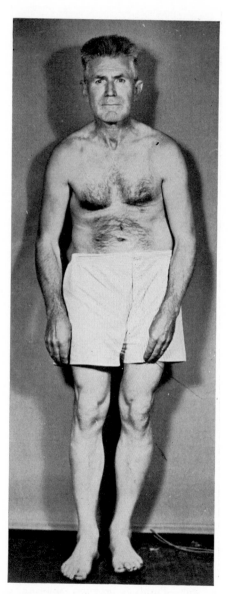

Fig. 201—*Paralysis agitans*, showing the typical flexed posture of the head and trunk, the flexion of the arms, and the pill-rolling position of the fingers.

cumstances has been said to run after his center of gravity. Sometimes a compulsive tendency to walk backward is found. In a typical case of paralysis agitans, the gait begins painfully slow, with short shuffling steps, increasing in rate as the walking proceeds (festinating gait). Running on the flat or upstairs is often much easier than walking.

The *facies* in paralysis agitans is usually described as immobile. Blinking and smiling are infrequent. There is little mobility in facial expression. The usual description of the facies of paraly-

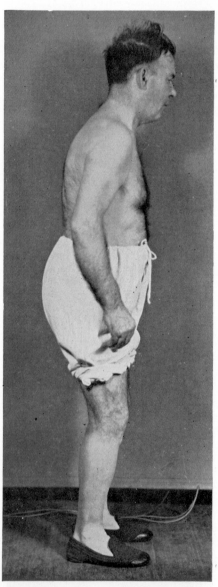 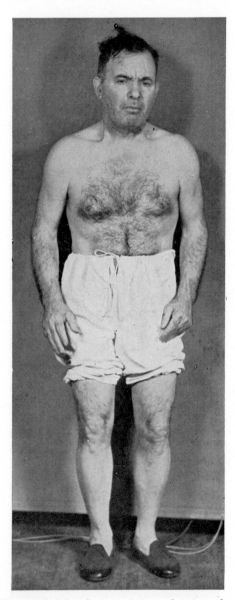

Fig. 202—*Paralysis agitans*, showing the typical flexion posture of the head, trunk and limbs.

Fig. 203—*Paralysis agitans*, showing the flexion posture of the arms and the pill-rolling position of the hands.

sis agitans as expressionless is inaccurate. On the contrary, the facies have an anxious, apprehensive quality. Loss of mobility of the facial muscles is usually present, but is not always found. Some patients with paralysis agitans have

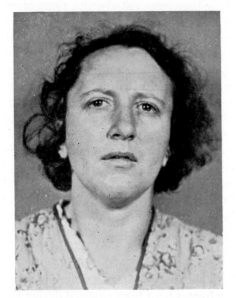

Fig. 204—*Paralysis agitans*, showing the smoothed-out, immobile, yet anxious facies.

relatively good facial appearance. The skin of the face in the postencephalitic type is oily and greasy.

The *handwriting* is tremulous and often micrographic. Movements are slow and deliberate. There is, in fact, a paucity of movement, usually referred to as *akinesis*. Extraneous movements, such as crossing the legs, gesturing, crossing the arms, and the many other such movements indulged in by the normal person are lost early in paralysis agitans. *Weakness* of movement is present in slight degree but never as great as in pyramidal tract disturbance. Decrease of power is a common complaint on the part of the patient. The reflexes are unchanged or may be slightly increased. A Babinski sign is not present in typical paralysis agitans. Cases of pallidopyramidal de-

generation combining features of pyramidal and extrapyramidal disease have been recorded and in such instances a Babinski sign is found.

Slowness of movement is constant. With this is associated a long latency between the desire to act and the initiation of the movement, as, for example, in walking. Sufferers from paralysis agitans are slow in arising from a chair, in walking, in sitting down, and in the numerous other voluntary acts of the normal person. The *mentality* is unaffected in the senile and encephalitic forms of paralysis agitans. There is no threat to intellectual functions, therefore, in these subjects. In

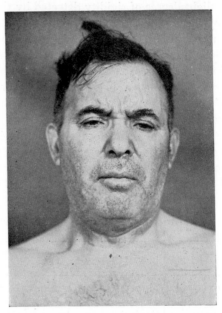

Fig. 205—*Paralysis agitans*, showing the anxious and smoothed-out facies with little mobility.

some instances, psychoses are found in the encephalitic form, usually in the acute stages of the disease, but at times also in the postencephalitic period. The arteriosclerotic forms of paralysis agitans, associated as they are with evidence of cortical damage, are not uncommonly accompanied by evidence of mental deterioration and even by psychoses.

Diagnosis: The diagnosis of paralysis agitans in its fully developed form is easy and can be made at a glance. The facial expression or lack of it, the flexed attitude, the tremor, the gait, are all so characteristic as to make error impossible.

Early diagnosis is essential, since the response to treatment is better in the early stages of the disease. Recognition is made by the history of slowing, fatigue, or tremor. On examination there is found an absence of blinking, a decrease in facial expressiveness as the patient recounts his illness, failure to swing the arm or arms in walking, the presence of a slight degree of rigidity detected by the cogwheel sign, a slight weakness of the voice and indistinctness of speech, and difficulty in repeating rapid movements. Some or all of these signs may be present and even in very early stages of the disease may be detected by the wary.

The encephalitic form of paralysis agitans occurs at any age but usually appears in the young, before forty years. A history of encephalitis may often be obtained by symptom (fever, diplopia, hypersomnolence), but in many cases no such history is obtainable, the disease occurring seemingly without precedent infection. In many instances, a history of "grippe" or influenza is obtainable; these may represent abortive types of encephalitis. Progress of the disease is often more rapid than in senile paralysis agitans and greasy skin and sialorrhea are common. Oculogyric crises may be found in the postencephalitic form. Tremor is less prominent than in the senile form of paralysis agitans and when present tends to be coarse in type. Rigidity is more prominent than tremor. *Pallilalia* (repetition of a word or phrase) and *echolalia* (repetition of words addressed to the patient) are more frequent than in senile paralysis agitans. Choreo-athetosis is sometimes encountered. The encephalitic form of paralysis agitans is practically always a sequel of encephalitis, but in rare instances, parkinsonism syndromes have been reported during the acute stages of the disease.

Table 58 summarizes the main means of distinguishing between the senile, en-

Table 58—Features of the Various Types of Paralysis Agitans

	Senile	*Encephalitic*	*Arteriosclerotic*
AGE	Fifty to sixty chiefly; not uncommonly over sixty	Any age; often in young under forty	Sixty or over
ONSET	Gradual	Gradual	Gradual
SPREAD	Usually general but partial involvement not uncommon (one arm, or arm and leg)	Same	Trunk and legs especially
TYPE	Tremor and rigidity usually; in some cases more tremor than rigidity and vice versa	Rigidity more pronounced than tremor as rule	Rigidity marked; tremor practically nil
SPECIAL FEATURES		Greasy skin, sialorrhea common	Pseudobulbar symptoms forced laughing or crying, pyramidal signs, aphasia and other indications of arteriosclerosis

cephalitic, and arteriosclerotic forms of paralysis agitans.

Paralysis agitans syndromes are produced by other conditions of various sorts but are never in as pure a form as in the senile and encephalitic forms of the disease. *Manganese poisoning*, seen especially in miners of the ore, produces symptoms of paralysis agitans. Parkinson-like symptoms are seen in senility. In such states a little rigidity and tremor is found but not a fully developed parkinsonian syndrome. *Carbon monoxide* has a special affinity for the basal ganglia, especially for the lenticular nucleus (pallidum, putamen). Nonfatal cases of the disease may show residual tremor and rigidity, but the total picture is not that of typical paralysis agitans. The facies are lacking, as well as the characteristic trunk and limb posturing, though rigidity is present. *Brain tumors* involve the basal ganglia area but do not usually produce a paralysis agitans syndrome. *Softenings* involving the basal ganglia area (putamen, caudate, pallidum) are common but do not in the vast majority of instances produce the typical symptoms of paralysis agitans. They are, as a rule, asymptomatic. The same is true of hemorrhage into this region.

Tremor due to various other causes must be differentiated from that of paralysis agitans. The tremor of *senility* is constant and fails to demonstrate the usual features of the parkinsonian case. It is usually but not always unassociated with rigidity, and is often accompanied by evidences of mental deterioration. *General paresis* may cause tremor of the hands, which is usually associated with facial and lingual tremors. It rarely reaches the degree of the parkinsonian tremor. The tremor of *alcoholism* is constant, often accompanied by facial tremors and mental deterioration. Rigidity is not present and other features of paralysis agitans are lacking. *Familial tremor* is at times mistaken for paralysis agitans. It occurs usually in males, is constant, increases with movement, and fails to respond to treatment.

The *course* of paralysis agitans is definitely downward. There is no recovery from the disease. The progression is usually slow in the senile and encephalitic forms and more rapid in the arteriosclerotic variety. The encephalitic form may develop rapidly for a time and then level off. Death is by an intercurrent disease, usually years after the onset of symptoms.

Treatment: There is no cure for paralysis agitans in any of its forms. The treatment is purely *symptomatic*. Treatment is directed largely toward relief of the tremor and rigidity, but fatigue and somnolence are also to be reckoned with.

General physical measures are important. *Rest* is essential. Special diets are of no help. The question is often propounded by the patient as to how much exercise may be indulged in, the idea being that exercise must help the muscles. It is difficult to advise on this point, but a safe rule is to tell the patient to avoid fatigue. Periods of rest during the day are advisable. Tobacco is best avoided. Alcohol should not be permitted even in the slightest degree.

Many forms of drug, vaccine, and serum therapy have been advocated for paralysis agitans. No single drug treatment is effective and the dosage and type must be worked out in every case individually. Comparative studies have shown that no single treatment is superior to any other. It is important as working principles to keep in mind (1) that large dosages of any of the effective drug vary from case to case; (2) that tolerance to one drug is often developed and that change or "staggering" of drugs is necessary from time to time; (3) that in changing from one drug to another in the treatment of paralysis agitans it is essential that the dosage of the new drug be as closely equivalent to that of the old as possible in order to avoid a letdown; (4) that such simple measures as rest and general hygiene must not be neglected; and (5) that psychotherapy is important.

It is difficult to advise on the choice of drugs in paralysis agitans. Many are available and it is often the experience that different cases react differently to the various drugs open to choice. No rigid rules can be laid down; the choice of drugs and their optimum dosage are matters which must be worked out individually.

The medical treatment of paralysis agitans is symptomatic. There are no drugs available which are capable of curing the disease, or which can be given with the understanding that they will hold the disease in check. Regardless of treatment, progression is the rule.

The available drugs consist of the belladonna group and its derivatives and antihistaminics. The drugs available for treatment are helpful in controlling the rigidity associated with the disease. There is no known drug at present which is capable of controlling tremor. *Atropine sulfate* in an aqueous solution (0.5 per cent) is effective in many cases. It is started at one drop daily for two or three days, then increased to one drop twice and then three times daily, with gradual increase of the dosage in gradual stages until the patient is taking from three to fifteen drops of the solution three times daily, depending on the tolerance. By gradual increase in the dose, the blurring of vision and gastrointestinal symptoms may be avoided, but if these develop, stopping the drug for a few days or decreasing the dose is usually effective.

The drug may be given in the tablet form, beginning with a dose of gr. $\frac{1}{200}$ two or three times daily, and gradually increasing to the point of tolerance.

Stramonium, either in the tincture or as the dried leaves, is useful in some cases. The fresh tincture should be given in doses of fifteen to seventy-five drops three times daily. In the case of the larger dosages, increase must be made gradually until the optimum dosage is reached. At times the tincture is not well tolerated or cannot be taken easily. In such cases, stramonium leaves (gr. $2\frac{1}{2}$) may be given two to five times daily. *Scopolamine* (hyoscine) *hydrobromide* is effective in doses of gr. $\frac{1}{200}$ to gr. $\frac{1}{100}$ or gr. $\frac{1}{50}$ several times daily, depending on the tolerance.

Synthetic belladonna-like compounds of many sorts have been used in the treatment of paralysis agitans. The most useful of these is *Artane* (trihexyphenidyl) which is given in doses of 2 mg. three times daily, increasing as necessary to 5 mg. three or four times daily. Dryness·of the mouth and blurring of vision are among the unpleasant side-reactions. The drug may be combined with others. It has relatively little effect on tremor. *Pagitane Hydrochloride* (cycrimine hydrochloride) is useful in dosages of 1.25 mg. three or four times daily, which can be increased in 1.25 mg. increments to a dosage of 2.5 mg. three or four times daily. As a rule, the drug is tolerated well. *Parsidol* (ethopropazine hydrochloride) is given in doses of 10 mg. and is more useful when used with Artane or some other drug than when used alone. It may be used alone, however, in doses of 10 to 20 mg. three or four times daily. *Cogentin* (benzotropine methanesulfonate) is very useful in the treatment of patients with great rigidity, but the drug cannot be tolerated in high doses. It is given as a 2 mg. tablet once or twice daily.

Antihistamines are useful as adjuncts in the treatment of paralysis agitans. They have relatively little value when used alone, but in conjunction with one of the compounds mentioned they appear to be helpful.

Amphetamine sulfate or *Dexedrine Sulfate* in dosages of 5 mg. two or three times daily is helpful in overcoming the fatigue of which these patients complain.

Barbiturates and the tranquilizing drugs are of no value in paralysis agitans.

Surgery: Surgical methods have been used in the treatment of paralysis agitans, especially for tremor, that most demoralizing of all the symptoms of the disease. There are many procedures available at present, but none appears to have reached the stage of maximum safety and results. Some are more reliable than others. Good results have been recorded, but the method of surgical relief of the tremor of paralysis agitans must at present be reserved for severe cases in which the patients are disabled or demoralized by their tremor. The operation cannot be recommended in our present state of knowledge because (1) the tremor recurs frequently after operation, and (2) hemiplegia or hemiparesis may result from the operation and may be persistent.

Psychotherapy: This is important. Parkinsonian patients as a class fail to adjust easily to their illness and are particularly demoralized by the tremor. They are easy prey for the designing and usually wander from one healer to another in search for a cure. Constant encouragement and reassurance are necessary. Sooner or later a realization of the incurable nature of the illness must be faced and proper adjustment made.

V. SYDENHAM'S CHOREA (*St. Vitus Dance, Chorea Minor*)

Sydenham's chorea is an acute disease occurring chiefly in children, characterized by involuntary movement and often associated with rheumatic disease.

Etiology: The disease occurs chiefly in childhood or early adolescence, and is rare in infancy. The usual age of onset is from five to sixteen years. It may appear in adults during pregnancy (chorea gravidarum), but in such instances a previous history of chorea in childhood is often obtainable. Girls are much more frequently affected than boys (two to one or three to one), for reasons which are not clear. Most cases occur during the spring. Race and heredity have no influence on the occurrence of the disease. Direct heredity is rare, but a family history of neuropathic tendencies is common—alcoholism, epilepsy, neuroses, tics, and insanity. The specific cause of chorea is not known, but there seems to exist a close relationship between chorea and rheumatic fever. Not all cases of chorea give evidence of rheumatic fever by heart and other signs at the time of examination, but in a large percentage a history of joint pains and other indications of the disease may be obtained. This leaves, however, a considerable percentage of cases in which there is neither history nor findings to indicate rheumatic infection.

The relationship between *chorea* and *rheumatic infection* has given rise to much discussion and the incidence of occurrence of rheumatic fever in chorea has been variously computed. A history of rheumatism was found in twenty-five per cent (Gowers); on the other hand, a rheumatic history has been found in as high as seventy-two per cent of cases (Tylden). In a series of one thousand cases of rheumatic fever and chorea followed over a period of eight years, it was found that the incidence of rheumatic heart disease in cases of rheumatic fever without chorea was eighty-six per cent as compared with fifty-four per cent in cases with chorea. It seems clear that chorea is not always associated with evidence of rheumatic heart disease but that it is frequently associated with rheumatic manifestations. Their precise occurrence is too variable to estimate. It has been suggested that those cases associated in the first episode with an increase erythrocyte sedimentation rate are probably due to rheumatic fever.

Fright, excitement, and worry are commonly said to be present preceding the onset of chorea, but it is doubtful whether these are of much importance in the development of the disease. In some cases, fear or excitement may precipitate chorea in patients predisposed to the disease. Tonsillitis has been accused in many instances and there is not infrequently a history of this disease preceding the onset of the chorea. It was found in 163 of 515 cases (Burr). Scarlet fever and diphtheria may precede the onset of chorea.

Pathology: The findings in the brain are not uniform. Necropsied cases are not numerous, but those which are available indicate that the cerebral hemispheres, basal ganglia, and brain stem may be affected, with, however, predominant involvement of the basal ganglia. The evidence for the pathological site of the lesions in Sydenham's chorea is founded on relatively few cases coming to necropsy. Infiltrations in the striatum have been found in Sydenham's chorea, in chorea gravidarum, and in symptomatic chorea. The small ganglion cells have been found involved predominantly. In the striatum particularly are found evidences of disease of the ganglion cells with perivascular infiltration and cell infiltration in the nerve tissue. The ganglion cells show no specific type of cell change; the vessels often show proliferative endarteritis, and there may be punctate hemorrhages in acute cases. Changes in the cerebral cortex similar to those

observed in the basal ganglia have been observed in some cases. Areas of ischemic cell disease, diffuse loss of ganglion cells in the third cortical layer, and ischemic necrosis have been described.

Symptoms: The *onset* of Sydenham's chorea is usually abrupt, but there is often a history to the effect that minor movements have been present for some time before serious movements began. These are usually mild and are likely to be regarded as mere habit movements which are of no consequence. They persist and spread, however, and eventually become pronounced. There is often a history of a *recent sore throat* or of repeated sore throats.

The movements of chorea are *involuntary*. They vary as to severity and frequency, in some cases being pronounced and almost constant; in others, mild and relatively infrequent. They involve particularly the proximal portions of the limbs and are more commonly seen in the arms than in the legs. The movements may be and often are confined to one side of the body or even to a single limb. The head is often affected. The movements are profuse, brief, discrete, abrupt, unsustained, and irregular, and are not stereotyped. Quick movements of the shoulder or arm, abrupt motion of the hand, tossing of the head, and similar movements are common, affecting first one part, then another in no fixed rotation. In mild cases there may be seen only an occasional involuntary movement of a shoulder or a hand, so slight at times as to require careful observation to detect them. Eventually in severe cases there is almost constant movement of first one part of the body and then another.

Even voluntary movements are performed abruptly and suddenly. When asked to extend the arms or tongue, the patient does so quickly as a rule.

Facial grimacing is common; grunting noises are frequent, and speech becomes indistinct, incoördinate, and even lost in severe instances. The movements cause simultaneous contraction of agonists and antagonists; they are increased invariably by emotional stress, and decreased by quiet repose and absence of excitement. They disappear during sleep. In most instances, a history of an emotional trauma of some sort will be offered by the parents, but it is doubtful whether this has a causal relationship to the disease. It may precipitate symptoms.

Muscular weakness is found not infrequently and may assume a hemiplegic form, with weakness involving one arm and leg. The limbs in such instances are flaccid and flaillike and show as a rule neither increase of reflexes nor pathological responses such as the Babinski sign. Weakness is found in other instances as well, but in many cases weakness, as evidenced by the dropping of objects, etc., is the result not of loss of power but of the involuntary movements. The muscles in general in chorea are hypotonic but tend to be even more so in paralytic cases. Incoördination is common and awkwardness in reaching for objects or in gauging distances is a common complaint. The reflexes are usually normal but may be decreased. Pendular knee jerks are seen at times. Of special interest is the choreic hand, which is best observed with the arms outstretched. This is characterized by flexion at the wrist and overextension at the metacarpophalangeal joints. This deformity of the hand is seen in most instances and may persist after the involuntary movements have disappeared. The pronator sign is also useful in diagnosis. It is best observed with the arms elevated above the head and is characterized by turning of the affected palm or palms outward, with overpronation of the arm at the elbow. With the arm outstretched horizontally, pronation of the hand is also seen but often not as clearly as with the arms elevated. The choreic handgrasp is said to be characteristic. "As the patient grasps the examiner's hand, the pressure is not steadily maintained, but waxes and wanes in strength" (Purves-Stewart).

The choreic facies is often more or less serene and has a tendency to a somewhat blank expression. Anxiety is not common, at least in the facial expression. Irritability is common. Mental symptoms are rare, but in adult forms confusion may be present, as well as other abnormal mental reactions. Irritability, peevishness, and forgetfulness are common. *Emotional instability* is common and most subjects are described as unreasonable and difficult to handle. Most patients are regarded as problems in schools, once symptoms develop. Sleep is poor. Incontinence is not found and consciousness is not disturbed during the disease. The tonsils are often diseased. The heart frequently reveals evidence of mitral disease due to rheumatic infection, but this is by no means constant and is often lacking. Pallor is common and secondary anemia often present.

The *duration* of choreiform attacks varies greatly. The average case lasts from six to eight weeks, but many last less than this and others continue for months. *Recurrences* are common and may develop over a number of months or years. They are so frequent, in fact, that they are looked upon as part of the natural history of the disease.

The personality of patients with Sydenham's chorea is of interest. In the majority of cases, the disease is found in youngsters with intense, conscientious make-ups, with a greater liking as a rule for intellectual rather than physical outlets, with a highly imaginative nature, often with a tendency to outlet through daydreaming, with good or superior school performances, and with a general tendency to introversion.

Diagnosis: The *diagnosis* of Sydenham's chorea offers no difficulties in a child with a history of recent sore throat, well-pronounced choreiform movements, and evidences of mitral disease. The greatest difficulty is offered by those mild cases in which there is a serious question whether the movements are choreiform or psychogenic in origin. The distinction is usually possible but in some cases it may be altogether impossible. In cases of psychogenic origin, there is a significant history of difficulty in adaptation, a personality make-up consistent with neurotic symptoms, and a stereotyped character to the movements which is not seen in true chorea. The choreic hand and the pronator sign are absent, but since these are not constant in chorea they are not absolute criteria. The absence of evidences of rheumatic infection is not helpful, since they are often absent in chorea.

Treatment: This is often difficult at home because of the special circumstances required. *Rest* and *absolute quiet* are essential, both of which are often impossible at home. Radio, reading, visitors, and any form of excitement are absolutely interdicted. Rest and quiet are essential even for mild cases, since proper handling of the situation in such instances may result in abortion of a more severe attack and in shortening the duration of the attack. A nutritious *diet* which requires no particular additions is desirable.

The use of drugs is not a matter of uniform opinion. *Iron* is often desirable because of the associated anemia. *Acetylsalicylic acid* is useful because of the relationship to rheumatic infection and

may be given in doses of 5 to 10 grains three times daily. *Fowler's solution* is often used in doses of three to five drops three times daily. It is tolerated in doses as high as ten drops three times daily. Beneficial effects are frequently seen with Fowler's solution, but these are probably the result of its tonic rather than of specific effects in Sydenham's chorea. Advice concerning the problem of sedatives is difficult to give. In most instances, it is unnecessary to use sedation. In severe cases, *phenobarbital*, gr. $\frac{1}{4}$ or gr. $\frac{1}{2}$, three times daily, may be given. *Sodium Amytal*, gr. 1, three or four times daily, is helpful. Bromides, chloral, and hyoscine have been used as sedatives in the disease. The value of ACTH and cortisone in the treatment of chorea is still undecided. Favorable and unfavorable results have been recorded. Use of the drugs is justifiable in severe, recurrent cases or in cases refractory to other methods of treatment.

In severe cases, *fever therapy* has been used successfully and has resulted in a shortening of the attack. It is usually induced by the intravenous injection of typhoid-paratyphoid vaccine (1000 million per cc.), giving an initial dosage of 25,000,000 bacteria and thereafter on alternate days doubling the last dosage given until a full cc. is administered. Seven to ten injections are necessary for a full course of treatment.

A difficult decision in treatment concerns the determination of the time when return to activity is permissible. As convalescence proceeds and the movements become fewer, pressure will be brought by the patient to permit a return to normal activities. This must never be allowed until all movements have ceased. Permission to get out of bed part of the day may be granted when the movements are greatly decreased. It is a safe rule that no return to activities should be allowed for two weeks after the movements have ceased. Even then return to full activity should be gradual in order to avoid recurrence of the attack. School activities, play, movies, radio, etc., must be returned to gradually.

The outlook in most cases of chorea is eventual cure, but recurrence is common. The prognosis for children is better than for adults, and more serious in cases following infectious diseases.

VI. HUNTINGTON'S CHOREA (Chronic Progressive Chorea)

Huntington's chorea is a disease of the basal ganglia and cerebral cortex characterized by chronic progressive chorea, mental deterioration, and a heredofamilial incidence.

Etiology: The disease is rare. It develops most frequently between the ages of thirty-five and forty, but it may develop from thirty to fifty and is not uncommonly found from twenty to thirty. Rare cases have been reported in childhood and during the second decade of life. It involves men and women equally. A *familial incidence* is characteristic of the disease but sporadic cases are known to occur. The average duration of the illness is fifteen years. Not all members of a stricken family develop the disease, roughly one-quarter to one-half being stricken. Huntington's chorea is transmitted as a single dominant gene not sex-linked. Rare cases are on record of patients who have twice married healthy partners and in each instance have given rise to choreic children. Monozygotic twins have in every instance developed the disease in both parties. In some families, all members develop the disease. Once the disease develops, it continues uninterrupted through one generation after another. Neurological disorders are common among the ancestors of the persons with Huntington's chorea, among them being alcoholism, mental deficiency, epilepsy, compulsive tics, migraine, and constitutional psychopathic traits. Congenital dislocation of the hips, Morquio's disease, and Sydenham's chorea have been found among afflicted families. Suicide is relatively common.

Pathology: The disease affects the basal ganglia and cerebral cortex. The caudate and putamen are most affected, the small ganglion cells being severely diseased, the large ganglion cells of the striatum suffering much less. The caudate and putamen are shrunken and become demyelinated. Gliosis is usually severe in the affected ganglia. The pallidum suffers much less than the striatum, but shows a mild loss or disease of its ganglion cells. Other parts of the basal ganglia system are normal or close to normal. The cerebral cortex shows severe damage, especially in the frontal areas, the outstanding features being cortical atrophy with loss of ganglion cells, especially in the lower layers (3, 5 and 6 particularly), associated with gliosis and not dependent on vascular disease.

The process is degenerative in character, though attempts have been made to demonstrate its dependence on a vascular factor.

Symptoms: The outstanding symptoms are the *chorea* and the *mental* deterioration occurring in an adult and pursuing a progressive course. The chorea is rapid and involves all muscles of the body. Facial grimacing is common, saluting movements of the arms, and irregular movements of various types are seen. The movements are unceasing. They are in constant process of changing, yet as one watches them there is a repetition of movements which, however, is not stereotyped. Movements of the arms are more active than those of the legs, but truncal movements are also active. They may remain confined largely to one limb or the face for some time before involving other portions of the body. Saluting movements are common; shrugging, flexion and extension of the limbs; twisting or turning movements of the head and trunk; and slow athetotic movements of the fingers, toes, head, and tongue are common. The athetoid movements are definite and pronounced in the fingers and toes, and are readily seen on careful scrutiny; slow twisting movements of the head are of a similar nature.

The muscular tone is increased in advanced stages of the disease, the limbs becoming hypertonic. The gait is clumsy because of the incessant choreiform movements. The speech is indistinct and dysarthric and may eventually become completely indistinct in the advanced stages. Loss of continuity of thought is common during speech and eventually speech becomes completely disintegrated. The movements are not controlled by effort and are increased by emotional factors. They disappear during sleep. The tendon reflexes are at first normal but later become overactive. Mental deterioration develops in every case and is characteristic of organic types of loss of intellectual power—loss of memory, concentration, attention, etc. It develops slowly at first and sets in some time after the chorea has been present. Mental deterioration is progressive and inexorable. It proceeds faster in some cases than in others but it is always found. Eventually dementia is profound and is most severe during the terminal portions of the disease. Huntington's chorea has been found in association with epilepsy, Friedreich's ataxia, migraine, myopathies, and myoclonic epilepsy. Mental symptoms are common during the course of the disease. Emotional instability is common, paranoid delusions, grandiose ideas, and hallucinations may be encountered. The course is progressive and incurable, the disease lasting as a rule from ten to twenty years.

Diagnosis and Treatment: The *diagnosis* of Huntington's chorea is not difficult. The main features on which tne diagnosis is made are (1) the hereditary features, (2) the onset in middle age (thirty-five to forty); (3) the occurrence of choreo-athetosis of a progressive nature, and (4) progressive mental deterioration. The hereditary features of the disease are rarely absent, but apparently sporadic cases may occur; in such instances, atypical mental features of various types are found in the family history. No difficulty is encountered in distinguishing Huntington's chorea from other forms of chorea.

No treatment is known. It has been suggested that *chlorpromazine* is helpful in Huntington's chorea, and that decrease in the movements follows dosages of the drug up to 200 to 300 mg. per day by mouth. *Reserpine* in doses of 4 to 10 mg. daily by mouth has been reported to help in the decrease of the involuntary movements.

VII. HEMIBALLISM (*Hemichorea*)

Hemiballism is a rare form of basal ganglia disease occurring for the most part in older people of sixty years or more, but sometimes between fifty and sixty. It affects women more than men. It is caused by a lesion involving the corpus or nucleus subthalamicum (body of Luys) of the opposite side. The syndrome has been found in association with hemorrhage, tuberculoma, metastatic carcinoma, infarct and softening involving the corpus subthalamicum. It has been reported with softening of the head of the caudate nucleus.

The symptoms develop abruptly and are quite dramatic. They consist of severe involuntary movements involving the arm and leg, but most particularly the arm. They resemble throwing movements. They are in reality very violent and excessive types of chorea and are of large amplitude and quite violent. The face is not usually affected. The symptoms are persistent and associated with severe exhaustion as the disease persists. The outlook is poor. The disease has been treated with good success by ablation of the opposite motor cortex and with complete cessation of the movements (Alpers and Jaeger).

VIII. SYMPTOMATIC CHOREA

The term "symptomatic chorea" is used for those cases in which the chorea appears as a symptom of some underlying condition. Included in this group are a number of ill-defined states, as well as others which are relatively better defined.

Senile chorea occurs, as the name implies, in old age, and is due to vascular lesions involving the striatum. It is in reality an arteriosclerotic form of chorea, the underlying condition being vascular disease of the brain. Mental deterioration and other evidences of cerebral arteriosclerosis are usually present.

Chorea is sometimes found in *intoxication* with lead, manganese, and mercury in particular. A special form of chorea is seen in hyoscine intoxication, associated usually with evidence of a toxic psychosis.

Infections of various sorts may be associated with chorea. Encephalitis lethargica may be associated with choreiform movements during the acute stages of the disease or as a late sequel. Diphtheria, epidemic encephalitis, smallpox, typhus, gonorrhea, scarlet fever, measles, syphilis, and influenza have been found at times to be associated with chorea (Lewy).

A special form of chorea, such as *electric chorea* (Henoch), has long been known, but it is rare. It is characterized by sudden involuntary contraction of a group of muscles, the result being a violent movement as if the muscles in question had been stimulated by an electrical current. The contractions occur at the rate of three to six per minute or as infrequently as once per minute and result in movements of the head, shoulders, arms, or legs, and even of tongue, glottis, and diaphragm. The disease tends to recover spontaneously in the course of a few days or weeks. A similar form of electric chorea known as *Bergeron's chorea* has been reported in children.

Another rare form is that known as *Dubini's chorea,* which has been described in northern Italy. The disease occurs at any age and is characterized by sharp muscle spasms involving first one arm and one side of the face, later the ipsilateral leg and finally the limbs of the opposite side (Keschner). Atrophy and decreased electrical excitability of the muscles follow. There are considerable pain and hyperesthesia of the skin associated with this form of chorea. High fever is common. Death occurs after days, weeks, or months. Recovery is rare.

There is considerable speculation as to whether the disease forms described as electric chorea are not in reality examples of myoclonus. They have many features of myoclonus as well as of chorea. The appearance of discrete muscular contractions is more characteristic of myoclonus than of chorea and there is much justification for placing these diseases in the myoclonus group.

IX. DYSTONIA MUSCULORUM DEFORMANS *(Torsion Spasm, Torsion Dystonia, Dystonia Lenticularis)*

Etiology: Dystonia is characterized by twisting, turning, or torsion movements of the trunk, the entire body, or of segments of the body, and is usually associated with increase of muscle tone,

Dystonia in general must be regarded as a symptom or syndrome and not as a specific disease. Careful attention to this principle will clarify understanding of the condition and will avoid difficulties in diagnosis. The following forms may be recognized (Keschner):

1. *Idiopathic dystonia of unknown origin.*
2. *Symptomatic dystonia, occurring in:*
    (*a*) Infections of the nervous system.
    (*b*) Vascular disease of the brain.
    (*c*) Toxic conditions (heavy metal poisoning, drugs, poison gases).
    (*d*) Tumors.

It appears in some instances in the idiopathic form without a specific cause, usually in children between seven and fifteen years of age, most commonly in Russian Jews. In such instances, it has a familial incidence. It occurs not uncommonly following epidemic encephalitis. It is also seen as a manifestation of progressive lenticular degeneration, since in some cases cirrhosis of the liver is found at necropsy.

The disease is associated with degeneration of the cells of the striatum (cau-

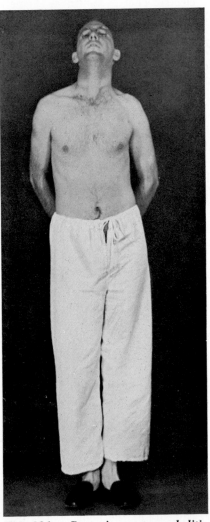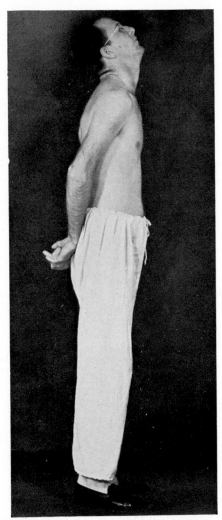

Fig. 206 — *Dystonia, postencephalitic,* showing marked dystonic movement of the head, intermittent in type, in a young man of 26 years.

date and putamen); changes have been found also in the pallidum, thalamus, corpus subthalamicum, inferior olives, pons, dentate nucleus, and cerebral cortex. Recent studies tend to emphasize the importance of the changes in the dentate nucleus, the cell loss and degenerations in the dentate nucleus.

Symptoms: The idiopathic variety is very rare and occurs chiefly in but is not confined to Jews. It develops from seven to fifteen years of age but it is not confined to children. Though several cases have been known to occur in a single family, the disease is not always familial.

The symptoms consist of *spasms* of twisting and torsion of the body and limbs. The spasms are not stereotyped and assume a variety of forms. They induce all sorts of bizarre distortions of the trunk and limbs.

The onset of the disease is gradual with the appearance of slow torsion movements. Walking becomes impaired because of a twisting or turning of a foot or leg or there may be an occasional jerking of an arm. Gradually the limbs become more involved. Implication of the neck muscles which is very constant gives a spasmodic torticollis effect, while involvement of the back and foot muscles is common. Clubfoot and other foot deformities are seen. The face usually escapes but facial grimacings and distortions occur. The hands and feet are not as much affected as the proximal parts of the limbs. The spasms are increased by movement; hence they appear particularly during walking, which is a series of contortions. The movements disappear in sleep. Associated with the spasms is a muscular *dystonia* characterized by rigidity of the musculature alternating with relaxation during the periods free of spasm. The rigidity may be persistent in some cases in which spasms are almost continuous, and muscle contractures may occur. While the disease involves all the limbs as a rule, it is seen at times in a single limb or confined to the limbs of one side. Despite the striking manifestations, the examination of the nervous system is negative.

Symptomatic dystonia is encountered more frequently than is the idiopathic variety. It is found not infrequently following *encephalitis,* either as an acute or chronic manifestation of the disease. As a rule, other evidences of postencephalitic sequelae are present, such as paralysis agitans or choreo-athetosis. The encephalitic variety of dystonia is more frequently confined to a single limb or even to the face or neck muscles, producing a picture of spasmodic torticollis. Dystonic movements may be encountered in *vascular disease* (hemorrhage, thrombosis, embolism) involving the basal ganglia. The movements are usually unilateral and may be confined to part of a limb, such as the hand. Similar movements are found following injuries to the basal ganglia in *intoxications,* particularly in carbon monoxide poisoning.

Diagnosis: The *diagnosis* is easy; the bizarre torsion movements of the neck, trunk, and pelvis are reproduced by no other disease. Almost invariably the disease is regarded as hysteria both early and late, due largely to the bizarre movements which are not recognized for their true significance. This tendency is a clear example of the propensity to regard as hysteria or as psychogenic those conditions which fail to correspond to one's conception or knowledge of organic syndromes.

It seems clear that dystonia must be regarded as a symptom which occurs in many diseases. It cannot be regarded as a disease entity. since little is as yet known concerning its underlying physiology and pathology. Dystonic movements and dystonia are observed in post-encephalitic conditions, torsion dystonia, spasmodic torticollis, athetosis, chronic progressive chorea, and related conditions. The dystonic movement, analyzed by means of motion pictures, reveals an excess of muscle tension as well as movement (Hery). Electromyogram studies of dystonic muscles reveal asynchronous, polyrhythmic discharges, with simultaneous innervation of agonists and antagonists (Hoefer and Putnam). The term "dystonia" should be reserved for cases with definite dystonic movements and postures, gradual in development and of uncertain cause. A study based on all available reported cases as well as on personal observations has led to the suggestion that the dystonias can be classified into three groups: "an early form, with an onset at or shortly after birth; the juvenile form, with an onset between the age of five and fifteen years; and the late form, with an onset after the age of fifteen" (Hery).

Spasmodic torticollis is in some cases an early and sometimes the only symptom of the disorders. In these instances it has been found to be associated with basal ganglia disease and is regarded by some as a fractional form of torsion spasm. There is great difficulty in determining whether spasmodic torticollis is the result of organic disease of the nervous system, of local irritative causes, or of psychogenic disturbances. It is safe to assert that spasmodic torticollis should not be regarded as being due to a dystonia unless (1) other evidences of a symptomatic dystonia are disclosed, as, for example, a history of onset after encephalitis, vascular or toxic disorders, or evidence of other manifestations of central nervous system disease are present, such as paralysis agitans, choreoathetosis, etc.: (2) other local or psychogenic causes have been excluded. Local causes, such as foci of infection in teeth, tonsils, or sinuses;

affections of the muscle; disease of the cervical spine are easy to exclude. Psychogenic factors are difficult to dispose of because of the almost constant history of increase of the movements by emotional factors and the evidences of emotional instability, which are invariably found in greater or lesser degree. In some cases the disease may persist for some time only as a torticollis and then later involve other muscles of the body. When torsion spasm is due to encephalitis, parkinsonian features are usually seen.

Prognosis and Treatment: The outlook in cases of idiopathic dystonia musculorum deformans is poor, since the disease is progressive. It is not unusual, however, for the disease to remain stationary for months or even years and even for remissions to take place. In the symptomatic variety little can be done to eradicate the symptom.

X. PROGRESSIVE LENTICULAR DEGENERATION (*Hepatolenticular Degeneration, Wilson's Disease*)

Progressive lenticular degeneration is a rare disease of the basal ganglia system characterized by a chronic progressive fatal course, a tendency to occur in families, and characterized by involuntary movements, rigidity, emotional disorders, dysarthria, and dysphagia.

Etiology: The disease occurs usually in adolescence (fifteen to twenty years), but onset in childhood (seven to ten years) has been seen, as well as later beginning of symptoms (thirty-five to forty). A familial tendency is common but there is little evidence that the disease is inherited. The precise cause of the disease is unknown.

Pathology: Changes are found in the nervous system and the liver. The liver is probably first affected, the lenticular lesions following from this (Wilson). Instances have been recorded in which the liver damage outstripped the cerebral process. In the brain, degeneration is most marked in the lenticular nucleus (putamen and pallidum), with the putamen much more affected than the pallidum. There is atrophy of both the putamen and pallidum, and often of the caudate. This is due to cell loss affecting particularly the cells of the putamen, associated with glial overgrowth. The pallidum is much less affected than the putamen. In some cases all the putamen cells are lost; in others, some cells escape. The putamen often shows evidence of cavitation (status spongiosus). Minor degrees of cell loss are sometimes found in the thalamus, red nucleus, corpus subthalamicum, and substantia nigra. The cerebellum may be affected in some cases, and the fibers coming from the pallidum (ansa lenticularis) are often involved.

Associated with the degeneration of the lenticular nucleus is the cirrhosis of the liver. The liver is small and shows typical hobnail cirrhosis both grossly and microscopically. The spleen is sometimes enlarged. The disorder is thought to be due to an inborn error of metabolism. There is increased copper in the liver and brain and increased urinary excretion of copper, as well as amino-aciduria. The plasma copper concentration is low, and excretion of copper in the feces is reduced. Amino-aciduria is present even in the absence of manifest liver disease. It is believed that the pathological changes in hepatolenticular degeneration could be due to copper accumulation in the tissues. There is no agreement on whether the copper deposits arise from a defect in copper metabolism, or from some error in amino-acid metabolism.

Cases have been reported with the typical clinical and pathological features of hepatolenticular degeneration but without amino-aciduria and abnormal copper storage and the typical Kayser-Fleisher ring. It is not yet clear whether these are to be regarded as a separate group.

Symptoms: The onset in most instances is gradual, but an acute rapid development has been observed in some cases. The disease is a combination of tremor and hypertonia, in varying degree. *Tremor* is often the first symptom and is present in every case. It is characterized by its constancy; by involvement more particularly of the distal segments of the limbs (hands, fingers, feet) early in the disease; by increase on movement, and emotional factors, but it is present also at rest. The tremor is fine, regular, and rhythmic (four to eight a second) and can be voluntarily inhibited for brief periods early in the disease. The head is not as a rule affected. The tremor becomes practically constant and generalized in the advanced stages and becomes a demoralizing factor. Spasmodic contractions, choreiform and athetotic movements occur but are not as frequent as the tremor.

Associated with the tremor is *hypertonia* or *rigidity* of the musculature. All the muscles of the body save the ocular muscles become affected eventually. The muscles reveal marked rigidity and are hard on palpation. The hypertonia involves chiefly the arm flexors and the leg extensors, giving the appearance roughly of the parkinsonian posture, but the trunk is not as a rule flexed as in paralysis agitans and the face is set in a stiff smile or vacant stare. Often the facial muscles are set in such fashion as to give a vacuous, silly appearance. Contractures develop as a result of the muscle rigidity. Muscle wasting occurs in some cases. Paralysis is not present, but movements become difficult due to the marked muscular rigidity. The gait is slow and difficult, due likewise to the rigidity, and later becomes impossible.

Mental symptoms are constant but vary in kind and degree. They may be slight or severe. Evidence of mental deterioration is found in many instances; in others, neurotic-like symptoms are found; in still others, infantile and childish reactions are outstanding. Involuntary laughter occurs and in some cases also psychotic states. Restlessness, euphoria, and emotional instability occur. Mental deterioration is usually present in the terminal stages.

Dysarthria is constant. It is at first characterized by slurring, but later becomes so marked as to make the speech unintelligible.

Dysphagia develops also, making swallowing difficult and later impossible, but there is no paralysis of the muscles of the palate or tongue.

The *Kayser-Fleischer* ring is found constantly. It appears as a green-brown ring in the cornea and is due to a deposit of pigment in Descemet's membrane. No changes are found in pupils, fundi, reflexes, or sensation. Sphincter control is lost late in the disease when deterioration is prominent, but not before this.

The *course* is progressive and fatal. The disease continues to advance and runs a course of four to five years, the tremors becoming more pronounced, and the rigidity increasingly greater.

Diagnosis: The diagnosis of progressive lenticular degeneration is easy in a fully developed case, the tremor, rigidity, dysphagia, dysarthria, emotional disturbances, and the progressive character of the malady in a young person being sufficient to establish the diagnosis.

The diagnosis should be considered in every case of tremor in a young person. Since tremor may be the first and only sign found early in the disease, the diagnosis must be made on findings other than those in a well-developed case. In this connection, the presence of a Kayser-Fleischer ring is sufficient to establish the diagnosis, though no other evidences of the disease may be present. The ab-

sence of this ring does not exclude the possibility of progressive lenticular degeneration since cases of the disease are on record without it.

Cirrhosis of the liver is constant at autopsy, yet liver function tests are of relatively little value in demonstrating disease of the liver in life. The cephalin flocculation test has been found most valuable, while hippuric acid synthesis, sulfobromphthalein excretion, and prothrombin time were often not significantly altered even in the presence of pronounced anatomic liver changes (Homburger and Kozol).

Pseudosclerosis (Westphal-Strümpell) is claimed by some to be a separate entity, but in all probability represents a variant of progressive lenticular degeneration. The age of onset is similar to that of progressive lenticular degeneration. The symptoms resemble so closely those of Wilson's disease (progressive lenticular degeneration) that the two conditions can hardly be separated. Tremor, rigidity, mental and emotional disturbances are present. The Kayser-Fleischer ring, which is said to be characteristic of pseudosclerosis, is found also in progressive lenticular degeneration. This consists of a greenish brown ring of pigment 1 to 2 mm. in width in the cornea. Pyramidal signs, which are said to be more characteristic of pseudosclerosis, are found rarely also in Wilson's disease. The claim for a separate entity distinct from Wilson's disease is based on the assumption that the lesions are more diffuse in pseudosclerosis, the symptoms less pronounced, and the fact that optic atrophy is sometimes found in the disease. As Wilson himself has shown, the lesions in progressive lenticular degeneration may be widespread though most pronounced in the lenticular nucleus.

A subvariety of the pseudosclerosis group has been recorded as an *acute degenerative striatal disease* (Woods and

Pendleton), described in three Chinese families characterized by abrupt onset, loss of equilibrium, speech defects, involuntary movements, and a general tendency to recover. In one case which came to necropsy, the pallidum and substantia nigra were necrotic.

Paralysis agitans may resemble the disease closely and may be very difficult to differentiate in early cases. The resemblance may be so close in such instances that some cases are undoubtedly regarded as parkinsonism. The onset of progressive lenticular degeneration in adolescence, the laughing facies, the increase of tremor on movement, the severe dysarthria and dysphagia, and the emotional and mental disturbances are different from paralysis agitans. The Kayser-Fleischer ring is of great importance in separating the two groups.

Pseudobulbar palsy may be confused because of the dysarthria and dysphagia, but can usually be differentiated by its much later age of onset (fifty or over), by the presence of pyramidal tract signs usually.

Multiple sclerosis must be separated but offers no great difficulties, since neither the tremors, the spasms, nor the rigidity are characteristic of multiple sclerosis.

Treatment: The treatment in general is unsatisfactory, but encouraging results in the control of the involuntary movements have been reported with BAL. This is given in a manner similar to that described for arsenic neuritis (p. 167).

XI. ATHETOSIS

Athetosis is a condition characterized by the occurrence of slow, irregular twisting movements, more commonly seen in the upper limbs, and more pronounced in the fingers and hands than in the proximal portions of the limbs (*v.* Chapter 3). It is a symptom which may occur in the course of many disorders:

1. *Congenital and Infantile Diseases:*
    (*a*) Status marmoratus (congenital double athetosis).
    (*b*) Status dysmyelinatus.
    (*c*) Infantile cerebral palsies.
2. *Symptomatic Athetosis:*
    (*a*) Encephalitis.
    (*b*) Porencephaly.
    (*c*) Progressive lenticular degeneration.
    (*d*) Cerebral arteriosclerosis with softening.
    (*e*) General paresis.
    (*f*) Tabes dorsalis.
    (*g*) Subacute combined degeneration.
    (*h*) Peripheral neuritis.

It may occur, therefore, under a wide variety of conditions. Of the congenital and infantile conditions, the occurrence is more common in the infantile cerebral palsies than in congenital disease. It is found not infrequently as an accompaniment of cerebral diplegia or in infantile hemiplegia. It develops also in cases of internal hydrocephalus in infants, in malformations of the brain, such as cerebral hemiatrophy, macrogyria, or microgyria, and in tuberous sclerosis.

In adults, athetoid movements may develop as the result of a number of vascular, encephalitic, and degenerative disorders.

Among the athetotic syndromes known to neurologists is *congenital double athetosis*. This is a disease which is found in infants in whom it is present from birth. It is associated with a pathological condition known as status marmoratus, characterized by a marbled appearance of the striatum (putamen and caudate). This is the result of an increase in the myelin architecture of these basal ganglia, resulting in a marbled appearance by the Weigert stain. Scattered among the normal structure of the striatum are small groups of fibers which when stained with a myelin sheath stain give a spotted appearance like marble (status marmoratus). This increased number of fibers in the striatum has a normal appearance as to myelin and nerve fiber structure. They are, therefore, normal myelinated nerve fibers. The condition is congenital and is the result of a prenatal developmental defect, but efforts have been made to attribute it to birth injury or to a febrile disease, such as encephalitis, early in life. In almost half the cases (forty-six per cent) a history of trauma at birth has been recorded. In addition to the findings in the striatum, damage is also observed in the thalamus, pallidum, and the cerebral cortex, the thalamus being affected more frequently than either the pallidum or cerebral cortex. The changes in these areas are similar to those found in the striatum.

Clinically, congenital double athetosis is characterized by involuntary movements which are present as a rule from birth, but may not become apparent until the child is several months of age. Development is often slow in these cases, with delay in sitting, walking, and talking. The movements are first noted when the child becomes active in the performance of voluntary movements, though they undoubtedly were present before. The athetotic movements which characterize the disease are featured by slow, sinuous movements which have a snake-like character and are more prominent in the distal portions of the limbs (fingers, toes, hands, forearms, feet) than in the proximal parts. Hyperextension and spreading of the fingers and toes are commonly seen. As the disease progresses, slow, snaky movements involve the limbs generally, the speech becomes dysarthric, and often unintelligible, there is facial grimacing, and the trunk and head participate in dystonic motions. The movements are increased by stress and emotional stimuli of many sorts. Bilateral paresis and spasticity, particularly of the lower extremities, are present in almost one-half the cases of double athetosis. Retarded speech development and/or dysarthria are present in eighty-per cent, and more than half the patients (fifty-eight per cent) are mentally defective (Carpenter).

Mental deficiency is usually present and convulsions are not uncommonly seen, though the latter are not a necessary part of the disease. The disease runs a course of variable duration, terminating at various periods after birth as the result of intercurrent infection. Congenital double athetosis must not be confused with the athetosis which is found associated with hemiplegias and other conditions resulting from birth injuries. These are not associated with a status marmoratus of the basal ganglia and will be considered under a discussion of cerebral birth conditions.

Medical treatment is of no avail. Surgical treatment of various sorts has been tried to control the athetosis, but these are still not sufficiently well worked out to determine their eventual efficacy. They consist of ablation of the motor and/or premotor cortex or section of the anterior columns in the cervical or thoracic portions of the spinal cord. Good results have been obtained by both methods and it is possible that the future will promise more relief through surgery.

Allied to status marmoratus is a disease known as *status dysmyelinatus*, which is extremely rare. It is a pathological entity characterized by failure or imperfection of development of the striopallidal fibers. It results also in the production of athetosis. The condition cannot be diagnosed clinically.

XII. MISCELLANEOUS AND ILL-DEFINED SYNDROMES

In addition to the well-defined syndromes found among the extrapyramidal disorders are others which are much less definite and some of which are open to question as clinical entities.

Progressive Pallidal Degeneration (*Syndrome of Hallervorden and Spatz*): This rare syndrome is associated with disease of the pallidum and substantia nigra, the cells of these ganglia being degenerated, the glial cells increased in number, and demyelination of the pallidum taking place. Degenerative changes have also been described in the cerebral cortex and striatum. The outstanding features of the disease are a familial occurrence, an onset in childhood between three and four years of age, progressive rigidity of all limbs, dysarthria, emotional disturbances and some degree of mental impairment amounting in some cases to dementia. The disease is difficult to diagnose clinically, but some suspicion of its presence may be aroused by the symptoms mentioned above as well as by the progressive rigidity without tremor. The disease is protracted in its course.

Spastic Pseudosclerosis (*Syndrome of Jakob*): This is a rare and ill-defined syndrome originally described as spastic pseudosclerosis, a poor term which should be discarded. Corticostriatospinal degeneration or diffuse encephalomyelopathy is a better term, since the symptoms are due to a combination of pyramidal and extrapyramidal disorders. The lesions are found in the pyramidal pathways, the cerebral cortex (frontal, motor), the striatum, pallidum, cerebellum, dentatum, and spinal cord. The symptoms appear from twenty to fifty-five years of age, but especially in the fourth and fifth decades. The suggestion has been made that spastic pseudosclerosis is a deficiency disease (Stengel and Wilson). The onset is gradual and the average duration one year. Remissions occur. Early symptoms are of a neurotic tinge with anxiety, depression, irritability, and insomnia. Later there develop tremors, rigidity, dysarthria, and disturbances of gait. Mental

symptoms of all sorts develop, with resulting severe dementia. The syndrome is almost impossible to diagnose clinically. Early in its course it is confused with multiple sclerosis; later, it is usually regarded as a vascular encephalopathy, and still later a presenile dementia (Alzheimer's or Pick's disease). The nature of the disease is unknown, as well as its cause, and it is still doubtful as to where it belongs in the group of pyramidal-extrapyramidal disorders. It is best regarded in our present state of knowledge as a degenerative encephalomyelopathy involving pyramidal, extrapyramidal, and spinal cord levels, not dependent so far as is known on vascular disease.

Extrapyramidal Syndromes Due to Exogenous Poisons: An extrapyramidal syndrome resembling paralysis agitans is seen in patients with chronic *manganese* poisoning, which produces degeneration of the striatum (caudate and putamen), pallidum and thalamus. The onset in such cases is usually gradual but may be acute. The general aspect is that of parkinsonism with the typical facies, rigidity of the limbs and trunk, tremor, monotonous voice, cramps in the calves and stiffness of the muscles, a peculiar slapping gait, and occasionally uncontrollable laughter and crying. The picture is that of a parkinsonism with evidences also of pyramidal pathway implication. Unlike typical paralysis agitans, however, pyramidal signs are present with hyperactive reflexes and Babinski's sign. Loss of libido and potentia are found and such rare symptoms as retrobulbar neuritis, difficulty in swallowing, and impairment of convergence.

Carbon disulfide intoxication in rayon workers particularly has been found to produce a paralysis agitanslike syndrome. According to reports, the syndrome produced by carbon disulfide resembles in all respects true paralysis agitans. The tremor is often general. The occurrence of paralysis agitans due to carbon disulfide poisoning is not common. A striatal-like syndrome is sometimes produced by *carbon monoxide* poisoning, but a pure picture of paralysis agitans is almost never seen despite the tendency to damage of the lenticular nucleus. Tremors, choreiform movements, dysarthria and rigidity alone or in unison are seen after carbon monoxide intoxication. Parkinsonlike syndromes have also been recorded in intoxication with *barbiturates* and in cases of *cyanide poisoning* which have recovered. Symmetrical necrosis of the pallidum has been observed in barbiturate poisoning.

XIII. SPASMODIC TORTICOLLIS

Torticollis is a condition characterized by deviation of the head due to contraction of the neck muscles by some irritative cause. It includes a number of conditions.

Etiology: Torticollis may occur at any age but is much more frequent in adults of middle or advanced ages. It may be found as part of a generalized or local dystonia, either as a local manifestation of dystonia musculorum deformans or as a symptomatic dystonia, due to encephalitis, cerebral arteriosclerosis, intoxications, or tumor. It is more commonly produced by local conditions, such as (1) myositis due to rheumatic infection or to foci of infection in the teeth, sinuses, or throat; (2) arthritis of the cervical vertebrae; (3) trauma of the cervical vertebrae; (4) congenital conditions, such as absence or fusion of the cervical vertebrae, the former being seen in the Klippel-Feil syndrome.

Symptoms: The torticollis may be spasmodic or constant. The movements are usually slow but may be abrupt. Though they are made to one side, they are associated with contraction of the muscles of both sides of the neck. The movements may be at first slight and may pass unnoticed, but they tend gradually to increase in severity, the head being pulled over with great force. The sternomastoid muscle is particularly involved, but contraction of the trapezius and the other neck muscles is common. The movements are aggravated by emotional factors of any sort and are relieved by supporting the head, either against the back of a chair, by lying down, or by resting the head in the hand. Early in the course of the disease, the movements may be relieved by rest, heat, or drugs, but these soon lose their effectiveness. There is great variability in the frequency of the spasms. They may be at first widely spaced or they may be frequent from the onset. Pain may be present in some forms but is not usually a prominent factor. Fatigue of the muscles involved is not usually seen, but irritability and demoralization develop from failure to control the movements and interference with work and social adjustments.

Diagnosis: The diagnosis of torticollis is easy. Great difficulties arise, however, in attempting to determine whether the disorder results from local, psychogenic, or central causes. The approach to this problem has already been referred to (*v.* Dystonia Musculorum Deformans).

Treatment: The treatment of torticollis is frequently a disappointing experience. The removal of foci of infection is advisable in cases due to local causes. In such cases also the use of salicylates, diathermy, or infrared applied to the neck muscles, massage, and bromides or barbiturates is helpful. In many instances, however, the use of local applications and drugs is of no avail. Such patients wander about as a rule, seeking help from many sources. In some instances, the use of a plaster cast to hold the head in proper position has been found helpful after application of the cast for many months. The method is often not successful. Surgical measures are usually disappointing. Various operations have been performed, among them being section of the spinal accessory nerve; section of posterior roots C2, 3, and 4 (Frazier); section of both anterior and posterior roots C2 to 4 bilaterally in addition to the spinal accessory nerve (Foerster). Surgical relief should be attempted only when other methods have failed since the results from sectioning the nerves and roots are often disappointing. Psychotherapy in those cases which result from emotional disorders is usually disappointing.

XIV. MYOCLONIAS

Myoclonus is characterized by the occurrence of sudden involuntary shocklike contractions of single muscles or muscle groups occurring regularly or irregularly in paroxysms, unassociated by movement of the limbs or other parts. Limb muscles are usually affected, particularly those of the lower limbs, the contractions being symmetrical as a rule but sometimes unilateral, and disappearing during sleep. The truncal, facial, ocular, pharyngeal, diaphragmatic, and laryngeal muscles may be involved.

Myoclonus is a symptom which may occur in the course of many conditions. It may be localized or general, and may occur at various times of life. Its detection gives no clue as to cause since in itself it represents merely an irritation of muscle contraction due to a nervous system process of some sort. The detection of myoclonus, therefore, must be followed by a search for its cause. Some of the forms of myoclonus are related to one another, as illustrated by a family of three brothers, two of whom had generalized myoclonus, while the third suffered from velopalatopharyngeal myoclonus (Van Leeuwen). In some instances, the myoclonus may exist for years without

other evidence of central nervous system involvement. The cause of the myoclonus cannot always be established.

The distinction between muscle fasciculations and myoclonus is not as a rule difficult, but a comparison of the two types of involuntary movements has been made and reveals the following features:

Similarities Between Fibrillation (*Fasciculation*) and Myoclonus (deJong and Jacobs)

Fibrillation (Fasciculation)	Myoclonus
Arrhythmic	Arrhythmic
Irregular incidence	Irregular incidence
Present after scopolamine hydrobromide	Present after scopolamine hydrobromide
Activated by impulses for voluntary movement	Activated by impulses for voluntary movement

Differences Between Fibrillation (*Fasciculation*) and Myoclonus (Modified After deJong and Jacobs)

Fibrillation (Fasciculation)	Myoclonus
Present during sleep	Disappears during sleep
Increased after prostigmine methylsulfate	Not affected by prostigmine methylsulfate
Present after nerve block	Not activated as a rule by direct tapping or electrical stimulation of muscle
Activated by mechanical stimulation of muscle	
Not affected by pin prick, emotion, or mental activity	Stimulated by pin prick, emotional, and mental activity
R D and increased chronaxia in some muscle fibers	No R D or increased chronaxia
Never a locomotor effect	Usually no locomotor effect

The involuntary movements known as myoclonus constitute a symptom which may occur in the course of several disorders.

Paramyoclonus Multiplex (Friedreich): This disease occurs in adults, chiefly in males, and is characterized by the presence of myoclonic twitchings involving the limb and trunk muscles particularly. It usually develops spontaneously, but has been found to start after fright, trauma, mental or physical exertion, infections (malaria, mumps, diphtheria), lead poisoning, general paresis, poliomyelitis, and in the course of Friedreich's ataxia (Keschner). It has been reported in three successive generations (Lindemulder). The contractions are brief, very rapid, irregular in their appearance, and may involve a whole muscle or only a part of it. The facial muscles are rarely affected, but the diaphragm and the laryngeal muscles may be involved, contraction of the latter producing a grunting noise. The movements are aggravated by emotional stimulation or by tapping the muscle, and disappear on motion and in sleep.

Familial Myoclonus (Unverricht): This form of myoclonus, referred to as myoclonic epilepsy, has been described in the discussion of Epilepsy (Chapter 14).

Encephalitic Myoclonus: Encephalitis lethargica is frequently followed by the occurrence of myoclonus, which, like dystonia, is usually associated with other evidences of postencephalitic sequelae, such as paralysis agitans, oculogyric crises, etc. The myoclonic twitchings may be widespread or may be confined to a single limb. Myoclonus may develop during the acute stages of encephalitis. A special form (Hunt, Sicard) occurring during encephalitis is characterized by an acute febrile onset with shooting pains in the trunk and limbs, followed in a few days by rhythmic myoclonus occurring synchronously in the affected muscles, involving first the abdominal muscles and simultaneously or shortly thereafter the limb muscles. During the acute stages, delirium and insomnia are present, associated with active delusions and hallucinations. The myoclonus subsides after the acute phase and is followed by a typical hypersomnolence with ocular palsies as in ordinary lethargic encephalitis. Death ensues in the course of two to three weeks.

Nystagmus Myoclonus: *Nystagmus myoclonus* is a rare congenital affection characterized by lateral nystagmus and myoclonic movements of the limbs or trunk. The movements are aggravated by cold or by tapping the muscles but can be controlled to some degree by will. The tendon reflexes are often exaggerated. Stigmata of degeneration are often found and include deformed teeth, hypospadias, facial asymmetry, persistent branchial cleft, local hyperhidrosis, circumscribed edema, etc. The disease is incurable but is not progressive.

Palatal Myoclonus: Of particular interest is a rare disorder referred to as palatal myoclonus. This is characterized by rapid repeated movements of the palate, varying from fifty to 180 per minute. The patient himself may be and often is unaware of the movement and may complain of twitching of the corner of the mouth or of a clicking noise in the ear when the eustachian tube is affected. The rapid movement may involve the palate alone, or it may implicate pharynx, larynx, tongue, fauces, mouth, and diaphragm. The movements are synchronous, interrupted by voluntary activity, do not interfere with the normal acts of swallowing, talking, or respiration, are uninfluenced by drugs, are decreased but not abolished during sleep, and are only partially abolished by local anesthesia. Evidences of underlying brain disease are usually present, the process varying in nature to include cerebral arteriosclerosis, multiple sclerosis, encephalitis, and tumor. Hysteria accounts for ten to twelve per cent of the cases. The disease is associated with hypertrophy and degeneration of the inferior olive and degeneration of the central tegmental tract.

16

Multiple Sclerosis

I. INTRODUCTORY

Multiple sclerosis is a peculiar and unpredictable disease. It is characterized by the occurrence of plaques of demyelination scattered without logical reason throughout the nervous system. It is not surprising, therefore, that its clinical manifestations are extremely variable and are dependent largely on the number, size, and distribution of the disseminated plaques. Hence an over-all description of the symptoms is extremely difficult and varies greatly from case to case. Its manifestations are described as protean. Difficult as is a comprehensive description of the symptomatology, this is relatively less certain than an account of the outcome of the disease. All in all, therefore, the disorder is characterized by great complexity in both diagnosis and prognosis.

Incidence and Distribution: Multiple sclerosis is unfortunately not an uncommon disease. Its *incidence* among all other neurological diseases ranges from six to ten per cent, but this is variable. Over a ten-year period of admissions to the neurological service of the Mt. Sinai Hospital in New York, the incidence of multiple sclerosis was 3.9 per cent. In a group of admissions in Philadelphia, its occurrence was found to be seven per cent. The incidence among draftees in World War I in the United States was 7.4 per cent. In England, the incidence was found to be 8.1 per cent (Brain) and in Northern Ireland 7.9 per 10,000 of population (Allison and Millar). The occurrence of the disease varies also in accordance with the geographical distribution. It is more common in Europe than in the United States. In England, it is the most common neurological disease of a nonsyphilitic nature; and on the continent of Europe it is also extremely frequent, especially in France, Germany, Scandinavia, and Austria. One in three to four thousand of the population of Switzerland is a victim of multiple sclerosis, giving an incidence of 360 cases per million of population. In the United States, it seems to be more commonly encountered in some areas than in others, and is distinctly less than in European countries. It is estimated that there are 200,000 people with multiple sclerosis in the United States, but this is an estimate and is probably inaccurate. Other estimates place the incidence at 35 to 64 per 100,000 population (Limburg). Multiple sclerosis is more frequent in colder climates. Statistical studies appear to indicate a greater incidence in the northern or colder parts of the United States (Ulett). No valid seasonal variations have been demonstrated. It has been suggested that the geographical incidence of multiple sclerosis may be related to the amount and nature of fat consumption. People in countries having high incidence of multiple sclerosis consume much fat; those in low incidence areas eat little fat (Swank). The disease seems to be more common among foreign-born than in native-born Americans. It is less frequent among Negroes than in the white population, but it occurs in colored people despite a prevalent impression to the contrary. Its incidence in this group has been estimated at 3.5 per cent.

Etiology: The specific cause of the disease is unknown. So little is known concerning this aspect of it that it is not even clear whether it is caused by an infectious agent or by some other process.

Males appear to be more frequently afflicted than females, but the preponderance in larger series of cases is not striking (fifty-two per cent in males). The *age* of onset is of importance. Most cases appear between nineteen and thirty years of age. This represents an average, however, and cases between forty and fifty are not uncommon. Less than ten per cent of patients with multiple sclerosis develop the disease at the age of forty or over (Müller). In older patients it has been found that the disease frequently is progressive, and that the first attacks occur at shorter intervals than in younger patients. A senile form occurring in the aged is recognized by some investigators. The occurrence of the disease in older subjects should be questioned and accepted with much caution, since multiple sclerosis may be simulated by diffuse processes of other sorts, among them being arteriosclerosis involving the brain and spinal cord. Authentic cases have been recorded, however, in older subjects of fifty or even over sixty.

Precipitating factors of various sorts are not infrequently described. These have been tabulated by von Hoesslin as follows:

	Per Cent
Injury and accident	11.4
Pregnancy and labor	5.8
Febrile diseases	4.2
Overexertion	3.9
Chilling	2.3
Fright and emotion	2.0
Poisoning	0.5

Pregnancy and the puerperium cause aggravation of the disease and each succeeding pregnancy appears to cause greater difficulty. The incidence of aggravation of the condition in pregnancy is high, but not all pregnant subjects suffer; some may come through pregnancy unaffected by the disease. The puerperium is a particularly hazardous time. It was found that 42.3 per cent of patients with known multiple sclerosis had exacerbations in the puerperium (Tillman). Multiple sclerosis may appear for the first time in pregnancy (6.2 per cent).

Infections such as colds, sore throat, and grippe may precede the onset of the disease and may cause aggravation of the symptoms of multiple sclerosis. They may cause a precipitation of symptoms in a latent case or in a patient in remission.

Fatigue and *emotional stress* may cause aggravation of symptoms. It is not uncommon to find that fatigue and general lack of energy for days or weeks may precede the onset of the disease. Loss of weight by dieting may at times precede the onset. *Trauma* may act in a similar fashion, or it may precipitate symptoms in a latent case. *Chilling* tends to precipitate multiple sclerosis, but on the other hand, sun *baths* or baths in hot water tend to produce a transitory increase in weakness in multiple sclerosis patients.

The disease has been described in *children,* but is rare. It is probable that most of the cases described in children are instances of postinfectious encephalitis, though it is undeniable that rare instances are found in children of six to ten years. Authentic examples in children have been confirmed by necropsy at times. About one hundred cases in children were recorded in the medical literature to 1922 (Wechsler). The diagnosis of multiple sclerosis in children is very difficult to establish. Many of those recorded are retrospective statistical diagnoses, symptoms of the disease having been found to be present early in life, in instances of well-established examples of the disease in adults.

The disease bears no relationship to *occupation,* all types and natures of occupations being represented. City dwellers appear to be more commonly afflicted than country folk. Social position also plays no rôle, both rich and poor being equally afflicted. A *familial* incidence has been reported in rare instances, involving two or three members of one family. Familial incidence of multiple sclerosis may not be as rare as it has seemed. Studies indicate that there is a familial vulnerability to multiple sclerosis and that a familial incidence occurs more fre-

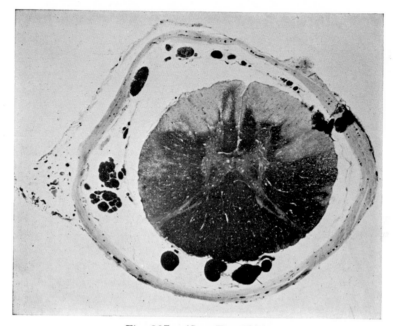

Fig. 207—*(See: Fig. 209.)*

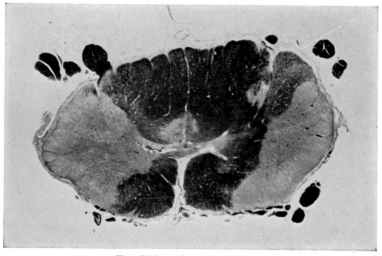

Fig. 208—*(See: Fig. 209.)*

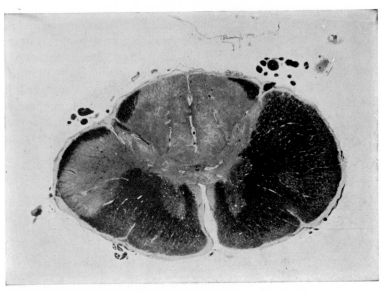

Fig. 209—*Multiple sclerosis.* Plaques of demyelination are seen in the posterior columns, lateral columns, and in the anterior columns of the spinal cord.

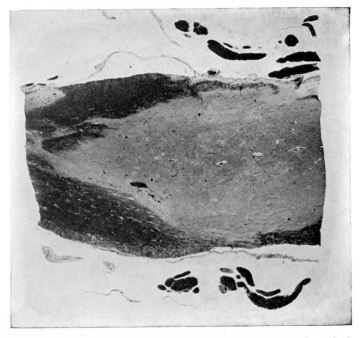

Fig. 210—*Multiple sclerosis.* A longitudinal section of the spinal cord showing an extensive area of demyelination involving almost the entire width of the cord substance.

quently than can be explained by chance. (Mackay). It has been estimated that 6.5 per cent of all cases may be familial. Evidences of degeneration are more frequent in families of patients with multiple sclerosis and include such conditions as deafness, tumor, tremor, stuttering, and psychopathic traits (Curtius). A special form of familial multiple sclerosis has been described, with a clinical picture of Friedreich's ataxia, but with the pathological characteristics of multiple sclerosis (Brommer). In rare instances, multiple sclerosis has been found in twins. Cases of multiple sclerosis occurring in families are rare and many which have been recorded have been confused either with Friedreich's ataxia or with family spastic paraplegia. A few authentic cases with necropsy studies are on record (Speigel and Keschner).

Pathology: Multiple sclerosis may involve any part of the neuraxis — the

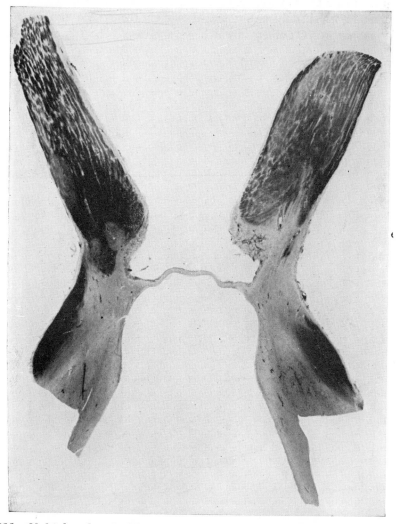

Fig. 211—*Multiple sclerosis.* Myelin sheath stain showing plaques, with demyelination of the optic nerves, chiasm, and optic tracts and great thinning of the optic chiasm. (Courtesy of Dr. Charles Davison.)

brain, brain stem, or spinal cord. It consists essentially of disseminated plaques of degeneration scattered about without logic in many parts of the nervous system. They involve almost exclusively the white matter of the brain and spinal cord, but involvement of the gray matter is not unusual in some areas. The number and distribution of the plaques vary so greatly that it is impossible to predict their location from case to case. It is apparent, therefore, why the symptoms of the disease are so variable. Cases are common in which only a few scattered plaques are present; others in which the entire nervous system is spattered with sclerotic areas; and still others between these two extremes. Moreover, the size of the sclerotic plaques varies greatly also from large to extremely small. Thus in some instances a well-placed large plaque may involve the spinal cord, causing great disability; in others, numerous small plaques may cause relatively little trouble.

Despite the illogical dissemination of lesions in multiple sclerosis certain areas are prone to be affected by the disease, though these need not be involved in every case. The spinal cord is particu-

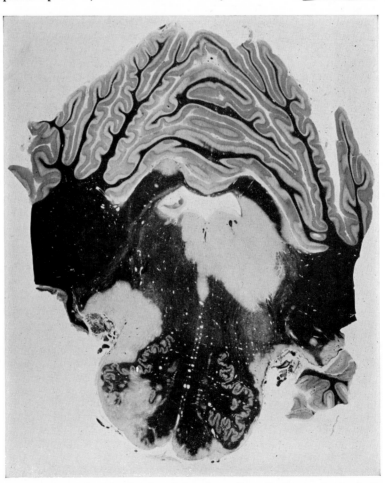

Fig. 212—*Multiple sclerosis,* showing large demyelinated plaques in the brain stem, involving the pyramids, inferior olive, superior and middle cerebellar peduncles, and tegmentum.

larly subject to involvement. The medulla, pons, optic nerves, internal capsule, and cerebrum are often involved. No part of the nervous system, in fact, is apt to escape.

The spinal cord may be involved anywhere along its course, the thoracic and lumbar levels suffering most heavily. The posterior and lateral columns are most commonly affected, but plaques may involve the anterior portion of the cord, or they may be found only in one-half of the cord at a given level. They may involve some pathways at one level and others at another. In some cases, the cord may be completely destroyed at a given segment by a single large plaque or a coalescence of plaques. As in other parts of the nervous system, the spinal cord may contain innumerable plaques or only a few. An occasional plaque may involve the gray matter of the anterior horns or the posterior or anterior roots.

In the medulla, the inferior cerebellar peduncle, the pyramids, and the medial fillet are most often involved; in the pons, the long corticocerebellar or corticospinal fibers; in the mesencephalon, the same fibers are most prone to be involved. Plaques in the cerebrum are found chiefly in the white matter, especially under the ependyma of the lateral ventricle. The cerebellum is not as often affected as its pathways.

The optic nerves, chiasm, or tracts are involved in a large percentage of cases, the nerves being particularly frequently involved.

Microscopic study of the affected areas reveals sharply demarcated areas or plaques devoid of myelin. They are clearly outlined by means of a myelin sheath stain. In areas of long standing, no myelin is seen; in more recent plaques, small balls of myelin are scattered through the degenerated areas. Axis cylinders are still visible in most of the areas, but they are decreased in number and may be almost totally absent in old plaques. Degenerative changes are commonly seen in the axones. Generally speaking, axis cylinders may be seen coursing through plaques of multiple sclerosis in varying numbers, numerous in some cases, moderately numerous in others, and scarce or absent in old plaques. In the older plaques, a heavy carpet of glial fibers is seen and in the more recent areas varying numbers of glial cells and fibers. In some instances, acute plaques are found, characterized by loss of myelin and axis cylinders and by the presence of large numbers of phagocytes and perivascular infiltration with lymphocytes and plasma cells. Changes in the vessels may be seen especially in fresh plaques, but they are demonstrable in chronic plaques as well. The relationship of plaques to blood vessels has been commented on by many observers, since they can often be seen in close proximity to blood vessels. Adventitial proliferation is seen in many vessels. Engorgement, tortuosity, and proliferation of veins in the vicinity of the plaque are commonly seen, according to Putnam. Fibrin clots and leukocytes can be found in veins of varying size and complete occlusion of vessels by fibrous tissue is encountered with considerable frequency (Putnam).

Pathogenesis: The *pathogenesis* of multiple sclerosis is almost as obscure as its cause and many concepts of its development have been proposed. These may be summarized as follows:

Vascular: According to Putnam and his co-workers, the plaques of multiple sclerosis are the result of occlusion of venules in the white matter by thromboses composed of fibrin, platelets, and leukocytes. Areas of destruction similar to those encountered in multiple sclerosis may be produced experimentally by the intravenous injection of tetanus toxin, a suspension of oil, and by carbon monoxide and chronic cyanide poisoning. Such areas are characterized by loss of myelin, relative intactness of the axis cylinders, perivascular infiltration, and gliosis just as those of multiple sclerosis. While obstructed vessels are not demonstrable in every plaque, the finding occurs with great frequency. Patent vessels, further-

induced fever, and other conditions is assumed to be associated with an increased tendency of the blood to clot in the cerebral venules under these conditions.

Further evidence that there may be a vascular component in multiple sclerosis is supplied by observed spasm of the retinal artery in cases of scotoma associated with the disease, sheathing of the

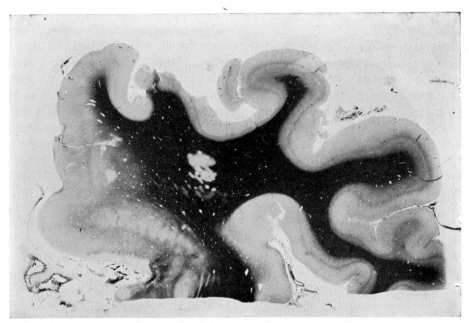

Fig. 213—*Multiple sclerosis.* A section of cerebral cortex showing a collection of small demyelinated plaques in the white matter.

more, are found in plaques which contain obstructed venules. Thrombi in venules and veins have been found in multiple sclerosis (Putnam). Their prevalence is not a matter of agreement; some deny their occurrence or assert that they are incidental to the disease. The concept of the production of plaques by thromboses is supported further by evidence of increased coagulability of the blood, and by a high blood fibrinogen in most cases of multiple sclerosis. The exacerbation of symptoms in multiple sclerosis during pregnancy, infections, trauma, artificially

retinal veins and increased capillary fragility. Clumping of red blood cells with sludging has been observed. Capillary resistance appears to be greater in multiple sclerosis patients than in normals.

Allergy: Owing to the production of areas of demyelination resembling multiple sclerosis by the injection of brain extract and other means, the view has arisen that multiple sclerosis may represent an allergic reaction in the brain and spinal cord. Demyelination, interpreted as encephalomyelitis or multiple sclerosis, has been observed after the administration of serum and vaccines, in the treatment of rabies, and after intramuscular injections of alcohol-ether extracts of normal rabbit brain. Repeated parenteral injections of heterologous emulsified brain tissue or extracts can produce demyelinating lesions in monkeys similar to multiple sclerosis. Homologous brain tissue in rabbits and monkeys produces demyelinizing lesions.

There are many points of similarity between the lesions of acute multiple sclerosis and those of allergic or anaphylactic reactions in the brain. These include the following: (1) the tendency in both instances for the demyelination to be found around the blood vessels, (2) the occurrence of hemorrhages in both conditions, (3) the presence of degenerative changes in the blood vessels in both conditions, (4) the disclosure of thrombus formation in both multiple sclerosis and brain anaphylaxis, and (5) the predominantly perivenous infiltration in the two processes. In all instances, many injections of emulsions of rabbit brain or other brain extracts were necessary, and a time interval of three to thirteen months was required for the appearance of symptoms. The response to the injected material probably involves an immunological response to the injected brain material. Adjuncts of various sorts have been added to the brain material with resulting response of the nervous system to injections. Because of this, it seems probable that an antigen-antibody reaction is involved in the formation of the lesions.

In humans there has been recorded a high incidence of allergic histories or of positive skin tests in patients with multiple sclerosis. No known instances of onset or exacerbation of multiple sclerosis has been known to follow contact with a substance, such as food, to which the patient has been known to be sensitive.

Virus: The resemblance of cases of acute disseminated encephalomyelitis to cases of acute multiple sclerosis has led some investigators to assume that the latter is due to a virus or to some infectious agent. This viewpoint assumes that encephalomyelitis disseminata is a distinct entity and that it differs from acute multiple sclerosis. There is good evidence to support the view that the two conditions are the same. Histologically, a distinction between the two conditions is impossible in the acute stages. While the eventual outcome of the acute areas of demyelination in disseminated encephalomyelitis is not universally agreed upon, a few observations point to the development of typical glial scars similar to those of multiple sclerosis. No infectious agent has ever been isolated in multiple sclerosis.

Ferment: The concept that multiple sclerosis is the result of a lipase ferment circulating in the blood is attractive but has little to support it. An increase in blood cholesterol has been found in some cases of multiple sclerosis and a great variability in others. Serum esterases are low in the active stages of the disease and high in the inactive phases.

Spirochete: Multiple sclerosis has been attributed to the action of a spirochete which has been demonstrated by Steiner, but the findings have been confirmed by no other investigators.

Toxic and Miscellaneous Factors: *Toxic* factors of many sorts have been implicated, but no clearcut evidence is available. Excessive amounts of lead have been found in the spinal fluid, brain, spinal cord, and bones of rare cases of multiple sclerosis, but lead poisoning cannot be demonstrated in most cases. The deficiency of *copper* and *molybdenum* in the soil in the geographic distribution of multiple sclerosis has been suggested. A *basal metabolic defect* has been proposed. Abnormal plasma proteins have been found during exacerbations of the disease, with return to normal during remission. *Brucellosis* has been connected with multiple sclerosis on the basis of positive skin tests in multiple sclerosis patients, but additional studies have failed to show a relationship between the two disorders. *Biochemical studies* reveal that in multiple sclerosis there is an abnormal response to oral glucose, with an elevation of pyruvic acid out of proportion to lactic acid. The fasting level of pyruvic acid is high in patients in relapse. Serum cholesterol is elevated; serum inorganic phosphorus is lower; inorganic phosphorus excretion is increased and uric acid/creatinine excretion is lower in patients in relapse·

II. SYMPTOMS

The clinical features of multiple sclerosis vary so widely that a description of a typical form of the disease would fail to include many variants which are equally characteristic. It is possible in a general sense to speak of predominant *types* of the disorder. While this is true, it must be remembered that in a disease such as multiple sclerosis, which affects so diffusely the central nervous system, types or forms of the disorder have only a relative meaning and refer really to predominant involvement of specific areas. These may be grouped as follows: (1) The classical form of Charcot, characterized by intentional tremor, slurring speech, and nystagmus. This is found in about ten per cent of cases and often appears late. Its place in the disease is discussed under diagnosis. (2) Spinal forms or predominantly spinal forms are very common. In such instances, the spinal cord is either predominantly or almost exclusively affected. Tabetic, spastic, and complete transverse myelitic varieties are encountered. (3) Bulbar varieties are less frequent, but

are common and are characterized by involvement predominantly of the brain stem (medulla, pons, midbrain). (4) Cerebellar forms are common, with almost exclusive involvement of the cerebellum or its pathways. (5) Cerebral forms with predominant implication of the cerebral hemispheres are encountered as well.

The *onset* of symptoms is usually slow and gradual, but in some forms is acute and apoplectiform. The specific complaints at the time of onset vary with the area affected. The duration of symptoms varies as greatly as the onset and is often inaccurate. Distinction must be drawn clearly between the immediate symptoms, which may extend back for a few weeks to a few years, and those which have developed in the dim past and have been completely forgotten. It is the latter, the transient symptoms, which assume great significance in the diagnosis of the disorder. Of the immediate symptoms, history of gradual loss of power of the legs is common; or there may be a gradual disturbance of coördination which is noticed as difficulty in maintaining equilibrium in walking or as numbness or clumsiness in the use of one or both arms. Among the transient symptoms encountered in a significantly large group, gradual loss of vision may be noted, or weakness or numbness in a single limb, difficulty in finding words, diplopia, or vertigo. Often such symptoms have been encountered during the life cycle of the patient, have disappeared after a varying length of time, and have been forgotten in the past history unless they are specifically sought after. Transient first symptoms of the type described were found in thirty-two of fifty-two patients having multiple sclerosis (Brown).

An acute or even explosive onset is not uncommon in some cases, and may simulate closely a febrile illness, even to the occurrence of fever. Such cases may develop with a single symptom, such as loss of vision, vertigo, or loss of speech; or they may develop with a variety of manifestations indicating a widespread involvement of the nervous system —

weakness, incoördination, tremor, numbness, visual disturbances, and other signs.

The symptoms, chronic or acute, may have been present for a variable length of time before help is sought. As a rule, they have persisted for months or years,

Table 59—Total Number of Cases Studied 141 (Male Cases 77, Female 64)
Symptoms and Signs Enumerated in the Order of the Frequency
of Their Occurrence in Multiple Sclerosis
(Sachs & Friedman) *

	Cases	Per cent
1. Abdominal wall reflexes were markedly diminished or absent in	118	83.7
2. The chief complaint was weakness and stiffness of one or both lower extremities	115	81.7
3. Nystagmus was present in	99	70.0
It was chiefly horizontal.		
Horizontal and vertical in	17	12.0
Horizontal and rotary in	3	2.0
4. Babinski's sign was present bilaterally in	94	67.0
Unilaterally in	16	11.3
5. Tremor was present in the extremities alone in	78	55.3
There was also tremor of the head in	31	22.0
6. Ataxia and adiadokokinesis were present in	66	47.0
7. Deep reflexes in the lower extremities were increased in	126	90.0
Ankle clonus was present in	61	43.0
Patellar clonus was present in	29	20.5
In 3 instances the knee jerks were diminished (tabetic type).		
8. There was a history of 1 or more remissions in	59	42.0
9. There were bladder symptoms in	57	40.0
Urgency was present in	18	12.6
Delay in starting urinary stream alone or in combination with urgency in 28 cases and incontinence in 21 cases.		
10. Speech was hesitant or otherwise disturbed in	51	36.0
11. The gait was spastic in	43	30.0
Spastic ataxic in	46	32.6
Ataxic alone in	15	10.6
12. There was evidence of facial weakness in	46	32.6
The other cranial nerves were very much less involved.		
The tongue deviated to the right in	14	10.0
There was difficulty in swallowing in	5	3.5
Uvula was drawn to one side in	4	2.8
The cochlear nerve was involved in	3	2.0
The vestibular nerve showed no response to stimulation in	2	1.4
Of the ocular muscles the internal rectus was involved in	6	4.3
There was ptosis in	2	1.4
The external rectus was involved in	3	2.8
13. Temporal atrophy was noted in	46	32.6
There was blurring of the disks or mild optic neuritis in	11	7.8
Vision was impaired without objective disk findings in	25	17.7

*From "General Symptomatology and Differential Diagnosis of Disseminated Sclerosis" by B. Sachs and E. Friedman. In: Multiple Sclerosis, Publication of the Association for Research in Nervous and Mental Disease, Paul B. Hoeber, Inc., Publishers.

	Cases	Per Cent
14. Pain, numbness and tingling were noted in.............................	43	30.0
Objective disturbances in posterior column sensation were present in.......	24	17.0
Mild changes in pain, temperature and touch perception were noted in.....	23	16.3
(Among these were cases with hyperalgesic zones.)		
Astereognosis was noted in....................................	5	3.5
15. There was a history of diplopia in..........................	31	29.0
16. Cremasteric reflexes were diminished in..........................	17	22.0
(Of the male cases.)		
17. Mental changes were noted in......................................	22	15.8
They were largely those of mental infantilism and signs of neurosis or neurasthenia. One patient was in a state hospital with the diagnosis of dementia praecox. One patient showed the picture of Korsakoff's psychosis.		
18. Emotional instability with explosive laughter occurred in.................	24	17.0
Defects of memory occurred in......................................	7	5.0
19. Spinal tenderness was present in.....................................	17	12.0
It was chiefly middorsal.		
20. There was a history of trauma in....................................	14	10.0
21. Pupillary disturbances were noted rarely.		
Pupils were irregular in...	6	4.3
They were slightly sluggish to light in..............................	12	8.5
Anisocoria was present in...	16	11.3
22. There was a history of marked dizziness in...........................	12	8.5
23. Disturbances of potency were noted in...............................	6	4.3
No disturbances in rectal control were seen in any of our cases.		

with intervals of freedom from symptoms or *remissions*. Such remissions are an important feature of the disease and are characteristic of multiple sclerosis. They occur in many but not in all cases. No good statistical studies are available of the percentage of remissions. Complete remissions were found in seventeen per cent of 516 cases (von Hoesslin). The remission of individual symptoms, however, is undoubtedly more frequent. Instances of multiple sclerosis without remissions are not uncommon. Two main types of the disease are recognized by some: the remittent and chronic progressive forms. The remittent form of the disease is more common and occurs six times as frequently as the chronic progressive form (Birley and Dudgeon). Instances of the disease with a steadily chronic progressive course are not uncommon and develop without a history of remissions. This uncontestable fact is

common experience in multiple sclerosis.

The remission of symptoms may be complete, with total freedom from symptoms of any sort, and may last for years; or it may result only in an incomplete remission of symptoms without total disappearance at any time. Single symptoms, such as diplopia, central scotoma, numbness of an extremity, tend to regress within a few months; whereas symptoms due to larger lesions, such as paraplegia, ataxia, and mental deterioration, tend to be permanent. Isolated symptoms tend to disappear in a far higher proportion of cases than do the same symptoms occurring in conjunction with others. First symptoms have a higher rate of recovery than the same symptoms occurring later in the disease (Brown and Putnam). Remissions of twenty-seven and thirty-nine years are known to the author. In the former instance, transient weakness of the left leg of one week's duration was followed by fully developed signs of multiple sclerosis twenty-seven years later. In the latter case, transient blindness of one eye was followed thirty-nine years later by unquestionable signs of multiple sclerosis. Both patients had been free of signs in the interim.

Examination of patients with multiple sclerosis reveals a variety of findings. General physical examination and routine laboratory studies of the blood, urine, etc., are without findings of any significance.

The diversity of the signs encountered in multiple sclerosis is demonstrated by Table 59, which shows also the difficulty of enumerating combinations of symptoms in the disease. The number of possible combinations is great.

Optic atrophy is a common finding and occurs early in the disease. It is found in a large percentage of multiple sclerosis patients. It is seen as a pallor of the temporal halves of the optic nerve heads, as a rule, but it may also be revealed as a complete optic atrophy, either primary or secondary. The temporal pallor, so-called, is often but not always associated with a central or paracentral scotoma. The incidence of atrophy of the temporal sides of the optic discs varies greatly in the many studies which have been made of multiple sclerosis. It has been found in 32.6 per cent (Sachs and Friedman); in thirty-two per cent (Obständer); in fifty per cent (Young); and in seventy-five per cent (Bonadurer). The probabilities are that temporal atrophy of the optic nerve occurs in close to thirty to thirty-five per cent of cases and may approach slightly higher figures. It has been found to be an early symptom in one-third of the cases of multiple sclerosis (Behr).

In a number of instances there is either a history of *retrobulbar neuritis*, or the patient may first present himself with this symptom as the earliest manifestation of the disease. The typical features of loss of or greatly reduced visual acuity, normal appearing optic nerves, and central or paracentral scotoma are present. The problem of retrobulbar neuritis in multiple sclerosis is one of great importance in the recognition of the disease. Attention has been called to the fact that of the many causes of retrobulbar neuritis, multiple sclerosis appears to take the leading rôle (Benedict). Among 223 cases of retrobulbar neuritis, fifty-one were due to multiple sclerosis (Gunn), while in another series of 176 cases multiple sclerosis was found to be the cause of the retrobulbar neuritis in seventy-five per cent of the patients and in still another the incidence was found to be fifty-five per cent (Marburg). Retrobulbar neuritis is not infrequently an early symptom or the first symptom of multiple sclerosis and the time interval between the occurrence of this symptom and the development of other features of multiple sclerosis may vary from a few days or weeks to ten or twenty years. Long intervals between the retrobulbar neuritis and other signs are not infrequent. The interval between the initial ocular symptoms of multiple sclerosis and other evidences of the disease may vary from less than one year to fourteen years (Yaskin). Patients between twenty and forty-four years of age who develop an episode of retrobulbar neuritis have a forty to fifty per cent chance of developing multiple sclerosis within ten to fifteen years (Taub and Rucker).

Spasm of the retinal arteries has been observed in patients with multiple sclerosis (Brickner) and sheathing and constriction of the retinal vessels have likewise been observed. Perivenous sheathing was found around the retinal vessels in ten (nineteen per cent) of fifty-two patients with multiple sclerosis (Truesch and Rucker). It was not related to a history of blurring of vision or the presence of temporal pallor of the optic nerves.

Choked disc is a rare finding, but that it may be found in multiple sclerosis is attested by the experience of many investigators. It is not, as a rule, of a high degree, usually measuring one to two diopters.

Homonymous hemianopsia is a rare symptom, but it has been reported in a number of instances, and in three cases with foci in the lateral geniculate body (Hermann). Its occurrence in multiple sclerosis has been denied by others. The *pupils* in multiple sclerosis are in the majority of cases normal, but in rare cases Argyll Robertson pupils have been described. Unequal, irregular, and sluggishly reacting pupils may be encountered.

The auditory nerve may be involved in multiple sclerosis, forty-three per cent of patients having been found with a measurable degree of deafness (Van Leden and Horton).

Oculomotor paralyses are sometimes encountered, usually as a weakness of a single ocular muscle, but sometimes as an extensive ophthalmoplegia. The incidence of oculomotor paralysis in multiple sclerosis has been variously computed. It has been found in twenty-five per cent (Berger); seventy per cent (Windmüller); twenty-nine per cent (Sachs and Friedman); forty per cent (Adie); and fifty per cent (Marburg). Diplopia is not uncommonly an early symptom and may be an isolated one. It may be lost in the dim past, and like retrobulbar neuritis, may have been forgotten by the patient. It should always be inquired after specifically in obtaining a history of the disease. The abducens nerve is most frequently affected, but isolated muscle involvement due to oculomotor nerve disease is not uncommon.

Trigeminal pain is occasionally encountered with characteristics typical of trigeminal neuralgia. Paresthesias along one or more divisions of the trigeminal nerve are also encountered.

Facial weakness is not uncommon. It is usually of a central type, but may at times be typically peripheral. It may be found alone or in association with hemiplegia. Peripheral facial paralysis may be an early symptom of multiple sclerosis.

Vertigo is a not uncommon feature of multiple sclerosis. In not a few cases it is a first symptom which may persist for a time and recur without other evidences of the disease. Vertigo has been found by many investigators to be an early or first symptom in multiple sclerosis (Berger, thirty per cent; Barre and Reys, fifty-six per cent; Charcot, seventy-five per cent). The vertigo is often of a typical vestibular type, characterized by recurrent episodes of dizziness: in other cases, it is more constant and simulates the central variety of vertigo. It is usually found with other evidences of multiple sclerosis, but may at times be found alone. In other instances, it is found with other well-marked evidences of the disorder.

Nystagmus is regarded as a characteristic feature of multiple sclerosis and has been described as one of its cardinal symptoms. It is found in seventy per cent of cases of multiple sclerosis (Sachs and Friedman). It is not present in every instance and may often develop late in the course of the illness. It is usually seen as a horizontal nystagmus which may be present on deviation of the eyes to one side and not to the other, or it may be found bilaterally. Vertical nystagmus is found alone in some instances, without horizontal nystagmus. True vertical nystagmus is probably most often due to multiple sclerosis. *Difficulty in swallowing, hoarseness* and *respiratory* difficulties, and paralysis of the *tongue* are rarely encountered.

Speech disturbances are common and are found in eleven to thirty-six per cent of patients. They may develop early in the disease or may not make their appearance until later. The speech is at first slightly slurred and indistinct, with occasional tripping over a syllable or word; later it becomes slowed and clearly indistinct, with frequent difficulties in enunciation. In advanced cases, the speech is completely dysarthric and may be difficult to comprehend. The speech difficulties are probably the result of cerebellar disturbances. *Aphasia* may be found in some cases.

Tremor has long been recognized as a special feature of the disorder, but it may not be found until long after the disease has developed. On the other hand, it may in some cases develop early. Its incidence varies (Sachs and Friedman, 55.3 per cent; Birley and Dudgeon, 42.6 per cent). It is usually referred to as an intention tremor and is characterized by appearance on movement, as, for example, in bringing the finger to the nose. It is usually not present at rest, is coarse (three or four per second), and may involve not only the arms but the legs as well. It may in some instances, however, be found even with the limb at rest. Like other tremors, it is aggravated by fatigue, exercise, emotions, etc. The intention tremor of multiple sclerosis has been described as one of the cardinal features of the disease, but it must be emphasized that the disease may run its course without the development of tremor and that the tremor may and often does develop late.

Motor disturbances are among the most common manifestations of multiple sclerosis. Weakness and stiffness were found in one or both lower extremities in 81.7 per cent of patients (Sachs and Friedman); motor disturbances were found in fifty-seven per cent (Obständer); thirty per cent (Adie); and in fifty-six of 152 subjects, 27.1 per cent (Marburg). The lower extremities are much more commonly affected than the arms. Paraplegia involving the legs is the most frequent motor symptom. It is often the earliest manifestation of the disease, with all the features of spastic weakness which may be at first slight and later pronounced, or which may be severe from the onset. Paraplegia in flexion is seen rarely. Hemiplegia may develop during the course of the disease, as well as monoplegias, involving arm or leg. Muscle atrophy due to a patch of sclerosis on one or more anterior horns is at times encountered but is rare. In rare instances, this may be symmetrical and give rise to signs resembling amyotrophic lateral sclerosis. Atrophy in multiple sclerosis is never widespread. In rare instances, weakness involving one or more peripheral nerve distributions may be encountered.

Convulsions are an infrequent accompaniment of multiple sclerosis. Epileptic attacks were found in thirteen out of 268 multiple sclerosis subjects (Bau-Prussak and Prussak). They may be of various types: generalized convulsions, jacksonian seizures, petit mal, epilepsia partialis continua, and psychic attacks. They may be the first symptom of the disease, other manifestations of multiple sclerosis not appearing for several years (ten to twenty-five) after the epileptic attack. In other instances, they may appear during the full expression of the disease.

Sensory disturbances in some form are an almost invariable accompaniment of the disease. Ataxia due to involvement of the posterior columns may involve both the arms and legs but is most common in the legs. There may be loss of both position and vibration senses, or a loss of vibration sense or of position sense alone. A single limb may at times be affected. Loss of vibration sense in the feet and legs is sometimes an early feature of the disease. Pain and temperature sensations may be lost or decreased either in segmental distribution due to a patch of sclerosis in the commissural gray matter of the cord, or it may be lost on one side of the body due to involvement of the anterolateral column in the spinal cord. Transverse syndromes with complete motor and sensory paralysis are also well known.

Cerebellar symptoms characterized by dyssynergia of the affected limbs, due to involvement of the spinocerebellar tracts in the cord, the cerebellar peduncles in the brain stem or the cerebellum are common. Pure cerebellar forms are not uncommonly seen.

Loss of the abdominal reflexes is frequently present but is not invariable. Instances are found in which the abdominal reflexes remain intact. Their loss comes early in the disease and in a young person with good abdominal muscles in whom multiple sclerosis is suspected, loss of the abdominal reflexes assumes great significance. They are lost in a high percentage of cases (83.7 per cent, Sachs and Friedman; seventy-seven per cent, Birley and Dudgeon). The abdominal reflexes are often lost early in the disease and may constitute one of the earliest findings. The cremasteric reflexes are usually lost and the plantar reflexes may also be absent. The tendon reflexes are usually overactive.

Emotional disturbances of some sort are usually present. Lability of emotional responses, with inability or decreased ability to inhibit emotional reactions, is probably the most common

manifestation. These affective disorders are part and parcel of the disease, are very frequent, and in a fair number of instances they precede the neurological signs. A sense of well-being is found in eighty-four per cent of patients (Wilson and Cottrell). Excessively easy laughing or crying is frequent. Euphoria, a sense of well-being despite obvious disabilities, and an unhealthy cheerfulness characterize many patients. Depressions of a mild degree are also found. Psychoses may develop during the course of the disease but are not common. Evidences of organic deterioration with memory loss and personality change are encountered in those patients with predominant involvement of the cerebrum.

Pain is uncommon in multiple sclerosis, but it may occur. Trigeminal pain or typical root pain may appear during the course of the disease. Trigeminal pain similar in all respects to trigeminal neuralgia may be one of the first symptoms. Paresthesias are common.

Bladder disturbances of one sort or another are frequently found. Urgency, delay in starting the stream of urine, and incontinence may develop during the course of the disease. Langworthy has found an incidence of urinary disturbance in sixty-two per cent of early cases of multiple sclerosis, the symptoms in order of occurrence being urgency, hesitancy, incontinence, frequency, dribbling, and acute retention. In a very small group of patients, disturbance of *potency* is encountered.

In very rare instances, *trophic ulcers* of the skin may develop. *Oscillopsia*, or the seeming movement of objects, has been described. At times the presence of *Lhermitte's sign* may be detected. This consists of a sensation of electricity radiating down the spine and/or limbs on active or passive flexion of the head. At times the sensation may radiate into the legs. The Lhermitte sign has been described in multiple sclerosis, Pott's disease, cervical tumor, head injury and cervical cord trauma. It has been induced by flexion of the head, bilateral jugular pressure and tapping of the cervical vertebrae. Among the less frequent manifestations associated with multiple sclerosis are paralysis agitans and muscle atrophies.

The *spinal fluid* in multiple sclerosis shows no pathogomonic changes. There is some abnormality in cell count, total protein, and/or colloidal gold in seventy-eight per cent of cases. There may be a moderate increase in cells in about twenty-five per cent of cases, usually under thirty cells per cu. mm. The protein may be increased. The colloidal gold curve is abnormal in seventy-one per cent of cases (Fremont-Smith and Merritt), showing a first zone (paretic) curve in twenty-five per cent, a midzone curve in twenty-two per cent, and a slight abnormality in twenty-four per cent.

The gamma globulin of the spinal fluid is elevated in eighty-five per cent of patients with multiple sclerosis and in ninety-five per cent the albumin content is normal. There is a high thymol turbidity reaction in the serum of multiple sclerosis patients.

The EEG has been found to be abnormal in forty-four to sixty-two per cent of patients, with no specific pattern discernible.

III. DIAGNOSIS

The diagnosis of multiple sclerosis presents many difficulties. In advanced cases recognition of the disease is easy, but early instances are more difficult to detect and sometimes hard to establish definitely, until further evidences of the disease are apparent. Early diagnosis is desirable in order to provide what relief may be expected from purely symptomatic treatment. Because of the disseminated nature of the disease, no permanent constellation of symptoms is found. Variety and variability are probably the outstanding features of multiple sclerosis.

Fundamentally, the recognition of multiple sclerosis depends upon the demonstration of involvement of multiple systems in the brain and spinal cord, due to disseminated lesions, sometimes numerous, sometimes few, ordinarily with a chronic background of symptoms, but sometimes with an acute story, and often with a history of remissions. The demonstration of disseminated lesions may be proved in one of two fashions: (1) By examination alone. The occurrence of lesions involving the optic nerves, the brain stem, cerebrum, and spinal cord in a single patient constitutes good proof of a disseminated process. The lesions may not always be numerous but they are disseminated. Optic atrophy, slurred speech, spastic paraplegia, or pallor of the temporal sides of the discs, absent abdominal reflexes, and spastic ataxic weakness are examples of some of the possible combinations. (2) By history and examination. The diagnosis of dissemination is not infrequently made on this basis, as, for example, in a patient with only spinal cord signs, such as posterolateral sclerosis, but with a history of previous episodes of numbness, transient blindness, or weakness. Having established the fact that the lesion is disseminated, the problem is then one of proving that the process is the result of multiple sclerosis. Here the age incidence of the disease and the tendency to remissions help in the diagnosis.

IV. TYPES

The demonstration of strict *types* is, of course, impossible in a disease so characteristically disseminated, but broad general categories may be designated.

In the *chronic remittent* form of the disease, there is ordinarily an account of waxing and waning of symptoms over a long period with remissions which are more or less complete but which are not invariably present. The development and recession of symptoms during the natural history of the illness may not be striking and must often be sought for in a careful survey of symptoms. With this background, the diagnosis is fortified by the disclosure of involvement of a multiplicity of areas in the nervous system—optic nerves, pyramidal tracts, posterior columns, etc., and upon the demonstration of such dissemination depends to a large extent the eventual diagnosis. Patients in this category may demonstrate spastic paraplegia, with involvement of posterior columns, optic atrophy, etc., or they may show primarily cerebellar involvement with slight involvement of other areas. There may be only mild evidences of disease of some systems, but the slightest indication of involvement of multiple systems is of importance. So great is the variety of possibilities that no detailed portrayal is possible.

Acute forms of multiple sclerosis are common. The onset, if sudden, often resembles a febrile disorder and is featured by loss of vision, hemiplegia, paraplegia, or other signs. No account of previous attacks is obtainable in such instances. Loss of vision due to a retrobulbar neuritis is relatively frequent and may be associated with slight indications of involvement of other parts—loss of abdominal reflexes, loss of vibration sense in the legs, hyperreflexia, an isolated Babinski sign, or other indications of disease of the nervous pathways. Frequently retrobulbar neuritis without assignable cause is the forerunner of multiple sclerosis, other evidences of the disease appearing months or years after the initial attack, which may be forgotten by the patient. In a small group of

patients, vertigo may be an isolated symptom which may be repeated before other evidences of the disease are disclosed.

Not a few cases of multiple sclerosis are characterized by a *chronic progressive* course without a history of remissions. Some of these may progress for some time with only spastic paraplegia, or cerebellar signs, and without indications of disseminated lesions. During their course, however, such evidences develop, making the nature of the illness clear.

Fatal attacks of multiple sclerosis may occur and are characterized by the rapid development of quadriplegia or bulbar symptoms, particularly disturbances in breathing (Cheyne-Stokes respiration or dyspnea) and swallowing. Severe respiratory failure may develop. The episodes occur usually in patients with well-established evidence of multiple sclerosis, but in rare instances the first episode of multiple sclerosis may prove to be fatal. The early use of a respirator may help avert a fatal outcome.

V. DIFFERENTIAL DIAGNOSIS

Because of its tendency to wide dissemination of symptoms, multiple sclerosis must be distinguished from a large variety of disorders. Among these are the following: There are many who regard *disseminated encephalomyelitis* and acute multiple sclerosis as identical, but the problem is still undecided (*v.* Encephalitis). Disseminated encephalomyelitis is acute, often abrupt in onset, with fever, weakness, or paralysis of the legs or of all the limbs, at times with hemiplegia, and with brain stem signs, such as cranial nerve palsies of various sorts (oculomotor paralyses, difficulty in swallowing, etc.). There is usually no history of antecedent symptoms or of remissions.

The dissemination of lesions responsible for scattered signs resembles closely multiple sclerosis. The febrile onset and the abrupt development differ from that of the usual case of multiple sclerosis.

It is doubtful whether *neuromyelitis optica* is a separate disease entity. Studies of the subsequent course of cases so diagnosed reveal characteristics of multiple sclerosis, such as the development of further symptoms and the involvement of other parts of the nervous system (Forster and Putnam). Blindness preceded or followed by a transverse myelitis are the outstanding features of this disorder. Remissions occur and the outcome may be fatal or may end in complete recovery.

Spinal cord tumor is sometimes confused with multiple sclerosis in those patients with the latter disease who develop a transverse spinal cord syndrome. The absence of subarachnoid block, the absence of increased protein in the spinal fluid, the absence of a history of pain, the presence of a story of previous symptoms with remissions, usually but not always in multiple sclerosis simulating a spinal cord tumor, the presence of other signs, such as temporal pallor of the discs, etc., suffice to differentiate the average case. The story of a progressive disability suggesting a tumor is helpful, but it is not always reliable, since it is precisely those cases of multiple sclerosis with a progressive history which give difficulties in diagnosis. A history of remission of the symptoms of the transverse lesion, such as the motor paralysis, tends to confirm a diagnosis of multiple sclerosis, but rare cases of tumor may be associated with such a history.

Subacute combined degeneration is usually easily distinguished by the clinical evidences of pernicious anemia, achlorhydria, and the characteristic blood findings. In patients without typical blood findings, the presence of achlorhydria and the clinical signs of anemia must suffice. The diagnosis may be confused by the tendency of subacute combined degeneration to be associated with optic atrophy, but in such instances the signs of pernicious anemia are well pronounced.

Meningovascular syphilis involving both brain and spinal cord may simulate multiple sclerosis closely, but is easily distinguished as a rule by the positive Wassermann reaction of blood and spinal fluid, and by other abnormalities of the spinal fluid.

Brain tumor requires differentiation in those patients with predominantly cortical symptoms, such as convulsions, mental and emotional disturbances. The absence of signs of increased intracranial pressure in multiple sclerosis makes the distinction not difficult, but is complicated by the occurrence rarely in multiple sclerosis of choked disc. Evidence of multiple foci and a history of remissions are very helpful. In some instances, multiple sclerosis must be distinguished from a tumor in the suprasellar area, but the occurrence of typical bitemporal hemianopsia associated usually with changes in the sella on roentgenologic examination is helpful. In some instances, suprasellar tumors may be associated with scotomas and optic atrophy, making the possibility of multiple sclerosis likely in some cases. Very difficult to differentiate may be a *pontile glioma* which develops slowly, involves cranial nerves, and usually pyramidal and cerebellar pathways and may even be associated with remissions. Tumors of this region usually occur in the young, are steadily progressive, and are usually but not always associated with signs of increased pressure.

Table 60—Differential Diagnosis of Multiple Sclerosis

Disseminated Encephalo-myelitis	Neuromyelitis Optica	Spinal Cord Tumor (Extramedullary)	Subacute Combined Degeneration	Meningo-Vascular Syphilis	Brain Tumor	Cerebellar Disease	Cerebral Arteriolo-sclerosis	Encephalitis
Onset acute, febrile	Onset acute	Onset gradual	Onset gradual	Readily differentiated on basis of blood and spinal fluid reactions	Onset gradual	Onset gradual or acute, depending on cause	Onset gradual	Onset acute, febrile
Paralyses: Cranial nerve palsies	Any age affected	Pain early and important feature	Paresthesias of hands and feet		Progressive history		Arteriosclerosis present in retina and in peripheral vessels	Evidence of encephalitis in community as rule
	Blindness, preceded or followed by transverse myelitis	Transverse cord syndrome	Signs confined to cord. No cranial nerve or brain stem involvement		Headache prominent	Degenerative or maldevelopmental types excluded by early age of onset and obviously congenital features		Specific type of encephalitis established by clinical and laboratory studies
No remissions	No remissions	Subarachnoid block present			Increased pressure (choked disc, high SF pressure)		Gradual mental deterioration	
Recovery: Incomplete but may be total	Recovery may follow	Proteins of spinal fluid elevated	No remissions				No remissions	
		No remissions	Clinical features of pernicious anemia		*Pontile Glioma:* Seen chiefly in young subjects. Slowly progressive course, often with nochoked disc or late in disease	Vascular type excluded by age of onset, evidence of arteriosclerosis	No evidence of disseminated cord lesions as rule and no cranial nerve or brain stem features	
			Blood picture usually but not always typical			Tumor excluded by signs of increased pressure		
			Achlorhydria present					

Cerebellar disease, such as tumor or softening, may be confused with those cases which are of a purely cerebellar type. The distinction is not difficult from tumor, due largely to the absence of signs of increased pressure. Softening may be more difficult to distinguish, but the presence of such features as generally overactive reflexes, absence of abdominal reflexes, and temporal pallor is helpful.

Cerebral arteriosclerosis may cause difficulty in older patients but may be distinguished by the demonstration of retinal arteriosclerosis, by the age of onset of the disease, and by the evidences of sclerosis of the peripheral vessels.

Encephalitis may be confused with cases which affect predominantly the brain stem. The febrile acute onset, the absence of a history of previous symptoms, the typical somnolence and rapid course of encephalitis, and the increase of lymphocytes in the spinal fluid in the acute stages of the disease are important distinguishing features. The history, furthermore, of sporadic cases of encephalitis in the community or of an epidemic is very helpful in diagnosis.

Hysteria is sometimes confused with multiple sclerosis in those instances in which there is a history of symptoms that have appeared and disappeared on many occasions, leaving no residual symptoms. The distinction may be impossible in some instances unless some residual sign or signs have persisted following one of the episodes. The diagnosis of multiple sclerosis as opposed to hysteria may be considered if (1) residual signs of central nervous system involvement are demonstrable, such as temporal pallor of the optic nerve, a Babinski sign, or impairment of position sense; or (2) there is no correlation between a presumed hysterical reaction and the personality adjustments of the patient.

VI. COURSE AND PROGNOSIS

The *course* of the symptoms in multiple sclerosis varies almost as much as the symptoms themselves. The disease need not become disabling and long survival is relatively frequent. The outlook for patients with multiple sclerosis is not as gloomy as it seems. The 10 year survival of a group of 418 subjects was seventy-nine per cent, as compared with eighty-five per cent in the normal population; the five year survival was ninety-three per cent as compared with ninety-five per cent for the normal population. Patients who are incapacitated when first seen appear to have a less malignant form of the disease and at the end of five and ten year periods a significant number (fifty-six per cent) are able to walk and work (MacLean and Berkson). Study of a group of patients after twenty years revealed seventy per cent had survived. Among the survivors the longest duration of illness was thirty-nine years and the average 27.8 years. It was found that a severe initial lesion was not incompatible with long survival (Allison).

Repeated attacks of symptoms at varying intervals may be followed by complete or almost complete recovery with each episode and may be associated with few or no residuals. Instances of this type are not infrequent. On the other hand, disabling symptoms (paralysis, blindness) may develop early in the disease, soon after initial symptoms, or not until many years have elapsed. Fatal forms of the disease are known to occur. Rarely, recovery seems to be permanent (Bramwell, McIntyre and McIntyre). As a rule, some scars are left after repeated attacks. Single symptoms, such as diplopia, retrobulbar neuritis, and vertigo are more favorable than combinations of symptoms. Spastic paralysis, ataxia, and cerebellar disturbances respond poorly. In the average case, the outlook in so far as life is concerned is not bad, but acute cases sometimes advance rapidly and may be over in the course of a year. Death ensues as a rule from an intercurrent disease.

VII. TREATMENT

No specific treatment of multiple sclerosis is available. Treatment consists, therefore, of purely symptomatic measures. The results are often discouraging and it is doubtful whether treatment has any specific influence on the course of the disease. It is decidedly open to debate whether those patients who make apparent complete or partial recoveries as a result of nonspecific treatment would not have developed remissions if left completely alone. Advanced cases rarely respond to treatment; early cases may do so. Despite this, some effort at treatment of the entire condition as well as of individual symptoms is justified.

Treatment of the disorder must begin with general hygiene measures which unfortunately are often neglected in management of the problem. *Fatigue* must be avoided, and conversely sufficient rest and relaxation are advisable. The symptoms of multiple sclerosis are aggravated by fatigue. *Exercise* is not contraindicated, but violent exercise should be avoided. *Tobacco* is not advisable in any form, and the same may be said of *alcohol*. No special *diet* is necessary, but a full and nutritious diet is desirable.

Drug treatment is of relatively little value. Sodium cacodylate has been given with good effect in some instances. Quinine hydrochloride has been advocated on the assumption that multiple sclerosis is due to the destruction of the lipoids of the myelin sheath, and quinine is said to inactivate lipases. It is given in doses of gr. 1 to 5 three times a day, depending on the tolerance, and should be withdrawn or reduced in amount if signs of cinchonism appear (tinnitus, deafness). Liver injections are sometimes helpful.

Nicotinic acid is one of the most useful agents in the treatment of muliple sclerosis because of its vasodilator effect. It is given by mouth in doses of 100 mg. three to six times daily. It is not necessary to give it intravenously except in acute cases when it may be given in doses of 100 mg. intravenously daily, in addition to the oral administration. It may be combined with thiamine chloride, 100 mg. intramuscularly daily.

Dicumarol has been advocated on the assumption that multiple sclerosis is the result of thrombosis of the venules in the nervous system. It is said to be of value in preventing progression of the disease. If the treatment is given, it must always be to hospitalized patients since hemorrhage requiring transfusions may develop from the nose, mouth, rectum, or uterus. It is given usually in an initial dose of 200 mg. in order to bring the prothrombin level down as quickly as possible, and thereafter in doses of 100 to 150 mg. daily, maintaining the prothrombin level at about 30. Prothrombin estimations must be performed daily. The treatment may be continued for long periods.

Histamine acid phosphate, given intravenously in doses of 2.75 mg. in 250 cc. of normal saline at a rate of 30 to 40 drops per minute, has been advocated. Twenty to forty treatments are necessary. The treatment has little to recommend it. Those patients who improve under it would probably improve by other methods.

Etamon chloride (tetraethyl ammonium chloride) offers help. It is given intramuscularly, beginning with 3 cc., advancing 1 cc. daily until the optimum dose is reached (7 to 12 cc.). It may be continued indefinitely at the optimum dose.

Sodium succinate has been used in the treatment of multiple sclerosis. Its value remains as yet undetermined. Succinates stimulate cellular respiration. Succinic acid acts as a catalyst in the metabolism of carbohydrates and fatty acids and is involved also in the oxidation reduction of cytochrome. Succinates increase the synthesis of acetylcholine. Sodium succinate may be given intravenously and orally. Intravenously it is given slowly by vein (20 ml. of a thirty per cent solution). Orally the drug is given as one teaspoonful (4.5 to 5 Gm.) of the powder in an ounce of water three times daily, followed by a glass of tomato juice. If no ill-effects are observed in 2 days the dose is doubled to two teaspoonsful three times daily.

Physiotherapy is valuable in patients with spasticity. Massage and passive muscle exercises may be helpful. Curare, in doses of 50 to 100 units intramuscularly daily, may be given in order to reduce spasticity and permit active muscle exercises. Reeducation and rehabilitation exercises are important.

Fever treatment is sometimes valuable in attacks of retrobulbar neuritis, but is of no value in other forms of the disease. This form of treatment should not be given during fulminating stages of the disease. It is best given in the form of injections of typhoid-paratyphoid vaccine (two thousand million per cc.) The initial dose should be fifty million intravenously, doubled every second or third day until a total of 1.5 cc. (three thousand million) is reached. Ten or twelve shocks suffice. The response varies, some patients developing marked fever with small doses, others little with large doses.

The treatment is severe and debilitates the patient. Iron is often necessary after a course of fever treatment. Artificial fever produced by the hypertherm machine is preferred by some.

High vitamin regimes containing large amounts of vitamins B_1, C, D, and E have been said to produce results in some cases, but the results are questionable. Large doses of vitamin B_{12} (1000 mg.) intramuscularly daily are said to help. No means have been found to prevent recurrent episodes of multiple sclerosis.

17

Intoxications and Injuries
by Physical Agents

The central nervous system may be attacked by many noxious agents as a result of (1) disturbance of appetite and personality (alcohol, morphine, marihuana); (2) industrial hazards (lead, carbon disulfide); (3) self-applied medication (bromides, barbiturates), and (4) suicidal intent (carbon monoxide, barbiturates, iodine). A knowledge of the characteristics, prevention, and treatment of the various noxious agents acting on the nervous system is therefore essential. Not all the noxious agents can be discussed even passingly, but the most commonly encountered in general practice merit some mention.

I. ALCOHOL

Alcohol may cause damage to the nerve structures in many areas. It may produce (1) alcoholic multiple neuritis; (2) alcoholic encephalopathies, characterized by many forms, among which are acute alcoholic hallucinosis, delirium tremens, Korsakoff's psychosis, and chronic alcoholism; (3) polioencephalitis hemorrhagica superior. "Alcoholic" neuritis has already been considered in the discussion of neuritis.

The *incidence* of alcoholism is appallingly high. "There are three arrests for drunkenness in every hundred people annually (Guthrie and Dayton, 1937); seven to nine out of every one hundred

thousand people die annually from alcoholism, about fifteen out of every one hundred thousand become first admissions with alcoholic psychoses to the state hospitals of the Commonwealth of Massachusetts each year" (Alexander). In the United States in 1938, alcoholism was diagnosed as the cause of death in 2569 persons, 0.2 per cent of the total death rate, or two per one hundred thousand of the population, as compared with six per one hundred thousand in 1900 (Schmid).

Alcohol is a narcotic and not a stimulant. Its supposed stimulating effect is the result of loss of inhibitory mechanisms from its narcotic effect on the cerebral cortex. Once ingested, it enters the blood stream quickly and there is a close correlation between the alcohol content of the blood, brain, spinal fluid, urine, and alveolar air. The degree of intoxication may be reliably determined by the concentration of alcohol in the blood. Slight intoxication is associated with blood alcohol values of 1 to 2 mg. per cc., severe intoxication with 2 to 4 mg. per cc., alcoholic coma with 4 to 5 mg. per cc., while values of 5 mg. or over may cause death from acute alcohol poisoning (Selesnick).

The *relationship* of alcohol to the various nervous system disorders with which it is associated is a problem of great interest and importance. Its mode of action is still under dispute but two main concepts stand out: (1) that alcohol has a direct toxic or injurious effect on the nervous system; (2) that its action is merely contributory and that the evidences of injury are the result of other actions, especially disturbances of metabolism. In the various types of psychosis associated with alcoholism there is always a history of prolonged use of alcohol, varying from five to forty-five years. Emphasis has come to be placed in recent years on vitamin deficiencies as the fundamental factor in the injurious effects of alcohol on the nervous system. In neuritis associated with alcohol, the assumption of a thiamine deficiency is made on the similarity of alcoholic multiple neuritis to beriberi (endemic) neuritis, as well as on other factors discussed in the section on neuritis. Similarly, in delirium tremens and Korsakoff's psychosis, a thiamine deficiency has been postulated (Wortis, Jolliffe). The production of Wernicke's polioencephalitis by many nonalcoholic conditions has led to the assertion that the fundamental factor in this disorder is not alcoholism itself but a thiamine deficiency. This concept is supported by the demonstration in animals of lesions similar to those seen in alcoholism, on the basis of a thiamine deficiency (Alexander). Present-day investigation, therefore, tends to minimize the direct action of alcohol on the nervous structures and to emphasize the rôle of vitamin deficiency, particularly of thiamine, though asserting that a multiple vitamin deficiency is probably present. The evidence of vitamin deficiency, however, in Korsakoff's psychosis and delirium tremens must be regarded as only suggestive and not yet firmly established.

The *pathology* of nervous system disorders associated with alcoholism is variable in kind and degree. In *acute alcoholic intoxication*, the brain is hyperemic and is severely edematous. Changes may be found in the cortical ganglion cells, especially of an edematous nature. Retrograde degeneration (axonal chromatolysis) of the cortical ganglion cells is found not only in acute alcoholism but in the chronic forms as well. The brain changes in *delirium tremens* are not specific and are, in fact, poorly defined. Brain edema is striking. The pia-arachnoid is often thickened and adherent to the cortex. The cortical ganglion cells show a variety of changes, none of them of a specific character—chronic sclerosis, axonal chromatolysis, etc. In *Korsakoff's psychosis* also no specific changes have been described. Ganglion cell changes in the cerebral cortex are common and at times in the basal ganglia. Glial reaction is scanty. Changes have been found in the corpora mamillaria. In *chronic alcoholism*, diffuse cortical ganglion cell damage, brain edema, and thickening of the pia-arachnoid are found. The findings in the case of Wernicke's *polioencephalitis hemorrhagica superior* are more definite. They consist of punctate hemorrhages, small foci of degeneration, varicose deformity of the blood vessels, and subacute necrosis of the parenchyma in the region of the collicular plate (Alexander), affecting largely the superior colliculi and oculomotor nuclei.

Acute Alcoholic Hallucinosis: This disorder represents an acute intoxication occurring in a chronic drinker. The onset is sudden, and the psychosis characterized by fear, anxiety, rich auditory hallucinations and misinterpretations. Visual hallucinations are not very common, but tactile hallucinations are found. Suicidal attempts are frequent, due to the conviction of a horrible end. The condition is thought by many to be closely related to delirium tremens, but in contrast to the latter, persons with acute alcoholic hallucinosis are well oriented and accessible, the duration is longer, and the sufferers from the condition, unlike those with delirium tremens, show a high incidence of psychopaths, psychosis, and suicide in their families. Others regard the condition as being closely allied to dementia precox, especially the catatonic form. The probabilities are that acute alcoholic hallucinosis is an acute schizophrenic reaction released by alcohol (Noyes).

Delirium Tremens: Alcoholic intoxications are at times associated with a severe psychosis in chronic drinkers, especially in middle-aged men. The disease is prone to occur as a result of (1) excessive prolonged drinking, (2) sudden withdrawal of alcohol, (3) bouts of overindulgence. Infection, trauma, intercurrent diseases of many sorts, may tend to precipitate symptoms in a chronic alcoholic.

The symptoms are dramatic in their fully developed state and are featured by active hallucinations and tremor. The onset is gradual over a course of two or three days with restlessness, anxiety, loss of sleep, increased irritability, and loss of appetite. This is followed suddenly by the development of delirium with active visual and auditory hallucinations, especially the former and sometimes with convulsions. Forms of all sorts — snakes, mice, rats, etc. — terrorize the sufferer, who shows an extreme degree of panic and terror as a result of the hallucinatory visions. Restlessness is extreme, and the reaction to the visual hallucinations is so great that restraints are necessary in order to keep the patient in bed and to prevent his escape from his imaginary experiences. Auditory hallucinations are not as common as those in the visual sphere; but voices, murmurs, and other auditory experiences are common. Suggestibility is a striking feature

so that patients with delirium tremens can be made to read from empty sheets of paper, etc.

Tremor is generalized, involving the face, tongue, and limbs. It is coarse, constant, and increased on movement. Associated with the terror and delirium is a constant tremor of body and limbs, ceaseless activity in an effort to escape, constant muttering, and often shrieking and yelling. The skin and tongue are dry, perspiration is profuse, the pulse rapid, the urine is scanty, and incontinence may be encountered. The tendon reflexes are usually absent, but there is no evidence of involvement of the nervous system apart from this. The delirium runs an average course of three or four days and disappears after a terminal sleep.

Most subjects recover in the course of five to seven days, but a mortality rate of about fifteen per cent is found. Dehydration and cirrhosis of the liver tend to increase the seriousness of the condition.

Korsakoff's Psychosis: This is characterized by multiple neuritis and psychosis, associated with alcohol indulgence. The condition has been reported in a variety of other conditions as well. Hence, it must be regarded as a symptomatic psychosis occurring chiefly in alcoholic intoxication, but in other states as well. The disease occurs chiefly between forty and fifty years of age and is more often found in women.

The psychosis develops rapidly as a rule and dominates the clinical picture. It is characterized by loss of memory, confabulation, and relatively good insight. Disorientation is striking, the gaps being filled in by confabulations of many sorts.

Associated with the mental picture is a multiple neuritis involving all the limbs as a rule. It may be severe or mild and need not parallel in severity the mental picture. Tenderness of the muscles and nerve trunks, absent reflexes, and loss of motor power are present. Sensory disturbances are difficult to evaluate during the psychosis. Cranial nerve palsies, especially of the face and eye muscles, are seen at times. The *outlook* is not, as a rule, good for complete recovery. Death occurs in about fifteen per cent of subjects.

Polioencephalitis Hemorrhagica Superior (Wernicke): This condition, associated at times with alcohol indulgence, is a form of hemorrhagic encephalitis involving the oculomotor nuclei. The condition is found not only in alcoholism but in a variety of other conditions including gastric carcinoma, pernicious anemia, macrocytic anemia following resection of the bowel, pregnancy, and bronchiectasis (Campbell).

The *clinical features* are characterized by a rapid onset of symptoms featured by headache, diplopia, and often by ataxic gait. The onset is almost always acute, sometimes with stupor. Outstanding are evidences of ocular paralyses with complete or incomplete ophthalmoplegias characterized by total inability to move the eyeballs or partial paralyses of varying degree. Weakness of the limbs and ataxia are not uncommon. The pupils may be irregular and respond sluggishly to light or there may be on rare occasions Argyll Robertson pupils. Though Argyll Robertson pupils are almost always the result of neurosyphilis, the experience of many investigators indicates that a true pupil of this type may occur in chronic alcoholism (Wilson, Nonne, Peter). The end result may be complete recovery, partial recovery, or death.

Treatment: The treatment of *delirium tremens* requires attention not only to the nervous symptoms but to the systemic condition as well. An adequate fluid and food intake reënforced by vitamins is essential. Feeding by nasal tube may be necessary, though it is often possible to feed by mouth even when great restlessness is present. Fluid (normal saline) by hypodermoclysis is often necessary. Carbohydrates should be given in large quantities. Care must be taken of the heart, and digitalis is therefore often required. Restraints should be avoided, but the restlessness must be combated by proper sedation. Morphine must be avoided. Paraldehyde is probably the best sedative and must be given in large quantities, drachms three or four at a dose. Large doses of thiamine (100 mg. intravenously daily) and nicotinic acid (500 to 600 mg. by mouth daily) have been advocated, and have been reported to be successful in many instances. Good results have been reported with small doses of insulin and with amphetamine (Benzedrine) sulfate. Lumbar puncture should be performed for diagnosis, but should not be used to reduce brain edema. Hypertonic solutions of sucrose (fifty per cent) or glucose (fifty per cent) are preferable for this purpose. The treatment of *Korsakoff's psychosis* is much the same as that of delirium tremens.

II. LEAD

Lead intoxication is responsible for many disorders of the nervous system. Among them are neuritis, encephalopathy, disease of the optic and oculomotor nerves, and myelopathy.

Lead encephalopathy is found as a rule in severe cases of lead poisoning. It is characterized pathologically by evidences of diffuse brain disease, seen as brain edema, widespread ganglion cell disease, endarteritis involving the cortical arterioles, at times foci of lymphocytic cells around the vessels, and in some instances by punctate hemorrhages.

Lead encephalopathy is more common in women than in men and appears to afflict Negroes more frequently than white subjects (6 to 8 per cent as compared with 1.3 per cent in whites). There is a high incidence of the disease in lower age groups, the symptoms of lead intoxication being more severe in children than in adults. Lead encephalopathy tends to occur most commonly in subjects exposed to relatively high concentrations of lead, especially in the dusty trades in which large quantities are absorbed through the respiratory tract.

The clinical features of lead encephalopathy are dominated in most instances by evidences of an organic brain syndrome which may be acute but is usually gradual in development. In the majority of instances, the picture is dominated by a slow deterioration of the mental functions with loss of memory and difficulty in concentration as early symptoms. Neurotic behavior, depression, and anxiety may appear early.

In the usual case, encephalopathy is preceded by other manifestations of lead poisoning and by a variety of symptoms, such as mental dullness, restlessness, irritability, loss of ability to concentrate, loss of memory, and insomnia. Headache is a common and distressing symptom and may be so severe as to compare with that of brain tumor. It may be persistent or intermittent, with frequent exacerbations. Mental symptoms may precede or accompany an attack of lead encephalopathy. In some instances, they may constitute the only manifestation of the disease. Acute psychotic episodes may be found, with confusion, delusions, and hallucinations. Delirium may be present. Convulsions are characteristic but are not constant. They may be generalized or focal, giving rise in the latter type to a picture closely resembling brain tumor. They may be preceded, accompanied, or followed by other manifestations of lead encephalopathy. Convulsions may be the first symptom of the disorder.

A large variety of symptoms have been observed during the course of lead encephalopathy. Among these are paralysis, tremor hemiplegia, hallucinations, paraplegias, blindness, hydrocephalus, convulsions, mental retardation, melancholia, and delirium. Little may be noted on examination save for tremor of the hands, face, and tongue, and evidence of intellectual deterioration or of an organic psychosis. Choked disc may be encountered in some instances.

Lead encephalopathy is common in children. Lesions are found in the cerebral hemispheres and cerebellum, and are characterized by serous inflammation associated with necrosis of capillaries and thrombi and tissue damage (Blackman). The onset in children is usually acute with headache and convulsions, and with signs of meningeal irritation and indications of increased intracranial pressure, such as choked disc. Cerebellar symptoms, such as awkwardness of movement and clumsiness of gait are common, and hemiparesis or hemiplegia may be found. The condition simulates brain tumor closely, especially cerebellar tumor, and the distinction between the two conditions can be made only if a history of exposure to lead is obtained and proper studies made to establish the diagnosis. Among the sequelae of lead encephalopathy in children who survive the acute stage may be mental retardation, convulsions, and hemiplegia or hemiparesis. In both children and adults, lead intoxication may simulate brain tumors.

Disease of the *optic nerve* is found at times in association with lead poisoning, either as an accompaniment of lead encephalopathy or with no other evidences of disease of the nervous system. The optic nerve changes may consist of (1) optic neuritis, (2) choked disc, (3) primary optic atrophy. The last condition is found only rarely in lead poisoning. *Oculomotor paralyses*, either single or multiple, may occur in lead poisoning.

Spinal cord disease, though uncommon, is at times a sequel of lead poisoning. Paraplegias of a spastic type and at times posterolateral sclerosis are encountered.

The central nervous system involvement by lead poisoning is usually associated with manifestations of systemic involvement, such as gastrointestinal symptoms, etc. This is not invariably the case, however. The *blood picture* is usually typical and excess of lead is demonstrable in the blood, urine, and feces. Lead is found deposited in the bones at the epiphyses in children, but not in adults. Lead may be found in minute quantities in the spinal fluid and may be recovered from the brain at necropsy.

The outlook in cases of lead encephalopathy in both adults and children is not good. Mortality rates have been estimated from twenty-five to seventy-five per cent and those patients who survive are prone to develop sequelae, such as convulsions.

The *treatment* is that of lead poisoning. In acute lead encephalopathy in children simulating brain tumor, decompression in order to conserve eyesight and relieve intracranial pressure may be required (Bucy and Buchanan).

III. CARBON MONOXIDE

Carbon monoxide poisoning may be responsible for a variety of conditions involving the nervous system. Among them are (1) neuritis, (2) encephalopathies of various types. The brain in fatal cases reveals changes in the cerebral cortex characterized by diffuse cell loss and, in some instances, by an elective destruction of the third and fourth cortical layers. Acute cases are characterized by hyperemia of the meninges and brain, and by punctate hemorrhages in the brain tissue, particularly in the cortex and pallidum. A selective destruction of the pallidum is particularly characteristic; this may be a complete liquefaction of this nucleus or only a partial destruction. At times the putamen and thalamus may be softened. Widespread ganglion cell disease is found in all parts of the nervous system.

The chief sources of carbon monoxide poisoning in civil life are (1) illuminating gas, (2) exhaust gas, and (3) coal gas. Carbon monoxide is a fertile source of poisoning, both accidental and intentional. Of 4794 cases of suicide in the United States in 1928, 2317, or forty-nine per cent, were by carbon monoxide poisoning, chiefly illuminating gas. The latter, however, is not composed exclusively of carbon monoxide (twenty to thirty per cent), but, in addition, of carbon dioxide, methane, acetylene, and other gases. A fertile source of poisoning by carbon monoxide is by means of the exhaust from gasoline motors which contains seven per cent of carbon monoxide (Beemke). Gas from blast furnaces is a frequent source of industrial poisoning and contains from twenty-four to thirty per cent of carbon monoxide. Coal dust explosions in mines, charcoal braziers, lime and brick kilns are also common sources.

Intoxication by carbon monoxide is due to the replacement of oxyhemoglobin by the carbon monoxide, which has an affinity for hemoglobin over two hundred times stronger than the affinity of hemoglobin for oxygen. The result of carbon monoxide inhalation is anoxia, the rate of development of which depends upon the volume of carbon monoxide inhaled per minute.

Percentage Saturation of the Blood with Carbon Monoxide and Corresponding Physiologic Effects (Henderson and Haggard)

Percentage of Hemoglobin in Combination with Carbon Monoxide — *Physiologic Effect*

Percentage of Hemoglobin in Combination with Carbon Monoxide	Physiologic Effect
10	No appreciable effect except shortness of breath on vigorous muscular exertion.
20	No appreciable effect in most cases except short wind even on moderate exertion; slight headache in some cases.
30	Decided headache; irritable, easily fatigued; judgment disturbed.
40 to 50	Headache, confusion, collapse, and fainting on exertion.
60 to 70	Unconsciousness; respiratory failure and death if exposure is long continued.
80	Rapidly fatal.
Over 80	Immediately fatal.

The symptoms of acute poisoning consist of headache, a sensation of tightness and throbbing about the forehead and in the temples, dizziness, dimness of vision, confusion, and in severe cases collapse and stupor. The inhalation of high concentrations of the gas results in immediate unconsciousness and death.

In patients who have survived a severe intoxication, or in those who inhale a constant small amount of the gas, numerous symptoms develop. Chronic poisoning may occur in persons exposed over long periods to low concentrations of carbon monoxide. In the latter, headache, anorexia, a feeling of general weakness, and anemia are found. In those patients who survive a nonfatal exposure to carbon monoxide, almost any neurological symptoms and signs may develop, depending upon the area of the brain destroyed.

Symptoms may develop immediately after exposure to the gas or they may be delayed for weeks or months after an apparent recovery. This is referred to as the relapsing form of the disease. Headache and vertigo are common. Loss of memory and difficulty in concentration, and mental deterioration which may be progressive are very frequent sequelae. Change in personality similar to that seen in other organic brain disease often occurs. Psychoses develop during the stage of acute intoxication and in the later stages after survival. In the acute phases, delirium and confusional psychoses predominate. The later psychotic manifestations vary in degree and content but are characterized by flattening of mood, loss of initiative, apathy, and severe disturbances of attention and memory. Convulsions may develop soon after exposure to the gas or they may not appear until some time later. Since the pallidum is often diseased in carbon monoxide poisoning, it is not unusual to find either well-developed parkinsonism or fragmentary parkinsonian syndromes characterized by tremor, rigid facies, and muscular rigidity of varying degree and extent. Aphasia, hemianopsia, and other evidences of focal brain damage have been recorded. Paraplegias and quadriplegias from extensive spinal cord damage have been described.

Habitual exposure to small quantities of carbon monoxide in the air results in the production of clinical symptoms (Beck, Roetman, and Suter). The symptoms occur under many circumstances, such as a mechanic in an automobile shop who breathes in small quantities of carbon monoxide from day to day, "or a workman at a blast furnace or gas plant, or a cook working in a small badly ventilated kitchen with a defective gas stove" (Henderson). The symptoms vary in intensity, depending on the quantity of carbon monoxide in the air breathed, the length of exposure, the amount of monoxide in the blood, the activity and previous condition of the patient, and other factors. The manifestations are purely subjective and consist of impairment of general health, nervousness, and ill temper.

IV. BROMIDES

Bromide intoxication is much more common than is usually recognized. Of one thousand consecutive patients admitted to a mental hospital, forty-four had mental symptoms which were due to or increased by bromide. The most frequent source is bromide medication, often self-administered. It is important to recognize the fact that bromide intoxication is practically always symptomatic and that there is almost always some underlying cause for the use of bromides, whether it be epilepsy, headache, pain, or some other specific disorder. The diagnosis is frequently obscured by the presence of the underlying condition for which bromides have been taken.

The level of *bromides in the blood* in patients with bromide intoxication varies greatly. Levels of 150 to 300 mg. are usually associated with evidences of bromidism, but lower levels may also cause intoxication and high levels are not infrequently unassociated with symptoms. There seems to be a wide variability, due probably to individual susceptibility to the drug. The *spinal fluid protein* has been reported to be frequently increased in bromidism.

A *bromide rash* is usually present, but is not always found. It may be seen with high or low bromide levels of the blood. Confusion and delirium are common, with disorientation, thick speech, and clouding of the sensorium. The clinical features of the mental syndrome are those of an organic reaction; that is, impairment of comprehension, interference with

the elaboration of impressions, defects in orientation and retention, difficulty in activation of memories, marked fluctuations in the level of attention, and emotional instability. Any type of organic reaction may be simulated; hence experience with bromide intoxication leads inevitably to a high respect for its capacity to mimic other diseases. This is portrayed vividly by the fact that bromide intoxication is frequently diagnosed encephalitis, taboparesis, general paresis, brain tumor, and paralysis agitans until the real nature of the disorder is revealed. The chief mental signs found in bromidism are listed as follows (Moore, Sobler, Alexander):

Drowsiness	Loss of memory
Insomnia	Impaired attention
Frightening dreams	Disorientation
Restlessness	Confabulation
Irrelevant conversation	Misidentification
Impaired comprehension	Sensory illusions
Interference with elaboration of impressions	Hallucinations (vision, sound, smell, touch)
Delusions (frequently of persecution)	Lability of affect

The *neurological findings* vary greatly and may simulate a wide variety of conditions. The face is often masklike, as in parkinsonism. The pupils may react sluggishly to light and accommodation, or they may simulate Argyll Robertson pupils. Coarse tremors of the tongue, face, and fingers are often encountered, simulating those of chronic alcoholism and general paresis. The speech is thick, slurred, and at times completely dysarthric. The gait is unsteady and ataxic and a positive Romberg's sign is common. Vertigo is common. The tendon reflexes are active or depressed. The condition may simulate chronic alcoholism, brain tumor, encephalitis, or general paresis.

The *diagnosis* depends upon a history of bromide ingestion, the demonstration of an acneform rash, and the presence of bromides in the blood. The condition must always be suspected in the presence of an organic mental reaction type of unexplained cause. The presence of the underlying condition for which bromides have been taken obscures the picture and makes diagnosis often difficult. After the bromidism has receded, the fundamental condition still remains to be dealt with.

Methyl bromide poisoning develops in subjects who work with it as a refrigerant, fumigant, or delousing agent. Nervous symptoms are typical of poisoning by this agent. They vary in intensity from case to case, but consist chiefly of headache, vertigo, lethargy, pareses, or paralyses, visual disturbances such as dimness of vision, delirium, mental disturbances, convulsions, and coma.

The *treatment* of bromidism requires attention to general physical needs, with free use of fluids. Intravenous fluids may be necessary. Sodium chloride tablets (gr. 5) may be given as often as necessary. Ammonium chloride (enteric-coated tablets) in a dosage of 5 to 8 grams daily has been found to be valuable. Treatment should always include efforts to eliminate the cause of the bromide habit.

V. SULFONAMIDES

In addition to neuritis, *the sulfonamides* may be responsible for central nervous system complications. Psychoses of various sorts have been reported after the use of *sulfanilamide*. Most of the reactions occur from three to ten days after the drug has been started, but in other instances abnormal mental reactions have developed after withdrawal of the drug. Depressions, confusional episodes, and toxic psychoses are the outstanding reactions. In addition, encephalitic pictures have been recorded, with aphasia, hemiparesis, etc. Dysmorphopsia, characterized by a distortion of visual images, has been found. Encephalo-

myelitis has been reported after the use of sulfanilamide.

Similar abnormal mental reactions have been found with *sulfathiazole,* but they are less frequent with this drug. Convulsions develop after the direct application of sulfathiazole to the brain but not with sulfanilamide, sulfapyridine, or sulfadiazine. A benign reaction is evoked by the latter drugs, with the development of scar formation after the drugs are applied to the brain. This scar is not, however, as a rule, extensive. Peripheral neuritis and transient blindness have been recorded with sulfathiazole. Encephalopathy associated with kidney disease has also been described.

Sulfapyridine has been found to produce confusion, restlessness, and irritability, all of which symptoms persisted after subsidence of the infection for which the drug was administered, and disappeared on withdrawal of the drug. Sciatica, polyneuritis, encephalomyelitis, and neuromyelitis have been recorded following the use of sulfapyridine. *Sulfadiazine* has been found to produce encephalopathy at times, as well as peripheral neuritis.

VI. ANTIBIOTICS

Under some circumstances, complications and sequelae may develop after the commonly used antibiotics.

Penicillin may cause convulsions when applied directly to the cerebral cortex. Convulsions may develop also after intrathecal use of the drug. Psychoses may occur. *Radiculitis* has been recorded after its intrathecal use, associated with paresthesias, urinary retention, sensory disturbances, and loss of power of the legs. Abnormal EEG tracings were found in 60 per cent of patients during the systemic administration of penicillin for non-neurological disorders (Johnson, Case, Walker, and Kollros). *Transverse myelitis* has been described following intrathecal administration, and *peroneal palsy* with foot drop has been observed after injections of penicillin into the buttocks. Anesthesia of the outer aspect of the thigh has been observed due to injury of the lateral femoral cutaneous nerve by direct injection of penicillin.

Streptomycin applied to the cerebral cortex of dogs and monkeys (1250 units) is capable of causing *convulsions*. In the human, its most serious sequel is *cerebellar dyssynergia* of varying degree, causing ataxic gait. The cerebellar disturbances may be transient or permanent. Their occurrence appears to be directly related to the total amount of drug used. *Kidney damage,* and a *sensitivity reaction* manifested by fever and skin eruption of varying severity, is a common evidence of toxicity. *Vertigo* is common. *Deafness* may result from the use of streptomycin or dihydrostreptomycin, but it is not as common as vertigo. The deafness may develop early in the course of use of the drug, or it may be delayed and appear weeks after its termination. The development of deafness appears to be related to the dosage of drug used. Intrathecal streptomycin has been found to be associated with many types of reactions, including shock-like states, convulsions, cerebellar signs, and rise in temperature.

VII. MANGANESE

Manganese poisoning occurs at times in miners of manganese ore and results probably from the inhalation and ingestion of manganese dust. Changes are found in the cerebral cortex and basal ganglia, consisting of ganglion cell loss in the pallidum and striatum particularly, and loss of cells in the cerebral cortex. The symptoms have been thoroughly summarized by Edsall and Drinker as follows: (1) a history of work in manganese dust for at least three months; (2) languor and sleepiness; (3) stolid, masklike facies; (4) low monotonous voice and economical speech; (5) muscular twitching, varying in degree from a fine tremor of the hands to gross rhythmical movements of the arms, legs, trunk, and head; (6) cramps in the calves, stiffness in the leg muscles, the cramps usually coming on at night and being worse after a day of exertion; (7) slight increase in tendon reflexes; (8) ankle and patellar clonus; (9) retropulsion and propulsion; (10) a peculiar slapping gait; (11) occasionally uncontrollable laughter; less frequently crying.

The total picture is that of paralysis agitans. The condition once developed is apt to persist, despite removal from exposure to the manganese dust, and the illness tends to hold on for years.

VIII. ARSENIC

Arsenic as a source of poisoning is found in industry and medicine and may give rise to intoxications by means of a variety of exposures. It is responsible for the production of (1) neuritis, (2) encephalopathies, and (3) myelopathies. Neuritis has already been considered. A not infrequent source of damage to the nervous system by arsenic results from the injection of arsphenamine and neo-arsphenamine. The brain in such cases reveals one of the following types of lesions: (1) diffuse petechial hemorrhages; (2) gross cerebral hemorrhage; (3) multiple symmetrical foci of softening in the gray and white matter of the brain, and (4) a combination of any of these lesions (Courville). It is essential to recognize the fact that the lesions are scattered and diffuse and that they are destructive, for upon this depends a clear conception of the varied symptomatology and the dubious outlook.

Reactions are reported to occur once in every 6500 cases and once in every 36,000 injections (Glaser, Imerman, and Imerman). They occur chiefly in patients with syphilis but are found also in non-syphilitic persons. In over fifty per cent of subjects, the disorder follows the second injection of the drug. The dosage of the drug has not been found responsible for the reaction. The reactions may occur any time within three days after injection, and often (thirty-three per cent) within twenty-four hours after administration of arsphenamine or neoarsphenamine.

The onset of symptoms is usually abrupt but may be gradual, with headache, vomiting, nervousness, and chills. Convulsions occur frequently (eighty per cent). Fever, tachycardia, increased respirations, ocular paralyses, changes in the reflexes, signs of meningeal irritation, delirium, and a variety of other signs may be found, depending on the areas of the brain which are damaged.

Recovery occurs in some cases. In others, the disorder is fatal. Death occurs within twenty-four hours in twenty-four per cent of the subjects.

A *myelitis* or *myelopathy* is found in rare instances following arsenic administration. The condition results from hemorrhage within the cord substance. The onset is sudden, with complete paralysis of the legs, and the findings are those of a complete transverse myelitis with motor and sensory paralysis and vesical disturbances. The outlook for recovery is poor.

IX. CARBON DISULFIDE

Intoxication with carbon disulfide occurs particularly in workers in rubber vulcanization and rayon manufacture. It may give rise to (1) neuritis, (2) psychoses, and (3) cerebral syndromes. The commonest form of carbon disulfide poisoning is *neuritis* (eighty-seven per cent), which involves most commonly the limbs and the optic and auditory nerves. Both motor and sensory disturbances are found. Paresthesias are common in the early stages and are usually associated with pain in the arms or legs

or both. The radial, ulnar, sciatic, and external peroneal nerves are most affected. Loss of muscle power, atrophy of the muscles, loss of reflexes, and objective sensory disturbances are found. Recovery is slow and may fall short of complete restitution of function.

Mental symptoms of more or less serious import are frequently found. The less serious disturbances consist of (1) extreme irritability and uncontrollable anger with rapid mood changes, (2) memory defects of rather severe degree, (3) severe insomnia, (4) loss of sexual libido and potentia. Psychotic reactions, such as manic episodes, depressions, and dementias, have been observed.

Optic neuritis and *optic atrophy* are not infrequently observed. Parkinsonian syndromes, usually of a mild or moderate degree but sometimes pronounced with all the features of parkinsonism, are sometimes found. In rare instances, carbon disulfide poisoning has given rise to symptoms simulating brain tumor—headache, vomiting, bradycardia, and blurred optic discs. Torsion spasm has been described after exposure to the gas.

X. ANTICONVULSANTS

Diphenylhydantoin sodium (*Dilantin Sodium*) is associated at times with somnolence, gum hypertrophy of varying degree, exfoliative dermatitis, vertigo, and cerebellar dyssynergia. The disturbances may occur singly or in combination, and may develop after short duration because of sensitivity to the drug or following prolonged medication. Withdrawal of the drug causes disappearance of all symptoms except the gum hypertrophy. The drug may be resumed with safety at a lower dosage.

Mesantoin causes exfoliative dermatitis at times. Gum hypertrophy, vertigo, and somnolence occur rarely. Death due to aplastic anemia has been recorded, and aplastic anemia with hypoplastic bone marrow terminating in recovery has also been observed.

Trimethadione (Tridione) is at times associated with photophobia and gastric disturbances. The symptoms disappear on reduction of dosage.

XI. MISCELLANEOUS INTOXICATIONS

Mercury poisoning is characterized largely by tremors affecting mainly the fingers and hands. These are fine, rapid, and constant. Tremors of the face are also encountered. Mental symptoms of a confusional nature have been described. Cerebellar symptoms are common, and in addition to tremor constitute the most striking feature of chronic mercury poisoning. The tremor is of the intentional type and is increased on movement. Dyssynergia, disturbance of equilibrium and gait, and a slow cerebellar type of speech are found. Evidences of intellectual deficit and even of deterioration have been described and rarely hemiplegia has been encountered. Choreiform movements, athetotic-like movements, and parkinsonian-like tremors are quite common; parkinsonian-like facies may develop.

Barbiturates taken in excess may give rise to psychoses, usually of a confusional type. In some instances, evidences of brain damage may develop, due to the presence of punctate hemorrhages, fatty degeneration of nerve cells and of the vascular endothelium. Acute barbiturate poisoning is characterized by confusion and later stupor, incoördination, indistinct speech, a weak and rapid pulse, low blood pressure. The reflexes are absent; there is often dilatation or contraction of the pupils; nystagmus is common, is usually horizontal but may be vertical as well; and there is almost always evidence of oculomotor paralysis of varying degree. The skin is often quite red but may be cyanotic. The

Table 61—Symptoms Found in Poisoning by Amanita Muscaria and Amanita Phalloides

	RAPID GROUP	DELAYED GROUP
	Amanita Muscaria	*Amanita Phalloides*
ONSET	Within a few minutes to three hours after ingestion	Six to fifteen hours after ingestion
SYMPTOMS	Excessive salivation and lacrimation; pupils contracted and fail to react to light or accommodation; nausea and vomiting; abdominal pains with profuse watery bowel movements; pulse often slow and irregular; dizziness and confusion; convulsions and coma in severe cases. Death within few hours in fatal cases	No symptoms for several hours; sudden onset with severe abdominal pain, nausea, vomiting, usually diarrhea; blood and mucus in stools and vomitus often; extreme thirst; anuria at times; jaundice in from two to three days; cyanosis and coldness of extremities; increasing prostration with coma and death. Fatal cases, death on the fifth to eighth day
PROGNOSIS	Good in mild cases; good in severe cases if treated with atropine	Grave; mortality fifty to seventy per cent; often one hundred per cent of a group

symptoms of chronic barbiturate intoxication are not as clearly defined. They are found in cases of barbiturate medication maintained for long periods of time. The mentality is dull and both concentration and memory are impaired. Nystagmus is common, as is incoördination of gait. Personality changes may develop with prolonged use of the drug.

Phosphorus is a rare source of poisoning, but it has a predilection for brain tissue as well as for the liver and blood vessels, causing a fatty degeneration of the affected organs. Neurological sequelae are of little significance, since they are almost always fatal. Phosphorus compounds, such as "Apiol" (triorthocresyl phosphate), give rise at times to neurological symptoms characterized by paresthesias, pains, weakness, and paralysis of the small hand muscles and the muscles of the legs and feet, absence of reflexes, without sensory disturbances.

Botulism is at times the cause of nervous system symptoms which may be the first manifestation of the disease. They are characterized by headache, diplopia, the development of ocular paralyses with ptosis and loss of movement of one or all the eyeball muscles, and difficulty in talking and swallowing. The clinical features are those of a rapidly progressive encephalitis with a history of onset after food ingestion, without fever and with clear mentality. The condition results from action of the botulinus toxin on the myoneural junctions. In some, but by no means all instances, there have been found evidences of polioencephalitis with acute degeneration of the cells in the affected brain stem nuclei, fatty cell degeneration, punctate hemorrhages and thromboses. In many cases the nervous system reveals no evidence of damage despite widespread neurological manifestations.

Mushroom poisoning is responsible for a small number of deaths and for clinical manifestations which include nervous system symptoms. There are over eighty species of poisonous mushrooms in the United States, of which the genus Amanita is responsible for practically all the severe cases of poisoning. Amanita phalloides causes over ninety per cent of the deaths from mushroom poisoning; some are due to Amanita muscaria. The symptoms found in the two groups are shown in Table 61 (Vanderveer and Farley).

Nervous system symptoms of various types accompany the systemic features of mushroom poisoning. They include convulsions, ocular paralyses, confusion, somnolence, blindness, paralysis of the bladder, paralysis of all the limbs, pupillary disturbances, tremors, twitchings of various sorts, Babinski's signs, signs of meningeal irritation and vasomotor paralysis. These may develop in varying combinations, depending on the area of the nervous system affected by the toxin.

Thallium is responsible at times for nervous complications. The drug is used in depilatory preparations. Polyneuritis is the most common complication and is associated with severe pains in the limbs. Excitement, irritability, and at times psychoses are produced by the drug. Other symptoms which have been found in thallium poisoning include somnolence, convulsions, choreiform movements, disturbances of hearing, retrobulbar neuritis. In mild cases of poisoning, recovery is good. Chronic cases are not as common as acute or subacute forms. They are characterized by loss of hair, polyneuritis, cerebral symptoms of the type described in the acute cases, retrobulbar neuritis, and eosinophilia.

Barium poisoning develops as the result of use of the drug in rat poisons. Acute poisoning is characterized by the development of an ascending flaccid paralysis involving all the limbs, associated with loss of reflexes but no sensory disturbances. The paralysis disappears in one or two days, leaving no residuals in favorable cases. Usually, however, the paralysis progresses to involve the brain stem nuclei and death ensues in a short time.

Gold preparations, particularly gold chloride used in the treatment of arthritis, may be associated with peripheral neuritis, psychoses, herpes zoster, meningitis, encephalitis, and cerebrovascular accidents.

Cyanide poisoning is rapidly fatal. Unconsciousness supervenes rapidly and death comes quickly. In persons who have recovered, neurotic symptoms have developed. Speech disturbances, weakness of the limbs, tremor, disturbance in equilibrium, paralysis of the limbs, and parkinsonism have been described as sequelae of poisoning with recovery. Chronic cyanide poisoning due to exposure in making of plastics is characterized by a variety of symptoms, such as generalized weakness, tinnitus, vertigo, and, in some instances, by peripheral paralyses with muscular atrophy and parkinsonianlike syndromes. Toxic psychosis has been observed in the use of thiocyanate for patients with hypertension, especially in the presence of renal damage. The clinical picture is that of a typical confusional psychosis, sometimes with delirium. Fatalities have been reported with potassium thiocyanate.

Benzene poisoning may be associated with retrobulbar neuritis, pseudomyasthenic syndromes, and neuritic manifestations. *Methyl chloride,* used in refrigeration, is characterized in states of intoxication by confusion, agitation, drowsiness, disturbances of vision, ocular paralyses, muscular twitchings, and chronic and tonic convulsions. *Tetrachlorethane,* used as a solvent and cleaning agent in many industries, is associated in some cases with neuritis, characterized by paresthesias, paralyses, sensory disturbances, and loss of reflexes. *Trichlorethylene* poisoning is characterized by disturbances of consciousness, retrobulbar neuritis in chronic cases, and at times convulsions.

Plant poisons of various sorts may be associated with involvement of the nervous system. Many of these are rare and of little practical value. *Ergotism* is characterized by headache, vertigo, and paresthesias. In its convulsive form, the prodromal symptoms mentioned are followed by muscular twitchings, and eventually by severe tonic convulsions. Epileptic seizures and psychoses develop. Tabeslike syndromes may be found. In *lathyrism,* nervous system symptoms are outstanding. The disease is developed as a result of ingestion of some types of peas. The symptoms are purely spinal. They are characterized by severe pains in the legs, followed in a short time by paralysis of the lower extremities, associated with circulatory disturbances (cyanosis, edema), and with incontinence and disturbances of sexual potency. Complete recovery is uncommon and spastic paralysis of the legs is a frequent residual.

Spinal anesthesia is in some instances associated with injuries to the nervous system. The incidence of such complications is low when compared with the total number of spinal anesthesias administered yearly, but the fact remains that residuals following the anesthesia have been recorded. These result from injuries to the axis cylinders and destruction of the myelin sheaths, degeneration of the anterior horn cells, and punctate hemorrhages within the spinal cord. The complications are found immediately or soon after use of the anesthetic but may be delayed for days or weeks. A variety of conditions have been found following spinal anesthesia. These include: headache; meningismus; abducens paralysis; involvement of the optic, oculomotor, trigeminal, facial, or hypoglossal nerves; lesions of the cauda equina; adhesive arachnoiditis with spinal cord involvement; myelitis; myeloradiculitis; encephalitis; causalgia. Internal hydrocephalus with symptoms suggestive of brain tumor has been recorded following spinal anesthesia, associated with extensive adhesive arachnoiditis of the spinal cord and brain stem. Pseudomonas aeruginosa meningitis has been found after spinal anesthesia, due to direct infection by the procedure. Other forms of meningitis have been reported, as well as extensive adhesive arachnoiditis with severe spinal cord syndromes. It is probable that some forms of spinal anesthesia are more often associated with nervous system complications than others. Headache is an extremely disabling symptom after spinal anesthesia and may persist for weeks. It results probably from loss of spinal fluid and the action of the anesthetic agent. Caffeine sodiobenzoate, gr. 7½ intravenously, gives temporary relief. The symptom disappears in time.

The reason for the development of sequelae in some cases of spinal anesthesia is not known. They are probably not related to the anesthetic agent. There is evidence to indicate that in some instances the detergents used in cleaning glassware and instruments may be responsible.

Intraspinal medication is not without its hazards. It is essential to bear in mind that the introduction of any foreign material into the subarachnoid space, whether it be serum, drugs, air, or oil, is followed by a sterile meningitis and an increase of proteins (Young and Alpers). These changes are transitory, but they are indicative of the fact that foreign material introduced into the spinal subarachnoid space causes a meningeal reaction. In some instances, when drainage accompanies the introduction of foreign material, changes are found in the spinal cord itself. Complications develop following the use of some drugs introduced into the spinal canal.

Magnesium sulfate given intrathecally has been followed by the development of transverse myelitis. Magnesium salts, given chiefly as magnesium sulfate by mouth or rectum, may not be harmless in their effects. Magnesium sulfate may be absorbed from the gastrointestinal tract in sufficient amounts to raise the level of magnesium in the blood and to produce depressant cerebral effects such as drowsiness, respiratory irregularities and depression. The same is true of *ammonium sulfate* introduced into the subarachnoid space to control pain. *Subarachnoid alcohol,* given to relieve pain, may cause destruction of axis cylinders and myelin in the cord and may be followed by incontinence of urine or paralysis of the legs. *Lipiodol* may be followed by severe pains which may last for a long time. It causes arachnoiditis due to its irritative action. *Pantopaque* is less irritative than lipiodol, but instances of arachnoiditis, sometimes extensive, have been recorded. Root pains may develop and rarely transverse spinal cord syndromes. The administration of *adrenocorticotropic hormone* (ACTH) has been associated with the production of seizures resulting at times in status epilepticus, as well as with coma and delirium. Convulsive seizures have also been reported with cortisone. The seizures reported after the use of both ACTH and cortisone have developed after prolonged use of the drug. They appear at varying intervals in the course of therapy. In three patients with seizures associated with ACTH, the seizures developed twenty, twenty, and ninety-two days after administration of the drug. In the case of cortisone, seizures were reported eleven and sixteen days after the use of the drug. Temporary and permanent nervous system damage have been reported with use of the drugs. Psychosis has been reported with prolonged use of an *antihistaminic,* prophenpyridamine (Trimeton). The psychosis was of a toxic type and disappeared with withdrawal of the drug.

Hemiplegia has been observed in the course of treatment with tetraethylthiuram (*Antabuse*).

Toxic encephalitis has been reported with *isoniazid* (isonicotinic acid hydrazine). Peripheral neuritis has been found also with prolonged use of isoniazid. Fatal toxic encephalitis has been recorded in *iproniazid*, the isopropyl derivative of isonicotinic acid hydrazide. Psychotic behavior has been observed with *reserpine*. Convulsions, hallucinations, and generalized tremors have been reported with *Asterol hydrochloride* when the drug was applied to large areas of the skin and scalp in large quantities.

Porphyria is a disease characterized by abnormal pigment metabolism resulting in the excretion of unusually excessive amounts of porphyrins and other pigments in the urine.

It is manifested in three main forms: (1) a congenital type, appearing in infancy, and characterized by lesions in the teeth, bones, and skin, the cutaneous lesions (hydroa aestivale) resulting from the photosensitizing properties of the porphyrins; (2) an acute idiopathic porphyria, occurring in early adult life, more commonly in females, with symptoms referable to the abdomen and the nervous system; (3) an acute toxic porphyria, resulting from the use of barbiturates.

The cause of the condition is not known. The congenital form points to a constitutional factor resulting in the faulty metabolism of porphyrins. In the acquired cases, a similar constitutional factor is assumed by some to be present, but evidence for this is lacking.

The pathology of the disorder is manifested largely in the nervous system. These are characterized chiefly by damage to the *peripheral nerves* which show typical parenchymatous neuritis, with dissolution of the myelin sheaths and destruction of the axis cylinders. The damage is widespread in severe cases. The anterior and posterior roots of the spinal cord are extensively diseased, but the cranial nerves are not as severely damaged as those of the limbs. The anterior horn cells of the spinal cord may be damaged severely, slightly or not at all. The nuclei of the brain stem may show similar changes. The cortical ganglion cells reveal toxic swelling and sometimes fatty deposits. The Purkinje cells of the cerebellum and those of the sympathetic ganglia may be diseased.

The *symptoms* of acute porphyria are characterized by the sudden onset of severe abdominal pain with vomiting resembling disease of the gallbladder, stomach, or intestines. The pain is extremely severe and is followed within varying periods of time, but usually quite rapidly by nervous system manifestations. Ascending or descending numbness or weakness of the limbs is common and may or may not be associated with pains in the arms or legs. The weakness may develop within a few hours or days, and often proceeds to complete paralysis. Respiratory paralysis develops in fatal cases. Transient blindness is common and striking. Mental symptoms of various sorts may develop. During the course of acute porphyria, an acute confusional psychosis may appear and often delirium. Manic excitements and depressions have been observed. Examination reveals a pure motor syndrome in most cases, with severe weakness or paralysis, little or no atrophy, absent reflexes, no tenderness of the muscles or nerve trunks and no sensory changes. Sphincter disturbances are usually present in some degree. The disease is afebrile as a rule. The spinal fluid may show an increase of proteins.

The *urine* is wine-colored or black, due to porphyrins and other pigments, among which are melanin, skatole, urofuscin, and urobilin. The urine may be normal in color in some instances, due to the presence of a colorless chromogen, but if the urine is allowed to stand or brought to a very acid reaction typical uroporphyrin will appear. Spectroscopic examination will reveal the pigments. The amount of porphyrins in the urine varies greatly in each case and disappears with the subsidence of an acute attack of porphyria.

The problem of *diagnosis* is that of an acutely developing motor neuritis in an adult, without sensory disturbances, with profound motor weakness, at times with respiratory difficulties late in the disorder, with transient blindness, and often with confusional episodes. The diagnosis is established by the wine-colored or dark urine which is free of blood and is found to contain porphyrins.

XII. ELECTRICAL INJURIES

Injuries due to the electrical current are common. The *voltage* necessary to produce damage varies. Death may be produced by currents of very low voltage and there are instances of death from alternating currents of 46 and 60 volts. High tension currents are less dangerous than low tension; hence the voltages in common daily use are most dangerous. An *amperage* of 70 to 110 ma. alternating at ordinary frequencies or a direct current of 200 to 250 ma. may be fatal if passed through the chest, but currents of much greater amperage are less often fatal. Alternating currents are three to four times more dangerous than direct currents. Induction coil currents are not dangerous to man, but spark discharges from condensers are capable of producing fatal effects.

The effect of the current on the body depends to a large extent on the *resistance* of the skin, since the resistance of other tissues, except for bone, is small in comparison (Pearl). Dryness, cleanliness, and thickness determine the degree of resistance; it is greater in a calloused palm and in a dry skin as compared with a moist one (5000 ohms as compared with 1000 ohms); perspiration reduces skin resistance. The point of exit is equally important as the point of entrance. Shoes have a high resistance when dry, but when wet their resistance is greatly reduced and a current may pass through the body and cause death. Shoes with iron nails are dangerous. The heart is the area of greatest danger in electrical shock. The central nervous system is a secondary danger zone. Currents from foot to foot are never fatal unless they traverse the chest. Currents from hand to hand or hand to foot are frequently fatal. The blood and lymph streams are the best conductors. There appears to be an *individual* susceptibility to the effects of the electrical current. Fatigue increases the susceptibility to current. It has been said that alertness, sleep, and anesthesia protect against currents. The greater the *duration* of contact the more serious the effect, regardless of type of current and nature of contact or resistance (Pearl).

Death from the electrical current may be due to (1) primary fibrillation of the ventricles, (2) failure of the respiratory center, (3) ventricular fibrillation combined with respiratory paralysis, (4) prolonged tetanus of the respiratory musculature, (5) *delayed death.*

Pathology: Damage to the nervous system is found in some degree in many cases of death from the electrical current. Damage to the nerve cells is common and is greatest in the parts traversed by the current. The degree and type of damage to the nerve cells varies. Parenchymatous changes are found in the peripheral nerves and the anterior horn cells of the spinal cord may show severe damage. Large splits or fissures in the cerebral cortex were found in an electrocuted criminal (Hassin), associated with swelling and chromatolysis of the ganglion cells and neuroglial changes. They were found in all layers of the cortex, were most marked in the basal ganglia, and less marked in the medulla and spinal cord. Punctate hemorrhages are found in the cerebrum and in the floor of the fourth ventricle when large currents are passed through the body. These are not found when death is produced by smaller currents.

Symptoms: Electrical shock results either in death or recovery, and in most of the latter instances no sequelae are encountered. Headache is common following the shock, but it is not persistent. Convulsions may develop in the acute stages. Peripheral nerve paralyses have been noted as sequelae and also hemiparesis or hemiplegia. Neurotic syndromes, anxiety, and organic mental syndromes have been encountered. Peripheral neuritis may follow. Choreo-athetosis has been recorded after electrical shock.

Treatment: Treatment consists first of all of freeing the victim from the current. If the patient is merely dazed with normal heart action and respirations, only fresh air and quiet are necessary. If he is unconscious, not breathing but with palpable pulse, or without pulse or heart beat, artificial respiration is immediately necessary. Ventricular fibrillation is common and if found to be present artificial respiration should be stopped. Potassium and calcium and cardiac massage are indicated for the cardiac condition, but are rarely effectual. Caffeine or epinephrine may be used.

XIII. HEAT EXHAUSTION AND HEAT STROKE

Heat exhaustion is characterized by extreme fatigue, vertigo, dimness of vision, and inability to make physical effort. The face is pale, the skin cold and clammy, the pulse weak and rapid, and the pupils dilated. The mouth temperature is usually normal but the rectal temperature is slightly increased.

Cramps develop frequently on exposure to heat in boiler or engine rooms where perspiration is excessive. Severe muscle cramps occur, often associated with nausea and vomiting and gastrointestinal cramps. Evidences of dehydration are present, seen in scanty urine and concentration of the blood. Salt is lost from the tissues rapidly. The condition may be prevented to a large extent by the ingestion of sodium chloride (gr. 5 to 10) as often as necessary to maintain the chloride balance. Once the condition develops, it may be combated by saline intravenously.

Heat stroke may develop on prolonged exposure to the sun or to heat in heated chambers. Headache may indicate onset of the disorder, followed soon by confusion or delirium, or by unconsciousness. The body temperature is high, the skin dry and hot, respirations deep and labored, and later irregular, and the pulse very fast (140 to 180). Petechiae may be seen. Treatment is unsatisfactory and the mortality high. Reduction of the temperature is important. This may be done by spraying the patient with water and cooling with fans. Massage to maintain circulation is important. Salt should be given in abundance. Plasma may be useful in patients showing evidence of shock.

18

Vegetative Nervous System and Endocrine Disorders

I. ANATOMY AND PHYSIOLOGY

A working knowledge of the anatomy and physiology of the vegetative nervous system is essential for an understanding of the various diseases which are associated with this portion of the neural mechanism.

The synonyms for the term autonomic nervous system are the vegetative nervous system and the involuntary nervous system. The autonomic nervous system is divisible anatomically, physiologically, and pharmacologically into two divisions: (1) the thoracolumbar or sympathetic, and (2) craniosacral or parasympathetic nervous system. The term sympathetic nervous system is also employed by some authors to include both divisions and thus may be used synonymously with the term autonomic nervous system.

The sympathetic or thoracolumbar division has its central neurons in the lateral horns of the gray matter of the thoracic and lumbar spinal cord. The fibers originating from these neurons leave by way of the anterior root and are myelinated. They leave the peripheral nerves in a group, which because of the myelination is known as the white ramus communicantes. These fibers are preganglionic and for the most part end in the paravertebral ganglia. This chain of ganglia, lying on either side of the vertebral column, is connected and extends from the coccyx into the cervical region. However, the fibers to the cervical ganglia come from the thoracic cord and the cervical spinal cord takes no part in the formation of the autonomic nervous system. The axones of the ganglion cells, the postganglionic fibers, are unmyelinated, and leave the ganglia in a group known as the gray ramus communicantes. These progress to the appropriate structures and terminate in the visceral ganglia, as, for example, the coeliac plexuses of the intestine. Many of the preganglionic fibers progress through the ganglia without synapse and terminate in the more peripheral ganglia.

The neurons giving rise to the craniosacral or parasympathetic division are situated in the brain stem and in the sacral cord. Their fibers progress without the intervention of ganglia (as in the thoracolumbar system) to the viscera and terminate in local ganglia, as, for example, Meissner's and Auerbach's plexuses of the intestine. The fibers are conducted by means of the sacral roots and the following cranial nerves: oculomotor, facial, glossopharyngeal, and vagus.

In addition to the peripheral mechanism and its connection with the gray matter of the spinal cord, there are control centers existing at higher levels in the cerebrospinal axis. In the medulla, especially in the areas about the dorsal motor nucleus of the vagus, are important areas concerned with vegetative functions, such as cardiac rate, blood pressure, and respiration. While these centers are not anatomically demarcated, the physiological evidence for their existence is unequivocal. At a still higher level, the hypothalamus presents a constellation of nuclear masses which are divisible into posterior and lateral groups which are primarily concerned with sympathetic functions and an anterior group subserving parasympathetic functions. Even the cerebral cortex is concerned to some extent with the maintenance of vegetative functions. Thus there have been demonstrated areas stimulation of which evoke cardiac acceleration and deceleration, increase or decrease of blood pressure level. These cortical areas, however, are not of primary importance.

The viscera and structures enervated by the autonomic nervous system are the recipients of fibers from both the craniosacral and thoracolumbar divisions. Thus the iris receives fibers from the thoracolumbar division by way of the cervical sympathetic ganglia and impulses propagated over these fibers lead to pupillary dilatation. In addition, the iris is enervated by fibers from the Edinger-Westphal component of the oculomotor nucleus and the impulses progressing over this pathway result in pupillary constriction.

The purpose of this dual innervation by the autonomic nervous system is the maintenance of homeostasis. This is best exemplified by the fact that mammals can adapt themselves to environmental changes, whereas cold-blooded animals are unable to do this. The thoracolumbar division can be considered as held in abeyance to meet emergencies. Discharge over this division occurs in states such as fear, rage, and pain. The parasympathetic, on the other hand, functions more constantly and is concerned primarily with the protection, conservation, and restoration of bodily resources. The

regulation of gastrointestinal normal functioning with peristalsis, the vegetative phenomena in the complex acts of defecation and urination, the maintenance of moderate cardiac rate and blood pressure; these are factors brought about by the functioning of the parasympathetic nervous system. When in response to threats from the environment the sympathetic nervous system functions predominate, bronchiolar dilation allows for greater respiratory exchange, thus meeting a greater oxygen demand; the blood supply of skeletal muscles is increased to supply greater metabolic needs; visceral peristalsis ceases and the sphincters remain closed. The individual is ready for defensive flight or aggression. A state of individual preparedness with mobilization of forces exists. In a general way, this presents the rôle of the sympathetic and parasympathetic nervous systems, and, like all generalizations, is open to exception.

The maintenance of homeostasis is further subserved by the operation of certain autonomic reflex mechanisms. The best known of these are concerned with cardiovascular regulation as, for example, the carotid sinus and aortic depressor mechanisms. These mechanisms consist essentially of sensory endings susceptible to blood pressure changes or alterations in the oxygen-carbon dioxide composition of the blood, and by the reflex production of changes in cardiac rate, blood pressure, and respirations serve to offset these alterations, thus maintaining constant or relatively constant blood supply of cerebral structures.

The afferent fibers of the autonomic nervous system conduct stimuli other than those beyond the realm of consciousness. Pain can undoubtedly be mediated by this system. This is indicated by the sensitivity of the viscera when the proper stimulus is employed.

While the hollow viscera are not sensitive to pin prick or thermal changes, dilatation of the lumen produces pain. Likewise ischemia of the cardiac muscle, as in anginal attacks or coronary occlusion, yields pain and since extirpation of the cervical sympathetic ganglia obviates this pain, the mediation must be over the sympathetic nervous system.

Pain other than visceral can likewise be mediated by the autonomic nervous system. Recent investigation has revealed that pain in the face in the distribution of the trigeminal nerve and following herpes zoster along that nerve's fibers can be relieved by extirpation of the cervical sympathetic ganglia.

Various and varied drugs affect the two divisions of the autonomic nervous system. Paralysis of one division produces a similar response to stimulation of the other. Thus paralysis of the parasympathetic by atropine produces pupillary dilation, bronchiolar dilation, decreased salivation and peristalsis, and increased cardiac rate. While therapeutically there are many pitfalls in the use of the drugs affecting the autonomic nervous system due to the production of side effects, the pharmacodynamics illustrate the divergence between the two divisions. Typical drug effects can be briefly summarized as follows: Effects of stimulation of the parasympathetic nervous system are produced by choline and acetylcholine; those of depression by atropine and allied drugs. The effects of sympathetic stimulation are induced by epinephrine and sympathin, those of depression by nicotine. An important exception in this scheme is the failure of sweat glands to follow the physiological plan.

This brief sketch of the autonomic nervous system presents in a general fashion the anatomical, physiological, and pharmacological differences between the two divisions of the autonomic nervous system and outlines the manner in which, by their interplay, the internal environment is maintained for the usual bodily functions and prepared for the emergencies inherent in environment. For more detailed accounts, reference should be made to the monographs by White and Kuntz.

II. FACIAL HEMIATROPHY

Facial hemiatrophy is a rare condition characterized by atrophy of the face, usually of one side. It is found chiefly in early life (ten to twenty years), but subjects younger than ten years are not unknown. The *cause* of the condition is not yet determined. Heredity plays no rôle in most cases. Previous infections (general or localized) have been held responsible in some cases (diphtheria, mastoiditis, tuberculous adenitis, infected teeth). Trauma has preceded some cases. The disease is probably the result of involvement of the vegetative nervous system and is regarded variously as resulting from (1) disease of the cervical sympathetic nerves, (2) vasospasm. The disease is regarded as a release phenomenon due to disturbances of higher centers, leading to increased and irregular activity of the lower centers (Wartenberg). By this concept, the disease is regarded as a heredodegeneration, but the irritation of the peripheral sympathetic nervous system which causes the hemiatrophy is not in the peripheral system itself, but comes from higher centers. Instances of facial hemiatrophy have been recorded in thyroid enlargement, cervical rib, cicatrix involving the neck, sarcoma of a cervical vertebra, and trauma following mastoidectomy.

Symptoms: They develop gradually at any point on the face—about the orbit, the angle of the mouth, the wing of the nose, or along the malar prominence. The process spreads out from this local atrophic center usually until the entire half of the face is involved, but it may stop anywhere in the course of its development, resulting in a focal or circumscribed atrophy. The skin, subcutaneous tissue, muscle, and bone are involved in the process. The face on the affected side assumes an atrophic appearance, the skin is smooth and shiny, the normal wrinkling of the skin is absent, the cheek is sunken, the muscles small, the bones of the face sharply outlined and covered by a tightly-drawn skin. The muscles are small due to the wasting of their fat and connective tissue elements. There may be in some instances an associated atrophy of the corresponding side of the tongue. Instances are known of extension of the process to the opposite side of the face. The process extends at times to involve the neck, shoulder, or even an entire half of the body. Falling out of the hair or blanching of the eyebrows may develop. Alopecia areata may be found. Sweating may be increased or decreased on the affected side. Pigmented nevi may be associated with the condition, as well as telangiectasis.

The condition must be differentiated from scleroderma and from all conditions causing facial hemiatrophy. The distinction between scleroderma and facial hemiatrophy may be impossible. The facial atrophies due to syringobulbia, amyotrophic lateral sclerosis, etc., are characterized by distinct evidences of anterior horn cell disease such as muscle fasciculations, reaction of degeneration, etc., and by other evidences of the diseases in question.

The disease is self-limited, burning itself out, as it were, leaving the face disfigured and atrophic.

Treatment: The only treatment which has proved of value thus far consists of plastic reconstruction of the atrophic face.

III. PROGRESSIVE LIPODYSTROPHY
(Lipodystrophia Progressiva, Lipodystrophy Cephalothoracica)

Progressive lipodystrophy is characterized by a symmetrical and progressive loss of subcutaneous fat from the face, neck, arms, thorax, and abdomen with complete or relative sparing of the pelvic girdles and lower limbs.

The disease appears most frequently between four and six years of age, affects females much more frequently than males, and has no familial or hereditary features. Its *cause* is not known. Hyperthyroidism has been reported in some cases and pituitary deficiency in others. A disorder of the vegetative nervous system resulting in disappearance of the fatty subcutaneous tissue is the most probable basic factor.

The development of *symptoms* is gradual, with a normal history of physical and mental growth prior to the onset. Fat disappears first from the face, the features assuming a thin, peaked appearance. This is not, as a rule, regarded as of significance at the onset, until it reaches a moderately advanced state. The process extends from the face to the neck, thorax, arms, and abdomen, with a resulting cachectic appearance in contrast to the well-preserved contour of the lower portions of the body. In some instances the process may be confined to the face; in others, it may involve only the face, neck, and arms. Not only do the lower limbs and pelvic girdles appear well preserved, but in some instances there may be an overdeposit of fat in these regions.

Examination reveals almost a total absence of subcutaneous fat in the affected parts. The skin is loose, and has lost its normal elasticity. The result is a cadaverous appearance which is frequently repulsive. The muscles, bones, hair, and sweat glands are normal. The disease may advance rapidly in one to two years or, in other instances, may take eight to ten years to unfold completely.

There is no impairment of muscle power and no loss of vigor resulting from the disturbance and patients with the disorder suffer no ill effects in regard to strength or ability to work. Emotional problems resulting from the need to adjust to the physical distortion resulting from the disease require careful treatment.

IV. RAYNAUD'S DISEASE

Raynaud's disease is a form of peripheral vascular disturbance caused by tonic contraction of the smaller arteries in the extremities, involving symmetrical areas in the hands and feet, causing periods of cyanosis or pallid asphyxia, associated with intermittent spasms of the terminal arteries, and occurring chiefly in young subjects.

The disease favors women much more than men, its incidence in females being about ten times that in males. The onset of symptoms occurs somewhere between puberty and the menopause and is rare in childhood or old age. The cause is probably a vasospasm affecting the terminal arteries, leaving the main branches unaffected, and is associated with a greatly exaggerated tendency to vasospasm in affected cases (Raynaud). Some maintain that vasomotor activity in Raynaud's disease is normal and that the peripheral spasm is due to local contraction of the smooth muscle in the digital arterioles (Lewis).

No changes are found in the peripheral vessels in early Raynaud's disease either on autopsy or by arteriographic studies. In the advanced stages, definite changes are found and are characterized by an obliterating endarteritis which is indistinguishable from Buerger's disease The capillaries in advanced cases are elongated, tortuous, and dilated. Ulcers appear in the skin at the tips of the fingers after prolonged periods of asphyxia. Later they may extend down to the bone. The subcutaneous tissue shows marked fibrotic changes in later stages. The sympathetic ganglia show vessel narrowing. edema of the connective tissue, and degenerative changes of the ganglion cells.

Symptoms: The symptoms develop gradually. *Pallor* of the affected fingers is noted, especially on exposure to cold or by strong emotional stimuli. This may involve all the fingers and toes, only some of them, or only the fingers or toes. The symmetry of the disease is one of its most striking features. Corresponding digits are involved almost always. The attacks of pallor are short and intermittent, lasting a few minutes only, and are followed or accompanied by cyanosis or redness. *Cyanosis* usually appears early and in advanced cases persists in greater or lesser degree. Repetition of the attacks is characteristic, at first infrequently, later much more frequently and with less complete recovery from the attacks as time goes on. Associated with the pallor are *numbness* and painful paresthesias, with a sensation of unpleasant burning or "pins and needles" sensation on recovery. Excessive sweating of the hands and feet is common and is likely to be increased by emotional upsets or excitement. As the disease develops and the recovery from the vasospasms is less complete, the fingers may remain permanently cyanosed and small areas of gangrene may develop on the ends of the digits. Ulcerations may occur. Sclerodermal changes frequently develop, and epilepsy has been found in some cases.

In the advanced stages of the disease, normal circulation is impossible and patients even in warm weather are forced to take steps to keep their fingers warm by gloves, muffs, etc.

Diagnosis: This is not difficult if the criteria demanded by Raynaud are followed. These are: (1) intermittent episodes of pallor, cyanosis, and redness; (2) bilateral and often symmetrical distribution; (3) absence of evidence of occlusion of the vessels.

Treatment: *Surgical.* Medical treatment is, on the whole, ineffective. Sympathectomy offers the most relief in early cases in which no changes in the vessels are present. The result is permanent vasodilatation and cure of the disorder. The operation must section preganglionic fibers to be successful. In the leg, excision of the second and third, or first, second, and third lumbar ganglia must be performed. The arm can be denervated by dividing the rami of the second and third thoracic ganglia and cutting the trunk below the third ganglion.

V. ACROCYANOSIS

Acrocyanosis is characterized by a *local asphyxia* involving the hands and the lower third of the forearms in typical cases. The feet and the lower third of the legs are often involved as well. The nose is sometimes involved. The affected portions of the limbs are cyanotic and colder than normal. Trophic changes in the form of hypertrophy of the soft parts are found, but the bones are unaffected. In a small number of cases, atrophy of the ends of the fingers is found. Subjective sensory disturbances are common in the form of numbness, pricking sensations, etc. Objectively, no sensory disturbances are usually found, but a decrease in sensory appreciation for all forms of superficial sensation (touch, heat, cold, pain), with greatest involvement of pain and cold, has been described in some cases.

The diseases affects women more frequently than men. It is particularly prone to develop at puberty, but may appear from puberty to menopause. Hereditary tendencies have been reported in some cases. Emotional factors may play a significant rôle in the production of the illness. The disease has followed infections of many sorts: osteomyelitis, encephalitis, tuberculosis, syphilis. The endocrine system has been accused of playing a causative rôle in the disorder, particularly involvement of the parathyroid, suprarenals, and hypophysis.

VI. ERYTHROMELALGIA

This is a rare disease, characterized by *redness* and *pain* in the extremities. It may develop at any age and appears to be more common in males. The cause is unknown. Trauma or use of the hands in strenuous occupations has preceded the onset in a number of cases. Infections appear to be of no significance.

The outstanding symptom is *paroxysmal pain,* a boring or sticking pain of great intensity, which is at first intermittent and then constant, aggravated by heat, constriction, and a dependent position of the limb, and relieved by cold. Redness and swelling appear after the pain has been present a varying length of time. Pressure causes disappearance of the redness. The surface temperature is increased.

The feet are most affected, but all four extremities may be involved. Hyperhidrosis may be found. Trophic disturbances of many sorts may be encountered, thickening of the skin, thickened and curved nails, etc. Atrophy of the skin may be present. Changes may be found in the joints. Gangrene is not usually encountered, but in rare instances it may develop.

Treatment consists of elevation of the limbs and cold applications. These may fail eventually to give relief. Sympathectomy has been advocated with some success.

VII. ACROPARESTHESIA

This is an ill-defined syndrome, occurring chiefly in females, most frequently about puberty and the menopause. It must be regarded as a symptom complex and not a disease *sui generis*. There appears to be a relationship, therefore, between sexual function and the development of symptoms in females. Alcoholism is a factor in males. Tuberculosis and trauma have been implicated in some cases.

The condition develops gradually and becomes more intense as it continues. It may develop acutely in some cases.

The *hands* are predominantly affected by sensations variously described as prickling, numbness, formication, etc. The affection is symmetrical, but one hand may be involved. The feet are rarely affected. The condition may spread into the forearms. The paresthesias are intermittent, appear chiefly at night, or on awakening in the morning, and are associated with a sensation of stiffness and lack of facility of movement of the fingers, which may be relieved by rubbing, vigorous massage, slapping, and movement of the fingers and hands. Pain may develop and may become so severe as to arouse the patient from sleep. Examination reveals nothing of significance in most cases.

The *diagnosis* is not difficult as a rule and is made on the basis of its occurrence in women, the absence of disease of the blood vessels and of objective neurological findings. Organic diseases of the nervous system may begin in similar fashion and it is here that greatest care must be taken. Cervical cord tumor, either intra- or extramedullary, may begin with paresthesia, as well as syringomyelia.

Acromegaly not infrequently begins in this fashion, but offers no difficulties. Tetany may be distinguished by increased muscle irritability and its acute onset. Multiple neuritis is easily distinguished by decreased motor power, decreased or absent reflexes, and nerve tenderness. Subacute combined degeneration of the cord will be manifested by varied combinations of posterior and lateral column disease, with disturbance of position and/or vibration sense, weakness of the limbs, Babinski's sign, etc.

The *treatment* is entirely symptomatic. Contrast baths may be helpful. Estrogenic substance by mouth or injection may relieve symptoms in menopausal cases, and is sometimes dramatically successful. Surgery is not indicated.

VIII. ANGIONEUROTIC EDEMA
(Quincke's Edema)

Angioneurotic edema is at times associated with nervous symptoms. It is characterized by *circumscribed swelling* of the skin and subcutaneous tissues and at times of the mucous membranes. Heredity plays a rôle in many cases and familial incidence is not uncommon. Allergic factors play an important part in causation; many sorts of foods and drugs have been implicated in the production of the symptoms. Infection, local trauma, and a neuropathic constitution are factors in causation of the disorder.

Attacks of edema develop acutely and rapidly and involve both skin and internal organs. They are painless and may involve a hand, forearm, the face, or, in rare instances, the entire body. The edema is firm and nonpitting. The mucous membranes of the larynx and pharynx are often affected, resulting in edema of the glottis, swelling of the uvula, tongue, etc. Effusions into the joints may be found, as well as edema involving the internal organs.

Involvement of the nervous system is common. Optic neuritis and choked disc have been observed frequently. Numerous subjective cerebral symptoms have been recorded — drowsiness, headache, mental disturbances, generalized convulsions, and loss of consciousness. Hemiplegia, aphasia, and even focal jacksonian convulsions have been recorded during the course of the disorder.

The *diagnosis* offers no difficulty in cases with typical edematous manifestations. More difficult is the relationship between cerebral symptoms and allergy without circumscribed skin edema. Headache, convulsions, transient hemiparesis or hemiplegia have all been observed and are regarded by some as occurring frequently in allergic states. The association between allergy and cerebral symptoms may be established with certainty when (1) allergy is definitely demonstrable; (2) cerebral manifestations develop in close association with allergic attacks.

IX. ADIPOSIS DOLOROSA (*Dercum's Disease*)

Adiposis dolorosa is a rare disease, occurring chiefly in women of middle age and characterized by painful subcutaneous fatty masses. A diffuse form is also known. The cause of the disease is not known, but endocrine dysfunction undoubtedly plays a rôle in the production of the disorder. Symptoms develop gradually, usually in women who are already obese. Nodular masses are noted in the skin, associated with pain and with tenderness on pressure. The tender, nodular masses become indurated with time. Pains in the joints are common. Pain may be so severe as to become paroxysmal. Weakness is an outstanding symptom, but is without organic basis in the nervous system. Neuritis is sometimes found in association with the condition, with tenderness along the nerve trunks. Mental symptoms are common but assume no specific type. Depression and intellectual deteriorations are common.

The treatment is purely symptomatic for the pain. The adiposity rarely responds to measures, endocrine or otherwise.

X. ENDOCRINE DISORDERS

Neurological and psychiatric disorders of various sorts may develop during endocrine diseases. Since many of these disorders are not primarily neurological in nature, no effort will be made to describe them in detail. Reference will be made rather to their neuropsychiatric manifestations.

Hyperinsulinism: Neuropsychiatric symptoms of many sorts are common in hyperinsulinism, but their incidence is difficult to define. They are common in

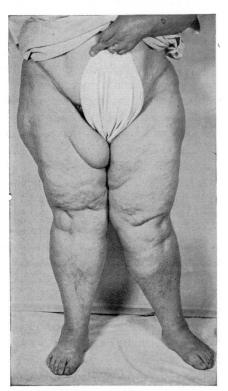

Fig. 214—*Adiposis dolorosa,* showing the heavy and characteristic deposit of fat.

hyperinsulinism, but hyperinsulinism as a cause of the neuropsychiatric symptoms listed below is not common. Most important is the recognition of the fact that nervous symptoms may be the first manifestation of the disease, as in the case of pernicious anemia. The onset of *symptoms* is gradual, often without awareness on the part of the patient of connection with food intake. Hunger pains, the development of symptoms on arising in the morning or in late morning or afternoon, their onset after exertion, are suggestive complaints. The neuropsychiatric symptoms may be divided into three groups (Wilder): (1) vegetative symptoms; (2) organic neurological symptoms; (3) psychiatric manifestations.

Vegetative symptoms consist of feelings of fatigue, drowsiness, hunger, sweating, or chills. Of these, fatigue is by far the most conspicuous. Other symptoms include flushing, pallor, tremors, acroparesthesias, salivation, nausea, bradycardia, and extrasystoles.

Organic neurological manifestations differ widely in variety and intensity. They may be mild or severe. They consist of headache, diplopia, speech disturbances, impairment of coördination, hemiplegia, aphasia, impairment of consciousness, involuntary movements of a choreiform nature, blindness, generalized or focal convulsions, petit mal episodes, and a number of other symptoms too numerous to mention. Forced laughing and crying, perseveration of speech, and amnesia have been found in some cases.

Among the *psychiatric manifestations* are maniacal outbursts, impulsiveness, sexual aggressiveness, depression, and a variety of complaints resembling neurosis.

The *pathological background* of the neuropsychiatric symptoms in hyperinsulinism reveals no uniform picture— studies both in experimental animals and humans reveal disease of the cortical ganglion cells, usually severe or moderately severe, of a nonspecific nature. Areas of focal cell loss may be found and in a few reported instances punctate hemorrhages were found. The pathological findings fail to explain adequately the clinical neuropsychiatric manifestations, since they are often milder than the clinical features. In some cases no significant brain changes have been found.

The symptoms have no direct relationship to the level of the blood sugar, severe manifestations occurring often with blood sugar levels higher than with milder symptoms. Interference with the oxidative processes of the brain cells is important in the production of symptoms. The early appearance of neuropsychiatric symptoms is accounted for by the fact that sugar is a most important constituent of nerve cell metabolism, and that nerve cells fail to store sugar; hence a deprivation of sugar is quickly felt.

Diagnosis: The *diagnosis* of neuropsychiatric symptoms due to hyperinsulinism is usually not easy. In typical instances, the condition may be suspected (1) with a history of onset of symptoms with hunger, after fasting, or following exertion; (2) relief of symptoms on feeding. With such a background, confirmatory studies can be made to establish definitely the diagnosis. As a rule, however, the indications are less decisive. A history of recurrent cerebral episodes, such as hemiparesis, convulsive attacks, etc., must always lead to a suspicion of hyperinsulinism. The lapses of consciousness and the petit mal episodes which occur during the disease are never as definite as in epilepsy. Even intelligent patients find great difficulty in describing them, and it is precisely this vagueness which should lead to suspicion of hyperinsulinism. In contrast, the epileptic has no difficulty as a rule in describing his petit mal episodes. The electroencephalogram may be helpful. In hyperinsulinism, the electroencephalogram appears to have been normal in the few cases in which it has been recorded.

The condition must be suspected in the presence of mental symptoms in a patient with no previous history of mental illness, in the atypical features of attacks, and in the presence of a well-integrated personality structure free from such episodes in the past and unlikely apparently on the basis of purely psychogenic factors to develop mental illness. *Hysteria* is not infrequently diagnosed in hyperinsulinism because of the bizarre nature of the petit mal episodes and even of the other neurological symptoms. The error serves but to emphasize once more the danger of a diagnosis of hysteria on such a basis. *Brain tumor* is a plausible diagnosis in the presence of focal brain manifestations, such as focal convulsions, aphasia, hemiparesis, etc., but manifestations of increased pressure are invariably lacking. *Cerebral vascular spasm* is at times diagnosed because of the recurrent attacks, but should not be entertained seriously in the absence of a labile vasomotor system, a labile blood pressure, or a hyperactive carotid sinus.

Hyperthyroidism: Hyperthyroidism may at times be associated with organic neurological symptoms, but psychiatric manifestations are more common. Ocular palsies are not common in patients with exophthalmos, but they are found at times. Impairment of lateral movements of the eyeballs is most common, but ophthalmoplegias of varying degree may be observed. Loss of convergence is sometimes seen. Optic atrophy has been observed. Progressive muscular atrophy may on rare occasions be simulated by exophthalmic goiter. The atrophy of the muscles is marked and is associated with fasciculations. It is more widespread, however, than in the classical form of progressive muscular atrophy, is not apt to be associated with bulbar symptoms, and is unassociated with reaction of degeneration. Hyperthyroidism may also simulate myasthenia gravis very closely. Paralyses of the facial, trigeminal, and hypoglossal nerves have been found in hyperthyroidism. Muscle cramps, choreiform movements, epileptic attacks, and multiple neuritis have been observed. Psychoses are not uncommon, but they have no specific features. As a rule, they are toxic psychoses with a coloring of the psychosis compatible with the premorbid personality. Depressed states and excitements are common. Neurotic manifestations, such as anxiety, nervousness, and phobias frequently occur.

Hypothyroidism: The hypothyroid patient is sluggish and slow as compared with the hyperthyroid subject. Organic neurological manifestations are uncommon. Posterolateral sclerosis has been described associated with myxedema, but is probably to be regarded as an incidental finding. Disturbances of hearing are quite common. Smell and taste are disturbed in about one-third of the cases. Cerebellar syndromes have been described and have disappeared with thyroid medication. Paresthesias are common. Headaches and vertigo are common.

Psychoses occur in about fifteen per cent of myxedema patients. Depressions predominate and slowness of thought and action are commonly found.

Hyperparathyroidism: On occasion, hyperparathyroidism is responsible for symptoms referable to the nervous system. It is rare, but its very rarity makes it necessary to consider it as a cause of unusual neurological syndromes.

The condition occurs usually as a result of hyperfunctioning of a parathyroid tumor with resultant overproduction of parathyroid hormone. Functional hyperparathyroidism may develop from the administration of parathyroid hormone. The *symptoms* which herald the onset of the condition are vague and nonspecific, and are, therefore, usually disposed of as neurotic. For some time there may be a complaint of paresthesias or of muscle cramps, often with a story of muscle twitchings as well. Pains are not uncommon and in some instances may dominate the picture. They may be typically radicular or peripheral nerve pains, but they are as often vague and ill defined, hence here, too, their disposal as neurotic in many instances. Weakness is a common symptom and may be the outstanding feature of the history. Increased tenseness and emotional instability are common features of the story, all of which adds to the impression of neurosis. In rare instances, convulsions occur during the course of the disease. Psychoses may occur. Diabetes insipidus has been reported in the course of the disease.

The typical manifestations of the disease are seen in the condition known as osteitis fibrosa cystica with demineralization of the bones, bowing of the legs, kyphosis of the spine, numerous tumors and bone cysts of varying size, hypotonia of the muscles and secondary anemia. In not a few instances, the fully developed condition of osteitis fibrosa cystica is not seen. Among the neurological conditions which may be found in hyperparathyroidism are asthenia and neuritis. In instances in which there has been collapse of a vertebra due to a pathological fracture, evidences of compression of the spinal cord may be found. This may be a complete transverse syndrome or there may be evidence of an incomplete transverse lesion. Cerebral symptoms are not common, but convulsions are known to occur in rare cases.

The blood calcium is increased, the blood phosphorus decreased, and the loss of calcium increased in the urine.

The diagnosis of *hyperparathyroidism* is dependent on the demonstration of the bony changes by roentgen examination, and the finding of the blood changes mentioned above. The importance of the condition neurologically lies in its resemblance to neurosis, neuritis, and other obscure conditions. In a doubtful case, not previously neurotic, with a history of weakness, pains, emotional tension, etc., particularly if there has been a previous history of muscular spasms and fractures, hyperparathyroidism must be suspected. Paget's disease, multiple myeloma, and osteoporosis must be distinguished from the condition.

The treatment consists of removal of a parathyroid tumor, which often results in symptomatic improvement.

Hypoparathyroidism: This condition is found most frequently in patients who have undergone thyroidectomy and have had unwittingly partial removal of the parathyroid gland. Idiopathic cases occur. The symptom-complex associated with parathyroid lack is characterized by *tetany*. The history is characterized by a long story of paresthesias of the extremities, muscle twitchings and cramps, and often convulsions. Muscle irritability is striking. Attacks of carpopedal spasm are common and are featured by attacks of sharp flexion of the wrist and ankle joints. Examination reveals (1) a positive Chvostek's sign, characterized by twitching of the mouth and face on tapping the face in the distribution of the facial nerve; (2) a positive Trousseau's sign, characterized by the production of carpopedal spasm on constriction of the arm or leg above the wrist or ankle; (3) a positive Erb's sign, consisting of increased electrical excitability of motor nerves. The serum calcium is low; there is a fall in urinary calcium excretion, a rise in serum phosphorus, and a fall in urinary phosphorus excretion.

Cerebral symptoms of various sorts may develop during hypoparathyroidism. Seizures, choked disc, psychiatric disorders, and mental retardation may be found. Choked disc is not an uncommon occurrence. Calcification of the basal ganglia may at times be seen in the roentgenogram.

The diagnosis both by symptoms and laboratory findings is not difficult, but a careful distinction must be made between idiopathic and secondary or symptomatic tetany.

Hypopituitary Syndromes: Decrease or loss of function of the pituitary gland gives rise to the Froelich syndrome or one of its fractions. The features of this syndrome have already been described (Pituitary Tumors). Associated with it are numerous neuropsychiatric symptoms, such as diabetes insipidus, fatigue, hypersomnolence, excessive susceptibility to cold, and excessive desire for sweets. Petit mal attacks and at times grand mal seizures may be encountered. Mental dullness is common but psychoses are rare. It is doubtful whether such symptoms as diabetes insipidus, hypersomnolence, and desire for sweets are due primarily to pituitary deficiency. The probabilities favor involvement of the adjacent hypothalamus as the cause of these symptoms.

Pituitary cachexia (Simmond's disease) is a rare manifestation of pituitary deficiency. It is associated with destruction of the anterior lobe of the pituitary gland, associated with carcinoma of the gland, tuberculosis or adenoma of the pituitary. It is characterized by severe emaciation, marked asthenia, loss of teeth and hair, achlorhydria, and secondary anemia, and in women with amenorrhea and sterility. Nervous symptoms are common and are characterized by anxiety, numerous somatic complaints, and an apparent absorption and introspection which stamps such patients as neurotic for long periods of time before the true nature of the condition is recognized. Psychoses develop frequently, especially in the later stages of the disease, but they have no specific features.

Dwarfism represents still another manifestation of destruction or lack of development of the anterior lobe of the hypophysis. It develops during the growth period, before full growth has been attained, and is due to a lack or absence of the growth factor. It is associated with no definite neuropsychiatric manifestations, except for a decreased mental capacity and reactive problems incident to the inferiority experienced as a result of the lack of physical and sexual development.

Hyperpituitary Syndromes: They are characterized by gigantism and acromegaly. In the former, mental retardation is common. In the latter, there are no striking neurological or mental features apart from those due to the presence of a pituitary tumor.

Hypothalamic Syndromes: While much is known concerning the physiological features of the hypothalamus, and much remains to be determined, relatively little is known concerning its clinical syndromes. Physiologically, it may be regarded as a chief vegetative center within the nervous system for the regulation of autonomic functions. It plays a significant rôle in *cardiovascular regulation* through partial control of vasoconstriction and vasodilatation, regulation of blood pressure, and to some extent of heart rate. Thus, heating or cooling the hypothalamus may produce vasodilatation or constriction, electrical stimulation may cause a rise or fall of blood pressure or of heart rate. It acts in unison with lower centers. It plays a significant rôle also in the regulation of *body temperature,* though the precise area of the hypothalamus concerned in this regulation is not yet known. Transection of the brain stem which leaves the hypothalamus intact produces no disturbance of temperature regulation, but destruction of the hypothalamus results in impairment or loss of temperature control. Separate areas exist for the control of heat loss and heat production through the production of panting, sweating, vasodilatation, etc. Loss of temperature regulation is associated with bilateral lesions of the hypothalamus, unilateral lesions causing little or no dysregulation.

The regulation of *water metabolism* is affected through the hypothalamus by means of its connection with the posterior lobe of the hypophysis. This is carried out through the supraoptico-hypophyseal fibers from the supraoptic nucleus in the hypothalamus to the hypophysis. The evidence is somewhat conflicting concerning the relative value of the hypothalamus and the hypophysis in the control of water metabolism, but the preponderance of evidence assigns the more important rôle to the former. *Carbohydrate metabolism* is reported to be influenced by hypothalamic activity, as well as *pilomotor regulation, fat metabolism, and gastrointestinal regulation.* It is probable that the hypothalamus also plays a part in the regulation of sleep. Lesions of this area result at times in hypersomnolence.

Clinically, the destruction of the hypothalamus by tumors or other destructive processes may result in the production of a *hyper-* or *hypothermia* with loss or impairment of the capacity to lose or retain heat in the body. Under rare circumstances, involvement of the hypothalamus may result in a type of epilepsy referred to as *diencephalic autonomic*

epilepsy, characterized by tonic spells and evidences of autonomic dysregulation, such as profuse perspiration, salivation, pupillary changes, tachycardia, etc.

Both clinical and experimental evidence is at hand to indicate that lesions of the hypothalamus may be associated with disturbance in *emotion.* Under such circumstances there is loss of the capacity to control emotions and it seems probable therefore that the hypothalamus plays a rôle in the expression of the emotions. Destruction of the hypothalamus in cats results in the production of a "sham rage" reaction on emotional stimulation, often of an insignificant nature. In some cases of brain tumor involving the hypothalamus, manic states, depression, and anxiety reactions have been observed. How important a rôle the hypothalamus plays in the expression of the emotions, or how it interacts with other areas concerned with the same function is not yet known; but it seems probable that for the expression of emotions, the hypothalamus is extremely important. Much uncertainty exists concerning the occurrence of disturbance of affect with the emotional disturbances of hypothalamic lesions, but in our present state of knowledge it is not possible to say what affect is involved in the process.

Emotional disturbances of various sorts, such as facetiousness, loss of emotional control, and various emotional states are found also with lesions involving the thalamus, and in diseases of the frontal lobes. How these correlate with the hypothalamus is not yet known.

XI. PUBERTAS PRECOX

This condition, characterized by premature bodily and sexual development, is important to recognize because it is associated usually with disease of the nervous system. It is characterized by precocious physical development in young males as a rule, the changes occurring before puberty is reached. The bodily habitus may be larger than normal for the age, the voice is deep, the genitals are much enlarged beyond their expected development, hairy growth in general is accelerated. In women there is enlargement of the breasts. Mental and physical development tends to lag behind the sexual precocity. The condition may be found in (1) tumors involving the pineal gland, under which conditions there is evidence of increased intracranial pressure (choked disc), and impairment or loss of upward gaze of the eyeballs (Parinaud syndrome); (2) tumors involving the hypothalamus; (3) tumors involving the suprarenal cortex, and (4) tumors of the testis.

19

Nuclear Amyotrophies and Myopathies

THE NUCLEAR AMYOTROPHIES

The nuclear amyotrophies include: (1) Progressive spinal muscular atrophy; (2) amyotrophic lateral sclerosis; (3) progressive bulbar paralysis.

All these seemingly different conditions are probably variants of the same process. All are degenerative processes with similar pathological substrates but with involvement of different areas of the nervous system. Whether they have the same cause cannot be stated, since the cause of none of them is known. Transitions between one group and another are quite common. Thus, progressive spinal muscular atrophy may develop features of amyotrophic lateral sclerosis in its clinical course and may show features of the latter under the microscope. So, too, progressive bulbar paralysis may show evidences of amyotrophic lateral sclerosis. The rigid separation of all these entities cannot, therefore, be maintained too strongly. All are probably part of a single group of nuclear amyotrophies.

There is grave doubt in the minds of some whether progressive spinal muscular atrophy is an entity or whether it does not represent the spinal form of amyotrophic lateral sclerosis, particularly in view of its tendency to develop pyramidal tract degeneration eventually. It seems best to regard it as an entity at present, since some cases run a longer and different course than amyothrophic lateral sclerosis.

The nuclear amyotrophies represent, therefore, a group of allied conditions characterized primarily by disease of the anterior horn cells with all the associated symptoms resulting from such disease (weakness or paralysis, atrophy, fasciculations, loss of reflexes, reaction of degeneration). In some forms of the disease (progressive spinal muscular atrophy), the involvement is almost exclusively of the anterior horn cells of the spinal cord; in others, it is exclusively that of the nuclei in the brain stem (progressive bulbar paralysis); in still other variants, the anterior horn cell disease is diffuse, involving spinal cord and brain stem (amyotrophic lateral sclerosis), and is accompanied by involvement of the pyramidal tracts. The fundamental process is essentially the same in all types of nuclear amyotrophies, the difference lying in the area of the neuraxis predominantly afflicted by the process—spinal cord, brain stem, or both. In this sense, the various nuclear amyotrophies are similar and may be regarded as variants of a single form. The key to the nuclear amyotrophies is regarded by some as amyotrophic lateral sclerosis, all other forms being regarded as variants or abortive types of the disease. Despite their similarity, there still remains differences in the main types, so that cases of progressive spinal muscular atrophy run their course without the development of either bulbar signs or evidences of pyramidal tract disease, as in cases of amyotrophic lateral sclerosis.

Until the subject is clarified further, it is best to regard the nuclear amyotrophies as having a common pathological background with minor variations, but with more or less distinct clinical features for the main forms. There is no conclusive evidence to assume a common cause for the various members of the group.

I. PROGRESSIVE SPINAL MUSCULAR ATROPHY

Etiology: The exact cause of progressive spinal muscular atrophy is not known. The disease affects males more commonly than females, and occurs most frequently at 35 to 45 years of age. Abiotrophy (Gowers) may be responsible, the cells of the anterior horns functioning to a certain age and then degenerating. Efforts have been made to distinguish two types, an idiopathic and a secondary type, the former due to no known cause, the latter to a wide variety of secondary causes. Secondary factors of many sorts have been accused of causing or influencing the disease. Extreme fatigue, exposure to cold, and many types of infections have been accused. Trauma is said to precipitate the symptoms in a small percentage of cases but cannot be looked upon as a cause (Turner). Syphilis is regarded as a cause in some cases. Lead poisoning and exposure to gasoline fumes have been found responsible at times.

Pathology: The muscles are atrophied, look pink or yellow, and microscopically show loss of striations, increase of fibrous tissue and sometimes of fat tissue. The anterior horn cells are particularly affected. Those of the cervical cord are most frequently diseased, but the thoracic and lumbar portions of the cord may also be affected. The process is degenerative. The anterior horn cells bilaterally undergo a slow, progressive degeneration with at first involvement of only some cells and eventually of all the cells of the affected anterior horns. The cells are shrunken and show typical chronic cell disease changes. No inflammatory evidences are found, except in the syphilitic form of the disease. The anterior horns shrink as a result of the cell atrophy, which is replaced by glial scar. The cells of the medulla may be affected. The pyramidal tracts of the spinal cord may frequently show evidences of demyelination when no signs of this are detectable clinically.

Symptoms: The onset of the disease is insidious and begins in the small hand muscles. Weakness and awkwardness of the hands are early symptoms, noticeable particularly in finer movements, such as buttoning clothes or picking up small objects. By the time awareness of this develops, however, atrophy of the small hand muscles is present and may be the first difficulty noticed. Weakness of the hands or arms is by far the most common complaint and the one which most often causes the patient to seek medical advice. Wasting of the muscles may, however, be the first noticeable symptom. Paresthesias of the fingers may be an early symptom. Pain is absent, the disease running characteristically a painless course. The weakness spreads from hands to forearms, arms, and shoulder girdles, and it may not be until these are affected that help is sought.

The small hand muscles are atrophied (thenar, hypothenar, lumbricals, interossei). The muscle atrophy may be slight at first, but it becomes intense eventually and is followed by atrophy of all the hand muscles, giving the appearance of a claw hand. The right hand is often affected first and more severely than the left. The thenar eminence and first interosseous muscle are first affected, followed by the other small muscles of the hands. Atrophy is usually present in the forearm, arm, and shoulder girdle muscles at the time of examination, but if not present, the process eventually affects these muscles. The process may spread from the small muscles of the hands to the shoulder girdle muscles, skipping the muscles of the forearm and arm, but in the usual instance it spreads from the hand to the forearm, arm, and shoulder girdle. The atrophy involves the leg muscles in the late stages of the disease, involving particularly the flexors of the foot and leg.

A special form of the disease, involving particularly the shoulder girdle, has been described as the scapulohumeral form and is to be distinguished from this form of myopathy. The process extends from the shoulder girdle to the hand muscles. In rare cases, the disease begins in the lower extremities (Dana). The atrophy is symmetrical, but involvement of one hand or arm for long periods of time is not uncommon before spread of the process to the other side. Fasciculations are found everywhere in the affected muscles. They may be very active in some muscles and absent in others. The biceps and triceps reflexes are absent and reaction of degeneration is present. Atrophy of leg and thigh muscles may develop later. Difficulties in swallowing and phonation from involvement of the nuclei of the medulla may develop. Probably in all cases, evidences of pyramidal tract involvement eventually develop. Sensory findings are absent. Reaction of degeneration is found in the muscles. The spinal fluid findings are normal.

An infantile form of the disease known as the *Werdnig-Hoffmann* type is found in infants during the first year of life, usually in the first few weeks or months of life. It is characterized by flaccid weakness of the trunk and leg muscles, shoulder and pelvic girdles with eventual complete flaccid paralysis and death within the first five years of life. Loose shoulders and hyperextensibility of the joints are found. The reflexes are absent. The leg muscles are affected first, particularly in their proximal segments. There is great variability, however, in this feature, since primary involvement of the arm and shoulder girdle muscles is known. The process spreads peripherally from the proximal portions of the limbs. Bulbar muscles may at times be affected. Atrophy is not always apparent, being hidden by the subcutaneous fat. Fibrillary twitchings may be seen but are usually lacking due to the subcutaneous tissue. Kyphoscoliosis is often present. In some instances, the disease becomes chronic and cases may go on for ten years.

In rare instances, a clinical picture similar to that of progressive muscular atrophy with generalized muscle atrophy, fasciculations, and weakness has been observed in association with pancreatic adenoma (hyperinsulinism).

Diagnosis: The diagnosis is not difficult. The symmetrical involvement of arm and hand muscles by atrophy, fasciculations, and loss of reflexes is sufficient to establish the diagnosis. The diagnostic problem appears usually in the form of a condition with atrophy of the small hand and arm muscles, associated with weakness, reflex loss, and absence of pain. The disturbances are, as a rule, symmetrical and the number of possibilities in such cases is limited—amyotrophic lateral sclerosis, syphilitic meningomyelitis, cervical cord tumor, bilateral cervical rib. In those instances in which the symptoms are unilateral, the problem is more difficult and distinction must be made between cervical rib, scalenus anticus syndrome, and brachial neuritis. The distinction between this and amyotrophic lateral sclerosis may be difficult in some cases, but the differentiation is academic.

Thenar neuritis may closely resemble progressive spinal muscular atrophy. It is usually unilateral, is most common in females with the atrophy confined to the thenar eminence and without fasciculations or evidences of atrophy elsewhere in the hand or arm muscles. It is due to neuritis of a branch of the median nerve and has a good outlook by virtue of its failure to progress.

Cervical rib and scalenus anticus syndrome may cause atrophy of the hand muscles and may be bilateral and symmetrical. Pain in the shoulder and arm, especially at night, coldness of the affected hand or hands, changes in pulse, and the roentgenological evidences of the disease in cervical rib are important factors. Pain is prominent and in this respect the disorder differs radically from progressive muscular atrophy. Muscle atrophy is much less prominent than pain.

Syringomyelia may cause atrophy of the small hand muscles and those of the arm, but is readily differentiated by the segmental loss of pain and temperature and the trophic disturbances.

Spinal cord syphilis may be distinguished by the positive spinal fluid serological findings. Among the conditions which may simulate progressive muscular atrophy, *hyperthyroidism* holds an important place. The wasting in this disease may be extensive and may pick out particularly the muscles involved in progressive muscular atrophy. Even muscle twitchings may be found, simulating fibrillations. Tremor, exophthalmos, and accelerated metabolism usually suffice, however, to differentiate the two conditions.

Cervical hypertrophic pachymeningitis

is featured by pain, paresthesias, and by evidences of cord compression.

Spinal cord tumor involving the anterior surface of the cord may cause atrophy of the hand muscles with or without pain. Evidences of cord compression are present after an interval history of pain.

Superior pulmonary sulcus tumor may be distinguished by the prominent history of shoulder pain, by the Horner's syndrome, the atrophy of the hand muscles and the tumor shadow in the apex of the lung.

Prognosis: The disease runs a slow, progressive course lasting ten to thirty years unless bulbar symptoms intervene, when the course is considerably shortened. Remissions of considerable length may occur during the course of the disease.

Treatment: The treatment is similar to that of amyotrophic lateral sclerosis and is discussed under that heading.

II. AMYOTROPHIC LATERAL SCLEROSIS

Etiology: The disease affects males more often than females. It is a disease of middle age, appearing usually between forty and fifty, but at times in subjects of twenty years or younger. The exact cause is not known. In the vast majority of cases, no assignable cause for the disease can be determined. Overexertion has been implicated in some instances, but this, like the other causes to be mentioned, must be regarded as an incidental factor. Alcohol, lead, and arsenic intoxication have been found in some cases. Previous infections may play a part. Syphilis and epidemic encephalitis may produce syndromes similar to amyotrophic lateral sclerosis; the same is true of typhus and influenza. Trauma has been regarded as a cause in some cases and as a precipitating factor in others. The symptoms in some cases appear in such close relationship to trauma that they are regarded as being directly related to the injury (Jelliffe). It is extremely doubtful whether it plays a part in the cause of the disorder. Most authorities agree that the disease is non-familial and not hereditary, but evidence has been presented that amyotrophic lateral sclerosis occurs as a hereditary disease and that heredity may account for a significant proportion of cases (Kurland). Familial forms may appear in the young and they may make their appearance in adults. The disease has been reported in three siblings with onset in all at fourteen years of age (Kreyenberg); in a father and three sons (Montanaro and Lopez); and in a mother and two daughters (Kalinowsky). Familial forms are not uncommon in the bulbar types.

Pathology: Amyotrophic lateral sclerosis is a systemic disease affecting the pyramidal or corticospinal system from cortex to periphery and the anterior horn cells of the spinal cord. The Betz cells of the motor cortex are often but not always diseased and may be completely diseased or only partially destroyed. The paracentral lobule containing the cells giving rise to the foot fibers are more affected than other portions, but all parts of the motor cortex are diseased. Secondary degeneration of the corticospinal system may be followed in the internal capsule, the peduncle, pons, pyramids of the medulla, and the lateral columns of the spinal cord. It may not be found extending through the entire length of the corticospinal tract, but may stop at various levels, in the pons, medulla, or cord (Davison). Degeneration of the pyramidal tract may be found, therefore, only in the spinal cord, or in the cord and brain stem, or may be followed from the motor cortex throughout

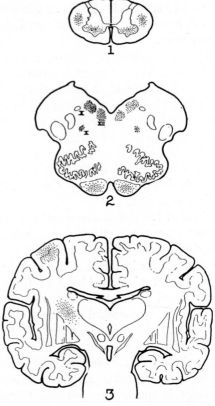

Fig. 215 — *Amyotrophic lateral sclerosis.* The dotted areas show the chief sites of predilection: (1) in the spinal cord (anterior horn cells and pyramidal tracts), (2) brain stem (cranial nerve nuclei and pyramids), (3) cortex (motor area and internal capsule).

the length of the pyramidal tract (Davison).

The nuclei of the brain stem show degeneration, especially the nuclei of the hypoglossal, vagus, facial, trigeminal, and oculomotor nerves. The cells of the anterior horns of the cord show changes similar to those of progressive muscular atrophy. The cervical segments are more affected than those of the thoracic and lumbar regions, but the entire cord is affected in some cases. The large nerve fibers in the anterior roots of the spinal cord are particularly affected, and the

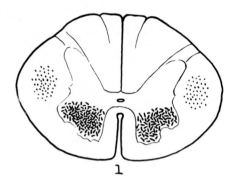

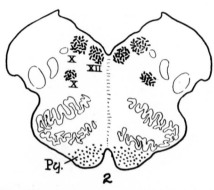

Fig. 216—*Amyotrophic lateral sclerosis.* The classical pattern, illustrating severe anterior horn cell and brain stem involvement with moderately severe pyramidal tract signs.

As in the case of progressive muscular atrophy, weakness and awkwardness in use of the hands or arms are probably the earliest and commonest symptoms. Imperceptible at first, the symptoms become gradually worse in the course of weeks or months until relief is sought. In some instances, weakness of the legs may be the presenting complaint. This is true particularly of those patients in whom spasticity of the legs outweighs the atrophy of the hand and arm muscles. In still others, bulbar symptoms constitute the presenting complaint—difficulty in swallowing and articulation or hoarseness being the most frequent

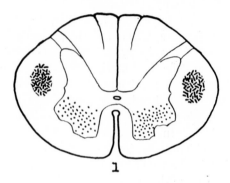

same is true of the large fibers in the pyramidal tracts of the spinal cord (Wohlfort and Swank).

Other fiber tracts may be affected. Among these are the cortical association tracts, posterior longitudinal bundle, rubrospinal tract, and other tracts in the brain stem and cord. The peripheral nerves and spinal roots show degenerative changes in some cases with myelin and axis cylinder loss.

Symptoms: The onset in cases of amyotrophic lateral sclerosis is similar to that of progressive muscular atrophy. The symptoms develop gradually, and are slow of development and recognition.

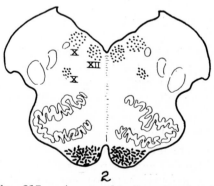

Fig. 217 — *Amyotrophic lateral sclerosis.* One of the many variants of the disease, showing moderate anterior horn cell disease and severe pyramidal tract involvement.

symptoms. In such patients, the duration of the illness before seeking medical
help is usually considerably shorter than
in other subjects because of the disabling nature of the symptoms. Bulbar
symptoms form an integral part of the
presenting illness in most patients with
amyotrophic lateral sclerosis. Sensory
symptoms such as pain around the
shoulder girdle region, are found not infrequently early in amyotrophic lateral
sclerosis, without evidences of objective
sensory disturbances. These occur more
frequently in the symptomatic types of
the disorder.

Atrophy of the hand muscles develops
first, usually bilaterally, but in some
instances unilaterally. The small hand
muscles are affected first, particularly
those of the thenar and hypothenar eminences, the interossei, lumbricals, and
other small hand muscles resulting in a
flat simian hand. Atrophy of the arm
and shoulder girdle muscles develops
quickly. In some cases atrophy may be
found not only in the arms and hands
but in the trunk and thigh and leg muscles as well. In rare cases, the process
may begin in the lower limbs and extend
from there to the arms. Fibrillations are
seen in the muscles everywhere and are
usually quite active in advanced or well-
pronounced cases, but they may be few and
difficult to find in early cases. They may
be localized around the shoulder girdle,
arms, hands or legs in symptomatic cases,
or few and diffuse in instances of true
amyotrophic lateral sclerosis. They bear
no relationship to the degree of atrophy or
weakness, but they are more pronounced
the more severe the degree of illness.

The arm and leg reflexes (biceps, triceps, patellar, Achilles) are overactive.
Babinski's sign is present bilaterally and
ankle clonus may be present. Babinski's
sign is not constant, however. It was
present in forty-three of 112 cases (Swank

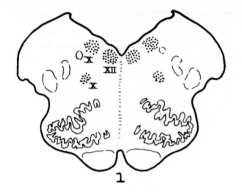

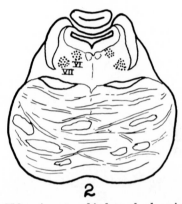

Fig. 218—*Amyotrophic lateral sclerosis.* One
of the variants of the disease, illustrating
pure bulbar involvement with little or no
spinal cord disease and no pyramidal tract
involvement. The clinical picture is that of
pure bulbar paralysis.

and Putnam). The abdominal reflexes
are decreased or absent. The first manifestation of pyramidal tract involvement
is usually hyperreflexia, followed by
Babinski's sign and absence of the abdominal and cremasteric reflexes (Swank
and Putnam). Sensory changes are not
found in the typical case. Subjective
sensory phenomena such as paresthesias
are common; pains may occur and are
not infrequent. Their nature varies.
Cramplike sensations due to spasticity
of the muscles are common. Dull muscle
aches are frequent, as are feelings of
numbness and coldness. Objective sensory changes are rare but have been re-

ported in some cases. Radicular sensory changes, central sensory disturbances of pain and temperature, and loss of position and vibration senses have been recorded. Optic atrophy occurs at times. In some cases there may be a hemiplegic form, with atrophy and fibrillations of the arm and spasticity of the leg. Mental symptoms, such as memory loss, difficulties in concentration and attention, are prominent, and psychoses may dominate the picture in some cases. Emotional instability and unmotivated laughing and crying are seen at times.

Mental symptoms may develop in amyotrophic lateral sclerosis. The mental picture is not uniform, a variety of reactions having been recorded. There is some question concerning the relationship of the mental symptoms to the disease. two concepts holding sway: (1) that the mental symptoms represent an organic syndrome directly related to brain changes in amyotrophic lateral sclerosis, and (2) that the relationship between the mental symptoms and the disease is fortuitous and not causal. They are not of a specific variety. Urgency of urination is not infrequent.

Bulbar symptoms are prominent in amyotrophic lateral sclerosis and develop as first symptoms in 25 to 35 per cent of the subjects. All the patients die eventually from bulbar involvement. The bulbar symptoms may appear as the first sign of the disease, they may develop with the arm and leg involvement early in the disease, or they may appear late in the disorder. They are characterized by difficulties in phonation with resulting indistinctness of speech; trouble in swallowing, especially liquids; hoarseness; and difficulty in chewing. Rarely there may develop ocular palsies. These consist of incomplete or complete ophthalmoplegia, with complete paralysis of ocular

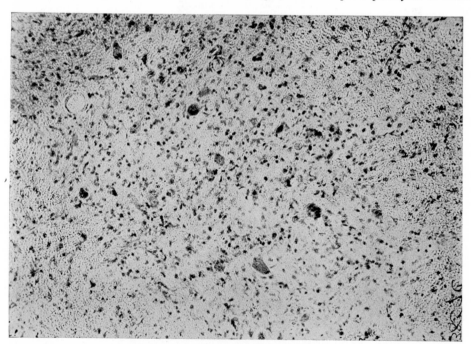

Fig. 219—*Amyotrophic lateral sclerosis.* Cell stain through the anterior horn of the spinal cord showing severe loss of ganglion cells and gliosis. (Courtesy of Dr. Charles Davison.)

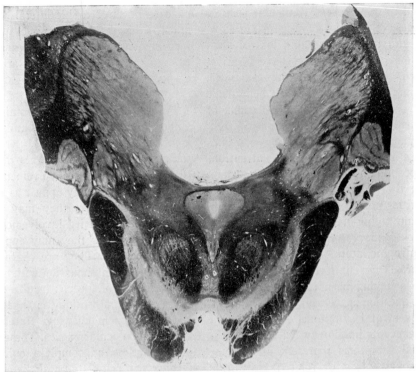

Fig. 220—(See: Fig. 222.)

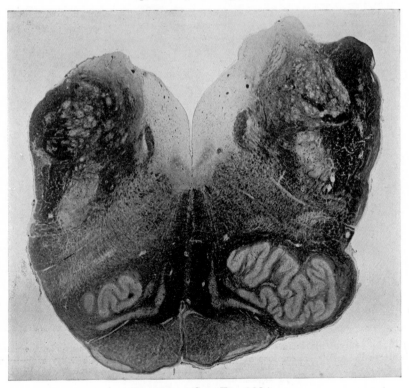

Fig. 221—(See: Fig. 222.)

movement in some instances. Paralysis of upward gaze (Parinaud's syndrome) has been observed. Changes in the reactions of the pupils even to complete lack of reaction to light has been found in rare instances (Spiller).

The manifestations of amyotrophic lateral sclerosis are so varied that a word picture covering all the forms is barely possible. The symptoms in all cases are a combination of amyotrophy (atrophy, weakness), fasciculations, and pyramidal tract involvement. The nature and degree of all these findings vary greatly. In the first place there is great variation in the intensity of involvement of the

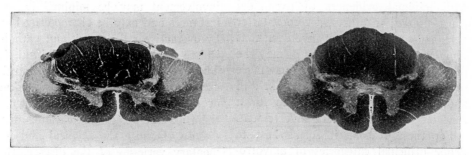

Fig. 222—*Amyotrophic lateral sclerosis.* Myelin sheath stains showing the demyelination of the pyramidal tracts in mesencephalon, medulla, and spinal cord. (Courtesy of Dr. Charles Davison.)

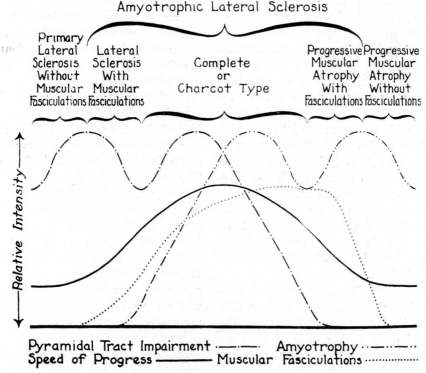

Fig. 223—*Amyotrophic lateral sclerosis.* A diagram showing the wide variation and extent of the amyotrophy, fasciculations, and pyramidal disease in the variants of the disease. (Swank and Putnam: Arch. Neurol. & Psychiat. 49:151, Feb. 1943.)

process; it is more marked in some patients in the medulla, in others in the cord, and in still others in both areas. In the second place there is wide variability in the involvement of the specific structures within the affected areas. In some cases severe anterior horn cell disease dominates the picture and is associated with minimal evidences of pyramidal tract disease; in others, severe anterior horn and pyramidal tract involvement is found; in still others, there may be relatively little anterior horn and more severe pyramidal tract disease; in still another category, there may be for a time only pyramidal tract involvement.

For these reasons it seems best to define principal categories of amyotrophic lateral sclerosis for the sake of clarity in clinical diagnosis. These include: (1) The classical form of Charcot, characterized by atrophy of the hand and arm muscles, accompanied by or followed later by spastic weakness of the legs, and bulbar symptoms. Atypical forms are not uncommon and include instances of involvement of one limb (monoplegic type); of one side of the body (hemiplegic type); of the shoulder girdle with involvement of one or both shoulder girdles; and of the legs, with involvement first of the legs, thighs, or pelvic girdle. Eventually, all the atypical forms develop into typical instances of the disease. (2) Bulbar type, with predominant involvement of the brain stem. (3) Incomplete type, including cases of lateral sclerosis with or without fasciculations.

Diagnosis: The diagnosis of amyotrophic lateral sclerosis offers few difficulties in a well-developed example. The gradual onset in later life of weakness of the limbs, especially the hands and arms, associated with evidence of muscle atrophy, fasciculations of the upper limbs and often of the lower, the occurrence of

bulbar signs, and the presence of pyramidal tract involvement, all seem to make a characteristic picture. The clinical manifestations, however, are not always uniform or stereotyped. Bulbar symptoms may predominate in some cases, with little evidence of involvement of the bodily musculature. Pyramidal tract involvement may be minimal in some instances and may be characterized only by overactive reflexes, without pathological responses such as the Babinski sign. The signs may be asymmetrical in other examples, with atrophy and weakness occurring only in one hand or arm, or there may be hemiplegic varieties of the disease. Despite the atypical and fragmentary varieties of the disease, there is usually enough in the entire clinical picture to establish a clinical diagnosis with certainty. The onset may be with leg symptoms—weakness and stiffness—in many instances, rather than in the arms. Unilateral symptoms—weakness of one arm and/or leg—may predominate for months or rarely for years, before the disease becomes generalized.

Electromyography may aid in the diagnosis of amyotrophic lateral sclerosis, in doubtful cases, but it is not possible in a questionable case to establish the diagnosis by means of the EMG alone. The findings of significance include: (1) the occurrence of fibrillation and fasciculation potentials in the limbs and head region, (2) a reduction in number and increase in size of motor-unit action potentials, and (3) normal excitability of the remaining fibers of motor nerves and a conduction velocity of motor nerves within normal range or not less than 75 per cent of average normal value (Lambert and Mulder).

In the diagnosis of amyotrophic lateral sclerosis, great care must be taken to differentiate the disease from amyotrophic syndromes which may resemble

Table 62—Differential Diagnosis of Diseases Causing Atrophy of the Hand and Arm Muscles

Progressive Muscular Atrophy	Amyotrophic Lateral Sclerosis	Cervical Rib	Scalenus Syndrome	Syringomyelia	Cervical Cord Tumor	Syphilitic Meningo-myelitis (Pachy-meningitis)	Hyperthyroidism	Thenar Neuritis	Superior Pulmonary Sulcus Tumor
Adults, thirty-five to forty-five	Adults, forty to fifty or over	Adults	Adults	Young adults	Adults	Adults	Atrophy of limb muscles may be prominent. No fasciculations	Adult females usually	Adults
Slowly progressive	Rapidly progressive	Pain prominent. Usually in arm but also arm and shoulder	Symptoms same as in cervical rib but due to hypertrophy of scalenus muscle	Symmetrical atrophy of hand muscles	Pain in back of neck, shoulders, arm — of root type	Pain prominent	No R. D.	Unilateral	Pain prominent in shoulder and arm
Symmetrical atrophy and weakness of hands. Extension to arms and shoulders	Atrophy of hands, arms, legs, but great variability in extent and distribution	Weakness of arm and/or hand common but atrophy not prominent		Loss of pain and temperature sensations, usually in affected areas, segmental in type	Atrophy of hand, arm, shoulder girdle muscles	Paresthesias prominent	Evidences of hyperthyroidism usually definite	No pain	Atrophy small hand muscles, usually interossei and hypothenars; forearm, arm, and shoulder girdle also at times
Bulbar symptoms rare	Bulbar symptoms practically always and may predominate	Radial pulse obliterated by special tests		Other sensory disturbances often—loss of position and vibration	Pyramidal tract signs	Atrophy of hand and arm muscles		Atrophy of the thenar eminence. No extension to other muscles	Horner's syndrome
No pain	Pyramidal signs constant; increased reflexes, Babinski's sign, etc.	Radial pulse weak on affected side		Pain may be present	Sensory level to area of lesion	Pyramidal tract signs			Roentgenogram shows tumor in apical region of lung; also erosion of vertebrae and ribs
No sensory disturbances	No pain	Blood pressure lower on affected side		Trophic changes in skin and joints prominent	Subarachnoid block and increased spinal fluid proteins	Sensory disturbances of many sorts			Progressive and fatal
No pyramidal signs as a rule	No sensory disturbances	Sensory disturbances often in hands		Very slow progression	Progressive, slow history, first of pain and upper limb weakness then of evidence of cord compression — by weakness, bladder disturbances, etc.	Spinal fluid Wassermann reaction positive and colloidal gold abnormal			
Course ten to twenty years	Course about 2 years in average case	Roentgenogram shows cervical ribs							

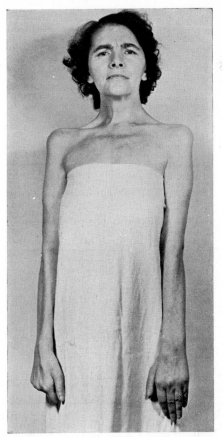

Fig. 224 — *Amyotrophic lateral sclerosis, showing the atrophy of the hand, forearm, and shoulder girdle muscles.*

stem. The atrophy and fasciculations are diffuse and not segmental. When they are, the diagnosis of amyotrophic lateral sclerosis must be in doubt.

Cervical cord tumor, either encapsulated or infiltrating, may simulate the disease, but sensory disturbances are usually present and pain is a common feature. Pain must always make one suspect a diagnosis of amyotrophic lateral sclerosis syndrome due to cord tumor. Difficulties in diagnosis may be offered especially by extramedullary tumors in the cervical region extending through the foramen magnum, causing involvement, usually asymmetrical, of hypoglossal and other nerves. In instances of cervical tumor, roentgenological studies may reveal erosion of the vertebrae; there may be evidence of subarachnoid block; the protein of the spinal fluid will be increased; and the progression will be considerably slower than in the case of amyotrophic lateral sclerosis. *Syphilitic*

it. These syndromes may be caused by a number of conditions. The distinction is important because of the invariably fatal course of amyotrophic lateral sclerosis. In general, two features must arouse the suspicion that an amyotrophic syndrome is present. These are: (1) The presence of root pain, especially in the region of the shoulder girdles and arms. Amyotrophic lateral sclerosis is, on the whole, a painless disorder. (2) The presence of segmental atrophy and fasciculations confined to the shoulder girdle and arm region. Amyotrophic lateral sclerosis is, on the whole, a diffuse process except in its predominantly bulbar form, and even here it is diffuse in the brain

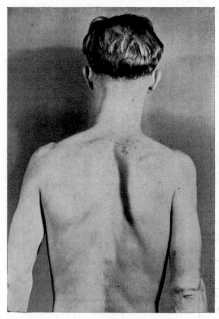

Fig. 225 — *Amyotrophic lateral sclerosis, showing atrophy confined to the right shoulder girdle.*

meningomyelitis may simulate the condition closely and may be indistinguishable from the classical amyotrophic lateral sclerosis. It occurs at an earlier age, is associated with pain quite frequently, and with positive serological reactions of the spinal fluid. The other conditions which may cause weakness and atrophy of the hand and arm muscles and may be confused therefore with amyotrophic lateral sclerosis have been considered in the diagnosis of progressive spinal muscular atrophy.

Under rare circumstances, *primary lateral sclerosis* requires separation from amyotrophic lateral sclerosis. The condition is found in adults, who give a history of painless loss of power of the legs, extending over a period of years, and characterized by all the features of a spastic paraplegia — overactive reflexes, spastic gait, Babinski sign, etc. The condition may involve one leg at times and spread to the other. Sphincter and sensory disturbances are not present. The disorder runs its course without evidence of involvement of other parts of the nervous system. It is regarded by some as an atypical form of amyotrophic lateral sclerosis.

There is some evidence to indicate that primary lateral sclerosis is a disease *sui generis* and that it may run its course without the development of other signs (Wechsler and Brody). Among 10,000 cases of neurolgical disease in the Mayo Clinic, 43 cases were found of what appeared to be true primary lateral sclerosis (Stark and Moersch). *In some cases, evidences of amyotrophic lateral sclerosis may eventually develop;* in others, multiple sclerosis may appear. It must not be assumed that every instance of pure spastic paraplegia is an example of primary lateral sclerosis, since other conditions may produce a spastic paraplegia during the course of their life cycles. Among these are extramedullary spinal cord tumor, Pott's disease, multiple sclerosis, and other disorders.

A syndrome resembling amyotrophic lateral sclerosis has been reported in persons with *chronic mercurial poisoning.* It has also been reported following gastrectomy and polyarthritis, and in triorthocresyl phosphate poisoning.

Prognosis: The disease is steadily progressive and fatal in one to six years. Most of the patients succumb within two to three years, but cases of ten years' duration have been recorded. "The prognosis increases in gravity as the clinical picture becomes more complete" (Swank and Putnam). The occurrence of many muscle fasciculations indicates that the disease is advancing rapidly. Predominantly bulbar forms of the disease are generally more rapidly fatal than others. Death is due to bulbar paralyses with respiratory failure or to intercurrent infections such as pneumonia.

Treatment: No specific treatment is known for the disease. The usual treatment is symptomatic, as in progressive spinal muscular atrophy. *Stomach tube* may be necessary early in the disease if bulbar symptoms appear early, in order to feed the patient. This should be kept in place and the patient fed with nourishing liquids reënforced with iron and vitamins. The tube may be removed at regular intervals for hygienic purposes. *Physiotherapy* in the form of general massage may help keep the patient comfortable. *Drugs* are of no avail. Recent investigators advocate the use of *vitamin E,* claiming stoppage of the progression of the disease. The regime is of little value. The regime of vitamin E consists of the following: (1) 250 mg. of synthetic vitamin E by mouth daily; (2) 200 mg. of alpha-tocopherol intramuscularly daily; (3) one ounce of wheat germ powder daily; (4) bile salts; (5) inclu-

sion in the diet of food rich in vitamin E,
such as lettuce, kale, whole wheat bread,
coarse cereals, butter, nuts, fat beef,
bananas, fresh corn, fresh green peas, and
yolks of eggs; (6) thiamine chloride by
mouth, or the B complex is also recommended. *ACTH* and *cortisone* have been
found to be of little value in the treatment
of the disease.

III. PROGRESSIVE BULBAR PARALYSIS

Etiology: Still another of the nuclear
amyotrophies is progressive bulbar paralysis, which, like progressive spinal muscular atrophy, is regarded by some as a
form of amyotrophic lateral sclerosis.
The disease occurs in older people, usually of the fifth and sixth decades, but
it may occur in younger patients. It has
been reported in families in some instances. The specific cause is unknown
and the general causes are the same
as for the other nuclear amyotrophies.
Bulbar paralysis occurs as a symptom
of involvement of poliomyelitis, arteriosclerosis, tumors, multiple sclerosis, etc.

Pathology: The disease affects the
motor nuclei of the hypoglossal (XII),
vagus (X), glossopharyngeal (IX), facial
(VII), and trigeminal (V) nerves. The
cells of the affected nuclei are reduced
in number, and show signs of degeneration, the nuclei being shrunken and pyk-
notic, and the cytoplasm being shrunken
also. Glial overgrowth is found in the
diseased nuclei. Degeneration of the
pyramidal tracts may be found in some
cases, just as in progressive spinal muscular atrophy.

Symptoms: The onset is almost always gradual, the presenting symptom
being difficulty in articulation, especially
in the use of the labials (p, b, f) or den-
tals (d, t), and linguals (l, n, r). This
slight indistinctness of speech may persist for some time and may excite little
attention until more severe dysarthria

develops, characterized by complete inability to emit words in advanced cases.
Swallowing difficulties are common, and
may occur early with the articulatory
troubles. The swallowing of liquids is
especially a problem and regurgitation
through the nose is common. Eventually,
solids cannot be swallowed either due to
palatal and/or pharyngeal paralysis. As
the disease advances, change in the timbre of the voice occurs, the voice becoming somewhat husky and hoarse, and
finally aphonic due to involvement of
the vagus nucleus in the medulla. Chewing may be difficult if the motor nucleus
of the trigeminus is concerned, but it is
not as commonly affected as other nuclei.
The muscles of the face are involved
early or late and result in difficulties in
facial movement and expression. The
lower facial muscles are much more
commonly affected than the upper. Possibly because of facial involvement, all
these patients have an expression of intense anxiety.

The affected muscles (facial, masseters,
tongue, larynx, pharynx) undergo atrophy. Fibrillations are seen in the face
and tongue and may be very active. The
vocal cords are in abductor paralysis in
patients with aphonia. The pharynx is
completely immobile, at least in its superior portion.

As a rule, no atrophy is seen in the
limbs; in some patients, atrophy and
fibrillations are present in the hands and
arms.

Chronic progressive ophthalmoplegia
has been regarded as one of the nuclear
amyotrophies. The onset is in childhood,
and less often in adult life. Familial
forms have been recorded. The symptoms develop gradually, ptosis being the
first and only symptom for a long time.
This is followed by gradual paralysis of
the other ocular muscles, sometimes
years elapsing between the onset and
complete paralysis. The end result is

total paralysis of the external ocular muscles, with complete immobility of the eyes. Necropsy studies reveal that the condition is a myopathy rather than a nuclear amyotrophy. Histological study of the ocular muscles in such instances reveals changes similar to those of progressive muscular dystrophy, with no changes of significance in the ocular nuclei.

Diagnosis: The diagnosis is easy in a pure case, but in patients with atrophy elsewhere the distinction between pure bulbar paralysis and progressive spinal muscular atrophy or amyotrophic lateral sclerosis is difficult. There is grave doubt in the minds of many as to whether progressive bulbar paralysis exists in a pure form. According to this view, there is always involvement of the pyramidal tract; hence the view that the condition is merely the bulbar manifestation of amyotrophic lateral sclerosis. *Myasthenia gravis* frequently has bulbar symptoms, often as the first sign. It occurs at a much earlier age, has no atrophy or fibrillations associated with it, gives a history of relief with rest and onset with fatigue, and reacts promptly to Prostigmin. *Pseudobulbar palsy* may give symptoms similar to those of true bulbar palsy, but no atrophy or fibrillations of the muscles are present, there is a previous history of strokes on one side and then the other, though this is not always present; compulsive crying and laughing are usually present, and almost always evidence of pyramidal tract involvement of one or both sides. Infiltrating *brain stem tumors* give signs of involvement of other systems, such as pyramidal and cerebellar, and less often sensory signs. Signs of increased pressure are not as a rule pronounced, and may appear late or not at all.

Prognosis and Treatment: The outlook is invariably poor and treatment is of no avail. The treatment used in amyo-trophic lateral sclerosis may be tried. Death occurs from respiratory paralysis or from intercurrent infections, such as pneumonia.

THE MYOPATHIES

In contrast to the nuclear amyotro-phies stand the myopathies which are due to primary involvement of the muscles. There are many forms of myopathy but all have many features in common, among which are the following:

(1) They are conspicuously congenital diseases, with a tendency to run in families. Sporadic cases without immediate familial tendencies are not infrequently encountered, however, despite the familial proclivity. The problem of heredity is not clearly defined. There is much evidence that the disease is familial and that those cases in which there is absence of familial alignment are characterized by the following: (a) the presence of sporadic cases; (b) inheritance by either a recessive or dominant factor, with the disease in abortive form in the parents and other members of the family; (c) inheritance by a sex-linked recessive factor; and (d) the transmission may possess multiple recessive factors requiring a certain number of these to be present before the disease becomes manifest (Milhorat and Wolff). The various types of muscular dystrophy appear to be transmitted in different ways: the pseudohypertrophic type as a sex-linked mendelian trait; the scapulohumeral form following no specific pattern; the facioscapulohumeral form as a dominant trait; and the distal form as a dominant trait. Evidence that progressive muscular dystrophy is a sex-linked heredofamilial disease is supplied by the occurrence, in two separate groups of nonidentical twins, of muscular dystrophy in the brother, with escape of the sister.

(2) They are characterized by muscle atrophy which is usually focal but may in

Table 63—Blood Analysis of the Dystrophies

Disease	Blood		Urine		Muscle	Other Chemical Constituents
	Creatinine	Creatine	Creatinine	Creatine		
PROGRESSIVE MUSCULAR DYSTROPHY			Decreased	Increased	Considerable diminution of the total acid-soluble phosphorus Diminution of inorganic phosphate, phosphagen, and glycogen	
AMYOTONIA CONGENITA		Normal	Decreased	Increased		
MYOTONIA CONGENITA (Thomsen's Disease)			High Normal	Normal	Low value for all phosphorus fractions; adenyl pyrophosphate especially low	Lowered cholinesterase in serum
MYOTONIA DYSTROPHICA		Normal	Decreased	Increased	Same as progressive muscular dystrophy, and decrease in potassium content of the muscle. Muscles sensitive to potassium	
MYASTHENIA GRAVIS		Decreased	Decreased	Increased	Very marked increase in potassium content, the phosphorus holding components normal	Slight decrease in serum potassium. Difference of opinion on cholinesterase values; reported normal by some and above normal by others
FAMILIAL PERIODIC PARALYSIS	Normal	Normal	Normal to slight increase	Normal	Diminution of total inorganic phosphate, low creatinine and considerable diminution of organic acid soluble phosphorus	Serum potassium and serum inorganic phosphorus lowered during attack

some forms become generalized or almost generalized. The atrophy of the myopathies differs from that of the nuclear amyotrophies in the absence of fasciculations; the absence of reaction of degeneration; the tendency to involve large muscle groups and to implicate the proximal muscle groups in contrast to the nuclear atrophies which involves primarily the small distal hand muscles, spreading later to other parts in the characteristic case: and finally the absence of involvement of the bulbar muscles. (3) There is no involvement of the nervous system. (4) The several types of myopathy often show a familial relationship with one another. (5) The course is one of progressive muscular weakness.

Transitional forms between one type of myopathy and another are not uncommon. Moreover, the occurrence of more than one form of the disease in families afflicted with myopathies bears testimony to the probable relationship of various types of the disease. Transitional forms are sometimes found also between myopathies and nuclear amyotrophies. In some instances, myopathies are associated with evidences of nervous system involvement, as in cases of myopathy associated with Friedreich's ataxia or other nervous system disorders.

No *classification* of the myopathies can be inclusive because of the transitional and borderline cases, but the following grouping includes the main types:

1. *Infantile type:*
   Amyotonia congenita
   Infantile muscular atrophy
2. *Progressive muscular dystrophy:*
   Pseudohypertrophic type
   True hypertrophic type
   Scapulohumeral type
   Facioscapulohumeral type
   Distal type
3. *Myotonia congenita* and *myotonia atrophica*
4. *Myasthenia gravis*
5. *Familial periodic paralysis*

These represent the well-defined forms; others less definitely stenciled types are not included.

I. AMYOTONIA CONGENITA

This is a rare form of myopathy, probably congenital. It is not hereditary. It has been described rarely in twins. It may occur in one of double ovum twins, or in both of identical twins, and it has been observed in triplets. Its cause is unknown. Symptoms are first noticed during the first year of life, but may be present from birth. The condition is characterized in general by atonic and small musculature, decreased motor power, and absent reflexes. It is first observed usually within the first year of life. The child is found to have difficulty in performing the usual motor acts which are regarded as normal in an infant. Lifting the head, turning the body, sitting up, standing, are all found to be impaired and serve to call attention to a disturbance in muscular power. Upon suspicion of a difficulty with muscular power, the patient is brought for examination, when it is found that the muscles are flaccid, the legs being more affected than the arms, and the trunk and face least of all. Due to the muscular atony, the limbs can be placed in all sorts of bizarre positions, hyperextension at the joints being pronounced. The muscles are small but not atrophic and fasciculations are not visible. They are soft, atonic, and lax. Motor movements lack power and vigor, but no true motor paralysis exists. The tendon reflexes are absent. Electrical excitability is diminished to both faradism and galvanism.

There is serious question whether amyotonia congenita (Oppenheim) and infantile spinal muscular atrophy (Werdnig-Hoffman) represent different syndromes. The former is said to be present at birth, while the latter develops in the second six months of life. Amyotonia congenita was reportedly characterized by a tendency to improvement, but it has been found that most babies with severe hypotonia at, or shortly after, birth showed the same downhill course as is observed in infantile spinal muscular atrophy. Pathologically, it has been found that the two conditions are identical.

It has been proposed that amyotonia congenita is a syndrome. "The diagnosis of amyotonia congenita, through common usage, is now generally taken to include all cases in which generalized weakness and hypotonia of the skeletal musculature is present at birth, or is noted within the first three months, and in which there is no clear evidence of any cerebral, skeletal or metabolic disorder" (Walton).

The syndrome is divided into three principal groups: (1) infantile spinal muscular atrophy and related syndromes, (2) symptomatic hypotonia, and (3) benign congenital hypotonia.

Symptomatic hypotonia has been found in (1) *neuromuscular* and *muscular disorders*—progressive muscular dystrophy, myasthenia gravis, polymyositis, and infantile polyneuritis; (2) *cerebral disorders*—diplegias, birth injury, kernicterus, cerebral lipoidosis; (3) *nutritional and metabolic disorders*—rickets, scurvy, cretinism, malnutrition, celiac disease, glycogen storage disease, chronic infection, or following an acute illness; (4) *skeletal disorders* — osteogenesis imperfecta, arachnodactyly; (5) *other disorders* — congenital heart disease, spinal cord birth injury (Walton).

II. PROGRESSIVE MUSCULAR DYSTROPHY

Included in this group are a number of forms, some of which involve a large part of the somatic musculature (pseudo-hypertrophic), while others affect predominantly only special groups (scapulohumeral and facioscapulohumeral).

It has been suggested that the muscular dystrophies may be divided into two main groups: (1) a childhood type and (2) a facioscapulohumeral type. The *childhood type* begins in early childhood; its victims are nearly always males; it is frequently inherited as a sex-linked recessive mendelian trait; it involves the axial and pelvic musculature initially, sparing the facial muscles; it is often accompanied by pseudohypertrophy; it is rapidly progressive and is seldom compatible with survival to adult life. The *facioscapulohumeral type* appears in late childhood or adolescence; it is inherited as a mendelian dominant, affecting both sexes; it involves facial and pectoral muscles initially; it is

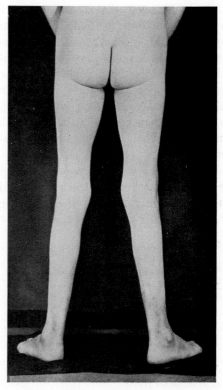

Fig. 226—(*See:* Fig. 228)

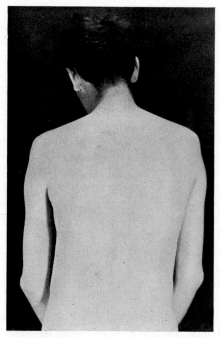

Fig. 227—(See: Fig. 228.)

rarely accompanied by hypertrophy (Tyler and Wintrobe).

Pathology: The pathology is characterized by atrophy and in some forms hypertrophy of the muscles. The atrophied muscles have a pale appearance and lose their normal striation. The hypertrophied fibers contain an increase of connective tissue and of sarcolemmal nuclei. Hyaline changes are found and eventually little is left of the muscle, which is replaced by connective tissue and fat. Some or all of the muscles may be affected, and even the heart muscle may be involved. A decreased output of creatinine and creatinuria is always found and is proportional to the extent of the muscular wasting. There is also a decreased creatine tolerance. Dystrophic muscles contain less creatine, acid-soluble phosphorus, phosphocreatinine, and adenosine triphosphate than do normal muscles. In progressive muscular dystrophy, large amounts of creatine are excreted, producing creatinuria. The level of the urine creatine and the impairment of the creatine tolerance are usually related to the amount of muscle disability. The ingestion of amino acids cause increase of creatine in the urine. Creatinuria and diminished excretion of creatinine are found also in patients with muscular wasting due to nervous disease (neuritis, peroneal muscular atrophy, poliomyelitis, progressive muscular atrophy, amyotrophic lateral sclerosis, etc.). The findings are, therefore, not pathognomonic of dystrophy. The diminution of creatinine excretion in the cases not due to dystrophy is directly proportionate to the reduction in muscle mass. The creatinuria is less than that found in the muscular dystrophies. Investigations have shown that in progressive muscular dystrophy there is a reduction in the amount of myoglobin and myosin and in nonheminbound iron.

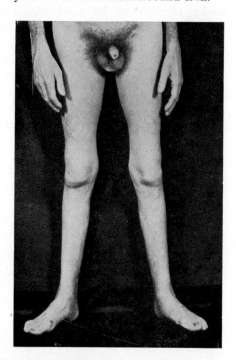

Fig. 228 — *Progressive muscular dystrophy in an adult with a history of twelve years' duration showing the wasting of the shoulder girdle, thigh and leg muscles.*

Muscular dystrophies have been produced in mice, rabbits, and chicks by the withholding of vitamin E from the diet. The active principle appears to be alpha-tocopherol. There is some doubt whether the experimental dystrophies so produced are similar pathologically to human cases. The addition of vitamin E as wheat germ oil or alpha-tocopherol to the diet prevents the development of experimental muscular dystrophies. The relationship of vitamin E to human muscular dystrophies is not as definite as in animals and thus far treatment of dystrophies by vitamins has been disappointing.

The endocrines have been accused of involvement in muscular dystrophy, but their relationship to the disease is unknown as yet. Hyperthyroidism, pituitary deficiencies, and other glandular disturbances are often found, but their precise relationship to the muscular dystrophy remains to be clarified. The androgenic hormone has been found to exert an influence on muscle metabolism, injections of the hormone resulting in changes in the creatine-creatinine excretion ratio.

Symptoms: The symptoms develop gradually in childhood or puberty, but may appear later. Attention is first called to them because of a lag in the anticipated normal functioning of the muscles. The specific symptoms depend largely on the muscles affected. The story of development of the illness is characterized by weakness of the body muscles noted in the performance of various functions, such as standing, walking, etc., with a delay in the development of these simple functions, and atrophy of the muscles. Children are brought to the physician, therefore, because of slowness in walking, awkwardness, or weakness. In generalized cases, difficulties are noted first in walking, in climbing stairs, in arising from a sitting or crouching posture, or getting up from the recumbent position.

The *gait* is found to be *waddling,* the trunk swinging from side to side in walking and the legs lifted high in typical steppage character. Arising from a chair or a crouch requires a push on the sides of the chair or on the thighs, in order to reach the erect posture. Climbing up on the body is required to get up from a recumbent position, the patient turning over, balancing on all fours, pushing himself up by bracing his hands on

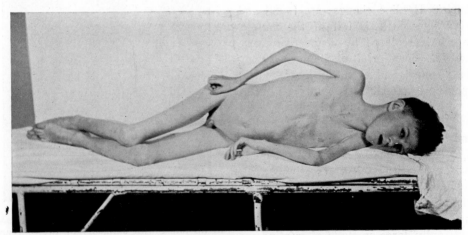

Fig. 229—*Myopathy.* **Marked wasting of the musculature in a boy with progressive muscular dystrophy.**

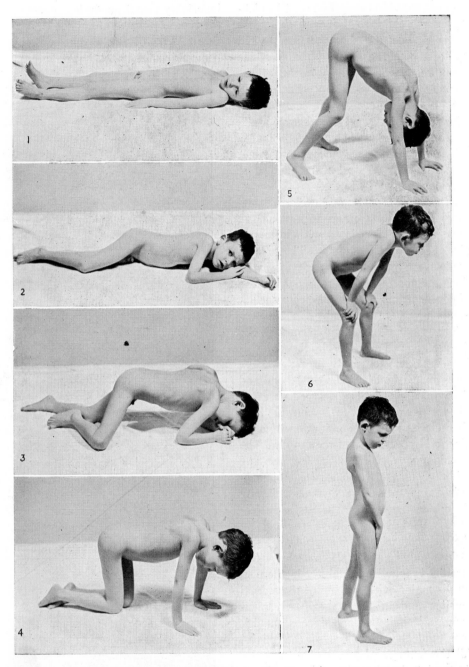

Fig. 230—*Progressive muscular dystrophy*, showing the characteristic method of arising from a prone posture by climbing up on the limbs.

his thighs and thrusting himself up by climbing up on his thighs.

Loose shoulders may be noted in picking up the child, so that with the hands in the axillae, the shoulders are pushed up loosely to the level of the ears, the trunk remaining fixed. Winging of the scapulae is noted in advanced cases.

Scoliosis and *lordosis* are present, and with them the typical protuberant abdomen and the backward slant of the trunk.

The *facies* becomes smoothed out and atonic and the typical transverse smile develops in advanced cases.

Atrophy of the muscles develops, sometimes generally, at others focally, and in some forms is associated with hypertrophy of some of the muscles. The reflexes are lost or diminished. Muscle fasciculations are absent and there is no reaction of degeneration. Abnormal electrocardiograms have been reported.

The PSEUDOHYPERTROPHIC FORM of the disease appears early in childhood and is found almost exclusively in males. Most cases appear first between the second and sixth years of life, but delayed onset up to twenty years of age is known. It is characterized by a combination of atrophy and hypertrophy of the muscles. The pseudohypertrophic muscles feel firm and rubbery but are weak despite their athletic appearance. The weakness, despite their size, is one of the striking features. The disease affects particularly the deltoid, triceps, infraspinatus, sartorius, glutei, and calf muscles. The atrophy is found particularly in the pectoralis major, with sparing of the sternal portion, and in the trapezius, serratus magnus, latissimus dorsi, biceps, quadriceps, and the adductors of the thighs. All the features of progressive muscular dystrophy already referred to are found in addition to the special characteristics of the hypertrophic form. The gait is waddling and steppage in character, loose

shoulders are present, climbing up to an erect posture from the prone position is invariably found, scoliosis is present, and the typical protuberant abdomen is prominent. As the disease advances, the hypertrophy disappears wholly or in part and

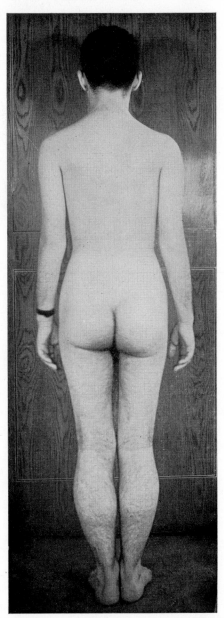

Fig. 231 — *Pseudohypertrophic muscular dystrophy,* showing the enlarged hypertrophic calves in a typical example of the disorder in a young man of sixteen.

is replaced by atrophy. Death usually occurs by the time adolescence is reached. Generally speaking, the earlier the onset, the shorter the survival.

TRUE HYPERTROPHY (hypertrophia musculorum vera) of the muscles is found in extremely rare cases in infants, giving the picture of the infant Hercules, with large and well-proportioned but weak muscles. The muscles are firm but fatigue easily, the reflexes are decreased or normal, and the course of the disease is slow, with little change from year to year (Spiller).

The SCAPULOHUMERAL FORM (juvenile type of Erb) begins in puberty or adolescence and is characterized by a heredofamilial incidence. Most cases occur in the second and third decades. The disease develops gradually and progresses slowly. Attention is first called to the disorder by the appearance of the drooping of the shoulders. The shoulders are typically loose. The shoulder girdle and upper arm are affected chiefly, the muscles of these parts being atrophic. Winging of the scapulae from involvement of the serrati is common. The arm muscles are affected first (biceps, triceps, supinator), followed later by the shoulder girdle group. Pseudohypertrophy is found especially in the triceps, deltoid, infraspinati, and teres major and minor muscles. It has been described rarely in the facial muscles. The pseudohypertrophy tends to disappear, however, the longer the disease persists. The process may extend later to other muscles, particularly those of the trunk and thighs, and in such instances affects particularly the glutei, quadriceps, adductors, and less often the hamstring muscles.

The FACIOSCAPULOHUMERAL FORM (Landouzy-Dejerine) is often familial and affects particularly the muscles of the face, arm, and shoulder girdle. It is much like the preceding form except for the involvement of the face. The time of onset in puberty or adolescence is similar to that of the scapulohumeral type. It differs from the latter in the involvement of the face, with the development of the typical myopathic facies—smoothed-out facial muscles, protuberant lower lip, loss of creases in the face, and a wide transverse smile. The involvement of the face may precede that of the arm and shoulder girdle muscles, sometimes by years, or it more commonly develops *pari passu* with the involvement of the other muscles.

There has been described a form of myopathy occurring predominantly in women during or after the climacteric period. This has been referred to as *menopausal muscular dystrophy*. It is characterized by progressive weakness, rapid or slow, of the hip and shoulder girdle muscles. The muscles are weak and have a "soft" consistency. Wasting of the muscles is unusual. The lower limbs are more affected than the upper. Difficulty in ascending stairs and in arising from a chair without help from the arms is common. The disease progresses to a point where a waddling gait is evident and the patient can no longer climb stairs. The bulbar muscles are not affected. The deep reflexes in the affected muscles may be decreased. Muscle biopsy is necessary for certain diagnosis and reveals evidence of dystrophy. The muscle is usually pale; microscopic examination shows patchy degeneration or necrosis of individual muscle fibers and usually proliferation of the sarcolemmal nuclei. The condition responds to cortisone which must be maintained to avoid relapse.

The DISTAL FORM (Gowers) is rare and is open to dispute. It is regarded by some as a form of peroneal muscular atrophy. This type of myopathy is not clearly etched. The recorded cases describe atrophy of the anterior tibial muscles with sparing of the peronei, involvement of the extensors of the hands, fingers, and toes, and the development of contractures. Absence of sensory disturbances is said to indicate distinction from peroneal muscular atrophy.

A LATE ADULT FORM of myopathy is found in rare instances in subjects over thirty years of age. In the recorded examples, the ages have varied from thirty to sixty years. The myopathy in such instances involves chiefly the face and shoulder girdle muscles and probably represents a late variant of the scapulohumeral and facioscapulohumeral forms of myopathy. Hypertrophy of other muscles is usually present. A histological study of the muscles in late cases of myopathy shows all the features found in the progressive muscular dystrophy.

CONGENITAL HYPERTROPHY of the muscles associated with extrapyramidal disease and mental deficiency (deLange) is a rare disorder. The condition occurs in infants and is characterized by generalized symmetrical muscular hypertrophy, which gives to the infant an athletic and Herculean appearance due to the bulging muscles; in addition there are permanent and paroxysmal hypertonicity of the muscles, mental deficiency of a severe degree, and arrested development. There may be considerable variation both in the degree of muscular hypertrophy and hypertonicity. The condition terminates fatally. The brain in such cases shows changes, particularly in the striatum, and porencephalic cysts in the cerebrum. The disease is confused chiefly with congenital myxedema. It is easily differentiated from myotonia congenita (Thomsen) by the age of onset and the absence of a myotonic reaction. Pseudohypertrophic muscular dystrophy is readily distinguished.

HEMIHYPERTROPHY is found in rare instances involving the muscles of one-half of the body. The condition is congenital, involves the right half of the body much more often than the left, and is often associated with mental deficiency. The muscles of the affected side are uniformly enlarged, and the bones participate in the process. The cause of the condition is unknown, but interrupted twinning is regarded as the most probable cause of the condition. The disease must be distinguished from Milroy's disease, which is a hereditary disorder characterized by edema of the lower extremities occurring in many members of the same family. The edema may affect one leg early in its course but both legs become involved later.

PARTIAL HYPERTROPHY of the body musculature is found in rare instances. Hemihypertrophy of the face occurs, either with or without other anomalies. In such instances, there is definite hypertrophy of the eyelid, cheek, and lips and, in some cases, associated ocular anomalies. The facial bones of the affected side are larger than those of the normal side.

Treatment: The treatment of most of the myopathies is a most unsatisfactory matter. Little can be done to restore the normal muscle bulk. *Massage* may help in maintaining muscle nutrition. *Heat* applied to the muscles in the form of infrared or diathermy may be helpful. Strychnine has been used in many cases with little effect. Activity within the limits of fatigue is desirable and normal use of the muscles is to be encouraged in contrast to enforced rest. *Glycine* in dosages of 2 to 4 drachms three or four times a day has been said to be beneficial, but is of no value. *Vitamin E* has recently evoked some enthusiasm and has been reported to produce good effects in restoring some of the muscle power. It should be given in the same fashion as for amyotrophic lateral sclerosis. It is of little value. The regime of vitamin E consists of the following: (1) 250 mg. of synthetic vitamin

E by mouth daily; (2) 200 mg. of alpha-tocopherol intramuscularly daily; (3) one ounce of wheat germ powder daily; (4) bile salts; (5) inclusion in the diet of foods rich in vitamin E, such as lettuce, kale, whole wheat bread, coarse cereals, butter, nuts, fat beef, bananas, fresh corn, fresh green peas, and yolks of eggs; (6) thiamine chloride by mouth, or the B complex is also recommended. *Ephedrine sulfate*, gr. ⅜ to ¾, is said to be effective in some instances.

III. PERONEAL MUSCULAR ATROPHY
(Charcot-Marie-Tooth Muscular Atrophy, Progressive Neural Muscular Atrophy)

This disease is not, strictly speaking, a myopathy, since it is due to a combination of peripheral nerve and spinal cord lesions, but it is considered here largely because it is manifested by muscular atrophy and its inclusion under the nuclear amyotrophies is much wider afield than its consideration here.

The specific *cause* of the disease is unknown. The disease is strongly hereditary and cases may as a rule be followed through several generations. The disease has been followed in as many as seven (Souques) and nine (Churchill) generations. "About fifty per cent of the children, one of whose parents is affected, may be expected not only to develop the malady, but to do so at the same age and to present the same typical or atypical distribution in the same sequence" (Purves-Stewart).

The disease may be transmitted as a dominant, recessive, or sex-linked characteristic. The following features have been determined by a study of the hereditary aspects of peroneal muscular atrophy (Allan): When the disease is transmitted as a dominant characteristic, it appears first about thirty years of age, continues for a long time and the atrophy is only moderate. When it is sex-linked,

recessive atrophy is noted about the middle of the second decade and by twenty-five years of age the patients are helpless and bedridden. When the atrophy is a simple recessive trait, it begins before eight years of age and in the second decade its victims become hopeless cripples.

The explanation offered is as follows (Allan): Those in whom the trait is dominant receive one defective gene from the affected parent and one normal gene from the unaffected parent and this combination of a pair of genes half good and half bad causes a late onset of the disorder. In the case of the sex-linked recessive trait, a defective gene is received from the mother without a corresponding normal gene from the father, the disease being therefore more severe and appearing earlier. When the atrophy is simple recessive, each parent supplies a defective gene and there is nothing to ameliorate the intensity of the disease, which appears early and develops severely. Isolated examples are uncommon, and cases in which the disease occurs in a single member of a family without obvious hereditary features should occasion no surprise. The disease usually occurs at the same age in all afflicted members of a family, this homochronicity being one of the features of the disease. Males are more commonly afflicted than females.

Pathology: The pathology of the disease is rather widespread and involves the muscles, the peripheral nerves, anterior horn cells and roots, the posterior roots, and the posterior columns. In some cases the spinal cord is not involved. The process is purely degenerative, the peripheral nerves showing a parenchymatous form of neuritis and the anterior horn cells a degenerative form of atrophy. The muscles are atrophic.

Symptoms: They develop as a rule gradually in childhood or later and are characterized by symmetrical involvement first of the peroneal muscles of the legs and the small muscles of the foot, especially the extensors and abductors. Difficulty in walking is the most common complaint and is accompanied by a noticeable inability to clear the foot from the ground, due to foot-drop. Pains and paresthesias in the legs are common and prominent early and late in the disease. The flexors of the foot are involved to a much less degree than the extensors. Claw foot and talipes equinovarus develop. The disease advances up the legs slowly, and involves eventually the entire leg and the lower third of the thighs, giving the typical rooster's leg appearance, with atrophy of the legs and lower thighs and well-preserved upper portions of the thighs. The hand muscles may become involved eventually, producing atrophy and a typical claw hand. The hip and shoulder girdles, face, and trunk are not involved.

The affected muscles are atrophied and often show fasciculations. Reaction of degeneration is present and the Achilles reflexes are lost. Diminution or loss of touch, pain, and temperature sensations is common; deep sensation, particularly vibration sense, is commonly lost in the legs. The spinal fluid reveals nothing of significance.

Diagnosis: It offers no difficulties in a typical instance. The early onset of weakness of the distal portions of the limbs, with weakness in dorsiflexion of the feet, resulting foot-drop, the strong hereditary trend, the atrophy of the legs and, in advanced instances, the "stork legs," the absent Achilles reflexes, the occurrence of pains, paresthesias and superficial sensory disturbances are characteristic. Difficulties occur in sporadic cases, but here, too, the features outlined stamp the condition clearly. Eventual extension to the hands and arms occurs. Few conditions simulate the atrophy of peroneal muscular atrophy. The *distal form of myopathy* is rare, occurs in older subjects, fails to show the same type of atrophy as peroneal muscular atrophy, and shows no fasciculations or sensory disturbances. *Friedreich's ataxia* is characterized by a familial incidence, with the typical Friedreich's foot, absence of reflexes, disturbance of posterior column function, and Babinski's sign. Superficial sensory disturbances are absent, and pains are not encountered. *Progressive muscular atrophy* may involve the legs primarily and cause atrophy of the foot extensors, but pains and sensory disturbances are totally lacking and there is no familial incidence. *Peripheral neuritis* may in some instances simulate peroneal muscular atrophy, but tenderness of the muscles and nerve trunks is striking and there is no familial incidence.

The disease runs a slow protracted course, often remaining stationary for long periods of time.

THE MYOTONIAS

Two main forms of myotonia are known: myotonia congenita (Thomsen) and myotonia atrophica or dystrophica. These two conditions, formerly separated, are now known to represent probably different stages of the same process. Myotonia as a symptom, moreover, is found in a variety of other conditions.

Myotonia is a symptom. It is characterized by delayed relaxation of the muscles after natural, mechanical, or electrical stimuli. The site of its occurrence is not precisely known. It may occur after blocking of the motor nerve. Some abnormality at the myoneural junction is presumed to be responsible for the condition. The "after-spasm" found in myotonic muscles which have been voluntarily contracted is characterized by discharge of the central motor neurons, but it is not found after nerve block. It is determined therefore by the myotonic condition of the muscles, probably a reflex contraction caused by some persistent effect in the proprioceptors of the intrinsic muscles (Denny-Brown and Nevin). The delayed relaxation of myotonic muscle appears to be the result of factors within the muscle itself and not of mechanisms within the nervous system or at the myoneural junctions. Curarization of myotonic muscle in goats (Brown and Harvey) and in man (Lanari) results in the persistence of the myotonia. The myotonic muscles are abnormally sensitive to potassium. Acetylcholine injected into the blood stream causes a painful prolonged muscular contracture in myotonic subjects; alcohol, calcium, insulin, and quinine relieve myotonia temporarily; neostigmine and potassium compounds increases myotonia. Myotonia appears to be abolished by the intravenous injection of procainamide. When given by mouth (0.25 gm. four times daily) the drug causes a decrease in myotonic symptoms maximal after one hour and diminishing after five to six hours.

Myotonia Congenita (Thomsen): This disease occurs as a rule in childhood, is strongly inherited, runs in families, often through several generations, and occurs most frequently in males. Sporadic cases are known to occur. There are probably no primary changes in the muscle in myotonia congenita, except for hypertrophy of the individual muscle fibers. No creatinuria is found, and the creatinine content of the urine is high normal.

Symptoms develop very early and appear gradually. The cardinal symptom is the *myotonic reaction,* characterized by an inability to relax the muscles readily after contraction due to abnormal persistence of contraction. Thus, shaking hands results in a prolonged handclasp until after several seconds relaxation becomes possible; similarly clenching the fist results in inability to relax the hand muscles. All muscle movements indeed are featured by difficulty in relaxation. Repetition of movement, however, results in easier relaxation until after several repeated movements relaxation approaches normal. Increased effort and force of contraction conversely cause greater myotonia. The myotonia is aggravated by rest, emotion, fever, forced effort, and cold. It is aided by warmth, mental relaxation, moderate amounts of alcohol, and repetition of movement. All muscles of the body participate, but some are more involved than others. The ocular and tongue muscles may be affected.

The muscles are very well developed, are hypertrophied, and the habitus athletic. The hypertrophy of the muscles is so deceiving as to give the patient the appearance of a well-developed athlete. No atrophy occurs. Stimulation of the muscles by mechanical stimulus results in the *myotonic response* characterized by a slow contraction which relaxes slowly. The reflexes are normal and no sensory disturbances are found. The outlook for life is good.

Myotonia Atrophica: This is much more common than the congenital form of the disease, and is characterized by occurrence in families, by atrophy and myotonia, by the frequent occurrence of cataract, by testicular atrophy, and other glandular disturbances.

The muscles show degeneration of the muscle fibers with replacement by connective tissue and sarcolemmal nuclei and fat. The nervous system is undamaged except in rare instances. Changes have been found in some cases in the thyroid gland, and testicular atrophy is common. The creatinine output of the urine is decreased and is proportional to the muscular wasting, as in muscular dystrophy.

The onset is gradual, usually between twenty and thirty-five years, but it may appear in childhood. Atrophy or myotonia may appear first, but myotonic symptoms usually are earlier to appear than atrophy. The symptoms on presentation consist, therefore, of difficulty in relaxation of muscles, weakness, atrophy, and loss of weight, with weakness the outstanding complaint

The *atrophy* is selective and affects particularly the facial muscles, muscles of mastication, sternomastoids, forearm and hand muscles, thigh and dorsiflexor muscles of the feet. The muscles of mastication and the muscles of the hand and forearm are affected early, and the temporal muscles are also involved early. The dorsiflexors of the feet are affected in fifty per cent of cases. Paralysis of the vocal cords occurs rarely. The result is a "hatchet" or "tapir" facies due to atrophy of the temporal, orbicularis oris, and oculi muscles. The gait is steppage in character due to weakness of the peronei.

The *myotonia* is also more or less selective and not as generalized as in myotonia congenita. Relaxation of the hand grips is difficult, and the myotonic reaction on mechanical percussion of a muscle is found in hand muscles, tongue, or other muscles. The reaction is less pronounced or absent in atrophied muscles. Muscle fasciculations are encountered rarely. *Cataract* is found in ten to thirty per cent of the subjects. *Frontal baldness* is common. *Atrophy of the testicles* occurs frequently, sexual function is decreased in both sexes, and childless marriages are frequent. The tendon *reflexes* are diminished or absent.

Personality deviations and mental retardation are common. Psychoses, mental deficiency, and disturbances of personality have been recorded during the course of the disease. It is not clear whether they are directly related to the myopathy. Bradycardia, hypotension, and electrocardiographic abnormalities are common. The disease is slowly progressive, death occurring before fifty of an intercurrent infection or exhaustion state.

Treatment: Myotonia congenita and atrophica are relieved by quinine in doses of 10 to 15 grains three times daily, the quinine serving to relieve the myotonic reaction. It is not effective in all cases. *Testosterone* may be given because of the testicular atrophy. Testosterone propionate, 25 mg. intramuscularly three times weekly, may be followed by methyl testosterone 10 to 30 mg. per day by mouth, if the response to injection is satisfactory. Subcutaneous implantation of testosterone pellets renewed at six to twelve month intervals may be used.

Myotonia Acquisita: This form occurs in adult life, has no hereditary features, is characterized by myotonic reaction of the muscles, and follows infections (typhoid, gastroenteritis), intoxications (alcoholism, lead poisoning), multiple neuritis, and, in rare instances, trauma. Hypertrophy of the affected muscles is found. The condition resembles myotonia congenita (Thomsen) in the presence of hypertrophy of the muscles, except for the tendency to improvement and even recovery. The condition begins usually with weakness, pain, and flaccid paresis of the limbs. Most of the reported cases have developed after a multiple neuritis.

Paramyotonia congenita is characterized by tonic spasms of the face, neck, and throat and to a lesser extent of the limbs. It is aggravated greatly by cold, so that the sufferer may become speechless or incapable of movement for minutes or hours which may be followed by generalized weakness. Warmth relieves the symptoms.

MYASTHENIA GRAVIS

This disease is characterized by excessive fatigability of the muscles with resultant weakness and paralysis. It is uncommon but is not rare.

Etiology: The cause of myasthenia gravis is not known. In the majority of cases, no specific cause can be assigned for the development of the disease. Associated disorders of the thymus gland have been recorded in about fifty per cent of necropsied cases of myasthenia gravis or in forty-one out of eighty-seven cases (Miller). Large or microscopic tumors may be found, and these may be benign or malignant. Hyperplasia or persistence of the gland is also found in some instances. Thymomas are found in fifteen per cent of cases in myasthenia gravis. Despite the frequent occurrence of thymic tumors in necropsied cases, no causative relationship between the two conditions has been demonstrated. Improvement of the disease following removal of the thymic tumor has been recorded by some investigators but not by others. No etiological relationship between myasthenia gravis and endocrine disturbances has been shown. Myasthenia gravis syndromes are sometimes seen following encephalitis, influenza, and in association with hyperthyroidism. It has been reported after electrical shock.

Pathology: The pathology is featured by the absence of changes in the nervous system and the absence of characteristic changes in the muscles. Lymphorrhages, or collections of lymphocytes, have been found in the muscles of some but not of all subjects. Apart from this, the muscles show nothing. The thymus gland shows the presence of hyperplasia or tumors in fifty per cent of necropsied cases. The tumors may be benign or malignant. No changes are found in the central nervous system or in the peripheral nerves. Endocrine disturbances have been recorded frequently, but their precise relation to the disease is unclear. Lymphorrhages are found at times in the thyroid, liver, suprarenals, kidneys, lungs, and pancreas. Hyperthyroidism is found in some cases, the clinical picture of this disease resembling myasthenia gravis very closely at times.

The *site* of the difficulty in myasthenia gravis is probably the myoneural junction in the muscle. Neostigmine causes an improvement in the myasthenia and it is assumed that it causes a delay in destruction of the acetylcholine at the myoneural junction; or there may be defective formation or mobilization of the acetylcholine which is corrected by neostigmine. Evidence is at hand to indicate that acetylcholine is formed within the axon as well as at the myoneural junction (Nachmansohn).

Neostigmine depends for its effectiveness in the treatment of myasthenia gravis partly on its inhibiting power on cholinesterase. By controlling the enzyme which splits acetylcholine, the transmission of the nerve impulse at the myoneural junction sufficient to create an adequate response in the muscle is made more certain. Other drugs which inhibit cholinesterase include tetraethylpyrophosphate (TEPP). Though the effects of this drug are more prolonged than those of neostigmine, it is more difficult to control.

Curare produces a picture similar to that of myasthenia, but it does not affect the liberation of acetylcholine. Myasthenic muscles are extremely sensitive to curare, responding quickly to doses well below the average normal (Bennett and Cash). Doses of curare of one fifth to one fiftieth of normal may be used to establish the diagnosis in latent cases. Since the test may produce symptoms in persons without myasthenia gravis, it is not specific. It is hazardous in patients with well-established myasthenia.

The possibility exists that the defect in myasthenia gravis is the result of some substance foreign to the myoneural junction or of failure of removal of some product of acetylcholine. The fundamental defect in myasthenia gravis appears to be some defect in the neuromuscular transmitting mechanism. The repair of this defect by neostigmine, which is known to protect the acetylcholine release of motor nerve endings from hydrolysis by cholinesterase, supports the hypothesis that in myasthenia gravis the normal metabolism of acetylcholine is deranged. There is evidence to suggest that an inhibitory substance is circulating in the blood stream and is responsible for the neuromuscular defect. This is suggested by the cure of myasthenia gravis by the removal of thymic tumors, suggesting that the hypothetical substance may arise in the thymus. Potassium chloride in large doses causes temporary relief. The infusion of amino acids has been reported to augment the muscle function in myasthenia gravis. Electromyogram studies reveal wide variations in the irregularity of the amplitude of response of single motor units, but that after the injection of neostigmine the responses become quite consistent and of uniform amplitude (Lindsley).

Chemical studies reveal a slight creatinuria in myasthenia gravis as well as a lowered excretion of creatinine. Myasthenic muscle is normal as to glycogen, lactic acid, and phosphorus compounds. The serum cholinesterase is slightly lowered.

Symptoms: The condition occurs more frequently in females and appears usually around twenty-five to thirty-five years of age. An onset in adolescence is not uncommon. Development in the aged occurs also, and cases rarely develop in infancy and childhood in the first two years of life. The majority of cases in children appear at about twelve years of age. Among thirty-four cases in children under seventeen, the average age was found to be 11.8 years, with only eight instances of the disease below ten years (Levethan, Fried, and Madonick). A familial occurrence is found in rare instances; in two sisters (Hart) and in two brothers (Rothbart). Myasthenia gravis has been observed in infants in the neonatal period, all born of mothers with myasthenia. In all the recorded instances the symptoms have been manifest by the third day, and in most of the recorded cases the diagnosis has been confirmed by neostigmine. The symptoms are transitory and have cleared up in varying periods of time (two weeks to four months). *Neonatal myasthenia gravis* is transient and differs from the rare cases of *congenital myasthenia gravis* in which the symptoms are persistent. The neonatal form is not altogether benign since deaths have been recorded in infants so afflicted.

The onset of symptoms is gradual but acutely developing cases are not unknown. The outstanding complaint is *weakness* or *fatigability,* which the intelligent patient will have noticed and is relieved by rest. The mode of development varies; in some instances, the complaints are confined largely to the muscles innervated by the cranial nerves; in others, the somatic musculature may be largely affected; in still others, a combination of bulbar and general somatic symptoms is found. The presenting complaint may be diplopia or drooping of the eyelids, or the development of strabismus; or difficulty in swallowing, talking, or aphonia may first call attention to the disease. These may appear alone or in combination with a general feeling of weakness. The significant feature of the history early in the disorder is the occurrence of easy fatigue which is relieved by rest. This feature may not be apparent even to intelligent patients and will often not be volunteered, but it can be elicited on direct questioning. Fatigue on walking, relieved by rest; fatigue on chewing, talking, or reading are striking and, until the disease becomes advanced, disappears on resting the affected parts. As the disease advances, the weakness becomes more and more pronounced so that the range and force of muscular movement is greatly decreased. Walking becomes difficult and can be carried out for only a short distance; chewing movements result in rapid fatigue so that mastication of food becomes difficult; swallowing becomes difficult and eventually impossible, the voice loses its timbre and clearing the throat impossible. The eventual outcome is that of complete or almost complete paralysis of bulbar, limb and truncal muscles.

Ocular symptoms frequently are among the first to appear, and are usually attributed to some other cause early in the disease. Diplopia, at first transient and later permanent, occurs early. Drooping of the eyelids may be noted on reading or at the moving pictures, and is found to be relieved by resting the eyelids by closing. Fatigue of the muscles of mastication on chewing and of the facial muscles on talking; disappearance of the voice during conversation; swallowing difficulties and regurgitation of food; all these may develop during the course of the illness. Speech and swallowing difficulties may be the first to appear. In a well-developed case, fatigue and weakness of the body musculature is present.

involving a large part of the body musculature or only isolated muscles. Here, too, the patient recounts fatigue in walking or in the performance of other motor acts, followed by weakness and paralysis of the involved muscles on continued use.

The affected muscles early in the disorder are relieved by rest. With the development of the disease, longer and longer rest periods are required to restore function, until finally rest is of no avail, the muscles remaining permanently paralyzed. Not all the muscles respond in the same degree; in a given case, paralysis may be found in some muscle groups while others still respond to rest. Most patients give a characteristic history of feeling stronger on arising in the morning and of being worse as the day proceeds. Palpitation has been recorded as a prominent symptom in myasthenia gravis.

The facies are characteristic in typical cases. The eyelids droop, the face is smoothed out and has a blank appearance, and the head is thrown back in order to clear the ptosed eyelids. Ocular paralysis of varying degrees may be found, from involvement of a single muscle to a complete ophthalmoplegia. Ocular paralyses vary in extent and degree. They may involve single ocular muscles or may cause complete external and internal ophthalmoplegia. The ocular paralyses are, as a rule, bilateral, but they are not necessarily symmetrical, and of equal degree in the two eyes. Unilateral ptosis or unilateral ocular paralysis, either complete or incomplete, is found at times. An analysis of twenty-six cases of myasthenia gravis reveals the frequency of ocular symptoms (Mattis): in twenty-five, ocular symptoms were found at some time during the course of the disease; in ninety per cent diplopia and in eighty-five per cent ptosis were present on one or more occasions; in forty-six per cent, ptosis was the first symptom; in four per cent, ptosis was present bilaterally; in nineteen per cent, ptosis involved only one lid throughout the course of the disease; in seventy-three per cent, ptosis was intermittent, involving the two lids singly in irregular alternation throughout the course of the disease; in seventy-seven per cent, ptosis and diplopia appeared simultaneously; and in sixty-five per cent some ocular symptom was the first indication of the disease.

The palate may be immobile and vocal cord movement may be impaired or lost. Hearing is often affected and tinnitus occurs at times. The facial muscles are weak and in severe cases may be paralyzed. Wrinkling of the forehead, closing of the eyelids, and movement of the muscles of facial expression are greatly impaired. In a well-developed case, the affected muscles are found to be weakened. In an advanced case, paralysis of the affected muscles is found, with inability to walk, to move the arms, or even to raise the head. Rapid fatigue of the eye muscles can be elicited early in the disease by simple maneuvers, such as having the patient fix his gaze on an object when drooping of the eyelids is observed; by clenching and unclenching the fists; by repeated chewing movements, etc. Muscle atrophy is not found or is very slight in some muscles and fasciculations are absent. The muscles often have a pudgy feel.

The *reflexes* are unaffected as a rule; later they become decreased. They tend to disappear on repeated stimulation but return on muscular rest. The pupillary reflex may be temporarily eradicated by repeated stimulation. Faradic stimulation of the affected muscles causes brisk contractions at first, but loss of excitability temporarily on repeated stimulation. This is known as the *myasthenic reaction*. It is readily demonstrable in a well-pronounced case; in some instances, it may be found only in isolated muscles. *Remissions* are quite characteristic of the disease. They may be complete and be associated with total recession of symptoms or only by partial

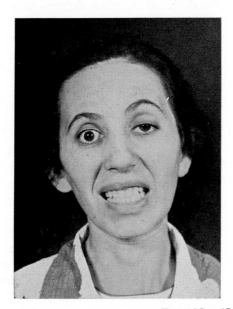 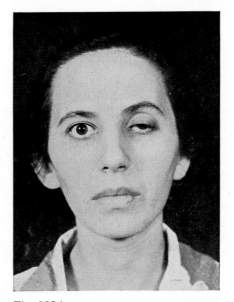

Fig. 232—*(See: Fig. 233.)*

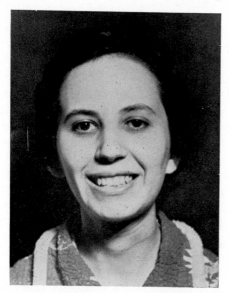

Fig. 233—*Myasthenia gravis,* showing ptosis and weakness of the facial muscles. Note the complete metamorphosis following the administration of neostigmine.

improvement. Their duration varies greatly from weeks to months or even years.

Diagnosis: The diagnosis of myasthenia gravis offers few difficulties in a typical case. The history of gradual onset of muscle weakness in a young or middle-aged person, usually a woman, with bulbar symptoms predominating in the early case; the history of improvement of the fatigue by rest; the demonstration of muscle weakness in eye, masticatory, swallowing or systemic muscles unassociated with atrophy, fasciculations or reflex changes; the production of the myasthenic reaction; and the elicitation of easy fatigue in the muscles on examination, are all striking evidences of the disease.

The problem of myasthenia gravis presents itself in many guises. In the majority of instances, the symptoms involve the bulbar muscles. Hence many patients present themselves either with ocular symptoms, such as ptosis, diplopia, or ocular weakness, or with difficulties in swallowing or phonation. In such instances, the history of fatigue and relief by rest, the myopathic facies, the fatigability of the affected muscles by use under test conditions, and the response to neostigmine are sufficient to establish the diagnosis. It is a safe rule that, in obscure instances of ocular or bulbar paralyses, myasthenia gravis must always be suspected and neostigmine given as a diagnostic test. The systemic musculature is often not involved early, or if involved may be overshadowed by the symptoms referable to the eyes and throat. The possibility of myasthenia gravis must not be discarded, therefore, in the absence of weakness of the limbs

In patients with only the ocular type of myasthenia, the longer the duration of the ocular symptoms alone the less is the possiblity of developing generalized myasthenia.

While myasthenia gravis is a disease primarily of adults, neonatal forms of the disease are known to occur rarely. These are transient, in contrast to the persistent congenital form. Congenital myasthenia gravis is characterized by diminished activity of the fetus in utero and the perfect symmetry of the muscular weakness. The condition is confused with nuclear aplasia and amyotonia congenita.

The use of *neostigmine* in diagnosis is extremely helpful. In every suspected case, neostigmine (2 to 3 cc. of a 1 to 2000 solution) with atropine, gr. $\frac{1}{150}$, should be injected intramuscularly. If myasthenia gravis is present, the muscular weakness will be greatly improved in the course of thirty to forty-five minutes as a rule and will disappear in the course of one or two hours, except in advanced cases, when it will be only partially relieved. The following test of the efficacy of neostigmine in the diagnosis of myasthenia gravis has been proposed (Schwab and Viets): Three cc. of neostigmine are injected intramuscularly, with 0.01 gr. of atropine sulfate. Thereafter, at intervals of ten minutes for one hour, the degree of objective improvement is noted in one column, with grading as follows: 0, no improvement; 1, slight improvement; 2, moderate improvement; 3, considerable improvement, and 4, complete recovery or marked improvement. In a second column with the same grading, the patient's subjective opinion of the improvement is scored. The figures in the two columns are added, and the total score obtained. The maximal score is forty-eight. If the total value is less than eight, the result of the test is negative and it is extremely unlikely that the patient has myasthenia gravis. If the total is from eight to eighteen, the outcome of the test is doubtful and it should be repeated or a trail of oral neostigmine given. If the score is more than seventeen, the result of the test is positive and the patient has myasthenia gravis.

Tensilon chloride (edrophonium chloride) is a short-acting anticholinesterase which is used in the diagnosis of myasthenia gravis. It is given intravenously in 1 cc. doses. If myasthenia is present the response of the weakened muscles will be similar to that of neostigmine, but much more rapid. A positive reaction is observed in one to three minutes.

The *curare sensitivity test* has been devised in order to aid in the diagnosis of myasthenia gravis (Bennett and Cash). The rationale of the test is based on the fact that curare neutralizes the action of acetylcholine at the myoneural junctions and produces an artificial form of myasthenia gravis. It is carried out as follows: About 1 mg. of curare per kilogram of body weight administered intravenously produces mild generalized curarization in a normal adult. One-tenth this estimated dosage is injected intra-

venously over a one-minute period in the suspected myasthenia patient. The peak reaction develops within two minutes. "If the patient has myasthenia, the existing myasthenic symptoms are aggravated, especially paralysis of the oculomotor muscles, weakness of the facial muscles and of the tongue, with dysarthria and dysphagia. New symptoms may appear, such as flaccid paresis of the trunk and extremities" (Bennett and Cash). Inability to speak or protrude the tongue may follow and the respiration may become labored. The test is terminated after two or three minutes by the intravenous injection of 1.5 mg. of neostigmine methylsulfate with $\frac{1}{100}$ gr. of atropine sulfate, all acute symptoms disappearing within one minute.

There seems to be no means at present of distinguishing precisely between some of the myopathies associated with acute or chronic thyrotoxicosis and myasthenia gravis. Forms of chronic thyrotoxicosis may resemble myasthenia gravis closely, associated as they are with fatigue, muscle weakness, and at times even cranial nerve involvement. A favorable response to neostigmine, in such cases, supports a diagnosis of myasthenia gravis, but it must be recognized that there is a type of thyrotoxic myasthenia which responds to prostigmine. In rare instances hyperthyroidism and myasthenia gravis may occur in the same patient. Thyroidectomy is hazardous in such patients. Because of the simultaneous existence of the two diseases, instances of this type will respond to neostigmine.

Roentgenograms of the chest reveal at times an enlargement in the mediastinum which is indicative of thymus involvement. In all cases of myasthenia gravis, routine chest films, if negative, should be followed by planograms in order to determine whether thymic enlargement is present.

The condition must be distinguished primarily from bulbar affections, none of which give the characteristic history of fatigue and weakness improved by rest. *Poliomyelitis* is easily differentiated by its acute, febrile onset and by evidences of meningeal irritation early in the disease, lymphocytosis of the spinal fluid, and by its stormy development and course. *Amyotrophic lateral sclerosis* and its bulbar syndromes are easily distinguished by the presence of muscle atrophy and fasciculations, and by evidence of systemic disease elsewhere. *Multiple sclerosis* is not readily confused, but may offer difficulties in rare instances. The history of remission of symptoms and the demonstration of optic atrophy, absent abdominal reflexes, and multiple system involvement will suffice to differentiate it.

The *course* of the disease is progressive. Despite treatment there comes a time when the muscles no longer respond. Death ensues as a result of cardiac or respiratory failure or by intercurrent infection.

Treatment: Proper care should be given to any physical abnormalities which may be present. Foci of infection should be sought and removed if present. The chest should be studied by the roentgen ray for the presence of a persistent thymus gland and irradiation given over this area if such a gland is present. Careful metabolic studies should be made; if evidences of hypothyroidism are found, thyroid extract should be given. In some instances, a myasthenic syndrome is seen with hyperthyroidism, which must be treated appropriately. Endocrine products should not be given indiscriminately unless there is a proper indication for their use.

In the administration of drugs for the treatment of myasthenia gravis it is necessary to distribute the dosage in accordance with the needs of the individual patient. In some instances it is necessary to give the drugs chosen for treatment as soon as the patient arises in the morning, especially in patients with bulbar symptoms, and to provide the main dosages before mealtime. In others the dose may be distributed evenly during the day. In still others, large doses may be necessary before retiring and the drug or drugs may be given during the night. Patients who understand their needs may be given some freedom in inserting dosages when they feel their need.

Formerly, *neostigmine* was by far the most effective drug in use for the treatment of myasthenia gravis. In severe cases, neostigmine must be administered by injection until a good dosage can be built up by mouth. In less severe cases the drug may be given by mouth just as effectively as by injection. It is given in tablets of 15-mg. dosage. The number of tablets per day will depend upon the severity of the disease and may vary from three to ten or twelve. The tablets should be distributed during those periods of the day when fatigue is most likely to develop and should be concentrated, therefore, at these times. In general, the tablets should be given at three to four hour intervals in well-pronounced cases. Some patients may require the drug on arising in order to enable performance of toilet. At times intramuscular injections of neostigmine methyl sulfate (0.25-0.5 mg.) may be required (1) to fortify the oral dosage, (2) to provide relief in crises of difficulty in swallowing or breathing.

Neostigmine has to a large extent been replaced by *Mestinon Bromide* (pyridostigmin bromide), a pyridine analogue of neostigmine. It has advantages over neostigmine in longer duration of action and mildness of side-effects. It is given as a tablet orally in 60-mg. doses. The total dosage varies with the severity of the disease, but as many as 25 to 30 tablets may be given daily. Mestinon has been found to be fully as effective as neostigmine in the treatment of myasthenia gravis. It is especially effective in patients with bulbar symptoms, and is particularly useful when the disease is resistant to neostigmine.

In some cases, the combined use of neostigmine and ephedrine appears to give better results than neostigmine alone. Ephedrine sulfate, gr. ⅜, is given two or three times a day with the neostigmine and seems to fortify its effect. Glycine has little or no value.

Operation for removal of a *thymus tumor* has yielded good results in some of the patients but not in all. The role of thymectomy is still difficult to assess. The results of thymectomy are still controversial, but large case studies indicate that the operation is indicated in patients with demonstrable thymomas and in those with poor response to neostigmine or Mestinon. The operation results are good in some cases, and indifferent or poor in others. The figures of reported improvement vary widely in different series. There appears to be no certain method of predicting the results of operation even in carefully selected cases. Few patients can do without neostigmine after operation. *Irradiation of the thymus gland* is beneficial in instances of hyperplasia of the gland but is without effect in cases of thymus tumor.

Adjuvant treatment may be supplied by the following drugs: *Guanidine hydrochloride,* in doses of 125 mg. three or four times a day by mouth. Unpleasant toxic symptoms are not infrequent and consist of nausea, abdominal cramps, muscular twitchings, and parethesias of the lips and finger tips. As a supplementary treatment, it is valuable in about 5 per cent of cases. *Potassium chloride* tends to prolong the effect of neostigmine in doses of 4 to 6 Gm., three times daily and even as high as six times daily. The gastric discomfort, nausea, diuresis, and at times diarrhea make its prolonged use difficult without interval. *Adrenocorticotropic hormone* (ACTH) appears at times to exert a beneficial effect on myasthenia gravis. The dosage varies, but a total dosage of 500 mg. (25 mg. a day) or more seems necessary to produce good results. This may be given in 25 mg. doses every six hours. The symptoms may be aggravated temporarily during treatment and there is often a relapse after the termination of treatment, usually not to the level prior to the institution of treatment. The type of patient benefited by this treatment is still ill-defined. *Cortisone* (corticotropin) appears to give results similar to ACTH. Both forms of treatment should be reserved for patients who appear to be responding inadequately to neostigmine and other forms of treatment.

Tetarethylpyrophosphate and similar compounds are effective inhibitors of anticholinesterase but are difficult to administer because of their unpleasant toxic reactions.

FAMILIAL PERIODIC PARALYSIS

This is a rare disease. It is regarded by some as a special form of the syndrome of periodic paralysis (Talbott). It is strongly inherited and appears in families extending through as many as six generations. It may be a dominant or recessive trait. Males are affected more frequently than females. The onset of symptoms occurs in the second and third decades, showing a tendency to diminish in frequency and intensity in middle life, and to disappear in late adult life. The cardinal symptoms are *periodic paralysis, loss of reflexes,* and *loss of electrical excitability* of the muscles. The onset is sudden, usually at night, the paralysis beginning peripherally in the legs and travelling centrally. It is usually symmetrical, but it may be unilateral; it is usually complete but it may be partial. The paralysis is flaccid and involves the bodily musculature. The bulbar muscles escape but in rare instances respiration, deglutition, and phonation may be involved. Consciousness is not affected. Electrocardiographic changes have been observed during an attack. Recovery occurs in six to eight hours. Attacks vary in frequency from several times a week to one or two in a year, decade, or lifetime. There are no signs or symptoms between attacks.

Periodic paralysis may appear as a syndrome in association with thyroid disease and malaria, and during excessive assimilation of desoxycorticosterone acetate in the treatment of Addison's disease. Exciting factors in attacks are strenuous exercise and a high carbohydrate meal.

The disease is associated with changes in the level of serum potassium and serum phosphate. During attacks, the serum potassium and phosphate levels are low; the more severe the attack, the greater the fall in serum potassium. The attacks can be terminated by feeding potassium chloride by mouth (2 to 5 gm.).

The serum potassium and phosphate levels are normal between attacks. Other blood constituents are normal. The reason for the decrease in concentration of serum potassium during paralysis is not clear, but the assumption is that there is a redistribution of potassium, the latter migrating from the serum into the intracellular spaces.

Attacks may prove fatal at times, but they are usually benign.

Treatment consists of the oral administration of potassium chloride, of from 2 to 10 gm. daily. This may be given by stomach tube in patients unable to swallow.

20

Degenerative Diseases

The degenerative diseases of the nervous system include a large number of disorders of unknown cause, some of them with hereditary tendencies, others of congenital origin. The designation degenerative disease refers to the pathological characteristics of the disorders rather than to their cause, since in most of the conditions included under this heading little or nothing is known of the precise cause of the disease. In a group so ill-defined it is inevitable that wide differences of opinion should exist concerning the disorders to be included under this heading. For the most part only those disorders have been included which have a congenital or hereditary background. No classification of the disorders so included appears to have sufficient cohesion to clarify the problem, for which reason a number of complicated classifications have been proposed, most of them too complex and confusing to help in the understanding of the problem.

A number of cases occur in which degeneration of the brain cells is associated with degeneration of the macula or with retinitis pigmentosa, and in which degeneration of the white matter is associated with optic atrophy. Since these have many pathological features in common, it has been suggested that they be grouped under the term neuronal lipidoses (Woltman).

I. AMAUROTIC FAMILY IDIOCY
(Cerebromacular Degeneration, Tay-Sachs Disease)

Amaurotic family idiocy is a rare, slowly progressive disease occurring in infants, characterized by severe mental impairment, paralyses, and blindness, and terminating fatally. The *cause* of the disease is unknown. In its infantile form it occurs almost exclusively among Jews, particularly among Polish and Russian Jews, but its occurrence among German Jews is not uncommon. It is found in non-Jews, especially in the juvenile and adult forms. The infantile and juvenile forms are characterized by the familial features of the disease, the parents acting as transmitters or carriers, the disease itself being transmitted as a recessive characteristic. Healthy children are found among afflicted families. "If two parents beget an amaurotic infant, the odds are that one-half of their progeny will carry the gene, and one-quarter exhibit it" (Wilson). Consanguinity occurs among the parents in about fifteen per cent of cases.

Several *forms* of the disease are known, these being: (1) the *infantile* form, by far the most common; (2) the *late infantile* form; (3) the *juvenile* form; (4) the *adult* form.

Pathology: Amaurotic family idiocy is one of a group of diseases associated with disturbance of lipoid metabolism. These disorders have been grouped as follows (Rothstein and Welt):

1. **Cerebroside lipoidosis (Gaucher's disease):**

2. **Phosphatide lipoidosis:**
   (a) Hand-Schüller-Christian disease.
   (b) Amaurotic family idiocy.

3. **Cholesterol lipoidosis:**
   (a) Hand-Schüller-Christian disease.
   (b) Xanthomatosis.

4. **Undetermined forms of lipoidosis:**
   (a) Lipoid cell hyperplasia of the spleen:
     (1) With diabetes mellitus.
     (2) Without diabetes mellitus.
   (b) Lipoid cell hyperplasia of the lymph
     nodes.

The brain may be smaller than normal and may weigh as little as 670 gm. Normal sized and even heavier than normal brains may be found. There may

It stains as a yellow granular material with routine hematoxylineosin and toluidin blue stains and it can be stained with special fat stains. The process is generalized, involving cerebrum, basal ganglia, brain stem, cerebellum, retina, and sympathetic ganglia. It may in some instances be confined to one or to a few areas. The neurofibrils are for the most part destroyed and the Nissl substance

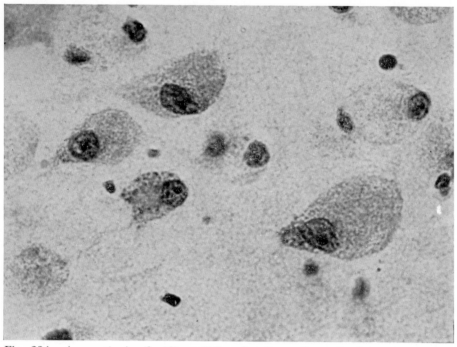

Fig. 234—*Amaurotic family idiocy.* Cell stain of ganglion cells from the cerebral cortex showing the typical pear-shaped ballooned-out cells filled with lipoid. (Courtesy of Dr. Charles Davison.)

be anomalies of the gyri, characterized by microgyria and pachygyria. The cerebellum is sometimes very small.

The outstanding feature of amaurotic family idiocy is a generalized disease of the ganglion cells characterized by a ballooning out and swelling of the cytoplasm, displacement of the nucleus, a loss of cell dendrites, and the presence of lipoid material in the cytoplasm. The lipoid fills the entire cell, giving it a characteristic ballooned-out appearance.

lost. The axones are preserved. The myelin sheaths are intact. The retinal ganglion cells show changes similar to those of the brain.

Two general concepts prevail concerning the *pathogenesis* of the disorder: (1) That amaurotic idiocy is a degenerative process of the nerve cells, the lipoid changes originating in the brain itself. It is regarded, therefore, as distinct from Niemann-Pick's disease. (2) That amaurotic idiocy is part of a generalized metabolic lipoid disorder affecting the entire body, that the lipoid in the brain tissue is similar to that of the lipoid deposit in the reticuloendothelial system of Niemann-Picks' disease, that the two diseases are identical and represent different phases of the same process.

Symptoms: In the *infantile* form (Tay-Sachs), birth is normal and devel-

of spasticity. *Difficulty in vision* is noted early, with a loss of response to visual stimuli of all sorts and a failure to follow objects with the eyes. The weakness becomes gradually more pronounced, fewer voluntary movements being made until the limbs are completely paralyzed and spastic. The reflexes are overactive as a rule, but may be decreased and are

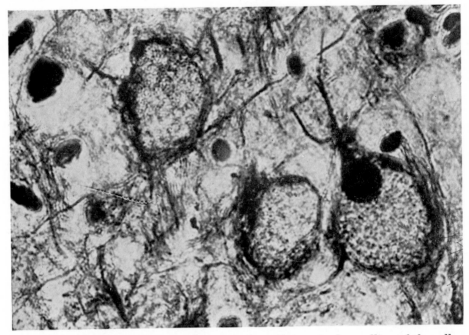

Fig. 235—*Amaurotic family idiocy,* showing in a silver stain the swelling of the cells, the eccentric nuclei, and the agglomeration of neurofibrils at the periphery of the cell. (Courtesy of Dr. Charles Davison.)

opment takes place without mishap for the first three to six months of life. One or more children in a family may be affected. After about six months, or between the third and sixth months, a gradual feebleness is noted. The infant becomes dull and apathetic, a state which is accompanied or soon followed by inability to hold up the head, difficulty in turning in bed, and inability to grasp objects. Weakness is apparent in many ways and the limbs may be limp and flaccid or may early exhibit some degree

even normal in some cases. The visual loss becomes progressively more pronounced until complete blindness ensues The *pupils* are usually inactive to light, but may respond normally; *optic nerve atrophy* is complete, and in the retina is a *cherry-red spot* occupying the position of the macula and surrounded by a white halo. *Mental development* is retarded and eventually completely stunted, and idiocy supervenes. Nystagmus may be seen; strabismus and deafness occur; hyperacusis is common. Epileptic seiz-

Table 64—Familial Retinocerebral Degeneration: The Neuronal Lipidoses (after Woltman).

Name	Sex	Age at Onset	Duration	Ophthalmologic	Comments
Tay-Sachs ..... (Infantile type)	F>M	3-16 mo.	2-3 yr.	Cherry spot ringed by lipid-laden ganglion cells and glia; optic atrophy; small vessels.	Also called (infantile) amaurotic (family) idiocy; cerebromacular degeneration. Usually Jewish parentage. Listless; flaccid, later spastic; amaurosis; dementia; nystagmus; hyperirritability to stimuli; convulsions. Brain deeply fissured, firm. Characteristic cell changes.
Spielmeyer-Vogt		2-4 yr.	1-3 yr.	In addition, may have retinal pigmentation.	Not only Jewish. Also cerebellar and athletic manifestations. Separate group hardly warranted.
Batten-Mayou.. (Juvenile type)	M=F	3½-15 yr.	10-15 yr. Average age death 18 yr.	Beaten silver macula; may appear late; retinal pigmentation; optic atrophy.	Also stammering and repitition; convulsive laughter and crying; flexed posture; may become psychotic. May be only cerebral or only macular. If no mental changes by age of ten, not likely to have any.
Kufs........... (Late or adult type)........		13-38 yr.	Years	May have retinal pigmentation; optic atrophy. Usually normal.	Also tremor, ataxia; usually no loss of vision; cold, cyanotic extremities.
Refsum		?	4-30 yr.	Retinal pigmentation; night blindness.	Called heredopathia atactica polyneuritiformis. Author's cases Norwegian. Deafness; ataxia; polyneuritis; ichthiosis; electrocardiographic changes; increased protein in spinal fluid. No mental deterioration. Fine, perinuclear granules of lipid in all nerve cells; fat-laden macrophages in meninges; interstitial hypertrophic neuritis.
				Lipidoses that Include Reticulo-endothelial System	
Niemann-Pick..	F>M	3-6 mo.	2 yr.	±cherry spot; may be blind and fundus normal.	Usually Jewish. Spasticity; convulsions; ±mental symptoms; ±blindness. Liver, spleen, lymph nodes enlarged. Foam cells (filled with lecithin, sphingomyelin) in organs and blood vessels. Neuronal changes as above. May have fever. Pick gives higher incidence in male.

Table 64 (Continued)

Name	Sex	Age at Onset	Duration	Ophthalmologic	Comments
Hand-Schüller-. Christian......	M>F	1st decade	Long	May have choked disks; secondary atrophy.	Seldom hereditary. Diabetes; dwarfism; hypogenitalism; mental deterioration; exophthalmos; xanthoma lids; fatty cornea. Changes secondary to infiltration of foam cells containing cholesterol and cholesterol esters into meninges, skull, long bones, etc.
Gaucher........					Cerebrosides (kerasin) deposited in reticuloendothelial system. This stands at end opposite Tay-Sachs disease.
Laurence-Moon-Biedl...	M>F	Childhood	Does not shorten life.	Retinitis pigmentosa; optic atrophy.	Nystagmus, cataract, opthalmoplegia; flaccidity or spasticity; ataxia; convulsions; mental impairment dystrophia adiposogenitalis; polydactylism; atresia ani. Neuropathologic findings? Retinitis suggests it may belong in this group.

ures may occur. In the last months of life the child becomes an inactive idiot. Death occurs before the second and at the latest before the completion of the third year with marked emaciation. The wasting which accompanies the disease is striking. Infants who at the onset of the illness are plump and chubby become gradually thinner until at the time of death they are markedly emaciated.

The *late infantile form* (Jansky-Bielschowsky) occurs at three to four years, the patient having been well before that time. Non-Jewish children are affected and the disease runs its course in three to four years. Blindness is present, but there is no cherry-red spot. Mental retardation develops and with it progressive paralysis. Convulsions occur. The outstanding diagnostic features are the occurrence of mental and physical retardation in the preschool child, blindness, convulsions, and paralyses.

The *juvenile* form (Vogt) occurs between six and twelve years of age, at the time of second dentition, is not confined to Jews, has no cherry-red spot, runs a somewhat slower course than the infantile type, is featured by retinitis pigmentosa, and in some but not all cases, by optic atrophy. In other respects the juvenile form is similar to the infantile type in its development of progressive paralyses, blindness, and mental deficiency.

The first symptom is usually impairment of vision, which progresses slowly to complete blindness. Gradual mental deterioration develops soon after the disturbance of vision and is characterized by dullness, silly behavior, and marked emotional lability. The process develops to the point of complete deterioration, with spasticity of the limbs, and imbecility. The pupils eventually lose their reaction to light. Convulsions, strabismus, cerebellar disturbances, decerebrate pictures, and parkinsonian syndromes have been found.

An *adult* form (Kufs) of amaurotic idiocy is known. It occurs between twenty-one and twenty-six years of age, has no racial predominance, and runs a protracted course of several years. Blindness is present, without a cherry-red spot but with retinitis pigmentosa. Marked mental disturbances develop during the course of the disease leading to dementia, but convulsions and paralyses do not appear. Involuntary movements and cerebellar disturbances have been observed. The most suggestive diagnostic features are the development of mental disturbances and dementia in a young adult, associated with blindness and retinitis pigmentosa.

Allied to amaurotic idiocy are a number of diseases. *Niemann-Pick's disease* is a congenital familial disorder which occurs in young children, is limited almost entirely to Jews, and is much more common in females than in males. The disease begins in the early months of life after a normal period at birth and is followed shortly thereafter by marked feeding disturbances, undernourishment, and evidence of mental retardation. Many infants fail to talk or walk; some have a mongoloid appearance. The weakness is less marked than in amaurotic idiocy and the mental retardation less profound. The spleen, liver, and lymph nodes are enlarged, the abdomen is protuberant, and the skin pigmented. A cherry-red spot may be found in the retina. Enlargement of the liver and spleen is found in the early months of life. The rapid increase in size of the abdomen, the pale and yellowish-brown discoloration of the skin of the face, arms, and sclerae, the slight ascites, the edema and bronchitis, are constant manifestations (Pick). The superficial lymph nodes are moderately to considerably enlarged. The red blood cells are moderately decreased. Occasionally there is a leukocytosis in the late stages and sometimes a leukopenia. Large vacuoles may be found in the lymphocytes and polymorphonuclear cells. The cholesterin content of the blood is markedly elevated; at times it is normal.

Progressive enlargement of the liver and spleen produces a very large abdomen which stands out in contrast to the general emaciation. The diagnosis can be made with certainty by puncture of the bone marrow or spleen and the demonstration of cells filled with lipoid. Large foamy cells are found throughout the reticuloendothelial system. "Combined forms" of Niemann-Pick's disease and amaurotic family idiocy have been described pathologically.

Hand-Schüller-Christian's disease, also allied to this general group of diseases, occurs in early childhood, affects males predominantly, has familial tendencies, and occurs racially more often among Jews, but it may develop in any race. It has a subacute course with onset of symptoms in childhood, most commonly in the first decade of life, but it may develop from the second to the fifth decades. It is associated with exophthalmos, diabetes insipidus, defects in the skull, xanthomatous masses in the skin, hyperglycemia, and normal lipoid, cholesterol, calcium, and phosphorus values. The disease is characterized chiefly but not exclusively by (1) bone lesions, (2) exophthalmos, (3) diabetes insipidus, all of which are found in a well-developed case. Any of them may be absent, however, depending on the degree of spread of the process. The *bone defects* are found in almost every case, usually in the parietal and sphenoid bones and the orbits, but any part of the skull may be involved. Other bones of the body show similar defects at times. *Diabetes insipidus* is quite constant and was present in thirty-six to forty-nine cases (Davison). Mental retardation, loss or decay of teeth, and pulmonary, cardiac, gastrointestinal, and renal complications may be found. Death ensues in two to four years, usually from intercurrent infection.

Gaucher's disease, xanthomatoma tuberosum multiplex, and *essential xanthomatosis* are other allied disorders. In xanthomatosis lipoid deposits may be found in the upper eyelids, skin, tendons, and joints, and in the internal organs. A hyperlipoidemia is present. The disorder is familial in some instances.

II. THE DIFFUSE SCLEROSES

Diffuse sclerosis is a poor term, applied as it is to a group of brain disorders of which the main paradigm is encephalitis periaxialis diffusa or Schilder's disease. It has no specific meaning and can be applied equally as logically to multiple sclerosis. As the term is used at present, it refers to a group of disorders of the brain, probably closely allied to one another both clinically and pathologically, characterized in general by areas of demyelination, relative intactness of axis cylinders, and by varied glial and mesodermal tissue response. The examples included under the grouping of diffuse sclerosis possess features common to all, together with more or less distinctive characteristics. The common clinical features which characterize them are: (1) familial tendency which is pronounced in some forms (Pelizaeus-Merzbacher disease) and less pronounced in others (Schilder's disease) ; (2) an early onset of symptoms, in infancy in some forms (Pelizaeus-Merzbacher and cerebral sclerosis of Krabbe), in childhood in others (Schilder's disease and encephalitis periaxialis concentrica) ; (3) a tendency to involve a number of systems and tracts; (4) an invariably fatal outcome, rapid in some forms (Schilder's disease; encephalitis periaxialis concentrica; cerebral sclerosis) and slow in others (Pelizaeus-Merzbacher disease).

The best-defined example of the group is encephalitis peraxialis diffusa (Schilder), but there are even doubts whether this should be regarded as a distinct entity, since it possesses features of multiple sclerosis. In any event, the limits of the group are poorly defined and the probabilities are that more entities will be added to it before it becomes more definitely delimited.

Encephalitis Periaxialis Diffusa (Schilder's Disease)

Encephalitis periaxialis diffusa, or Schilder's disease, is a relatively rare disorder occurring chiefly in children, characterized by an acute or subacute onset and course, and by blindness, convulsions, motor weakness, and mental symptoms. It is invariably fatal.

Etiology: Most cases occur in children or adolescents, but adult incidence is by no means uncommon. The precise cause is not known. It was regarded by Schilder as due to infection and examples of the disease are recorded in which it appears to have developed after an upper respiratory infection. Familial forms have been described. Trauma has been associated with the onset of the disease in a few instances.

Pathology: The disease is characterized generally by predominant involvement of the white matter, symmetrical in character, and usually extensive. In the majority of instances, the process implicates chiefly the white matter of the occipital lobes, extending forward into the parietal or frontal lobes. In others, the disease attacks chiefly the frontal lobes, extending into the deeper subcortical structures, such as the internal capsule, corpus callosum, and brain stem. The pathological process consists of a demyelination with relative preservation of the axis cylinders. The U fibers connecting adjacent gyri escape. Associated with the demyelination is a proliferation of the neuroglia and frequently evidence of perivascular infiltration with lymphocytes and plasma cells. The cortex is intact. The familial forms of the disease are associated chiefly with an abundance of regressive forms of neuroglia and absence of lymphocytic exudate in the perivascular spaces. Spinal cord lesions of a patchy nature have been recorded in some cases. The process is probably degenerative, but instances are recorded in which toxic-infectious processes seem to be at work.

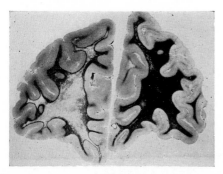

Fig. 236 — *Encephalitis periaxialis diffusa.* (Schilder's disease.) Myelin sheath stain showing the complete demyelination of the white matter and the intact arcuate fibers. (Courtesy of Dr. Charles Davison.)

Symptoms: The onset is often acute but may be insidious, with indiscriminate symptoms of various sorts. The history very often concerns disturbance of vision, with loss or impairment of vision a common complaint. In those cases which involve first the frontal areas, a loss of mental function, convulsions, or weakness of one side of the body are frequent complaints. The course is usually progressive, without remissions in the typical case, but remissive features are found in some cases. Progressive *blindness* is a feature of many cases, and is characterized by features of cortical blindness with a loss of vision, with intact pupillary reflexes, and normal appearing optic nerves. A homonymous hemianopsia may be observed early in the disease, later extending to involve all the fields of vision.

Mental retardation and slowing of the mental processes are found in cases involving primarily the frontal lobes. *Convulsions* appear not infrequently. They are usually generalized but may be focal. *Hemiplegia, monoplegia,* or *hemiparesis* are not uncommon and with convulsions may constitute the first symptoms. The optic nerves, as a rule, show no changes, but optic neuritis and choked disc may occur in some instances. *Aphasia* occurs in some instances. *Mental symptoms,* characterized by disturbance of memory and evidences of mental deterioration, are frequent in some forms. Basal ganglia symptoms, such as involuntary movements, involuntary laughing and crying, are found in some forms of the disease.

Diagnosis: The disease is difficult to diagnose in many instances. It may be suspected in children or young people with acute or subacute onset, with evidence of cortical blindness of a progressive nature, with no indication of pupillary or optic nerve involvement. In such instances, the diagnosis may be made with assurance during life. In cases involving particularly the frontal lobes and adjacent structures, the diagnosis is not as definite as in instances involving primarily the occipital lobes. In such instances, the course is featured by mental deterioration, convulsions, hemiplegia or hemiparesis, and by less common symptoms of various sorts. In some cases, the disease affects first the temporal lobes, the onset being with deafness, visual loss, and aphasia in such instances. The onset is more commonly of the frontal lobes than of the occipital or temporal lobe types.

Since the disease is progressive in nature, the condition is confused frequently with *brain tumor,* and in other cases with *encephalitis* and *multiple sclerosis.* Brain tumor is confused because of the progressive course in young adults, associated often with evidences of a frontal lobe or occipital syndrome. If choked disc is present, the distinction may be almost impossible. The bilaterality of the process is a distinction of great importance in favor of Schilder's disease, especially if there is no evidence of increased pressure. *Multiple sclerosis* may be confused in cases which show a multiplicity of symptoms, such as blindness, hemiplegia, mental symptoms, and other signs which indicate a widespread process. The differentiation is especially difficult in cases which show a tendency to remissions, but the latter are more characteristic of multiple sclerosis. Mental symptoms are more prominent in Schilder's disease.

Other Types of Diffuse Sclerosis

A very rare form of diffuse sclerosis sometimes confused with Schilder's disease is *aplasia axialis extracorticalis* or *Pelizaeus-Merzbacher disease*. This is a heredofamilial disease with a strong familial tendency, occurring in the first six months of life, and characterized by a combination of cerebral and cerebellar symptoms, such as head tremor, nystagmus, weakness of the limbs and trunk with spastic paraplegia, incoördination of the trunk and limbs, intention tremor, and at times a masklike facies. Optic atrophy and blindness may develop. Progress of the disease is slow. Head tremor is noticed early, followed somewhat later by spasticity of the legs and later of

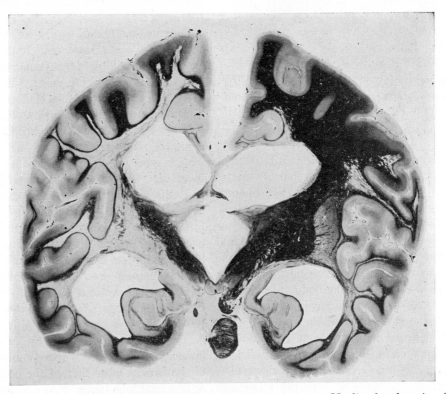

Fig. 237—*Encephalitis periaxialis diffusa* (Schilder's disease). Myelin sheath stain of the brain showing demyelination of the white matter extending into the internal capsule and cerebral peduncle. The arcuate fibers connecting adjacent cortical gyri are intact and there is internal hydrocephalus. (Courtesy of Dr. Charles Davison.)

the arms, and still later by incoördination of gait, intention tremor, slow speech, and finally after five to six years by evidences of mental deterioration. The disease is associated with a demyelination of the white matter of the cerebrum and cerebellum with relative escape of the internal capsule and brain stem, and with relative intactness of the axis cylinders. Not all the brain is affected, so that areas of normal myelin structure are found in the affected regions. The disease runs a slow, protracted course, death occurring in adult life.

A confusing number of syndromes associated with a diffuse sclerosis has been described. The syndrome of *cerebral sclerosis* (Krabbe) is claimed by its author to be a special form of brain sclerosis, but appears rather to be an acute type of Pelizaeus-Merzbacher disease. The disease is familial, the symptoms appearing at four to six months with fretfulness and constant crying, followed by apathy and stupor, rigidity of the musculature developing to the point of helplessness, tonic fits, and clonic convulsions. Swallowing difficulties develop, blindness may develop associated with optic nerve atrophy or without it, and deafness may occur. The disease runs a rapid course and lasts only about one year.

Probably a special form of Schilder's disease is a rare condition known as *encephalitis periaxialis concentrica* (Balo). This is characterized pathologically by concentric circles of gray and white, the gray portions representing degenerated tissue, the white being normal white matter. The white substance of the cerebral hemispheres is involved, the cerebral cortex, basal ganglia, brain stem, and spinal cord remaining uninjured. The microscopic picture in the degenerated areas is similar to that of Schilder's disease. The clinical features are not specific. The onset is at any age, usually with focal manifestations, such as aphasia, hemiparesis, or hemianopsia. Eventually, bilateral pyramidal signs, pseudobulbar palsy, convulsions, mental deterioration, and choked disc appear. The disease is invariably fatal and the diagnosis has been made only at necropsy.

A type of diffuse sclerosis different from the more common forms has been described by Greenfield as *progressive cerebral sclerosis in infants associated with primary degeneration of the interfascicular glia*. In the two reported cases, development was normal in the first two years of life except for a condition of diplegia in one case. Thereafter there developed mental and physical regression, with loss of the powers of walking and talking, and then of sight, hearing, and recognition. Death occurred at the age of three years. Necropsy showed a diffuse sclerosis of the cerebral hemispheres sparing the optic tracts and, to a lesser extent, the pyramidal tracts. The absence of myelin was associated with a complete or almost complete absence of oligodendroglia, not only in the affected areas, but in the neighboring myelinated tracts.

The combination of hemangioma of the face, buphthalmos, congenital glaucoma, and hemangioma of the brain is referred to as *Sturge-Weber's disease*. In typical instances, the four conditions occur together. Not infrequently one or more features are lacking. In order to make a diagnosis of the disorder, at least two of the characteristic factors must be present.

The hemangioma of the face is usually unilateral but may rarely be bilateral. It may extend over the shoulder or large parts of the body. The cerebral hemangioma is often calcified. Convulsions are a common symptom of the brain hemangioma. Hemiplegia occurs frequently.

III. TUBEROUS SCLEROSIS
(Epiloia)

Tuberous sclerosis is a rare disease, but it is found with surprising frequency in institutions for the feebleminded. It is associated with both visceral and brain changes and with mental deficiency and convulsions.

Etiology: A familial incidence is found in many but not in all instances, abortive forms and isolated examples being quite common. The family history often shows a high incidence of epilepsy and alcoholism, and psychoses are not uncommon among the forebears. The precise cause is not known.

Pathology: The skin of the face shows collections of typical adenoma sebaceum, with a winglike distribution over the cheeks. Tumors are found in the kidneys, liver, heart, and other viscera.

The brain changes are characterized by scattered hard nodules in the cortex and in the walls of the ventricles, the latter having a verrucose appearance. The number of foci varies from few to many, scattered in all parts of the brain. The affected gyri are broad, widened, show a dimple in the center, and are extremely firm to palpation. The affected cerebral cortex shows a number of abnormal nerve and glial cells with a reduction or severe loss of ganglion cells. The ganglion cells are often large, their shape variable, and their structure abnormal. The glial cells are often large, and are usually greatly increased in number. Demyelination and loss of axis cylinders are found in the diseased areas.

The condition is regarded as a developmental condition affecting both ganglion cells and glial elements, probably allied to neurofibromatosis (von Recklinghausen's disease).

Symptoms: The age of onset varies widely. In the true tuberous sclerosis case, the onset is in infancy or early childhood. Later onset occurs in many instances, however. The onset is gradual, attention being called first to *delay in development*. Crawling, walking, and talking are late. *Mental development* is retarded, the rate of its occurrence varying widely from case to case. In some instances, the retardation is apparent by the second and third years; in others, not until five or six years of age. *Skin manifestations* appear some time within the first decade and are apparent first as an adenoma sebaceum over the nose and cheeks. Development continues to be retarded, so that by the fifth to sixth year increasing *mental dullness, emotional outbursts*, and *disturbances of speech* develop. *Convulsions* occur frequently *pari passu* with the mental deficiency. Generalized seizures are common, but minor and focal attacks are not uncommon. The frequency of attacks varies widely, some patients experiencing several attacks a day, others only two to four attacks a year. Long remissions from epileptic seizures may occur frequently.

Examination in the typical case reveals an adenoma sebaceum over the face. The patients are usually undersized and show stigmata of degeneration frequently, such as the simian hand, shortening and incurving of the little finger, and misshapen, asymmetrical, or excessively large ears. Other stigmata include hemihypertrophy, epicanthus, high palate, supernumerary digits, syndactyly, and hydrocephalus. "Drusen" or phakomata are found in the retina. Retinal tumors are found in some cases. Paralyses of various types may be encountered (monoplegia, hemiplegia, paraplegia). Speech is usually impaired. Mental defectiveness, usually of a severe degree (imbecility or idiocy), is usual. In less severe cases the degree of mental defect is less pronounced.

Diagnosis: The diagnosis of tuberous sclerosis is easy in characteristic cases with onset in infancy, a history of delayed development, convulsions, mental deficiency, and adenoma sebaceum. Many abortive forms of the disease are known, however. Among these are cases of adenoma sebaceum with convulsions, with no evidence of mental deficiency; adenoma sebaceum with epilepsy and signs of increased intracranial pressure; and finally cases of adenoma sebaceum alone or visceral tumors alone without convulsions or mental deficiency have been regarded as abortive forms of tuberous sclerosis in some instances.

Treatment: The treatment is purely symptomatic.

IV. CEREBRAL DIPLEGIA
(Little's Disease)*

There is probably no more heterogeneous and ill-defined group in neurology than that collection of conditions commonly referred to as cerebral diplegia or *Little's disease*. Though the clinical features are well stated in Little's description, almost any form of cerebral birth palsy has come to be designated cerebral diplegia or Little's disease. The result has been a profound confusion which is far from being resolved even at the present time. Much of the difficulty seems to have arisen from a desire to attribute all diplegias to a common cause, a tendency which is hardly in accord with the facts. Cerebral diplegia may occur congenitally at birth, or it may become apparent in the postnatal period. The clinical features remain the

*The present tendency to group the cerebral diplegias, infantile hemiplegias, monoplegias, and paraplegias under the unitary heading of "Cerebral Palsy" appears to me to be undesirable, and I have therefore avoided use of the term. To classify these various conditions in a single group is to assume that they have a common pathological background and cause. Since this assumption cannot be sustained by the facts, I have chosen to group them under separate headings.

same, despite minor variations of onset. Hence it seems best to designate two main groups of cases: (1) congenital or Little's disease; (2) acquired, occurring early in the postnatal period. The present confusion can be minimized by adhering to this grouping, reserving the term Little's disease for the cases occurring before or at birth and designating the rest as acquired diplegias. If it is clearly recognized that no single cause is assignable to all cases, the problem becomes clearer.

Etiology: No single cause covers all the cases. *Intrauterine factors* play an important rôle in some cases, especially in the congenital type, but their precise nature cannot be designated. Toxemias and infections transmitted across the placental membranes may account for some examples of the disease; maldevelopment for others. The importance of the rôle of intrauterine disease in the production of the congenital cases of cerebral diplegia is difficult to assess, since proof of intrauterine disease is often difficult to obtain. Evidence appears to be accumulating, however, that the transmission of disease from mother to fetus may be more common than is generally recognized, and a number of conditions have been shown recently to be capable of intrauterine transmission. It is possible and even probable that next to birth injury, intrauterine processes are the most important causative factors in the production of the congenital form of cerebral diplegia (Little's disease).

More evidence is accumulating to support the belief that cerebral diplegia and the cerebral palsies result often from intrauterine factors. *Rubella* occurring in the mother in the first three months of pregnancy has been found to be associated with congenial anomalies, among which are deaf-mutism, cataract, microphthalmia and buphthalmos, congenital heart disease, and congenital dental abnormalities, such as "sharklike" and "pointed" incisors and enamel hypoplasias. No good figures are available, but it has been estimated that "the risk of anomalies in the infant may be upward of 25 per cent following rubella during the first three months of pregnancy" (Aycock and Ingalls). Reports have been made of anomalous development following maternal infection with rubella in the eighth or ninth month of pregnancy.

In *poliomyelitis* also, the risk to the infant appears to be high if the disease occurs in the mother during the first three months of pregnancy.

Suggestive evidence is at hand that *dietary deficiency* in the mother may cause congenital anomalies. Diets deficient in vitamin A caused litters from sows to be born blind or without eyeballs, or with bare lips, misplaced kidneys, and other defects. Skeletal deformities in rats were produced by dietary deficiency and prevented by riboflavin. The evidence is not yet clear in regard to humans.

Infectious mononucleosis occurring in pregnancy may cause congenital defects. *Fetal irradiation* is also a cause of anomalous development in the offspring of laboratory animals.

Trauma at birth has been assigned an important rôle in many instances and doubtless is an important factor, but its significance has been overemphasized. Punctate hemorrhage or larger effusions are produced by tearing of dural veins from the application of forceps which produce a shearing action of the easily molded skull bones. Septal tears may occur by the shearing action in the process of molding of the head. Breech deliveries are prone to be associated with a high percentage of tears. Diplegias are known to occur in cesarean births and an easy uncomplicated labor is frequently encountered in diplegics. Difficult and precipitate

labor occurs, however, in not a few cases. *Asphyxia* during the course of labor is said to be significant in many instances, but the rôle of asphyxia and of cerebral anoxemia has not been definitely demonstrated. It may, however, be a factor in the causation of the disease. Windle attempts to supply experimental evidence of the C. N. S. changes associated with asphyxia at birth. He tied off the uterine arteries in pregnant guinea pigs and delivered the fetuses which he then resuscitated. He states that asphyxial changes can produce severe changes in the nervous system. Many sets of symptoms were produced. He believes the findings are comparable to those produced in humans with asphyxia during birth and that asphyxia may produce inferior mentality and mental dullness. The rôle of analgesics, such as barbiturates, in the production of cerebral anoxemia and asphyxia has been stressed recently as a factor of importance. Anoxia at critical stages of prenatal development in the mouse may result in acquired malformations of the fetus. *Subarachnoid hemorrhage* may be a factor but its rôle is difficult to assess. It has been found in some cases of cerebral diplegia, but its rôle in the production of diplegia has been challenged.

Prematurity is associated with diplegia not infrequently. Maternal illness has a direct bearing on prematurity. In white women, the incidence of prematurity without maternal illness was 5.5 per cent and rose to 13.5 per cent with illness. In Negro women, the respective percentages were 9.2 and 16.6. Approximately 80 per cent of stillborn infants of both sexes were the offspring of mothers who had some illness during pregnancy (Brown, Ayon, Anderson).

Pathology: The pathological background of cerebral diplegia is as varied as the causative factors and should serve to emphasize the fact that there is no single cause or pathological basis for the disease. The pathological process, whatever its type, may moreover produce changes in many parts of the brain, accounting, therefore, for the variety of clinical syndromes encountered. Among the brain findings are: (1) Cerebral agenesis, which accounts for not a few cases. It may vary widely in type and extent and may be featured by microcephaly, absence of the pyramidal tracts, and other anomalies. The conditions in this group are probably the result of intra-uterine factors. (2) Atrophic lobar sclerosis, consisting of a focal atrophy of brain substance and associated with moderate or severe loss of ganglion cells and myelin and overgrowth of glia. It is probably due to extrauterine causes, such as trauma, meningeal hemorrhage, vascular occlusion, or encephalitis, and must be regarded as associated with the acquired diplegias. (3) Porencephaly is found in some cases, and may be due to intrauterine or extrauterine conditions. (4) Meningeal hemorrhage. (5) Status marmoratus.

In a surprising number of cases of cerebral diplegia, the brain appears normal both grossly and microscopically.

Symptoms: The disease manifests itself as a diplegia or paraplegia predominantly. There is no familial tendency in most cases, but the affliction of two members of a family and the occurrence of the disease in twins has been recorded. The birth history is often normal, but a history of precipitate or prolonged labor, especially in a first-born, is common. Prematurity is also a frequent accompaniment.

Symptoms are noted at birth in the severe congenital conditions, or they may not be observed until several months after birth, the child being described as normal up to this time. Many of the histories of normal development are doubtless due to inaccurate observations by the parents. The child is usually fretful and irritable and in severe cases may be cyanotic, and may have feeding and breathing difficulties.

Paralysis is present in varying degree. In the severe cases there is almost complete paralysis and spasticity of the arms and legs, affecting more severely the legs. In less advanced cases, the paralysis and spasticity are less pronounced. The mild cases show chiefly involvement of the legs with slight implication of the arms. These are the cases usually referred to as paraplegic. In some instances, the weakness may be hemiplegic in type. The tendon reflexes are overactive and pathological reflexes are present. The gait is characterized by the "scissors" position, the legs being strongly adducted and often crossing over in front of one another in attempted progression. Walking is slow in development, never normal, and in severe cases totally impossible.

Involuntary movements occur in almost every case. These are of a choreoathetotic nature as a rule. Athetoid movements of the fingers and toes are common, associated at times with grimacing movements, sometimes quite pronounced.

Mental deficiency is not a frequent accompaniment of the motor disturbances of cerebral diplegia. When it occurs it may be pronounced to the degree of idiocy or imbecility, or it may be relatively mild. It is by no means constant, however, and a normal mentality is often encountered in cerebral diplegia. Many a diplegic has overcome his physical handicaps and has lived a useful intellectual life. Sixty-five to 70 per cent of patients with cerebral diplegia have a normal mentality.

Convulsions, usually generalized, are not common and may occur early or late in the disease. Focal convulsions are not as frequent as generalized seizures.

Pseudobulbar symptoms, such as dysarthria and dysphagia, are so pronounced in some cases that a special pseudobulbar form of the disease has been designated in some cases. Speech, like walking, is usually delayed in the average case of cerebral diplegia and may never acquire normal features.

Cerebellar ataxia is striking in some forms of the disease, and a special cerebellar form has been described.

Diagnosis: The diagnosis of cerebral diplegia offers few difficulties as a rule. The typical *spastic* case shows symptoms from the time of birth, with paralysis of the arms and legs, most severe in the legs, mental deficiency usually but not always, choreoathetotic movements, and often convulsions. In some cases, the onset may be delayed. The cause and the pathological background vary.

Recognition must be made of a *cerebellar* type of cerebral diplegia. This form of diplegia is characterized by cerebellar dyssynergia of severe degree, associated with disturbances of speech, gait, station, and incoördination of the extremities. Cases of this type have no paralysis or spasticity, are free from mental defect or epilepsy, and show a tendency toward recovery. An *atonic type* of diplegia has also been described, characterized by motor paralysis with flaccidity. There is inability to stand or walk, great difficulty in articulation, often mutism, and a marked mental defect.

A disease of the basal ganglia which may be considered at this point has been designated as *kernicterus.* This disease tends to attack several members of a family. The birth history is normal and the child is apparently born healthy. Severe jaundice develops within the first few days, usually before the second day. The pathogenesis of kernicterus is not clearly understood, but study of a fatal case forty-eight hours after birth revealed the blood vessels of the brain to be filled with agglutinated masses of erythrocytes and suggested the following theory (Wiener and Brody): The antibodies in the maternal serum in kernicterus are almost always agglutinins, suggesting that maternal Rh agglutinins in the infant circulation combine with the Rh + erythrocytes, causing agglutination of the red cells. which plug arterioles and produce agglutination thrombi and ischemic infarcts with loss of ganglion cells. Nervous symptoms then appear within the next twenty-four hours and are characterized by tonic and clonic movements which develop later into convulsions. Between these attacks there is a tendency to a generalized spasticity and opisthotonus. Choreoathetoid movements develop at or about the fourth week in children who survive the immediate illness, and emotional instability follows. Most cases terminate fatally by the fifth day after the onset of the jaundice, but longer survivals have been reported.

The disease takes its name from a yellow icteric staining of the basal ganglia, particularly the subthalamic nuclei, the striatum and pallidum, the thalamus, dentate nucleus, cornu Ammonis, inferior olives, and some of the nuclei of the cranial nerves of the medulla. The ganglion cells are degenerated in varying degrees in all the pigmented areas. Demyelination in the putamen and pallidum is usually found; there is a marked dropping out of cells in the subthalamic nuclei. Patchy degeneration of the optic nerves and demyelination of the lateral columns have been recorded.

The jaundice in cases of kernicterus is regarded chiefly as due to a primary dysfunction of the blood. Erythroblastosis is commonly found in the condition but is regarded by many as secondary to hemolysis of toxic origin. Fetal septicemia and maternal toxemia are regarded as other causes of the jaundice.

A *familial cerebral degeneration* (Paterson and Carmichael) has been described, characterized clinically by a familial incidence, mental deficiency, blindness, and muscular weakness, but without paralysis or abnormal movements. Children live from two to six months and usually die before two years of age. There is severe degeneration of the cortex, the lenticular nuclei, the caudate, and the genu of the internal capsule.

A syndrome of *congenital muscular hypertrophy, extrapyramidal motor disturbances, and mental deficiency* has been described by deLange. The condition is present from birth. The muscular hypertrophy is generalized and the extrapyramidal disturbances consist chiefly of muscular rigidity.

Cerebral diplegia must be distinguished from other cerebral birth palsies, particularly hemiplegias. The occurrence of the condition at birth or shortly thereafter serves to separate the cases from cerebral conditions due to encephalitis or vascular disorders.

Children with severe cases, associated with marked brain damage, often fail to survive the first two years of life. Those with less severe cases tend to level off, regain some of their lost ground in development, and may survive for years, succumbing eventually to intercurrent disease. Epilepsy tends to persist but may respond well to medical treatment.

Treatment: Nothing constructive can be done in the mentally defective cases. In those with normal or almost normal mentality, *physiotherapy* is often valuable. Active and passive exercises and massage are helpful. Tenotomy and the overcoming of deformities by orthopedic operations, such as muscle transplants, may be performed, followed later by massage and exercise. *Surgical procedures* for athetosis may be performed (*v.* Extrapyramidal Diseases). The *convulsions* so common in the disorder may be controlled by the use of Dilantin Sodium, phenobarbital, or bromides (*v.* Epilepsy).

V. INFANTILE CEREBRAL HEMIPLEGIA

This group of cases is often erroneously included among the diplegias but requires separate consideration.

Etiology: The causes of the condition are similar to those of diplegia. The disease may be congenital or acquired. Birth injury is probably the most common cause, but congenital defects which are developed *in utero* are significant factors. The acquired cases result frequently from encephalitis associated with a febrile disease, such as measles, chickenpox. mumps, German measles, etc. Syphilis may be a factor but is rare.

Pathology: Among the congenital conditions which may be found is *porencephaly,* characterized by a cavity formation, unilateral or bilateral, and usually connecting with the lateral ventricle. *Hemiatrophy of the brain* may be found in some instances. The affected cerebral hemisphere is much smaller than its mate and in some instances may be almost absent. The cerebral cortex is poorly developed and the motor system of the affected hemisphere is rudimentary. Acquired conditions associated with the hemiplegia include softenings of the brain tissue due to thrombosis or embolism, thrombosis of the dural sinuses, trauma, and brain tumor.

Symptoms: The clinical features are easy to detect. In the congenital hemiplegias the condition is present from birth; in acquired cases it develops at some time during infancy. The limbs of one side are paralyzed, are usually spastic, but may be flaccid. Congenital hemiplegias are associated with a loss of muscle bulk in the affected limbs, which are smaller than those of the healthy side. The hemiplegia may be complete or mild, the latter cases manifesting themselves as a slight awkwardness in the use of the hand and arm, and a slight dragging of the leg. In congenital cases, speech, walking, and training habits are greatly delayed. Convulsions are frequent and occur more often than among diplegics. Mental deficiency of some degree is usually present. Involuntary movements may be found.

Severe cases show little tendency to improvement; milder cases may recover completely or be only moderately handicapped by the condition.

VI. PORENCEPHALY

Porencephaly is not uncommonly encountered in neurological disorders as a cause of epilepsy or hemiplegia in children. For this reason it deserves more than the passing mention customarily given to it. Porencephaly is a defect in the cerebral hemispheres as a rule, appearing as a cystlike cavity communicating with the ventricles or separated from them only by a thin layer of brain tissue, covered on the outside by a thin layer of cortex and thickened pia arachnoid and containing a clear colorless fluid.

Etiology: Porencephaly may be found at any age, but it is more frequent in young subjects, particularly up to fifteen years. It may manifest its presence in adults of forty or over.

The condition may be congenital or acquired and has been ascribed to a number of causes. Among the congenital causes assigned are anoxia of the brain tissue and defects of fetal development. The acquired causes include circulatory disturbances (thrombosis, embolism, hemorrhage); inflammatory lesions (tuberculosis, syphilis, encephalitis); trauma.

Pathology: Porencephalic cysts may be large or small, unilateral or bilateral, and may be encountered in any part of the brain. They are most frequently situated in the parietal and occipital areas. They are usually but not always connected with the ventricle and may at times communicate with the subarachnoid space. The roof of the cyst is composed usually of a thin layer of cerebral cortex and fibrotic pia arachnoid. The cortex shows a considerable loss of ganglion cells and a marked hyperplasia of glial cells. In some instances, the cap

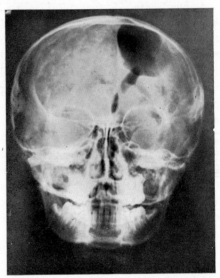

Fig. 238—*Porencephalic cyst,* showing the cyst and its connection with the lateral ventricle in a child of 10 years with a right hemiparesis.

of the cyst is composed only of a cortex filled with glial scar. The gyri adjacent to the porencephalic cyst may show evidence of atrophy.

Symptoms: The symptoms of porencephaly may make their appearance early in life before the tenth year, or they may not be apparent until adult life. The presenting symptom is usually convulsions, but weakness of one side of the body is not uncommon. Symptoms have usually been present for months or years

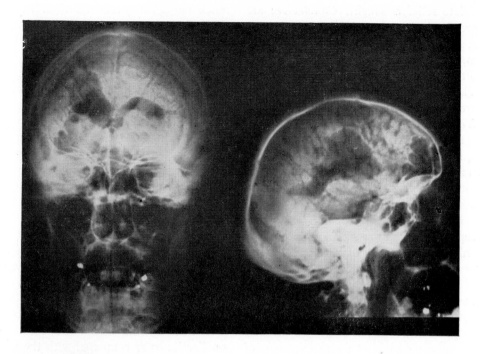

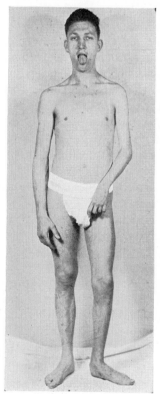

Fig. 239—*Porencephaly*, associated with long-standing left hemiplegia and showing the porencephalic cyst in the right frontoparietal area.

before relief is sought. *Convulsions* are present in practically all cases and constitute the outstanding symptom. They may be generalized or focal but are more often focal jacksonian motor convulsions. The onset of the convulsions varies greatly and may appear at various ages. *Hemiparesis* or *hemiplegia* is commonly present. Other focal symptoms, such as aphasia or hemianopsia, may be encountered. *Mental retardation* is sometimes found. *Hydrocephalus* is occasionally associated with porencephaly.

Diagnosis: The diagnosis of porencephaly must always be suspected in a child with a history of focal convulsions, or in a child or pubescent with a history of focal convulsions and hemiplegia or hemiparesis or with some other evidences of focal damage. It should be suspected also in patients with generalized convulsions, but with indications of focal lesions, such as hemiparesis, etc. While the diagnosis may be suspected on clinical grounds, it can be established with certainty only by either encephalography or ventriculography. By these means it is seen as a cyst, communicating with the lateral ventricle, associated often with dilatation of the subarachnoid pathways. There is no displacement of the midline structures except in exceptional instances, when the midline structures may be pulled over to the side of the cyst. Changes in the skull are not infrequently seen in x-ray films. Thinning of the skull on the side of the lesion is common (Pendergrass and Perryman). These changes include thickening or compensatory hypertrophy of the skull bones, elevation of the petrous ridge, and increased pneumatization of the petrous pyramid, and mastoid, frontal, and ethmoid sinuses (Pendergrass and Perryman). Calcification is rarely seen.

The condition must be distinguished from *hemiatrophy of the brain,* which is much more uncommon than porencephaly. This condition is characterized by mental retardation or deficiency; epilepsy, either focal or generalized, but more usually focal, and hemiplegia. It is due to atrophy of a cerebral hemisphere, which may be congenital or acquired, the former being due to agenesis of the brain, the latter to a number of conditions, such as thrombosis, encephalitis, hemorrhage, and trauma. The condition may be suspected by the detection of facial and cranial asymmetry, the presence of smaller cranial bones of one side of the skull by x-ray; it may be established by encephalogram, which reveals a smaller hemisphere on one side of the brain. Thickening of the skull on the atrophied side, smaller sinuses, and lack of development of the muscles and bones of the hemiplegic limbs with resultant smaller limbs as compared with the normal side of the body are other features.

Other conditions confused with porencephaly include the many causes of epilepsy. *Brain tumor* is not often a problem, since it occurs infrequently in the cerebral hemispheres in children and is associated with signs of increased pressure. *Encephalitis* can be established readily by a history of infection, a febrile onset, the known presence of encephalitis in the community, and the demonstration as a rule of widespread damage in the nervous system.

Treatment: The treatment of porencephaly resolves itself usually into the treatment of convulsions and hemiplegia. For the convulsions, a rigid medical program is preferred in an effort to control the convulsive attacks. Dilantin Sodium, phenobarbital, and other anticonvulsive remedies (*v.* Epilepsy) should be tried. If these prove unsuccessful after a good trial period, operation should be considered. The effects of operative removal of the porencephalic cyst are successful in only about one-third of the cases, so that medical management of the case is necessary even after operative removal of the cyst. Little can be gained by operation in an attempt to relieve a hemiplegia associated with porencephaly, since the paralysis not only is not as a rule relieved but is sometimes aggravated by operation.

VII. CEREBELLAR DEGENERATIONS

A number of clinical conditions is associated with primary cerebellar manifestations. Some of these are well defined, as, for example, Friedreich's ataxia (*v.* Diseases of Spinal Cord) and hereditary cerebellar ataxia (Marie). Other forms, such as olivopontocerebellar atrophy and parenchymatous degeneration of the cerebellum are difficult to detect clinically. Transition and mixed forms are common.

Olivopontocerebellar Atrophy: This is thus far a well-defined pathological syndrome, with indistinct clinical correlations. Anatomically, it is characterized by a system atrophy of the inferior olives in the medulla, atrophy of the cerebellar cortex, and the middle cerebellar peduncle, together with partial atrophy of the inferior cerebellar peduncle due to loss of the olivocerebellar fibers. Cortical disease is found at times. Involvement of the basal ganglia has been recorded in a few cases, especially the pallidum, putamen, and substantia nigra. The red nucleus and the dentate nuclei have been found involved. Degeneration of cranial nerve nuclei has been found in some cases.

Symptoms: The *symptoms* are not distinctive and diagnosis during life is tentative. Thus far the diagnosis is distinctly a pathological matter. The disease is not hereditary or familial, but both features have been disclosed in some cases. Syphilis and alcoholism have been reported in some cases. The onset is in adult life and progression slow, patients living for many years with the disease. The outstanding symptoms are cerebellar; they are slowly progressive and bilateral. They include loss of equilibrium, slow dysarthric speech, tremor, and dyssynergias of various sorts. Parkinsonian features have been found in some cases, with rigidity an outstanding symptom. The reflexes are at times overactive and incontinence of urine occurs at times. Death occurs after several years from intercurrent disease.

Parenchymatous Atrophy of Cerebellum: This is a well-defined pathological entity, difficult of diagnosis during life. It is characterized by reduction in size of the cerebellar hemispheres and an almost total loss of the Purkinje cells. The granular layer shows mild indications of cell loss. The cerebellar fiber systems are intact and the other ganglion cells of the cerebellum are little involved. The dentate nucleus has been found to be damaged at times. The cause of such a selective degeneration of the Purkinje cells is not known. It has been regarded as due to abiotrophy, chronic alcoholism, syphilis, virus infection, and interference with blood supply to the organ in the various cases reported.

Symptoms: The symptoms develop in adult life, between forty and eighty, but frequently in the sixth and seventh decades. Males are more affected than females. No hereditary or familial incidence is found in most cases, but a familial incidence has been recorded in a few examples of the disease. The symptoms are purely cerebellar. The onset is slow, symptoms developing first in the lower extremities. Difficulty in walking appears first and progresses slowly. Thereafter, other signs of cerebellar disease develop, such as tremor, slow and slurred speech, incoordination of the limbs and trunk. Nystagmus is not found. Intellectual functions are not impaired in the usual case, but deterioration has been recorded in some instances. The process develops slowly for ten to fifteen years, death ensuing from intercurrent disease.

The disease may be suspected in an adult who develops evidence of bilateral cerebellar disturbances, slowly progressive, without evidence of tumor or vascular disease, and with no indication of an infectious onset. The slow procession of symptoms over a period of years will help fix the diagnosis, but only necropsy findings can establish it definitely.

VIII. PRIMARY DEGENERATION OF THE CORPUS CALLOSUM (*Marchiafava's Disease*)

This is a rare disorder, largely a pathological entity. All the cases recorded thus far have been in Italian males. The disease occurs in the latter half of life. Excessive use of alcohol has been found in practically all cases. Marchiafava's disease is considered a form of chronic alcoholic encephalopathy, for which an inadequate diet and prolonged alcoholism are necessary antecedents.

Pathologically, the disease is characterized by symmetrically placed lesions in the corpus callosum, especially in the genu and anterior third of this region of the brain. Other areas of degeneration have been found in the anterior commissure, the centrum ovale of the cerebral hemispheres, the middle cerebellar peduncle, and the optic nerves. The symptoms of the disease are not explainable on the basis of the callosal involvement alone, but require postulation of a more diffuse cerebral disorder (Merritt and Weisman). The microscopic picture consists of demyelination of the affected areas, persistence of axis cylinders, absence of gliosis and inflammation.

The symptoms are not definite and a diagnosis during life is not possible with certainty. The onset is slow and the development of symptoms insidiously progressive. The condition is confused in its early stages with alcoholic intoxication. Mental symptoms are frequent and are often the first indications of disease. They consist of excitement, aggression, apathy, moral perversions, sexual misdemeanors, and intellectual deterioration. Convulsions are almost constant and may occur frequently or at widespread intervals. Tremors, dysarthria, transitory hemiparesis, brief attacks of weakness without loss of consciousness, paresis of the legs and variable reflex changes have been reported (King). Remissions and exacerbations occur during the course of the disease, which terminates after three to six years with extreme weakness and gradual loss of consciousness leading to coma, often preceded by convulsions.

Agenesis of the corpus callosum is a rare condition, practically always disclosed at necropsy. It may be discovered at any age, but is more frequently encountered in children. It is associated with a large number of developmental defects of the brain, such as radial arrangement of the fissures on the internal surface of the brain, failure of union of the parietal-occipital and calcarine fissures, microgyria, enlargement of the anterior commissure, absence of the olfactory bulbs, hydrocephalus, and microcephaly.

The clinical syndrome associated with agenesis of the corpus callosum is not specific and diagnosis during life impossible. Mental deficiency is common, but normal mentality has been frequently encountered. A variety of neurological symptoms has been recorded, depending largely on other areas of the brain involved in the process of agenesis. These include hemiplegia, paraplegia, and other motor disturbances, as well as convulsions.

21

Congenital and Developmental Disorders

I. CLASSIFICATION

The nervous system, like other parts of the body, is subject to a number of congenital and developmental disorders which may involve any part of the neuraxis—the cerebral hemispheres, brain stem and cerebellum, the cranial nerves, spinal cord, and even the bones of the skull and vertebrae. The more common developmental disorders include the following:

1. **Disorders of the Brain:**
   (a) Dysgenesis:
      (1) Anencephaly.
      (2) Microcephaly.
      (3) Megalencephaly.
   (b) Encephalocele.
   (c) Hydrocephalus.
   (d) Cranial nerve agenesis.
2. **Disorders of the Spinal Cord:**
   (a) Spina bifida.
   (b) Meningocele.
   (c) Meningomyelocele.
   (d) Diplomyelia.
3. **Disorders of the Skull, Vertebrae, and Skeleton:**
   (a) Craniostenoses.
   (b) Cleidocranial dysostosis.
   (c) Hypertelorism.
   (d) Congenital elevation of the scapula.
   (e) Congenital absence of vertebrae.

Congenital Anomalies: The problem of cause has been clarified and has tended to show the increasing importance of environmental factors. Causal factors include the following (Behrman)

1. *Genetic*
2. *Environmental*

These include nutritional, chemical, endocrine, irradiation, infective, mechanical and delay or defects in fertilization. The critical period for the development of fetal abnormalities appears to be the first two months of development.

Genetic factors may be dominant, recessive or sex-linked. Of the environmental factors, some are of greater significance than others. Maternal *nutritional* disturbances, such as general starvation, vitamin or mineral deficiencies may cause malformations, but only if the malnutrition occurs in the critical period of the first two months. The deficiency must lie within narrow limits. "If the deficiency is not quite enough, the development of the embryo is not affected; and if too much, it will result in embryonic death and abortion" (Behrman). *Irradiation* factors act by interrupting embryonic differentiation or fetal growth and the effects depend on the amount of exposure and at what stage of development the exposure occurred. Mental or physical abnormalities have been found in 37.3% of offspring after post-conceptional radium or x-ray irradiation (Goldstein and Murphy). Among the infectious factors rubella has acquired increasing importance. Rubella in the mother in the first two months of gestation is associated with fetal abnormalities of various sorts in almost all instances (80%). Evidence has accumulated to indicate that deformities such as amputations previously attributed to mechanical factors may result from the mating of certain strains. Rh incompatibility has been shown to have a higher incidence of fetal abnormality.

II. DISORDERS OF THE BRAIN

1. Hydrocephalus

Hydrocephalus refers to an excessive accumulation of cerebrospinal fluid within the brain or the meningeal spaces. It is of two types: internal and external. The customary classification of hydrocephalus into obstructive and communicating types is not used here, since the problem is well covered by the two groups indicated.

Internal hydrocephalus refers to an accumulation of fluid within the ventricles of the brain. It is associated chiefly with an obstruction to the outflow of the cerebrospinal fluid. This obstruction may be anywhere within the ventricular system (obstructive hydrocephalus) or it may be outside this system and produce dilatation of both ventricular and subarachnoid spaces (communicating hydrocephalus). Obstruction to the outflow of fluid may occur at the foramen of Monro, connecting the lateral and third ventricles, causing a dilatation of one or both lateral ventricles, depending on whether the obstruction is unilateral or bilateral. Obstruction at this site is rare. More commonly the obstruction is in the third ventricle, the aqueduct of Sylvius or in the fourth ventricle, all the cavities anterior to the block becoming dilated and filled with fluid. Obstruction in the third ventricle causes dilatation of both lateral ventricles; obstruction in the aqueduct of Sylvius causes dilatation of the lateral and third ventricles; obstruction in the fourth ventricle causes dilatation of the lateral and third ventricles, and the aqueduct of Sylvius.

Internal hydrocephalus may be slight or pronounced and may develop rapidly or slowly. It is not always the result of obstruction. Thus it may occur with congenital defects of the brain. It is found in mild degree in association with degeneration and atrophy of brain tissue, as in general paresis, cerebral arteriosclerosis, senile dementia, etc., and is referred to as hydrocephalus exvacuo.

It is associated with brain changes of varying degree. The choroid plexuses are atrophic and show degenerative changes in the congenital forms. The cerebral cortex undergoes a varying degree of compression. In severe instances, it may be greatly thinned, there may be a marked loss of cells, and gliosis of the cortex. The progression of cortical atrophy in infantile hydrocephalus is slow in the ordinary case. As the hydrocephalus progresses, it becomes more pronounced, but it is possible that severe degrees of cortical atrophy in early cases of infantile hydrocephalus are the result of agenesis rather than of pressure.

Developmental anomalies are found in some instances—agenesis of the corpus callosum, spina bifida, meningocele, cerebellum, etc. In congenital hydrocephalus, the entire ventricular system is dilated; in acquired cases, the extent of the dilatation will depend upon the site of the obstruction to the flow of fluid. A special and rare form of local accumulation of fluid is seen in the *dilatation* of the *cavum septi pellucidi* and the *cavum Vergae*. Neither of these cavities are connected with the ventricular system, though the space between the leaflets of the septum pellucidum has been referred to as the fifth ventricle. The *cavum Vergae* constitutes the posterior part of the *cavum septi pellucidi*. Both these cavities may become filled with fluid at times. No characteristic symptoms are produced and the origin of the fluid is not known.

The causes of internal hydrocephalus are numerous. *Congenital cases* result usually from failure of the cerebrospinal fluid pathways to open *in utero* when the fluid begins to form. It is associated with a variety of structural malformations, some of which have already been mentioned. One of the special forms of developmental anomalies is the *Arnold-Chiari malformation*. This is a condition characterized by displacement of the medulla and tonsils of the cerebellum through the foramen magnum into the upper portion of the cervical canal. It is usually found in association with spina bifida and less frequently with platybasia. The condition may occur without spina bifida or bony deformities of any sort (Chiari; Bucy and Lichtenstein: Mc-Comwell and Parker). It causes signs of intracranial disorder, characterized by headache, often choked disc, cerebellar and pyramidal tract signs, and involvement of the lower cranial (X to XII) and upper cervical nerves. Hydrocephalus is usually present. It may produce a picture resembling syringomyelia. Operation results usually in good relief of the symptoms.

Acquired causes of internal hydrocephalus include brain tumor, which may block off the cerebrospinal fluid circulation anywhere along its course in the ventricular system; atresia of the aqueduct of Sylvius; inflammatory exudate, resulting in closure of the cerebrospinal fluid pathways, especially the foramina of Luschka and Magendie in the roof of the fourth ventricle.

External hydrocephalus refers to an accumulation of fluid outside of the ventricles, confined to the subdural or subarachnoid spaces. Fluid accumulation under the dura is found following trauma and is referred to as *subdural hydroma*. This has already been discussed (*v.* Cranial Trauma). It is by far the most important type of external hydrocephalus. Another form is seen as fluid accumulation in the subarachnoid space. usually referred to as serous meningitis. This is in reality an external hydrocephalus resulting from head injury, and associated often with infection of the mastoids and sinuses, allergy, and other causes. Accumulations of fluid in the subarachnoid space are found in many conditions associated with atrophy of cerebral gyri, such as arteriosclerosis, senile dementia, and other diseases. This is not external hydrocephalus, gives rise to no symptoms, and should not be regarded as external hydrocephalus.

Clinically, hydrocephalus may be infantile (congenital) or acquired. The acquired cases are characterized by the specific conditions giving rise to the hydrocephalus and require no extended consideration. *Infantile hydrocephalus* is present from birth, but often fails to be recognized until somewhat later. Enlargement of the head is the first noticeable feature of the condition. Parents note an abnormal size of the head, the significance of which is not grasped often until it is noted that associated with it are manifestations of slow development. It is noted also that the infant becomes fussy or dull and feeds poorly. Sitting, walking, and talking are slowed and mental development is retarded in many cases. As the head enlarges the sutures separate, the fontanels bulge, and the superficial veins of the frontal and temporal regions stand out. Motor development is frequently retarded, with resulting development of paralyses, spasticity, and even decerebrate rigidities.

Many of the associated neurological manifestations are the result not of the hydrocephalus but of the accompanying disorders of brain development. A cracked-pot sound is present on percussion of the skull. Choked disc is occasionally found, but is not usually present if the hydrocephalus has developed before closure of the skull sutures. The spinal fluid and interventricular pressures are increased. Incoördination in movement of the limbs and trunk is often found because of failure of development of the cerebellum. Mental development is retarded, at times to the point of severe mental deficiency. Normal mental powers are not uncommon, however. The development of the hydrocephalic child is slow and retarded. Motor powers never reach normal, and for the most part infants so afflicted die before reaching full development due to the progressive development of the hydrocephalus. In some, the hydrocephalus becomes chronic and may persist for years.

Treatment: The surgical treatment of hydrocephalus is composed of two steps: (1) the location and nature of the block in the circulation of the fluid; (2) the choice of treatment for its relief.

Location of the occlusion may be determined by injection of dye into the ventricles. If dye is recovered in the spinal fluid a communicating hydrocephalus is assumed to be present; if none is obtained, obstructive hydrocephalus is present. The results, unfortunately, are not always clean cut, for dye may penetrate past an obstruction and give misleading results. The method is, therefore, of questionable value. Ventriculography may be used in other cases, but it must be recognized that this procedure bears with it a high mortality in hydrocephalic infants. Combined ventricular and lumbar puncture is of doubtful help.

The choice of cases for operation is difficult. Factors of importance in the decision to operate are the presence of increased intracranial pressure, which can be measured by direct ventricular tap, and the presence of a normal mentality in the infant. Patients with acute hydrocephalus due to brain tumor or to atresia of the aqueduct require, of course, operation for the specific cause of the block.

Several methods have been advocated for the relief of infantile hydrocephalus: (1) Endoscopic coagulation of the choroid plexus (Putnam, Scarff), the object of the operation being to destroy the source of the cerebral spinal fluid. This appears to be the best procedure thus far evolved for the treatment of hydrocephalus. The operation relieves intracranial pressure sufficiently to prevent death from pressure. Putnam states that "those patients who show a reasonably normal mentality at the time of operation usually make a good operative recovery, and have an excellent chance of growing up normally." (2) Short-circuiting operations, the object of which is to bypass the fluid from the ventricles to the subarachnoid space or cisterns. A number of such methods have been advanced—puncture of the corpus callosum, section of the floor of the third ventricle, catheter bypass from the lateral ventricle to the cisterna magna.

Postural dehydration (Penfield) is advocated for those cases in which there is a close balance of absorptive capacity and fluid formation. By this method the head is elevated as high as possible, the diet concentrated as much as possible, and fluid restriction maintained. Good results are said to be obtained by this method in mild cases of hydrocephalus.

Lumbar puncture as a means of relief of pressure is hazardous and as a method for relief of the hydrocephalus has no value.

2. Cerebral Dysgenesis

A number of clinical conditions emerge as a result of maldevelopment of all or part of the brain structure. Most of them present no difficulties in diagnosis.

Anencephaly: Many types of anencephalic monster are seen and are of greater theoretical than practical value. Infants with this deformity are usually premature. The skull reveals a defect of varying size and the face is badly formed. Hemicephaly, meningoencephalocele, complete rachischisis are found in the condition.

The brain is often visible through the skull defect, the nature and degree of the cerebral malformation varying from case to case. The cerebral hemispheres are absent or are represented only by rudimentary tissue. Movements of the limbs are possible and automatic functions such as swallowing and crying are retained. Death occurs as a rule within a few days, though the majority of anencephalic monsters are born dead.

Microcephaly: This is a condition characterized by the presence of a small brain in a small head. The brain in such cases varies widely in size, from extremely small specimens of 125 to 150 grams to others weighing 900 to 1000 grams. The cerebral hemispheres are small and show microgyria and often a simplification of the cortical pattern. The cortex is thin, maldeveloped, and shows heterotopic formations. The white matter is decreased in amount. The cerebellum and brain stem are proportionately small. The condition is due to a defect of development.

The skull is small in all diameters. The forehead recedes, the occiput is flat, and the vertex is angular or ridged. The sutures and fontanels often close early. The chin is often receding, the ears large, and the face simianlike in appearance. Development is slow and usually retarded. The general stature is small, microcephalics hardly ever reaching a height beyond five feet. The limb and truncal structure is underdeveloped. The mental defect varies from idiocy to high-grade feeblemindedness, but, as a rule, severe amentia is present. There may be no neurological defects associated with the condition, or diplegia or paraplegias may be found. Marked restlessness and frequently great destructiveness characterize microcephalics.

Megalencephaly or Macrocephaly: A symmetrical enlargement of the brain associated with an increase in the size of the nerve cells and a general increase in number of all the cellular elements. Megalencephalic brains weigh 2000 to 2200 grams, about 500 to 700 grams more than normal brains. The brain configuration and cortical pattern are normal; the cerebral hemispheres are greatly enlarged, but the brain stem and cerebellum may be proportionately smaller in some instances; the cerebral cortex is wider than normal, whereas the white matter appears relatively thinned; the ventricles are relatively small. Histologically, the number of nerve and glial cells is found to be increased; many large oversized nerve cells are found in the cerebral cortex; and embryological defects may be found in the cortex.

The large brain is associated with mental deficiency, usually idiocy, but instances of normal mentality have been recorded. General physical development is retarded, the subjects revealing a curious disproportion between the size of the head and the mental and physical development. Convulsions are commonly present. Death occurs before adult life.

Mongolian Idiocy: A special form of amentia characterized by mental deficiency, and a peculiar facial appearance resembling the mongol facies. The brain is smaller than normal, the cortical pattern simplified, and the cortical gyri frequently small. The cerebellum is often small. The cortex is thin and shows a loss of nerve cells. Heterotopias are often present. The cause of mongolism is not known. The condition is probably due to defective development. Mongolism occurs frequently in the offspring of elderly mothers, the last child being usually affected. The significant factors in the production of mongolism in women over forty-one years of age are changed ovarian activity and uterine responsiveness. In the younger age group (twenty-one to thirty years) the important factors are inability to become pregnant, impaired hormonal regulation, bleedings during pregnancy, menstrual irregularities, previous abortions, and uterine and ovarian anomalies (Benda).

The condition can usually be recognized at birth. The head is small, the face flat and small, the eyes slanted and the palpebral fissures narrow, the nose small and short. The hair is scanty and dry and the skin coarse and dry. The tongue protrudes between the lips, is thick and contains transverse fissures. The limbs are short as compared with the trunk and the abdomen protuberant. The hands are short and broad and the fingers stubby. The feet are small, flat. and may be deformed. Muscular hypotonia is present in all cases and is a characteristic feature of the disease. Strabismus, nystagmus, cataract, and speckled iris are among the ocular defects.

Development is retarded and slow. Talking and walking are very slow in development. Walking develops at about the third and often as late as the fifth year. Talking is similarly slow and always remains imperfect. Mental deficiency is always present, usually of a severe degree.

Encephalocele: This is a condition characterized by a protrusion of part of the cranial contents through a defect in the skull. This may be composed of meninges (menigocele) or meninges and brain tissue (meningoencephalocele). Defects of this type are most commonly found in the occipital region in the midline or close to it. Other types are found at the base of the nose, in the region of the orbit, or presenting within the nose or pharynx. Other anomalies are often present — hydrocephalus, spina bifida, cerebral agenesis, etc. The size varies from a small enlargement (1 cm.) to very large swellings several centimeters in diameter. The symptoms are merely those of an obvious defect involving the skull, consisting of an abnormal swelling in the occiput, at the base of the nose, the side of the orbit or the base of the skull, presenting in the midline in the nose or pharynx. The diagnosis offers no difficulties, but the problem as to whether such a swelling is a meningocele or has no connection with the cranial contents can be shown by pressure on the meningocele with subsequent increase in bulging of the anterior fontanel; by increase in tension and size of the defect on increasing intracranial pressure as in crying; and finally by demonstration of a defect in the cranial bone by roentgenogram.

III. CONGENITAL DEFECTS OF THE CRANIAL NERVES

These are found rarely. Three types have been described, depending on the nerves involved. The first involves only the oculomotor nuclei; the second involves the facial nerves and sometimes the trigeminal and acoustic nerves; the third type affects the hypoglossal and glossopharyngeal nerves. Combinations of the main types occur. The condition is associated with an absence or great decrease of cells in the cranial nerve nuclei which are affected, due to congenital failure of development. Prenatal degeneration due to undisclosed causes has been held responsible. but intrauterine infections may be the cause at times. The disorder occurs at times in families, in which case it is hereditary, and is often associated with other congenital anomalies, such as spina bifida. Psychoses and other neuropathic defects are not uncommon among other members of afflicted families.

Symptoms are present from birth or soon thereafter. One or more nerves may be affected and the condition may be unilateral or bilateral, usually the latter. Not all the nerves may be affected in a single subject. Ophthalmoplegia may be found without other cranial nerve involvement, or there may be multiple cranial nerve palsies.

In the *oculomotor type,* complete paralysis of the ocular muscles is present in some forms, with ptosis of the eyelids and inability to move the eyeballs, giving the face a vapid appearance not supported by the normal intellect usually found in these cases. The pupillary reflexes are retained. Partial paralyses are found more often involving only some of the ocular muscles. Congenital ptosis of the eyelids is probably the most common form of the disorder. Unilateral partial ocular paralyses are not uncommon. The external rectus muscles alone are infrequently affected.

Facial paralysis is usually bilateral and involves all parts of the facial musculature. The result is a characteristic peripheral facial paralysis, which is often more pronounced in the upper portions of the face. Wrinkling the forehead, closing the eyes, blowing out the cheeks, and other movements of the face are greatly weakened or paralyzed. The face in these instances has a masklike appearance. Associated with the facial palsy may be involvement of the hypoglossal, abducens, and auditory nerves. Deafness is found in some cases. *Lingual* paralysis associated with unilateral or bilateral atrophy and weakness of the tongue occurs rarely. It is associated often with paralysis of the pharynx.

IV. DISORDERS OF THE SPINAL CORD

1. *Spina Bifida*

Spina bifida is a condition characterized by an incomplete closure of the vertebral column, associated usually with an accompanying defect involving the spinal cord or its membranes. It is often associated with hydrocephalus and with other evidences of maldevelopment, such as syndactylism, clubfeet, harelip, encephalocele, etc. Spina bifida is an expression of inadequate fusion of the embryonal tissues in the dorsal median region of the developing embryo, and the resulting pathological states are manifested in cutaneous, mesodermal, and neural derivatives (Lichtenstein). Hence, skin, bone, and spinal cord take part in the disorder. Associated usually with spina bifida is some degree of myelodysplasia ranging from complete rachischisis or araphia and diplomyelia to minor cord deformities. A number of abnormal conditions have been recorded by Lichtenstein in association with spina bifida. These include short cauda equina and low-lying conus medullaris; Arnold-Chiari malformation; dysplasia of the cerebellum; stenosis of the aqueduct of Sylvius: hydromyelia of the uppermost levels of the cervical cord; syringomyelia in the cervical cord.

The condition is found most commonly in the lumbar or lumbosacral region and uncommonly in the upper cervical area. A defect in the bony structure of the spine is present, involving one or more of the vertebrae due to a failure of closure of the vertebral arches during embryonic life. Through this projects a mass of varying size which is covered with a thick layer of skin under which project meninges and spinal cord or its roots (*meningomyelocele*); in other instances, only membranes project through the opening, covered with a very thin layer of skin or no skin at all (*meningo-cele*); in still other instances, no external swelling is seen, but the vertebrae may be defective for a few or several spines and the cord, represented by a defective, flattened ribbon of tissue, lies exposed (*complete rachischisis* or araphia); finally, the most common of all is *spina bifida occulta,* which is also associated with no external swelling but with a defective bony closure. Overlying the defect may be a dimple, a small collection of coarse hair, a large or small fat pad or telangiectasis. This defect is most common in the lumbar or lumbosacral region and is, as a rule, associated with no neurological disturbances; in some cases, however, there may be an accompanying lack of development of the lower portion of the spinal cord.

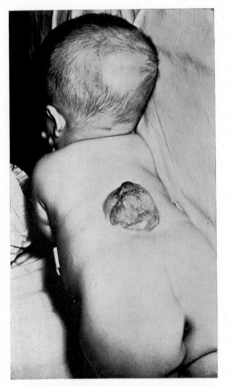

Fig. 240 — *Spina bifida* and *meningocele* shown in an infant with hydrocephalus.

Symptoms: The appearance of symptoms, apart from the swelling, varies greatly, depending on the nature of the defect. In cases of meningomyelocele, severe neurological symptoms may be present from birth; in meningocele, the same may hold true or they may be unapparent until later; in spina bifida occulta, no symptoms may be present or they may be delayed until late infancy or childhood.

The neurological features of *meningo-myelocele* are serious and are usually apparent from birth. Their extent will depend on the degree of maldevelopment of the spinal cord; hence the symptoms may vary from case to case. Enlargement of the head is almost always found, but attention may not be directed to it because of the more obvious spinal defect. The afflicted infant is small and underdeveloped. Development is slow. Movement of the legs is impaired or greatly reduced in extent and power. A flaccid paralysis is often present, with atrophy of the muscles of the lower limbs, especially in those cases in which the cauda equina roots are caught in the sac. The reflexes are usually absent. Spastic paralysis is found in cases of complete rachischisis, in which the spinal cord is exposed over several segments. Sensory findings are of little value because of the age of the subjects, but loss of pain sensation can be demonstrated. Trophic ulcers of the feet, abnormal thickening of the nails, clubfeet, trophic and necrotic changes of the bones occur. Incontinence of both urine and feces is usual. Meningomyelocele involving the cervical region is associated with atrophy and weakness of the forearm and hand muscles, and often spastic paralysis of the legs, giving a combination of an amyotrophic lateral sclerosis syndrome. Trophic ulcers are found in the fingers, sometimes associated with loss of terminal phalanges. Sensory changes of many sorts may be found, from segmental sensory dissociations, as in syringomyelia, to transverse sensory levels.

Meningocele frequently produces symptoms only of a local tumor associated with evidence of hydrocephalus. Paralyses are not as a rule present unless included in the sac are spinal roots. In such instances, there may be local paralyses of the leg or legs and less frequently of the arms. The symptoms which invite attention are the meningocele sac, which is present at birth, and the gradually developing hydrocephalus, which becomes apparent during development. Growth is slow and retarded.

Spina bifida occulta in the majority of instances gives rise to no symptoms and is found frequently in routine x-ray examination of the back in adults. In some cases, however, it is associated with an underlying maldevelopment of the cord, usually of minor degree, but occasionally severe. Myelodysplasia associated with spina bifida occulta gives rise to symptoms and signs similar to those described in cases of meningomyelocele. Minor types of disorder associated with it include foot drop, eneuresis, equino valgus and varus, scoliosis, incontinence of urine, atrophy of the leg, and edema.

Diagnosis: The diagnosis of spina bifida offers few difficulties. In cases of meningomyelocele and meningocele, the presence of the sac is obvious. For purposes of treatment, a distinction between the one and the other is important. Meningomyelocele is established by the presence of a sac associated with indications of myelodysplasia as seen in paralyses of the legs or arms. A meningocele may be assumed to be present when no such changes are demonstrable. The problem is more difficult in cases of spina bifida occulta associated with maldevelopment of the cord. Such cases

present themselves with weakness of the legs, atrophies, etc., the true nature of the disorder being established by the presence of an overlying area of hypertrichosis, a heavy fat pad or dimple, and by roentgen demonstration of a defect in the vertebral arches. In such instances, the assumption of an associated myelodysplasia with the spina bifida occulta is justified. Less obvious are the cases of this defect associated with minor paralyses, such as foot-drop, incontinence, etc. While such disorders may develop in occult spina bifida, every effort should be made in instances of this sort to exclude other causes. The assignment of spina bifida occulta as a cause of some cases of eneuresis with which it is associated is highly problematical. The association is probably fortuitous. On the other hand, rare cases of incontinence may be attributable to this condition.

Prognosis and Treatment: Most patients with meningomyelocele succumb in infancy; a few survive, only to die later. Meningocele patients survive somewhat longer. The sac in all patients with spina bifida enlarges gradually, becomes more tense, and becomes associated with a progressively developing hydrocephalus. Rupture of the sac with escape of spinal fluid and subsequent infection occurs.

Surgical treatment is the only measure of value. Operation should not be performed on patients with definite myelodysplasia. It should be deferred until after the third year if possible, unless there is obvious danger of rupture of the sac, in which case immediate operation is necessary. Acute hydrocephalus develops frequently after the removal of the sac, but this has been prevented in some degree by Penfield's operation of replacement of the inner lining of the sac and repair of the defect, on the assumption that this membrane contains spaces capable of absorbing spinal fluid. The problem of treatment, however, is so definitely surgical that reference must be made to surgical treatises for details of the various operations available.

2. Diplomyelia

Duplication of the spinal cord occurs rarely and has relatively little clinical significance. It may be found in the fetus, in association with spina bifida, or it may be encountered in adults. It is practically always a post-mortem finding and, so far as is known, it is associated with no symptoms of significance. It is characterized by a doubling of the spinal cord, usually in the lumbar and lumbosacral segments, the two portions being as a rule symmetrical. The spinal roots in the affected areas may be doubled and there is duplication of the spinal canal. The condition has never been reported in the entire length of the spinal cord.

In very rare cases, absence of the spinal cord (amyelia) is found in association with anencephaly.

V. DISORDERS OF THE SKULL, VERTEBRAE, AND SKELETON

1. Craniostenoses

The craniostenoses are deformities of the skull associated with early closure of the sutures and with neurological symptoms of varied nature.

Oxycephaly: *Oxycephaly* is probably the most common of the craniostenoses. It is characterized by the presence of an unusually high head and a steeply rising forehead, a relative decrease in the transverse and a shortening of the antero-posterior diameters of the skull. The supraorbital ridges, glabella, frontal eminences, and the entire relief of the forehead are smoothed out. The only constant feature of the skull deformity is the disproportionate height of the skull, the

other characteristics varying from case to case.

Associated with the skull deformity are signs referable to the cranial nerves. Disturbances of eyesight predominate. The eyes are prominent and some degree of exophthalmos is constant due to reduction in size of the orbits. In some cases, the exophthalmos may be very severe. Optic atrophy is almost always found, but is not constant. It is usually a secondary atrophy of the optic nerve, but may be primary. Papilledema has been found early in the condition. Loss of vision is, therefore, a common symptom and total blindness may develop in

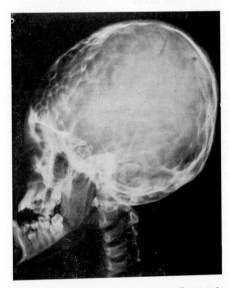

Fig. 241—*Oxycephaly*, showing the typical shape of the skull, the closure of the cranial sutures, and the hammered silver appearance of the inner table of the skull.

severe cases. In some cases, disturbances of hearing are found and in others loss of smell. Strabismus is often encountered. Increased intracranial pressure is often present, as indicated by the papilledema and the increased digital skull markings. In some instances, headache, vomiting, and a rise in spinal fluid pressure have been found. Epileptic attacks occur. The intellectual level of oxycephaly patients is average normal in many instances, but all degrees of feeblemindedness may be found in the condition. Syndactylism is often associated with the disorder.

The condition is due to a premature stenosis of the skull sutures. The coronal suture is prematurely closed in all cases. Other sutures may be affected early, but sooner or later all sutures become affected, with resulting premature closure of coronal, sagittal, and other sutures of the skull.

Roentgenograms of the skull reveal characteristic changes, consisting of closure of the skull sutures, shortening and deepening of the cranial fossae, shortening of the superior orbital fissure, and thinning of the bones of the skull. The middle fossa is markedly deepened, and the posterior fossa may form one-half to two-thirds of the base of the skull. The widening of the sutures and the erosion of the dorsum sellae seen in increased intracranial pressure is not found in oxycephaly.

The cause of the condition is not known. The skull deformity is assumed to develop as a result of expansion of the growing brain in a skull without elasticity or expansibility due to premature closure of the sutures.

Treatment of the condition is surgical and is directed toward the preservation of vision. Subtemporal decompression has been performed for this reason in cases diagnosed before the development of optic atrophy, or in those in which atrophy was early.

Acrobrachycephaly: This disorder is similar to oxycephaly. It is characterized by an abnormally high skull, by flattening of the head in the anteroposterior diameter, but unlike oxycephaly, a great widening of the skull in the transverse diameter is present. As a result, the head is high, short, and broad, the forehead wide, and the eyes widely separated. The head is actually and relatively broad so that a true brachycephaly exists. The eyeballs protrude and the eyes are obliquely set. Optic neuritis and optic atrophy may be present. Syndactylism, polydactylism, and deformities of the feet are found in some cases. Intelligence is normal in the majority of cases.

Scaphocephaly: This is characterized by a high head of excessive length in the anteroposterior diameter and flattened laterally. Further characteristics are bulging of the forehead and a large, full occiput. The deformity is the result of premature obliteration of the sagittal, parietotemporal, sphenoparietal, and sphenotemporal sutures (Pancoast, Pendegrass, and Schaeffer). Exophthalmos, strabismus, optic neuritis, and optic atrophy may be found.

Craniofacial Dysostosis (Crouzon): It is closely allied to oxycephaly, from which it must be separated in diagnosis. It is associated with premature closure of the sutures. The condition is usually familial and hereditary, but isolated instances occur. It is characterized by (1) cranial deformity consisting of a high, domelike, thin skull associated with obliteration of the sutures, a marked bony prominence at the site of the anterior fontanel and often a ridge or crest of bone along the midline of the skull; (2) facial deformity consisting of underdevelopment of the bones of the face, prognathism, flattening of the bridge of the nose, a parrotlike nose, and micrognathia of the upper jaw; (3) ocular difficulties, such as exophthalmos, optic atrophy, papilledema, and strabismus. Optic atrophy is not always present but when found may progress to full blindness. Intelligence is unimpaired. Headache may be quite pronounced. Roentgenograms show a domelike formation of the vault with obliteration of the sutures. The skull is very thin.

The condition is distinguished from oxycephaly by its hereditary characteristic, by the more pronounced involvement of facial deformities, and by a less pronounced tower skull than is found in oxycephaly.

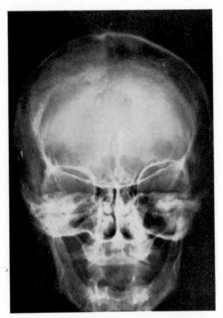

Fig. 242—*Hypertelorism,* showing the widened distance between the eyes.

2. *Other Deformities*

Hypertelorism: A condition characterized by excessive distance between the eyes, its outstanding feature, by broadening of the bridge of the nose, by a brachycephalic head, flattening of the occiput, and bulging of the temporal regions. The skull presents a low forehead and pronounced vertex. The orbits are circular and deep. The nasal bones are short. Strabismus is usually present. Mental deficiency is present in most cases. The deformity is the result of enlargement of the lesser wings of the sphenoid bone, with decrease in size of the greater wings.

Cleidocranial Dysostosis: Cleidocranial dysostosis is a rare syndrome affecting persons of both sexes and all ages and occurring in diverse racial and national groups. In a typical case, the head is large, especially in comparison to the face, and it is wide and flat with protruding cranial bosses and bulging frontal region. The bones of the cranial vault are slow to develop so that the fontanelles and sutures are widely separated at birth and may remain apart into adulthood. Usually there is a depression at the fontanelles, and sometimes a pulse may be felt there if the bone is absent. The frontal sinuses are absent or much reduced, and brow ridges are frequently absent. The mastoids are often virtually lacking, a trait which finds a possible explanation in the absence of the clavicles and consequent maldevelopment of the sternocleidomastoid muscles. The base of the skull is frequently poorly developed (which may contribute to the brachycephaly), and platybasia with a downward bending of the occiput is mentioned in some cases. The sella turcica has been noticed to be large by some authors, but was reported as normal in other cases and small in one.

The face is usually poorly developed. The bridge of the nose is cartilaginous, the nasal, and sometimes the lacrimal, bones being deficient or completely absent. The root of the nose is therefore regularly depressed, but it is often wide so that a Mongoloid fold may cover the inner canthus of the eye. The orbits are relatively high, but a tendency towards exophthalmos is sometimes reported. The palate is typically highly arched and narrowed, and may be defective, leaving a cleft. The mandible is frequently disproportionate to the rest of the face.

The dentition is usually markedly affected. The milk teeth appear later than is normal in infants. They are not replaced at the proper time by the permanent dentition, and there is virtually never a full complement of teeth in the mouth despite a tendency to supernumerary anterior teeth. Unerupted teeth are found in the mandible and maxilla of most subjects, and the eruption of teeth in older persons is frequently reported. The teeth are usually very irregular in position, and the occlusion is so bad that many have their teeth extracted and wear dentures.

The dysostotic person is often very short. In children, as in adults, dwarfing may be very common in this condition. The short stature is usually, at least in part, the result of curvatures of the vertebral column: kyphosis, lordosis, and scoliosis are mentioned. Scoliosis is the most frequent and has been reported in more than thirty cases. Wedging of the vertebral bodies is common. Spina bifida occulta is very frequent and often occurs in the cervical and upper dorsal regions. Cervical meningocele has been reported. The thorax is sometimes funnel-shaped, sometimes flattened from side to side.

Defective clavicles are the most characteristic trait of this condition. Both bones may be completely lacking, or one or both may be imperfect. Very frequently, there is a sternal bony rudiment or even an only slightly shortened bone attached to the sternum. Occasionally, there is also an acromial rudiment, which may be widely separated from the other fragment or may form a pseudarthrodial joint. Especially when one only of the clavicles is divided, the differential diagnosis of an ununited fracture may be of practical importance.

Other defects of the shoulder girdle have been reported. The scapula is frequently small, and the superior fossa and the coracoid process may be absent. Anomalies of the musculature have been variously described in numerous cases,

but these are apparently secondary to the lack of clavicles. There are occasional anomalies of the humeral head, and congenital dislocation of the humerus has been reported.

The most prominent symptom is the unusual motility of the shoulders, which in some cases can be voluntarily approximated in front. There is usually no functional loss in the arms. Many persons do heavy work.

The pelvic girdle frequently is affected. The pelvic inlet may be unduly narrow and distorted. The most common pelvic anomaly is a gap at the symphysis pubis.

Anomalies of the legs, to which some of the reduction in stature may be ascribed, are extremely common. These consist of genu valgum, coxa vara, pes planus, and many other types of deformity of the lower extremities.

The disease is hereditary, but sporadic forms occur.

Platybasia (*Basilar Impression*): This is a term used to designate a deformity of the bony structures about the foramen magnum. It is characterized essentially by a settling down of the skull on the spine. The first cervical vertebra is often rudimentary and its posterior arch may be fused with the occiput; the foramen magnum is deformed. The spinous processes of the second and third cervical vertebrae may be fused. The condition is caused by a variety of disorders — hydrocephalus, rickets, Paget's disease, and congenital anomaly, most of the cases being associated with the last-named condition. Cases have been recorded in age ranges of seventeen to seventy years.

The disorder is often present without symptoms, but when symptoms are present they may be extremely variable. The neck is usually short, with the head shifted downward between the shoulders and tilted backward. The neurological symptoms vary greatly, depending on the structures involved. Compression of the cervical roots and the spinal cord may cause pain in the neck or over the back of the head, atrophy of the hand muscles, and weakness of the limbs, suggesting an amyotrophic lateral sclerosis syndrome. In other instances of cord involvement, partial transverse syndromes may be produced.

Headache, choked disc, and cerebellar disturbances may develop in cases of blockage of the subarachnoid space by the odontoid process. Cranial nerve palsies involving the accessory and hypoglossal nerves as well as other nerves of the posterior fossa have been recorded, due to an arachnoiditis associated with the bony deformity.

The symptoms of platybasia are the result of pressure of the foramen magnum and the upper cervical spine on the upper portion of the cervical cord, the medulla, pons, and cerebellum. Not all the symptoms of the disorder are attributable to pressure. Some of them are the result of torsion of the affected portions. Arachnoiditis, which is associated with the condition, also accounts for some of the symptoms, as well as compression of the vertebral arteries and interference with fluid escape from the foramina of Luschka and Magendie due to cerebellar herniation into the cervical canal. Projection of the odontoid process into the cervical canal may cause pressure on the brain stem or cervical cord in some cases.

The diagnosis is made by roentgenogram. On a lateral view of the skull, a line drawn from the posterior edge of the hard palate to the posterior lip of the foramen Magnum should normally find the odontoid process below this line. If it lies above this line, basilar impression is present. Decrease in size and distortion of the foramen Magnum are constantly present. The condition tends to be progressive. Basilar impression or platybasia may simulate multiple sclerosis, amyotrophic lateral sclerosis, spinal cord tumor, or brain tumor.

The treatment consists of *operation*, either high cervical laminectomy or suboccipital craniectomy.

Klippel-Feil Syndrome: This syndrome is a condition characterized by reduction in number of the cervical vertebrae and fusion of the cervical spine.

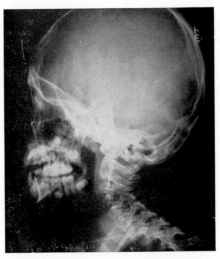

Fig. 243 — *Klippel-Feil syndrome,* showing fusion of the cervical vertebrae.

Many variants are known. Complete or partial absence of the cervical vertebrae are found and a bewildering variety of fusions occur, from complete fusion of the entire cervical spine to partial fusion of many sorts. In typical cases the cervical spine is a solid mass of bone. The condition is present at birth and is at times familial.

Spina bifida is frequently found. It is usually of the false type. The spinal cord is usually normal, but diplomyelia has been recorded.

Fusion and deformity of the ribs are often present. Other abnormalities occur.

These include torticollis, facial asymmetry, kyphosis and thoracic scoliosis, abnormal dentition, cleft palate, hydrocephalus, micrognathia, strabismus, platybasia, pulmonary stenosis, and patent foramen ovale and interventricular septum. The etiology is probably a disorder of segmentation due to intrauterine or external disorders.

It is not hereditary or familial, but cases have been recorded in parent and offspring. Males and females are equally affected. Numerical reduction of the vertebral axis is not necessary for a diagnosis of Klippel-Feil syndrome. The anomaly has a genetic basis.

The outstanding clinical feature is the shortness of the neck with a low hairline on the back of the neck; the shoulders are high and the chin close to the sternum, the occiput prominent, the trapezii flaring, stretching at times from the mastoid processes to the shoulders, giving rise to the appearance of a web neck. Associated with the condition are scoliosis or kyphoscoliosis, elevation of the scapula, torticollis, facial asymmetry, spina bifida, and limb abnormalities, such as clubhand or clubfoot. A number of neurological disorders have been described with the condition, including mental deficiency, quadriplegia, syringomyelia, myopathy, mirror movements, Marie's cerebellar ataxia, and Friedreich's ataxia.

Congenital Elevation of the Scapula (Sprengel's Deformity): A rare condition characterized by the presence of a high scapula, due to its failure to descend during fetal development. It is associated at times with the Klippel-Feil syndrome, cervical ribs, syringomyelia, and other abnormalities. The deformity is unilateral. The scapula is fixed, in some cases a bony ridge running from the lower cervical vertebrae to the scapula. Scoliosis is usually present.

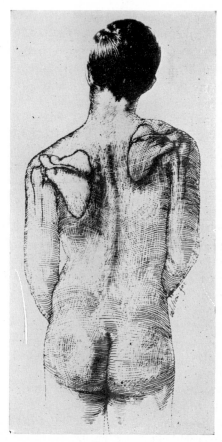

Fig. 244—*Sprengel's deformity*, showing the characteristic elevation of the scapula, shortness of the neck, tilting of the head and scoliosis.

22

Diseases of the Skull and Vertebrae

I. DISEASES OF THE SKULL

The skull and vertebrae may be the seat of primary or secondary disease of many types. Some of these have already been considered in the sections on Developmental and Congenital Disorders — oxycephaly, scaphocephaly, craniofacial dystosis, spina bifida, etc. In addition to these are acquired disease forms which require description.

1. Osteomyelitis of the Skull

Etiology: Osteomyelitis of the skull bones occurs chiefly between twenty and thirty years of age and is less common in older subjects, probably due to increasing density of the bone with age. By far the greatest number of cases follow disease of the frontal sinuses, a few resulting from disease of the ethmoid cells and antrum. It may result also from infection of the sphenoid sinus. The disease usually follows acute sinusitis, but it may develop during an acute exacerbation of a chronic infection, or even without acute manifestations whatever.

Infections of various sorts in the sinuses precede the osteomyelitis, the staphylococcus being the most common offending organism. The streptococcus and other bacteria may at times be responsible for the condition. Any of the common infections which produce frontal sinusitis may be complicated by osteomyelitis — the common cold, influenza, scarlet fever, etc. Swimming has been held responsible

in some cases. Some cases of osteomyelitis of the skull follow operation on the frontal sinuses.

Pathology: Infection in the bones of the skull extends by the diploe of the bone, producing a thrombophlebitis and an accompanying bone infection. The bone in its early stages shows engorgement of the vessels of the diploe and the formation of pus in the interspaces. Thrombosis of the vessel is present. The infection spreads to the inner or outer surface of the bone, the inner table being more affected than the outer. Rupture through the outer table may result in a subperiosteal abscess and swelling of the soft tissues of the forehead. If the infection breaks through the inner table, an extradural or subdural abscess, or a brain abscess, may follow. Microscopic study of the bone reveals polynuclear cells, bacteria, osteoclasts, and osteoblast formation in varying amounts, depending on the acuteness of the process.

Symptoms: In the usual case, there is a history of sinus infection of relatively short duration, often acute and fulminating in character, either with no previous history of sinus disease, or with a background of chronic sinus infection. The usual accompaniments of sinus infection are present—headache, fever, malaise. A history of an acute infection preceding the sinus infection is often obtainable, or there may be a history of onset after swimming. In some instances, however, a clear-cut history of sinus infection is lacking or may be so mild as to make a diagnosis of sinusitis doubtful.

The first symptom of osteomyelitis of the skull associated with frontal sinusitis is often swelling of the frontal region, associated with headache and usually with fever. The latter often reaches 103° to 104° F., but in some cases it may be normal or almost normal throughout the course of the illness. Systemic symptoms, such as malaise, chills, etc., may be severe in some cases and mild in others. The swelling of the soft tissues of the forehead stops usually at the hairline and may be associated with redness of the skin and fluctuation. Roentgenograms reveal a typical destruction of the bone.

Treatment: The treatment is surgical, and consists of wide removal of the diseased bone. Strong support may be given surgical treatment by the use of sulfonamide drugs. The prognosis depends on the virulence of the infection, the rapidity with which diagnosis is made and treatment instituted, and the absence of serious complications, such as brain abscess or extradural abscess.

2. Benign Frontal Hyperostosis (Stewart-Morel Syndrome)

This condition is characterized by a hyperostosis involving the frontal bones, associated with which are obesity, mental disturbances, and a number of neurological symptoms, such as headache, epileptic seizures, and other manifestations.

Etiology: The disease occurs preponderantly in women, over ninety-five per cent of cases being recorded in females. The average age incidence is from thirty to forty-five years, but older patients are not uncommon. Symptoms appear frequently at the time of menopause. The exact cause is not known. The disorder has been found in association with senile dementia, Pick's lobar atrophy, Alzheimer's presenile psychosis, and cerebral arteriosclerosis.

Pathology: The outstanding feature consists of a hyperostosis involving the inner tables of the frontal bones; the external surface of the bone is unchanged. The condition is confined entirely to the frontal bones, but instances of extension to the parietal bone and the orbital plates are on record. The frontal bones become progressively thickened and dense, with resulting decrease in capacity of the anterior portion of the cranial cavity. The underlying dura is adherent to the thickened inner table and the arachnoid may be adherent to the underlying brain. Atrophy of the frontal convolutions is sometimes seen.

Symptoms: The symptoms develop gradually, persist and become progressive. Headache is usually the first and often the most persistent feature. It is almost always frontal in location, and is described as constant, dull, and often severe. Pain in the face is sometimes present but is not the typical pain of trigeminal neuralgia. Obesity is an almost constant accompaniment of the syndrome and with headache constitutes the most prominent clinical symptom. It is characterized by fat accumulation of the trunk, especially of the breasts, without involvement of the face or limbs except for the proximal portions of the latter. Generalized convulsions occur in a small percentage of cases. Mental symptoms of various sorts have been described, including depression and evidences of intellectual deterioration. The latter is often severe and may progress to marked deterioration, but many grades of loss of mental function are observed. Muscular weakness, fatigue, and vertigo are frequent complaints. Hirsutism is often present in women.

Diagnosis: The diagnosis of hyperostosis frontalis interna may be suspected in a middle-aged woman who complains of intractable headache, who is obese, and who may have in addition indications of mental disturbances. It may be postulated tentatively also in patients with a history of headache and vertigo; in other instances, with face pain or convulsions. Headache is common to all the subjects and with it obesity; other symptoms are not found consistently, save for the mental disturbances, which may vary greatly in form and intensity. While the condition may be suspected under the conditions mentioned, the diagnosis can be made with certainty only by roentgenological examination, which reveals a characteristic picture of thickening of the frontal bones and evidences of bony excrescences involving the inner table of the skull.

There is grave doubt concerning the recognition of hyperostosis frontalis interna as a disease entity. A review of 700 cases reveals that the condition is not uncommon in women and that it is unrelated to whatever clinical state may accompany it (Schneeberg, Woolhandler, and Levine). The condition has been reported with obesity, psychoneurosis or psychosis, headache, hirsutism, mental retardation or deterioration, weakness, vertigo, menstrual disorders, tinnitus, hypertension, neurolgical disorders, visual disturbances, convulsions, somnolence, lethargy, fatigue, epilepsy, narcolepsy, diabetes mellitus, and diabetes insipidus. The contention that it bears no relation to the clinical condition which accompanies it is based on the following facts: (1) the clinical features said to be associated with it are found as frequently in control patients without hyperostosis frontalis interna, (2) examples of the condition without symptoms are not infrequent, and (3) no constant group of symptoms can be found related to the disorder.

The disease pursues a chronic course. The headache is persistent and other symptoms tend to become chronic.

Treatment: The treatment is purely symptomatic. The headache is particularly stubborn and responds poorly as a rule to the usual analgesics. The same is true of the face pain. Epileptic attacks may be controlled by Dilantin Sodium, phenobarbital, or other measures used in the treatment of epilepsy. Subtemporal decompression has been used to relieve persistently stubborn headaches.

3. Osteitis Deformans (Paget's Disease)

Neurological symptoms of many sorts have been recorded in the course of osteitis deformans or Paget's disease. The disease is too well known to require description here; hence only its neurological consequences will be mentioned.

Osteitis deformans is characterized by proliferation and destruction of bone. which is probably not of inflammatory origin. All parts of the skeleton are affected, but the skull and vertebrae are particularly prone to be involved. The disease may on rare occasions involve only the atlas and axis, and cause spinal cord compression in the cervical region. The symptoms produced in the nervous system in the course of osteitis deformans result from one or more of several processes: (1) There may be narrowing of the foramina at the base of the skull by the proliferating bone, thus causing symptoms due to pressure on the nerves traversing the foramina. (2) There may be symptoms resulting from distortion of the shape of the skull and crowding of its contents. The base of the skull, particularly, becomes flattened, the posterior fossa crowded, the ventrolateral dimension becomes decreased and symptoms result from torsion and stretch on the nerves in the posterior fossa and compression of the contents of the posterior fossa. (3) Symptoms may result from cerebral arteriosclerosis, which is always present and often severe. The brain shows moderate to severe arteriosclerosis, and the cerebral cortex areas of ischemia and cell loss. Softenings of the cerebrum and cerebellum are found.

The neurological *symptoms* which accompany the disease are rather varied. They are gradual in development and progressive in character. Progressive loss of vision is found and is associated with primary or secondary optic atrophy. Retinal hemorrhages have been reported. Choroiditis is also found. Headache occurs frequently. Deafness is found in a small percentage of cases, but its relationship to Paget's disease is not definitely established. Ocular paralyses sometimes develop. Epileptic attacks, almost always generalized, have been reported in a small number of instances. Whether these result from the metabolic disturbances associated with osteitis deformans, or from the associated cerebral arteriosclerosis and its attendant brain changes, or from both factors, is not known. Cerebellar disturbances have been recorded in rare instances. Mental symptoms are not uncommon and may precede or accompany changes in the bones. They are probably the result of the cerebral arteriosclerosis which is so common in the disorder. Organic mental syndromes predominate, but depression and excited states have been encountered. Brain tumor has been reported rarely in Paget's disease. Though the relationship of the two conditions is probably fortuitous, it emphasizes the fact that the cerebral signs in Paget's disease are not always the result of this condition.

Spinal cord symptoms may develop from narrowing of the spinal canal, or by collapse, dislocation, or fracture of the diseased vertebrae. In the former instance, symptoms are slow in appearance and, in the latter, rapid. The symptoms are those of spinal cord compression with pain, weakness of the legs, often urinary incontinence, and sensory disturbances. Subarachnoid block is usually present. Laminectomy for relief of the cord compression is recommended in such cases.

II. TUMORS OF THE SKULL AND OTHER CONDITIONS

Primary tumors of the skull are often associated with neurological symptoms. Hemangioma, osteoma, osteochondroma, and other tumor types may cause cerebral symptoms. Cholesteatoma of the skull may encroach on the underlying brain tissue and produce headache, dizziness, mental symptoms, hemiparesis, and hemianopsia, depending upon the location of the tumor.

Osteitis fibrosa cystica involving the skull may at times be associated with headache, neuralgias, epileptic attacks, and hemianopsia. The condition may at times involve the spine and produce evidences of spinal cord compression indistinguishable from tumor.

Involvement of the skull occurs frequently in polyostotic *fibrous dysplasia*, but in some instances the skull is involved exclusively. Children and adolescents are affected. Localized clinical symptoms may develop especially when the base of the skull is affected. Ocular symptoms such as unilateral exophthalmos and optic atrophy are prominent. A calcified mass in the anterior fossa may be seen in roentgenograms. The disorder is usually confused with tumors around the sella turcica.

Eosinophilic granuloma of bone is a rare entity of undetermined cause. It afflicts young persons of either sex and has a predilection for flat bones; though any bone may be affected. There are no systemic symptoms, the patient seeking help because of swelling on the bone due to the growth of the tumor. There may be local tenderness. Pathologically, the medulla of the bone is found to be replaced by a granuloma composed of eosinophils, eosinophilic myelocytes, fibroblasts, and large mononuclear cells.

Roentgenograms reveal a localized, sharply punched-out area of rarefaction with no surrounding bone reaction. The lesions usually appear to be cystic; the cortex is not involved as a rule. The lesions may be single or multiple and usually involve the ribs, vertebrae, pelvis, skull, humerus, and femur. Leukocytosis is occasionally present and rarely moderate eosinophilia. The blood calcium, phosphorus, phosphatase, cholesterol, and protein levels in the blood are normal.

Rarely, eosinophilic granulomas are associated with neurological complications. These include headache, vertigo, vomiting, and cranial nerve signs, especially seventh nerve involvement (Osborne, Freis, and Levin).

Index

NOTE: Words in *italics* refer to therapeutic agents.
Page numbers in *italics* refer to illustrations.

A

Abdominal
migraine, 132
reflex, 18, 61
Abducens nerves, in disease, 214
Abscess
brain. *See:* Brain, abscess
cryptogenic, 585
extradural, 349
spinal, 243
vs. abscess, brain, 595
meningeal, headache in, 126
Accessory movement, 50
Accommodation reflex, test of, 12
Acetylsalicyclic acid. See: Acid, acetylsalicyclic
Achilles reflex
in neuritis, diabetic, 172
in sciatica, 205
in tabes dorsalis, 279
tests of, 17, 205
Achlorhydria in degeneration, combined,
subacute, 343
Achondroplastic dwarfs, 306
Achylia gastrica in degeneration, combined.
subacute, 343
Acid
acetylsalicyclic
in chorea, Sydenham's, 688
in headache, migraine, 134
in paralysis, facial, peripheral, 222
base equilibrium in epilepsy, 641
hydrochloric
in ischemia, cerebral, 515
in neuritis
alcoholic, 170
pellagra, 174
in polyneuritis, 167
isonicotinic
in meningitis, tuberculous, 370
hydrazide, toxic effect of, 179
nicotinic
in headache, migraine, 134
in neuritis
pellagra, 174
retrobulbar, 214
in sclerosis, multiple, 724
in spasm, cerebral, vascular, 515
para-aminosalicylic in tuberculous meningitis,
370

Acidosis in epilepsy, 641
Acoustic
nerve. *See:* Nerves, acoustic
nystagmus, reflex, 38
tumors, 540, 565
Acrobrachycephaly, 827
Acrocyanosis, 749
Acromegaly, adenoma and, *573, 575*
Acroparesthesia, 750
ACTH
in chorea, Sydenham's, 688
in myasthenia gravis, 794
in optic neuritis, 214
toxic effects of, 740
Actinomycosis, meningitis in, 376
Activation technics in electroencephalography,
67
Adductor reflex of thigh, test of, 18, 62
Adenoma
acromegaly and, 573
pancreatic, *vs.* progressive muscular atrophy,
760
pituitary, 536, *537,* 570
sebaceum, 807
treatment in, 582
Adhesive spinal arachnoiditis, 245
Adie's syndrome
in tabes dorsalis, 283
pupil in, 33
Adiposis dolorosa, 751, *751*
Adrenal cortex extract
in meningitis, meningococcic, 355
in meningococcic infection, fulminating,
356
Adrenocorticotropic hormone. See: ACTH
Agenesis of corpus callosum, 816
Agnosia, 121
clinical significance of, 122
forms of, 122
tactile, in cortical syndrome disease, 108
Air-borne infection, poliomyelitis due to,
251
Air myelography, 80
Akinesis in paralysis agitans, 681
Akinetic syndrome, 96
Alcohol
and nervous system, 726
injection
in causalgia, 234

837

—

Index